SCIENTIFIC BASIS of TRANSFUSION MEDICINE

SECOND
EDITION

SCIENTIFIC BASIS of TRANSFUSION MEDICINE

Implications for Clinical Practice

EDITED BY

KENNETH C. ANDERSON, M.D.

Associate Professor of Medicine
Harvard Medical School
Medical Director, Kraft Family Blood Donor Center
Department of Adult Oncology
Dana-Farber Cancer Institute
Boston, Massachusetts

PAUL M. NESS, M.D.

Professor
Pathology and Medicine
Johns Hopkins University School of Medicine
Director, Transfusion Medicine
Johns Hopkins Hospital
Senior Medical Director, Greater Chesapeake and Potomac Region
American Red Cross, Blood Services
Baltimore, Maryland

W.B. SAUNDERS COMPANY
A Division of Harcourt Brace & Company
Philadelphia London Toronto Montreal Sydney Tokyo

W.B. SAUNDERS COMPANY
A Division of Harcourt Brace & Company

The Curtis Center
Independence Square West
Philadelphia, Pennsylvania 19106

Library of Congress Cataloging-in-Publication Data

Scientific basis of transfusion medicine: implications for clinical practice / [edited by] Kenneth C. Anderson, Paul M. Ness.—2nd ed.

p. cm.

Includes bibliographical references and index.

ISBN 0–7216–7684–7

1. Blood—Transfusion. 2. Hematology. I. Anderson, Kenneth C. II. Ness, Paul M. [DNLM: 1. Blood Transfusion. 2. Blood Physiology. WB 356 S4165 2000]

RM171.S36 2000 615′.39—dc21

DNLM/DLC 99–37690

SCIENTIFIC BASIS OF TRANSFUSION MEDICINE:
Implications for Clinical Practice ISBN 0–7216–7684–7

Printed in the United States of America.

Last digit is the print number: 9 8 7 6 5 4 3 2 1

CONTRIBUTORS

CHESTER A. ALPER, MD
Professor of Pediatrics, Harvard Medical School, Boston, Massachusetts; Vice President, The Center for Blood Research, Boston, Massachusetts; Senior Associate in Hematology and Oncology, Department of Medicine, Children's Hospital, Boston, Massachusetts

BARBARA ALVING, MD
Professor of Medicine, Uniformed Services University of the Health Sciences, Bethesda, Maryland; Director, Division of Blood Diseases and Resources, National Heart, Lung, and Blood Institute, National Institutes of Health, Bethesda, Maryland

KENNETH C. ANDERSON, MD
Associate Professor of Medicine, Harvard Medical School, Boston, Massachusetts; Medical Director, Kraft Family Blood Component Laboratory, Dana-Farber Cancer Institute, Boston, Massachusetts

JOHN A. J. BARBARA, MA, MSc, PhD, FRCPath
Honorary Senior Lecturer, Royal Free and University College Medical School, London, United Kingdom; Microbiology Consultant to National Blood Service (NBS) Authority and Lead Scientist in Transfusion Microbiology, London and S. E. Zone, NBS, North London, Colindale, London, United Kingdom

WILLIAM R. BELL, MD
Professor of Medicine, Radiology, and Nuclear Medicine, The Johns Hopkins University School of Medicine, Baltimore, Maryland; Clinical Director, Division of Hematology, Department of Medicine, The Johns Hopkins University Hospital, Baltimore, Maryland

ERNEST BEUTLER, MD
Chairman, Department of Molecular and Experimental Medicine, The Scripps Research Institute, La Jolla, California

DAVID H. BING, PhD
Scientific Director, Genomics Collaborative, Cambridge, Massachusetts

NEIL BLUMBERG, MD
Professor, Pathology and Laboratory Medicine, University of Rochester, Rochester, New York; Director, Transfusion Medicine, Strong Memorial Hospital, Rochester, New York

J. M. BOWMAN, MD
Professor of Pediatrics (Retired) and Senior Scholar, Department of Pediatrics and Child Health, Faculty of Medicine, University of Manitoba, Winnipeg, Manitoba, Canada

HAL E. BROXMEYER, PhD
Chairman and Mary Margaret Walther Professor of Microbiology and Immunology; Professor of Medicine; and Scientific Director of the Walther Oncology Center, Indiana University School of Medicine, Indianapolis, Indiana

SILVANA Z. BUCUR, MD
Assistant Professor, Department of Pathology and Laboratory Medicine, and Instructor in Medicine, Division of Hematology and Oncology, Emory University, Atlanta, Georgia; Assistant Director, Emory University Hospital Blood Bank, Emory University Hospital, Atlanta, Georgia

MICHAEL P. BUSCH, MD, PhD
Adjunct Professor, Department of Laboratory Medicine, University of California School of Medicine, San Francisco, San Francisco, California; Vice President, Research and Scientific Services, Blood Centers of the Pacific, San Francisco, California; Blood Systems, Inc., Scottsdale, Arizona

RICHARD A. CARTER, MD
Assistant Professor, Division of Hematology and Oncology, Emory University, Atlanta, Georgia

DAVID B. CLARK, PhD
Manager, Technology Transfer, American Red Cross, Washington, D.C.

MARY E. CLAY, MS, MT(ASCP)
Administrative Scientist, Division of Transfusion Medicine, University of Minnesota, Minneapolis, Minnesota; Manager, Research and Development Department, American Red Cross, North Central Blood Services, St. Paul, Minnesota

CATHY CONRY-CANTILENA, MD
Medical Officer, National Institutes of Health, Bethesda, Maryland; Medical Director, Greater Chesapeake and Potomac Region of the American Red Cross, Baltimore, Maryland

KENNETH CORNETTA, MD
Associate Professor of Medicine, Microbiology and Immunology and Medicine and Molecular Genetics, Indiana University, Indianapolis, Indiana; Director, Bone Marrow Transplantation, Indiana University School of Medicine, Indianapolis, Indiana

GEOFF DANIELS, PhD
Senior Research Fellow, Bristol Institute for Transfusion Sciences, Bristol, United Kingdom

RICHARD J. DAVEY, MD
Chief Medical Officer, American National Red Cross Blood Services, Roslyn, Virginia

LOUIS DePALMA, MD
Professor of Pathology and of Anatomy and Cell Biology, George Washington University School of Medicine, Washington, D.C.; Director, Division of Clinical Pathology, George Washington University Hospital, Washington, D.C.

GEORGE DESPOTIS, MD
Assistant Professor of Anesthesiology and Pathology, Washington University School of Medicine, St. Louis, Missouri; Barnes-Jewish Hospital, St. Louis, Missouri

DANA V. DEVINE, PhD
Associate Professor of Pathology, University of British Columbia, Vancouver, British Columbia, Canada; Senior Scientist, Canadian Blood Services, Vancouver, British Columbia, Canada

RICARDO SOBHIE DIAZ, MD, MsC
Director of Retrovirology Laboratory, Infectious Diseases Division, Federal Medical School of Sao Paulo, Sao Paulo, Brazil

ROGER Y. DODD, PhD
Head, Department of Transmissible Diseases, American Red Cross, Jerome H. Holland Laboratory, Rockville, Maryland

WILLIAM N. DROHAN, PhD
Professor, Graduate Program in Genetics, George Washington University, Washington, D.C.; Adjunct Professor, Department of Chemistry and Biochemical Engineering, University of Maryland, Baltimore, Maryland; Senior Director, Plasma Development, American Red Cross, Rockville, Maryland

SUNNY DZIK, MD
Assistant Professor of Internal Medicine, Harvard Medical School, Boston, Massachusetts; Co-Director, Blood Transfusion Service, Massachusetts General Hospital, Boston, Massachusetts

JOSEPH C. FRATANTONI, MD
Vice President, Biologics, C. L. McIntosh & Associates, Rockville, Maryland; Clinical Professor of Medicine, Uniformed Services University of the Health Sciences, Bethesda, Maryland

JANICE L. GABRILOVE, MD
Professor of Medicine; Chief, Division of Neoplastic Diseases; Deputy Director for Clinical Affairs of the Derald H. Ruttenberg Cancer Center, Mt. Sinai Medical Center, New York, New York

JEREMY A. GARSON, MD, PhD, MRCP, FRCPath
Senior Clinical Lecturer in Virology, Department of Virology, Royal Free and University College Medical School, University College, London, United Kingdom; Honorary Consultant in Medical Virology, University College London Hospitals, National Health Service Trust, London, United Kingdom

TERRENCE L. GEIGER, MD, PhD
Associate Research Scientist, Yale University School of Medicine, New Haven, Connecticut; Attending Physician, Yale–New Haven Hospital, New Haven, Connecticut

LAWRENCE T. GOODNOUGH, MD
Professor of Medicine and Pathology, Department of Pathology, Washington University School of Medicine, St. Louis, Missouri; Director of Transfusion Services, Barnes-Jewish Hospital, St. Louis, Missouri

F. CARL GRUMET, MD
Professor of Pathology, Stanford University School of Medicine, Stanford, California; Director, Histocompatibility Laboratory, Stanford University Blood Center, Palo Alto, California

EMANUEL HACKEL, PhD
Professor Emeritus, Department of Medicine and Zoology, Michigan State University, East Lansing, Michigan

LAURENCE A. HARKER, MD
Blomeyer Professor of Medicine and Director, Division of Hematology and Oncology, Emory University School of Medicine; Consultant, Emory University Hospital and Grady Memorial Hospital, Atlanta, Georgia

JOANNA M. HEAL, MBBS, MRCP
Clinical Associate Professor, Department of Medicine, University of Rochester, Rochester, New York

CHRISTOPHER D. HILLYER, MD
Associate Professor, Department of Pathology and Laboratory Medicine; Assistant Professor of Medicine, Division of Hematology and Oncology; and Director, Emory University Transfusion Medicine Program, Emory University, Atlanta, Georgia

BRUCE HUG, MD
Resident, Department of Pathology and Laboratory Medicine, University of Pennsylvania Medical Center, Philadelphia, Pennsylvania

K. J. KAO, MD, PhD
Professor, Department of Pathology, College of Medicine, University of Florida, Gainesville, Florida; Director, Blood Bank and Hematology Laboratory, Shands Hospital at the University of Florida, Gainesville, Florida

ANNE KESSINGER, MD
Professor of Medicine and Chief, Section of Oncology/Hematology, University of Nebraska Medical Center, Omaha, Nebraska

THOMAS S. KICKLER, MD
Professor of Pathology and Medicine, Johns Hopkins University School of Medicine, Baltimore, Maryland; Director, Hematology and Coagulation Division, and Director, Platelet Immunology, Johns Hopkins Hospital, Baltimore, Maryland

KAREN E. KING, MD
Assistant Professor, Department of Pathology, Johns Hopkins University School of Medicine, Baltimore, Maryland; Associate Medical Director, Transfusion Medicine, and Medical Co-Director, Hematopoietic and Therapeutic Support Service, Johns Hopkins Hospital, Baltimore, Maryland

HARVEY G. KLEIN, MD
Chief, Department of Transfusion Medicine, Warren G. Magnuson Clinical Center, National Institutes of Health, Bethesda, Maryland

THOMAS A. LANE, MD
Professor, Department of Pathology, University of California, San Diego, School of Medicine, San Diego, California; Medical Director, Transfusion Service, and Medical Director, Stem Cell Laboratory, University of California, San Diego, Medical Center Hospitals, San Diego, California

NAOMI L. C. LUBAN, MD
Professor of Pediatrics and Pathology and Vice Chair, Pediatrics, George Washington University School of Medicine, Washington, D.C.; Director, Transfusion Medicine, and Vice Chair, Laboratory Medicine, Children's National Medical Center, Washington, D.C.

JEANNE LUMADUE, MD, PhD
Assistant Professor of Pediatrics and Pathology, George Washington University School of Medicine, Washington, D.C.; Director, Hematology and Stem Cell Processing Laboratories, Children's National Medical Center, Washington, D.C.

THOMAS J. LYNCH, PhD
Senior Staff Fellow, Center for Biologics Evaluation and Research, Food and Drug Administration, Bethesda, Maryland

MICHAEL McHEYZER-WILLIAMS, PhD
Assistant Professor, Department of Immunology, Duke University Medical Center, Durham, North Carolina

JAY E. MENITOVE, MD
Clinical Professor of Medicine, University of Missouri–Kansas City School of Medicine, Kansas City, Missouri; Clinical Professor of Medicine, Kansas University School of Medicine, Kansas City, Kansas; Executive Director and Medical Director, Community Blood Center of Greater Kansas City, Kansas City, Missouri

ALISON R. MOLITERNO, MD
Instructor, Division of Hematology, Department of Medicine, Johns Hopkins University School of Medicine, Baltimore, Maryland

THOMAS MORITZ, MD
Universitat—GH Essen, Essen, Germany; Staff Member, Innere Klinik and Poliklinik (Tumorforschung) Westdeutsches Tumorsentrum, Essen, Germany

HERBERT A. PERKINS, MD
Clinical Professor of Medicine, University of California School of Medicine, San Francisco, California; Senior Medical Scientist, Blood Centers of the Pacific, San Francisco, California

PATRICIA T. PISCIOTTO, MD
Professor of Laboratory Medicine, University of Connecticut School of Medicine, Farmington, Connecticut; Director of Blood Bank, John Dempsey Hospital, Farmington, Connecticut

FRED V. PLAPP MD, PhD
Clinical Associate Professor, University of Missouri–Kansas City School of Medicine, Kansas City, Missouri; Medical Director, Saint Luke's Regional Laboratories, Kansas City, Missouri

JANE M. RACHEL, MA
Manager, Molecular Diagnostics and Flow Cytometry, Saint Luke's Regional Laboratories, Kansas City, Missouri

JEFFREY J. RADE, MD
Assistant Professor, Division of Cardiology, Department of Medicine, Johns Hopkins University School of Medicine, Baltimore, Maryland; Staff and Interventional Cardiologist, Johns Hopkins University Hospital, Baltimore, Maryland

JOHN D. ROBACK, MD, PhD
Assistant Professor, Department of Pathology, Emory University School of Medicine, Atlanta, Georgia

MARIA LUZ DEL ROSARIO, MD
Pediatric Hematology Fellow, College of Medicine, University of Florida, Gainesville, Florida

SCOTT D. ROWLEY, MD
Associate Professor, Department of Medicine, University of Washington School of Medicine, Seattle, Washington; Associate Member, Fred Hutchinson Cancer Research Center, Seattle, Washington

R. SUE SHIREY, MS, MT(ASCP) SBB
Technical Specialist, Transfusion Medicine Division, Johns Hopkins Hospital, Baltimore, Maryland

DON L. SIEGEL, PhD, MD
Assistant Professor of Pathology and Laboratory Medicine, University of Pennsylvania School of Medicine, Philadelphia, Pennsylvania; Attending Physician, Blood Bank/Transfusion Medicine Section, Department of Pathology and Laboratory Medicine, University of Pennsylvania Medical Center, Philadelphia, Pennsylvania

LESLIE E. SILBERSTEIN, MD
Professor of Pathology and Laboratory Medicine, University of Pennsylvania School of Medicine, Philadelphia, Pennsylvania; Director, Blood Bank/ Transfusion Medicine Section, Department of Pathology and Laboratory Medicine, University of Pennsylvania Medical Center, Philadelphia, Pennsylvania

KENNETH J. SMITH, MD
Professor of Medicine, Emory University School of Medicine, Atlanta, Georgia; Interim Director, Division of Hematology and Oncology, Emory University School of Medicine, Atlanta, Georgia

EDWARD L. SNYDER, MD
Professor, Laboratory Medicine, Yale University School of Medicine, New Haven, Connecticut; Director, Blood Bank, Yale–New Haven Hospital, New Haven, Connecticut

JERRY L. SPIVAK, MD
Professor of Medicine and Oncology, Johns Hopkins University School of Medicine, Baltimore, Maryland; Active Staff, Johns Hopkins Hospital, Baltimore, Maryland

RONALD G. STRAUSS, MD
Professor of Pathology and Pediatrics, University of Iowa College of Medicine, Iowa City, Iowa; Medical Director, University of Iowa DeGowin Blood Center, University of Iowa Hospitals and Clinics, Iowa City, Iowa

DAVID F. STRONCEK, MD
Chief, Laboratory Services Section, Department of Transfusion Medicine, Warren G. Magnuson Clinical Center, National Institutes of Health, Bethesda, Maryland

THOMAS F. TEDDER, PhD
Associate Professor, Department of Immunology, Duke University Medical Center, Durham, North Carolina

MARILYN J. TELEN, MD
Professor of Medicine, Duke University, Durham, North Carolina; Chief, Division of Hematology, and Co-Director, Transfusion Service, Duke University Health System, Durham, North Carolina

IAIN J. WEBB, MD
Instructor in Medicine, Harvard Medical School, Boston, Massachusetts; Medical Director, Cell Manipulation, Gene Transfer and Cryopreservation Laboratories, Dana-Farber Cancer Institute, Boston, Massachusetts

KEVIN P. WHITBY, PhD
Research Fellow in Virology, Department of Virology, Royal Free and University College Medical School, University College, London, United Kingdom

DAVID A. WILLIAMS, MD
Associate Investigator, Howard Hughes Medical Institute, and Kipp Professor of Pediatrics, Indiana University School of Medicine, Indianapolis, Indiana

ROBERT M. WINSLOW, MD
Adjunct Professor of Medicine, University of California, San Diego, School of Medicine; Staff Hematologist, University of California San Diego Medical Center, San Diego, California

YUAN ZHUANG, PhD
Assistant Professor, Department of Immunology, Duke University Medical Center, Durham, North Carolina

PREFACE
TO THE SECOND EDITION

When we prepared the first edition of *Scientific Basis of Transfusion Medicine: Implications for Clinical Practice,* we understood that the field would continue to evolve rapidly, making subsequent revisions of our text mandatory to retain currency with the discipline. We are therefore delighted that W.B. Saunders and our many contributing colleagues have agreed to support this second edition, which you now have the opportunity to inspect.

We were gratified that the published reviews of the first edition were generally favorable. The many encouraging comments from individual readers also indicated to us that the project had met its intended goals, attempting to integrate "the advances in heterogeneous fields of scientific exploration that provide the basis for rational and safe transfusion practice." The high levels of interest expressed by international readers and many colleagues who do not traditionally align their interests with transfusion medicine gave us additional indications of our initial success.

Although we elected to maintain the general structure that we used in the first edition, a number of changes in authorship and topics have upgraded the content of this edition. We are particularly grateful to Drs. Daniels, Dzik, Geiger, Hillyer, and Kao for providing new chapters for this edition. Two of our senior contributors, Drs. Hackel and Perkins, were able to continue their commitment to the book, enhancing their chapters with the assistance of Drs. Daniels and Grumet. Other contributors from the first edition have enlisted new colleagues who have also added substantially to the value of the new text. In some areas, we deleted topics that have not evolved in major ways since publication of the first edition, although the chapters from the first edition still remain as authoritative references.

Mr. Marc Strauss and his able associates at Saunders provided excellent support to the continuation of this project. The continuing love and patience of our families, now including some transfusion recipients, makes our continuing professional development possible.

PREFACE
TO THE FIRST EDITION

Advances in multiple fields of research are broadening the scientific basis for evolving principles and practices within transfusion medicine. In particular, enhanced understanding of hematopoiesis, immunology, molecular genetics, immunohematology of cellular and plasma proteins, intrauterine and neonatal physiology, transplantation biology, immunomodulating effects of transfusion, and biology of infectious diseases has influenced transfusion practices. It is the goal of *Scientific Basis of Transfusion Medicine: Implications for Clinical Practice* to relate these scientific developments to their current and future impacts on transfusion practices.

This text reviews the influence of molecular genetics and growth factors on our understanding of the basic biology of hematopoiesis. An up-to-date discussion of cellular and humoral immunity, complement, and genetics provides the basis for understanding the immunohematology of transfusion. New developments in the structure, function, and immunology of cellular and protein components further enhance this understanding and have implications for their utility. The rapidly evolving field of transplantation immunology has facilitated intrauterine and neonatal transfusion as well as transplantation of bone marrow, peripheral blood, and umbilical cord stem cells.

Much attention has appropriately been directed toward the prevention of observed and potential adverse effects of transfusion. Our text defines the pathogenesis as well as the modes for prevention and treatment of immunomodulatory complications of transfusion, focusing on transfusion-associated alloimmunization, graft-versus-host disease, and immunosuppression. Immunological and molecular technologies have increased our understanding of the biology and pathogenesis of transfusion-related infection. Most importantly, these technologies suggest new strategies for identification and prevention of such an infection.

These developments have fostered the emerging diagnostic and therapeutic technologies applied to transfusion. Refinements in immunoassays, cell kinetics, flow cytometry, and molecular biology, such as polymerase chain reaction methodology, provide more sensitive and accurate diagnoses. Derivative therapeutic strategies include alternatives to homologous transfusions, recombinant growth factors, viral inactivation techniques, and gene therapy.

This is not a standard textbook on blood banking, and no effort has been made to exhaustively describe methods for the collection and provision of blood components. Rather, emphasis is on the integration of the advances in heterogeneous fields of scientific exploration that provide the basis for rational and safe transfusion practice. We believe strongly that there is no other discipline in which advances in both technology and biology have more directly influenced medical practice. Thus an opportunity exists for a comprehensive text to encompass this emerging field as it relates to the management of patients who require transfusion. This book is not intended only for physicians who specialize in transfusion medicine. It is likely to be of general interest to students and physicians who care for patients who need transfusions.

To accomplish our goals, we have been fortunate to recruit many colleagues, with primary interests in transfusion medicine, who have specific research expertise in the clinical or basic science areas. We were also able to enlist many who work in basic sciences or applied areas of clinical medicine for whom transfusion medicine is not their primary concern. Each of these individuals is an expert in a field related to transfusion medicine. They were encouraged to describe the status of their field in a manner relevant to transfusion issues. As a result, some of the chapter content may be more challenging to the traditional blood banker. We would encourage readers to increase their knowledge in these rapidly evolving areas.

The editors are also grateful to the contributors whose scholarship defines the quality of this book. We are grateful to Richard Zorab of the W.B. Saunders Company for his expertise and commitment to this project. We also express our appreciation to Sandra Valkhoff, for her expert editorial assistance.

The editors are indebted to their patients, students, laboratory coworkers, and other colleagues for their continued teaching and inspiration. We are most grateful for the loving support and patience of our families while much time and effort was devoted to this undertaking.

NOTICE

CONTENTS

SECTION

I Hematopoiesis

CHAPTER 1

Erythropoiesis

Alison R. Moliterno
Jerry L. Spivak

Erythropoiesis is the orderly, continuous process by which committed erythroid progenitor cells proliferate and differentiate into the mature red blood cells that are responsible for the transport of oxygen from the lungs to the tissues. Under normal circumstances, erythropoiesis must be ultimately responsive to tissue oxygen demands, as reflected by changes in production of erythropoietin, the primary regulator of erythropoiesis. In this chapter, the anatomy, physiology, and regulation of erythropoiesis are discussed.

ANATOMY OF ERYTHROPOIESIS

The term *erythron* has been used to describe the physiologically collective organ that encompasses the full complement of erythroid cells from the earliest committed erythroid progenitor cell to the mature circulating erythrocyte.[1] The erythron has three compartments: primitive progenitor cells, some of which are self-renewing; differentiating cells, recognizable morphologically as red cell precursors; and circulating erythrocytes. The pool size and proliferation of erythroid progenitor cells are responsive to tissue oxygen requirements through the mediation of the glycoprotein hormone erythropoietin.

Hematopoiesis may occur in a variety of sites, including the liver and spleen during fetal development and in certain clinical disorders in adults; normally, however, it is anatomically confined to the bone marrow of the axial skeleton. The trabecular bones of the pelvis and sternum are the primary sites of hematopoiesis in the adult, although in states of extreme stress, erythropoiesis will expand into the long bones and then into the liver and spleen, recapitulating its ontogeny. If the process is sufficiently exuberant, hematopoietic cells may spill into the paravertebral space and elsewhere, creating masses that can produce symptoms if they intrude on vital structures.[2]

Bone marrow consists of trabecular bone, containing a sinusoidal network of venous channels with hematopoietic cells encased among fat cells and stromal cells in the spaces between the venous sinuses.[3] The luminal surface of the sinuses is made up of a layer of endothelial cells. The adventitial or extraluminal surface of the vascular sinuses consists of a sheath of reticular cells that extend reticulin fibers throughout the hematopoietic compartments, contacting many types of cells. The supportive tissue between the vascular channels is known as *stroma*. It provides the microenvironment required for hematopoietic cell growth and includes, in addition to reticulin, collagen and other proteins such as laminin, proteoglycans, and fibronectin, to which hematopoietic cells and certain hematopoietic growth factors adhere.[4] Fibronectin is a large, multidomain molecule through which erythroid precursors attach to the supportive stroma by interacting with a specific receptor.[5, 6] Hemonectin is another protein constituent of the extracellular matrix of bone marrow that appears to have specific binding sites for granulocytic cells.[7] In addition to providing a framework for growth of hematopoietic cells, stromal elements also bind growth factors that regulate hematopoiesis,[8] may assist in enucleation, and may have other regulatory functions as well.

Hematopoietic Stem Cells

The hematopoietic cells that exist in the bone marrow stroma have variable capacities for self-renewal and propagation. In general, as hematopoietic cells acquire properties of differentiated cells, they lose their ability to self-renew and are eventually capable only of terminal differentiation and maturation. The maturation of erythrocytes from primitive hematopoietic cells occurs in an orderly manner through several stages, as shown in Figure 1–1.

The pluripotent hematopoietic stem cell (PHSC) can both renew itself and supply the populations of cells that are destined to differentiate along all of the hematopoietic lineages. The existence and characterization of the PHSC is demonstrated by studies that assess the capacity of bone marrow fractions to provide long-term engraftment to lethally irradiated recipients.[9] The PHSC is not distinguishable morphologically from other stem cells in the marrow, and its frequency among the marrow stem cells is less than 1%.[10] In addition, antigens specific only to the

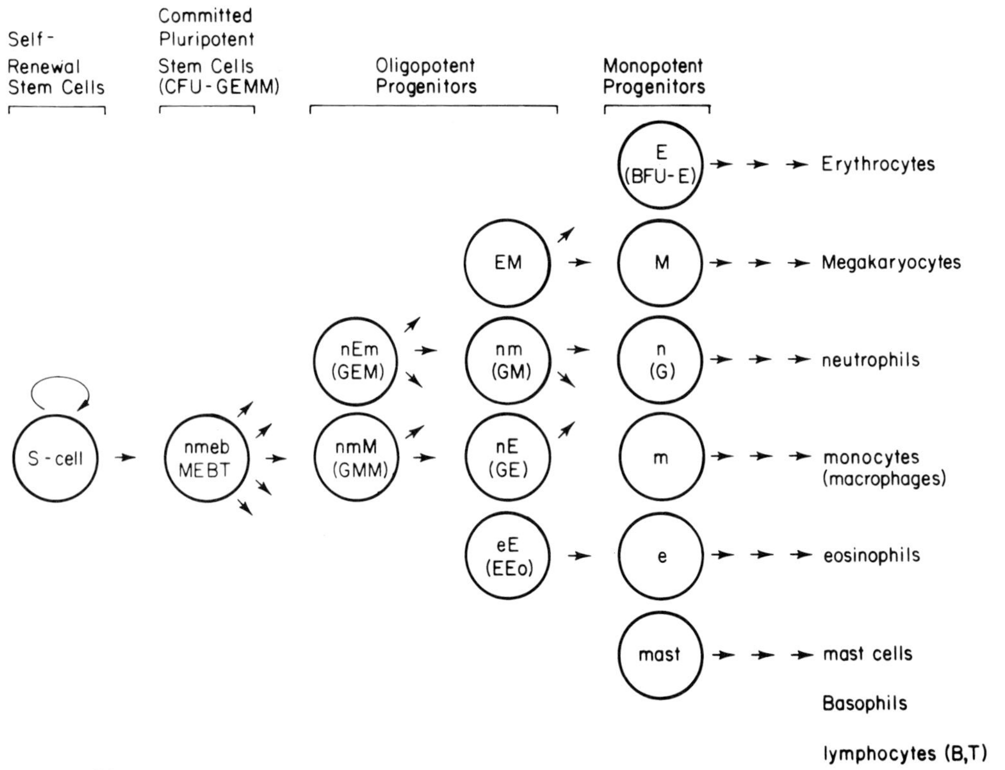

Figure 1–1. Sequence of lineage-specific commitment of hematopoietic progenitor cells based on a model of random commitment. Lymphoid progenitor cells also derive from the pluripotent stem cell but have been omitted from the diagram. Abbreviations reflect the potential for differentiation to a particular end-stage cell. (Adapted from Ogawa M, Porter PN, Nakahata T. The renewal and commitment to differentiation of hematopoietic stem cells. Blood 1983; 61:823–829.)

PHSC have not been identified; this situation makes the purification of the PHSC difficult. Incorporation of both size differences among progenitor populations (the PHSC is small and can be separated by counterflow elutriation)[11] and expression of certain membrane proteins ($CD34^+/CD38^-$)[10] have allowed the identification of a very small subset of the marrow stem cell pool capable of long-term multilineage engraftment.

The exact mechanism defining the direction of maturation of the PHSC seems to be a random process,[12] and hematopoietic growth factors appear to be permissive rather than instructive with regard to the proliferation and commitment of primitive progenitor cells to different cell lines. However, certain hematopoietic growth factors are required by committed progenitor cells of both the erythroid and myeloid lineages during specific stages of maturation. The PHSC may reproduce themselves or may differentiate into either lymphoid or mixed myeloid progenitor cells (colony-forming unit for granulocytes, erythroid cells, monocytes or macrophages, and megakaryocytes [CFU-GEMM]). The CFU-GEMM has a limited capacity to self-renew, or it may differentiate along the erythroid, myeloid, or megakaryocytic line.

The erythroid burst-forming unit (BFU-E) has very high proliferative capacity but limited self-renewal capacity and is named for the burst-like colonies that it forms in vitro in viscous medium.[13] These colonies may ultimately contain hundreds or thousands of nucleated cells.[14] The BFU-E is the earliest erythroid progenitor and can itself be divided into early and late forms; the early form has a higher proliferative capacity.[15] Early BFU-E may reside in the marrow or circulate in peripheral blood[16] and, at least in vivo, demonstrates a requirement for growth factors such as interleukin-3 (IL-3)[17–19] and granulocyte-macrophage (monocyte) colony-stimulating factor (GM-CSF)[20, 21] and for other factors such as stem cell factor,[22] interleukin-9,[23] and insulin-like growth factor-1.[24] Like the PHSC, the BFU-E constitutes only a small fraction of the marrow cell population. The majority are not in active cell cycle.[25] They appear to acquire the erythropoietin cell receptor as they mature and become responsive to erythropoietin.[26, 27]

The early BFU-E is responsible for replenishing the late, or mature, BFU-E pool,[25, 27] which then replenishes the population of erythroid precursors that terminally differentiate. The late BFU-E appears to represent a crucial transition phase in erythroid differentiation; at this stage, endotoxin interrupts erythropoiesis,[28] clonal suppression arises in polycythemia vera,[29] and infection with certain viruses occurs.[30]

Erythroid colony-forming units (CFU-E), the progeny of the BFU-E,[31] are completely dependent on erythropoietin for both proliferation and viability.[32] These are committed cells that differentiate into morphologically recognizable erythroblasts.[31] They are found mainly in the bone marrow, and the majority are in active cell cycle.[25] CFU-E form colonies of 4 to 64 hemoglobin-containing cells that enucleate spontaneously in tissue culture. CFU-E are the most erythropoietin dependent of all the erythroid progenitors and do not survive without it.[25] A late form of the CFU-E has been identified on the basis of a migration behavior during sedimentation that is different from the behavior of classic CFU-E.[33] Late CFU-E require only 24 hours for terminal differentiation and extrusion of the nucleus in vitro.[34] Presumably, these cells represent erythroid progenitors that have passed through the colony-forming stage and are committed to terminal differentiation at the time of harvest.

The earliest morphologically recognizable red cell precursor in the bone marrow is the proerythroblast (corresponding to a late CFU-E cell in clonogenic assays), which is approximately 10 times the size of a mature red cell. These cells reside in the bone marrow for approximately 5 to 7 days and progress through four stages. Proerythroblasts divide into basophilic erythroblasts, then into polychromatophilic erythroblasts, and finally into orthochromatic erythroblasts. These last cells extrude their nuclei and become reticulocytes, which enter the peripheral blood pool. After metabolizing residual RNA, they circulate for approximately 120 days before being removed by the reticuloendothelial system.

Erythropoiesis in the marrow occurs anatomically in units called *erythroblastic islands*, which consist of one or two macrophages surrounded by erythrocyte precursors in various stages of maturation.[35] These units are not apparent on examination of bone marrow films, because aspiration disrupts them, but they can be visualized in biopsy specimens.[36]

Ontogeny and Hemoglobin Production

During embryogenesis, the first differentiated hematopoietic cells can be detected in the blood islands of the yolk sac. Pluripotent and committed cells—BFU-E, CFU-E, and granulocyte-macrophage colony-forming units (CFU-GM)—are present in the yolk sac, but their numbers decline around the fifth week of gestation as the liver becomes the major site of hematopoiesis.[37, 38] Beginning approximately in the fifth month of gestation, the site of hematopoiesis gradually shifts to bone, and by birth, hepatic hematopoiesis has ceased. Because intramedullary capacity is limited, however, hepatic and splenic hematopoiesis, although ineffective, may resume in the setting of hematopoietic stress.[39] The earliest circulating erythroid cells are large and nucleated but are gradually succeeded by a population of nonnucleated cells.[40]

Studies in avian and amphibian embryos indicate hematopoietic stem cell activity within the embryo proper, which challenges the assumption that the yolk sac is the source of the PHSC for the fetal liver and, subsequently, the adult bone marrow.[41, 42] Mammalian hematopoietic activity has been identified in the yolk sac and the aorta-gonad-mesonephros (AGM) region at the prehepatic stage of hematopoiesis. Transplantation studies show that the AGM region precedes the yolk sac in embryonic hematopoietic stem cell development and that the AGM has a much higher frequency of PHSC. These observations indicate that the AGM is the first tissue initiating PHSC and that the yolk sac stem cells may be the result of stem cell migration from the AGM.[43]

Yolk sac erythropoiesis is characterized by the production of the embryonic hemoglobin chains and the hemoglobins Gower I ($\zeta_2\epsilon_2$), Gower II ($\alpha_2\epsilon_2$), and Portland ($\zeta_2\gamma_2$).[44] As erythropoiesis shifts to the liver, hemoglobin F ($\alpha_2\gamma_2$) becomes the major hemoglobin produced, although some hemoglobin A production also starts during this time. Around 30 weeks of gestation, there is a major switch from γ- to β-chain synthesis.[45] With regard to the shift from embryonic to adult hemoglobins, this may reflect the progression of primitive erythropoiesis in the yolk sac to definitive erythropoiesis in the liver, a hemoglobin shift that therefore may result from a change in precursor cell rather than from a switch in the transcription of the globin gene in a single common precursor.[46]

Membrane Assembly During Erythrogenesis

The unique shape of the erythrocyte and its ability to withstand many cycles of shearing, folding, and unfolding during its life span of 120 days depend largely on the red cell membrane and its associated cytoskeleton. The erythrocyte membrane consists of a lipid bilayer, integral membrane proteins that span the bilayer, and peripheral proteins that lie immediately beneath the cytoplasmic surface of the bilayer. Cholesterol and phospholipid, which are asymmetrically distributed between inner and outer portions of the bilayer, constitute about half of the overall membrane mass, and proteins constitute the other half. The erythrocyte membrane is schematically represented in Figure 1–2.

The protein components of the red cell membrane are named according to their migration during polyacrylamide gel electrophoresis (PAGE). When membranes are completely solubilized in an ionic detergent such as sodium dodecyl sulfate (SDS), approximately 10 major protein bands are distinguished when the resultant mixture is separated by PAGE and stained with Coomassie blue, although more than 100 minor proteins are apparent when more sensitive stains are used. Four major glycoproteins are revealed by periodic acid–Schiff staining.

Spectrin, the largest and most abundant protein of the membrane skeleton, is a large filamentous protein consisting of two distinct polypeptide chains—the α chain (240,000 Da, band 1) and the β chain (225,000 Da, band 2)—which are arranged antiparallel to form a heterodimer approximately 100 nm in length. The α chain of one dimer associates with the β chain of another dimer in a head-to-head manner to produce tetramers and higher molecular weight oligomers. Tail associations of multiple spectrin tetramers form and are stabilized by junctional complexes of actin (band 5) and protein 4.1.

Interaction of the spectrin-actin meshwork with the overlying lipid bilayer is mediated by ankyrin (band 2.1) and by protein 4.1. Ankyrin appears to bind the membrane to the bilayer by linking to the intrinsic membrane band 3 protein, the anion transporter. Protein 4.1 seems to link the skeleton to the membrane through associations with the cytoplasmic domains of the membrane glycophorins[47] and the anion channel.[48] The glycophorins span the bilayer and have extracellular domains containing a large number of oligosaccharide chains that express the speci-

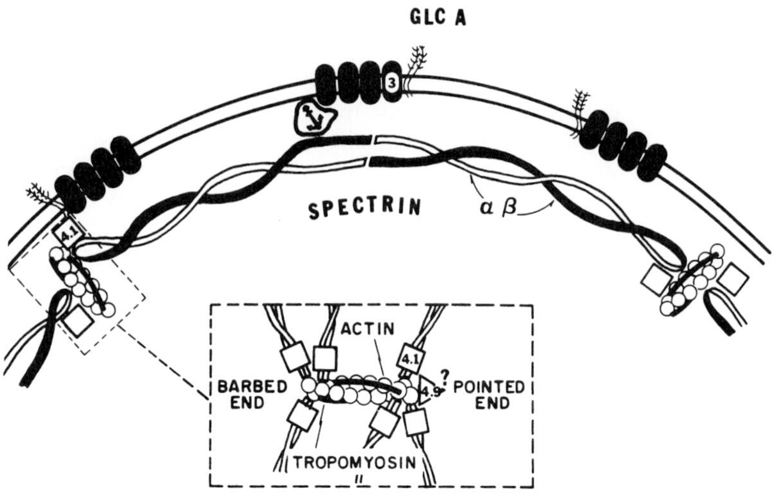

Figure 1–2. Schematic diagram of the human erythrocyte membrane skeleton. (Reproduced with permission from Bennett V. The membrane skeleton of human erythrocytes and its implications for more complex cells. Annu Rev Biochem 1985; 54:273–304.)

ficities for the MNS blood group system[49, 50] and apparently contain a receptor for the influenza virus.[51] The anion transporter accounts for 25% of the total membrane protein, spans the lipid bilayer, and plays an important role in respiration by exchanging chloride for bicarbonate and by permitting the movement of water. It may be involved in removal of senescent red cells, because hemoglobin denaturation during red cell aging leads to the clustering of band 3 and its coating by circulating immunoglobulin.[52] The ABO blood group antigens are contained in carbohydrate moieties on the extracellular domain of this protein.[53] The blood group P antigen serves as the receptor for parvovirus B19, which preferentially replicates in human erythroid progenitor cells.[54]

Because the membrane cytoskeleton confers shape and mechanical stability on the erythrocyte, deficiencies or functional abnormalities of any of the major membrane proteins including band 3 protein, ankyrin, protein 4.2, β spectrin and α spectrin, can cause defects in erythrocyte shape and mechanical stability.[55] Spectrin deficiency has been associated with spherocytosis,[56] and abnormal spectrins may result in pyropoikilocytosis.[57] Deficiency or functional abnormality of protein 4.1 can also result in elliptocytosis.[58, 59] Loss of glycosylphosphatidylinositol anchoring of proteins such as decay-accelerating factor and membrane inhibitor of reactive lysis (the pathophysiological basis of the acquired stem cell disorder paroxysmal nocturnal hemoglobinuria), result in hemolysis because of the unregulated action of complement on the red cell surface.[60]

During erythropoiesis, biogenesis of the membrane skeleton proceeds by protein synthesis, followed by assembly of the components. Assembly appears to proceed by attraction of newly synthesized proteins to high-affinity binding sites previously incorporated into the membrane.[61, 62] In vitro studies of developing avian[63] and mammalian[62, 64, 65] erythroid cells have defined the mechanism of membrane assembly during erythropoiesis. Although there are variations among species, it appears that undifferentiated erythroid progenitor cells constitutively synthesize major components of the membrane skeleton—specifically, α and β spectrin and ankyrin—as well as other membrane proteins. The anion transporter is synthesized earliest in red cell development and is inserted into the bilayer, followed by ankyrin and then by spectrin. The β subunit of spectrin is critical to membrane assembly because it contains the ankyrin-binding site; α spectrin is synthesized in excess of β spectrin, although the rate of synthesis of β spectrin may be increased 1.3- to 1.5-fold during stimulation with erythropoietin.[66] The assembly of α spectrin is limited by the amount of β spectrin synthesized, because the subunits are unstable as monomers. Assembly is completed within minutes of synthesis, and unassembled proteins are degraded. Protein 4.1 apparently is synthesized later and very rapidly, suggesting that its assembly is controlled by synthesis rather than by availability of protein 4.1–binding sites.[63]

During the nucleated stage of erythropoiesis, erythroid progenitor cells contain vimentin filaments that anchor the nucleus to the plasma membrane[64]; these filaments disappear as the cells enter the erythroblastic stage.[62] It has been postulated that enucleation during mammalian erythroid development is facilitated by the loss of vimentin filaments.[62] Although spontaneous extrusion of the nucleus can be observed in vitro, there may be some anatomical facilitation as well, because enucleation appears to take place chiefly in certain sites in marrow, spleen, or liver.[4]

Release of reticulocytes from the marrow may be facilitated by loss of the red cell fibronectin receptor. This receptor is a 140,000-Da protein that mediates selective binding of erythrocytes to fibronectin fibers in the stroma of the marrow.[5, 6] During differentiation, the fibronectin receptor vanishes from the membranes of erythroid cells, principally as they reach the reticulocyte stage of maturation in the marrow and through additional remodeling during passage through the spleen.[67] In a study of CFU-E and more mature cells purified from human marrow, more than 50% of CFU-E adhered to fibronectin. There was progressive loss of binding through maturation until reticulocytes were unable to adhere to fibronectin, which suggests that adhesion to fibronectin is developmentally regulated during erythropoiesis.[68] Although loss of the receptor obviously facilitates release of cells from the marrow, the presence of small amounts of fibronectin receptor on reticulocyte membranes may also facilitate the recognition and remodeling of young erythrocytes in the spleen.

During erythroid differentiation, a number of other membrane proteins expressed prominently on erythroid progenitors, such as the transferrin receptor and the human leukocyte antigen (HLA)–DR, are eliminated through different mechanisms.[69] The transferrin receptor is lost by shedding of membrane vesicles, and other proteins are lost during enucleation. Conversely, expression of the blood group antigens D,[70] A,[71] and Tn[72] progressively increases with erythroblast maturation.

NUTRITIONAL ASPECTS OF ERYTHROPOIESIS

Lack of iron or of vitamins such as cyanocobalamin (B_{12}) and folic acid results in anemias with well-recognized clinical features as well as characteristic morphological, biochemical, and proliferative abnormalities of cells in the bone marrow and peripheral blood. However, only a few studies have investigated the effects of these nutritional deficiencies on erythroid progenitor cells. With the advent of techniques enabling isolation of highly purified populations of erythroid progenitor cells, additional information on the effect of these deficiency states on erythropoiesis has been acquired.

Iron Deficiency

Iron-deficiency anemia has been classically described as a hypoproliferative anemia; however, when iron deficiency was experimentally induced in rats, the number of CFU-E in marrow increased 3.5 times over the level in control animals.[73] There were no significant differences in the numbers of BFU-E or CFU-GM. Iron deficiency appeared therefore to block terminal differentiation of pronormoblasts and their progeny without inhibiting the maturation of less mature cells. In another study of CFU-E proliferation with in vitro cultures of marrow cells from iron-overloaded or iron-deficient rats, the cultures from the iron-deficient animals grew large numbers of CFU-E, which responded to hemin (the oxidized form of heme), in contrast to the cultured CFU-E from the iron-overloaded marrow, which did not.[74] The biological basis for these observations may rest in the interplay of iron status and erythropoietin physiology. Altered intracellular iron balance, whether induced by chelators or by treatment with anti–transferrin receptor antibodies, resulted in elevations of serum erythropoietin levels in human subjects.[75] These observations suggest that intracellular iron balance regulates erythropoietin production. Further evidence of the relationship of erythropoietin biology to iron metabolism comes from studies of the effect of erythropoietin on the function of iron regulatory protein (IRP)–1. In human and murine cell lines, erythropoietin enhanced the binding of IRP-1 to the iron-responsive elements, resulting in increased transferrin receptor expression and increased iron uptake into cells.[76] The iron-deficient state induces erythropoietin production, which in turn increases iron uptake into cells.

Megaloblastic Anemias

Both folic acid and transcobalamin II are important in erythropoiesis, and erythroid progenitor cells express receptors for both of these nutritional factors. Interestingly, anti–folate receptor antibodies arrest erythropoiesis but do not prevent the proliferation of early erythroid progenitor cells, the BFU-E.[77]

Less information is available concerning erythropoiesis during vitamin B_{12} deficiency. In marrow taken from patients with vitamin B_{12} deficiency, there was a fourfold increase in the number of erythroid colonies formed during culture with erythropoietin in comparison with marrow from normal controls.[78] In another study using marrow from 11 megaloblastic patients and 14 normal controls, the megaloblastic marrows showed significant elevations in the binding of anti-human immunoglobulin but not in the binding of anti–crystallizable fragment (Fc) receptor to polychromatophilic erythroblasts; this observation suggests that abnormal immunological epitopes are expressed during megaloblastic development, mediating autoantibody binding. It was postulated that this antibody binding might also play a role in the premature destruction of these cells during megaloblastic erythropoiesis.[79]

In these nutritional deficiency states, the cells most affected are apparently those entering terminal differentiation, whereas more primitive cells are less affected and may accumulate to the degree permitted by the ambient concentration of growth factors such as erythropoietin.

Pyridoxine-Responsive Sideroblastic Anemia

Although categorized here as nutritional deficiencies, these disorders are not true deficiency states; rather, they are hematopoietic stem cell disorders that respond to pyridoxine supplementation. The common feature of these anemias is microcytosis with ringed sideroblasts, associated with mutations of the δ-aminolevulinate synthase (ALAS2) gene.[80] Mutations of ALAS2 that affect the binding of its cofactor, pyridoxal 5′-phosphate, results in loss of function of ALAS2, a critical enzyme in the heme biosynthetic pathway. Supplementation with pyridoxine stabilizes the function of ALAS2 and results in improved, although perhaps not completely normal, erythropoiesis. Although typically a heritable disorder with expression in early adulthood, manifestations in the older population that are responsive to pyridoxine have been reported.[81] Therefore, this process should be considered in all patients with sideroblastic anemia.

REGULATORS OF ERYTHROPOIESIS

Erythropoiesis appears to be regulated by a number of humoral and cell-associated factors that may stimulate or inhibit erythropoiesis. Erythropoietin is the most extensively studied and clinically important. However, erythropoietin is not the only growth factor that interacts with erythroid cells; other factors(such as GM-CSF, granulocyte colony-stimulating factor [G-CSF], and thrombopoietin), interleukins (such as interleukin [IL]–1, [IL]-3, [IL]-6, and [IL]-9), stem cell factor, and certain stromal proteins have been found to have important roles in promoting or inhibiting erythropoiesis. These act chiefly on the more primitive cells, before and including the BFU-E, whereas later erythroid progenitor cells (CFU-E and beyond) appear to respond mainly to erythropoietin.

Colony-stimulating factors (CSFs) are a group of glycosylated proteins that target a range of cell types and are increasingly recognized as clinically useful agents, especially in patients with impaired myelopoiesis. In addition to stimulating the proliferation and maturation of erythroid and myeloid cells, these proteins may stimulate the function of mature cells. GM-CSF is glycoprotein produced by macrophages and endothelial cells.[82, 83] In addition to affecting BFU-E, it influences the proliferation and behavior of granulocyte and monocyte precursors.[21]

Thrombopoietin is a 45,000-Da glycoprotein produced primarily in the liver and, to a lesser extent, in the kidney, smooth muscle, spleen, and bone marrow. Although thrombopoietin is the lineage-specific factor for the proliferation and differentiation of megakaryocyte progenitors,[84] thrombopoietin also acts directly on hematopoietic stem cells in vitro,[85] and mice with targeted disruption of the thrombopoietin gene have reduced numbers of both multilineage and committed progenitor cells.[86] Thrombopoietin has been demonstrated to have particular significance in the development of erythroid progenitors, inasmuch as hematopoietic progenitor cells cultured in the presence of erythropoietin and thrombopoietin produce greater numbers of erythroid colonies than observed in cultures with erythropoietin alone. This effect may be derived either from direct proliferative effects of thrombopoietin on erythroid progenitors[87, 88] or by thrombopoietin's promoting survival of hematopoietic stem cells,[89] which subsequently increase the pool of erythroid progenitors.

Interleukins are a family of proteins with molecular weights ranging from 15,000 to 30,000 Da, generally produced by lymphocytes. IL-3 is a 28,000-Da glycoprotein required for development of hematopoietic cells, chiefly by providing a permissive environment for maturation to early progenitor cells.[90] Of erythroid precursors, the BFU-E are most sensitive to IL-3.[19] Interleukins IL-1 and IL-6 appear to have some effect in promoting colony formation,[90–92] and IL-9 may have a similar role.[23] IL-6 appears to require stem cell factor to promote the proliferation of erythroid progenitors.[93]

Stromal factors include the stromal proteins to which erythroid progenitors adhere. *Stem cell factor* (SCF), or *kit*-ligand (denoting its identity as the protein binding to the transmembrane tyrosine kinase receptor encoded by the c-*kit* oncogene), may affect the migration and stromal adhesion of the hematopoietic stem cell and acts to stimulate CFU-GEMM and BFU-E proliferation.[94–96] A deficiency of the stromal protein hemonectin has been demonstrated in a strain of mice with decreased hematopoiesis[97] and is believed to be the molecular defect in these animals.

A variety of hormones (including glucocorticoids, androgens, estrogens, progesterones, growth hormones, prolactins, thyroid hormones, and insulin and insulin-like growth factors) and other agents such as prostaglandins have variable effects on the behavior of erythropoietic cells in vivo and in vitro, although isolating specific effects attributable to these agents is even more difficult than in the case of more specific hematopoietic growth factors. Glucocorticoids may be inhibitory or stimulatory, depending on experimental conditions.[98, 99] Androgens enhance erythropoiesis[100] but do not appear to affect erythropoietin levels under normal circumstances.[101] Of these various growth factors, insulin-like growth factor-1 appears to be the most important physiologically.[24]

Inhibitors of erythropoiesis may prevent the recruitment of stem cells into cycle or may interfere with maturation, and may be homeostatic or pathological. For example, locally active factors such as IL-1, tumor necrosis factor, or transforming growth factor-β may suppress the production of erythropoietin,[102, 103] and because these inhibitors of erythropoietin production may also directly inhibit the effects of erythropoietin on erythroid progenitor proliferation,[104, 105] their contribution to suppression of erythropoiesis overall is greatly magnified. Interestingly, transforming growth factor-β–induced inhibition of erythroid progenitor cell proliferation appears to be associated with enhancement of erythroid cell differentiation.[106] A differentiation-inhibiting protein (DIP) has been isolated from the blood of a woman with pure red cell aplasia, which suggests that erythropoietic inhibitors may have roles in certain disease states.[107]

Finally, certain transcription factors involved in the regulation of erythropoiesis have been defined. TAL-1, a basic helix-loop-helix protein, is essential for embryonic hematopoiesis, whereas GATA-2, a zinc finger protein, is required for both primitive and definitive embryonic erythropoiesis.[108] GATA-1 is another zinc finger protein that transactivates a number of erythroid-specific genes, including the globin genes[109, 110] and the erythropoietin receptor gene.[111] Although its expression is not limited to erythroid cells, GATA-1 is necessary for the completion of primitive and definitive embryonic erythropoiesis. An important aspect of its function appears to be suppression of apoptosis;[112] GATA-2, in fact, appears to promote erythroid cell proliferation. The mechanisms involved in the sequential expression of these transcription factors during development are not currently known.

Erythropoietin

Erythropoietin is the principal hormone regulating red cell production and is an obligatory growth factor for erythroid cells from the level of the CFU-E through the basophilic erythroblast stage. Production of this hormone appears to be regulated primarily by tissue oxygen demand, and it seems to function as the primary means of feedback from the tissue to the bone marrow concerning oxygen requirements. Erythropoietin is never absent from plasma, even in the anephric state or in states of extreme erythrocytosis. Interestingly, except in states of severe hypoxic exposure, hormone levels do not remain significantly above normal, although they may remain somewhat higher than normal in individual cases.[113, 114] The humoral regulation of erythropoiesis in response to hypoxia was first demonstrated in 1950,[115] and the first bioassay for this activity was described in 1953.[116] The serum erythropoietin concentration is primarily related to the rate of production in the kidney; however, regulation may also occur as a consequence of the rate of use. For a given hemoglobin concentration, serum erythropoietin levels were lower in patients with proliferative anemias than in patients with hypoproliferative anemias, which indicates an inverse relationship between red blood cell precursor mass and the serum erythropoietin level.[117]

Erythropoietin is a heavily glycosylated protein with a molecular weight of 30,400 Da and a carbohydrate content of 30% to 40%.[118, 119] The carbohydrate structure, consisting mainly of tetra-antenary branching units,[120] is rich in sialic acid. The carbohydrate moiety is essential for secretion from the cells that produce erythropoietin, for hormone survival in the circulation, and for its biological activity. Desialated erythropoietin is rapidly cleared from the circulation and metabolized in liver,[121, 122] and incompletely glycosylated erythropoietin has reduced biological activity.[123, 124]

The gene for human erythropoietin has been localized to human chromosome 7 (7q11–22)[125] and consists of a single copy with five exons that encode a 193–amino acid peptide. The final active peptide remains after cleavage of a 27–amino acid N-terminal leader sequence and consists of 166 amino acids with a predicted molecular weight of 18,400 Da.[119] The mature, functionally active hormone lacks arginine 166, apparently as a result of post-translational modification.[126] The secreted protein is hydrophobic, and because it is a pharmacological reagent, albumin is necessary to prevent its adsorption to glass surfaces. Its structure is highly conserved with a remarkable degree of homology among human, murine, and primate erythropoietins; and cross-reactivity is the rule among mammalian species.[127, 128]

Erythropoietin Receptor

Erythropoietin interacts with its target cells through specific cell surface receptors. Once the erythropoietin gene was cloned, it was possible to identify the gene for its receptor by expression cloning.[129] The gene consists of 8 exons and 7 introns and contains a promoter region with defined transcription factor binding sites (CACCC, GATA-1, Sp1) and one inhibitory and two enhancer regions 5′ to the ATG initiation site. Erythroid specific expression of the gene appears to be provided by elements both 5′ and 3′ prime to the promoter that can exert a negative effect in nonerythroid tissues. The receptor is expressed primarily by erythroid progenitor cells, but also by embryonal stem cells, multipotent hematopoietic progenitor cells, endothelial cells, and neural cells.[130–132] The biological role of this receptor in nonerythroid cells has not been established.

The erythropoietin receptor gene codes for a 508–amino acid glycoprotein located on human chromosome 19.[133] The receptor is a member of the hematopoietic growth factor receptor superfamily that includes the receptors for IL-2 (β-chain), IL-3, IL-4, IL-5, IL-6, IL-7, GM-CSF, G-CSF, thrombopoietin, leukemia inhibitory factor (LIF), ciliary neurotrophic factor (CNTF), oncostatin M, growth hormone, and prolactin.[134] They share in common four positionally conserved cysteines in their extracellular domain, as well as a tryptophan-serine-X-tryptophan-serine (WSXWS) motif or its homolog located near the transmembrane region, and each lacks kinase motifs in their intracellular domain. These receptors also contain shared homologous regions in the proximal portion of their intracellular domain that are responsible for mitogenesis and for association with members of a specific cytoplasmic tyrosine kinase family: the Janus kinases (JAKs). An important characteristic of receptors in this superfamily is ligand-induced dimerization or hetero-oligomerization. In addition, soluble forms of many of these receptors, including the erythropoietin receptor, have been identified; with the exception of the soluble IL-6 receptor, the function of these soluble receptors is undefined.

Binding of erythropoietin causes its receptor to dimerize, leading to the approximation of two JAK2 molecules. Once associated, the JAK2 molecules intramolecularly autophosphorylate, become activated, and phosphorylate some or all of the eight tyrosines in the receptor's cytoplasmic domain. This permits receptor docking by cytosolic proteins with SH2 domains, where they can be phosphorylated, presumably by JAK2, and also associate with other cytosolic proteins to form signal-transducing complexes. In addition to JAK2 and the erythropoietin receptor, other proteins phosphorylated on tyrosine after receptor-ligand binding include SHIP, STAT5, SHP1, SHP2, shc, PLC, Vav, Ras GAP, fes, Raf, PI-3 kinase, and MAPK.[135]

The tyrosine phosphorylation of cytosolic proteins after binding of erythropoietin by its receptor activates a number of biochemical pathways. For example, phosphorylation of STAT5 permits its homodimerization and rapid translocation to the nucleus, where it is involved in the activation of a number of genes, including c-fos and cis,[136] whereas phosphorylation of Shc and Ras GAP leads to activation of the RAS-MAPK pathway. How these pathways, as well as others, are integrated into erythroid cell proliferation and differentiation has not yet been established and is likely to be complex. Thus both the JAK2 and the PI-3 kinase pathways have been independently linked to erythroid cell proliferation.[137] The redundancy of signal transduction pathways between the various receptors expressed in a single cell, coupled with the complexity of signal regulation of the receptors, render predictions of functional consequences of receptor abnormalities challenging. For example, inherited mutations of the erythropoietin receptor associated with erythrocytosis that are the result of carboxyl-terminal truncations implicate hypersensitivity of the erythropoietin receptor to erythropoietin, because this domain of the receptor functions in its downregulation.[138] However, in vitro studies of such mutations indicate that the hypersensitivity may be not to erythropoietin but rather to insulin-like growth factor-1.[135] Furthermore, there is evidence of cross talk between the receptors of different growth factors. For example, SCF stimulation of c-kit leads to tyrosine phosphorylation and activation of the erythropoietin receptor.[139]

The specific genes activated after exposure to erythropoietin are currently under scrutiny, but it is well established that expression of c-myc, in contrast to c-fos or c-jun, is rapidly upregulated by erythropoietin in erythroid progenitor cells.[140] C-myc expression is correlated with the proliferative behavior of erythroid progenitor cells but with not their differentiation; this correlation is not surprising, inasmuch as erythroid cell differentiation can take place in the absence of proliferation and most CFU-E are in active cell cycle in the absence of erythropoietin. STAT5 is not involved in the upregulation of c-myc expression and does not appear to be required for the proliferation of erythroid progenitor cells.[141]

Hematopoietic growth factors are involved not only in the regulation of the proliferation of their target cells but also in maintaining their viability. This contention is correct with regard to erythropoietin, but only to the extent that it is progenitor cell stage–specific. Erythropoietin acts as a survival factor for late-stage erythroid progenitor cells such as the CFU-E, which are actively cycling.[142] However, for early erythroid progenitor cells that are largely quiescent, erythropoietin acts as both a mitogen and a survival factor.[143] An important corollary of this is the requirement for erythropoietin to prevent apoptosis in erythroid progenitor cells through the upregulation of Bcl-x expression,[144] in contrast to terminal differentiation, which occurs in the absence of erythropoietin. At pharmacological doses, the hormone may have other functions, such as promoting hemoglobin F synthesis.[145] The expression of the erythropoietin receptor varies throughout erythroid progenitor cell maturation, with maximal expression at the CFU-E stage and decreased expression during terminal differentiation.[146]

Erythropoietin Physiology

Erythropoietin is produced constitutively in peritubular interstitial fibroblastoid cells in the inner cortex of the kidney near the proximal convoluted tubules.[147] These cells appear to contain the renal oxygen sensor as well.[148] With increasing anemia, the number of renal interstitial cells staining for erythropoietin messenger RNA rises exponentially, along with increases in serum erythropoietin. These data suggest that the rise in serum erythropoietin is caused by the production of the hormone by larger numbers of cells rather than to a higher rate of erythropoietin production by cells already producing the erythropoietin.[149] Thus, in states of hypoxia, more peritubular cells may be recruited to erythropoietin production, but neither anemia nor hypoxia appears to affect the rate or net synthesis of hormone in cells that produce it constitutively.[149] Erythropoietin is also produced in hepatocytes, but a greater degree of hypoxia appears to be necessary to initiate its production in the liver.[150] In contrast to kidney cells, hepatocytes can vary their rate of erythropoietin production.[151] In addition to hepatocytes, liver cells of interstitial nonepithelial morphology, which resemble the erythropoietin-producing cells of the kidney, also produce erythropoietin.[151] In states of extreme hypoxia, a substantial fraction of total body erythropoietin may be produced in the liver.[152]

There are no preformed stores of erythropoietin in either the kidneys or the liver to meet higher demand for this hormone. New synthesis occurs in states of greater need. Animals that have been pretreated with inhibitors of RNA synthesis do not respond to hypoxia with increased erythropoietin production.[153] Although the level of erythropoietin production initially reflects the degree of anemia or hypoxia,[149] high initial levels are not usually maintained, probably because immediate compensatory mechanisms—such as changes in ventilation, heart rate, and stroke volume; redistribution of blood flow; and changes in oxygen-hemoglobin affinity—reduce the degree of tissue hypoxia except in extreme cases. Although elevated production of erythropoietin is not sustained, increases in red cell production and red cell mass in hypoxic states appear to be maintained by lower concentrations of hormone. For example, a state of hypobaric hypoxia results in detectable increases in circulating erythropoietin within 2 hours.[154] If elevated erythropoietin production is sustained, an increase in red cell mass results, satisfying tissue oxygen demands. Erythropoietin production is subsequently suppressed, by the increased red cell mass, which can be sustained by hormone levels in the normal range, although slightly higher than baseline.[98, 99]

It is likely that the initial burst of erythropoietin production triggered by tissue hypoxia serves to recruit early erythroid progenitor cells into a maturing pool of erythropoietin-responsive cells and that thereafter only small quantities of hormone are required for their support and differentiation. However, because patients with end-stage renal disease and anemia usually have normal levels of erythropoietin, it appears that factors other than the level of erythropoietin are important in maintaining a normal rate of red cell production. The clearance of the hormone from plasma has been studied in experimental animals.[121, 155, 156] The level of the hormone influences neither its production nor its clearance,[121] but its clearance is influenced by the cellularity of the bone marrow, in which erythropoietin is metabolized by its target cells.[117]

Erythropoietin can be measured with a sensitive radioimmunoassay. The normal serum level varies from 4 to 26 mU/mL. In general, serum immunoreactive erythropoietin reflects the amount of biologically active hormone,[157] and in normal states there is a loglinear relationship between hemoglobin level and the serum immunoreactive erythropoietin. Because of the wide range of "normal" erythropoietin levels, it is only after the hematocrit declines below 10.5 g/dL that an unequivocal rise in serum erythropoietin is evident. Blood donors who are repeatedly phlebotomized become anemic, but their serum erythropoietin levels do not rise substantially unless the hematocrit falls below 35 g/dL.[158] In renal disease, correlation between the immunoreactive erythropoietin level and hemoglobin concentration is lost when the serum creatinine level exceeds 1.5 mg/dL.[157] A number of other conditions, such as rheumatoid arthritis,[159] cancer,[160] infection,[157] sickle cell disease,[161] acquired immunodeficiency syndrome (AIDS),[162] bone marrow transplantation,[163] and pregnancy,[164] can affect the relationship between hemoglobin and erythropoietin levels. In polycythemia vera, the erythropoietin level is usually low or normal. An elevated erythropoietin level may reflect ectopic hormone production or tissue hypoxia.[165] In some patients with secondary erythrocytosis and an increased level of erythropoietin, multiple measurements may be necessary to establish a diagnosis, because erythropoietin production may fluctuate.[165] Unless tissue hypoxia is severe, both the elevated red cell mass and the attendant state of hyperviscosity actually tend to suppress erythropoietin production and normalize the serum erythropoietin level. Thus the serum erythropoietin level cannot be considered a surrogate measure of tissue oxygenation.

REFERENCES

1. Boycott AE. The blood as a tissue: hypertrophy and atrophy of the red corpuscles. Proc R Soc Med 1929; 23:15.
2. Papavasiliou C, Sandilos P. Effect of radiotherapy on symptoms due to heterotopic marrow in β-thalassemia. Lancet 1987; 1:13.
3. Lichtman MA. The ultrastructure of the hematopoietic environment of the marrow: a review. Exp Hematol 1981; 9:391.
4. Hanspal M. Importance of cell-cell interactions in regulation of erythropoiesis. Curr Opin Hematol 1997; 4:142.
5. Patel VP, Lodish HF. The fibronectin receptor on mammalian erythroid precursor cells: characterization and developmental regulation. J Cell Biol 1986; 102:449.
6. Tsai S, Patel V, Beaumont E, et al. Differential binding of erythroid and myeloid progenitors to fibroblasts and fibronectin. Blood 1987; 69:1587.
7. Campbell AD, Long MW, Wicha MS. Haemonectin, a bone marrow adhesion protein specific for cells of the granulocytic lineage. Nature 1987; 329:744.
8. Gordon MY, Riley GP, Watt SM, et al. Compartmentalization of a hematopoietic growth factor (GM-CSF) by glycosaminoglycans in the bone marrow microenvironment. Nature 1987; 326:403.
9. Orlic D, Bodine DM. What defines a pluripotent hematopoietic stem cell (PHSC): will the real PHSC please stand up! Blood 1994; 84:3991.
10. Civin CI, Almeida-Porada G, Lee MJ, et al. Sustainable, retransplantable, multilineage engraftment of highly purified adult human bone marrow stem cells in vivo. Blood 1996; 88:4102.
11. Jones RJ, Wagner JE, Celano P, et al. Separation of pluripotent haematopoietic stem cells from spleen colony-forming cells. Nature 1990; 347:188.
12. Ogawa M, Porter PN, Nakahata T. The renewal and commitment to differentiation of hematopoietic stem cells. Blood 1983; 61:823.
13. Axelrod AA, McLeod DL, Shreeve MM, et al. Properties of cells that produce erythrocytic colonies in vitro. *In* Robinson WA (ed): Proceedings of the Second International Workshop on Hematopoiesis in Culture. Washington, DC: U.S. Government Printing Office, 1974, pp 226–234.
14. Gregory CJ, Eaves AC. Human marrow cells capable of erythropoietic differentiation in vitro: definition of three erythroid colony responses. Blood 1977; 49:855.
15. Humphries RK, Eaves AC, Eaves CJ. Characterization of a primitive erythropoietic progenitor found in mouse marrow before and after several weeks in culture. Blood 1979; 53:746.
16. Clark BJ, Housman D. Characterization of an erythroid precursor cell of high capacity in normal human peripheral blood. Proc Natl Acad Sci U S A 1977; 74:1105.
17. Iscove NN, Roitsch CA, Williams N, Guilbert LJ. Molecules stimulating early red cell, granulocyte, macrophage and megakaryocyte precursors in culture: similarity in size, hydrophobicity and charge. J Cell Physiol 1982; 1(suppl 1):65.
18. Goldwasser E, Ihle JN, Prystowsky MB, et al. The effect of interleukin 3 on hemopoietic precursor cells. *In* Golde DN, Marks PA (eds): Normal and Neoplastic Hematopoiesis. New York: Alan R Liss, 1983, pp 301–309.
19. Goodman JW, Hall EA, Miller KL, Shinpock SG. Interleukin 3 promotes erythroid burst formation in "serum free" cultures without detectable erythropoietin. Proc Natl Acad Sci U S A 1985; 82:3291.
20. Donahue RE, Emerson SG, Wang EA, et al. Demonstration of burst-promoting activity of recombinant GM-CSF on circulating erythroid progenitors using an assay involving the delayed addition of erythropoietin. Blood 1985; 66:1479.
21. Donahue RE, Wang EA, Stone DK, et al. Stimulation of haematopoiesis in primates by continuous infusion of recombinant human GM-CSF. Nature 1986; 321:872.
22. Dai CH, Krantz SB, Zsebo KM. Human burst-forming units–erythroid need direct interaction with stem cell factor for further development. Blood 1991; 78:2493.
23. Donahue RE, Yang YC, Clark SC. Human P40 T-cell growth factor (interleukin-9) supports erythroid colony formation. Blood 1990; 75:2271.
24. Sawada K, Krantz SB, Dessypris EN, et al. Human colony-forming units–erythroid do not require accessory cells but do require direct interaction with insulin-like growth factor I and/or insulin for erythroid development. J Clin Invest 1989; 83:1701.
25. Iscove NN. The role of erythropoietin in regulation of population size and cell cycling of early and late erythroid precursors in mouse bone marrow. Cell Tissue Kinet 1977; 10:323.
26. Sieff CA, Emerson SG, Mufson A, et al. Dependence of highly enriched bone marrow progenitors on hematopoietic growth factors and their response to recombinant erythropoietin. J Clin Invest 1986; 77:74.
27. Gregory CJ. Erythropoietin sensitivity as a differentiation marker in the erythropoietic system: studies of three erythropoietic colony responses in culture. J Cell Physiol 1976; 89:289.
28. Udupa KB, Reissmann KR. In vivo and in vitro effect of bacterial endotoxin on erythroid precursors (CFU-E and ERC) in the bone marrow of mice. J Lab Clin Med 1977; 89:278.
29. Adamson JW, Singer JW, Catalano P, et al. Polycythemia vera: further in vitro studies of hematopoietic regulation. J Clin Invest 1980; 66:1363.
30. Kost TA, Koury MJ, Hankins WD, Krantz SB. Target cells for Friend virus–induced erythroid bursts in vitro. Cell 1979; 18:145.
31. Stephenson JR, Axelrod AA, McLeod DL, Shreeve MM. Induction of colonies of hemoglobin-synthesizing cells by erythropoietin in vitro. Proc Natl Acad Sci U S A 1971; 68:1542.
32. Hara H, Ogawa M. Erythropoietic precursors in mice under erythropoietic stimulation and suppression. Exp Hematol 1977; 5:141.
33. Misiti J, Spivak JL. Separation of erythroid progenitor cells in mouse bone marrow by isokinetic-gradient sedimentation. Blood 1979; 54:105.
34. Ouellette PL, Monette FC. Erythroid progenitors forming clusters in vitro demonstrate high erythropoietin sensitivity. J Cell Physiol 1980; 105:181.
35. Bessis, M. Living Blood Cells and Their Ultrastructure. Berlin: Springer-Verlag, 1973.
36. Bessis M, Lessin LS, Beutler E. Morphology of the erythron. *In* Williams WJ, Beutler E, Erslev AJ, Lichtman MA (eds): Hematology, 3rd ed. New York: McGraw-Hill, 1983, p 257.
37. Migliaccio G, Migliaccio AR, Petti S, et al. Human embryonic hemopoiesis. Kinetics of progenitors and precursors underlying the yolk sac–liver transition. J Clin Invest 1986; 78:51.
38. Moore MAS, Metcalf D. Ontogeny of the haematopoietic system; yolk sac origin of in vivo and in vitro colony forming cells in the developing mouse embryo. Br J Haematol 1970; 18:279.
39. Brannon D. Extramedullary hematopoiesis in anemia. Bull Johns Hopkins Hosp 1927; 41:104.
40. Jones OP. Cytology of pathogenic marrow cells with special reference to bone marrow biopsies. *In* Downey H (ed): Handbook of Hematology. New York: Hoeber, 1938, p 2043.
41. Lassila O, Eskola J, Tiovanen P, et al. The origin of lymphoid stem cells studied in chick yolk-sac embryo chimeras. Nature 1978; 272:353.
42. Turpern JB, Knudson CM, Hoefen PB. The early ontogeny of hematopoietic cells studied by grafting cytogenetically labeled tissue analgen: localization of a prospective stem cell compartment. Dev Biol 1981; 85:112.
43. Medvinsky A, Dzierzak E. Definitive hematopoiesis is autonomously initiated by the AGM region. Cell 1996; 86:897.

44. Peschle C, Mavilio F, Care A, et al. Haemoglobin switching in human embryos: asynchrony of ζ and ε globin switches in primitive and definitive erythropoietin lineage. Nature 1985; 313:235.
45. Bunn HF, Forget BG. Hemoglobin: Molecular, Genetic, and Clinical Aspects. Philadelphia: WB Saunders, 1986.
46. Nakano T, Kodama H, Honjo T. In vitro development of primitive and definitive erythrocytes from different precursors. Science 1996; 272:722.
47. Anderson RA, Lovrien RE. Glycophorin is linked by band 4.1 to the human erythrocyte membrane skeleton. Nature 1984; 307:665.
48. Pasternak GR, Anderson RA, Leto TL, Marchesi VT. Interactions between protein 4.1 and band 3. An alternative binding site for an element of the membrane skeleton. J Biol Chem 1985; 260:3676.
49. Furthmayr H. Glycophorins A, B, and C: a family of sialoglycoproteins. Isolation and characterization of trypsin-derived peptides. J Supramol Struct 1978; 9:79.
50. Anstee DJ. The blood group MNSs-active sialoglycoproteins. Semin Hematol 1981; 18:13.
51. Marchesi VT. Functional proteins of the human red blood cell membrane. Semin Hematol 1979; 16:3.
52. Low PS, Waugh SM, Zinke K, Drenckhahn D. The role of hemoglobin denaturation and band 3 clustering in red blood cell aging. Science 1985; 227:531.
53. Low PS. Structure and function of the cytoplasmic domain of band 3: center of erythrocyte membrane-peripheral protein interactions. Biochim Biophys Acta 1986; 864:145.
54. Brown KE, Young NS. Parvoviruses and bone marrow failure. Stem Cells 1996; 14:151.
55. Wichterle H, Hanspal M, Palek J, Jarolim P. Combination of two mutant alpha spectrin alleles underlies a severe spherocytic hemolytic anemia. J Clin Invest 1996; 98:2300.
56. Agre P, Casella JF, Zinkham WH, et al. Partial deficiency of spectrin in hereditary spherocytosis. Nature 1985; 314:380.
57. Knowles WJ, Morrow JS, Speicher DW, et al. Molecular and functional changes in spectrin from patients with hereditary pyropoikilocytosis. J Clin Invest 1983; 71:1019.
58. Tchernia G, Mohandas N, Shohet SB. Deficiency of skeletal membrane protein band 4.1 in homozygous hereditary elliptocytosis. J Clin Invest 1981; 68:454.
59. McGuire M, Smith BS, Agre P. Distinct variants of erythrocyte protein 4.1 inherited in linkage with elliptocytosis and Rh type in three white families. Blood 1988; 72:200.
60. Rosse WF. Hematopoiesis and the defect in paroxysmal nocturnal hemoglobinuria. J Clin Invest 1997; 100:953.
61. Lazarides E, Moon RT. Assembly and topogenesis of the spectrin-based membrane skeleton in erythroid development. Cell 1984; 37:354.
62. Lazarides E. From genes to structural morphogenesis: the genesis and epigenesis of a red blood cell. Cell 1987; 51:345.
63. Staufenbiel M, Lazarides E. Assembly of protein 4.1 during chicken erythroid differentiation. J Cell Biol 1986; 102:1157.
64. Koury ST, Repasky EA, Eckert BS. The cytoskeleton of isolated murine primitive erythrocytes. Cell Tissue Res 1987; 249:69.
65. Nijhoh W, Wierenga PK. Biogenesis of the red cell membrane and cytoskeletal proteins during erythropoiesis in vitro. Exp Cell Res 1988; 177:329.
66. Hanspal M, Kalraiya R, Hanspal J, et al. Erythropoietin enhances the assembly of spectrin heterodimers on the murine erythroblast membranes by increasing spectrin synthesis. J Biol Chem 1991; 266:15626.
67. Patel VP, Ciechanover A, Platt O, Lodish HF. Mammalian reticulocytes lose adhesion to fibronectin during maturation to erythrocytes. Proc Natl Acad Sci U S A 1985; 82:440.
68. Vuillet-Gaugler MH, Breton-Gorius J, Vainchenker W, et al. Loss of attachment to fibronectin with terminal human erythroid differentiation. Blood 1990; 75:865.
69. Robinson J, Sieff C, Delia D, et al. Expression of cell-surface HLA-DR, HLA-ABC and glycophorin during erythroid differentiation. Nature 1981; 289:68.
70. Rearden A, Masouredis SP. Blood group D antigen content of nucleated red blood cell precursors. Blood 1977; 50:981.
71. Reyes F, Lejonc JL, Gourdin MF, et al. Human normoblast A antigen seen by immunoelectron microscopy. Nature 1974; 247:461.
72. Vainchenker W, Vinci G, Testa U, et al. Presence of the Tn antigen on hematopoietic progenitors from patients with Tn syndrome. J Clin Invest 1985; 75:541.
73. Kimura H, Finch CA, Adamson JW. Hematopoiesis in the rat: quantitation of hematopoietic progenitors and the response to iron deficiency anemia. J Cell Physiol 1986; 126:298.
74. Abraham NG, Lutton JD, Levere RD. Heme metabolism and erythropoiesis in abnormal iron states: role of delta-aminolevulinic acid synthetase and heme oxygenase. Exp Hematol 1985; 13:838.
75. Kling PJ, Dragsten PR, Robert RA, et al. Iron deprivation increases erythropoietin production in vitro, in normal subjects and patients with malignancy. Br J Haematol 1996; 95:241.
76. Weiss G, Houston T, Kastner S, et al. Regulation of cellular iron metabolism by erythropoietin: activation of iron-regulatory protein and upregulation of transferrin receptor expression in erythroid cells. Blood 1997; 89:680.
77. Antony AC, Bruno E, Briddell RA, et al. Effect of perturbation of specific folate receptors during in vitro erythropoiesis. J Clin Invest 1987; 80:1618.
78. Hoffman R, Zanjani ED, Zalusky R, Wasserman LR. Erythroid colony growth in disorders of erythropoiesis [Abstract]. Blood 1975; 46:1023a.
79. Wiener E, Wickramasinghe SN. Natural autoantibodies may play a role in ineffective erythropoiesis during megaloblastic hematopoiesis. Clin Exp Immunol 1991; 83:121.
80. Cotter PD, Baumann M, Bishop DF. Enzymatic defect in "X-linked" sideroblastic anemia: molecular evidence for erythroid-aminolevulinate synthase deficiency. Proc Natl Acad Sci USA 1992; 89:4028.
81. Cotter PD, May A, Fitzsimons EJ, et al. Late onset X-linked sideroblastic anemia. Missense mutations in the erythroid delta-aminolevulinate synthase (ALAS2) gene in two pyridoxine-responsive patients initially diagnosed with acquired refractory anemia and ringed sideroblasts. J Clin Invest 1995; 96:2090.
82. Clark SC, Kamen R. The human hematopoietic colony-stimulating factors. Science 1987; 236:1229.
83. Sieff CA, Niemeyer CM, Faller DV. The production of hematopoietic growth factors by endothelial accessory cells. Blood Cells 1987; 13:65.
84. Kaushansky K. Thrombopoietin: the primary regulator of platelet production. Blood 1995; 86:419.
85. Ku H, Yonemura Y, Kaushansky K, Ogawa M. Thrombopoietin, the ligand for the Mpl receptor, synergizes with steel factor and other early acting cytokines in supporting proliferation of primitive hematopoietic progenitors of mice. Blood 1996; 87:4544.
86. Carver-Moore K, Broxmeyer HE, Luoh SM, et al. Low levels of erythroid and myeloid progenitors in thrombopoietin- and c-mpl–deficient mice. Blood 1996; 88:803.
87. Papayannopoulou T, Brice M, Farrer D, Kaushansky K. Insights into the cellular mechanisms of erythropoietin-thrombopoietin synergy. Exp Hem 1996; 24:660.
88. Kieran MW, Perkins AC, Orkin SH, Zon LI. Thrombopoietin rescues in vitro erythroid colony formation from mouse embryos lacking the erythropoietin receptor. Proc Natl Acad Sci USA 1996; 93:9126.
89. Ratajczak MZ, Ratajczak J, Marlicz W, et al. Recombinant human thrombopoietin (TPO) stimulates erythropoiesis by inhibiting erythroid progenitor cell apoptosis. Br J Haematol 1997; 98:8.
90. Ikebuchi K, Wong GG, Clark SC, et al. Interleukin 6 enhancement of interleukin 3–dependent proliferation of multipotential hematopoietic progenitors. Proc Natl Acad Sci U S A 1987; 84:9035.
91. Ikebuchi K, Ihle JN, Hirai Y, et al. Synergistic factors for stem cell proliferation; further studies of the target stem cells and the mechanism of stimulation by interleukin-1, interleukin-6, and granulocyte colony-stimulating factor. Blood 1988; 72:2007.
92. Leary AG, Ikebuchi K, Hirai Y, et al. Synergism between interleukin-6 and interleukin-3 in supporting proliferation of human hematopoietic stem cells: comparison with interleukin-1 alpha. Blood 1988; 71:1759.
93. Sui X, Tsuji K, Tajima S, et al. Erythropoietin-independent erythrocyte production: signals through gp130 and c-kit dramatically promote erythropoiesis from human CD34+ cells. J Exp Med 1996; 183:837.
94. Nocka K, Buck J, Levi E, et al. Candidate ligand for c-kit transmembrane kinase receptor: KL, a fibroblast derived growth factor, stimulates mast cells and erythroid progenitors. EMBO J 1990; 9:3287.

95. McNiece IK, Langley KE, Zsebo KM. Recombinant human stem cell factor synergizes with GM-CSF, CT-CSF, IL-3 and Epo to stimulate human progenitor cells of the myeloid and erythroid lineages. Exp Hematol 1991; 19:226.
96. Dai CH, Krantz SB, Zsebo KM. Human burst-forming units-erythroid need direct interaction with stem cell factor for further development. Blood 1991; 78:2493.
97. Anklesaria P, Greenberger JS, Fitzgerald TJ, et al. Hemonectin mediates adhesion of engrafted murine progenitors to a clonal bone marrow stromal cell line from S1/S1d mice. Blood 1991; 77:1691.
98. Billat CL, Felix JM, Jacquot RL. In vitro and in vivo regulation of hepatic erythropoiesis by erythropoietin and glucocorticoids in the rat fetus. Exp Hematol 1982; 10:133.
99. Leung P, Gidari AS. Glucocorticoids inhibit erythroid colony formation by murine fetal liver erythroid progenitor cells in vitro. Endocrinology 1981; 108:1787.
100. Shahidi NT. Androgens and erythropoiesis. N Engl J Med 1973; 289:72.
101. Weber JP, Walsh PC, Peters CA, Spivak JL. Effect of reversible androgen deprivation on hemoglobin and serum immunoreactive erythropoietin in men. Am J Hematol 1991; 36:190.
102. Fandrey J, Jelkmann WE. Interleukin-1 and tumor necrosis factor-alpha inhibit erythropoietin production in vitro. Ann N Y Acad Sci 1991; 628:250.
103. Faquin WC, Schnieder TJ, Goldberg MA. Effect of inflammatory cytokines on hypoxia-induced erythropoietin production. Blood 1992; 79:1987.
104. Means RT, Dessypris EN, Krantz SB. Inhibition of human erythroid colony-forming units by interleukin-1 is mediated by gamma interferon. J Cell Physiol 1992; 150:59.
105. Means RT, Krantz SB. Inhibition of human erythroid colony-forming units by tumor necrosis factor requires beta interferon. J Clin Invest 1993; 91:416.
106. Krystal G, Lam V, Dragowska W, et al. Transforming growth factor beta 1 is an inducer of erythroid differentiation. J Exp Med 1994; 180:851.
107. Durkin JP, Biquard JM, Blanchet JP, et al. Characterization of a novel erythropoiesis-inhibiting human protein. Ann N Y Acad Sci 1991; 628:233.
108. Shivdasani RA, Orkin SH. The transcriptional control of hematopoiesis. Blood 1996; 87:4025.
109. Martin DIK, Tsai S-F, Orkin SH. Increased-globin expression in a nondeletion HPFH mediated by an erythroid-specific DNA-binding factor. Nature 1989; 338:435.
110. Evans T, Felsenfeld G. The erythroid-specific transcription factor Eryf1: a new finger protein. Cell 1989; 58:877.
111. Youssoufian H, Zon L, Orkin SH, et al. Structure and transcription of the mouse erythropoietin receptor gene. Mol Cell Biol 1990; 10:3675.
112. Weiss MJ, Orkin SH. Transcription factor GATA-1 permits survival and maturation of erythroid precursors by preventing apoptosis. Proc Natl Acad Sci U S A 1995; 92:9623.
113. Abbrecht PH, Littel JK. Plasma erythropoietin in men and mice during acclimatization to different altitudes. J Appl Physiol 1972; 32:54.
114. Milledge JS, Cotes PM. Serum erythropoietin in humans at high altitude and its relation to plasma renin. J Appl Physiol 1985; 59:360.
115. Reissmann KR. Studies on the mechanism of erythropoietic stimulation in parabiotic rats during hypoxia. Blood 1950; 5:372.
116. Erslev AJ. Humoral regulation of red cell production. Blood 1953; 8:349.
117. Cazzola M, Guarnone R, Cerani P, et al. Red blood cell precursor mass as an independent determinant of serum erythropoietin level. Blood 1998; 91:2139.
118. Davis JM, Strickland TW, Yphantis DA. Characterization of recombinant human erythropoietin produced in Chinese hamster ovary cells. Biochemistry 1987; 26:2633.
119. Lai PH, Everett R, Wang FF, et al. Structural characterization of human erythropoietin. J Biol Chem 1986; 261:3116.
120. Sasaki H, Bothner B, Dell A, Fukada M. Carbohydrate structure of erythropoietin expressed in Chinese hamster ovary cells by a human erythropoietin cDNA. J Biol Chem 1987; 262:12059.
121. Spivak JL, Hogans BB. The in vivo metabolism of recombinant human erythropoietin in the rat. Blood 1989; 73:90.
122. Goldwasser E, Kung CKH, Eliason J. On the mechanism of erythropoietin-induced differentiation: XIII. The role of sialic acid in erythropoietin action. J Biol Chem 1974; 249:4202.
123. Dordal MS, Wang FF, Goldwasser E. The role of carbohydrate in erythropoietin action. Endocrinology 1985; 116:2293.
124. Takeuchi M, Takasaki S, Shimada M, Kobata A. Role of sugar chains in the in vitro biologic activity of human erythropoietin produced in recombinant Chinese hamster ovary cells. J Biol Chem 1990; 265:12127.
125. Law ML, Cai GY, Lin FK, et al. Chromosomal assignment of the human erythropoietin gene and its DNA polymorphism. Proc Natl Acad Sci U S A 1986; 83:6920.
126. Recny MA, Scoble HA, Kim Y. Structural characterization of natural human urinary and recombinant DNA–derived erythropoietin. J Biol Chem 1987; 262:17156.
127. McDonald J, Lin FK, Goldwasser E. Cloning, sequencing and evolutionary analysis of the mouse erythropoietin gene. Mol Cell Biol 1986; 6:842.
128. Shoemaker CB, Mitsock LD. Murine erythropoietin gene: cloning, expression, and gene homology. Mol Cell Biol 1986; 6:849.
129. D'Andrea AD, Lodish HF, Wong GG. Expression cloning of the murine erythropoietin receptor. Cell 1989; 57:277.
130. Schmitt RM, Bruyns E, Snodgrass HR. Hematopoietic development of embryonic stem cells in vitro: cytokine and receptor gene expression. Genes Dev 1991; 5:728.
131. Anagnostou A, Lee ES, Kessimian N, et al. Erythropoietin has a mitogenic and positive chemotactic effect on endothelial cells. Proc Natl Acad Sci 1990; 87:5978.
132. Masuda S, Nagao M, Takahata K, et al. Functional erythropoietin receptor of the cells with neural characteristics. J Biol Chem 1993; 268:11208.
133. Winkelmann JC, Penny LA, Deaven LL, et al. The gene for human erythropoietin receptor: analysis of the coding sequence and assignment to chromosome 19p. Blood 1990; 76:24.
134. Bazan JF. Structural design and molecular evolution of a cytokine receptor superfamily. Proc Natl Acad Sci U S A 1990; 87:6934.
135. Damen JE, Krystal G. Early events in erythropoietin-induced signaling. Exp Hemat 1996; 24:1455.
136. Sawyer ST, Penta K. Association of JAK2 and STAT5 with erythropoietin receptors. J Biol Chem 1996; 271:32430.
137. Klingmuller U, Wu H, Hsiao JG, et al. Identification of a novel pathway important for proliferation and differentiation of primary erythroid progenitors. Proc Natl Acad Sci U S A 1997; 94:3016.
138. Sokol L, Luhovy M, Guan Y, et al. Primary familial polycythemia: a frameshift mutation in the erythropoietin receptor gene and increased sensitivity of erythroid progenitors to erythropoietin. Blood 1995; 86:15.
139. Wu H, Klingmuller U, Acurio A, et al. Functional interaction of erythropoietin and stem cell factor receptors is essential for erythroid colony formation. Proc Natl Acad Sci U S A 1997; 94:1806.
140. Bondurant MC, Yamashita T, Muta K. C-myc expression affects proliferation but not terminal differentiation or survival of explanted erythroid progenitor cells. J Cell Physiol 1996; 168:255.
141. Quelle FW, Wang D, Nosaka T, et al. Erythropoietin induces activation of STAT5 through association with specific tyrosines on the receptor that are not required for a mitogenic response. Mol Cell Biol 1996; 16:1622.
142. Koury MJ, Bondurant MC. Erythropoietin retards DNA breakdown and prevents programmed death in erythroid progenitor cells. Science 1990; 248:378.
143. Spivak JL, Pham T, Isaacs M, et al. Erythropoietin is both a mitogen and a survival factor. Blood 1991; 77:1228.
144. Silva M, Grillot D, Benito A, et al. Erythropoietin can promote erythroid progenitor survival by repressing apoptosis through Bcl-X_l and Bcl-2. Blood 1996; 88:1576.
145. Al-Khatti A, Veith RW, Papayannopoulou T, et al. Stimulation of fetal hemoglobin synthesis by erythropoietin in baboons. N Engl J Med 1987; 317:415.
146. Sawada K, Krantz SB, Dai CH, et al. Purification of human blood burst-forming units–erythroid and demonstration of the evolution of erythropoietin receptors. J Cell Physiol 1990; 142:219.
147. Lacombe C, Da Silva JL, Bruneval P. Peritubular cells are the site of erythropoietin synthesis in the murine hypoxic kidney. J Clin Invest 1988; 81:620.
148. Shuster SJ, Badiavas EV, Costa-Giomi P, et al. Stimulation of

erythropoietin gene transcription during hypoxia and cobalt exposure. Blood 1989; 73:13.
149. Koury ST, Koury MJ, Bondurant MC, et al. Quantitation of erythropoietin-producing cells in kidneys of mice by in situ hybridization: correlation with hematocrit, renal erythropoietin mRNA, and serum erythropoietin concentration. Blood 1989; 74:645.
150. Bondurant MC, Koury MJ. Anemia induces accumulation of erythropoietin mRNA in the kidney and liver. Mol Cell Biol 1986; 6:2731.
151. Koury ST, Bondurant MC, Koury MJ, Semenza GL. Localization of cells producing erythropoietin in murine liver by in situ hybridization. Blood 1991; 77:2497.
152. Erslev AJ, Caro J, Kausu E, Silver R. Renal and extrarenal erythropoietin production in anemic rats. Br J Haematol 1980; 45:65.
153. Schooley JC, Mahlmann LJ. Evidence for de novo synthesis of erythropoietin in hypoxic rats. Blood 1972; 40:662.
154. Caro J, Erslev AJ. Biologic and immunologic erythropoietin in extracts from hypoxic whole rat kidneys and their glomerular and tubular fractions. J Lab Clin Med 1984; 103:922.
155. Steinberg SE, Garcia JF, Matzke GR, Mladenovic J. Erythropoietin kinetics in rats: generation and clearance. Blood 1986; 67:646.
156. Emmanuel DS, Goldwasser E, Katz AI. Metabolism of pure human erythropoietin in the rat. Am J Physiol 1984; 247:F168.
157. Spivak JL, Hogans BB. Clinical evaluation of a radioimmunoassay for serum erythropoietin using reagents derived from recombinant erythropoietin. Blood 1987; 70:143a.
158. Kickler TS, Spivak JL. Effect of repeated whole blood donations on serum immunoreactive erythropoietin levels in autologous donors. JAMA 1988; 260:65.
159. Hochberg MC, Arnold CM, Hogans BB, Spivak JL. Serum immunoreactive erythropoietin in rheumatoid arthritis: impaired response to anemia. Arthritis Rheum 1988; 31:1318.
160. Miller CB, Jones RJ, Piantadosi S, et al. Decreased erythropoietin response in patients with the anemia of cancer. N Engl J Med 1990; 322:1689.
161. Sherwood JB, Goldwasser E, Chilcote R, et al. Sickle cell anemia patients have low erythropoietin levels for their degree of anemia. Blood 1986; 67:46.
162. Spivak JL, Barnes CD, Fuchs E, Quinn TC. Serum immunoreactive erythropoietin in HIV-infected patients. JAMA 1989; 261:3104.
163. Schapira L, Antin JH, Ransil BJ. Serum erythropoietin levels in patients receiving intensive chemotherapy and radiotherapy. Blood 1990; 76:2354.
164. Beguin Y, Lipscei G, Thoumsin H, Fillet G. Blunted erythropoietin production and decreased erythropoiesis in early pregnancy. Blood 1991; 78:89.
165. Cotes PM, Dore CJ, Yin JAL, et al. Determination of serum immunoreactive erythropoietin in the investigation of erythrocytosis. N Engl J Med 1986; 315:283.

CHAPTER 2
Granulopoiesis

Janice Gabrilove

Granulocytes play an essential role in the immune response to tissue injury and are primarily responsible for host defense against microorganisms and exposure to foreign antigen. The granulocytic series encompasses three morphologically distinct cell lines: the neutrophil, the eosinophil, and the basophil (Fig. 2–1). These three lineages are distinguished by their respective secondary granules, nuclear morphology, primary location, and function.

The first recognizable cell of the granulocytic series is the myeloblast. After division and differentiation, the following sequence of cells may be seen: promyelocyte, myelocyte, metamyelocyte, band cell, and segmented or mature granulocyte. Specific or secondary granules appear from the promyelocyte stage onwards. In line with the dominance of neutrophils among the granulocytes of the peripheral blood, neutrophil precursors form the majority of granulocyte precursors in the marrow, with few eosinophil precursors and rare basophil precursors present (Table 2–1).

NEUTROPHIL GRANULOCYTES

Neutrophil granulocytes arise from a committed progenitor cell referred to as the *colony-forming unit for granulocyte-macrophage (CFU-GM),* under the influence of specific regulatory proteins (Fig. 2–2). Human neutrophilic

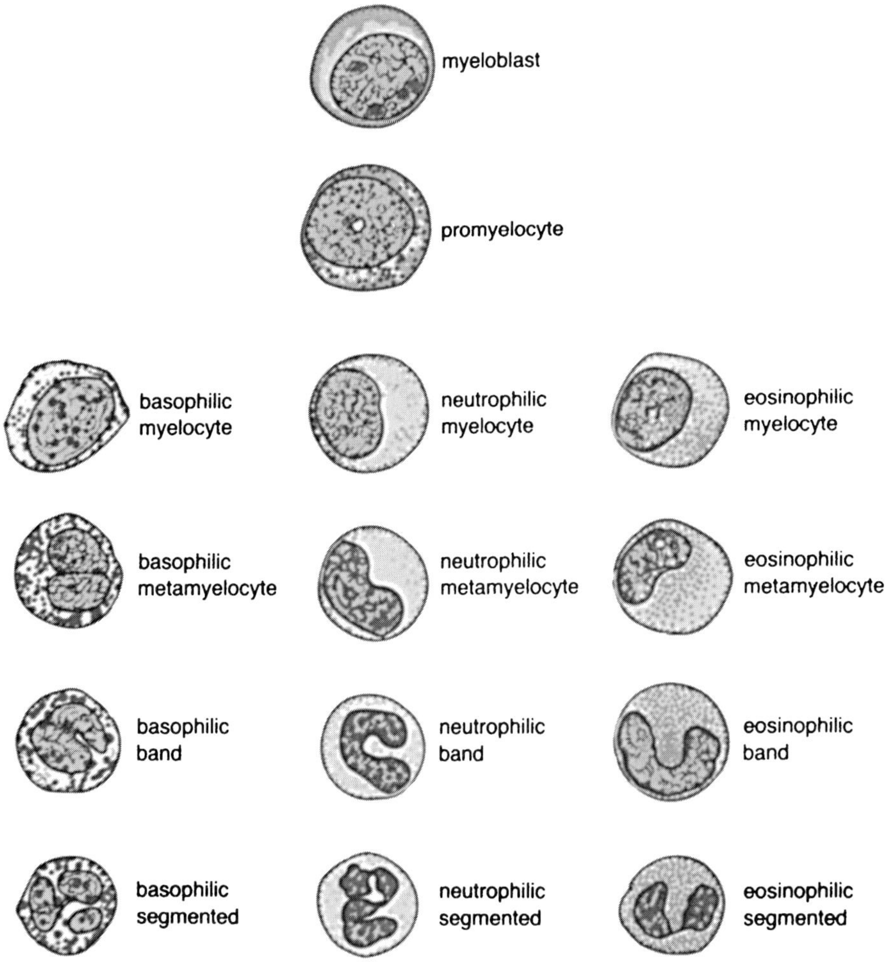

Figure 2–1. Granulocyte differentiation and maturation: the myeloblast and promyelocyte give rise to three different cell lines, according to the type of secondary granules and nuclear morphology. (From Hoffrand AV, Pettit JF. Clinical Hematology. London: Gower Publishing Company, 1988, p 12.)

Table 2–1. Differential Counts of Bone Marrow Aspirates From 12 Healthy Men

Cell Type(s)	Mean (%)	Observed Range (%)	95% Confidence Limits (%)
Neutrophilic series (total)	53.6	49.2–65.0	33.6–73.6
	0.9	0.2–1.5	0.1–1.7
Myeloblasts	3.3	2.1–4.1	1.9–4.7
Promyelocytes	12.7	8.2–15.7	8.5–16.9
Myelocytes	15.9	9.6–24.6	7.1–24.7
Metamyelocytes	12.4	9.5–15.3	9.4–15
Band	7.4	6.0–12.0	3.8–11.0
Segmented			
Eosinophilic series (total)	3.1	1.2–5.3	1.1–5.2
	0.8	0.2–1.3	0.2–1.4
Myelocytes	0.9	0.2–2.4	0–2.7
Band	0.5	0–1.3	0–1.1
Segmented			
Basophilic and mast cells	0.1	0–0.2	
	25.6	18.4–33.8	15.0–36.2
Erythrocytic series (total)			
Pronormoblasts	0.6	0.2–1.3	0.1–1.1
Basophilic	1.4	0.5–2.4	0.4–2.4
Polychromatophilic	21.6	17.9–29.2	13.1–30.1
Orthochromatic	2.0	0.4–4.6	0.3–3.7
Lymphocytes	16.2	11.1–23.2	8.6–23.8
Plasma cells	1.3	0.4–3.9	0–3.5
Monocytes	0.3	0–0.8	0–0.6
Megakaryocytes	0.1	0–0.4	
Reticulum cells	0.3	0–0.9	0–0.8
M:E ratio	2.3	1.5–3.3	1.1–3.5

Modified from Wintrobe MM. Clinical Hematology, 8th ed. Philadelphia, Lea & Febiger, 1981, p 189.

polymorphonuclear granulocytes (PMN) are produced by the bone marrow at a base-line rate of 1600 million cells/kg/d. Another way of quantifying the tremendous number of cells this represents is that the granulocytes in 25 liters of whole blood would be needed to replace the PMNs normally lost every day; this fact reveals why successful PMN transfusions have been problematic.[1]

PMNs constitute approximately 65% of the total white blood cell population (Table 2–2). PMN precursors multiply and mature in the bone marrow, circulate briefly in the peripheral blood, and, in the event of an inflammatory stimulus, migrate from the blood stream between the endothelial cells of the postcapillary venules and collect in tissues as part of the inflammatory cell exudate (Fig. 2–3). Neutrophil production and differentiation in the bone marrow take 14 days and consist of a mitotic portion and a nonmitotic portion (see Fig. 2–3).[2, 3] Cells of the neutrophil lineage that possess mitotic capability are the myeloblast, promyelocyte, and myelocyte (see Figs. 2–1 and 2–3). The myeloblast is a large undifferentiated cell with an eccentric nucleus containing large nucleoli and prominent cytoplasm devoid of granules. This stage of development is followed by the promyelocyte and myelocyte stages, during which two types of granules develop (Tables 2–3 and 2–4). The primary granule, the azurophil, is formed during promyelocyte development and contains myeloperoxidase as well as lysosomal enzymes, neutral proteases, acid mucosubstances, cationic bactericidal proteins, and lysozyme.[4] The secondary granule, the specific granule, is formed in the Golgi complex, beginning with the myelocyte stage of differentiation, and is peroxidase-negative (see Tables 2–3 and 2–4). These granules consist of lactoferrin, vitamin B_{12}–binding proteins, and lysozyme.[5, 6] The metamyelocyte and band forms are nonsecretory, nonproliferating cells that give rise to the mature PMN. These terminally differentiated cells contain both azurophilic and specific granules in a ratio of 1:2. The azurophilic granules at this stage of differentiation are not normally observed with routine staining, because they lose their metachromasia and are recognized only on electron microscopy.

The transit times within the mitotic and postmitotic compartments, previously determined by isotope-labeling studies, are 7.5 and 6.5 days, respectively, under normal physiologic, steady-state conditions.[2] In the setting of infection, the regulatory protein granulocyte colony-stimulating factor (G-CSF) reduces these times dramatically[8–10] in order to maintain host integrity. Large numbers of band and segmented neutrophils are held in the marrow as a reserve pool, which under normal conditions contains 10 to 15 times the number of neutrophils within the circulating compartment. Following their release, cells spend from 6 to 12 hours in the circulation before migrating into the tissues (see Fig. 2–3; Fig. 2–4).[2, 3] Once in the blood, approximately 50% of the neutrophils are freely circulating, and 50% are in a marginated pool. In the tissues, they survive 1 to 2 days before being destroyed during defense or by senescence,[2] and they are lost via the oral cavity.[11]

The neutrophil granulocyte is an important component of the immune system. Through its ability to identify and destroy foreign pathogens, it serves as a general and primary defense mechanism against various organisms, particularly bacteria. Neutrophils function predominantly via phagocytosis.[12] Intracellular organisms are destroyed by lysosomal enzymes and the production of toxic oxygen radicals. Neutrophils can also kill target cells bound by antibodies in a process called antibody-dependent cellular cytotoxicity.[13]

Table 2–2. Normal Values of Blood Leukocyte Concentration

Cell Type	Mean (Cells/mm³)	Mean (%)	95% Confidence Limits (Cells/mm³)
Neutrophils	4300	55.3	1800–6700
Eosinophils	230	3.0	0–570
Basophils	40	0.5	0–120

Modified from Boggs DR: The kinetics of neutrophilic leukocytes in health and in disease. Semin Hematol 1967; 4:359.

EOSINOPHIL GRANULOCYTES

The circulating eosinophils comprise 2% to 5% of normal peripheral blood leukocytes. Less is known about the kinetics of eosinophil production, differentiation, circulation, and migration.[3] Eosinophils are derived from primitive colony-forming cells situated within the bone marrow, under the influence of granulocyte-macrophage colony-stimulating factor (GM-CSF),[14, 15] interleukin-3 (IL-3),[16]

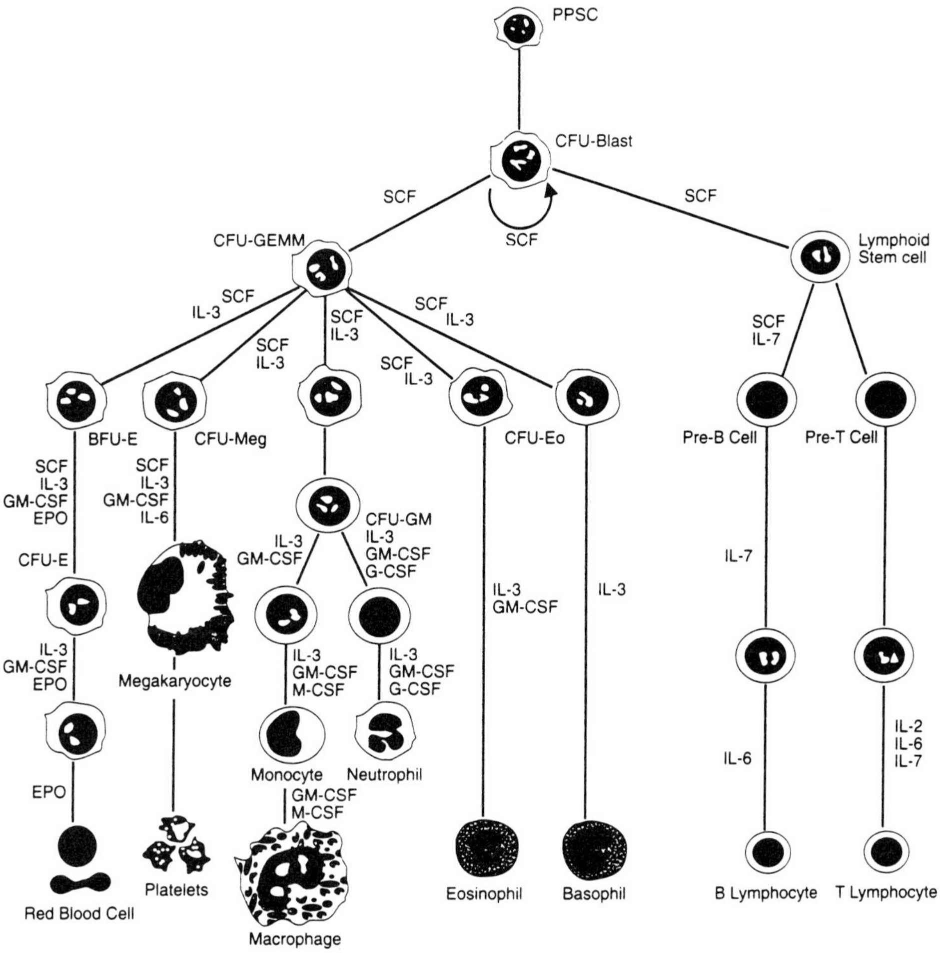

Figure 2–2. The regulation of hematopoiesis. (From AMGEN Investigator's Brochure. Recombinant-methionyl human stem cell factor r-metHuSCF. Thousand Oaks, CA: AMGEN, 1992, 2.)

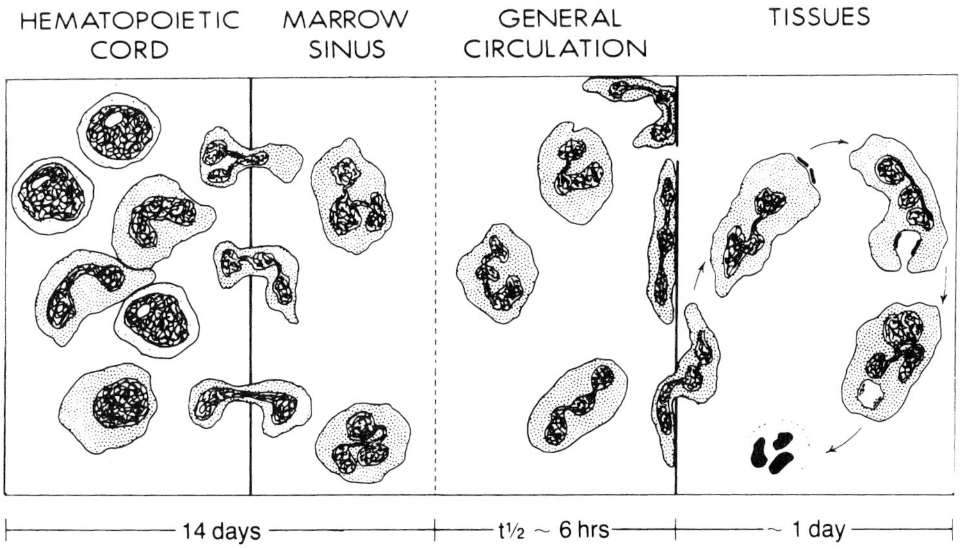

Figure 2–3. Diagrammatic representation of the compartments of the PMN cycle. (From Bainton DF. Anatomy and physiology of neutrophilic granulopoiesis. *In* Lichtman MA (ed). Hematology and Oncology. The Science and Practice of Clinical Medicine Series, vol 6. New York: Grune & Stratton, 1980, p 124.)

Table 2–3. Enzyme and Protein Content of Neutrophil, Eosinophil, and Basophil Granules

Cell Type	Granules	Function
Neutrophil	Azurophilic (primary)	Bacterial and fungal infection
	Myeloperoxidase	
	Lysosomal enzymes	
	Neutral proteases	
	Acid mucosubstances	
	Cationic bactericidal proteins	
	Lysozyme	
	Specific (secondary)	
	Lysosomal	
	Lactoferrin	
	Vitamin B_{12} binders	
Eosinophil	Histaminase	Allergic and parasitic disease
	Arylsulfatase	
	Major basic protein	
	Eosinophil-derived neurotoxin	
	Eosinophil cationic protein	
	Cyanide-insensitive peroxidase	
Basophil	Slow reacting substance of anaphylaxis	Allergic and parasitic disease
	Histamine	

Table 2–4. Enzyme and Protein Content of Neutrophil Granules

Substance	Primary Granules (Azurophilic)	Secondary Granules (Specific)
Acid phosphatase	+	−
N-Acetyl–glucosaminidase	+	−
Cathepsin B	+	−
Cathepsin D	+	−
Cathepsin G	+	−
β-Glucuronidase	+	−
β-Glycerophosphatase	+	−
α-Mannosidase	+	−
Elastase	+	−
Collagenase	−	+
Gelatinase	−	−
Proteinase 3	+	−
Lysozyme	+	+
Peroxidase	+	−
Arylsulfatase	+	−
Alkaline phosphatase	−	−
Lactoferrin	−	+
Vitamin B_{12}–binding protein	−	+

+, present; −, absent.

and IL-5.[17–19] They can be distinguished from PMNs by their unique granules, which can be initially detected by electron microscopy at the promyelocyte stage. These granules are distinguished by Wright-Giemsa staining at the myelocyte stage of differentiation, when they are vividly apparent. Eosinophil granules under electron microscopy are ellipsoidal, membrane-bound organelles. They contain a dense lamellated crystalloid core encapsulated by a less dense matrix.

The matrix contains peroxidase, arylsulfatase, and other hydrolytic enzymes. The dense crystalloid structure also contains basic proteins rich in arginine and lysine (accounting for the eosin staining) as well as phospholipid and melanin. The major basic protein, which constitutes 50% of the core, binds to acidic macromolecules, including heparin, which it neutralizes. Eosinophils are also signified by their unique nuclear segmentation; 80% of

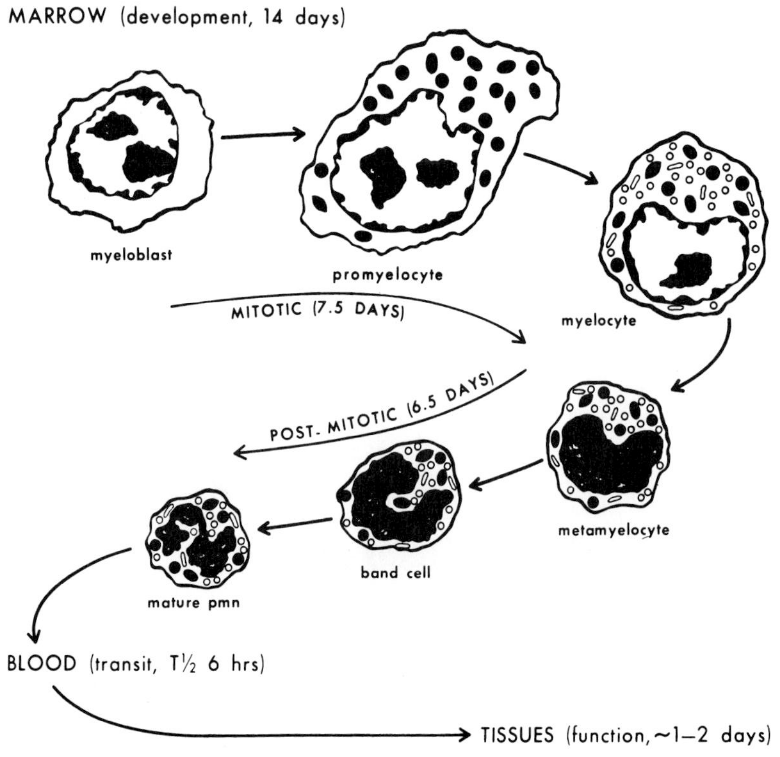

Figure 2–4. Diagrammatic representation of PMN life cycle and stages of PMN maturation. Out of every 100 nucleated cells in bone marrow, 2 are myeloblasts, 5 are promyelocytes, 12 are myelocytes, 22 are metamyelocytes and bands, and 20 are mature PMNs, yielding 60% developing neutrophils. (From Bainton DF. The development of neutrophilic polymorphonuclear leukocytes in human bone marrow. J Exp Med 1971; 134:907, by copyright permission of the Rockefeller University Press.)

the nuclei have two large round or ovoid lobes containing heavily condensed chromatin. Eosinophils are thought to persist in the circulation, with a half-life of 6 to 12 hours, and then to enter the marginated pool (along the blood vessel wall) or to infiltrate tissues.

At the site of inflammation, eosinophils secrete the granule components, including major basic protein, eosinophil cationic protein, and eosinophil-derived neurotoxin,[19, 20] which is toxic to parasites. Because eosinophils express receptors for the Fc (crystallizable fragment) of IgG, IgE, and complement components C4, C3b, and C3d, they are capable of phagocytosing immune complexes.[20] In vitro data also suggest that eosinophils can ingest and kill microorganisms. Many of the functional activities of eosinophils are accomplished through the release of specific substances, including toxic oxygen metabolites, a cyanide-insensitive peroxidase, a variety of other enzymes, membrane-derived leukotriene C4, and platelet-derived growth factor.[21]

BASOPHIL GRANULOCYTES

Basophil granulocytes (basophils) constitute up to only 2% of the white blood cell count (20 to 60 cells/μL of blood) and 0.3% of bone marrow elements.[22] Basophils arise from an independent progenitor cell (see Fig. 2–2). The basophilic granulocyte may be first recognized at the promyelocyte stage of development. It is smaller than the neutrophil or eosinophil promyelocyte and has a higher nuclear-to-cytoplasmic ratio. Maturation of this cell is not accompanied by a noteworthy change in its size; the terms *myelocytic* and *metamyelocytic* refer primarily to a change in the shape of the cell's nucleus. The mature basophil possesses a brioche-shaped nucleus without distinct segmentation. In addition, basophil maturation is accompanied by an increase in metachromasia and a decrease in the activity of chloroacetate esterase, with the mature basophil being invariably negative for this reaction. Human basophils can be generated in vitro from cord blood, fetal liver, or bone marrow in the presence of T cell–conditioned medium[22]; basophil production has been shown to be optimized when cells are grown in the presence of IL-4 plus IL-3,[22, 23] nerve growth factor,[24] *kit*-ligand[22] (KL; also known as stem cell factor, mast cell growth factor, and Steele's factor), or GM-CSF.[23, 24] The circulating basophil is subject to circadian rhythms, as is the eosinophil. The basophil spends little time in the circulation; instead, the cells migrate rapidly into barrier tissues, including mucosal membranes, skin, and serosal structures.[22]

REGULATION OF GRANULOPOIESIS

Cells of the granulocyte series arise from specific committed progenitors, unique to each of the respective lineages. These include CFU-GM, eosinophils, and basophils. These committed progenitor cells, in turn, are the progeny of uncommitted stem cells, which are induced to proliferate and differentiate under the influence of specific hematopoietins, including IL-1,[25] IL-3,[26] IL-6,[27] and KL.[28]

The regulation of granulopoiesis is designed to respond rapidly to invasion by microorganisms and to deliver to the periphery functional effector cells required to maintain host defense. The production of granulocytes is a complex and dynamic process during which a small number of self-renewing stem cells give rise to lineage-specific progenitors that proliferate and mature in the bone marrow, subsequently entering the blood as mature neutrophil, eosinophil, and basophil granulocytes. The regulatory molecules that have been shown to be involved in granulocyte development are depicted in Figure 2–2, and their respective biochemical and biologic features are outlined in Tables 2–5 to 2–8. These cytokines, working alone and together, constitute the inflammatory response to injury by foreign pathogens and control the number and availability of phagocytes required to protect the host.

GRANULOCYTE COLONY-STIMULATING FACTOR

G-CSF is a glycoprotein that regulates the production and function of neutrophil granulocytes. G-CSF was originally identified as a leukemia differentiation factor that could be detected in murine serum or lung-conditioned medium following endotoxin administration. Purification re-

Table 2–5. Biochemical and Molecular Characteristics, Cell Sources, and Targets of the CSFs

Factor or Cell Lineage	Chromosomal Location	mRNA Size (kb)	Protein Size (kDa)	Cell Source	Granulocyte Target
GM-CSF	5q23–32	1.0	14–35	Monocytes, fibroblasts, endothelial cells, T lymphocytes, epithelial cells	N, E, and B
G-CSF (n)	17q11–123	2.0	18	Monocytes, endothelial cells, epithelial cells	N
IL-3 (multi-CSF)	5q23–31	1.0	14–28	T lymphocytes	N, E
IL-5	5q31		45	T lymphocytes	E, B
IL-8	4q12–21		8	Monocytes, fibroblasts, hepatocytes, endothelial cells	N
KL^{248}	12p	18	Stromal cells	N, B	
KL^{164}		36 (dimer)			

N, neutrophil; m, monocyte; e, eosinophil; b, basophil, E, erythrocyte; M, megakaryocyte.

Table 2–6. Biological Properties of G-CSF on Cells of the Neutrophil Granulocyte Lineage

Cell	Effects
Precursor cell	Stimulates the proliferation of committed progenitors for neutrophil granulocytes Stimulates the growth and transient clonal proliferation of promyelocytes and myelocytes Reduces the transit time (from 96 hours to 24 hours) required for a neutrophil granulocyte to develop from a mitotic precursor
Mature, terminally differentiated cells	Primes neutrophils to produce superoxide Augments neutrophil-mediated ADCC and phagocytosis Enhances neutrophil migration and specific binding of the chemotactic bacterial peptide FMLP Induces myeloperoxidase, alkaline phosphatase, and high-affinity receptors for IgA Fc on neutrophils Functions as a weak chemoattractant for neutrophil granulocytes

Table 2–8. Biologic Effects of GM-CSF on Granulocyte Development

Cell	Effects
Precursor cells	Proliferation of CFU-GM
Mature terminally differentiated cells	
Neutrophils	Survival and protein synthesis Migration inhibition Oxidative metabolism Degranulation Cytokine secretion Recruitment IgA-mediated phagocytosis Uptake and destruction of parasites, bacteria Cytotoxicity (ADCC) Changes in cell surface receptors Arachidonic acid release, leukotriene, and platelet-activating factor synthesis
Eosinophils	Survival Cytotoxicity Leukotriene synthesis
Basophils	Histamine release

Modified from Gasson JC: Molecular physiology of granulocyte-macrophage colony-stimulating factor. Blood 1991; 77:1131.

vealed that this leukemia differentiation factor was identical to a colony-stimulating factor that exclusively supported the growth of neutrophil granulocyte precursors.[29]

Human G-CSF was first purified to homogeneity from the human bladder carcinoma cell line 5637[30]; subsequently, the gene for human G-CSF and its cDNA was cloned molecularly.[31] The gene for G-CSF is single-copy and has been localized to the long arm of chromosome 17 (17q11–23), a region that contains other genes involved in neutrophil granulocyte development.

In vitro, G-CSF is produced by a variety of cell types, including neutrophil granulocytes,[32] endothelial cells,[33] fibroblasts,[34] and bone marrow stromal cells,[35] following stimulation by endotoxin, tumor necrosis factor, IL-1, or GM-CSF. The cell type representing the most important source of this factor under physiological conditions in vivo remains unknown. In normal adults, circulating levels of immunoreactive G-CSF range between 20 and 95 pg/mL, are unrelated to age or sex, and exhibit no diurnal variation. There is controversy regarding the relationship between circulating levels of G-CSF and the neutrophil count under physiological conditions. Although the precise role of G-CSF in the maintenance of steady-state neutrophil granulopoiesis is uncertain, Hammond and colleagues (see reference 73) showed that normal dogs can develop neutralizing antibodies to canine G-CSF after receiving human G-CSF and thereafter develop profound neutropenia. This result suggests that G-CSF is critical for the day-to-day regulation and production of neutrophil granulocytes. In bacteremia, in which the characteristic leukocytosis is neutrophil in type, G-CSF levels have been found to exceed 2000 pg/mL,[8] providing additional evidence that G-CSF is a systemic regulator of neutrophil production.

Table 2–7. Effect of CSFs on Neutrophil Granulocyte Development

Factor	Effects
GM	CSF
Circulating half	Life of neutrophil extended from 6 to 12 hours to up to 4 days Significant proliferation of committed myeloid progenitors No effect on transit time from mitotic to postmitotic compartment
G	CSF
No effect on circulating half	Life of neutrophil Proliferation of committed myeloid progenitors Decreased transit time of neutrophil precursors from mitotic to postmitotic compartment, with subsequent release to mature cells within 24 hours

Low numbers of high-affinity receptors for G-CSF exist on normal immature and mature neutrophil granulocytes.[36] The molecular weight of the receptor observed in crosslinking experiments is 150,000 D.[36] The high-affinity receptor for human G-CSF has been cloned and found to have an amino-terminal immunoglobulin domain, three fibronectin type III regions, and four conserved cysteine residues characteristic of the cytokine receptor superfamily. A portion of the extracellular domain of the G-CSF receptor exhibits a striking similarity to the neural cellular adhesion molecules family of adhesion molecules.[36]

G-CSF promotes the survival and stimulates the growth and expansion of immature neutrophil granulocyte precursors, enriched promyelocytes, and myelocytes (see Table 2–6).[37] G-CSF has also been shown to enhance the effector-cell capability of neutrophil granulocytes and to function as a weak chemoattractant for these cells.

Early preclinical studies demonstrated the ability of G-CSF to augment the number of functionally normal neutrophils in healthy[38] and tumor-bearing rodents[39] and in nonhuman primates.[40] This neutrophil granulocytosis results from an augmentation in the number of divisions and a reduction (from 96 hours to 24 hours) in the time required for maturing neutrophil granulocyte precursors to develop into terminally differentiated cells released into the circulation (see Tables 2–6 and 2–7).[10] This particular biological effect is unique to G-CSF.

GRANULOCYTE-MACROPHAGE COLONY-STIMULATING FACTOR

GM-CSF controls the proliferation of neutrophil, eosinophil, and basophil progenitor cells and stimulates the functional activity of their respective terminally differentiated cells. Human GM-CSF was first purified by Gasson and associates[41] from a human T cell leukemia virus–infected T-lymphoblastoid cell line. The purified protein was found to be identical to the previously described T-lymphocyte–derived lymphokine referred to as neutrophil migration inhibition factor.[41] Human GM-CSF is highly and variably glycosylated, accounting for the wide range of molecular weights reported. The complementary cDNA encoding the human GM-CSF protein was molecularly cloned by Wong and colleagues.[42] In vitro, GM-CSF is produced by activated T lymphocytes, B lymphocytes, endothelial cells, mast cells, fibroblasts, macrophages, mesothelial cells, and osteoblasts in response to specific activating agents.[43] Unlike G-CSF, GM-CSF is not detectable in serum under physiological conditions, suggesting that GM-CSF normally acts in a paracrine fashion.

Receptors for GM-CSF exist on normal neutrophils, their precursors, and eosinophil granulocytes.[35] These cells normally express low numbers of high-affinity binding sites, with dissociation constants (K_d) of 30 to 100 pM.[35] The low-affinity human GM-CSF receptor (alpha subunit) has been cloned, sequenced, and localized to the pseudoautosomal region of the sex chromosomes. A 120-transmembrane adapter protein (beta subunit), which confers high affinity to the GM-CSF receptor, is a component shared with the receptors for two other growth factors that stimulate the proliferation and activation of eosinophil granulocytes, IL-3 and IL-5.[36]

GM-CSF stimulates the production of neutrophil, eosinophil, and basophil granulocytes (see Table 2–8). In addition, it enhances the function of the terminally differentiated cells of these respective lineages. The more profound effects of GM-CSF on effector cell function compared with G-CSF may reflect the critical role of GM-CSF in host defense and the inflammatory response. GM-CSF has been shown to directly affect neutrophil expression of cellular adhesion molecules, locomotion, responsiveness to chemotactic factors, biosynthetic function, and tumoricidal and phagocytic activities. Priming effects of GM-CSF have also been described; they include the stimulation of the respiratory burst, degranulation, enhanced synthesis of mediators of inflammation such as leukotrienes and platelet-activating factor, and elaboration of cytokines. In the presence of GM-CSF, eosinophils exhibit enhanced tumoricidal and phagocytic activities.

INTERLEUKIN-3

Murine IL-3 was first described as a multilineage colony-stimulating factor produced by mitogen-stimulated T lymphocytes.[26] Murine IL-3 was first purified, isolated, and characterized by Ihle and coworkers.[44] Gibbon and human IL-3 have been cloned using expression-cloning techniques.[45] IL-3 is a complex glycoprotein ranging in size from 14 to 28 kD. It has been shown to support the growth of early multilineage progenitor cells and, in particular, eosinophil precursors. In addition, IL-3 stimulates the functional activity of mature eosinophil and neutrophil granulocytes.

INTERLEUKIN-5

IL-5 is the product of activated T lymphocytes.[46] It was initially observed that culture supernatants from T cells stimulated with parasite-specific antigens induced eosinophil colony formation. This eosinophil differentiation factor was found to be distinct from IL-3, appearing as a single band of 45 kD on gel filtration.[47] Independently, others identified a B cell growth factor (BCGF II) produced by T cells that was distinct from IL-4. These two activities were subsequently demonstrated to be derived from the same protein. IL-5 exists as a dimer and exhibits species cross-reactivity. The gene for IL-5 encodes a 134–amino acid polypeptide that includes a terminal leader sequence. The core protein contains at least two glycosylation sites.

kit-LIGAND

KL is a glycoprotein that acts on primitive hematopoietic multilineage blood cell progenitors.[48] Endogenous *kit*-ligand is the ligand for the proto-oncogene *c-kit*, a cell surface tyrosine kinase receptor, which is found on 1% to 3% of normal human bone marrow cells.[49] The naturally occurring form of the KL is a 165–amino acid polypeptide, heavily N- and O-glycosylated, and normally exists as a dimer. The initial gene product is a 248–amino acid precursor that is subsequently cleaved during processing to form the mature protein. Alternate splicing of the gene also results in a membrane-bound form of KL.[50] Unlike most hematopoietic growth factors, KL circulates at relatively high concentrations in human plasma (mean, 3.5 ± 1.6 ng/mL, n = 180).

A synthetic gene for human KL has been constructed and transfected into *Escherichia coli;* this nonglycosylated form of KL exhibits biological activity similar to that of the native glycosylated moiety.

KL alone has little ability to stimulate the growth of CFU-GM; however, it is a potent permissive factor, significantly augmenting the proliferative action of other colony-stimulating factors for the growth of erythroid, myeloid, megakaryocyte, and uncommitted progenitor cells.[51, 52] KL promotes the activation of purified human skin mast cells and basophils; in addition, in the presence of anti-IgE, KL induces the release of histamine and prostaglandin D2 from mast cells and basophil granulocytes.[22] CD34-positive cells cultured in the presence of both KL and IL-3 give rise to cultures containing increased numbers of basophil granulocytes as well as mast cells.[22, 51]

INTERLEUKIN-8

IL-8, also known as monocyte-derived neutrophil chemotactic factor, is generated as a 99–amino acid precursor with a 22–amino acid leader sequence.[53] Several mature forms have been characterized; however, the major form consists of 72 amino acids. IL-8 has considerable sequence homology with peptides from platelet alpha granules. IL-8 induces the activation of the motile apparatus and directional margination; expression of cellular adhesion molecules; release of gelatinase, vitamin B_{12}–binding protein, beta-glucuronidase, and elastase; and stimulates the production of oxygen metabolites. IL-8 is produced by many cells of the appropriate structure in response to IL-1α or IL-1β, IL-2, IL-6, lipopolysaccharide, or interferon.

ABNORMALITIES OF GRANULOPOIESIS

Abnormalities of granulopoiesis can be divided into quantitative (both increases and decreases) and qualitative disorders. Granulocytopenia can occur when the rate of removal from the circulation of granulocytes exceeds the rate of production. The most common and clinically most significant syndromes are due primarily to a decrease in neutrophil numbers.

NEUTROPENIA

Neutropenia is a neutrophil count of less than 1000 cells/μL of blood. In humans, there can be some variation in the normal value for neutrophil number. These variations are believed to be secondary to differences in distribution between the circulating and marginated pools of cells, not a deficiency in production. The primary complication of neutropenia is infection. The relative risk of infectious complications is highly dependent on the circulating number of neutrophils at the time in question. Data extracted by Bodey and colleagues[54] from patients receiving myelosuppressive chemotherapy for myeloid leukemia indicate a 20% rise in infectious complications as the neutrophil count drops to below 1000 cells/μL. As the count falls below 500 cells/μL, the risk of infection rises to 50%; with neutrophil counts below 200 cells/μL, the risk reaches 100%. In addition to the level of neutropenia, the rate of decline in neutrophil count and the duration of neutropenia affect the likelihood of infection. Concomitant mucositis may further increase the rate of infection by providing additional portals of entry for infectious organisms. This link between neutrophil number and risk of infection has also been shown to hold for patients with nonhematological malignancies,[55] demonstrating the wide applicability and importance of these initial observations.

Many disorders can cause neutropenia (Table 2–9).

Table 2–9. Clinical Syndromes of Neutropenia

Absolute neutropenia	
Primary disorders	
Congenital	Kostmann's syndrome
	Shwachman-Diamond syndrome
	Neutropenia with dysgammaglobulinemia or agammaglobulinemia
	Reticular dysgenesis
	Chédiak-Higashi syndrome
Cyclic	Congenital
	Acquired
Idiopathic	
Secondary disorders	
Malignant	
Lymphoid	Hairy cell leukemia
	Chronic lymphocytic leukemia
	Hodgkin's disease
	Non-Hodgkin's lymphoma
	Multiple myeloma
	Acute lymphoblastic leukemia
Myeloid	Acute myeloid leukemia
	Myelodysplastic syndrome
	Refractory anemia with excess blasts
	Refractory anemia with excess blasts in transformation
Nonmalignant	Autoimmune disease
	Felty's syndrome
	Systemic lupus erythematosus
	Rheumatoid arthritis
	T lymphocytosis (T-gamma disease)
	AIDS/HIV infection
	Aplastic anemia
Induced by drugs or therapy	Chemotherapy
	Antibiotics (penicillin, sulfas, chloramphenicol)
	Antithyroid drugs
	Antidepressants
	Anticonvulsants (carbamazepine, phenytoin)
	Radiation therapy
	Organic solvents
Functional neutropenia	Drug-related (steroids, ethanol)
	Chédiak-Higashi syndrome
	Chronic granulomatous disease
	Autoimmune disease
	Thermal damage
	Diabetes mellitus

Modified from Gabrilove J. Neutropenia. *In* Rakel RE (ed). Conn's Current Therapy 1991. Philadelphia: WB Saunders, 1991, p. 324.

They may be subdivided into three major categories: underproduction, including primary and secondary disorders; excessive destruction; and abnormal distribution.

Primary Disorders

Three primary disorders of neutropenia have been described. The first is *congenital neutropenia,* which can be divided into two major syndromes: Kostmann's syndrome and Shwachman-Diamond syndrome. In Kostmann's syndrome (infantile agranulocytosis), an autosomally recessive disease, patients present with profound neutropenia (fewer than 500 cells/μL), eosinophilia, monocytosis, and hypergammaglobulinemia.[56] The disorder is associated with a maturation arrest in the bone marrow at the promyelocyte-myelocyte stage, recurrent bacterial infections, and oral ulcerations. Shwachman-Diamond syndrome, inherited as an autosomal-recessive trait, is characterized by chronic neutropenia in the first decade of life, normal monocyte counts, bone marrow granulocyte hyperplasia, hypergammaglobulinemia, and exocrine pancreatic insufficiency.[57]

Cyclic neutropenia may be congenital or acquired.[58] The congenital type is of autosomal-dominant transmission with varying penetrance. Both types are characterized by oscillations of the absolute neutrophil count (ANC) from low-normal ranges to nadir values of 0 to 200 cells/μL. The periodicity of the cycling phenomenon is 14 to 21 days. Review of peripheral blood reveals a monocytosis during the period of greatest neutropenia. Coincident with this, the bone marrow examination usually indicates a myeloid maturation arrest. Many affected patients also have mild cycling of erythroid and megakaryocytic lines. They suffer from chronic, recurring bacterial infections and exhibit a high incidence of mucosal ulceration involving the oropharyngeal, anorectal, and vaginal regions. The occurrence of these ulcers is linked to the cycling of the neutrophils, worsening as neutropenia becomes more severe and clearing as neutrophil counts improve. As in some of the congenital neutropenias, there is a compensatory hypergammaglobulinemia. Occasional spontaneous remissions have occurred in both types of cyclic neutropenia.

Idiopathic neutropenia manifests as mild to moderate neutropenia (ANC values of 500 cells/μL or fewer).[59] This disorder probably represents a spectrum of etiologies and is characterized by a normocellular or hypocellular bone marrow with a decrease in mature myeloid cells, occasional peripheral monocytosis, hypergammaglobulinemia, and usually only a slight increase in infectious complications.

Secondary Disorders

The secondary disorders of neutropenia are most often the result of an underlying malignant or nonmalignant disease. Among the *malignant disorders,* the majority are of hematological origin. Lymphoid malignancies such as acute lymphoblastic leukemia have been shown to produce transforming growth factor-β (TGF-β), which is known to have an inhibitory effect on normal myeloid progenitor growth.[60] Such "inhibitory factors" may play an etiological role in the neutropenia seen in the setting of acute lymphoblastic leukemia (ALL), hairy cell leukemia (HCL), chronic lymphocytic leukemia (CLL), non-Hodgkin's lymphoma, Hodgkin's disease, multiple myeloma, and myeloid malignancies such as acute myeloid leukemia and myelodysplastic syndromes—refractory anemia with excess blasts and refractory anemia with excess blasts in transformation. In the last two disorders, neutropenia also results from a relative maturation arrest of myeloid elements.

Autoimmune diseases such as systemic lupus erythematosus and rheumatoid arthritis are the most frequently encountered *nonmalignant disorders* associated with neutropenia. Felty's syndrome, with its constellation of arthritis, neutropenia, ulcers, and splenomegaly, is a major treatment problem. Affected patients often have high titers of antineutrophil antibodies.

T-lymphocytosis or T-gamma disease is a disorder characterized by a true peripheral blood and bone marrow lymphocytosis (greater than 5000 cells) due to an increase in peripheral blood large granular lymphocytes (more than 50% of the total lymphocyte count) with T suppressor–natural killer phenotype.[61] These cells have a potentially suppressive effect on myeloid maturation associated with the marrow lymphocytosis. The disease is characterized by mild neutropenia with few infectious complications, except for a slight increase in frequency of viral syndromes. Neutropenia associated with human immunodeficiency virus (HIV-1) infection is believed to be secondary to viral suppression of normal myeloid progenitor growth or an immune etiology.[62] Infectious complications are frequently due to nonopportunistic organisms whose growth is secondary to the overall immunocompromised state of the host, rather than due to the neutropenia.

Aplastic anemia is a state of hypoproduction of all hematopoietic cell lines. Its precise cause is unknown, but alterations in the marrow microenvironment, loss of stem cells, and constitutive production of negative regulators (specifically, constitutive production of interferon-γ by polyclonal populations of suppressor cells in response to unknown antigens) are the most investigated potential causes. In this condition, severe neutropenia is one component of pancytopenia.

Infections such as viral (e.g., hepatitis), rickettsial, and gram-negative sepsis have been known to cause transient neutropenia. In the case of endotoxemia, bone marrow suppression may be due to excessive production of specific negative regulator(s) such as tumor necrosis factor.[63]

The final group of neutropenic syndromes are those related to various *drug and other therapies.* Chemotherapy characteristically causes neutropenia 10 to 14 days after infusion of the drug. In some circumstances, the nadir of blood counts occurs 3 to 4 weeks after administration. The extent and duration of neutropenia depend on the dose of the drug, the presumed marrow progenitor level on which the drug acts, and concomitant administration of other chemotherapeutic agents. A variety of medications have been implicated in the development of other forms of neutropenia. Among these are antithyroid drugs (propylthiouracil),[64] antidepressants (tricyclics),[65] anticonvulsants (carbamazepine and phenytoin),[66] and antibiotics (penicillins, sulfas, and chloramphenicol).[67, 68] Mechanisms include antibody production (e.g., cephalosporins) and progenitor cell injury (chloramphenicol). Resolution of iatrogenic neutropenia varies. For cephalosporins, it typically occurs within 7 days; for other drugs, recovery occurs gradually after the drug is withdrawn.

Radiotherapy, particularly gamma radiation, can cause suppression of peripheral blood counts, on the basis of toxicity to both circulating and intramedullary hematopoietic progenitors. Exposure to radiation in large enough doses (more than 200 cGy of total-body irradiation) can cause syndromes of pancytopenia related to marrow aplasia.

Table 2–10. Evaluation of Neutropenia

Review of previous blood counts	
History	Exposure Radiation Organic solvents Infectious complications Periodicity of symptoms
Physical examination	Ulcers Lymphadenopathy Splenomegaly Signs of infection
Review of peripheral blood smear	Evidence of dysmyelopoiesis Pelger-Hüet neutrophils Lymphocytosis Large granular lymphocytes Abnormal cells Hairy cells Myeloblasts Lymphoblasts
Bone marrow aspiration and biopsy	Morphological features Cytogenetics Cell surface markers Lymphoid versus myeloid Special stains Sideroblast Periodic acid–Schiff stain Sudan black stain Naphthol esterase
Complete blood counts every other day for 1 month	Rule out cyclic component
Peripheral blood studies	Antineutrophil antibody HIV antibody Autoimmune work-up Rheumatoid factor Antinuclear antibody Complement (C3, C4, CH50) Vitamin B_{12} and folate Chemistries Liver function tests, including lactate dehydrogenase Renal function Uric acid Serum protein electrophoresis Immunoelectrophoresis

Modified from Garbrilove J. Neutropenia. *In* Rakel RE (ed). Conn's Current Therapy 1991. Philadelphia: WB Saunders, 1991, p 325.

Clinical Evaluation of the Patient With Neutropenia

Evaluation of patients with neutropenia (Table 2–10) begins with a thorough history and review of laboratory data.[69, 70] In particular, previous blood counts can aid in defining the duration of the abnormality in question. History-taking must concentrate on any previous exposure to radiation or organic solvents as well as a full drug and medication screening. Previous signs or symptoms of infection should be elicited and their periodicity noted. Any possible related illnesses must be elaborated. A complete physical examination, with particular attention paid to mucosal ulcerations, lymphadenopathy, splenomegaly, and any signs of infection, should be performed.

Hematological evaluation should begin with a review of the peripheral blood smear, with particular attention to abnormal cells that may be indicative of disorders such as HCL, CLL, the acute leukemias, and other hematological disorders. Complete blood count with differential should be obtained every other day for a period of 1 month to rule out a cyclic component. Bone marrow aspiration and biopsy must be performed with special studies for cytogenetics, cell markers (lymphoid and myeloid), sideroblast stain, and standard morphologic features. Peripheral blood should be analyzed for antineutrophil and HIV antibodies, autoimmunities (including rheumatoid factor, antinuclear antibody, and complement studies), vitamin B_{12}, folate, liver and renal function, lactate dehydrogenase, uric acid, serum protein electrophoresis, and immunoelectrophoresis.

Treatment

Treatment of neutropenia depends on the suspected cause. Acute neutropenia must further involve a search for possible offending drugs or signs and symptoms of infection. In general, these types of neutropenia require either the cessation of implicated drugs or the prompt identification of complicating disorders. Resolution of neutropenia in these instances is typically rapid.

Various therapies have been tried for the primary neutropenic disorders. In the congenital disorders, minimal response has been noted to steroids, γ globulin, lithium salts, splenectomy, and plasmapheresis.[56, 57] Allogeneic bone marrow transplantation has resulted in partial as well as complete remissions.[56] Therapy with growth factors has also yielded varying responses. Granulocyte colony-stimulating factor (G-CSF) has resulted in improved neutrophil counts associated with fewer infectious episodes.[56, 59, 70, 72] On the other hand, GM-CSF has been shown to have no clinical benefit.[71]

Cyclic neutropenia, both congenital and acquired, may exhibit spontaneous clinical remissions.[58] Various therapies, such as γ globulin, plasmapheresis, splenectomy, and corticosteroids, have proved to be without benefit. Lithium carbonate therapy has caused some increases in neutrophil counts, although its exact mechanism of action is unknown.

The gray Collie model for cyclic neutropenia has allowed studies to explore the therapeutic role of hematopoietic growth factors.[73, 74] On the basis of the benefits seen with CSF in this model, a pilot study was conducted by Hammond and associates[75] in humans with cyclic neutropenia. The initial findings have been further substantiated in the setting of a phase III randomized clinical trial.[72] Results of therapy for idiopathic neutropenia are essentially the same as noted for the cyclic states, with the exception that reports indicate that GM-CSF as well as G-CSF may produce increases in neutrophil counts and clinical improvement.[76]

Neutropenia secondary to underlying illness responds best to treatment of the primary disorder. Among the malignant states, CLL, ALL, multiple myeloma, non-Hodgkin's lymphoma, and Hodgkin's disease are best managed with appropriate combination chemotherapy regimens. In HCL, the interferons,[77] pentostatin,[78] and 2-chlorodeoxy adenosine[79] appear to be most effective in inducing clinical remission. Studies with G-CSF in HCL have resulted in improvement in neutrophil counts and concomitant infections previously unresponsive to antibiotic therapy, without significant effect on the underlying disease.[80] Clinical trials of G-CSF in combination with interferon-α are currently under way.

Traditional chemotherapy for patients with myeloid leukemia remains the "gold standard" for its treatment. Studies with G-CSF and GM-CSF are being conducted to evaluate the ability of these cytokines either to induce cycle leukemia cells into S-phase to improve cell kill of chemotherapy[81–83] or, in the case of G-CSF, to evaluate the potential differentiating effect on myeloid blasts.

In the myelodysplastic syndromes, low-dose cytosine arabinoside has resulted in complete response rates of approximately 30%.[84] Intensive chemotherapy and vitamins have yielded lower response rates. Results of allogeneic bone marrow transplantation suggest that 30% to 40% of patients with myelodysplastic syndromes who have HLA-matched donors can achieve a durable long-term disease-free remission when treated in this fashion.[85] Attempts at differentiation therapy with hexamethylbisacetimide[86] and *cis*-retinoic acid[87] have resulted in few significant responses. Because the major complications of these disorders are the cytopenias that accompany them, treatment with various growth factors has been studied. Trials with both G-CSF[88, 89] and GM-CSF[90–92] have resulted in significant improvements in total white blood cell count and neutrophil counts; however, no clear benefit in overall survival has yet been shown.

In secondary neutropenia associated with autoimmune disorders, γ globulin and plasmapheresis have been used without success.[93] Corticosteroids have been effective in systemic lupus erythematosus and, in conjunction with other appropriate medications, have yielded responses in the rheumatoid arthritides.[94] Splenectomy in patients with Felty's syndrome has produced transient increases in neutrophil counts with subsequent declines to preoperative levels.

T-lymphocytosis has been noted to respond to γ globulin with partial, but no complete, responses. Alternative treatment with steroids and plasmapheresis has been ineffective. Cyclosporin alone,[95] G-CSF,[72] or the combination of cyclosporin and hematopoietic growth factor(s) may prove effective, and all are being evaluated.

In patients with neutropenia associated with HIV-1 infection, G-CSF and GM-CSF used alone and in conjunction with antiviral therapy (i.e., zidovudine) have improved neutrophil counts.[96, 97]

Various therapies have been utilized in aplastic anemia. Corticosteroids, androgens, antithymocyte globulin, and allogeneic bone marrow transplantation have become the mainstays of therapeutic intervention. Various cytokines and growth factors, including G-CSF, GM-CSF, and, in one study, IL-3, have also shown some initial promise in improving neutrophil counts in selected patients.

Neutropenia due to drugs or medications is best treated by removal of the offending agent; resolution of neutropenia most often occurs within 48 hours. Both G-CSF and GM-CSF have been used on a compassionate basis in drug-related neutropenia, with an acceleration of recovery noted. Prospects in the treatment of neutropenia secondary to chemotherapy have been buoyed by favorable results in trials using both G-CSF and GM-CSF. Other cytokines (IL-1 and IL-3), whose actions occur in early stages of hematopoiesis, are currently being studied with the hope of improving the deficiencies of other cell lineages associated with chemotherapy as well as further augmenting myeloid reconstitution.

GRANULOCYTOPATHY

Abnormalities of neutrophil function (regardless of the absolute number) may occur in some diseases, yielding a state of "relative neutropenia." Neutrophil dysfunction can involve defects in degranulation (Chédiak-Higashi syndrome), superoxide production (chronic granulomatous disease), or chemotaxis (thermal burns, diabetes mellitus, drugs such as ethanol and steroids) (Tables 2–11 and 2–12).[98]

The possibility of a defect in neutrophil function should be considered in any patient suffering from repetitive infections. If these infections are in several anatomical sites and caused by pyogenic bacteria of low virulence, the likelihood of phagocytic dysfunction increases. In evaluating such a patient, sex, age, onset of illness, family history, physical findings, and type of organisms causing infection are all helpful distinguishing points (Fig. 2–5).[98] The management of patients with granulocytopathies in-

Table 2–11. Pathogenesis of Microbicidal Defects of Polymorphonuclear Neutrophilic Leukocytes

Abnormality	Associated Conditions
Decreased cell numbers	Myeloproliferative disorders Granulocytopenia induced by chemical (including drug) and physical agents Congenital granulocytopenias Granulocytopenia associated with infiltration of marrow by microorganisms or abnormal cells
Defective cell migration	Glucocorticoid treatment
Defective chemotaxis*	Genetic deficiencies of complement Chédiak-Higashi syndrome Malignancies Lazy leukocyte syndrome Diabetes mellitus Uremia Rheumatoid arthritis Hyperimmunoglobulinemia E Increased concentration of chemotactic inhibitors in Hodgkin's disease and Bruton-type agammaglobulinemia
Defective opsonization	Congenital and acquired hypogammaglobulinemia Complement abnormalities (deficiency or hypermetabolism of C3) Sickle cell disease Tuftsin deficiency
Defective ingestion	Neutrophil dysfunction
Defective intracellular killing	Chédiak-Higashi syndrome Total deficiency of glucose-6-phosphate dehydrogenase in the granulocytes Myeloperoxidase deficiency Lipochrome histiocytosis

*Enhanced and depressed chemotaxis have been reported in patients with severe bacterial infections. A family with abnormal chemotaxis attributed to a dysfunction of C5 has been described.

From Steigbigel RT. Microbicidal defects in polymorphonuclear leukocytes. *In* Lichtman MA (ed). Hematology and Oncology. The Science and Practice of Clinical Medicine Series, vol 6. New York: Grune & Stratton, 1980, p 137.

Table 2–12. Disorders Associated With Defective Granulocyte Intracellular Killing

Defect	Clinical Problem	Mode of Inheritance	Physical Findings	Laboratory Findings
Chronic granulomatous disease (CGD)	Recurrent and poorly resolving infection of the integument, lungs, bones, and lymphoreticular organs due to catalase-positive organisms. Granuloma and abscess formation in viscera.	Majority are X-linked–recessive. Approximately 1/7 show autosomal-recessive inheritance.	Eczematoid lesions. Adenopathy Hepatosplenomegaly	Defective granulocyte and monocyte intracellular killing of catalase-positive bacteria. Lack of granulocyte response to ingestion of bacteria: no increase in O_2 consumption, hexose monophosphate shunt activity, H_2O_2, or O_2 production; failure of activation of NADPH oxidase. Chemotaxis has very rarely been found to be abnormal in patients with CGD-like defects.
Chédiak-Higashi syndrome	Recurrent, severe infection due to both catalase-positive and catalase-negative organisms. Bleeding tendency associated with platelet storage pool defect.	Autosomal-recessive	Oculocutaneous albinism, photophobia, nystagmus, localized adenopathy during infection. Accelerated phase associated with hepatosplenomegaly and diffuse lymphadenopathy.	Enlarged granules in leukocytes and melanocytes, vacuoles in bone marrow granulocytes. Granulocytes demonstrate increased baseline hexose monophosphate shunt activity and normal response to stimulus with increased O_2 consumption and H_2O_2 production and NBT dye reduction. Intracellular killing of bacteria is delayed but not absent, possibly owing to impaired lysosomal fusion with phagocytic vacuoles.
Total glucose-6-phosphate dehydrogenase (G-6-PD) deficiency	Hemolytic anemia; increased susceptibility to severe infection caused by catalase-positive bacteria.	Evidence for X-linked recessive pattern in one family; also reported in a female.	Adenopathy with infections. Can manifest in adults.	The oxidative metabolism and microbicidal abnormalities in granulocytes are similar to those seen in CGD; however, NADPH oxidase activity is normal, and G-6-PD is completely absent.
Myeloperoxidase deficiency	Increased susceptibility to disseminated *Candida albicans* infection noted in one patient.	Autosomal-recessive	No distinguishing features.	Decreased killing of *C. albicans* and delayed killing of bacteria by granulocytes. Absence of myeloperoxidase H_2O_2 production and hexose monophosphate shunt activity after stimulation of patient's granulocytes are greater than normal.
Lipochrome histocytosis	Recurrent infections, especially pneumonia, arthritis.	Unknown	Splenomegaly Hepatomegaly	Diffuse nodular densities on chest roentgenogram. Positive latex fixation. Decreased bacterial killing by granulocytes associated with diminished NBT dye reduction and hexose monophosphate shunt response to stimuli. Depressed lymphocyte transformation response to mitogenic stimulation.

Modified from Steigbigel RT. Microbicidal defects in polymorphonuclear leukocytes. *In* Lichtman MA (ed). Hematology and Oncology. The Science and Practice of Clinical Medicine Series, vol 6. New York: Grune & Stratton, 1980, p 138.

NBT, nitroblue tetrazolium.

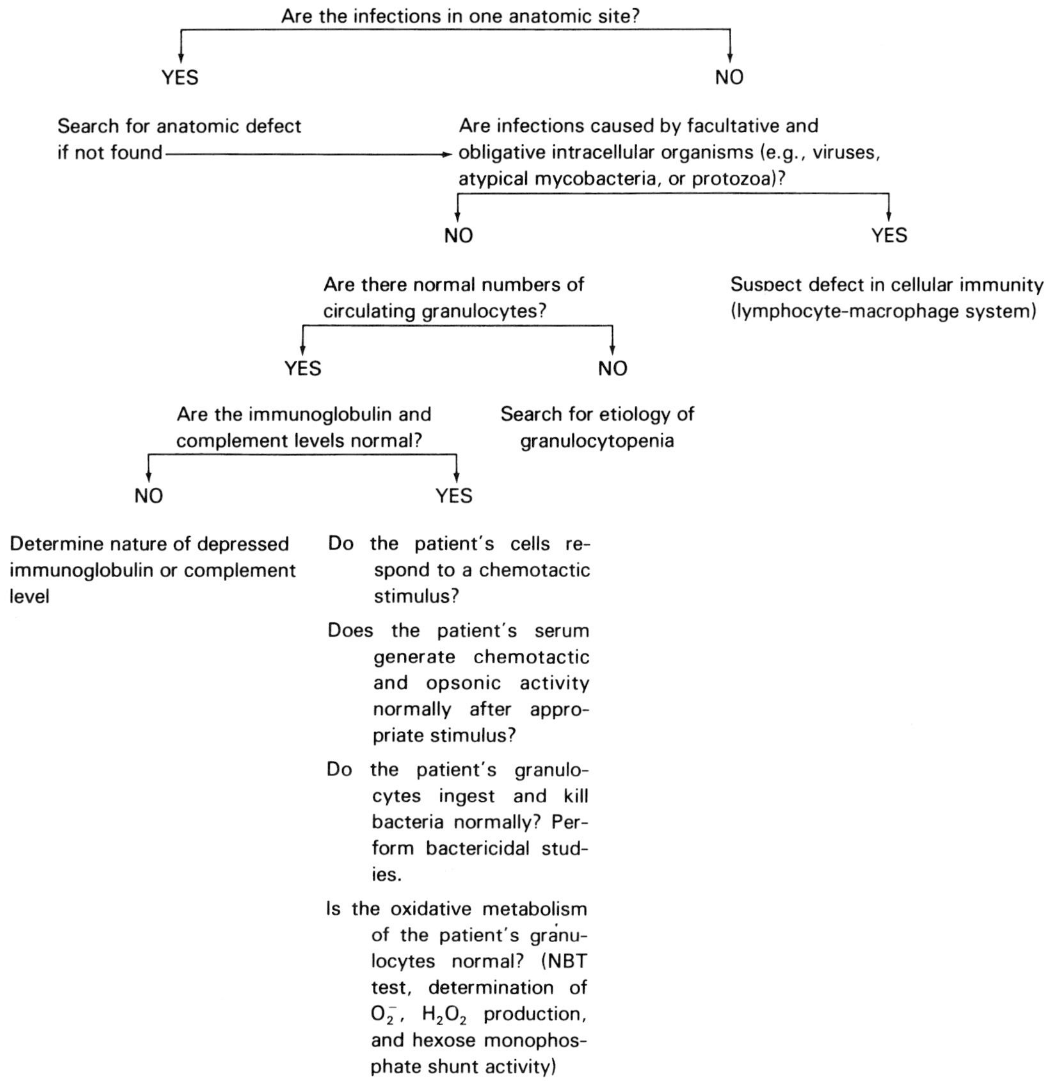

Figure 2–5. Approach to the patient with frequent infections. (From Steigbigel RT. Microbicidal defects in polymorphonuclear leukocytes. *In* Lichtman MA (ed). Hematology and Oncology. The Science and Practice of Clinical Medicine Series, vol 6. New York: Grune & Stratton, 1980, p 139.)

volves the prevention and early treatment of infection. Prophylactic antibiotics, such as synthetic penicillin to prevent *Staphylococcus aureus* infection in chronic granulomatous disease has been successful in reducing the incidence of infection in these patients. Gamma interferon has also been shown to be effective in reducing infection in patients with this disease.[99] The mechanism of this effect is unknown.

GRANULOCYTE TRANSFUSION

Granulocyte transfusions must be reserved for those neutropenic patients with documented life-threatening bacterial or fungal infections refractory to antibiotic therapy. These transfusions must be blood groups ABO-compatible. Provision of granulocytes to such patients has long been a desirable goal that has been hampered by the inability to collect adequate numbers of cells from appropriate donors. Investigators have, however, reported on the ability of G-CSF to allow for the collection of large numbers of granulocytes from normal donors.[100–102] The feasibility of procuring such effector cells[100–102] will enable investigators to test whether this therapeutic modality offers benefit either to neutropenic patients with refractory infections or to patients with defects of polymorphonuclear leukocytes.

LEUKOCYTOSIS

Leukocytosis refers to a rise in the leukocyte count above the upper limit of normal. The most common cause of leukocytosis is an absolute increase in neutrophilic granulocytes. An elevated white blood cell count can also occur from an increase in eosinophils (eosinophilia) and, although rarely, from an increase in basophils (basophilia).

An increase in circulating neutrophils above 8000 cells/μL is generally taken as the numerical definition of neutrophilia (Table 2–13). The most common cause of

Table 2–13. Causes of Neutrophilia

Infections	Bacterial Viral Fungal Parasitic Protozoal	Malignant tumors (with or without evidence of marrow invasion)	Bronchogenic carcinoma Renal cell carcinoma Gastric carcinoma
Hormones	Epinephrine Corticosteroids Etiocholanolone	Nonmalignant hematological disorders	Hemorrhage Hemolytic anemias Postsplenectomy reaction Recovery from agranulocytosis Therapy of megaloblastic anemias Transfusion reactions
Drugs, toxins	Lithium Chlorpropamide Endotoxin Lead Mercury	Physical stimuli	Burns Electric shock Prolonged exposure to cold Exercise Pregnancy
Metabolic derangements	Diabetic ketoacidosis Thyroid storm Eclampsia	Miscellaneous	Anoxia Certain cardiac arrhythmias Familial neutrophilic conditions
Inflammatory conditions	Rheumatoid arthritis Acute gout Thyroiditis Colitis		
Hematological malignancies	Myeloproliferative disorders (e.g., chronic myelogenous leukemia, polycythemia vera, myelofibrosis) Hodgkin's disease		

Modified from Golde DW, Belzer MB. Neutrophilia and leukemoid reactions. *In* Lichtman MA (ed). Hematology and Oncology. The Science and Practice of Clinical Medicine Series, vol 6. New York: Grune & Stratton, 1980, p 129.

neutrophilia is bacterial infection. Neutrophilia is also associated with certain endocrine, inflammatory, malignant (nonhematopoietic), and nonmalignant conditions (see Table 2–13). An elevation in white blood cell count in the absence of obvious infection (leukemoid reaction) needs to be distinguished from chronic myelogenous leukemia. The characteristics used to distinguish between these conditions include spleen size, history of fever, presence of anemia, leukocyte alkaline phosphatase value, cytogenetics (Philadelphia chromosome), and BCR/ABL gene rearrangement (Table 2–14).

A number of diseases are associated with an increase

Table 2–14. Differentiation of Leukemoid Reaction (in the Absence of Hematopoietic Growth Factor Administration) From Chronic Myelogenous Leukemia

Features	Leukemoid Reactions	Chronic Myelogenous Leukemia (CML)	Myeloproliferative Disorder
Symptoms			
Abdominal fullness	Not common	Very helpful if present; caused by increased size of spleen	Can be present
Fever	Usually present	Usually absent	Can be present
Physical findings			
Lymphadenopathy	Depends on underlying process	Unusual before accelerated phase	Can be present
Splenomegaly	Depends on underlying process	Present in 90%; spleen may be very large	Often present
Signs of infection	Often present	Usually absent	Usually absent
Laboratory findings			
White blood cell count* (cells/μL)	<75,000	>75,000	Varies: wide range in elevation
Presence of immature white blood cells	Occasional myelocytes may be seen	Myelocytes common; promyelocytes and blast cells usually present	Same as in CML
Anemia	May be present; usually mild unless associated with hemolysis or hemorrhage	Presenting hemoglobin usually 9.0 to 11.0 gm/dL	Can have leukoerythroblastic picture
Basophilia	Rare	Common	Rare
Leukocyte alkaline phosphatase	Increased	Usually very low	Low
Philadelphia chromosome and/or breakpoint cluster region	Absent	Present	Absent

*The total white blood cell count is nearly always above 30,000 cells/μL at the time of diagnosis and may be between 30,000 and 75,000 cells/μL. If the count is over 75,000 cells/μL, a leukemoid reaction is very unlikely. Thus, in the range of 30,000 to 75,000 cells/μL, the white blood cell count alone is not a discriminating factor.

Modified from Golde DW, Belzer MB. Neutrophilia and leukemoid reactions. *In* Lichtman MA (ed). Hematology and Oncology. The Science and Practice of Clinical Medicine Series, vol 6. New York: Grune & Stratton, 1980, p 131.

Table 2-15. Conditions Associated With Eosinophilia

Frequent association	Metazoan infestation. Atopic states. Drug allergy. Pulmonary eosinophilias: Löffler syndrome, pulmonary infiltration with eosinophilia. Skin diseases: pemphigus, pemphigoid. Eosinophilic myeloproliferative disease. Hypereosinophilic syndromes. Treatment with IL-2, GM-CSF, and IL-3.	Less frequent association	Neoplastic disorders Hodgkin's disease Lymphoma Lung cancer Gastrointestinal cancer Radiation treatment Angiitis Rheumatoid arthritis Immune deficiency syndromes Congenital defects Cardiovascular defects Thrombocytopenia with absent radius Familial reticuloendotheliosis with eosinophilia Ulcerative colitis

Modified from Kellermeyer RW. Eosinophilia. *In* Lichtman MA (ed). Hematology and Oncology. The Science and Practice of Clinical Medicine Series, vol 6. New York: Grune & Stratton, 1980, p 132.

in eosinophils (Table 2–15). In addition, treatment with IL-2, IL-3, and GM-CSF is associated with eosinophilia. Data have demonstrated that the eosinophilia seen in conjunction with Hodgkin's disease is due to the production of IL-5 by Reed-Sternberg cells.[103] The eosinophilia in autoimmune disease and drug allergy is probably due to production and secretion of lymphokines (i.e., IL-3, GM-CSF, or IL-5) by activated T lymphocytes.

REFERENCES

1. Bainton DF. Neutrophils, eosinophils, basophils and monocytes. *In* Lichtman MA (ed): Hematology and Oncology. The Science and Practice of Clinical Medicine Series, vol 66. New York: Grune & Stratton, 1980.
2. Bainton DF. The development of neutrophilic polymorphonuclear leukocytes in human bone marrow. J Exp Med 1971; 134:907.
3. Cline MJ. The normal granulocyte. *In* Cline MJ (ed): The White Cell. Cambridge, MA: Harvard University Press, 1975.
4. Bainton DF, Farquhar MG. Differences in enzyme content of azurophil and specific granules of polymorphonuclear leukocytes. I: histological staining of bone marrow smears. J Cell Biol 1968; 39:286.
5. Baggiolini M. The enzymes of the granules of polymorphonuclear leukocytes and their functions. Enzyme 1972; 13:132.
6. DeDuve C. Lysosomes, a new group of cytoplasmic particles. *In* Hiyachi T (ed): Subcellular Particles. New York: Ronald Press, 1959.
7. Bainton D, Farquhar MG. Origin of granules in polymorphonuclear leukocytes: two types derived from opposite Golgi complex in developing granulocytes. J Cell Biol 1966; 28:277.
8. Kawakami M, Tsutsumi H, Kumakawa T, et al: Levels of serum granulocyte with colony-stimulating factor in patients with infections. Blood 1990; 76:1962–4.
9. Moore MAS, Gabrilove JL, Sheridan AP. Therapeutic implications of serum factors inhibiting proliferation and inducing differentiation of myeloid leukemia cells. Blood Cells 1983; 9:125–37.
10. Lord BI, Molineux G, Pojda Z, et al. Myeloid cell kinetics in mice treated with recombinant interleukin-3, granulocyte colony-stimulating factor (CSF) or granulocyte-macrophage CSF, in vivo. Blood 1991; 77:2154.
11. Isaacs R, Danielian AC. A study of the white blood corpuscles appearing in the saliva and their relation to those in the blood. Am J Med Sci 1927; 174:70.
12. Stossel T. Phagocytosis. N Engl J Med 1974; 290:717.
13. Platzer E, Oez S, Welte K, et al. Human pluripotent hematopoietic colony-stimulating factor: activities on human and murine cells. Immunobiology 1986; 172:185.
14. Gabrilove JL, Welte K, Harris P, et al. Pluripoietin: a second human hematopoietic colony-stimulating factor produced by the human bladder carcinoma cell line 5637. Proc Natl Acad Sci U S A 1986; 83:2478.
15. Tomonaga M, Golde DW, Gasson JC. Biosynthetic (recombinant) human granulocyte-macrophage colony-stimulating factor: effect on normal bone marrow and leukemia cell lines. Blood 1986; 67:31–6.
16. Warren DJ, Moore MAS. Synergism among interleukin-1, interleukin-3, and interleukin-5 in the production of eosinophils from primitive hemopoietic stem cells. J Immunol 1988; 140:94.
17. Lopez AF, Sanderson CJ, Gamble JR, Campbell HD, Young JG, et al. Recombinant human interleukin-5 is a selective activator of human eosinophil function. J Exp Med 1988; 167:219.
18. Yamaguchi Y, Suda T, Suda J, et al. Purified interleukin-5 supports the terminal differentiation and proliferation of murine eosinophilic precursors. J Exp Med 1988; 167:43.
19. Clutterbuck EJ, Hirst EMA, Sanderson CJ. Human interleukin-5 regulates the production of eosinophils in human bone marrow cultures. Blood 1989; 73:1504.
20. Tai PC, Spry CJF. Studies on blood eosinophils. I: patients with a transient eosinophilia. Clin Exp Immunol 1976; 24:415.
21. Kay AB, Anwar ARE. Proceedings of the Eosinophil Centennial. *In* Mahmoud AAF, Austen KF (eds): The Eosinophil in Health and Disease. New York: Grune & Stratton, 1980.
22. Denburg JA. Basophil and mast cell lineages in vitro and in vivo. Blood 1992; 79:846.
23. Denburg JA, Richardson M, Telizyn S, Bienenstock J. Basophil/mast cell precursors in human peripheral blood. Blood 1993; 61:775.
24. Tsuda T, Wong DA, Dolovich J, et al. Synergistic effects of nerve growth factor and granulocyte-macrophage colony-stimulating factor on human basophilic cell differentiation. Blood 1991; 77:971.
25. Dinarello CA. Biology of interleukin-1. FASEB J 1988; 2:108.
26. Leary AG, Yang YC, Clark SC, et al. Recombinant gibbon interleukin-3 supports formation of human multilineage colonies and blast cell colonies in culture: comparison with recombinant human granulocyte-macrophage colony-stimulating factor. Blood 1987; 70:1343.
27. Kishimoh T. The biology of interleukin-6. Blood 1989; 74:1.
28. Martin FH, Suggs SV, Langley KE, et al. Primary structure and functional expression of rat and human stem cell factor DNAs. Cell 1990; 63:203.
29. Burgess A, Metcalf D. Characterization of a serum factor stimulating the differentiation of myelomonocytic leukemic cells. Int J Cancer 1980; 26:647.

30. Welte K, Platzer E, Lu L, et al. Purification and biological characterization of human pluripotent hematopoietic colony-stimulating factor. Proc Natl Acad Sci U S A 1985; 82:1526.
31. Souza LM, Boone TC, Gabrilove J, et al. Recombinant human granulocyte colony-stimulating factor: effects on normal and leukemic myeloid cells. Science 1986; 232:61.
32. Lindemann A, Reidel D, Oster W, et al. Granulocyte-macrophage colony-stimulating factor induces cytokine secretion by human polymorphonuclear leukocytes. J Clin Invest 1989; 83:1308.
33. Zsebo KM, Yuschenkoff NV, Shiffer S, et al. Vascular endothelial cells and granulopoiesis: interleukin-1 stimulates release of G-CSF and GM-CSF. Blood 1988; 71:99.
34. Munker R, Gasson J, Ogawa M, et al. Recombinant human tumor necrosis factor induces production of granulocyte-macrophage colony-stimulating factor. Nature 1986; 323:79.
35. Fibbe WE, Damme J, Billiau A, et al. Interleukin-2 induces human marrow stromal cells in long-term culture to produce G-CSF and M-CSF. Blood 1988; 71:430.
36. Kaczmarski RS, Mufti GJ. The cytokine receptor superfamily. Blood Rev 1991; 5:193.
37. Begley CG, Nicola NA, Metcalf D. Proliferation of normal human promyelocyte and myelocytes after a single pulse stimulation by purified GM-CSF or G-CSF. Blood 1988; 71:640.
38. Warren DJ, Moore MAS. Synergism among interleukin-1, interleukin-3, and interleukin-5 in the production of eosinophils from primitive hemopoietic stem cells. J Immunol 1988; 140: 94.
39. Moore MAS. Hematologic effects of interleukin-1, granulocyte colony-stimulating factor, and granulocyte-macrophage colony-stimulating factor in tumor-bearing mice treated with fluorouracil. J Natl Cancer Inst 1990; 82:1031.
40. Welte K, Bonilla MA, Gillio AP, et al. In vivo effects of recombinant human G-CSF in therapy induced neutropenias in primates. Exp Hematol 1987; 15:72.
41. Gasson JC, Weisbart RH, Kaufman S, et al. Purified human granulocyte macrophage colony-stimulating factor: direct action on neutrophils. Science 1984; 226:1339.
42. Wong GG, Witek JS, Temple P, et al. Human GM-CSF, molecular cloning of complementary DNA and purification of the natural and recombinant proteins. Science 1985; 228:810.
43. Gasson J. Molecular physiology of granulocyte macrophage colony-stimulating factor. Blood 1991; 77:1131.
44. Ihle J, Keller J, Oroszlan S, et al. Biologic properties of homogeneous interleukin-3. J Immunol 1983; 131:282.
45. Fung MC, Hapel AJ, Ymer S, et al. Molecular cloning of cDNA for murine interleukin-3. Nature 1984; 307:233.
46. Yokota T, Lee F, Rennick D, et al. Isolation and characterization of a mouse cDNA clone that expresses mast-cell growth factor activity in monkey cells. Proc Natl Acad Sci U S A 1981; 81:1070.
47. Sanderson CJ, O'Garra A, Warner DJ, et al. Eosinophil differentiation factor also has B cell growth factor activity: proposed name interleukin-4. Proc Natl Acad Sci U S A 1986; 83:437.
48. Williams DE, Eisenman J, Baird A, et al. Identification of a ligand for the *c-kit* proto-oncogene. Cell 1990; 63:167.
49. Lerner NB, Nocka KH, Cole SR, et al. Monoclonal antibody YB5.B8 identifies the human *c-kit* protein product. Blood 1991; 77:1876.
50. Anderson DM, Lyman SD, Baird A, et al. Molecular cloning of mast cell growth factor, a hematopoietin that is active in both membrane bound and soluble forms. Cell 1990; 63:235.
51. Bernstein ID, Andrews RG, Zsebo KM. Recombinant human stem cell factor enhances the formation of colonies by $CD34^+$ and $CD34^+ lin^-$ cells, and the generation of colony-forming cell progeny from $CD34^+ lin^-$ cells cultured with interleukin-3, granulocyte colony-stimulating factor, or granulocyte-macrophage colony-stimulating factor. Blood 1991; 77:2316.
52. Brandt J, Briddell RA, Srour EF, et al. Role of *c-kit* ligand in the expansion of human hematopoietic progenitor cells. Blood 1992; 79:634.
53. Baggiolini M, Walz A, Kunkel SL. Neutrophil-activating peptide-1/interleukin 8, a novel cytokine that activates neutrophils. J Clin Invest 1989; 84:1045.
54. Bodey GP, Buckley M, Sathe YS, Freireich EJ. Quantitative relationships between circulating leukocytes and infection in patients with acute leukemia. Ann Intern Med 1966; 64:328.
55. Crawford J, Ozer H, Stoller R, et al. Reduction by granulocyte colony-stimulating factor of fever and neutropenia induced by chemotherapy in patients with small-cell lung cancer. N Engl J Med 1991; 325:163.
56. Bonilla MA, Gillio AP, Ruggiero M, et al. Effects of recombinant human granulocyte colony-stimulating factor on neutropenia in patients with congenital agranulocytosis. N Engl J Med 1989; 320:1574.
57. Shwachman H, Diamond LK, Oski FA, Khaw KT. The syndrome of pancreatic insufficiency and bone marrow dysfunction. J Pediatr 1964; 65:645.
58. Dale DC, Hammond WP IV. Cyclic neutropenia: a clinical review. Blood Rev 1988; 1:178.
59. Jakubowski AA, Souza L, Kelly F, et al. Effects of human granulocyte colony-stimulating factor in a patient with idiopathic neutropenia. N Engl J Med 1989; 320:38.
60. Nitsu Y, Urushizaki Y, Koshida Y, et al. Expression of TGF-beta gene in adult T-cell leukemia. Blood 1988; 71:263.
61. Chan WC, Link S, Mawle A, et al. Heterogeneity of large granular lymphocyte proliferations: delineation of two major subtypes with distinct origins, immunophenotypes, functional and clinical characteristics. Blood 1986; 68:1142.
62. Zon LI, Arkin C, Groopman JE. Haematologic manifestations of human immunodeficiency virus (HIV) infection. Br J Haematol 1987; 66:251.
63. Lu L, Welte K, Gabrilove JL, et al. Effects of recombinant human tumor necrosis factor, recombinant human-interferon, and prostaglandin E on colony formation of human hematopoietic progenitor cells stimulated by natural human pluripotent colony-stimulating factor, pluripoietin, and recombinant erythropoietin in serum-free cultures. Cancer Res 1986; 46:4357.
64. Bartels EC. Agranulocytosis during propylthiouracil therapy. Am J Med 1948; 5:48.
65. Goodman HL. Agranulocytosis associated with Tofranil. Ann Intern Med 1961; 55:321.
66. Abbott JA, Schwals RS. The serious side effects of the newer antiepileptic drugs: their control and prevention. N Engl J Med 1950; 242:943.
67. Spain DM, Clark TB. A case of agranulocytosis occurring during the course of penicillin therapy. Ann Intern Med 1946; 25:732.
68. Britton CJC, Howkins J. Action of sulphanilamide on leucocytes. Lancet 1938; 2:718.
69. No reference.
70. Gabrilove JL, Gordon MS. Neutropenia. *In* Rakel RE (ed). Conn's Current Therapy 1991. Philadelphia: WB Saunders, 1991, pp 323–326.
71. Welte K, Zeidler C, Reuther A, et al. Correction of neutropenia and associated clinical symptoms with rhG-CSF in children with severe congenital neutropenia. Blood 1988; 72:465.
72. Dale DC, Bonilla MA, Davis MW, et al. A randomized controlled phase III trial of recombinant human granulocyte colony-stimulating factor (filgrastim) for treatment of severe chronic neutropenia. Blood 1993; 81:2496.
73. Hammond WP, Donahue RE, Dale DC. Purified recombinant human granulocyte-macrophage colony-stimulating factor stimulates granulocytopoiesis in canine cyclic hematopoiesis. Blood 1986; 68(suppl):165a.
74. Lothrop CD Jr, Warren DJ, Souza LM, et al. Correction of canine cyclic hematopoiesis with recombinant human granulocyte colony-stimulating factor. Blood 1988; 72:1324.
75. Hammond WP, Price TH, Souza LM, Dale DC. Treatment of cyclic neutropenia with granulocyte colony stimulating factor. N Engl J Med 1989; 320:1306.
76. Ganser A, Ottmann O, Erdmann H, et al. The effect of recombinant human granulocyte-macrophage colony-stimulating factor on neutropenia and related morbidity in chronic severe neutropenia. Ann Intern Med 1989; 111:887.
77. Quesada JR, Reuben J, Manning JT, et al. Alpha interferon for induction of remission in hairy-cell leukemia. N Engl J Med 1984; 310:15.
78. Spiers ASD, Moore D, Cassileth PA, et al. Remissions in hairy-cell leukemia with pentostatin (2-deoxycoformycin). N Engl J Med 1987; 316:825.
79. Piro LD, Carrera CJ, Carson DA, Beutler E. Complete remissions in hairy cell leukemia after treatment with 2-chlorodeoxyadenosine [Abstract]. Blood 1988; 72(suppl):220a.

80. Glaspy JA, Baldwin GC, Robertson PA, et al. Therapy for neutropenia in hairy cell leukemia with recombinant human granulocyte colony-stimulating factor. Ann Intern Med 1988; 109:789.
81. Jakubowski A, Andreeff M, Tafuri A, et al. In vivo and in vitro studies of rhG-CSF in acute nonlymphocytic leukemia. Blood 1989; 74:1034.
82. Bettelheim P, Valent P, Andreef M, et al. Recombinant human granulocyte-macrophage colony-stimulating factor in combination with standard induction chemotherapy in de novo acute myeloid leukemia. Blood 1991; 77:700.
83. Estey EH, Dixon D, Kantarjian HM. Treatment of poor-prognosis newly diagnosed acute myeloid leukemia with ara-C and recombinant human granulocyte-macrophage colony-stimulating factor. Blood 1990; 75:1766.
84. Cheson BD, Simon R. Low-dose ara-C in acute nonlymphocytic leukemia and myelodysplastic syndromes: a review of 20 years' experience. Semin Oncol 1987; 14(suppl 1):126.
85. Appelbaum FR, Storb R, Ramberg RE, et al. Treatment of preleukemic syndromes with marrow transplantation. Blood 1987; 69:92.
86. Kizaki M, Koeffler HP. Differentiation-inducing agents in the treatment of myelodysplastic syndromes. Semin Oncol 1992; 19:106.
87. Gabrilove JL. Differentiation factors. Semin Oncol 1986; 13:228.
88. Negrin RS, Haeuber DH, Nagler A, et al. Treatment of myelodysplastic syndrome with recombinant granulocyte colony-stimulating factor. Ann Intern Med 1989; 110:976.
89. Negrin NR, Haeuber DH, Nagler A, et al. Maintenance treatment of patients with myelodysplastic syndromes using recombinant human granulocyte colony-stimulating factor. Blood 1990; 76:36.
90. Vadhan-Jaj S, Keating M, LeMaistre A, et al. Effects of recombinant human granulocyte-macrophage colony-stimulating factor in patients with myelodysplastic syndromes. N Engl J Med 1987; 317:1545.
91. Baser A, Volkers B, Greher J, et al. Recombinant human granulocyte-macrophage colony-stimulating factor in patients with myelodysplastic syndromes: a phase I/II trial. Blood 1989; 73:31.
92. Thompson JA, Lee DJ, Kidd P, et al. Subcutaneous granulocyte-macrophage colony-stimulating factor in patients with myelodysplastic syndromes. J Clin Oncol 1989; 7:629–37.
93. Jandl JH. Leukocyte anomalies. *In* Blood, Textbook of Hematology. Boston: Little, Brown, 1987, pp 571–588.
94. Reynolds CW, Foon KA. Tγ: lymphoproliferative disease and related disorders in humans and experimental animals: a review of the clinical, cellular, and functional characteristics. Blood 1984; 64:1146.
95. Pastor E, Sayas MJ. Severe neutropenia associated with large granular lymphocyte lymphocytosis: successful control with cyclosporin A. Blut 1989; 59:501.
96. Pluda JM, Yarchoan R, Smith PD, et al. Subcutaneous recombinant granulocyte-macrophage colony-stimulating factor used as a single agent and in an alternating regimen with azidothymidine in leukopenic patients with severe human immunodeficiency virus infection. Blood 1990; 76:463.
97. Scadden DT, Bering HA, Levine JD, et al. Granulocyte-macrophage colony-stimulating factor mitigates the neutropenia of combined interferon-alfa and zidovudine treatment of acquired immune deficiency syndrome–associated Kaposi's sarcoma. J Clin Oncol 1991; 9:802.
98. Steigbigel RT. Microbicidal defects in polymorphonuclear leukocytes. *In* Littmann MA (ed). Hematology and Oncology. The Science and Practice of Clinical Medicine Series, vol 6. New York: Grune & Stratton, 1980.
99. The International Chronic Granulomatous Disease Cooperative Study Group. A controlled trial of interferon gamma to prevent infection in chronic granulomatous disease. N Engl J Med 1991; 324:509.
100. Bensinger WI, Price TH, Dale DC, et al. The effects of daily recombinant human granulocyte colony-stimulating factor administration on normal granulocyte donors undergoing leukapheresis. Blood 1993; 81:1883.
101. Casper CB, Seger RA, Burger J, Gmur J. Effective stimulation of donors for granulocyte transfusions with recombinant methionyl granulocyte colony-stimulating factor. Blood 1993; 81:2866.
102. Strauss RG. Therapeutic granulocyte transfusions in 1993. Blood 1993; 81:1675.
103. Samoszuk M, Nansen L. Detection of interleukin-5 messenger RNA in Reed-Sternberg cells of Hodgkin's disease with eosinophilia. Blood 1990; 75:13.

CHAPTER 3

Megakaryocytopoiesis and Platelet Kinetics

Richard A. Carter
Kenneth J. Smith
Laurence A. Harker

In normal persons, blood platelets circulate at a concentration of 250 × 10^9/L (range, 150 to 400) with a lifespan of 9 to 10 days. Megakaryocytes give rise to platelets through a process of progenitor mitogenesis, as well as through megakaryocyte proliferation, endo-reduplication differentiation, and final release into the circulation of cytoplasmic elements as platelets. Thrombopoietin induces loglinear expansion of early progenitors, as well as proliferating and endo-reduplicating megakaryocytes through thrombopoietin receptor–initiated mitogenesis. Because receptor-bearing platelets compete for unbound thrombopoietin, the peripheral concentration of platelets diminishes the stimulus for megakaryocytopoiesis, thereby mediating compensatory changes in platelet production. Thrombocytopenia results from impaired production, increased destruction, altered intravascular distribution, or a combination of these abnormalities. Megakaryocytic cytoplasmic mass is the marrow substrate destined to become circulating platelets, and the effective delivery of that substrate as viable platelet product into the peripheral blood is estimated as platelet turnover (peripheral concentration of platelets divided by the average platelet lifespan and corrected for the extent of platelet pooling in the spleen).

In the absence of injury or disease, spontaneous bleeding is usually averted by peripheral platelet levels of 5000/μL to 10,000/μL. Patients undergoing cardiopulmonary bypass surgery, in contrast, may require 100,000 platelets/μL to maintain normal hemostasis. Platelet transfusions are usually successful in restoring platelet counts and hemostatic function in patients with transient thrombocytopenia secondary to myelosuppressive chemotherapy. Thrombopoietin therapy may be useful in the future in sustaining platelet hemostasis. In this chapter, the quantitative alterations in marrow megakaryocytopoiesis and platelet kinetics found in states of health and disease are reviewed.

MEGAKARYOCYTOPOIESIS

Development and Maturation of Megakaryocytes

Megakaryocyte Generation

Megakaryocytes give rise to circulating platelets (thrombocytes) through a process of proliferation, endo-reduplication, differentiation, and delivery of preformed cytoplasmic fragments into the circulation (Fig. 3–1). This process involves the mitotic expansion of four components—(1) hematopoietic progenitor cells, (2) megakaryocyte progenitors, (3) diploid megakaryocytes, and (4) polyploid megakaryocytes—together with the acquisition of cytoplasmic mass corresponding to cell ploidy and with inherent functional and structural constituents that make up peripheral platelets.[1–6]

Multipotent hematopoietic stem cells undergo progressively restrictive development, becoming, in turn, committed megakaryocyte progenitors, diploid megakaryoblasts (cells with basophilic undifferentiated cytoplasm incapable of cell division), and polyploid megakaryocytes (cells undergoing three to five sequential synchronous doublings of DNA within a common cytoplasm of corresponding mass). The expanding cytoplasm forms the ultrastructural and biochemical machinery characteristic of functional platelets. Marrow megakaryocytes are morphologically large, granular, and polyploid cells, averaging 16N, but ranging from 8N to 128N.[7–12]

Megakaryocyte progenitors are $CD34^+$ cells having the appearance of small, immature, mononuclear marrow cells that produce megakaryocyte colony-forming units (CFU-MKs) in semisolid media in vitro.[6, 13] The existence of multipotent stem cells has been demonstrated in humans through studies of pathological states, as illustrated by the finding of the Philadelphia chromosomal translocation coincidentally in megakaryocyte, erythroid, and myeloid lineages, indicating a common precursor to be the source of the mutation.[14] Similarly, studies of patients heterozygous at the locus for glucose-6-phosphate dehydrogenase (G6PD) who have chronic myeloproliferative disorders demonstrate equal proportions of G6PD isoenzymes A and B in skin fibroblasts; however, platelets, red cells, and granulocytes all contain only one isoenzyme type,[15–18] which implies a single stem cell origin for these three hematopoietic lineages. Results of bone marrow transplantation studies also confirm the pluripotent stem cell source of megakaryocytic lineage studies.[19]

Measurements of Megakaryocytopoiesis

Because platelets are derived from megakaryocytic cytoplasm, it follows that the megakaryocyte cytoplasmic mass represents the substrate available for platelet production.

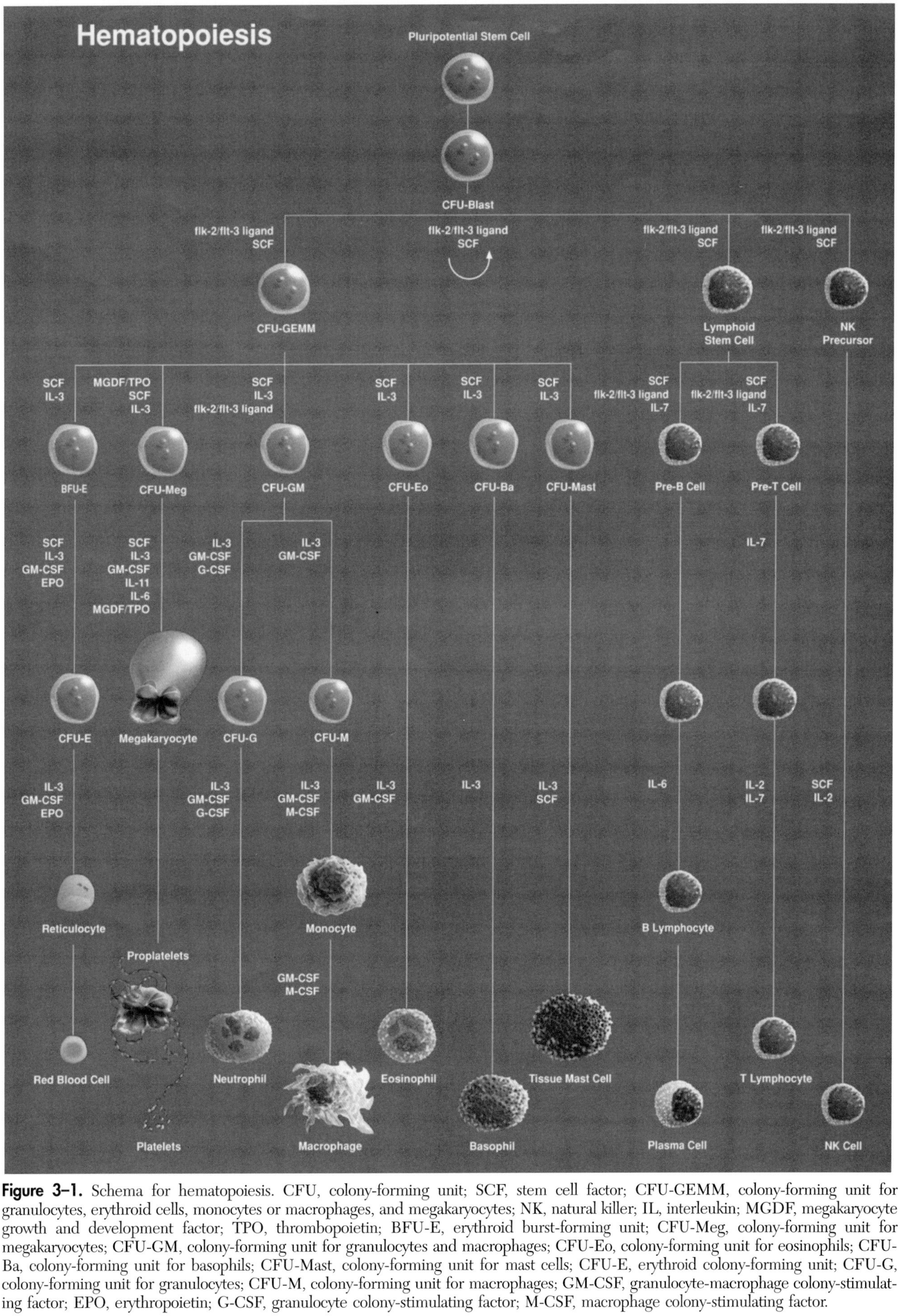

Figure 3–1. Schema for hematopoiesis. CFU, colony-forming unit; SCF, stem cell factor; CFU-GEMM, colony-forming unit for granulocytes, erythroid cells, monocytes or macrophages, and megakaryocytes; NK, natural killer; IL, interleukin; MGDF, megakaryocyte growth and development factor; TPO, thrombopoietin; BFU-E, erythroid burst-forming unit; CFU-Meg, colony-forming unit for megakaryocytes; CFU-GM, colony-forming unit for granulocytes and macrophages; CFU-Eo, colony-forming unit for eosinophils; CFU-Ba, colony-forming unit for basophils; CFU-Mast, colony-forming unit for mast cells; CFU-E, erythroid colony-forming unit; CFU-G, colony-forming unit for granulocytes; CFU-M, colony-forming unit for macrophages; GM-CSF, granulocyte-macrophage colony-stimulating factor; EPO, erythropoietin; G-CSF, granulocyte colony-stimulating factor; M-CSF, macrophage colony-stimulating factor.

The megakaryocyte cytoplasmic mass may be calculated as the product of the mean megakaryocyte cytoplasmic volume and the total number of megakaryocytes.[20] However, some megakaryocytic cytoplasm may not undergo fragmentation into platelets. This failure to undergo release represents a measure of ineffective thrombocytopoiesis. In pathological states, thrombocytopoiesis may be increasingly ineffective because megakaryocytes may undergo early apoptosis, may fail to interact with the sinus wall, or are deficient in the mechanisms forming or delivering proplatelets.[21]

Antibodies to platelet integrin $\alpha_{IIb}\beta_3$ (GPIIb/IIIa) fibrinogen receptors stain small "lymphoid" marrow cells[22] as well as small cells present in colonies derived from CFU-MK (promegakaryoblasts).[23, 24] These cells are detected in culture by day 4 or 5.[24] Ploidy measurements of these cells show that they are 2N or 4N. At the ultrastructural level, these cells do not exhibit platelet organelles, such as demarcation membranes or platelet α granules, but they do express the cytochemical marker platelet peroxidase.[25]

During differentiation, GPIb appears slightly later than platelet integrin $\alpha_{IIb}\beta_3$. In double-labeling experiments, an anti-GPIb monoclonal antibody does not stain all the small cells labeled by antiplatelet integrin $\alpha_{IIb}\beta_3$ monoclonal antibodies. GPIX, which exists as a heterodimer complex with GPIb in the platelet membrane, is concomitantly expressed with GPIb during megakaryocytic differentiation. In contrast, platelet glycoprotein GPIV, also called GPIIIb and described as the thrombospondin (TSP) receptor, appears at a later stage of differentiation.[26, 27] After platelet activation, the platelet integrin $\alpha_{IIb}\beta_3$ receptors undergo conformational change, expressing receptor function for adhesive proteins (fibrinogen, fibronectin, vitronectin, and von Willebrand factor [vWF]).

Quantitative analysis of megakaryocyte cellular differentiation markers may be useful in studying mechanisms regulating platelet production. However, the study of the cellular differentiation of megakaryocytes has proved difficult, partly because of their rarity (constituting about 0.05% of all nucleated bone marrow cells), fragility, and tendency to aggregate.[7, 28, 29] Thus a large number of marrow cells and a highly selective method for megakaryocytic identification are needed for suitable analysis. Early studies of isolated megakaryocytes used marrow flushed or scraped from the bones of experimental animals to achieve high cell yield with little admixture with blood and activated coagulation factors.[30–32]

To overcome some of the technical limitations associated with methodology based on physical separation, flow cytometry has been developed for the analysis of animal megakaryocytes.[31, 33–36] This method has been shown to be sensitive and rapid for the analysis of infrequent cell populations, even in complex cell mixtures such as bone marrow.[37] By employing fluorescence-activated cell sorting on bone marrow aspirates, it is possible to prepare, on a routine basis, highly purified (>98%) viable human megakaryocytes expressing a lineage marker identified by specific monoclonal antibodies.[10–12] DNA content is concomitantly measured by staining with propidium iodide.

Measurements of megakaryocyte cell size present additional problems. Originally, megakaryocyte size was measured directly by light microscopy. A mean diameter of 36 μm in marrow smears was reported by Levine and associates.[8] Berkow and coworkers[38] reported a diameter of 50 ± 15 μm in centrifugal-elutriated megakaryocytes fixed on slides, and Tomer and colleagues[11] reported a mean diameter of 33 ± 22 μm, with a range of 12 to 50 μm, in megakaryocyte preparations isolated by cell sorting and then fixed and analyzed by laser-based computerized image analysis. Using direct microscopic analysis of megakaryocytes in unfractionated marrow suspension, Levine[7] reported a mean diameter of 24 μm and a range of 10 to 48 μm. Employing both flow cytometry and light microscopy, Tomer and colleagues[11] reported a mean diameter of 28 μm and a range of 10 to 46 μm. The observation by Levine and associates[8] that cells more than 20 μm in diameter are morphologically recognizable megakaryocytes was also confirmed by cell sorting in that study.

In all animals studied, ploidy classes are identified as geometric progressions of 2N (diploid), 4N, 8N, 16N, and so forth. In normal guinea pigs, rats, and nonhuman primates, 16N is most common.[39–44] Earlier results of the distribution of ploidy levels have been confirmed with the use of flow cytometric analysis of bone marrow.[33, 36] The distribution of normal human megakaryocytes also has a modal ploidy of 16N.[45–50] The ploidy distribution obtained by flow cytometry on a large number (1200 to 3000) of cells in fractionated and unfractionated normal marrow demonstrates 16N for about half of the megakaryocytic population; 23% of cells demonstrate 8N or less, and 22% demonstrate 32N or more.[12]

Although changes in cell size, cytoplasmic granularity, and ploidy have been observed by direct microscopy,[7, 8, 48] quantitative analysis of large numbers of cells is more readily accomplished by flow cytometry. The relationships among the cellular characteristics of size, fine internal structure (granularity), expression level of membrane glycoproteins, and ploidy have been carried out by flow cytometric estimates of DNA fluorescence.[11, 51] With the slit-scan technique (time of flight) for direct measurement of cell diameter, the calculated cell volumes appear to correlate directly with cell DNA content for each of the ploidy classes of 8N or higher.[52] This observation is in agreement with observations in previous studies performed by histology or cytology on limited numbers of cells.[8, 53–55] The total surface membrane immunofluorescence (for platelet integrin $\alpha_{IIb}\beta_3$ complex) was correlated with cell size and cell ploidy, indicating enhanced membrane integrin $\alpha_{IIb}\beta_3$ expression with cell maturation. However, the expression of GPIb is disparately low for cells of 8N or less, indicating that the acquisition of this protein occurs later in maturation.[28, 56]

Flow cytometric analysis of marrow aspirates may be used to estimate megakaryocyte volume, on the basis of measurement of cell diameters, and to estimate megakaryocyte:erythroid ratio, from relative cell frequencies.[51, 52, 57] The time-of-flight technique[58] can be used to directly measure diameter of marrow megakaryocytes in suspension, from which the mean megakaryocyte volume can then be determined.[52, 57] The frequency of megakaryocytes in relation to total nucleated marrow cells may also be estimated from marrow aspirates by quantifying the marrow ratio of megakaryocytes to nucleated erythroid elements. Nucleated erythroid precursors are discriminated from other marrow cells by simultaneous labeling with fluoresceinated monoclonal antibodies against human glycophorin A and supravital staining of cell DNA with hydroethidine.[57] This procedure does not require fixation or permeabilization, thereby minimizing the manipulations and obviating any selective cell loss. Fluoresceinated monoclonal antibodies against megakaryocyte-platelet integrin $\alpha_{IIb}\beta_3$ are used to estimate megakaryocyte frequency. This technique reveals that the mean megakaryocyte number in normal subjects is $11.2 \pm 2.1 \times 10^6$/kg. The average megakaryocyte volume is $28 \pm 4.5 \times 10^3$ μL. The derived megakaryocyte mass is $31 \pm 5.3 \times 10^{10}$ μL/kg, similar to previous estimates.[59]

Increases in DNA synthesis have been recognized as early as 12 hours after induction of thrombocytopenia.[60] By 24 to 48 hours, there is also an increase in the proportion of cells with 32N and 64N ploidy levels.[33, 43, 61, 62] DNA synthesis and ploidy level may be increased within 18 hours when thrombocytopenia is severe. By 48 hours, the increase in ploidy may be associated with an increase in the size of the marrow megakaryoblasts.[33, 43, 54, 61–64] The maturation process of the megakaryocytes may be assessed by changes in the transit time through the four maturational stages or the transit times of cytoplasmic protein labels with the use of sulfate-35 or selenomethionine-75.[60, 65] The number of megakaryocytes increases only after days of thrombocytopenic stimulation.

Increase in megakaryocyte ploidy in response to accelerated platelet consumption has been observed in humans, in agreement with the observations in experimental animals.[9, 11, 20, 66] Although some studies have reported no change in ploidy of megakaryocytes in immune thrombocytopenic purpura (ITP) patients,[49, 67] flow cytometric analysis of relatively large numbers of megakaryocytes clearly demonstrates an increased proportion of high-ploidy cells in ITP.[12] In all patients, megakaryocyte ploidy is significantly shifted toward high ploidy classes (right shift) with an increased proportion of 32N or higher cells. This shift in ploidy is accompanied by an increase in cell size and granularity. The shift to the right is also associated with a reciprocal decrease in the 16N cells, without a change in the relative frequency of cells of 8N or less.

It is of interest that an analysis of the ploidy distribution pattern in 12 thrombocytopenic patients with megakaryocytic hypoplasia showed a shift toward the low-ploidy cells (left shift),[12] similar to the shift observed in experimental animals hypertransfused with platelets.[33, 43] A shift to the left may reflect selective damage to more mature megakaryocytes or interference with the maturation process in these patients.

Thus the limited results in humans suggest that human megakaryocytes respond to altered platelet demand in a manner similar to that found in experimental animals and that these changes are mediated by thrombopoietin.

Platelet Formation

The process by which mature megakaryocytes release platelets is not fully understood. Quantitative electron microscopic analysis demonstrates megakaryocytes to be parasinusoidal in location: that is, less than 1 μm away from a marrow sinus wall.[68] In 1910, Wright[69] reported that mature megakaryocytes extend filaments of cytoplasm into sinusoidal spaces, where they detach and fragment into individual platelets. Later studies using phase-contrast microscopy in tissue culture[70] and electron microscopy[71] confirmed this interpretation. Long cytoplasmic extensions of human megakaryocytes containing platelet-specific organelles within areas defined by constriction points (proplatelets) have been studied in vitro.[72] On the basis of these data, Choi[72] hypothesized that platelet-specific granules cluster within megakaryocyte cytoplasm, followed by massive reorganization of cytoskeletal structures into proplatelets separated by constriction points and cytoplasmic extensions between endothelial cells into vascular sinusoids, with final cytoplasmic separation into proplatelet masses within flowing blood.[72] Because entire megakaryocytes may pass through transendothelial apertures with diameters of 6 μm, some megakaryocytes may reach the lungs via the circulation.[73]

Platelets vary in size under certain circumstances. For example, large platelets occur in genetic syndromes, such as Bernard-Soulier syndrome, May-Hegglin anomaly, and Mediterranean macrothrombocytopenia.[74–76] In these syndromes, platelet size is inversely related to the circulating count, similar to the changes observed in human volunteers developing thrombocytosis induced by injections of Mpl ligands. In addition, Wistar-Furth rats exhibit a deficiency in platelet proteins that may be related to the genetic macrothrombocytopenia in these animals.[77] These findings demonstrate that platelet number and size are inherently determined during megakaryocytopoiesis. Acquired thrombocytopenia may also manifest large platelets, with restoration of platelet size when the platelet count returns to normal. For example, flow cytometric studies of marrow aspirates demonstrate increased megakaryocyte size and ploidy in destructive thrombocytopenia with compensatory increases in platelet production (i.e., "stress" thrombocytopoiesis) both in humans[12, 78] and in experimental animals.[61] Thus the size of cytoplasmic fragments may depend on the degree of megakaryocytic maturation and the intensity of the stimulus driving platelet production.

Thrombopoietin Regulation of Megakaryocytopoiesis

Platelet production is regulated to meet changing requirements for peripheral blood platelets by altering megakaryocytopoiesis. In experimental conditions, modifications are concurrently produced in the proliferation of committed precursor and immature diploid megakaryocytes, as well as in endoreduplication and cytoplasmic differentiation of polyploid megakaryocytes and in platelet release.[33, 60–64, 79–81]

The hematopoietic growth factor activity specific for the growth and development of megakaryocyte lineage cells is produced by endogenous thrombopoietin (TPO, also referred to as a Mpl ligand, analogous to erythropoietin for cell of the erythroid lineage). Endogenous TPO regulating megakaryocytopoietic activities has been concurrently isolated, cloned, and functionally characterized by several different groups of investigators.[82–86] The complementary DNA for human and murine thrombopoietin belongs to the cytokine family of genes encoding for a glycoprotein homologous with erythropoietin that binds with its receptor (Mpl) on megakaryocytes and selectively initiates proliferation, maturation, and cytoplasmic delivery of platelets into the circulation. This coincident discovery stems from the report by Souyri and colleagues of a cellular gene (c-Mpl) homologous with genes encoding for a family of hematopoietic growth factor receptors,[87] and the ability of excess Mpl antisense oligodeoxynucleotide to selectively abolish megakaryocyte colony formation. Subsequent cloning of the Mpl receptor from engineered cell lines provided the essential tool for isolating and cloning thrombopoietin, the Mpl ligand. The ligand was subsequently purified from thrombocytopenic plasma, sequenced, cloned, and characterized.[82, 83, 85, 86] One group successfully isolated and characterized thrombopoietin from transfected cell clones that produced the growth factor.[83, 84] The identical molecule has been isolated and cloned by all four groups of investigators.

Thrombopoietin is produced as a recombinant protein, recombinant human thrombopoietin (rHuTPO). Both colony-stimulating activity and platelet-elevating activity in thrombocytopenic plasma are neutralized by the addition of Mpl receptor in excess.[85] The complementary DNA for Mpl ligand codes for a protein comprising 353 amino acids.[82, 83, 86] Thrombopoietin constitutes a 154-residue amino-terminal erythropoietin-like functional domain (21% sequence identity with erythropoietin and 25% additional similarity), and a 178-residue carboxy-terminal domain without homology to any known proteins and without known function. The gene for thrombopoietin is located on chromosome 3 (bands 26 to 28). Interestingly, abnormalities in chromosome 3 (inversion or deletion) are associated with megakaryocytic leukemia.[88] TPO-specific messenger RNA is found in the liver, kidneys, and marrow stroma.[82, 83, 86]

The full-length glycosylated recombinant human thrombopoietin is designated rHuTPO, whereas the polyethyleneglycol (PEG)–derivitized 163-residue amino-terminus of the recombinant human polypeptide produced in *E. coli* is known as PEG–recombinant human megakaryocyte growth and development factor (PEG-rHuMGDF). In suspension culture, rHuTPO and PEG-rHuMGDF induce TPO receptor signaling of $CD34^+$ murine and human marrow cells to undergo hematopoietic stem cell differentiation into megakaryocyte progenitors,[81, 89] and they stimulate the replication of megakaryocyte lineage cells and megakaryocyte endoproliferative enlargement,[11, 90] thereby amplifying the cytoplasmic substrate generating circulating platelets.[82, 83, 83–85, 91–94] These two Mpl ligands, rHuTPO and PEG-rHuMGDF, are the most potent agents inducing megakaryocytopoiesis in nature,[82–84, 86] and exhibit synergy with other cytokines known to influence megakaryocyte growth in culture: namely, interleukin (IL)–3, IL-6, IL-11, stem cell factor (SCF), and erythropoietin.[95–97]

Endogenous TPO maintains peripheral platelet concentrations physiologically constant by modulating megakaryocytopoiesis to compensate for changing peripheral requirements.[54, 90, 98–101] Megakaryocytopoiesis is regulated by plasma levels of unbound TPO. The level in normal subjects is 95 ± 6 pg/L.[102–104] For example, endogenous TPO levels increase several orders of magnitude in patients with thrombocytopenia after marrow ablative chemotherapy as the platelet counts drop, and then they return to baseline after the peripheral platelet counts normalize by platelet transfusional therapy or hematopoietic recovery.[86, 105]

Feedback modulation of plasma TPO levels does not depend primarily on gene transcriptional regulation,[106] as shown by the observations that TPO and TPO receptor messenger RNA in heterozygote "knockout" mice remain at half the levels found in normal mice,[107–109] despite thrombocytopenia. On the other hand, thrombocytopenia has been reported to induce marrow stromal expression of TPO messenger RNA,[110, 111] which implies a regulatory mechanism of unclear importance.

One important feedback mechanism modulating plasma levels of unbound Mpl ligand involves competitive binding of unbound TPO with TPO receptor–bearing peripheral platelets, marrow megakaryocytes, and possibly plasma-soluble TPO receptor,[92, 106, 112] leading to reciprocal changes in plasma-unbound TPO levels and peripheral platelet counts and/or number of marrow megakaryocytes.[102–104] The plasma level of thrombopoietin is elevated in patients with thrombocytopenia due to marrow hypoplasia and falls after platelet counts are restored by transfusions.[103, 104] Thrombopoietin avidly binds to the Mpl receptors on platelets (about 200 receptors per platelet). In summary, it is reasonable to postulate that circulating levels of unbound thrombopoietin induce concentration-dependent receptor-mediated proliferative and endoproliferative maturation of early megakaryocyte progenitors and that negative feedback regulation is produced by the circulating concentration of platelets via binding of thrombopoietin with receptor-bearing peripheral platelets and shed soluble Mpl receptor in plasma.

Several pleiotropic human growth factors exert stimulatory activity on megakaryocytes, both in vivo and in vitro, including IL-3 (multi–colony-stimulating factor [CSF]), IL-6, IL-11, granulocyte-macrophage colony-stimulating factor (GM-CSF), and leukemia inhibitory factor (LIF).[10, 113–127] IL-1 may stimulate megakaryocytopoiesis indirectly,[114, 115, 128] and erythropoietin exhibits colony-stimulating activity in animal studies.[129, 130] Stem cell factor (also referred to as mast cell growth factor, steel factor, or c-kit ligand) promotes both megakaryocyte burst-forming unit (BFU-MK) with IL-3 and megakaryocyte colony-forming unit (CFU-MK) in synergy with both IL-3 and GM-CSF[131] in clonogenic assays and long-term bone marrow cultures.[114, 115, 121, 122, 128] GM-CSF may induce megakaryocytic maturation in vivo, as shown in humans[124] and in nonhuman primates,[126] although there is no corresponding increase in the circulating platelet counts.[132] The direct stimulatory effect of GM-CSF on megakaryocytes is also evident in cultures of megakaryocytes purified directly from human marrow aspirates.[11, 125] IL-6 affects primarily megakaryocyte maturation,[113, 118, 123, 128] although the combination of IL-6 and IL-3 promotes megakaryocyte proliferation.[115, 123] The administration of IL-6 to primates markedly increases platelet counts and megakaryocytic size and ploidy.[117, 127] IL-11 and LIF also affect both megakaryocytic size and ploidy.[116, 119, 120] In addition, combined effects have been demonstrated for IL-6 and IL-3,[115, 123] IL-3 and GM-CSF,[114, 115, 122, 128] and IL-3 and IL-11.[119, 120] Thus the effects of these growth factors on different stages of megakaryocytes may modulate the effects of endogenous TPO or recombinant Mpl ligands. There is also evidence for negative control of megakaryocytopoiesis.[133–135] In addition, megakaryocytes appear to be capable of synthesizing and secreting human growth factors, including IL-1, IL-6, and GM-CSF,[113, 136–138] and the expression of cell surface membrane receptors for IL-6 and GM-CSF.[113, 124, 136–138]

Thrombopoietin Therapy

PEG-rHuMGDF or rHuTPO increases the concentration of circulating platelets in a loglinear dose-dependent manner in baboons, reaching peak values 2 weeks after daily subcutaneous injections are initiated (Fig. 3–2).[139] On a molar basis, rHuTPO produces equivalent effects to those reported for PEG-rHuMGDF (Fig. 3–3). Although the mean platelet volume decreases as the platelet count increases (8.0 ± 1.2 versus 6.6 ± 0.8 fL; $p < 0.01$), there is no relationship between the extent of change in mean platelet volume and the dose of PEG-rHuMGDF administered. After discontinuing therapy, platelet counts fall to baseline values and mean platelet volumes normalize within 2 weeks (see Fig. 3–2). Platelet lifespan is normal during therapy with PEG-rHuMGDF or rHu-MGDF in baboons. Platelet mass turnover, a steady-state measure of the rate at which platelet mass enters the peripheral circulation, increases in a loglinear dose-dependent manner. Platelet ultrastructure is not affected by Mpl ligands.

PEG-rHuMGDF or rHuTPO also increases megakaryocyte number, size, and ploidy in a loglinear dose-dependent manner, in comparisons of basal measurements with findings obtained after 3 and 14 days of PEG-rHuMGDF treatment.[139] Because mean megakaryocyte volumes and ploidy attain predictable maximum values within 3 days of the beginning of therapy, megakaryocyte ploidy is an accurate measure reflecting Mpl ligand stimulation of megakaryocytopoiesis.[139] Peripheral leukocyte, neutrophil, or erythrocyte counts do not change significantly during PEG-rHuMGDF or rHu-MGDF administration in baboons or rabbits.[139]

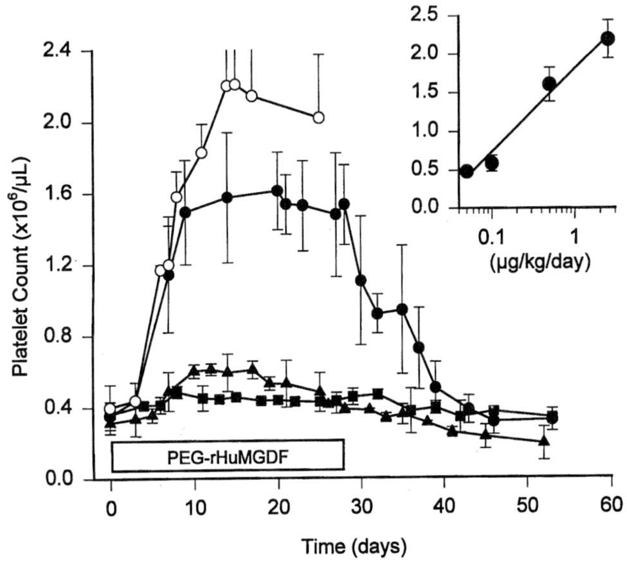

Figure 3–2. Dose-response effects of polyethyleneglycol-derived recombinant human megakaryocyte growth and development factor (PEG-rHuMGDF).

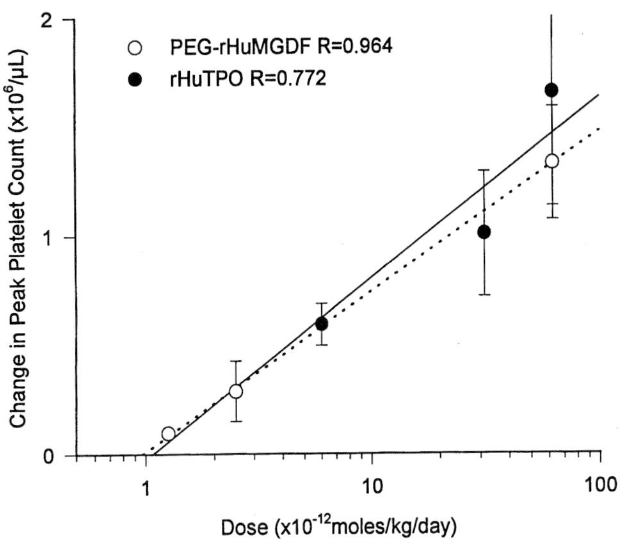

Figure 3–3. Equivalence of recombinant human thrombopoietin (rHuTPO) and polyethyleneglycol-derived recombinant human megakaryocyte growth and development factor (PEG-rHuMGDF).

In comparison with other megakaryocyte-stimulating growth factors, thrombopoietin increases platelet production to previously unattainable levels. Under the assumption that recombinant thrombopoietin has lineage specificity and negligible toxicity, similar to what is observed for the other two late-acting hematopoietic growth factors erythropoietin and G-CSF, thrombopoietin is expected to have considerable application in patients with platelet transfusion–dependent thrombocytopenia or other thrombocytopenic disorders responsive to exogenously stimulated platelet production.[140–142]

PLATELET KINETICS

Mechanisms of Platelet Production and Destruction

The overall rate of platelet production in normal humans ranges from 35,000 to 44,000 platelets/µL/day.[20, 143–147] These estimates of platelet production have been measured indirectly by determining the turnover of circulating platelets (the platelet count divided by the platelet lifespan and corrected for splenic pooling) under steady-state conditions. This estimation assumes that platelet removal is equivalent to platelet production when the platelet count is constant.[20] Platelet turnover has been used as a measure of the delivery of viable platelets into the general circulation.[20] As expected, megakaryocyte mass generally correlates directly with platelet turnover in normal persons. However, intramedullary destruction of platelets or intrinsic abnormalities of platelet formation by megakaryocytes may result in defective delivery of cytoplasmic mass as viable platelets. This discrepancy between marrow substrate megakaryocyte cytoplasmic mass and circulating platelet product is referred to as ineffective thrombocytopoiesis.

The reliability of platelet turnover measurements depends on the accuracy with which each of the three variables used in calculating platelet turnover can be determined: namely, mean concentration of circulating platelets, platelet lifespan, and the distribution of platelets in the systemic versus splenic circulation (recovery of labeled platelets in the systemic circulation). The summation of errors associated with these three determinations may be considerable, as illustrated in ITP patients.[145]

In normal humans, approximately two thirds of the platelets are in the general circulation, and the remaining platelets are reversibly sequestered in a second vascular pool, primarily in the spleen. The difference in proportions between the systemic and the splenic platelet pools may be determined by measuring the proportion of radiolabeled platelets remaining in the systemic circulation after infusion. The size of the splenic pool has been estimated to be about 30% of the whole-body platelet mass.[20, 148] In asplenic persons, approximately 100% of the infused platelets are recovered. In patients with splenomegaly, as much as 90% of total-body platelet mass may be sequestered in the splenic circulation.[148] Studies performed by Heyns, Wessels, and colleagues[144, 149] showed that platelet accumulation in the spleen reached 90% of the maximum activity within about 15 minutes after reinjection of labeled platelets. Although the role of the spleen in the regulation of the platelet count has remained controversial, the splenic pool appears to be fully exchangeable. For example, intravenous infusion of epinephrine, which reduces blood flow to the spleen and causes the organ to empty passively into the circulation, normally causes platelet levels to increase 30% to 50% but does not affect platelet concentrations in asplenic persons.[148] Hepatic pooling of labeled platelets is also significant initially, reaching a maximum of about 16% of the whole-body radioactivity 6 to 8 minutes after injection of labeled platelets and attaining steady state approximately 45 minutes after the reinfusion of the platelets. At equilibrium, hepatic radioactivity is 10% or less of the total-body radioactivity.[144, 149]

The platelet lifespan in normal persons is 9.5 ± 0.6 days.[20] Platelet disappearance is generally linear over the first week of circulation, reflecting primarily platelet senescence.[150] However, in patients with thrombocytopenia due to enhanced peripheral destruction, the platelet lifespan is shorter and the disappearance pattern becomes exponential, reflecting primarily random platelet removal.[151]

Because senescence is the principal physiological mechanism for removal of circulating platelets, the elimination kinetics of platelets in normal subjects are nearly zero order: that is, a linear decay curve extends to 9 to 10 days for mixed-age platelet cohorts under steady-state conditions.[90, 146, 152, 153] Slight curvilinearity in the normal platelet elimination pattern is attributable to random loss by some extrinsic process involving 10% to 15% of the circulating platelets and to the variance of intrinsic platelet longevity.[90, 146, 152, 153] It has been postulated that this random loss results from a fixed rate of platelet use in the maintenance of normal vascular hemostasis.[146 146, 152] The average time that platelets remain in the circulation (i.e., platelet lifespan) is approximated by the intersect axis of the tangent to the platelet disappearance curve with time and is computed by means of gamma function analysis.[146, 152] Gamma analysis of platelet kinetics allows quantification of random and senescent mechanisms of platelet destruction, accounts for dynamic changes in platelet age distributions after alterations of platelet production rate, and permits modeling of platelet loss specific to pathological conditions (e.g., immune destruction). Gamma model predictions of platelet survival probabilities and platelet tracer decay curves are illustrated for normal subjects, patients with marrow hypoplasia, and immune thrombocytopenic patients in Figure 3–4. The gamma model incorporates an elimination rate constant for random platelet use.[1] As evident in the shape of the survival probability curve, platelet loss in normal subjects

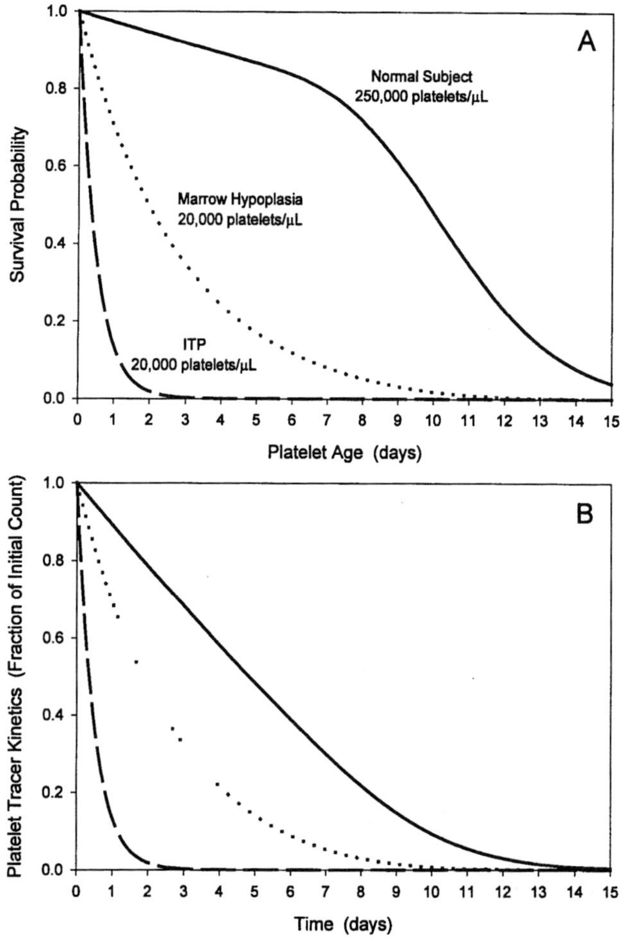

Figure 3–4. Gamma model predictions of *(A)* platelet survival probability and *(B)* platelet tracer kinetics in normal subjects *(solid line)*, patients with marrow hypoplasia *(dotted line)*, and patients with idiopathic thrombocytopenic purpura (ITP) *(dashed line)*.

is determined primarily by senescence, which is depicted by a nearly linear platelet decay curve. However, when fractional vascular use is increased by thrombocytopenia or random elimination is increased by immune destruction, platelet elimination occurs randomly, and the decay curve is exponential. It is important that platelet survival models account for additive factors specific to pathological conditions, as illustrated by the example of platelet kinetics in ITP.

According to gamma function analysis of radionuclide-labeled platelet disappearance patterns, platelet lifespan in normal subjects averages 232 ± 38 hours (9.6 ± 1.5 days).[152–154] Intrinsic platelet longevity (platelet viability in absence of random use) is estimated after accounting for loss due to random platelet use and approximates 11 days. It is expected that during thrombocytosis induced by Mpl ligand, the platelet lifespan more closely approaches the intrinsic lifespan of 11 days.

Measurement of Platelet Lifespan

At present, platelet survival studies are usually performed to (1) evaluate thrombocytopenic patients; (2) discriminate between disorders of decreased production and increased platelet destruction (destructive or consumptive thrombocytopenia); (3) determine the rate and the site of platelet consumption associated with thrombotic disease or evaluate the efficacy of antiplatelet drugs interfering with platelet-thrombogenic surface interaction; and (4) assess platelet viability in platelet concentrates after storage.

When platelets disappear from the circulation, they are taken up by the mononuclear phagocytic system.[149, 155–160] The accumulation of platelet radioactivity in the spleen and liver has been quantified, and it is evident that these organs are major sites of removal of the labeled platelets. Heyns, Wessels, and others[144, 149] showed that after the injection of indium-111–labeled platelets, the radioactivity in the liver increased significantly and linearly with time from a level of 9.6% equilibrium to 28.7% of the total-body radioactivity. The mean splenic radioactivity also increased significantly from 31.1% to 35.6% during the clearance of labeled platelets. After labeled platelets are removed from circulation (about 10 days), 30.3% of the whole-body platelet radioactivity is neither in the liver nor in the spleen. Platelets not removed by these two organs are presumably removed by the mononuclear phagocytic cells of the bone marrow. In nonhuman primates, it has been demonstrated by the quantification of organ radioactivity that about 15% of labeled platelets are destroyed in the bone marrow.[161]

A number of different methods have been used to measure platelet lifespan.[162] The procedure most commonly used in humans is the measurement of the disappearance time of platelets labeled isotopically in vitro.

Theoretically, a labeled cohort of cells would provide the most accurate survival data. In human beings, selenomethionine-75 has been proposed as a platelet cohort label.[163, 164] This analog of the amino acid methionine is incorporated directly into a component of megakaryocytic proteins, including thrombosthenin.[165] In rats, measurement of the specific activity of isolated platelet thrombosthenin after selenomethionine-75 administration provided a reproducible but imperfect cohort survival curve.[165] This complex method has not been practical for human studies. Because cohort survival studies are generally not feasible, labeling of a random platelet population (autologous or homologous) has been widely used for platelet survival measurements in humans. To be suitable for random platelet labeling in vitro, the ideal radiolabel should have the following characteristics: (1) platelet specificity; (2) efficient incorporation; (3) intracellular retention without significant reuse; (4) a half-life long enough to permit the measurement of the entire lifespan of the labeled cell but short enough to eliminate unnecessary irradiation; (5) no effect on the viability or function of the labeled cell; and (6) sufficient energy to emit radiation for external imaging. Unfortunately, not one of the commercially available radiolabels is platelet specific. Therefore, in vitro labeling must be carried out on isolated platelet preparations. Manipulations involved in the separation of platelets from other blood cells and plasma proteins have potential adverse effects on the test platelets ("collection injury").[144, 166–168] Currently, most of platelet survival studies are performed by using indium-111–oxine.

Chromium-51 (^{51}Cr). ^{51}Cr was first introduced as a tracer for platelet labeling by Robertson et al.[169] The platelet uptake of ^{51}Cr is rapid; up to 50% of the binding occurs in 30 minutes[170, 171] at 37°C. The extent of ^{51}Cr elution from labeled platelets and the reuse of the isotope in vivo are controversial.[145–172] The method for platelet labeling with ^{51}Cr was the standard method for platelet survival measurement for many years.[173] The radionuclide, however, has several drawbacks, including the relatively long half-life (28 days), low incorporation rate into platelets (low labeling efficiency: 10% on the average), and photon emission not well suited for external imaging. Therefore, body localization by external detection is inefficient, and accurate data cannot be obtained unless large quantities of radioactivity are used.[162] This requirement demands that a large volume of blood (200 to 500 mL) be obtained to provide sufficient numbers of platelets.[172] For these reasons, ^{51}Cr has largely been replaced by ^{111}In-oxine.

Indium-111–Oxine (^{111}In-Oxine). ^{111}In-oxine as a platelet label was introduced by Thakur and associates in 1976[174, 175] and is now firmly established as the preferred isotope.[149, 158, 176–178] This isotope forms a stable lipophilic chelate with oxine (8-hydroxyquinoline), which is readily incorporated into platelets (and other cells) by passive processes. ^{111}In has a half-life of 2.8 days, which is long enough for platelet survival measurements, and its photon emissions are suitable for external detection. Labeling with ^{111}In-oxine has not been shown to affect platelet function,[149, 162, 174, 177–179] and no significant portion of the ^{111}In taken up is subsequently lost from platelets.[174, 178] The isotope is incorporated efficiently into platelets, and the labeling efficiency in normal preparations reaches the levels of 80% to 95%.[144, 145, 173, 179, 180] Consequently, ^{111}In-oxine is commonly used for platelet kinetic studies, especially in thrombocytopenia.[145–166] The major drawback of the labeling technique with ^{111}In-oxine is the lack of specificity for platelets and the high avidity for plasma proteins, particularly transferrin.[157, 160, 175] Therefore, high labeling efficiency requires not only that platelets are isolated by differential centrifugation but also that plasma proteins be eliminated. This procedure results in a loss (that may be preferential) of up to 40% of platelets[157, 181] and manipulation of platelets in the absence of protein that may cause "collection injury."[176–178] Indium-111–mercaptopyridine-N-oxide (^{111}In-Merc) and indium-111–tropolone have been shown to allow relatively efficient cell labeling in plasma,[182–184] but the data to recommend these agents over ^{111}In-oxine are insufficient.[185] Indium-111 permits an accurate estimation of the size of the splenic pool through quantitative imaging.[145, 149, 186]

The recommended method for the use of ^{51}Cr as a platelet radiolabel was published by the International Committee for Standardization in Hematology (ISCH) in 1977.[173] Although several different procedures involving ^{111}In have been proposed as an alternative,[144, 145, 177, 187] a consensus regarding a standard method appeared only as recently as 1986, when the Ad Hoc Committee of the Symposium on Radiolabeling of Stored Platelet Concentrates proposed the use of a standard procedure to facilitate comparison of results from different laboratories.[185] This protocol was recommended for platelet survival studies performed on normal persons by using fresh platelets or for studies using stored platelet concentrates. The ISCH-recommended method for platelet survival study with the use of ^{111}In was published in 1988.[188] The recommended method for calculation of platelet lifespan is the gamma function model for nonlinear estimation.[185–188]

Whereas several different ^{111}In-labeling methods appear to be adequate for patients with normal or moderately reduced platelet counts, the direct application of these methods to patients with platelet counts below 50,000 platelets/μL is less suitable. The ISCH protocol recommends that the volume of blood required for the study of patients with platelet counts of 20,000 to 30,000 platelets/μL be increased from 43 to 200 mL and indicates that lesser platelet counts may be too low for study. Heyns and coworkers[145, 166] studied autologous platelet labeling in patients with moderate to severe thrombocytopenia. Although the results obtained were satisfactory, it appeared that harvesting efficiency was dependent on the initial platelet count (mean harvest of 55% ± 21%, in comparison with 87% ± 74% in normal subjects) and that the labeling efficiency was markedly reduced (48% ± 24%, in comparison with 80% ± 3% in normal subjects). The reduced labeling efficiency was attributed to the decreased platelet concentration in the labeled platelet preparation, with an increase in contaminating plasma.

Employing a modified method for thrombocytopenic patients (platelet counts reduced to 10,000), high uptake of ^{111}In-oxine (91% ± 2.1%) by autologous platelets has been achieved.[152] The high labeling efficiency permitted the decrease in the blood volume required for survival studies and the elimination of the pellet formation and of the resuspension step after the incubation with the radioisotope, thereby decreasing the possibility of producing a "collection injury." The recovery of the labeled platelets in circulation at equilibrium was normal, and the survival time in patients with near-normal platelet counts was also normal. When platelet lifespan measurements were prospectively studied in patients with moderate to severe thrombocytopenia (10,000 to 150,000 platelets/μL),[152] the results in patients with megakaryocytic hypoplasia were predicted by the platelet count. However, platelet lifespan in patients with ITP was much shorter than predicted values. Thus measurement of platelet survival time in thrombocytopenic patients is useful for discriminating between patients with megakaryocyte hypoplasia and patients with thrombocytopenia caused by increased platelet destruction. In thrombocytopenic patients with equivocal clinical manifestations, the measurement of platelet lifespan, together with assays for antiplatelet glycoprotein autoantibodies[189, 190] and flow cytometric analysis of marrow megakaryocytes,[12] may be useful in characterizing pathogenetic mechanisms of thrombocytopenia.

Platelet Transfusion Therapy

Platelet survival shortens progressively as peripheral platelet counts fall below 100,000/μL, because fixed platelet hemostatic use becomes progressively more important in determining the lifespan of platelets in thrombocytopenic patients with impaired platelet production.[155, 191, 192] In preliminary observations, platelet lifespan is normalized in thrombocytopenic patients when circulating platelet concentrations are normalized, either by transfusion or after increasing platelet production by administration of an Mpl ligand, such as PEG-rHuMGDF (unpublished observations).

These platelet kinetic findings have relevance in the transfusion management of patients with severe thrombocytopenia. By transfusing sufficient platelets to raise the peripheral concentration from approximately 10,000/μL to 75,000 to 100,000/μL, the calculated platelet lifespan is predicted to increase severalfold: from 2 to 8 days. Consequently, the period of protection provided by the transfused platelets would be prolonged several additional days, and the required frequency of platelet transfusions would be significantly decreased. In preliminary reports of administration of PEG-rHuMGDF to platelet donors, it has been shown that transiently elevating peripheral platelet counts two- to threefold proportionally amplifies platelet yields in the corresponding apheresis products.[193, 194] This strategy for producing high-dose platelet concentrates may provide the means for raising platelet counts in thrombocytopenic recipients to levels that normalize platelet lifespan and hemostatic function: namely, more than 75,000 platelets/μL.

In a preliminary report, post-transfusion platelet increments in recipients of high-dose platelet concentrates were proportionally higher than in recipients of standard-dose platelet concentrates.[193] After transfusion of high-dose concentrates, platelets would be predicted to initially disappear from the circulation at normal rates in the absence of antiplatelet antibodies, widespread tissue damage, or systemic infection. Consequently, the peripheral platelet count would be expected to exceed 75,000 platelets/μL for several days after the transfusion of a high-dose platelet product. Thus platelet hemostatic protection can be provided by transfusing approximately the same number of platelets one-half to one-third as often. In addition, larger, less frequent platelet transfusions appear to confer more effective platelet hemostatic function. Therefore, transfusing high-yield platelet concentrates may provide hemostatic protection more effectively and more efficiently than conventional platelet concentrates given more frequently. Although administration of high-dose platelet concentrates might be anticipated to increase total platelet use in a thrombocytopenic patient, this effect may be largely offset by the increased platelet lifespan at higher platelet counts. In addition, vascular damage related to chemotherapy may increase endothelial use, and the benefits of administering high-dose concentrates may be greater than anticipated by current utilization models. Thus high-dose platelet concentrates may provide an effective and efficient means for supporting platelet hemostatic function in severe thrombocytopenia, which argues against splitting high-dose concentrates into either conventional-dose or mini-dose packs.

SUMMARY

Abnormal circulating platelet counts result from quantitative alterations in megakaryocytopoiesis and platelet kinetics. Megakaryocytopoiesis involves the commitment, proliferation, and differentiation of the megakaryocytic cell lineage, together with the cytoplasmic acquisition of functional and structural properties of platelets. Megakaryocytes respond to increased demand for peripheral blood platelets by modifying the progenitor cell compartment, cellular replication, endoreduplication, cytoplasmic differentiation, and platelet shedding. Flow cytometry of aspirated marrow is a powerful technique for quantitative characterization of megakaryocyte number, size, ploidy, and cytoplasmic differentiation. The regulation of megakaryocytopoiesis is mediated primarily by endogenous thrombopoietin. Stimulated megakaryocytopoiesis typically manifests increased megakaryocytic number, size, increased ploidy, and a shortened cytoplasmic maturation time.

Platelet production may also be measured indirectly by determining platelet turnover (the circulating concentration divided by platelet survival time, corrected for splenic pooling). In general, platelet turnover correlates directly with the megakaryocytic cytoplasmic mass. A discrepancy between the available megakaryocytic cytoplasmic substrate and platelet turnover reflects ineffective thrombocytopoiesis. Autologous platelet survival time may be reliably measured for even thrombocytopenic patients with the use of ^{111}In-oxine labeling. Normally, platelets survive approximately 9 to 10 days in the circulation, and approximately one third of the blood platelets are pooled within the splenic circulation. To discriminate between disorders of platelet production and platelet destruction, platelet kinetic measurements in patients with low platelet counts are interpreted by relating the measured survival time to the circulating concentration. Treatment for thrombocytopenia will involve the administration of recombinant thrombopoietic growth factor (rHuTPO or PEG-rHuMGDF, when they become available) or the transfusion of platelet concentrates.

ACKNOWLEDGMENT

This work was supported, in part, by grant RR 00039 supporting the Emory General Clinical Research Center from the National Institutes of Health.

REFERENCES

1. Burstein SA, Harker LA. Control of platelet production. *In* Harker LA, Zimmerman TS (eds): Clinics in Haematology. Philadelphia: WB Saunders, 1983:3.
2. Gewirtz AM. Human megakaryocytopoiesis. Semin Hematol 1986; 23:27.
3. Vainchenker W, Kieffer N. Human megakaryocytopoiesis: In vitro regulation and characterization of megakaryocytic precursor cells by differentiation markers. Blood Rev 1988; 2:102.
4. Breton-Gorius J, Vainchenker W. Expression of platelet proteins during the in vitro and in vivo differentiation of megakaryocytes and morphological aspects of their maturation. Semin Hematol 1986; 23:43.
5. Schick BP, Schick PK. Megakaryocyte biochemistry. Semin Hematol 1986; 23:68.
6. Jackson CW, Arnold JT, Pestina TI, et al. Megakaryocyte biology. *In* Kuter DJ, Hunt P, Sheridan W, Zucker-Franklin D (eds): Thrombopoiesis and Thrombopoietins: Molecular, Cellular, Preclinical, and Clinical Biology. Totowa, NJ: Humana Press, 1997, p 3.
7. Levine RF. Isolation and characterization of normal human megakaryocytes. Br J Haematol 1980; 45:487.
8. Levine RF, Hazzard KC, Lamberg JD. The significance of megakaryocyte size. Blood 1982; 60:1122.
9. Mazur EM, Lindquist DL, de Alarcon PA, et al. Evaluation of bone marrow megakaryocyte ploidy distributions in persons with normal and abnormal platelet counts. J Lab Clin Med 1988; 111:194.
10. Tomer A, Harker LA, Burstein SA. Purification of human megakaryocytes by fluorescence-activated cell sorting. Blood 1987; 70:1735.
11. Tomer A, Harker LA, Burstein SA. Flow cytometric analysis of normal human megakaryocytes. Blood 1988; 71:1244.
12. Tomer A, Friese P, Conklin R, et al. Flow cytometric analysis of megakaryocytes from patients with abnormal platelet counts. Blood 1989; 74:594.
13. Mazur EM. Historical perspective and overview. *In* Kuter DJ, Hunt P, Sheridan W, Zucker-Franklin D (eds): Thrombopoiesis and Thrombopoietins: Molecular, Cellular, Preclinical, and Clinical Biology. Totowa, NJ: Humana Press, 1997, p 95.
14. Whang J, Frei E, III, Tjio JH. The distribution of the Philadelphia chromosome in patients with chronic myelogenous leukemia. Blood 1963; 22:664.
15. Adamson JW, Fialkow PJ. Polycythemia vera: Stem cell and probable clinical origin of the disease. N Engl J Med 1976; 245:913.
16. Fialkow PJ, Jacobson RJ, Papayannopoulos T. Chronic myelocytic leukemia: clonal origin in a stem cell common to the granulocyte, erythrocyte, platelet and monocyte/macrophage. Am J Med 1977; 63:125.
17. Jacobson RJ, Salo A, Fialkow PJ. Agnogenic myeloid metaplasia: A clonal proliferation of hematopoietic stem cells with secondary myelofibrosis. Blood 1978; 51:189.
18. Fialkow PJ, Faguet SB, Jacobson RJ. Evidence that essential thrombocythemia is a clonal disorder with origin in a multipotent stem cell. Blood 1981; 58:916.
19. Fauser AA, Messner HA. Identification of megakaryocytes, macrophages and eosinophils in colonies of human bone marrow containing neutrophilic granulocytes and erythroblasts. Blood 1979; 53:1023.
20. Harker LA, Finch CA. Thrombokinetics in man. J Clin Invest 1969; 48:963.

21. Lichtman MA, Brennan JK. Megakaryocyte structure, maturation and ecology. *In* Colman RW, Hirsh J, Marder VJ, Salzman EW (eds): Hemostasis and Thrombosis: Basic Principles and Clinical Practice, 2nd ed. Philadelphia: JB Lippincott, 1987, p 395.
22. Rabellino EM, Nachman RL, Williams N, et al. Human megakaryocytes: 1. Characterization of the membrane and cytoplasmic components of isolated marrow megakaryocytes. J Exp Med 1979; 149:1273.
23. Mazur EM, Hoffman R, Chasis J, et al. Immunofluorescent identification of human megakaryocyte colonies using an antiplatelet glycoprotein antiserum. Blood 1981; 57:277.
24. Vinci G, Tabilio A, Deschamps JF, et al. Immunological study of in vitro maturation of human megakaryocytes. Br J Haematol 1984; 56:589.
25. Breton-Gorius J, Reyes F. Ultrastructure of human bone marrow cell maturation. Int Rev Cytol 1986; 46:251.
26. Asch AS, Barnwell J, Silverstein RL, et al. Isolation of the thrombospondin membrane receptor. J Clin Invest 1987; 79:1054.
27. Edelman P, Vinci G, Villeval JL, et al. A monoclonal antibody against an erythrocyte ontogenic antigen identifies fetal and adult erythroid progenitors. Blood 1986; 67:56.
28. Rabellino EM, Goodwin L, Bussel JB, et al. Studies of human marrow megakaryocytes. *In* Evatt R, Levine RF, Williams N (eds): Megakaryocyte Biology and Precursors: In Vitro Cloning and Cellular Properties. New York: Elsevier, 1981, p 233.
29. Nakeff A. Megakaryocytic cells. Bibl Haematol 1984; 48:131.
30. Levine RF, Fedorko ME. Isolation of intact megakaryocytes from guinea pig femoral marrow. Successful harvest made possible with inhibitors of platelet aggregation: Enrichment achieved with a two-step separation technique. J Cell Biol 1976; 69:159.
31. Nakeff A, Valeriote F, Gray JW, et al. Application of flow cytometry and cell sorting to megakaryocytopoiesis. Blood 1979; 53:732.
32. Ishibashi T, Burstein SA. Separation of murine megakaryocytes and their progenitors on continuous gradients of Percoll. J Cell Physiol 1985; 125:559.
33. Jackson CW, Brown KL, Somerville BC, et al. Two-color flow cytometric measurement of DNA distributions of rat megakaryocytes in unfixed, unfractionated marrow cell suspensions. Blood 1984; 63:768.
34. Levine RF, Bunn PA, Hazzard KC, et al. Flow cytometric analysis of megakaryocyte ploidy. Comparison with Feulgen microdensitometry and discovery that 8N is the predominant ploidy class in guinea pig and monkey marrow. Blood 1980; 56:210.
35. Jackson CW, Steward SA, Brown LK, et al. Inverse relationship between megakaryocyte buoyant density and maturity. Br J Haematol 1986; 64:33.
36. Worthington RE, Nakeff A, Micko S. Flow cytometric analysis of megakaryocyte differentiation. Cytometry 1984; 5:501.
37. Parks DR, Herzenberg LA. Fluorescence-activated cell sorting: Theory, experimental optimization, and applications in lymphoid cell biology. Methods Enzymol 1984; 108:197.
38. Berkow RL, Straneva JE, Bruno ED, et al. Isolation of human megakaryocytes by density centrifugation and counterflow centrifugal elutriation. J Lab Clin Med 1984; 103:811.
39. Levin J. Thrombopoiesis. *In* Colman RW, Hirsh J, Marder VJ, Salzman EW (eds): Hemostasis and Thrombosis: Basic Principles and Clinical Practice, 2nd ed. Philadelphia: JB Lippincott, 1987, p 418.
40. Odell T-T Jr, Jackson CW, Gosslee DG. Maturation of rat megakaryocytes studied by microspectrophotometric measurement of DNA. Proc Soc Exp Biol Med 1965; 119:1194.
41. Odell T-T Jr, Jackson CW. Polyploidy and maturation of rat megakaryocytes. Blood 1968; 32:102.
42. Paulus JM. DNA metabolism and development of organelles in guinea pig megakaryocytes: a combined ultrastructural, autoradiographic and cytophotometric study. Blood 1970; 35:298.
43. Pennington DG, Olsen TE. Megakaryocytes in states of altered platelet production: cell numbers, size and DNA content. Br J Haematol 1970; 18:447.
44. Tanum G, Engeset A. Low ploidy megakaryocytes in steady-state rat bone marrow. Blood 1983; 62:87.
45. DeLeval M. Etude cytochimique quantitative des acides desoxyribonucleiques au cours de la maturation megacaryocytaire. Nouv Rev Fr Hematol 1968; 8:392.
46. Kinet-Denoel C, Bassleer R, Andrien JM, et al. Ploidy histograms in ITP. *In* Paulus JM (ed): Platelet Kinetics: Radioisotopic, Cytological, Mathematical and Clinical Aspects. Amsterdam: North-Holland, 1971, p 280.
47. Penington DG, Weste SM. Ploidy histograms in ITP. *In* Paulus JM (ed): Platelet Kinetics: Radioisotopic, Cytological, Mathematical and Clinical Aspects. Amsterdam: North Holland, 1971, p 284.
48. Ishibashi T, Ruggeri ZM, Harker LA, et al. Separation of human megakaryocytes by state of differentiation on continuous gradients of Percoll: size and ploidy analysis of cells identified by monoclonal antibody to glycoprotein IIb/IIIa. Blood 1986; 67:1286.
49. Queisser U, Queisser W, Spiertz B. Polyploidization of megakaryocytes in normal humans, in patients with idiopathic thrombocytopenia and with pernicious anaemia. Br J Haematol 1971; 20:489.
50. Lagerlof B. Cytophotometric study of megakaryocyte ploidy in polycythemia vera and chronic granulocyte leukemia. Acta Cytol 1972; 16:240.
51. Tomer A. Flow cytometry as a universal tool in megakaryocyte research. National Heart, Lung, and Blood Institute Workshop, August 1994.
52. Tomer A, Harker LA. Quantitative cytometric measurement of normal human megakaryocytes. J Exper Clin Hematol 1989; 31:37.
53. Dupon H, Dupon M-A, Bricaud H, et al. Megakaryocyte separation in homogeneous classes by unit gravity sedimentation: Physicochemical, ultrastructural and cytophotometric characterizations. Biol Cell 1983; 49:137.
54. Harker LA. Kinetics of thrombopoiesis. J Clin Invest 1968; 47:458.
55. Penington DG, Streatfield K, Roxburgh AE. Megakaryocytes and the heterogeneity of circulating platelets. Br J Haematol 1976; 34:639.
56. Vainchenker W, Deschamps JF, Bastin JM, et al. Two monoclonal anti-platelet antibodies as markers of human megakaryocyte maturation: Immunofluorescent staining and platelet peroxidase detection in megakaryocyte colonies and in in vivo cells from normal and leukemic patients. Blood 1982; 59:514.
57. Tomer A, Harker LA. Effects of anagrelide on human megakaryocytopoiesis. Clin Res 1991; 39:40a.
58. Shapiro HM. Practical Flow Cytometry, 3rd ed. New York: Wiley-Liss, 1995.
59. Mollace V, Salvemini D, Anggard E, et al. Nitric oxide from vascular smooth muscle cells: regulation of platelet reactivity and smooth muscle cell guanylate cyclase. Br J Pharmacol 1991; 104:633.
60. Ebbe S, Stohlman F Jr, Overcash J, et al. Megakaryocyte size in thrombocytopenic and normal rats. Blood 1968; 32:383.
61. Corash L, Chen HY, Levin J, et al. Regulation of thrombopoiesis: effects of the degree of thrombocytopenia on megakaryocyte ploidy and platelet volume. Blood 1987; 70:177.
62. Odell TT, Murphy JR, Jackson CW. Stimulation of megakaryocytes by acute thrombocytopenia in rats. Blood 1976; 48:765.
63. Rolovic Z, Baldini M, Dameshek W. Megakaryocytopoiesis in experimentally induced immune thrombocytopenia. Blood 1970; 35:173.
64. Burstein SA, Adamson JW, Erb SK, et al. Megakaryocytopoiesis in the mouse: response to varying platelet demand. J Cell Physiol 1981; 109:333.
65. Odel TT, Jackson CW, Friday TJ. Megakaryocytopoiesis in rats with special reference to polyploidy. Blood 1970; 35:775.
66. Bessman JD. The relation of megakaryocyte ploidy to platelet volume. Am J Hematol 1984; 16:161.
67. Nomura T, Kuriya S, Dan K. Characteristics of megakaryocytes in relation to platelet production in idiopathic thrombocytopenic purpura. Acta Haematol Jpn 1983; 46:1541.
68. Lichtman MA, Chamberlain JK, Simon W, et al. Parasinusoidal location of megakaryocytes in marrow: a determinant of platelet release. Am J Hematol 1978; 4:303.
69. Wright JJ. The histogenesis of the blood platelets. J Morphol 1910; 21:203.
70. Theiry JP, Bessis M. Mecanisme de la plaquettogenese: etude in vivo par la microcinematographie. Rev Hematol 1956; 11:162.
71. Behnke O. An electron microscopic study of the rat megakaryocyte: II. Some aspects of platelet release and microtubules. J Ultrastruct Res 1969; 26:111.
72. Choi E. Regulation of proplatelet and platelet formation in vitro. *In* Kuter DJ, Hunt P, Sheridan W, Zucker-Franklin D (eds): Thrombopoiesis and Thrombopoietins: Molecular, Cellular, Pre-

clinical, and Clinical Biology. Totowa, NJ: Humana Press, 1997, p 271.
73. Tavassoli M, Aoki M. Migration of entire megakaryocytes through the marrow blood barrier. Br J Haematol 1981; 48:35.
74. Godwin HA, Ginsburg AD. May-Hegglin anomaly: a defect in megakaryocyte fragmentation? Br J Haematol 1974; 26:117.
75. Von Behrens WE. Mediterranean macrothrombocytopenia. Blood 1975; 46:199.
76. Paulus JM, Casals FJ. Platelet formation in Mediterranean macrothrombocytosis. Nouv Rev Fr Hematol 1978; 20:151.
77. Jackson CW, Hutson NK, Steward SA, et al. Platelets of the Wistar Furth rat have reduced levels of alpha-granule proteins: an animal model resembling Gray. J Clin Invest 1991; 87:1985.
78. Tomer A, Scharf RE, McMillan R, et al. Bernard-Soulier syndrome: Quantitative characterization of megakaryocytes and platelets by flow cytometric and platelet kinetic measurements. Eur J Haematol 1994; 52:193.
79. Williams N, McDonald TP, Rabellino EM. Maturation and regulation of megakaryocytopoiesis. Blood Cells 1979; 5:43.
80. Williams N, Egger RR, Jackson HM, et al. Two-factor requirement for murine megakaryocyte colony formation. J Cell Phys 1982; 110:101.
81. Greenberg SM, Kuter DJ, Rosenberg RD. In vitro stimulation of megakaryocyte maturation by megakaryocyte stimulatory factor. J Biol Chem 1987; 262:3269.
82. deSauvage FJ, Hass PE, Spencer SD, et al. Stimulation of megakaryocytopoiesis and thrombopoiesis by the c-Mpl ligand. Nature 1994; 369:533.
83. Lok S, Kaushansky K, Holly RD, et al. Cloning and expression of murine thrombopoietin cDNA and stimulation of platelet production in vivo. Nature 1994; 369:565.
84. Kaushansky K, Lok S, Holly RD, et al. Promotion of megakaryocyte progenitor expansion and differentiation by the c-Mpl ligand thrombopoietin. Nature 1994; 369:568.
85. Wendling F, Maraskovsky E, Debili N, et al. c-Mpl ligand is a humoral regulator of megakaryocytopoiesis. Nature 1994; 369:571.
86. Bartley TD, Bogenberger J, Hunt P, et al. Identification and cloning of a megakaryocyte growth and development factor that is a ligand for the cytokine receptor Mpl. Cell 1994; 77:1117.
87. Souyri M, Vigon I, Penciolelli JF, et al. A putative truncated cytokine receptor gene transduced by the myeloproliferative leukemia virus immortalizes hematopoietic progenitors. Cell 1990; 63:1137.
88. Pinto MR, King MA, Goss GD, et al. Acute megakaryoblastic leukaemia with 3q inversion and elevated thrombopoietin (TSF): an autocrine role for TSF? Br J Haematol 1985; 61:687.
89. Hoffman R. Human hematopoietic stem cells: potential use as tumor-free autografts after high-dose myeloablative cancer therapy. Am J Med Sci 1995; 309:254.
90. Paulus JM. Platelet Kinetics: Radioisotopic, Cytological, Mathematical and Clinical Aspects. Amsterdam: North-Holland, 1971.
91. Choi ES, Hokom M, Bartley T, et al. Recombinant human megakaryocyte growth and development factor (rHuMGDF), a ligand for c-Mpl, produces functional human platelets in vitro. Stem Cells 1995; 13:317.
92. Kuter DJ, Beeler DL, Rosenberg RD. The purification of megapoietin: A physiological regulator of megakaryocyte growth and platelet production. Proc Natl Acad Sci U S A 1994; 91:11104.
93. Kaushansky K. Thrombopoietin: the primary regulator of platelet production. Blood 1995; 86:419.
94. Kato T, Ogami K, Shimada Y, et al. Purification and characterization of thrombopoietin. J Biochem 1995; 118:229.
95. Broudy VC, Lin NL, Kaushansky K. Thrombopoietin (c-Mpl ligand) acts synergistically with erythropoietin, stem cell factor, and IL-11 to enhance murine megakaryocyte colony growth and increases megakaryocyte ploidy in vitro. Blood 1995; 85:1719.
96. Ku H, Yonemura Y, Kaushansky K, et al. Thrombopoietin, the ligand for the Mpl receptor, synergy with steel factor and other early-acting cytokines in supporting proliferation of primitive hematopoietic progenitors of mice. Blood 1996; 87:4544.
97. Kobayashi M, Laver JH, Kato T, et al. Thrombopoietin supports proliferation of human primitive hematopoietic cells in synergy with steel factor and/or interleukin-3. Blood 1995; 88:429.
98. Odell TT, McDonald TP, Detwiler TC. Stimulation of platelet production by serum of platelet-depleted rats. Proc Soc Exp Biol Med 1961; 108:428.
99. Evatt BL, Shreiner DP, Levin J. Thrombopoietic activity of fractions of rabbit plasma: studies in rabbits and mice. J Lab Clin Med 1974; 83:364.
100. Mazur E, South K. Human megakaryocyte colony-stimulating factor in sera from aplastic anemia dogs: partial purification, characterization and determination of hematopoietic cell lineage specificity. Exp Hematol 1985; 13:1164.
101. Tayrien G, Rosenberg RD. Purification and properties of a megakaryocyte stimulatory factor present both in the serum-free conditioned medium of human embryonic kidney cells and in thrombocytopenic plasma. J Biol Chem 1987; 262:3262.
102. Kuter DJ. The regulation of platelet production in vivo. *In* Kuter DJ, Hunt P, Sheridan W, Zucker-Franklin D (eds): Thrombopoiesis and Thrombopoietins: Molecular, Cellular, Preclinical, and Clinical Biology. Totowa, NJ: Humana Press, 1997, p 377.
103. Nichol JL. Serum levels of thrombopoietin in health and disease. *In* Kuter DJ, Hunt P, Sheridan W, Zucker-Franklin D (eds): Thrombopoiesis and Thrombopoietins: Molecular, Cellular, Preclinical, and Clinical Biology. Totowa, NJ: Humana Press, 1997, p 359.
104. Nichol JL. Endogenous TPO (eTPO) levels in health and disease: possible clues for therapeutic intervention. Stem Cells 1998; 16(suppl 2):165–175.
105. Nichol JL, Hokom MM, Hornkohl A, et al. Megakaryocyte growth and development factor. Analyses of in vitro effects on human megakaryopoiesis and endogenous serum levels during chemotherapy-induced thrombocytopenia. J Clin Invest 1995; 95:2973.
106. Stoffel R, Wiestner A, Skoda RC. Thrombopoietin in thrombocytopenic mice: evidence against regulation at the mRNA level and for a direct regulatory role of platelets. Blood 1996; 87:567.
107. Gurney AL, Carver-Moore K, de Sauvage FJ, et al. Thrombocytopenia in c-Mpl–deficient mice. Science 1994; 265:1445.
108. de Sauvage FJ, Luoh S-M, Carver-Moore K, et al. Deficiencies in early and late stages of megakaryocytopoiesis in TPO-KO mice [Abstract]. Blood 1995; 86:255a.
109. deSauvage FJ, Carver-Moore K, Luoh SM. Physiologic regulation of early and late stages of megakaryocytopoiesis by thrombopoietin. J Exp Med 1996; 183:651.
110. McCarty JM, Sprugel KH, Fox NE, et al. Murine thrombopoietin mRNA levels are modulated by platelet count. Blood 1995; 86:3668.
111. Sungaran R, Markovic B, Chong BH. Localization and regulation of thrombopoietin mRNA expression in human kidney, liver, bone marrow and spleen using in situ hybridization. Blood 1997; 89:101.
112. Kuter DJ, Rosenberg RD. Appearance of a megakaryocyte growth-promoting activity, megapoietin, during acute thrombocytopenia in the rabbit. Blood 1994; 84:1464.
113. Navarro S, Debili N, LeCouedic J-P, et al. Interleukin-6 and its receptor are expressed by human megakaryocytes: in vitro effects on proliferation and endoreplication. Blood 1991; 77:461.
114. Bruno E, Miller ME, Hoffman R. Interacting cytokines regulate in vitro human megakaryocytopoiesis. Blood 1989; 73:671.
115. Bruno E, Cooper RJ, Briddell RA, et al. Further examination of the effects of recombinant cytokines on the proliferation of human megakaryocyte progenitor cells. Blood 1991; 77:23.
116. Metcalf D, Nicola NA. Leukemia inhibitory factor can potentiate murine megakaryocyte production in vitro. Blood 1991; 77:21.
117. Stahl CP, Zucker-Franklin D, Evatt BL, et al. Effects of human interleukin-6 on megakaryocyte development and thrombocytopoiesis in primates. Blood 1991; 78:1467.
118. Kimura H, Ishibashi T, Uchita T, et al. Interleukin 6 is a differentiation factor for human megakaryocytes in vitro. Eur J Immunol 1990; 20:19.
119. Bruno E, Briddell RA, Cooper RJ, et al. Effects of recombinant interleukin-11 on human megakaryocyte progenitor cells. Exp Hematol 1991; 19:378.
120. Burstein SA, Mei R, Henthorn J, et al. Recombinant human leukemia inhibitory factor (LIF) and interleukin-11 (IL-11) promote murine and human megakaryocytopoiesis in vitro. Blood 1990; 76(suppl 1):450a.
121. Debili N, Hegyi E, Navarro S, et al. In vitro effects of hematopoietic growth factors on the proliferation, endoreplication, and maturation of human megakaryocytes. Blood 1991; 77:23.
122. Robinson BE, McCrath HE, Quesenberry PJ. Recombinant murine granulocyte macrophage colony-stimulating factor has mega-

karyocyte colony stimulating activity and augments megakaryocyte colony stimulation by interleukin 3. J Clin Invest 1987; 79:1648.
123. Imai T, Koike K, Kubo T, et al. Interleukin-6 supports human megakaryocytic proliferation and differentiation in vitro. Blood 1991; 78:1969.
124. Aglietta M, Monzeglio C, Sanavio F, et al. In vivo effect of human granulocyte-macrophage colony-stimulating factor on megakaryocytopoiesis. Blood 1991; 77:1191.
125. Tanaka H, Ishida Y, Kaneko T, et al. Isolation of human megakaryocytes by immunomagnetic beads. Br J Haematol 1989; 73:18.
126. Stahl CP, Winton EF, Monroe MC, et al. Recombinant human granulocyte-macrophage colony-stimulating factor promotes megakaryocyte maturation in nonhuman primates. Exp Hematol 1991; 19:810.
127. Asano S, Oakno A, Ozawa K. In vivo effect of interleukin 6 in primates: stimulated production of platelets. Blood 1990; 75:1602.
128. Hoffman R. Regulation of megakaryocytopoiesis. Blood 1989; 74:1196.
129. Vainchenker W, Bouguet J, Guichard J, et al. Megakaryocyte colony formation from human bone marrow precursors. Blood 1979; 54:940.
130. Dessypris EN, Gleaton JH, Armstrong OL. Effect of human recombinant erythropoietin on human marrow megakaryocyte colony formation in vitro. Br J Haematol 1987; 65:265.
131. Briddell RA, Bruno E, Cooper RJ, et al. Effect of c-kit ligand on in vitro human megakaryocytopoiesis. Blood 1991; 78:2854.
132. Tomer A, Stahl CP, McClure HM, et al. Effects of recombinant human granulocyte-macrophage colony-stimulating factor on platelet survival and activation using a nonhuman primate model. Exp Hematol 1993; 21:1577.
133. Karpatkin S, Garg SK, Freedman ML. Role of iron as a regulator of thrombopoiesis. Am J Med 1974; 57:521.
134. Levin J, Conley CL. Thrombocytosis associated with malignant disease. Arch Intern Med 1964; 114:497.
135. Marchasin S, Wallerstein RO, Aggeler PM. Variation of the platelet count in disease. Calif Med 1964; 101:95.
136. Fuse A, Kakuda H, Shima Y, et al. Interleukin 6, a possible autocrine growth and differentiation factor for the human megakaryocytic cell line, CMK. Br J Haematol 1991; 77:32.
137. Brach MA, Lowenberg B, Mantovani L, et al. Interleukin-6 (IL-6) is an intermediate in IL-1–induced proliferation of leukemic human megakaryoblasts. Blood 1990; 76:1972.
138. Avraham H, Vannier E, Chi S, et al. Cytokine gene expression and synthesis by human megakaryocyte cell lines. Blood 1990; 76(suppl 2):446a.
139. Harker LA, Marzec UM, Hunt P, et al. Dose-response effects of pegylated human megakaryocyte growth and development factor (PEG-rHuMGDF) on platelet production and function in nonhuman primates. Blood 1996; 88:511.
140. Jones DV Jr, Ashby M, Vadhan-Raj S, et al. Recombinant human thrombopoietin clinical development. Stem Cells 1998; 16(suppl 2):199–206.
141. Kuter DJ. The use of PEG-rHuMGDF in platelet apheresis. Stem Cells 1998; 16(suppl 2):231.
142. Schiffer CA. Opportunities for the use of thrombopoietic growth factors. Stem Cells 1998; 16(suppl 2):249.
143. Branehog I, Kutti J, Ridell B, et al. The relation of thrombokinetics to bone marrow megakaryocytes in idiopathic thrombocytopenia purpura (ITP). Blood 1975; 45:551.
144. Wessels P, Heyns ADP, Pieter H, et al. An improved method for the quantification of the in vivo kinetics of a representative population of 111-In–labelled human platelets. Eur J Nucl Med 1985; 10:522.
145. Heyns ADP, Badenhorst PH, Lotter MG, et al. Platelet turnover and kinetics in immune thrombocytopenic purpura: results with autologous 111-In–labeled platelets and homologous 51-CR–labeled platelets differ. Blood 1986; 67:8692.
146. Hanson SR, Slichter SJ. Platelet kinetics in patients with bone marrow hypoplasia: evidence for a fixed platelet requirement. Blood 1985; 66:1105.
147. Paulus JM, Aster RH. Platelet kinetics: Production, distribution, life-span, and fate of platelets. *In* Williams N, Beutler E, Erslev O, Lichtman MA (eds): Hematology, 2nd ed. New York: McGraw-Hill, 1983, p 1185.
148. Aster RH. Pooling of platelets in the spleen: role in the pathogenesis of "hypersplenic" thrombocytopenia. J Clin Invest 1966; 45:645.
149. Heyns ADP, Lotter MG, Badenhorst PN, et al. Kinetics, distribution and sites of destruction of indium-111–labelled human platelets. Br J Haematol 1980; 44:269.
150. Peters AM, Lavender JP. Platelet kinetics with indium-111 platelets: comparison with chromium-51 platelets. Semin Thromb Hemost 1983; 9:100.
151. Harker LA. The kinetics of platelet production and destruction in man. Clin Haematol 1977; 6:671.
152. Tomer A, Hanson SR, Harker LA. Autologous platelet kinetics in patients with severe thrombocytopenia: discrimination between disorders of production and destruction. J Lab Clin Med 1991; 118:546.
153. Harker LA. Platelet survival time: its measurement and use. Prog Hemost Thromb 1978; 4:321.
154. Cole JL, Marzec UM, Gunthel CJ, et al. Ineffective platelet production in thrombocytopenic HIV-infected patients. Blood 1998; In press.
155. Davey MG. The survival and destruction of human platelets. Bibl Haematol 1966; 22:1.
156. Aster RH. Studies of the fate of platelets in rats and man. Blood 1969; 34:117.
157. Kotilainen M. Platelet kinetics in normal subjects and haematologic disorders with special reference to thrombocytopenia and to the role of the spleen. Scand J Haematol 1969; 5(suppl):9.
158. Klonizakis I, Peters AM, Fitzpatrick ML, et al. Radionuclide distribution following injection of In-111–labelled platelets. Br J Haematol 1980; 46:595.
159. Robertson JS, Dewanjee MK, Brown ML, et al. Distribution and dosimetry of In-111–labeled platelets. Radiology 1981; 140:169.
160. Scheffel U, Tsan MF, Mitchell G, et al. Human platelets labeled with In-111–8-hydroxyquinoline: kinetics, distribution and estimates of radiation dose. J Nucl Med 1982; 23:149.
161. Heyns ADP, Lotter MG, Kotze HF, et al. Quantification of in vivo distribution of platelets labeled with indium-111–oxine. J Nucl Med 1982; 23:943.
162. Shulman NR, Jordan JV Jr. Platelet kinetics. *In* Colman RW, Hirsh J, Marder VJ, Salzman EW (eds): Hemostasis and Thrombosis. Basic Principles and Clinical Practice, 2nd ed. Philadelphia: JB Lippincott, 1987, p 431.
163. Ardaillou N, Najean Y, Eberlin A. Study of platelet kinetics using 75-Se-selenomethionine. *In* Paulus JM (ed): Platelet Kinetics. Amsterdam: North Holland, 1971, p 131.
164. Brodsky I, Ross EM, Petkov G, et al. Platelet and fibrinogen kinetics with 75-Se-selenomethionine in patients with myeloproliferative disorders. Br J Haematol 1972; 22:179.
165. Dassin E, Najean Y. The use of 75-Se-methionine as a tracer of thrombocytopoiesis. In vivo incorporation of the tracer into platelet proteins: a biochemical study. Acta Haematol 1979; 61:61.
166. Heyns ADP, Badenhorst PN, Wessels P, et al. Indium-111–labelled human platelets: a method for use in severe thrombocytopenia. Thromb Haemost 1984; 52:226.
167. Kelton JG. Platelet survival studies; An overview of the factors affecting the efficiency and reliability of platelet radiolabeling. Transfusion 1986; 26:19.
168. Slichter SJ. Post-storage platelet viability in thrombocytopenic recipients is reliably measured by radiochromium-labeled platelet recovery and survival measurements in normal volunteers. Transfusion 1986; 26:8.
169. Robertson JS, Milne WL, Cohn SH. Labeling and tracing of rat blood platelets with chromium-51. *In* Proceedings of the 2nd International Radioisotopic Congress, July 19–22, 1954. London: Butterworth Scientific Publications, 1954, p 205.
170. Tsukada T, Steiner M, Baldini M. Mechanism and kinetics of chromate transport in human platelets. Am J Physiol 1971; 221:1697.
171. Abrahamsen AF. A modification of the technique for 51-Cr–labelling of blood platelets. Scand J Haematol 1968; 5:53.
172. Heaton WAL. Indium-111 (111-In) and chromium-51 (51-Cr) labeling of platelets. Are they comparable? Transfusion 1986; 26:16.
173. International Committee for Standardization in Hematology, Panel for Standardization in Hematology. Recommended methods of radioisotope platelet survival studies. Blood 1977; 50:1137.
174. Thakur ML, Welch MJ, Joist JH. Indium-111–labeled platelets: Studies on preparation and evaluation of in vitro and in vivo function. Thromb Res 1976; 9:345.

175. Thakur ML. Radioisotopic labeling of platelets: an historical perspective. Semin Thromb Hemost 1983; 9:79.
176. Thakur ML, Walsh LJ, Malech HL, et al. Indium-111–labeled human platelets: improved method, efficacy and evaluation. J Nucl Med 1981; 22:381.
177. Hawker RJ, Hawker LM, Wilkinson AR. Indium (111-In) labeled human platelets: Optimal methods. Clin Sci 1980; 58:243.
178. Joist JH, Baker RK, Thakur ML, et al. Indium-111–labeled human platelets: Uptake and loss of label and in vitro function of labeled platelets. J Lab Clin Med 1978; 92:829.
179. Schmidt KG, Rasmussen JW. Labelling of human and rabbit platelets with 111-indium–oxine complex. Scand J Haematol 1979; 23:97.
180. Vigneron N, Dassin E, Najean Y. Double radioactive labeling for the simultaneous study of autologous and homologous human platelets' life span. Nouv Presse Med 1980; 9:1835.
181. Corash L, Shafer B, Perlow M. Heterogenicity of human whole blood platelet subpopulation: II. Use of subhuman primate model to analyze the relationship between density and platelet age. Blood 1978; 52:726.
182. Thakur ML, McKenney SL, Park CH. Simplified and efficient labeling of human platelets in plasma using indium-111–2-mercaptopyridine-*N*-oxide: Preparation and evaluation. J Nucl Med 1985; 26:510.
183. Thakur ML, McKenney SM. Indium 111–mercaptopyridine *N*-oxide–labeled human leukocytes and platelets: mechanism of labeling and intracellular location of 111-indium and mercaptopyridine *N*-oxide. J Lab Clin Med 1986; 107:141.
184. Dewanjee MK, Wahner HW, Dunn WL, et al. Comparison of three platelet markers for measurement of platelet survival time in healthy volunteers. Mayo Clin Proc 1986; 61:327.
185. Snyder EL, Moroff G, Simon TS, et al. Recommended methods for conducting radiolabeled platelet survival studies. Transfusion 1986; 26:37.
186. Heyns AP, Lotter MG, Badenhorst PN. Methodology of platelet imaging. *In* Harker LA, Zimmerman TS (eds): Methods in Hematology: Measurements of Platelet Function, 8th ed. New York: Churchill Livingstone, 1983, p 216.
187. Schmidt KG, Rasmussen JW. Kinetics and distribution in vivo of 111-In–labelled autologous platelets in idiopathic thrombocytopenic purpura. Scand J Haematol 1985; 34:47.
188. International Committee for Standardization in Hematology Panel on Diagnostic Applications of Radionuclides. Recommended method for indium-111 platelet survival studies. J Nucl Med 1988; 29:564.
189. McMillan R, Tani P, Millard F, et al. Platelet-associated and plasma anti-glycoprotein autoantibodies in chronic ITP. Blood 1987; 70:1040.
190. Tomer A, Schreiber AD, McMillan R, et al. Menstrual cyclic thrombocytopenia. Br J Haematol 1989; 71:519.
191. Tsukada T, Tango T. On the methods calculating mean survival time in 51-CR–platelet survival study. Am J Hematol 1980; 8:281.
192. Branehog I, Kutti J, Weinfeld A. Platelet survival and platelet production in idiopathic thrombocytopenic purpura (ITP). Br J Haematol 1974; 27:127.
193. Kuter D, McCullough J, Romo J, et al. Treatment of platelet (PLT) donors with pegylated recombinant human megakaryocyte growth and development factor (PEG-rHuMGDF) increases circulating PLT counts (CTS) and PLT apheresis yields and increases platelet increments in recipients of PLT transfusions [Abstract]. Blood 1997; 90:579a.
194. Goodnough LT, Dipersio J, McCullough J, et al. Pegylated recombinant human megakaryocyte growth and development factor (PEG-rHuMGDF) increases platelet (PLT) count (CT) and apheresis yields of normal PLT donors: initial results [Abstract]. Transfusion 1997; 37(suppl 9S):67S.

CHAPTER 4

Hematopoietic Growth Factors

Silvana Z. Bucur
John D. Roback
Christopher D. Hillyer

OVERVIEW OF HEMATOPOIESIS AND CYTOKINE BIOLOGY

Hematopoiesis is a multifaceted process leading to the formation and release of different types of mature blood cells. This process requires the interaction of stem cells, the bone marrow microenvironment (bone marrow stroma and extracellular matrix), and various cytokines that perform important regulatory functions. Since 1990, many hematopoietic cytokines have been identified, their genes cloned, and their recombinant forms employed in clinical practice.

Multipotent stem cells, the majority of which exist in the resting stage (G_0) of the cell cycle, possess self-renewal capacity and the capability to proliferate and differentiate into more mature progenitors committed to specific cell lineages. The hematopoietic stem cell constitutes a very small percentage (<0.01%) of all bone marrow mononuclear cells.[1] Phenotypic characterization of the early hematopoietic progenitors is defined by their cell surface antigenic profile. Most notably, the CD34 antigen, a 115-kD glycoprotein, is expressed on approximately 1% to 3% of bone marrow cells and 0.1 to 0.5% of peripheral blood mononuclear cells.[2] Approximately 5% to 20% of the bone marrow $CD34^+$ population expresses Thy-1^{low} and does not express CD38, human leukocyte antigen (HLA)–DR, or lineage-specific antigens. These cells ($CD34^+$, Thy-1^{low}, $CD38^-$, lin^-) represent a more immature progenitor subpopulation in which multipotent stem cells are found.[3, 4] Currently, indirect functional assays (e.g., long-term culture–initiating cell [LTC-IC] assays) are the only means of studying their characteristics and reconstitution potential.[1] In semisolid colony assays, $CD34^+$ bone marrow cells give rise to colony-forming units (CFUs) of various lineages, including erythroid (CFU-E), granulocyte-macrophage (CFU-GM), megakaryocyte (CFU-Meg), and granulocyte-erythroid-macrophage-megakaryocyte (CFU-GEMM), and to burst-forming erythroid units (BFU-E)[2, 5, 6] (Fig. 4–1).

The bone marrow microenvironment, or stroma, is composed of elements essential for sustaining hematopoiesis, including endothelial cells, fibroblasts, macrophages, adipocytes, and the extracellular matrix. These stromal cells express several classes of adhesion molecules, including integrins, selectins, sialomucins, and members of the immunoglobulin gene superfamily. The adhesion molecules facilitate cell-cell and cell-matrix contact, modulate the interaction between cytokines and hematopoietic cells, and are involved in the signaling mechanism required for the localization of the hematopoietic stem cells to the bone marrow. In addition, stromal cells secrete a variety of hematopoietic cytokines that are involved in the regulatory process of hematopoiesis. The interaction among stromal adhesion molecules, stem cells, and cytokines provides the signals necessary for proliferation, differentiation, maturation, and survival of the hematopoietic cells.[7–9]

Alone or through synergistic interactions, cytokines can stimulate cellular developmental processes and maintain the integrity of cells. They may enhance the functional activity of the mature progeny, regulate apoptosis, or possess inhibitory functions.[10–12] During steady-state hematopoiesis, these regulatory cytokines are produced

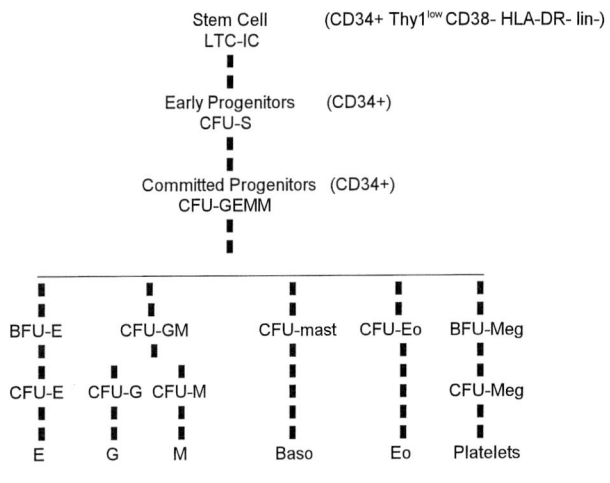

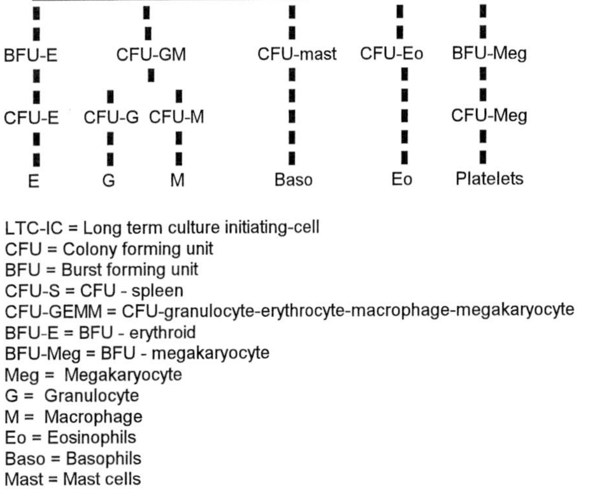

Figure 4–1. Hematopoiesis.

locally in the bone marrow and at distant sites, exerting their effects through autocrine/paracrine and endocrine routes. During states of increased demand, their effect is exerted predominantly through the endocrine route.[13, 14]

Hematopoietic cytokines can be categorized as *early-acting*—such as stem cell factor, Flt-3 ligand, interleukin (IL)–3, granulocyte-macrophage colony-stimulating factor (GM-CSF), and IL-6—or *late-acting,* including erythropoietin (EPO), granulocyte colony-stimulating factor (G-CSF), macrophage colony-stimulating factor (M-CSF), and thrombopoietin (TPO). Early-acting cytokines act locally and are lineage-nonspecific, affecting the immature stages common to each lineage. In contrast, late-acting cytokines are lineage-specific and affect late maturational stages by promoting the release of mature cells from the bone marrow and increasing the survival of cells in circulation (by preventing apoptosis). The role of cytokines is not limited to hematopoiesis. They exert immunomodulatory effects by regulating lymphocyte development and activation. They can effect macrophage and natural killer cell function, promote endothelial cell activation, and upregulate major histocompatibility complex (MHC) and adhesion molecule expression. Cytokines are also involved in inflammatory responses and angiogenesis and may possess antitumor effects. The gamut of effects that cytokines exert on hematopoietic and nonhematopoietic cells requires a complex network of interactions among cytokines, their receptors, and the responsive cells.[15–17] (Table 4–1 lists the major biological activities of other hematopoietic cytokines.)

The activity of hematopoietic cytokines is mediated by specific receptors expressed on the surface of target cells. This receptor-ligand interaction triggers intracellular signals that translate into developmental changes within the cell. Structurally, cytokine receptors are integral membrane glycoproteins, composed of an extracellular ligand-binding domain, a transmembrane segment, and a C-terminal intracellular domain. The presence or absence of a tyrosine kinase domain distinguishes two cytokine receptor families. Receptors in the *cytokine receptor family* are devoid of intrinsic enzymatic activity and demonstrate a high degree of homology with one another. On the basis of similarities in the signal transducer domain, these receptors can be divided into three groups: one group consists of the receptors for GM-CSF, IL-3, and IL-5, which share a common β chain; a second group is composed of receptors for IL-6 and IL-11, among others, which share a common signal transducer, gp130; the third group is composed of the IL-2, IL-4, IL-7, IL-9, and IL-15 receptors, which share the β chain and the γ chain (γ-c). In contrast, receptors in the *tyrosine kinase receptor family* possess intrinsic tyrosine kinase activity within the cytoplasmic domain and contain a common extracellular immunoglobulin-like domain.[18–21]

In general, receptor-ligand interactions result in oligodimerization of the receptor, activation of a receptor-specific tyrosine kinase, receptor transphosphorylation, and subsequent phosphorylation of downstream signaling proteins. The phosphorylated receptor provides binding sites for signaling proteins containing an Src homology 2 (SH2). The specific signal transduction pathway activated is dependent on the cytokine, the type and maturational stage of cell, and the interaction with other cytokines and their receptors. The end result is a signal that modulates development, differentiation, and/or survival of the target cell.[18–21]

ERYTHROPOIETIN

EPO, a 166–amino acid (aa) glycoprotein, has a molecular weight of approximately 35 kD.[22] The gene for EPO is found on chromosome 7 (7pter–q22). EPO displays considerable homology among primate and nonprimate species.[23, 24] EPO is produced mainly by the peritubular cells of the renal cortex[25] and, to a lesser extent, by the liver.[26] EPO is synthesized constitutively by the kidney, thus maintaining a sustained serum level. The oxygen tension in the blood is sensed by the renal cortex; when hypoxemia ensues, an increased number of peritubular cells are induced to synthesize EPO.[27] Although there is no feedback inhibition mechanism based on plasma levels, in pathological conditions the production of EPO may be inhibited by other cytokines, including tumor necrosis factor (TNF)–α and IL-1.[28, 29] The secretion, biological activity, and plasma kinetics of EPO are affected by its carbohydrate moiety, composed predominantly of sialic acid.[30]

EPO regulates red blood cell production through its interaction with the EPO receptor, whose gene has been localized to chromosome 19(p). The EPO receptor is expressed at a density inversely proportional to the degree of maturity of the cell; thus, it is present at high density on CFU-E and proerythroblasts but undetectable on reticulocytes. Qualitative differences among EPO receptors have been described as correlating with receptor functional capacity as well as with the maturational stage of the erythroid cell. Thus, EPO exerts its maximum effect on CFU-E and proerythroblasts, which express the greatest number of highly functional, full-length receptors.[31, 32]

Although the EPO receptor does not possess tyrosine kinase activity, a number of intracellular proteins (SHIP, JAK2, STAT5, SHP1, SHP2), including the EPO receptor itself, are tyrosine phosphorylated after the receptor-ligand interaction. Two major signal transduction pathways are subsequently activated: the *ras* pathway and the JAK2/STAT5 pathway.[33] These signaling pathways stimulate intracellular processes, including synthesis of DNA and RNA, post-translational modification of nuclear proteins, synthesis of hemoglobin, alterations in calcium flux, and increased iron uptake. These processes subsequently translate into specific cellular responses in the target cells (proliferation, differentiation, maturation, and inhibition of apoptosis).[34]

EPO regulates constitutive erythropoiesis and stimulates the production of red blood cells in response to hypoxemia. It does not influence lineage commitment; rather, it facilitates the transition of the less EPO-responsive BFU-E (or other precursors) into the more EPO-responsive CFU-E, in a manner not involving altered cell cycle kinetics. It stimulates the proliferation and enhances the maturation rate of CFU-E and prolongs their survival by inhibiting apoptosis[35, 36] (see Table 4–1).

Recombinant human erythropoietin (rHuEPO) re-

Table 4–1. Biological Activities of Hematopoietic Cytokines

Factor	Source	Major Target Cells	Principal Biological Effects
EPO	Liver Kidney	CFU-E/proerythroblast	Stimulates erythrocyte production in response to hypoxia
GM-CSF	Mast cells T lymphocytes Endothelial cells Fibroblasts	Myeloid, erythroid, megakaryocytic lineage	Stimulates proliferation and differentiation of multilineage progenitors Stimulates growth of CFU-G, CFU-M, CFU-Eo Enhances function of mature cells Stimulates growth of malignant cells
G-CSF/M-CSF	Monocytes Macrophages Endothelial cells Fibroblasts	Granulocyte, monocyte	Stimulates proliferation of granulocyte/monocyte-committed progenitors Stimulates maturational processes in granulocytes Activates phagocytic and secretory function of granulocytes/macrophages
TPO	Liver Kidney	Megakaryocyte, other lineages	Stimulates the production of platelets Synergizes with other cytokines to effect other lineages
SCF	Fibroblasts Endothelial cells	Early progenitors	Modest proliferative effect (alone) Synergizes with other cytokines
Flt-3 ligand	Bone marrow stroma	Early progenitors	Modest proliferative effect (alone) Synergizes with other cytokines
IL-3	Mast cells T lymphocytes	Granulocyte, monocyte, erythrocyte, eosinophil, basophil, megakaryocyte	Stimulates multilineage colony growth Stimulates lymphocyte proliferation and differentiation Synergizes with other cytokines
IL-1	Monocytes Macrophages	Monocytes, neutrophils, stromal cells	Induces inflammatory responses Synergizes with IL-3 to effect early progenitor proliferation
IL-2	T lymphocytes	T cells	Stimulates proliferation and activation of lymphocytes, NK cells
IL-4	Mast cells Basophils	Myeloid lineage, T and B cells	Stimulates the proliferation of T and B lymphocytes Induces immunoglobulin secretion Inhibits release of IL-1 Inhibits function of LAK cells
IL-5	T lymphocytes	Eosinophils	Activates cytotoxic lymphocytes Stimulates production of eosinophils
IL-6	Macrophages Endothelial cells Fibroblasts	B and T cells, myeloma cells, myeloid precursors, megakaryocytes	Synergizes with other cytokines Induces acute-phase responses Induces acute-phase protein synthesis Stimulates megakaryocytopoiesis
IL-7	Bone marrow stroma	B cells, megakaryocytes	Stimulates growth of lymphocytes Induces expression of other cytokines in monocytes
IL-8	Various cells	Granulocytes	Enhances neutrophil function Stimulates chemotaxis
IL-9	T lymphocytes Leukemic cells lines	$CD4^+$ cells, erythroid progenitors	Synergizes with EPO and IL-3
IL-10	Lymphocytes	Lymphocytes	Inhibits Th1 and Th2 cytokine response Inhibits proinflammatory cytokines and other cytokine synthesis
IL-11	Bone marrow stroma Fibroblasts	B cells, megakaryocytes, blasts	Synergizes with SCF and IL-3 Increases cycling activity of committed progenitors Stimulates production of acute-phase proteins
IL-12	Monocytes Macrophages	T cells, macrophages	Stimulates Th1 response Enhances functional activity of NK cells Enhances antifungal activity of macrophages

EPO, erythropoietin; CFU-E, colony-forming unit–erythroid; GM-CSF, granulocyte-macrophage colony-stimulating factor; CFU-G, colony-forming unit–granulocyte; CFU-M, colony-forming unit–macrophage; CFU-Eo, colony-forming unit–eosinophil; TPO, thrombopoietin; SCF, stem cell factor; IL, interleukin; LAK, lymphokine-activated killer; NK, natural killer.

quires post-translational glycosylation for clinical efficacy and thus is manufactured in mammalian cells. It has been evaluated in a variety of clinical conditions associated with absolute or relative EPO deficiency (Table 4–2). The role of rHuEPO in the correction of anemia of chronic renal insufficiency is well established[37]; rHuEPO has also proved efficacious in the treatment of anemia associated with zidovudine (AZT) therapy in patients with acquired immunodeficiency syndrome (AIDS), in whom it has been demonstrated that serum EPO levels, specifically levels below 500 mU/mL, predict responsiveness to exogenous administration of rHuEPO.[38] Certain cases of cancer-associated anemia and chemotherapy-induced anemia may also be responsive to exogenous EPO administration.[39–42] Although rHuEPO administration reduces the red blood cell requirement after bone marrow transplantation (BMT), it does not appear to be cost effective in this setting.[43, 44]

In the perioperative period, the administration of rHuEPO has been found to be beneficial in the collection of autologous blood from anemic or alloimmunized patients. It has also been used prophylactically in Jehovah's Witness patients (whose religious beliefs do not prohibit its use, in contrast to other blood products) and in normal bone marrow donors. In surgical patients at risk for significant perioperative bleeding, as well as those who exhibit signs of anemia preoperatively, the administration of rHuEPO has been shown to reduce allogeneic blood transfusion requirement.[45–53]

In other clinical situations, the role of rHuEPO, either alone or in combination with other cytokines, is still under investigation.[54–62] Whereas in most cases of anemia the exogenous administration of rHuEPO replenishes an endogenous deficiency, in sickle cell anemia the goal of rHuEPO therapy is to enhance the production of hemoglobin F, which in synergy with hydroxyurea subsequently reduces sickling.[58]

Table 4–2. Indications for Recombinant Human Erythropoietin Administration

FDA-Approved Indications

- Chronic renal insufficiency[37]
- Malignancy and chemotherapy–induced[38–41]
- Zidovudine (AZT)–induced with EPO, <500mIU/mL[42]
- Anemia of chronic disease with EPO deficiency[51]
- Preoperative autologous blood donation[51–53]
- Preoperative anemia[51–53]

Relative Indications

- Myelodysplastic syndromes[48, 49]
- Aplastic anemia[50]

Investigational Use

- Bone marrow transplantation[47, 55, 56, 62]
- Sickle cell anemia[58]
- Thalassemia[60]
- Rheumatoid arthritis[54]
- Anemia of prematurity[57, 61]
- Mobilization of iron stores in certain patients with hemochromatosis[59, 60]

FDA, (U.S.) Food and Drug Administration; EPO, erythropoietin.

MYELOID COLONY-STIMULATING FACTORS

The development of the myeloid lineage is primarily regulated by four hematopoietic growth factors: IL-3, GM-CSF, M-CSF (or CSF-1), and G-CSF. IL-3 and GM-CSF are early-acting cytokines, inducing the proliferation and differentiation of early progenitors, whereas M-CSF and G-CSF act late during the developmental stage, promoting cellular maturation.[63]

The effect of these cytokines is mediated through specific receptors that exist in high- and low-affinity forms.[64, 65] The high-affinity receptors are expressed at a density directly proportional to the degree of maturation of the cell. Receptor-ligand interaction results in the internalization and degradation of the ligand with accompanying loss of the high-affinity receptor for the specific ligand. Receptor transmodulation can occur directly, through the specific receptor-ligand interaction, or indirectly, through the action of other ligands and their receptors and through the effect of regulatory proteins on non–cytokine-binding domains of the receptor.[66–69] A similar phenomenon, termed *cross-competition,* has been observed between GM-CSF, IL-3, and IL-5 and takes place on the membrane surface of cells that bind more than one cytokine with high affinity.[70]

Granulocyte-Macrophage (Monocyte) Colony-Stimulating Factor

GM-CSF is an *N*-glycosylated, 127-aa polypeptide with a variable carbohydrate content. The gene has been localized to the long arm of chromosome 5 (5q21–32) and is closely linked to the gene encoding for IL-3.[71] GM-CSF is synthesized by T cells and stromal cells, including macrophages/monocytes, endothelial cells, and fibroblasts. In normal persons, GM-CSF is rarely detected in the serum, and levels do not vary with the absolute neutrophil count. However, variations in serum GM-CSF levels may occur during infection (increased levels) and in the presence of interferon-1β (decreased levels). GM-CSF is cleared from circulation by its receptor on mature granulocytes with less than 40% renal clearance.[72]

Gearing and associates cloned the human GM-CSF receptor, a member of the cytokine receptor family with a molecular weight of approximately 45 kD.[73] The high-affinity receptor is represented by the α/β complex, in which the β subunit modulates the ligand affinity of the α subunit (low-affinity receptor).[74] The GM-CSF receptor is expressed at highest density on mature granulocytes and with variable density on diverse normal nonhematopoietic cells and malignant cells.[73, 75–79] Upon binding its ligand, heterodimerization and rapid phosphorylation of the β subunit occurs, which in turn initiates intracellular signal transduction. Four known signal transduction pathways—*ras*-MAPK (*m*itogen-*a*ctivated-*p*rotein *k*inase); JAK2/STAT5; PI 3-kinase; and a pathway involving the activation of c-fes, c-yes, pim, CREB, and protein kinase C—are triggered by GM-CSF, leading to specific cellular responses.[80]

In vitro assays have demonstrated that GM-CSF promotes the growth of multilineage colonies, including

CFU-GEMM, CFU-GM, colony-forming unit (CFU-Eo), BFU-E, and CFU-Meg, and stimulates their proliferation and differentiation into mature myeloid elements, including neutrophils, macrophages, and eosinophils. In the murine system, the hematopoietic activity of GM-CSF seems to be concentration-dependent: low concentrations give rise to macrophage colonies, intermediate concentrations induce neutrophil and mixed granulocyte/macrophage colonies, and the highest concentrations stimulate the growth of megakaryocytic and multipotential progenitor colonies.[80–83] GM-CSF mobilizes neutrophils, monocytes, and eosinophils into the peripheral blood and, through inhibition of apoptosis, prolongs their survival in the circulation.[84] GM-CSF also affects the function of mature myeloid elements, decreasing random motility and increasing neutrophil chemotaxis.[85] Neutrophil and monocyte phagocytosis and cytotoxicity are also enhanced in the presence of GM-CSF, through both antibody-dependent and antibody-independent mechanisms.[86–88] GM-CSF modulates neutrophil cell-surface adhesion molecules: expression of CD11b (complement C3bi) is upregulated, whereas leukocyte adhesion molecule-1 (LAM-1) is downregulated in the presence of GM-CSF.[89]

GM-CSF exerts an antitumor effect against certain malignant cell lines, which appears to be mediated through increased production of TNF. In other solid tumor cell lines and myeloid leukemic cells, however, GM-CSF can exhibit a stimulatory effect.[78, 79, 90] GM-CSF also induces the proliferation and migration of vascular endothelium, suggesting a role in inflammatory response and wound healing.[76, 91, 92]

In vivo administration of human recombinant GM-CSF (rhGM-CSF) is associated with an initial decline in circulating granulocytes secondary to margination, followed by demargination and mobilization of marrow neutrophils within 36 to 48 hours of administration, after which a sustained increase in the production rate of neutrophils is observed.[93] Administration of rhGM-CSF is indicated (Table 4–3) for severe neutropenic states associated with the post-BMT period and for the treatment of graft failure after BMT. GM-CSF, either alone or in combination with other cytokines, has been shown to produce a 10- to 100-fold increase in the peripheral blood progenitors (both $CD34^+$ and CFUs) after chemotherapy; thus, it is an effective agent for peripheral blood stem cell mobilization in the autologous and allogeneic BMT setting. In acute myelogenous leukemia (AML), the administration of rhGM-CSF postinduction chemotherapy has reduced the treatment-associated morbidity and neutrophil recovery time. Although in vitro data suggested that GM-CSF can induce leukemic cells to cycle and thus possibly prove beneficial before induction chemotherapy, this "priming" effect has not been supported by in vivo studies. In the treatment of solid tumors, GM-CSF reduced the myelosuppressive effect of high-dose chemotherapy regimens.[94–106]

In patients with neutropenia secondary to myelodysplastic syndrome with recurrent infections, GM-CSF with or without concurrent administration of EPO has been found to reduce the degree of neutropenia and the number of episodes of infection. Although there are few data to support a definite clinical benefit, a small number of patients with drug-induced neutropenia, aplastic anemia, and hairy cell leukemia have responded to GM-CSF. The use of GM-CSF in combination with other hematopoietic cytokines for ex vivo expansion of progenitor cells is under investigation.[106]

Table 4–3. Indications for rhGM-CSF and rhG-CSF Administration

Approved Indications[103]
Myelosuppressive chemotherapy[95, 97, 98]
As primary prophylaxis of febrile neutropenia[114]
To prevent recurrence of febrile neutropenia and maintain dose intensity[114–117]
Myeloablative chemotherapy with autologous, allogeneic, or syngeneic bone marrow rescue[94, 96, 99, 118–124]
Bone marrow graft failure or delay after allogeneic, autologous, or syngeneic BMT
Autologous peripheral blood progenitor cell mobilization and collection[100–105]
Induction chemotherapy for acute myelogenous leukemia
Myelodysplastic syndromes with recurrent infections[95]
Relative Indications[103]
AIDS-associated neutropenia (rhG-CSF)
Drug-induced neutropenia
Aplastic anemia[128]
Severe chronic neutropenia[127, 128]
Investigational Indications[103]
Normal granulocyte donors[125, 126]
Visceral leishmaniasis
Severe community-acquired pneumonia

rhGM-CSF, human recombinant granulocyte-macrophage colony-stimulating factor; rhG-CSF, human recombinant granulocyte colony-stimulating factor; BMT, bone marrow transplantation; AIDS, acquired immunodeficiency syndrome.

Granulocyte Colony-Stimulating Factor

G-CSF is a 174-aa, *O*-glycosylated, single-chain polypeptide with a molecular weight of approximately 25 kD. Human G-CSF is encoded by a single gene, located on chromosome 17 (17q11–22) and is highly homologous with the murine G-CSF gene.[107] Numerous agents (e.g., GM-CSF, IL-1, IL-3, and IL-4) can induce a variety of cells, including macrophage/monocytes, fibroblasts, endothelial cells, and mesothelial cells, to produce G-CSF and downmodulate its receptor. Detectable plasma G-CSF levels have been demonstrated only in conditions associated with the presence of multiple inflammatory cytokines (TNF-α, IL-1). During states of neutropenia, plasma G-CSF levels are inversely proportional to the absolute neutrophil count.[108]

G-CSF exerts its biological effects through specific high-affinity receptors expressed on cells of myeloid lineage. The gene for human G-CSF receptor is located on chromosome 1p32–35. The receptor is a single-chain, 812-aa polypeptide. A 759-aa variant that lacks an endogenous kinase domain is also expressed. The extracellular domain of the G-CSF receptor contains an immunoglobulin-like region, three fibronectin type III domains, and a cytokine receptor homologous (CRH) domain. The intracellular domain contains a region homologous to the gp130 component of the IL-6 receptor. Alternative splicing gives rise to five G-CSF receptor isoforms, including a soluble form. The various receptor isoforms have a common extracellular domain, but their transmembrane and cytoplasmic regions differ. The G-CSF receptor is expressed on a variety of cells, including myeloid leukemia cells. The biological significance of the presence of the G-CSF receptor on various cells of nonhematopoietic origin is unclear.[109]

The early events in the G-CSF signaling cascade are similar to those of other cytokines and are followed by the activation of JAK1, JAK2, and Tyk2, with subsequent phosphorylation and activation of STAT1 and STAT3 proteins. The signal transduction pathways activated by G-CSF are dependent on the proliferating status of the target cells. The JAK/STAT pathway and the Rel pathway are activated in mature, nonproliferating cells, whereas the *ras*/MAPK pathway regulates these proliferative processes. The role of the Lyn/Syk pathway is not known as yet.[20, 109]

The biological activity of G-CSF is restricted to hematopoietic cells of the granulocytic lineage. In vitro, it stimulates the proliferation and differentiation of CFU-G and can induce quiescent progenitor cells to enter the G_1-to-S phase of the cell cycle. G-CSF administration produces neutrophil demargination and release of mature and immature neutrophils from the bone marrow into the peripheral blood. G-CSF increases the production rate of neutrophils 10-fold by decreasing the maturation time, increases their survival, and decreases the motility and skin window migration of granulocytes. G-CSF enhances the phagocytic function of mature granulocytes by increasing superoxide generation, stimulating endocytosis, and increasing the expression of crystallizable fragment γ receptor I (FcγRI) on the neutrophil cell surface. Antibody-dependent cellular cytotoxicity and chemotaxis are also stimulated by G-CSF. G-CSF alone does not influence the sustained growth of pluripotent progenitor cells, although it modulates their response to other cytokines, such as IL-3, IL-1α, IL-1β, and IL-6.[110–113]

Administration of human recombinant G-CSF (rhG-CSF; see Table 4–3) in cancer patients receiving various myelosuppressive chemotherapy regimens accelerates neutrophil recovery and decreases the incidence, severity, and duration of febrile neutropenia. In the setting of autologous and allogeneic BMT, the administration of rhG-CSF significantly reduces the duration of severe neutropenia (absolute neutrophil count, $<500/mm^2$) and the duration of febrile episodes. Only a nonsignificant downward trend in the length of hospital stay and antibiotic use has been observed. After rhG-CSF administration, there is a 10-fold increase in progenitor cell content of the peripheral blood. The use of rhG-CSF–mobilized peripheral blood progenitor cells after myeloablative therapy has shortened the time to hematological recovery as well as decreased the severity of some BMT-related toxicities.[114–126] In severe chronic neutropenic states, whether idiopathic, congenital, or cyclic, rhG-CSF administration has been effective in reducing the incidence and duration of infection and subsequent hospitalization, although the development of myelodysplasia after treatment has been reported.[127, 128] The use of rhG-CSF for priming of normal donors to increase the number of granulocytes harvested is under investigation.[114–126]

Macrophage (Monocyte) Colony-Stimulating Factor

M-CSF is a 47- to 90-kD, glycosylated polypeptide. The human M-CSF gene has been localized to the long arm of chromosome 5 at band q33.1. Alternative splicing of the principal gene transcript gives rise to several messenger RNAs encoding for M-CSF precursors of similar structure. Two identical protein subunits are linked by disulfide bonds to form the biologically active, homodimeric form. Various forms of M-CSF are produced through proteolysis of the intracellular domain, proximal to the membrane-anchoring segment. With the aid of mammalian expression systems, two different precursors have been identified. The principal soluble growth factor is 223 aa residues in length and is produced through proteolysis of a larger 554-aa precursor molecule. A second, biologically active precursor is a 256-aa membrane-bound protein.

The biological effects of M-CSF are facilitated through the interaction with its receptor, the product of c-Fms proto-oncogene (c-Fms).[129–133] The c-Fms receptor is an integral transmembrane glycoprotein containing intrinsic tyrosine kinase activity. The receptor is expressed with a density directly proportional to the degree of cellular differentiation. M-CSF receptor binding leads to internalization of the complex through a series of events. First, noncovalent receptor dimerization leads to transphosphorylation of specific residues on the receptor, followed by interaction with signaling proteins containing SH2 domains. This in turn leads to covalent dimerization and conformational changes, followed by tyrosine dephosphorylation and, finally, internalization of the receptor. In murine and human systems, the ligand-receptor interaction leads to tyrosine phosphorylation of other proteins, including PI-3 kinase, cCbl, SHP-1, and Tyk2, which subsequently activate various intracellular signaling pathways, including *ras*-dependent and *ras*-independent and JAK/STAT pathways. In human monocytes, M-CSF activates protein kinase C and phospholipase A_2 and increases GTPase activity. In addition, in murine macrophages, M-CSF enhances the activity of Na^+/H^+ exchange activity and cyclin D1 expression involved in cell cycle modulation.[132–144]

M-CSF is produced by bone marrow stromal cells. It promotes monocyte/macrophage proliferation and differentiation. It stimulates phagocytic and secretory functions of macrophages, enhances macrophage fungicidal and bactericidal activity, and stimulates antibody-dependent cytotoxicity. Although M-CSF increases intracellular production of TNF and IFN in monocytes, this activity does not seem related to its fungicidal activity.[145–148]

Administration of human recombinant M-CSF (rhM-CSF) to rats and nonhuman primates produces a significant increase in the number of circulating monocytes, and in monkeys an increase in monocyte antitumor antibody-dependent cell-mediated cytotoxicity (ADCC) activity has been demonstrated as well.[149] Administration of rhM-CSF to humans after chemotherapy led to increases in monocytes, neutrophils, and platelets, and a survival benefit was demonstrated in post-BMT patients with fungal disease. Because of overlap of major effects with GM-

CSF, M-CSF has no current clinical indication; however, its potential uses remain under investigation.[150, 151]

THROMBOPOIETIN

TPO is the physiological regulator of megakaryopoiesis. The protein contains 332 aa residues and a 21-aa signal peptide. The single-copy gene for human TPO has been localized to chromosome 3q26–27 and has structural similarities to the EPO gene, which suggests a common ancestral origin. TPO is synthesized primarily in the liver (small amounts may also be produced by the kidney) as a 38-kD protein that undergoes significant post-translational *O*-glycosylation and is secreted as a 90-kD glycoprotein. The N-terminal half of TPO contains an EPO-like domain that is 23% identical (50% homologous) with EPO and shares some similarity with α and β interferons. The C-terminal does not display significant sequence similarity to that of other proteins in the database. The EPO domain is responsible for the biological activity of TPO, and the heavily glycosylated C-terminal confers its stability in circulation. As platelets express high-affinity TPO receptors (c-mpl), which bind and clear TPO from the circulation, serum TPO levels are determined directly by the circulating platelet mass.[152–156]

Although much is known about the biological effects of TPO, there is very little information about the intracellular events triggered by the interaction of TPO with its receptor, c-mpl. It has been demonstrated that the binding of TPO to c-mpl induces tyrosine phosphorylation of several intracellular proteins, including JAK2, Shc, Tyk2, and c-mpl itself, as well as STAT3 and STAT5 proteins.[157, 158]

TPO has been shown to increase the number, size, and ploidy of megakaryocytes. It stimulates the production of lineage-specific progenitor cells (CFU-Meg), as well as precursors of other lineages (BFU-E and CFU-GEMM). Although it stimulates the growth of both early megakaryocyte progenitors and late megakaryocytes, it is not involved in the "shedding" of platelets from megakaryocytes, and in high enough concentrations, it may actually inhibit this process. Along with other cytokines, including GM-CSF, IL-3, IL-6, and EPO, TPO stimulates the proliferation and increases the survival of pluripotent stem cells. This synergy induces a multilineage effect: with EPO, it stimulates BFU-E and CFU-E proliferation; with GM-CSF, it effects early myeloid progenitor growth; and synergy with IL-3 increases the production of CFU-Meg, as well as megakaryocytic endomitosis and cytoplasmic maturation.[159–162]

The administration of TPO to nonhuman primates has been shown to increase CFU-Meg production in the bone marrow, followed by up to a 10-fold increase in circulating platelets. No significant effects on peripheral blood leukocyte or erythrocyte counts were noted. Although TPO produces dramatic increases in peripheral blood platelets, it only has a mild effect on platelet function; therefore, thrombogenesis is not enhanced by TPO administration.[163–165] Similarly, in human clinical trials, the administration of TPO produced increases in platelet production.[166, 168] There is a wide range of potential uses for thrombopoietin: TPO may reduce chemotherapy- and radiation-related thrombocytopenia[168]; it may aid in the treatment of hematological disorders with inherent thrombocytopenia, such as myelodysplastic syndromes, aplastic anemia, or other bone marrow failure states; and it may also decrease platelet requirements in patients with liver disease or in patients undergoing cardiovascular bypass or liver transplantation. In transfusion medicine, the use of TPO in donors could increase the yield of platelets in plateletpheresis and increase the yield of peripheral blood progenitors through synergism with other cytokines. Ex vivo, TPO could be used to increase platelet production and survival, as well as to enhance the expansion of peripheral blood or cord blood progenitors.[169]

OTHER HEMATOPOIETIC STIMULATORY CYTOKINES

Stem Cell Factor

Human stem cell factor (SCF) is encoded by a gene on chromosome 12q22–24. Alternative splicing at a key cleavage site gives rise to either the soluble (cleaved) form of SCF or the membrane-bound (noncleaved) form of SCF. Both forms of SCF are biologically active. Soluble SCF, a glycoprotein of approximately 18 kD, possesses a complex secondary structure and circulates as a dimer.[170, 171] Fibroblasts and endothelial cells both synthesize and release soluble SCF and express membrane-bound SCF. SCF is also produced by other cells, including intestinal epithelial cells, keratinocytes, and thymocytes.[172]

SCF exerts its hematopoietic activity through the interaction with its receptor, c-kit (CD117). The c-kit receptor is a 145-kD glycoprotein, possessing tyrosine kinase activity within its cytoplasmic tail. The binding of SCF to c-kit leads to receptor dimerization and tyrosine autophosphorylation, creating binding sites for SH2-containing proteins. A protein tyrosine phosphatase, SHP1, modulates the phosphorylation of substrates in the signal transduction pathway of SCF.[173–175]

The c-kit receptor is widely expressed on hematopoietic cells with the greatest density on immature cells. The hematopoietic progenitor cells expressing the c-kit receptor give rise to increased numbers of multilineage CFUs and long-term bone marrow culture–initiating cells (LTBMC-IC).[176] In vitro, SCF demonstrates synergy with other hematopoietic growth factors, including GM-CSF, G-CSF, and IL-3, stimulating the proliferation and differentiation of all lineages.[177, 178]

The synergistic activity of SCF has also been observed in animal models, in which cytokine combinations that include SCF increased the number of peripheral blood progenitor cells and enhanced engraftment in transplanted animals. In phase I and II clinical trials, the administration of cytokine combinations produced a higher yield of peripheral blood progenitors than did SCF alone. The use of SCF has been limited because of its significant adverse effects: mast cell degranulation, severe allergic reactions, and increased skin pigmentation. SCF-primed hematopoietic cells are more easily transduced by retroviral vectors; thus, it may be potentially useful in gene therapy. Ex vivo expansion of progenitor cells could also be enhanced by exposure to SCF alone or in combination with other cytokines.[179–182]

Flt-3 Ligand

Flt-3 ligand exerts its effects on hematopoietic cells through a tyrosine kinase receptor, Flt-3 (also Flk-2, Stk-1), in much the same way as SCF interacts with c-kit and M-CSF with c-Fms. Flt-3 receptors are expressed only on the surface of $CD34^+$ bone marrow progenitors. The gene for Flt-3 ligand has been mapped to chromosome 13q12–13.[183–185]

In vitro, the greatest effect of Flt-3 ligand is exerted on the primitive hematopoietic progenitors with only a moderate effect on lineage-committed progenitors. On primitive progenitors, it exerts an expansion effect, whereas the effect on more differentiated progenitors is limited to an increase in CFU-GM and monocytic precursors and enhanced growth of B cell precursors. The administration of Flt-3 ligand to mice produced a dramatic increase in bone marrow and peripheral blood CFUs, specifically CFU-GM, CFU-GEMM, and BFU-E. In vivo, Flt-3 ligand exhibits synergy with other cytokines, including IL-3, SCF, IL-11, IL-6, and IL-7, to further enhance lymphohematopoiesis. In mice, synergy of Flt-3 ligand with G-CSF increases peripheral blood stem cell (PBSC) mobilization, and Flt-3 ligand in combination with either G-CSF or GM-CSF may exert an antiapoptotic effect by preventing upregulation of Bax. The capability of Flt-3 ligand to expand hematopoietic progenitors ex vivo may be of benefit in the transplantation setting. In addition, its ability to recruit early progenitors into cell cycle could increase the efficiency of retroviral transduction of hematopoietic progenitors.[186–197]

Interleukin-3

Human IL-3 is a 140-aa glycoprotein with a molecular weight between 14 and 28 kD, depending upon the degree of glycosylation. The gene encoding human IL-3 has been mapped to chromosome 5q, just upstream of the gene for GM-CSF. Disulfide bonds stabilize the molecule, which possesses two active sites for binding with its receptor. In humans, activated T cells are the major source of IL-3.[198, 199]

Like the IL-5 and GM-CSF receptors, the IL-3 receptor is a heterodimer that binds the ligand with high affinity. It is expressed on a variety of normal hematopoietic cells of varying degrees of maturation, with the exception of mature neutrophils and malignant hematopoietic cells.[200] The signal transduction pathway involves the activation of the JAK2 tyrosine kinase and STAT5 proteins (and, to a lesser degree, STAT1 and STAT3) and the induction of c-myc, as well as the activation of the *ras* pathway. IL-3 signaling regulates the cell cycle, triggering DNA synthesis and inhibiting apoptosis.[201]

IL-3 has been shown to have a multilineage effect, stimulating erythropoiesis, myelopoiesis, and megakaryocytopoiesis in animal models and in human clinical trials.[202, 203] The synergism of IL-3 and GM-CSF was initially observed in primates and later demonstrated in clinical trials with humans.[204, 205] The in vivo synergism and cross-competition for receptor sites lead to development of a GM-CSF/IL-3 fusion protein known as PIXY321. PIXY321, in both preclinical studies and clinical trials, demonstrated more hematopoietic activity than did either cytokine alone.[206, 207]

Interleukin-6

The gene for human IL-6 has been localized to chromosome 7. Human IL-6, a single-chain 212-aa glycoprotein, has a molecular weight of 26 kD and shows significant genetic and structural homology with G-CSF.[208, 209] The receptor for IL-6 contains an α and a β subunit. The structure of the ligand-binding chain (gp80) is unique to IL-6, whereas the β subunit (gp130) is common to the cytokines in this group (IL-11 and others). IL-6 receptor is expressed on various cells of hematopoietic and nonhematopoietic origin. The signal transduction cascade involves accessory intracellular kinases and JAK-Tyk that may lead to the activation of STAT3 proteins.[210, 211]

The effect on the differentiation of the myeloid lineage is primarily synergistic with other cytokines, including IL-3, GM-CSF, and M-CSF. IL-6 synergizes with IL-1 and IL-2 to induce T cell proliferation, control the development of memory T cells, and enhance the cytotoxicity of natural killer cells. It induces the differentiation of B cells into plasma cells and increases their immunoglobulin secretion. The anti-inflammatory activity of IL-6 results from several effects: inhibition of IL-1– and TNF-α–induced synthesis of lipopolysaccharide; induction of tissue inhibitor of metalloproteinase (TIM) synthesis, which has anti-inflammatory activity; inhibition of phospholipase A_2; and induction of glucocorticoid synthesis.[212, 213] IL-6 may possess osteoclastic activity,[214] and there is evidence that it may function as a cachectin.[215] In animal models, IL-6 administration has produced an increase in platelet production and enhanced the recovery of hematopoietic and immune systems in mice treated with 5-fluorouracil. Phase I and II clinical trials of IL-6, either alone or in combination with G-CSF, demonstrated a hastened platelet recovery time in cancer patients receiving chemotherapy. With the development of human recombinant TPO and IL-11, the IL-6 effect on platelet production may be of less clinical significance than its other biological effects, including immunomodulatory and antitumor effects.[216–220]

IMMUNOMODULATORY CYTOKINES

It is well recognized that a variety of cytokines regulate the immune system through numerous mechanisms. Cytokines stimulate the proliferation and differentiation of hematolymphopoietic cells, activate and enhance the function of effector cells, induce primary T and B cell responses, facilitate antigen presentation, and modulate the expression of cellular adhesion molecules. IL-2 induces the proliferation and activation of T and B lymphocytes and natural killer cells and, together with IL-1, induces T lymphocytes to express interferon-γ. Mutation of IL-2 receptor leads to an immunodeficiency state with lymphocytopenia.[221–223] IL-7 is produced by thymic and bone marrow stroma and is essential in the proliferation and differentiation of T lymphocytes.

IL-7 has been shown to accelerate thymic reconstitution in mice after BMT.[224, 225] IL-4 is produced by T cells, mast cells, and basophils. IL-4 promotes the growth of B cells and modulates antigen presentation. IL-4 also increases the proliferation of T cells and induces differentiation toward the Th2 phenotype, which in turn modulates allergic and cell-associated immune responses.[226–228] IL-13 stimulates B cell growth and immunoglobulin isotype switching, as well as modulating the activity of adhesion molecules.[229] IL-16 promotes proliferation and chemotaxis of T cells, monocytes, and eosinophils; induces cytokine synthesis in target cells; and modulates cell adhesion molecule interactions and expression of certain cell surface receptors.[230]

IL-12 is a 75-kD heterodimer composed of two chains: p35 and p40. It is produced constitutively by macrophages, dendritic cells, and B cells and is also induced by a variety of pathogens, including *Leishmania major, Mycobacterium tuberculosis,* and *Toxoplasma gondii.*[231] The β_1 chain of the IL-12 receptor has low-affinity ligand-binding activity; however, when coupled with the β_2 chain, it forms the high-affinity IL-12 receptor. The signal transduction pathway involves the interaction of one chain with JAK2 and β2 subunit with Tyk2 and subsequent tyrosine and serine phosphorylation of STAT3 and STAT4 proteins.[232]

IL-12 is an important regulator of cell-mediated immune responses. It promotes the differentiation of Th1 cells and enhances the production of interferon-γ while inhibiting Th2 responses. In murine tumor models, IL-12 reduced the tumor burden and slowed the growth of tumor.[233, 234] Phase I and II human clinical trials with IL-12, however, have demonstrated serious toxic effects.[235]

REFERENCES

1. Dexter T, Testa N. Differentiation and proliferation of hematopoietic cells in culture. Methods Cell Biol 1976; 14:387.
2. Civin IC, Strauss LC, Brovall C, et al. Antigenic analysis of hematopoiesis: III. A hematopoietic progenitor cell surface antigen defined by monoclonal antibody raised against KG-1a cells. J Immunol 1984; 133:157.
3. Uchida N, Weissman IL. Searching for hematopoietic stem cells: evidence that Thy 1-1^{lo} Lin-Sca 1$^+$ cells are the only stem cells in C 57 BL/Ka-Thy 1.1^{lo} bone marrow. J Exp Med 1992; 175:175.
4. Sovalat H, Liang H, Wunder E, Henon P. Flow cytometry characterization of CD34$^+$ cells in bone marrow, cytopheresis products and cord blood at birth. Int J Cell Cloning 1992; 10(suppl 1):20.
5. Civin IC, Loken MR. Cell surface antigens on human marrow cells: dissection of hematopoietic development using monoclonal antibodies and multiparameter flow cytometry. Int J Cell 1987; 5:267.
6. Andrews RG, Singer JW, Bernstein ID. Monoclonal antibody 12-8 recognizes a 115-kd molecule present on both unipotent and multipotent hematopoietic colony-forming cells and their precursors. Blood 1986; 67:842.
7. Hemler ME. Adhesive protein receptors on hematopoietic cells. Immunol Today 1988; 9:109.
8. Albelda SM, Buck CA. Integrins and other cell adhesion molecules. FASEB J 1990; 4:2868.
9. Springer TA: Adhesion receptors of the immune system. Nature 1990; 346:425.
10. Whetton AD, Dexter TM. Influence of growth factors and substrates on differentiation of hemopoietic stem cells. Curr Opin Cell Biol 1993; 5:1044.
11. Jacobsen SEW, Ruscetti FW, Ortiz M, et al. The growth response of Lin-Thy-1$^+$ hematopoietic progenitors to cytokines is determined by the balance between synergy of multiple stimulators and negative cooperation of multiple inhibitors. Exp Hemat 1994; 22:985.
12. Metcalf D. Hematopoietic regulators: redundancy or subtlety? Blood 1993; 82:3515.
13. Pech N, Hermine O, Goldwasser E. Further study of internal autocrine regulation of multipotent hematopoietic cells. Blood 1993; 82:1502.
14. Cluitmans FHM, Esendam BHJ, Veenhof WFJ, et al. The role of cytokines and hematopoietic growth factors in the autocrine/paracrine regulation of inducible hematopoiesis. Ann Hematol 1997; 75:27.
15. Metcalf D. Hematopoietic regulators: redundancy or subtlety? Blood 1993; 82:3515.
16. Cosman D, Lyman SD, Rejean L, et al. A new cytokine receptor superfamily. Trends Biochem Sci 1990; 15:265.
17. Testa U, Pelosi M, Gabbianelli M, et al. Cascade transactivation of growth factor receptors in early human hematopoiesis. Blood 1993; 81:1442.
18. Miyajima A, Mui AL, Ogorochi T, Sakamaki K. Receptors for granulocyte-macrophage colony stimulating factor, interleukin-3 and interleukin-5. Blood 1993; 82:1960.
19. Woodcock JM, Bagley CJ, Lopez AF. Receptors of the cytokine superfamily: mechanisms of activation and involvement in disease. Ballière's Clin Haematol 1997; 10:507.
20. O'Shea JJ. Jaks, STATs, cytokine signal transduction, and immunoregulation: are we there yet? Immunity 1997; 7:1.
21. Pellegrini S, Dusanter-Fourt I. The structure, regulation and function of the Janus kinases (JAKs) and the signal transducers and activators of transcription (STATs). Eur J Biochem 1997; 248:615.
22. D'Andrea AD, Lodish HF, Wong GG. Expression cloning of the murine erythropoietin receptor. Cell 1989; 57:277.
23. Law ML, Cai GY, Lin FK, et al. Chromosomal assignment of the human erythropoietin gene and its DNA polymorphism. Proc Natl Acad Sci U S A 1986; 83:6920.
24. Shoemaker CB, Mitsock LD. Murine erythropoietin gene: cloning, expression and gene homology. Mol Cell Biol 1986; 6:849.
25. Koury ST, Bondurant MC, Koury MJ. Localization of erythropoietin synthesizing cells in murine kidneys by in situ hybridization. Blood 1988; 71:524.
26. Bondurant MC, Koury MJ. Anemia induces accumulation of erythropoietin mRNA in the kidney and liver. Mol Cell Biol 1986; 6:2731.
27. Schuster SJ, Badiavas EV, Costa-Giomi P, et al. Stimulation of erythropoietin gene transcription during hypoxia and cobalt exposure. Blood 1989; 73:1316.
28. Koury ST, Koury MJ, Bondurant MC, et al. Quantitation of erythropoietin-producing cells in kidneys of mice by in situ hybridization: correlation with hematocrit, renal erythropoietin mRNA, and serum erythropoietin concentration. Blood 1989; 74:645.
29. Erslev AJ. Erythropoietin titers in health and disease. Semin Hematol 1991; 28:2.
30. Goldwasser E, Kung CKH, Eliason J. On the mechanism of erythropoietin-induced differentiation: XIII. The role of sialic acid in erythropoietin action. J Biol Chem 1974; 249:4202.
31. Krantz SB. Erythropoietin. Blood 1991; 77:419.
32. Youssoufian H, Longmore G, Neumann D, et al. Structure, function, and activation of the erythropoietin receptor. Blood 1993; 81:2223.
33. Klingmuller U. The role of tyrosine phosphorylation in proliferation and maturation of erythroid progenitor cells. Signals emanating from the erythropoietin receptor. Eur J Biochem 1997; 249:637.
34. Spivak JL. The mechanisms of action of erythropoietin. Int J Cell Cloning 1986; 4:139.
35. Kelley LL, Koury MJ, Bondurant MC, et al. Survival or death

of individual proerythoblasts results from differing erythropoietin sensitivities. A mechanism for controlled rates of erythrocyte production. Blood 1993; 82:2340.
36. Papayannopoulou T, Finch CA. On the in vivo action of erythropoietin: a quantitative analysis. J Clin Invest 1972; 51:1179.
37. Eschbach JW, Egrie JC, Downing MR, et al. Correction of the anemia of end-stage renal disease with recombinant human erythropoietin. Results of a combined phase I and II clinical trial. N Engl J Med 1987; 316:73.
38. Miller CB, Platanias LC, Mills SR, et al. Phase I–II trial of erythropoietin in the treatment of cisplatin-associated anemia. J Natl Cancer Inst 1992; 84:98.
39. Oster W, Herrmann F, Gamm H, et al. Erythropoietin for the treatment of anemia of malignancy associated with neoplastic bone marrow infiltration. J Clin Oncol 1990; 8:956.
40. Pangalis GA, Poziopoulos C, Panayiotidis P, et al. Treatment of anemia in B–chronic lymphocyte leukemia (B-CLL) with recombinant human erythropoietin. Blood 1993; 82(S1):574a.
41. Platanias LC, Miller CB, Mick R, et al. Treatment of chemotherapy-induced anemia with recombinant human erythropoietin in cancer patients. J Clin Oncol 1991; 11:2021.
42. Fischl M, Galpin JE, Levine JD, et al. Recombinant human erythropoietin for patients with AIDS treated with zidovudine. N Engl J Med 1990; 322:1488.
43. Klaesson S, Ringden O, Ljungman P, et al. Reduced blood transfusion requirements after allogeneic bone marrow transplantation: results of a randomized double-blind study with high-dose erythropoietin. Bone Marrow Transplant 1994; 13:397.
44. Steegmann JL, Lopez J, Otero MJ, et al. Erythropoietin treatment in allogeneic BMT accelerates erythroid reconstitution: results of prospective controlled randomized trial. Bone Marrow Transplant 1992; 10:541.
45. Guadiani VA, Mason HD. Preoperative erythropoietin in Jehovah's Witnesses who require cardiac procedures. Ann Thorac Surg 1991; 51:823.
46. Mercuriali F, Zanella A, Barosi G, et al. Use of erythropoietin to increase the volume of autologous blood donation by anemic rheumatoid arthritis patients undergoing major orthopedic surgery. Transfusion 1993; 33:55.
47. Mitus AJ, Antin JH, Rutherford CJ, et al. Use of recombinant human erythropoietin in allogeneic bone marrow transplant donor/recipient pairs. Blood 1994; 83:1952.
48. Bernell P, Hippe E, Wallvik J, et al. Erythropoietin resistant myelodysplastic syndromes may respond when erythropoietin is used in combination with granulocyte-macrophage colony-stimulating factor. Br J Haematol 1994; 87(S1):152a.
49. List AL, Noyes W, Power J, et al. Combined treatment of myelodysplastic syndromes (MDS) with recombinant human interleukin-3 (IL-3) and erythropoietin (EPO). Blood 1993; 82(S1):377a.
50. Ishibashi T, Noji H, Nakazato K, et al. Erythropoietin increased platelet count in two patients with severe aplastic anemia. Blood 1993; 82(S1):501a.
51. de Andrade JR, Jove M. Baseline hemoglobin as a predictor of risk of transfusion and response to epoetin alpha in orthopedic surgery patients. Am J Orthop 1996; 25:533.
52. Goldberg MA, McCutchen JW. A safety and efficacy comparison study of two dosing regimens of epoetin alpha in patients undergoing major orthopedic surgery. Am J Orthoped 1996; 25:544.
53. Faris PM, Ritter MA. The effects of recombinant human erythropoietin on perioperative transfusion requirements in patients having a major orthopaedic operation. J Bone Joint Surg 1996; 78:62.
54. Pincus T, Olsen NJ, Russell IJ, et al. Multicenter study of recombinant human erythropoietin in correction of anemia in rheumatoid arthritis. Am J Med 1990; 89:161.
55. Steegmann JL, Lopez J, Otero MJ, et al. Erythropoietin treatment in allogeneic BMT accelerates erythroid reconstitution: results of prospective controlled randomized trial. Bone Marrow Transplant 1992; 10:541.
56. Vannucchi AM, Bosi A, Grossi A, et al. Stimulation of erythroid engraftation by recombinant human erythropoietin in ABO-compatible, HLA-identical, allogeneic bone marrow transplant patients. Leukemia 1992; 6:215.
57. Phibbs RH, Keith JF. Recombinant human erythropoietin stimulates erythropoiesis and reduces transfusions in preterm infants. Pediatr Res 1994; 35:248a.
58. Rodgers GP, Dover GJ Uyesaka N, et al. Augmentation by erythropoietin of the fetal-hemoglobin response to hydroxyurea in sickle cell disease. N Engl J Med 1993; 328:73.
59. Rodgers GP, Lessin LS. Recombinant erythropoietin improves the anemia associated with Gaucher's disease. Blood 1989; 73:2228.
60. Rachmilewitz EA, Goldfarb A, Dover G. Administration of erythropoietin to patients with β-thalassemia intermedia: a preliminary trial. Blood 1991; 78:1145.
61. Messer J, Haddad J, Donato L, et al. Early treatment of premature infants with recombinant human erythropoietin. Pediatrics 1993; 92:519.
62. Ayash LJ, Elias A, Hunt M, et al. Recombinant human erythropoietin for the treatment of the anaemia associated with autologous bone marrow transplantion. Br J Haematol 1994; 87:153.
63. Weisbart RH, Golde DW. Physiology of granulocyte and macrophage colony-stimulating factors in host defense. Hematol Oncol Clin North Am 1989; 3:401.
64. Kaushansky K, Karplus PA. Hematopoietic growth factors: understanding functional diversity in structural terms. Blood 1993; 82:3229.
65. Miyajima A, Mui AL-F, Ogorochi T, et al. Receptors for granulocyte-macrophage colony-stimulating factor, interleukin-3, and interleukin-5. Blood 1993; 82:1960.
66. Li W, Stanley ER. Role of dimerization and modification of the CSF-1 receptor in its activation and internalization during the CSF-1 response. EMBO J 1991; 10:277.
67. DiPersio JF, Hedvat C, Ford CF, et al. Characterization of the soluble human granulocyte-macrophage colony-stimulating factor receptor complex. J Biol Chem 1991; 266:279.
68. Walker F, Nicola NA, Metcalf D, Burgess AW. Hierarchical down-modulation of hematopoietic growth factor receptors. Cell 1985; 43:269.
69. Lopez AF, Eglinton JM, Lyons AB, et al. Human interleukin-3 inhibits the binding of granulocyte-macrophage colony-stimulating factor and interleukin-5 to basophils and strongly enhances their functional activity. J Cell Physiol 1990; 145:69.
70. Lopez AF, Elliott MJ, Woodcock J, et al. GM-CSF, IL-3 and IL-5: cross-competition on human haematopoietic cells. Immunol Today 1992; 13:495.
71. Yang YC, Kovacic S, Kriz R, et al. The human gene for GM-CSF and IL-3 are closely linked in tandem on chromosome 5. Blood 1988; 71:958.
72. Layton JE, Hockman H, Sheridan WP, Morstyn G. Evidence for a novel in vivo control mechanism of granulopoiesis: mature cell–related control of a regulatory growth factor. Blood 1989; 74:1303.
73. Gearing DP, King JA, Gough NM, Nicola NA. Expression cloning of a receptor for human granulocyte-macrophage colony-stimulating factor. EMBO J 1989; 8:3667.
74. Hayashida K, Kitamura T, Gorman DM, et al. Molecular cloning of a second subunit of the receptor for human granulocyte-macrophage colony-stimulating factor (GM-CSF): reconstitution of a high-affinity GM-CSF receptor. Proc Natl Acad Sci U S A 1990; 87:9655.
75. Cannistra S, Grosheck P, Garlick R, et al. Regulation of surface expression of the granulocyte/macrophage colony-stimulating factor receptor in normal human myeloid cells. Proc Natl Acad Sci U S A 1990; 87:93.
76. Bussolino F, Wang J, Defilippi P, et al. Granulocyte and granulocyte-macrophage colony-stimulating factor induce human endothelial cells to migrate and proliferate. Nature 1989; 337:471.
77. Baldwin G, Gasson J, Kaufman S, et al. Non-hematopoietic tumor cells express functional GM-CSF receptors. Blood 1989; 73:1033.
78. Berdel W, Danhauser-Riedl S, Steinhauser G, et al. Various human hematopoietic growth factors (interleukin-3, GM-CSF, G-CSF) stimulate clonal growth of nonhematopoietic tumor cells. Blood 1989; 73:80.
79. Dedhar S, Gaboury L, Galloway P, et al. Human granulocyte-macrophage colony-stimulating factor is a growth factor active on a variety of cell types of nonhematopoietic origin. Proc Natl Acad Sci U S A 1988; 85:9253.
80. Gomez-Cambronero J, Veatch C. Emerging paradigms in granulocyte-macrophage colony-stimulating factor signaling. Life Sci 1996; 59:2099.
81. Metcalf D, Johnson G, Burgess A. Direct stimulation by purified

GM-CSF of the proliferation of multipotential and erythroid precursors cells. Blood 1980; 55:138.
82. Metcalf D, Burgess A, Johnson G, et al. In vitro actions on hematopoietic cells of recombinant murine GM-CSF purified after production in *Escherichia coli:* comparison with purified native GM-CSF. J Cell Physiol 1986; 128:421.
83. Walker F, Nicola N, Metcalf D, et al. Hierarchical down-modulation of hematopoietic growth factor receptors. Cell 1985; 43:269.
84. Brach MA, deVos S, Gross H, et al. Prolongation of survival of human polymorphonuclear neutrophils by granulocyte macrophage colony-stimulating factor is caused by inhibition of programmed cell death. Blood 1992; 80:2920.
85. Gasson J, Weisbart R, Kaufman S, et al. Purified human granulocyte-macrophage colony-stimulating factor: direct action on neutophils. Science 1984; 226:1339.
86. Griffin J, Spertini O, Ernst T, et al. Granulocyte-macrophage colony-stimulating factor and other cytokines regulate surface expression of leukocyte adhesion molecule-1 on human neutrophils, monocytes and their precursors. J Immunol 1990; 145:576.
87. Fleischmann J, Golde D, Weibart R, et al. Granulocyte-macrophage colony-stimulating factor enhances phagocytosis of bacteria by human neutrophils. Blood 1986; 68:708.
88. Villalta F, Kierszenbaum F. Effects of human colony-stimulating factor on the uptake and destruction of a pathogenic parasite *(Trypanosoma cruzi)* by human neutrophils. J Immunol 1986; 137:1703.
89. Arnaout M, Wang E, Clark S, et al. Human recombinant granulocyte-macrophage colony-stimulating factor increases cell-to-cell adhesion and surface expression of adhesion-promoting surface glycoproteins on mature granulocytes. J Clin Invest 1986; 78:597.
90. Cannistra S, Vellenga E, Groshek P, et al: Human granulocyte-monocyte colony-stimulating factor and interleukin-3 stimulate monocyte cytotoxicity through a tumor necrosis factor–dependent mechanism. Blood 1988; 71:672.
91. Schwartz EL, Maher AM. Enhanced mitogenic responsiveness to granulocyte-macrophage colony-stimulating factor in HL-60 promyelocytic leukemia cells upon induction of differentiation. Cancer Res 1988; 48:2683.
92. Bussolino F, Ziche M, Wang J, et al. In vitro and in vivo activation of endothelial cells by colony-stimulating factors. J Clin Invest 1991; 87:986.
93. Cebon J, Layton JE, Maher D, Morstyn G. Endogenous haematopoietic growth factors in neutropenia and infection. Br J Haematol 1994; 86:265.
94. Spitzer G, Adkins DR, Spencer V, et al. Randomized study of growth factors post–peripheral-blood stem-cell transplant: neutrophil recovery is improved with modest clinical benefit. J Clin Oncol 1994; 12:661.
95. Estey E, Thall P, Andreef M, et al. Use of granulocyte colony stimulating factor before, during, and after fludarabine plus cytarabine induction therapy of newly diagnosed acute myelogenous leukemia or myelodysplastic syndromes: comparison with fludarabine plus cytarabine without granulocyte colony-stimulating factor. J Clin Oncol 1994; 12:671.
96. Gulati SC, Bennett C. Role of granulocyte-macrophage colony-stimulating factor (GM-CSF) after autologous BMT for Hodgkin's disese. Ann Intern Med 1992; 116:177.
97. Hornung RL, Longo DL. Hematopoietic stem cell depletion by restorative growth factor regimens during repeated high-dose cyclophosphamide therapy. Blood 1992; 80:77.
98. Brugger W, Bross K, Fisch J, et al. Mobilization of peripheral blood progenitor cells by sequential administration of interleukin-3 and granulocyte-macrophage colony-stimulating factor following polychemotherapy with etoposide, ifosfamide, and cisplatin. Blood 1992; 79:1193.
99. Nemunaitis J, Rosenfeld C, Ash R, et al. Phase III double-blind trial of rhGM-CSF (sargramostim) following allogeneic bone marrow transplant (BMT). Blood 1993; 82(S1):286a.
100. Triozzi PL. Autologous bone marow and peripheral blood progenitor transplant for breast cancer. Lancet 1994; 344:418.
101. Tarella C, Ferrero D, Bregni M, et al. Peripheral blood expansion of early progenitor cells after high-dose cyclophosphamide and rhGM-CSF. Eur J Cancer 1991; 27:22.
102. Socinski MA, Cannistra S, Elias A, et al. Granulocyte-macrophage colony-stimulating factor expands the circulating haematopoietic progenitor cell compartment in man. Lancet 1988; 1(8596):1194.
103. Goodnough LT, Anderson KC, Kurtz S: Indications and guidelines for the use of hematopoietic growth factors. Committee report. Transfusion 1993; 33:944.
104. Haycock DN, To LB, Dowse TL, et al. Ex vivo expansion and maturation of peripheral blood stem and progenitor cells for transplantation [Abstract]. Blood 1993; 82(S1):483a.
105. Holyoake TL, Franklin IM. Bone marrow transplants from peripheral blood. BMJ 1994; 309:4.
106. Ketley NJ, Newland AC. Haemopoietic growth factors. Postgrad Med J 1997; 73:215.
107. Le Beau M, Lemons R, Carrino J, et al: Chromosomal localization of the human G-CSF gene to 17q11 proximal to the breakpoint of the t(15;17) in acute promyelocytic leukemia. Leukemia 1987; 1:795.
108. Pauksen K, Elfman L, Ulfgren AK, Venge P. Serum levels of granulocyte-colony stimulating factor (G-CSF) in bacterial and viral infections, and in atypical pneumonia. Br J Haematol 1994; 88:256.
109. Demetri GD, Griffin JD. Granulocyte colony-stimulating factor and its receptor. Blood 1991; 78:2791.
110. Nathan CF. Respiratory burst in adherent human neutrophils: triggering by colony-stimulating factors CSF-GM and CSF-G. Blood 1989; 73:301.
111. Lieschke GJ, Burgess AW. Granulocyte colony-stimulating factor and granulocyte-macrophage colony-stimulating factor (Part I). N Engl J Med 1992; 327:28.
112. Lieschke GJ, Burgess AW. Granulocyte colony-stimulating factor and granulocyte-macrophage colony-stimulating factor (Part II). N Engl J Med 1992; 327:99.
113. Ikebuchi K, Ihle JN, Hirai Y, et al. Synergistic factors for stem cell proliferation: further studies of the target stem cells and the mechanism of stimulation by interleukin-1, interleukin-6, and granulocyte colony-stimulating factor. Blood 1988; 72:2007.
114. Crawford J, Ozer H, Stoller R, et al. Reduction by granulocyte colony-stimulating factor of fever and neutropenia induced by chemotherapy in patients with small-cell lung cancer. N Engl J Med 1991; 315:164.
115. Gabrilove JL, Jakubowski A, Scher H, et al. Effect of granulocyte colony-stimulating factor on neutropenia and associated morbidity due to chemotherapy for transitional cell carcinoma of the urothelium. N Engl J Med 1988; 318:1414.
116. Miles DW, Fogarty O, Ash CM, et al. Received dose intensity: a randomized trial of weekly chemotherapy with and without granulocyte colony-stimulating factor in small-cell lung cancer. J Clin Oncol 1994; 12:77.
117. Neidhart J, Mangalik K, Kohler W, et al. Granulocyte colony-stimulating factor stimulates recovery of granulocytes in patients receiving dose-intensive chemotherapy without bone-marrow transplantation. J Clin Oncol 1989; 7:1685.
118. Gisselbrecht C, Prentice HG, Bacigalupo A, et al. Placebo-controlled phase III trial of lenograstim in bone marrow transplantation. Lancet 1994; 343:696.
119. Schuening FG, Lilleby K, Clift RA, et al. Phase I study of rhG-CSF after marrow transplantation from HLA-identical siblings. Blood 1993; 82(S1):349a.
120. Sheridan WP, Morstyn G, Wolf M, et al. Granulocyte colony-stimulating factor and neutrophil recovery after high-dose chemotherapy and autologous bone marrow transplantation. Lancet 1989; 2:891.
121. Sheridan WP, Morstyn G, Wolf M, et al. Granulocyte colony-stimulating factor and neutrophil recovery after high-dose chemotherapy and autologous bone marrow transplantation. Lancet 1989; 2:891.
122. Duhrsen U, Villeval JL, Boyd J, et al. Effects of recombinant human granulocyte colony-stimulating factor on hematopoietic progenitor cells in cancer patients. Blood 1988; 72:2074.
123. Peters WP, Rosner G, Ross M, et al. Comparative effects of granulocyte-macrophage colony-stimulating factor (GM-CSF) and granulocyte colony-stimulating factor (G-CSF) on priming peripheral blood progenitor cells for use with autologous bone marrow after high dose chemotherapy. Blood 1993; 81:1709.
124. Bensinger W, Singer J, Applebaum F, et al. Autologous tranplantation with peripheral blood mononuclear cells collected after administration of recombinant granulocyte stimulating factor. Blood 1993; 81:3158.

125. Bensinger WI, Price TH, Dale DC, et al. The effects of daily recombinant human granulocyte colony-stimulating factor administration on normal granulocyte donors undergoing leukapheresis. Blood 1993; 81:1883.
126. Caspar CB, Seger RA, Del Ferro E, et al. Effective stimulation of donors for granulocyte transfusions with recombinant methionyl granulocyte colony-stimulating factor. Blood 1993; 81:2866.
127. Dale DC, Bonilla MA, Davis MW, et al. A randomized controlled phase III trial of recombinant human granulocyte colony-stimulating factor (filgrastim) for treatment of severe chronic neutropenia. Blood 1193; 81:2496.
128. Hashimi IA, Wang H, Saunders EF, et al. G-CSF therapy, congenital neutropenia and the development of myelodysplastic syndrome with monosomy 7. Blood 1993; 82(suppl 1):551a.
129. Das S, Stanley E. Structure-function studies of a colony-stimulating factor (CSF-1). J Biol Chem 1982; 257:13679.
130. Pettenati M, Le Beau M, Lemons R, et al. Assignment of CSF-1 to 5q33.1: evidence for clustering of genes regulating hematopoiesis and for their involvement in the deletion of the long arm of chromosome 5 in myeloid disorders. Proc Natl Acad Sci U S A 1987; 84:2970.
131. Ladner MB, Martin GA, Noble JA, et al. Human CSF-1: gene structure and alternative splicing of mRNA precursors. EMBO J 1987; 6:2693.
132. Rettenmier CW, Roussel MF. Differential processing of colony-stimulating factor 1 precursors encoded by two human cDNAs. Mol Cell Biol 1988; 8:5026.
133. Sherr C, Rettenmier C, Sacca R, et al. The c-fms proto-oncogene product is related to the receptor for the mononuclear phagocyte growth factor, CSF-1. Cell 1985; 41:665.
134. Li W, Stanley ER. Role of dimerization and modification of the CSF-1 receptor in its activation and internalization during CSF-1 response. Eur Mol Biol J 1991; 10:277.
135. Imamura K, Dianoux A, Nakamura T, et al. Colony-stimulating factor 1 activates protein kinase C in human monocytes. Eur Mol Org J 1990; 9:2423.
136. Nakamura T, Lin L-L, Kharbanda S, et al. Macrophage colony stimulating factor activates phosphatidylcholine hydrolysis of cytoplasmic phospholipase A_2. Eur Mol Biol Org J 1992; 11:4917.
137. Vairo G, Argyriou S, Bordun A-M, et al. Na^+/H^+ exchange involvement in colony-stimulating factor-1–stimulated macrophage proliferation. Evidence for a requirement during late G_1 of the cell cycle but not for early growth factor responses. J Biol Chem 1990; 265:16929.
138. Vadiveloo PK, Vairo G, Novak U, et al. Differential regulation of cell cycle machinery by various antiproliferative agents is linked to macrophage arrest at distinct G_1 checkpoints. Oncogene 1996; 13:599.
139. Yusoff P, Hamilton JA, Nolan RD, Phillips WA. Haematopoietic colony stimulating factors CSF-1 and GM-CSF increase phosphatidylinositol 3 kinase activity in murine bone marrow-derived macrophages. Growth Factors 1994; 10:191.
140. Kanagasundaram V, Jaworowski A, Hamilton JA. Association between phosphatidylinositol-3 kinase, Cbl and other tyrosine proteins in CSF-1 stimulated macrophages. Biochem J 1996; 320:69.
141. Sengupta A, Liu WK, Yeung DC, et al. Identification and subcellular localization of proteins that are rapidly phosphorylated in tyrosine response to colony stimulating factor 1. Proc Natl Acad Sci U S A 1988; 85:8062.
142. Chen HE, Chang S, Trub T, et al. Regulation of colony-stimulating factor-1 receptor signaling by the SH2 domain-containg tyrosine phosphatase SHPTP1. Mol Cell Biol 1996; 16:3685.
143. Novak U, Harpur AG, Paradiso L, et al. CSF-1-induced STAT1 and STAT3 activation is accompanied by phosphorylation of Tyk2 in macrophages and Tyk2 and JAK1 in fibroblasts. Blood 1995; 86:2948.
144. Buscher D, Hipskind RA, Krautwald S, et al. Ras-dependent and independent pathways target the mitogen-activated protein kinase network in macrophages. Mol Cell Biol 1995; 15:466.
145. Guilbert L, Stanley E. Specific interaction of murine colony stimulating factor with mononuclear phagocytic cells. J Cell Biol 1980; 85:153.
146. Stein J, Borzillo GV, Rettenmier C. Direct stimulation of cells expressing receptors for macrophage colony-stimulating factor (CSF-1) by a plasma membrane-bound precursor of human CSF-1. Blood 1990; 76:1308.
147. Karbassi H, Becker J, Foster J, et al. Enhanced killing of *Candida albicans* by murine macrophages treated with macrophage colony-stimulating factor: evidence for augmented expression of mannose receptors. J Immunol 1987; 139:417.
148. Warren MK, Ralph P. Macrophage growth factor CSF-1 stimulates human monocyte production of interferon, tumor necrosis factor, and colony stimulating activity. J Immunol 1986; 148:2281.
149. Khwaja A, Johnson B, Addison IE, et al. In vivo effects of macrophage colony-stimulating factor on human monocyte function. Br J Haematol 1991; 77:25.
150. Motoyoshi K. Macrophage colony-stimulating factor for cancer therapy. Oncology 1994; 51:198.
151. Nemunaitis J, Myers JD, Buckner CD, et al. Phase I trial of recombinant macrophage colony-stimulating factor in patients with invasive fungal infections. Blood 1991; 78:907.
152. Kaushansky K. Thrombopoietin: the primary regulator of platelet production. Blood 1995; 86:419.
153. Sohma Y, Akahori H, Seki N, et al. Molecular cloning and chromosomal localization of human thrombopoietin gene. FEBS Lett 1994; 353:57.
154. de Sauvage FJ, Hass PE, Spencer SD, et al. Stimulation of megakaryopoiesis and thrombopoiesis by the c-mpl ligand. Nature 1994; 369:533.
155. Bartley TD, Bogenberger J, Hunt P, et al. Identification and cloning of a megakaryocyte growth and development factor that is a ligand for the cytokine receptor mpl. Cell 1994; 77:1117.
156. Fieler PJ, Gurney AL, Stefanich E, et al. Regulation of thrombopoietin levels by c-mpl–mediated binding to platelets. Blood 1996; 87:2154.
157. Gurney Al, Wong SC, Henzel WJ, de Sauvage FJ. Distinct regions of c-mpl cytoplasmic domain are coupled to the JAK-STAT signal transduction pathway and Shc phosphorylation. Proc Natl Acad Sci U S A 1995; 92:5292.
158. Miyakawa Y, Oda A, Druker BJ, et al. Thrombopoietin induces tyrosine phosphorylation of STAT3 and STAT5 in human blood platelets. Blood 1996; 87:439.
159. Kuter DJ, Beeler DL, Rosenberg RD. The purification of megapoietin: a physiological regulator of megakaryocyte growth and platelet production. Proc Natl Acad Sci U S A 1994; 91:11104.
160. Angchaisuksiri P, Carlson PL, Dessypris EN. Effects of recombinant thrombopoietin on megakaryocyte colony growth and megakaryocyte ploidy by human $CD34^+$ cells in a serum free system. Br J Haematol 1996; 93:13.
161. Broudy VC, Lin NL, Kaushansky K. Thrombopoietin (c-mpl ligand) acts synergystically with erythropoietin, stem cell factor, and interleukin-11 to enhance murine megakaryocyte colony growth and increases megakaryocyte ploidy in vitro. Blood 1995; 85:1719.
162. Kobayashi M, Laver JH, Kato T, et al. Recombinant human thrombopoietin (Mpl-ligand) enhances proliferation of erythroid progenitors. Blood 1995; 86:2494.
163. Winton EF, Thomas GR, Marian ML, et al. Prediction of threshold and optimally effective thrombocytopoietic dose of rTPO in nonhuman primates based on murine pharmacokinetic data. Exp Hematol 1995; 23:879a.
164. Farese AM, Hunt P, Boone T, MacVittie TJ. Recombinant human megakaryocyte growth and development factor stimulates thrombopoiesis in normal nonhuman primates. Blood 1995; 86:54.
165. Harker LA, Hunt P, Marzec YM, et al. Regulation of platelet production by megakaryocyte growth and development factor in non-human primates. Blood 1996; 87:1833.
166. Begley G, Baseer R, Clarke K, et al. Randomized, double-blind, placebo-controlled phase I trial of pegylated megakaryocyte growth and development factor administered to patients with advanced cancer after chemotherapy [Abstract 719]. Proc Am Soc Clin Oncol 1996; 15:271a.
167. Basser R, Rasko JE, Clarke K, et al. Thrombopoietic effects of pegylated recombinant human megakaryocyte growth and development factor (PEG-MGDF) in patients with advanced cancer. Lancet 1996; 348:1279.
168. Fanucchi M, Glaspy J, Crawford J, et al. Safety and biological effects of pegylated megakaryocyte growth and development factor in lung cancer patients receiving carboplatin and paclitaxel: randomized, placebo-controlled phase I study [Abstract 720]. Proc Am Soc Clin Oncol 1996; 15:271a.
169. Kuter DJ. Thrombopoietin: biology, clinical applications, role in the donor setting. J Clin Apheresis 1996; 11:149.

170. Zsebo KM, Wypych J, McNiece IK, et al. Identification, purification and biological characterization of hematopoietic stem cell factor from buffalo rat liver–conditioned medium. Cell 1990; 63:195.
171. Martin FH, Suggs SV, Langley KE, et al. Primary structure and functional expression of rat and human stem cell factor cDNAs. Cell 1190; 63:203.
172. Linenberger ML, Jacobsen FW, Bennett LG, et al. Stem cell factor production by human marrow stromal fibroblasts. Exp Hematol 1995; 23:1104.
173. Lorenz U, Bergemann AD, Steinberg HN, et al. Genetic analysis reveals cell type-specific regulation of receptor tyrosine kinase c-kit by the protein tyrosine phosphatase SHP1. J Exp Med 1996; 184:1111.
174. Reith AD, Ellis C, Lyman AD, et al. Signal transduction by normal isoforms and W mutant variants of the Kit receptor tyrosine kinase. EMBO J 1991; 10:2451.
175. Rosnet O, Birnbaum: Hematopoietic receptors of class III receptor-type tyrosine kinases. Crit Rev Oncogenesis 1993; 4:595.
176. Petzer AL, Hogge DE, Lansdorp PM, et al. Self-renewal of primitive human hematopoietic cells (long-term culture-initiating cells) in vitro and their expansion in defined medium. Proc Natl Acad Sci U S A 1996; 93:1470.
177. Bernstein ID, Andrews RG, Zsebo KM. Recombinant human stem cell factor enhances the formation of colonies by $CD34^+$ and $CD34^+lin^-$ cells, and the generation of colony-forming cell progeny from $CD34^+lin^-$ cells cultured with interleukin-3, granulocyte colony-stimulating factor, or granulocyte-macrophage colony-stimulating factor. Blood 1991; 77:2316.
178. de Haan G, Dontje B, Nijhof W, Loeffler M. Effects of continuous stem cell factor administration on normal and erythropoietin-stimulated murine hematopoiesis: experimental results and model analysis. Stem Cell 1995; 13:65.
179. Wu D, Nayar R, Keating A. Synergistic effect of stem cell factor with interleukin-3 or granulocyte-macrophage colony-stimulating factor on the proliferation of murine primitive hematopoietic progenitors. Exp Hematol 1994; 22:495.
180. McNiece IK, Briddel RA. Stem cell factor. J Leuk Biol 1995; 57:14.
181. Morstyn G, Brown S, Gordon M, et al. Stem cell factor is a potent synergistic factor in hematopoiesis. Oncology 1994; 51:205.
182. Dale DC, Rodger E, Cebon J, et al. Long-term treatment of canine cyclic hematopoiesis with recombinant canine stem cell factor. Blood 1995; 85:74.
183. Lyman SD, James L, Vanden BT, et al. Molecular cloning of a ligand for the flt3/flk2 tyrosine kinase receptor: a proliferative factor for primitive hematopoietic cells. Cell 1993; 75:1157.
184. Carow CE, Kim E, Hawkins AL, et al. Localization of the human stem cell tyrosine kinase-1 gene (FLT-3) to 13q12-q13. Cytogenet Cell Genet 1995; 70:255.
185. Small D, Levenstein M, Eunkyung K, et al. STK-1, the human homolog of the Flk-2/Flt-3, is selectively expressed in the $CD23^+$ human bone marrow cells and is involved in the proliferation of early progenitor/stem cells. Proc Natl Acad Sci U S A 1994; 91:459.
186. Rosnet O, Birnbaum D. Hematopoietic receptors of class III receptor-type tyrosine kinases. Crit Rev in Oncogenesis 1993; 4:595.
187. Gabbianelli M, Pelosi E, Montesoro E, et al. Multi-level effects of flt3 ligand on human hematopoiesis: expansion of putative stem cell and proliferation of granulocytic progenitors/monocytic precursors. Blood 1995; 86:1661.
188. McKenna HJ, de Vries P, Brasel K, et al. Effect of flt3 ligand on ex vivo expansion of human $CD34^+$ hematopoietic progenitor cells. Blood 1995; 86:3413.
189. Hirayama F, Lyman SD, Clark SC, Ogawa M. The flt3 ligand supports proliferation of lymphohematopoietic progenitors and early B-lymphoid progenitors. Blood 1995; 85:1762.
190. Brasel K, McKenna HJ, Morrissey PJ, et al. Hematologic effects of flt3 ligand in vivo in mice. Blood 1996; 88:2004.
191. Hudak S, Hunte B, Culpepper J, et al. Flt3/flk2 ligand promotes the growth of murine stem cells and the expansion of colony-forming cells and spleen colony-forming units. Blood 1995; 85:2747.
192. Haylock DN, Horsfall MJ, Dowse TL, et al. Increased recruitment of hematopoietic progenitor cells underlies the ex vivo expansion potential of FLT3 ligand. Blood 1997; 90:2260.
193. Lisovsky M, Estrov Z, Zhang X, et al. Flt3 ligand stimulates proliferation and inhibits apoptosis of acute myeloid leukemia cells: regulation of Bcl-2 and Bax. Blood 1996; 88:3987.
194. Sudo Y, Shimazaki C, Ashihara E, et al. Synergistic effect of FLT-3 ligand on the granulocyte colony-stimulating factor–induced mobilization of hematopoietic stem cells and progenitor cells into blood in mice. Blood 1997; 89:3186.
195. Molineux G, McCrea C, Qiang X, et al. Flt-3 ligand synergizes with granulocyte colony-stimulating factor to increase neutrophil numbers and to mobilize peripheral blood stem cells with long-term repopulating potential. Blood 1997; 89:3998.
196. Dao MA, Hannum CH, Kohn DB, Nolta JA. FLT3 ligand preserves the ability of human $CD34^+$ progenitors to sustain long-term hematopoiesis in immune-deficient mice after ex vivo retroviral-mediated transduction. Blood 1997; 89:446.
197. Gabbianelli M, Pelosi E, Montersoro E, et al. Multi-level effects of flt3 ligand on human hematopoiesis: Expansion of putative stem cells and proliferation of granulocytic progenitors/monocytic precursors. Blood 1995; 86:1661.
198. Yang Y-C, Ciarletta AB, Temple PA, et al: Human IL-3 (multi-CSF). Identification by expression cloning of a novel hematopoietic growth factor related to murine IL-3. Cell 1986; 47:3.
199. Niemeyer CM, Sieff CA, Mathey-Prevot B, et al. Expression of human interleukin-3 (multi-CSF) is restricted to human lymphocytes and T-cell tumor lines. Blood 1989; 73:945.
200. Sato N, Caux C, Kitamura T, et al. Expression and factor-dependent modulation of the interleukin-3 receptor subunits on human hematopoietic cells. Blood 1993; 82:752.
201. Hara T, Miyajima A. Function and signal transduction mediated by the interleukin 3 receptor system in hematopoeisis. Stem Cell 1996; 14:605.
202. Oster W, Firsch J, Nicolay U, Schulz G. Interleukin-3. Biologic effects and clinical impact. Cancer 1991; 67:2712.
203. Ottmann OG, Ganser A, Seipelt G, et al. Effects of recombinant human interleukin-3 on human hematopoietic progenitor and precursor cells in vivo. Blood 1990; 76:1494.
204. Donahue RE, Seehra J, Metzger M, et al. Human IL-3 and GM-CSF act synergistically in stimulating hematopoiesis in primates. Science 1988; 241:182.
205. Fay JW, Lazarus H, Herzig R, et al. Sequential administration of interleukin-3 (rhIL-3) and rhGM-CSF following autologous bone marrow transplantation: an update of phase I/II trial. Blood 1993; 82(S1):287.
206. Vadhan-Raj S: PIXY321 (GM-CSF/IL-3 fusion protein). Biology and early clinical development. Stem Cells 1994; 12:253.
207. Vadhan-Raj S, Broxmeyer HE, Andreef M, et al. In vivo biologic effects of PIXY321, a synthetic hybrid protein of a recombinant human granulocyte-macrophage colony-stimulating factor and interleukin-3 in cancer patients with normal hematopoiesis: a phase I study. Blood 1995; 86:2098.
208. Kishimoto T. The biology of interleukin-6. Blood 1989; 74:1.
209. Taga T, Hibi M, Hirata Y, et al. Interleukin-6 triggers the association of its receptor with a possible signal transducer, gp 130. Cell 1989; 58:573.
210. Hirano T, Matsuda T, Nakajima K. Signal transduction through gp 130 that is shared among the receptors for the interleukin 6 related cytokine subfamily. Stem Cells 1994; 12:262.
211. Kishimoto T, Akira S, Taga T. Interleukin-6 and its receptor: a paradigm for cytokines. Science 1992; 258:593.
212. Leary AG, Ikebuchi K, Hirai Y, et al. Synergism between interleukin-6 and interleukin-3 in supporting proliferation of human hematopoietic stem cells: comparison with interleukin-1α. Blood 1988; 71:1759.
213. Caracciolo D, Clark SC, Rovera G. Human interleukin-6 supports granulocytic differentiation of hematopoietic progenitor cells and acts synergistically with GM-CSF. Blood 1989; 73:666.
214. Bot FJ, Van Eijk L, Broeders L, et al. Interleukin-6 synergizes with M-CSF in the formation of macrophages colonies from purified human marrow progenitor cells. Blood 1989; 73:435.
215. Udagawa N, Takahashi N, Katagiri T, et al. Interleukin (IL)-6 induction of osteoclast differentiation depends on IL-6 receptors expressed on osteoblastic cells but not on osteoclast progenitors. J Exp Med 1995; 182:1461.
216. Oldenburg HS, Rogy MA, Lazarus DD, et al. Cachexia and the acute-phase response in inflammation are regulated by interleukin-6. Eur J Immunol 1993; 23:1889.

217. Takatsuki F, Okano A, Suzuki C, et al. Interleukin 6 perfusion stimulates reconstitution of the immune and hematopoietic systems after 5-fluorouracil treatment. Cancer Res 1990; 50:2885.
218. Ishibashi T, Kimura H, Shikama Y, et al. Interleukin-6 is a potent thrombopoietic factor in vivo in mice. Blood 1989; 74:1241.
219. Crawford J, Figlin R, Chang A, et al. Phase I/II trial of recombinant human interleukin-6 (rhIL-6) and granulocyte colony-stimulating factor (G-CSF) following ifosfamide, carboplatin and etoposide (ICE) chemotherapy in patients with advanced non–small cell lung carcinoma (NSCLC). Blood 1993; 82:367a.
220. Schrezenmeier H, Spath-Schwalbe E, Drechsler S, et al. Phase I trials of interleukin-6 (IL-6) in patients with advanced renal cell carcinoma (RCC) and patients with aplastic anemia (AA): effects of long-term application and differences of hematopoietic response to IL-6 in patients with normal hemopoieis versus patients with aplastic anemia. Blood 1993; 82:368a.
221. Kundig TM, Schorle H, Bachmann MF, et al. Immune responses in interleukin-2–deficient mice. Science 1993; 262:1059.
222. Willerford DM, Chen J, Ferry JA, et al. Interleukin-2 receptor alpha chain regulates the size and content of the peripheral lymphoid compartment. Immunity 1995; 3:521.
223. Sharfe N, Dadi HK, Shahar M, Roifman CM. Human immune disorder arising from mutation of the chain of the interleukin-2 receptor. Proc Natl Acad Sci U S A 1997; 94:3168.
224. He YW, Malek TR. Interleukin-7 receptor alpha is essential for the development of gamma delta$^+$ T cells, but not natural killer cells. J Exp Med 1996; 184:289.
225. Bolotin E, Smogorzewska M, Smith S, et al. Enhancement of thymopoiesis after bone marrow transplant by in vivo interleukin-7. Blood 1996; 88:1887.
226. Piccinni M-P, Macchia D, Parronchi P, et al. Human bone marrow non-B, non-T cells produce IL-4 in response to cross linkage of Fce and Fcg receptors. Proc Natl Acad Sci U S A 1991; 88:8656.
227. Paul WE. Interleukin-4: a prototypic immunoregulatory lymphokine. Blood 1991; 77:1859.
228. Kopf M, Le Gros G, Bachmann M, et al. Disruption of the murine IL-4 gene blocks Th2 cytokine responses. Nature 1993; 362:245.
229. McKenzie ANJ, Culpepper JA, de Wala Malefyt R, et al. Interleukin-13, a novel cell-derived cytokine that regulates human monocyte and B cell function. Proc Natl Acad Sci U S A 1992; 5:815.
230. Center DM, Kornfield H, Cruikshank WW. Interleukin 16 and its function as a CD4 ligand. Immunol Today 1996; 17:476.
231. D'Andrea A, Gengaraju M, Valiante NM, et al. Production of natural killer cell stimulatory factor (interleukin-12) by peripheral blood mononuclear cells. J Exp Med 1992; 176:1387.
232. Lamont AG, Adorini L. IL-12: a key cytokine in immune regulation. Immunol Today 1996; 17(5):214.
233. Manetti R, Parronchi P, Giudizi MG, et al. Natural killer cell stimulatory factor (interleukin 12 [IL-12]) induces T helper (Th1)-specific immune response and inhibits the development of IL-4-producing Th cells. J Exp Med 1993; 177:1199.
234. Germann T, Gately MK, Schoenhaunt DS, et al. Interleukin-12/T cell stimulating factor, a cytokine with multiple effects on T helper type 1 (Th1) but not Th2 cells. Eur J Immunol 1993; 23:1762.
235. Brunda MJ, Luistro L, Warrier RR, et al. Antitumor and antimetastatic activity of interleukin 12 against murine tumors. J Exp Med 1993; 178:1223.

SECTION

II Immunology and Genetics

CHAPTER 5

T Lymphocytes and the Adaptive Immune Response

Terence L. Geiger

INTRODUCTION: THE NOTION OF SELF

The idea that the immune system can distinguish self from nonself has been central to immunology for nearly one hundred years.[1] Paul Ehrlich, in the late 19th century, studied antibody responses to an array of substances, foreign and native. Whereas antibodies were readily produced against foreign substances, they could not be induced against self constituents. This finding led him to develop the notion of *horror autotoxicus:* that the immune system is restricted to responding against foreign antigens. Karl Landsteiner further developed this concept by serologically classifying people on the basis of the presence of specific agglutinins in their blood. People failed to produce self-specific agglutinins. This work defined the ABO blood group system and formed the foundation for modern transfusion medicine.

In the 1940s and 1950s, experimental work attempted to decipher the mechanics underlying the restriction of immune responses to foreign antigens. Owen observed that dizygotic cattle twins with chimeric blood cells become cross-tolerant. This observation led Burnet and Fenner to hypothesize that any antigen present during a critical embryonic period would be perceived by the immune system as self and induce a state of tolerance.[2] Billingham and colleagues experimentally documented such a critical period. Antigen injected into a fetus or neonate produced tolerance. After this time, it produced immunity.[3] These studies led to the concept of immunological education: that the immature immune system learns what self is and that this knowledge guides future immune responses.

Since the 1950s, much effort has been directed at attempting to understand the nature of self and of immunological education. The current view of immunological self differs from earlier views. Ehrlich's version of the biological self consists of the sum of proteins, lipids, carbohydrates, and other components that determine physical makeup. However the immune system's antigen receptors have the capability of perceiving only a fraction of this biological self. It is this limited self, the immunological self, that directs immunological education.

The concept of immunological education has also evolved dramatically. The idea that a critical embryonic period exclusively defines the immune system's view of self is no longer accepted. Rather, immunological education has been found to be a continuous process extending from fetal through adult life and involving both immature and mature lymphocytes. Both the time during development that the immune system is exposed to antigen and the context in which antigen is presented determine the nature of an immune response.[4, 5] The immune system relies on molecular signals signifying danger to guide its antigen-specific responses.[6] In the presence of such danger signals, lymphocytes specific for either foreign or self antigens can be activated. In their absence, tolerance may occur.

T lymphocytes and the antigen-presenting cells (APCs) with which they interact are fundamental to antigen-specific immune responses. This chapter focuses on T cells, how they come to recognize and respond to antigens, and the immunological consequences of this recognition. The specific consequences of antigen recognition in relation to transfusion, including alloimmunization, antibody production, graft-versus-host disease, and immunomodulation are discussed in other chapters. Because of the breadth of the topic covered, most aspects of the T cell response can be dealt with here only in a rather superficial manner. Nevertheless, some excellent reviews are referenced in each section for the reader interested in additional detail. The reader is also referred to several well-written basic texts for additional information.[7–9]

INNATE VERSUS ADAPTIVE IMMUNITY

The immune system is broadly divided into two subsystems: innate and adaptive. The innate immune system is composed of invariant structures that have evolved to assist in the defense against pathogens.[10] Critical to this task are receptors that recognize stereotyped molecular patterns, some of which have been termed *pattern recognition receptors* (PRRs).[11] PRRs are either soluble, such as complement or lipopolysaccharide binding protein, or cell associated, such as mannose binding receptors or major histocompatibility complex (MHC)–specific receptors on natural killer (NK) cells. Detection of pathogens or pathogenic processes by PRRs initiates responses aimed at their neutralization. For example, double-stranded RNA is a molecular motif characteristic of some RNA viruses. It is absent from the host. Receptors for double-stranded RNA initiate a cascade of responses, particularly through the secretion of interferon (IFN)–α and IFN-β, aimed at neutralizing the offending virus.[12]

Adaptive immunity uses nonstereotyped receptors. Unlike PRRs that are genetically encoded in the germ line, adaptive receptors are formed through genetic recombination during the development of B and T lymphocytes.[13] A virtually limitless array of antigen-binding receptors results. Two receptor types are found: B cell receptors (BCRs or immunoglobulins), and T cell receptors (TCRs). These receptors are antigen-specific, although the gene rearrangements that result in their formation occur without knowledge of or influence from the antigens to which they respond. Because of the diversity of such antigen-specific receptors, the frequency of B or T cells expressing any single receptor is low. It is estimated that fewer than 1:100,000 T cells will respond to any single peptide antigen.[14] Consequently, adaptive immunity requires the expansion of antigen-specific lymphocytes to generate an effective response. This expansion is slow. Whereas innate responses are immediate or induced within a brief time period, adaptive responses require days to develop.

Although the innate and adaptive parts of the immune system have long been scientifically segregated, their intimate interrelationship is now beginning to be appreciated.[10, 11] Because adaptive immunity is slow to arise, the innate immune system must form a front guard against pathogens. Its activation results in an inflammatory response that is a required prelude to the development of adaptive responses. Thus it has long been known that effective immunization with proteins generally requires an adjuvant. The role of adjuvant appears to be the initiation of an inflammatory response to permit adaptive immunity. The interrelationship between innate and adaptive immunity is also evident in the fact that mice deficient in complement components C3 or C4 or the complement receptor CR1 have impaired antibody responses to T cell–dependent antigens.[15–17] The understanding of the complex web of interactions that link the innate and adaptive immune systems is in its infancy. Nevertheless, the data currently available clearly define these interactions as critical in all immune responses.

ADAPTIVE RESPONSES TO ANTIGEN: TOLERANCE, IGNORANCE, AND IMMUNITY

Exposure to antigen may lead to an adaptive immune response. Immunizing responses include antibody production, delayed-type hypersensitivity, and cytotoxic T cell responses.[18–20] Exposure to antigen, however, may also lead to immunological unresponsiveness, or tolerance. Tolerance must also be considered an adaptive response. By limiting the range of immune responses, it minimizes the potential for the immune system to harm the host. As mentioned earlier, Billingham and colleagues found that by injecting strain disparate cells into fetal or neonatal mice, they could induce tolerance. Skin from the corresponding disparate strain of mice grafted into neonatally tolerized adult mice was accepted indefinitely. Skin grafts from other strains were rapidly rejected. Later studies demonstrated that the susceptibility to tolerance induction by this technique waned rapidly after birth.[21]

Although tolerance induction is facile in the neonate, it can also be achieved in the adult. Early studies of induced tolerance in the adult analyzed antibody response after antigen injection. Two forms of tolerance to many antigens were noted. In low-zone tolerance, injection of a small dose of antigen induced tolerance. In high-zone tolerance, injection of a large dose of antigen induced tolerance. For bovine serum albumin, these dosages differ by a magnitude of 10^4. The precise requirements for achieving low-zone or high-zone tolerance vary with antigen. For some antigens, prior immunosuppression is necessary to generate tolerance.[22, 23]

Immunosuppression can also permit the long-term acceptance of completely allogeneic grafts. Immunosuppression may be facilitated by whole body irradiation,[24] total lymphoid irradiation,[25] chemotherapy,[26] antilymphocyte antisera,[27] and antibodies against cell surface molecules critical for immune responses, such as adhesion molecules.[28]

Experimental models of donor specific transfusion have demonstrated that the intravenous administration of allogeneic APC-depleted splenocytes[29] or whole splenocytes[30, 31] can induce tolerance. Cytolytic T lymphocyte response is eliminated by the T cell fraction.[32] This is termed the veto effect.[33, 34] $CD4^+$ T cell response is eliminated by the B cell fraction.[32] B cells can also tolerize T cells to soluble protein antigens.[35–37]

The studies just described demonstrate that tolerizing processes operate in the adult and the fetus. Dresser and Mitchison first suggested that the capacity for tolerance induction is identical in neonate and adult. Whereas the immune competence of the adult normally masks this tolerance, the incompetence of the neonate highlights it.[22]

Tolerance and immunity have long been considered the yin and yang of immune responses. Less appreciated is a third response to antigens: ignorance. Immunological ignorance differs from immunological tolerance. Whereas a tolerized immune system lacks the capacity to respond to antigen, an ignorant immune system is capable of responding to antigen but elects not to. Recognition of immunological ignorance as a distinct entity is largely derived from studies of how the immune system responds to self antigens. Studies in the 1980s demonstrated that T cells specific for self antigens can be isolated, even in the absence of autoimmune disease.[38–42] These T cells were fully antigen responsive in vitro. Furthermore, immunization with self antigens is sufficient to elicit autoimmunity in several experimental models. Autoreactive T cells are present, but they are activated only after immunization in vivo.[43–45]

One of the more enlightening models of T cell ignorance involved the generation of mice transgenic for both the lymphocytic choriomeningitis virus (LCMV) glycoprotein expressed on pancreatic β-islet cells and a rearranged TCR that recognizes this protein. The rearranged TCR imparts a specificity for LCMV glycoprotein that is expressed on virtually all T cells in these mice. These T cells are ignorant. They are fully responsive to antigen in vitro and yet do not respond to it in vivo.[46, 47] That they are indeed not tolerant is apparent because immunization with antigen by LCMV infection provokes a rejection of the transgenic islets and the onset of diabetes.

Tolerance, ignorance, and immunity are all possible consequences of antigenic exposure in the setting of transfusion. The benefits of transfusion in promoting tolerance in renal transplant recipients has long been recognized. Simultaneously, many of the most difficult situations that arise in transfusion medicine result from the immunization of a recipient to donor antigens. Yet virtually every transfusion of homologous blood involves the administration of alloantigen. Fortunately, the most frequent response to these alloantigens seems to be ignorance.

HOW T CELLS SEE ANTIGEN: THE T CELL RECEPTOR

The TCR senses antigen for the T cell. TCRs are heterodimers, of which there are two types: αβ and γδ.[48] A substantial majority of T cells express αβ TCRs. Because αβ T cells have been most extensively studied, further discussion is limited largely to them. However, the basic principles of TCR formation and antigen recognition by γδ T cells are similar.

The universe of antigenic structures that the immune system may encounter is virtually limitless. The diversity of TCRs expressed by T cells must mirror this antigenic diversity. If the repertoire of TCRs is not sufficiently diverse, pathogens may evolve so as to be effectively invisible to the adaptive immune system.

Generation of TCR diversity is a product of the genomic organization of TCR genes (Fig. 5–1). These genes are composed of multiple segments that somatically recombine. In the germ line, these segments include variable (V), diversity (D), joining (J), and constant (C) regions. The D region segments are present only in the β and δ genes and are absent from α and γ. Rearrangement of the TCR links a V region, sometimes a D region, and a J region gene segment together. This creates a transcription unit that, together with the downstream C region, encodes a TCR chain.[49]

The random association of V, D, and J segments generates substantial diversity; the number of possible recombinatorial products is the product of the number of each of these segments. Additional diversity is, however, generated at each recombination site. This results from nucleotide addition by the enzyme terminal deoxynucleotide transferase and/or nucleotide removal by nucleases, a process termed *N-region diversification*. Changes in the genetic code at these recombinatorial sites alters the amino acid sequence of the resulting TCR chain. Not surprisingly, the sites where V and D, D and J, or V and

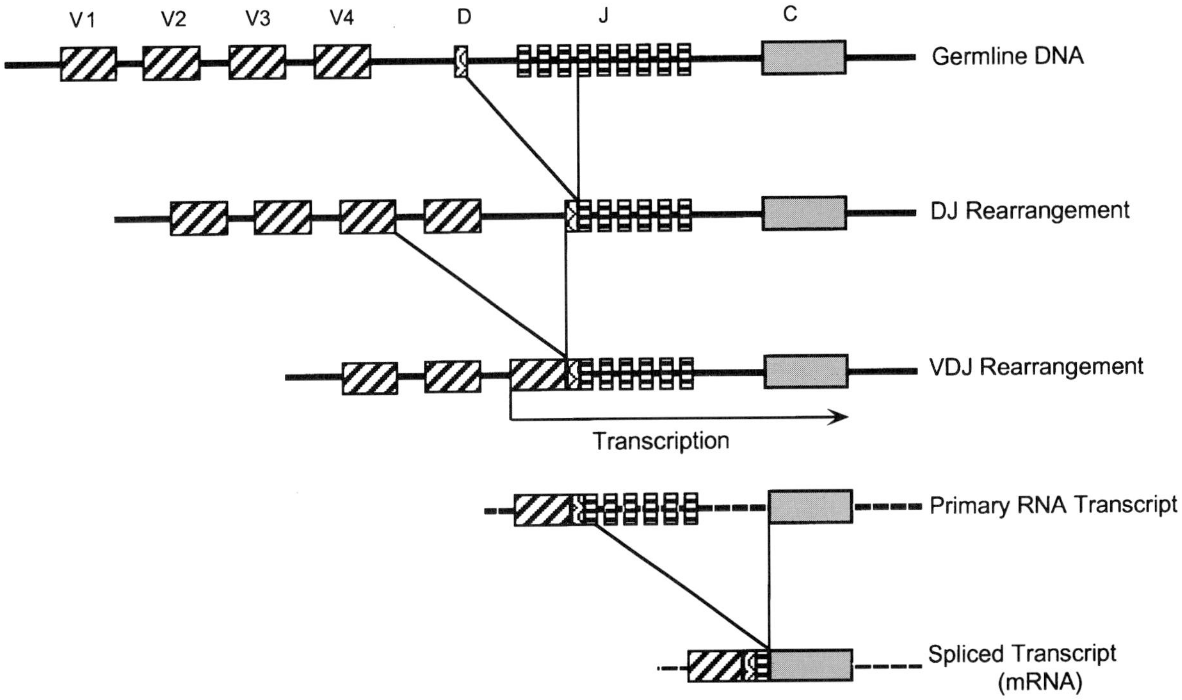

Figure 5–1. T cell receptor (TCR) gene rearrangement. The germ line genetic sequence consists of multiple variable, diversity (β chain only), and junctional segments (V, D, J, C). Rearrangement juxtaposes these elements. Completion of rearrangement brings the necessary elements for RNA transcription in proximity, enhancing the transcription of the rearranged gene. This figure is illustrative and does not reflect the full complexity of the TCR loci.

J segments unite are the most diverse regions within the TCR. The potential amino acid sequence diversity of the αβ TCR as a consequence of the combination of recombinatorial diversity and N-region diversification has been estimated at 10^{16}.

The mechanics of TCR gene rearrangement, though not entirely elucidated, are well studied. Somatic cell gene rearrangement with the elimination of portions of germ line genetic sequence is unique to lymphoid cells. A search for lymphoid-specific genes necessary for VDJ recombination yielded two products: recombination activating genes 1 and 2 (RAG-1, RAG-2).[50, 51] RAG-1 and RAG-2 encode protein products that dimerize, forming part of a multiprotein complex termed a recombinase. The rag-1 and rag-2 proteins recognize nucleotide signal sequences consisting of a conserved heptamer and nonamer separated by a 12– or 23–base pair spacer that flank V, D, and J region gene segments.[52] They cleave the DNA adjacent to the signal sequences. The rag-1 and rag-2 proteins are not, however, sufficient to ligate the clipped segments of DNA together. Conserved proteins known to be involved in DNA repair are important in this task.

Although lymphoid specific, the rag proteins are not sufficient to provide cell-type specificity in rearrangement; rag-1 and rag-2 are necessary for antigen receptor recombination in both T and B cell precursors. Thus they cannot independently discriminate BCR signal sequences from TCR signal sequences. Studies support a role for chromatin accessibility in ensuring that only the appropriate antigen receptor is rearranged.[53]

The TCR's primary structure places it in the immunoglobulin superfamily of proteins.[54, 55] It has thus long been physically modeled on the basis of the immunoglobulin molecule. High-resolution x-ray crystallographic studies affirm this structural assignment.[56] The variable domains of the α and β chains form an immunoglobulin-like structure. Although the scaffolding is well conserved, the upper surface, consisting of peptide loops termed *complementarity determining regions* (CDRs), is less conserved. Three CDRs are present on each TCR chain: CDR1, CDR2, and CDR3. Whereas CDR1 and 2 are encoded in the germ line V region gene, CDR3 is formed where the V, D, and J segments combine. The CDR3 hence forms the most variable portion of the surface of the TCR and is therefore most significant in providing antigen specificity.

Although the α and β chains and the γ and δ chains form the antigen recognition unit of the TCR, they are not independently expressed on T cells. Several other proteins are required for TCR surface expression and intracellular signaling. These include the CD3 γ, δ, and ϵ chains and a dimer of the ζ chain or its splice variant η (Fig. 5–2).[57] The invariant chains of the TCR associate with the α and β chains through noncovalent interactions.

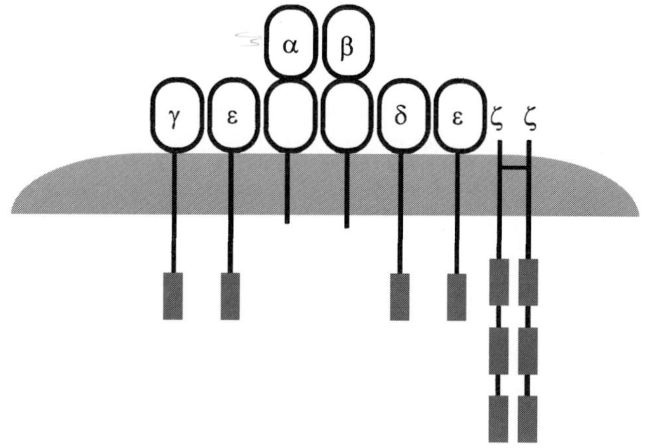

Figure 5–2. The TCR/CD3 complex consists of eight polypeptide chains. Specificity is determined by the αβ chains (or, in some T cells, by TCR γδ chains). Expression of the CD3 chains γ, δ, and ϵ, as well as ζ or its splice variants are necessary for surface expression and signaling. Signaling occurs with phosphorylation of the CD3 and ζ immune tyrosine activation motif (ITAM) tyrosines. ITAMs are indicated by gray boxes in the diagram.

T CELLS RECOGNIZE ANTIGEN FRAMED BY MHC MOLECULES

The first recognition of the importance of the MHC came in the 1930s and 1940s with the work of Peter Gorer and then George Snell, who were studying graft rejection in mice.[1] The MHC that they defined is the window that T cells have to the world. T cells do not "see" antigen alone, they "see" it in the context of MHC molecules. Antigen and MHC are unified. T cells do not recognize even antigen presented by different alleles of the same MHC molecule.[58]

As the genetics of immune responses were studied, it became clear that MHC genes not only were of paramount importance in graft rejection, but also were critical to all types of immune responses. The capacity to produce antibodies to specific antigens was mapped to MHC genes, defining them as "immune response" genes. These genes also proved critical for graft-versus-host disease and all manners of cellular immunity. Two major types of MHC molecules are found.[59] Class I MHC molecules are heterodimers consisting of a 44-kD α (or heavy) chain, which is encoded within the MHC locus on chromosome 6, and a 12-kD β chain, called β_2-microglobulin, encoded on chromosome 15. Class II MHC molecules are also heterodimers, composed of a 32- to 34-kD α chain and a 29- to 32-kD β chain, both encoded within the MHC locus.

Attempts to demystify the antigen-MHC singularity culminated in the late 1980s with x-ray crystallographic structures of several MHC molecules (Fig. 5–3). These structures demonstrate how T cells see a union of antigen and MHC. The upper surface of the MHC molecule is composed of a β sheet over which lies two parallel α helices. This sheet serves as a platter on which peptide antigens are presented. In class I molecules, peptide antigens are sandwiched in an approximately 10 Å wide and 25 Å–long groove between the α helices.[60–63] A similar structure is observed for class II MHC molecules. However, two major differences between class I and class II are seen. First, whereas the antigen-binding region of class II molecules is derived from both the α and β chains, this region on the class I molecule is formed

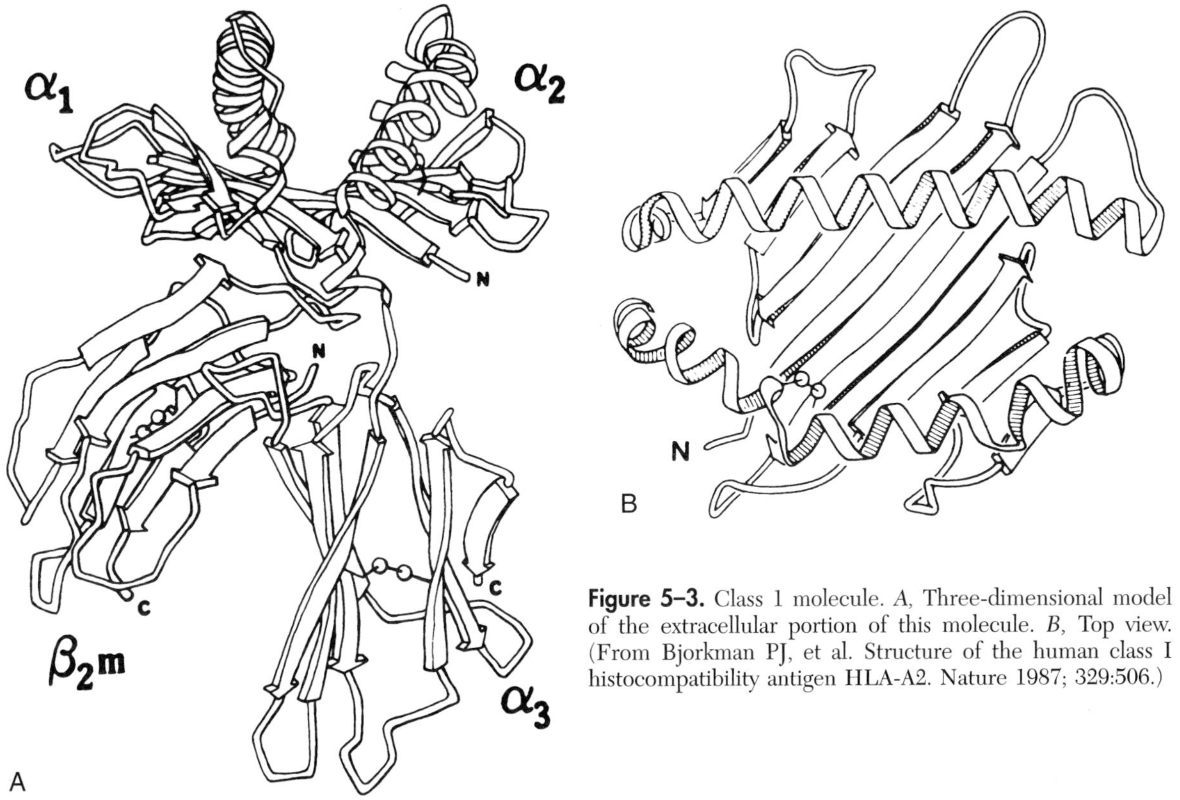

Figure 5–3. Class 1 molecule. *A,* Three-dimensional model of the extracellular portion of this molecule. *B,* Top view. (From Bjorkman PJ, et al. Structure of the human class I histocompatibility antigen HLA-A2. Nature 1987; 329:506.)

only by the α (heavy) chain. Second, the antigen-binding groove is closed at either end of the class I molecule, whereas it is open in class II molecules. As a result, antigenic peptides bound to class I molecules are limited to approximately 8 to 10 amino acid residues in length. Class II binding peptides can be significantly longer and are commonly in the range of 13 to 24 amino acids.

When MHC molecules are crystallized with their native peptide content, an amorphous mass (suggestive of a large variety of peptide structures) is observed in the peptide-binding groove. Indeed, a large array of peptide antigens can be directly eluted from isolated MHC molecules. Among these peptides, minimal antigenic determinants capable of activating T cells can be found.[64–68] Analysis of these peptides reveals how such an abundant array can bind within the invariant MHC binding sites. Peptides eluted from each MHC molecule contain anchor residues that are fairly conserved in their nature.[69–70] These anchor residues lock the peptide in place. For example, peptides binding to the class II human leukocyte antigen (HLA)–DR3 molecule have a negatively charged glutamic or aspartic acid at position 4 and a hydrophobic residue at position 9.

Peptides can be removed from the MHC peptide binding groove and replaced with a single antigenic peptide. Structural, biochemical, and functional studies of such MHC-peptide complexes have clarified the chemistry of peptide binding.[71] Pockets are present within the MHC binding groove. Peptide side chains fit snugly into these pockets, providing sufficient free energy to hold the peptide in place. The peptides do not necessarily protrude out of the top of this binding groove. In some cases they are buried within, largely enveloped by the MHC molecule. Some structural studies show that less than 25% of the MHC molecule's surface that the TCR interacts with is derived from peptide. With each peptide bound a unique antigenic surface is presented to T cells. This uniqueness not only is a result of the physical structure of the peptide itself but also results from surface residues of the MHC molecule adjusting so as to optimize the peptide-MHC complex's stability.

X-ray crystallographic analysis has also been conducted on TCR cocrystallized with MHC-peptide.[72, 73] The TCR Vα interacts primarily with the MHC region containing the N-terminus of the bound peptide (the "left hand" surface). The Vβ domain interacts predominantly with the MHC region containing the carboxyl terminus of the peptide (the "right hand" surface). Although crystallographic analysis is limited, the two available structures of TCR with MHC-peptide show that the precise fit and orientation of TCR with peptide-MHC varies.

MHC POLYMORPHISM AND POLYGENICITY

The MHC is unique among cellular proteins in its variability (Fig. 5–4). No other human genetic locus is as polymorphic as the MHC.[74] In humans in which the MHC is termed the HLA, hundreds of different HLA alleles have been identified. This number will undoubtedly increase as more individuals from different ethnic groups are HLA typed by molecular means, particularly DNA sequencing. In addition to its polymorphism, the MHC is noteworthy for its polygenicity. The class I region

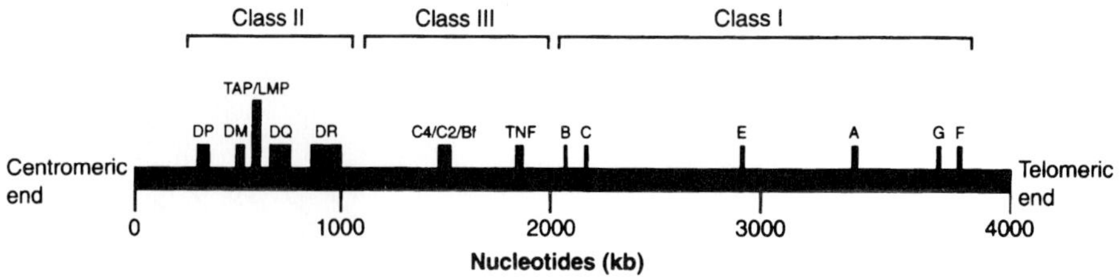

HLA class II alleles

Locus	Number of alleles
HLA-DRA	2
HLA-DRB	179
HLA-DQA	18
HLA-DQB	29
HLA-DPA	8
HLA-DPB	69
HLA-DMA	4
HLA-DMB	5
Total	314

HLA class I alleles

Locus	Number of alleles
HLA-A	67
HLA-B	149
HLA-C	39
HLA-E	5
HLA-F	1
HLA-G	6
Total	266

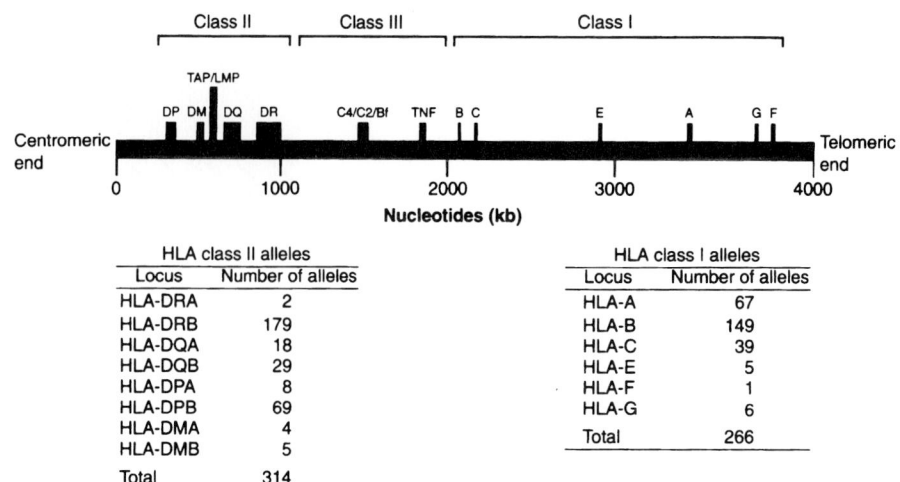

Figure 5–4. Human leukocyte antigen (HLA) polymorphism. Linear diagram of the HLA region showing the relative positions of the major loci involved in antigen presentation. TAP/LMP are the genes encoding the transporter for antigen processing (TAP), which transports peptides from the cytoplasm to the endoplasmic reticulum, and two low-molecular-weight polypeptides (LMP) of the proteasome, which produces peptides in the cytoplasm. The locations of the C4, C2, and factor B (Bf) complement loci and the tumor necrosis factor (TNF) genes in the class III region are also indicated. Tabulated beneath the class I and class II regions is the number of alleles for each locus defined on the basis of nucleotide sequence as of 1996. The definition of class II allelic sequence is more advanced than that of class I, and the number of class I alleles can be expected to exceed that of class II. (From Parham P, Outa T. Population biology of antigen presentation by MHC class I. Science 1996; 272:67.)

of the HLA is divided into class Ia and class Ib gene products. Three class Ia (A, B, and C) and several additional less polymorphic class Ib genes are encoded per haploid set of chromosomes. The class II region is likewise polygenic. Three categories of class II genes have been identified: DR, DQ, and DP. The DR region can encode one or two gene product per haploid genome. Although only a single DP and DQ α and β chain pair are found per HLA locus, in a heterozygote the α and/or β chain encoded by one chromosome can dimerize with the reciprocal chain from either the *cis* or *trans* chromosome, increasing the numbers of possible class II structures expressed by an individual.

The clinical difficulties resulting from polymorphism and polygenicity are all too evident in bone marrow transplantation and in transfusion with alloimmunized patients. Finding blood components with acceptable matches requires databases of thousands of prospective donors. Yet clearly MHC polymorphism did not arise to hinder transfusionists and transplanters. The high degree of polymorphism likely results from selective pressures arising from specific pathogens. If the MHC is invariant pathogens would be expected to evolve into forms not recognized by the MHC. With MHC polymorphism no selective advantage can be so obtained. Alternative MHC alleles will always be available to present pathogen derived antigens. Polygenicity ensures that an individual will always express some MHC alleles capable of presenting antigenic peptides.

Some epidemiological evidence supports this view of polymorphism and polygenicity. For instance, strains of Epstein-Barr virus in Papua New Guinea, where the HLA-A11 allele is common, contain mutations that prevent HLA-A11 molecules from binding antigenic viral peptides.[75] This may provide some survival advantage to the virus. As a result of HLA polymorphism and polygenicity, however, the majority of people will not be homozygous for HLA-A11 and will also express alternative HLA-A alleles (as well as B and C alleles) capable of presenting viral peptides. The idea that a population's complement of HLA alleles is influenced by specific pathogens is also suggested by studies of West Africans. Populations with high rates of exposure to *Plasmodium falciparum* also include a high frequency of the HLA-B53 allele.[76] This allele is in turn associated with an expedited recovery from *P. falciparum*–induced malaria.

DISTINCT FUNCTIONS FOR DISTINCT CLASSES OF MHC MOLECULES

Class I MHC Is Recognized by CD8 T Cells and Class II MHC by CD4 T Cells

Although class I and class II MHC molecules fold into similar structures, they are functionally distinct. Three differences in the biology of MHC account for their functional specialization. First, class I and class II molecules are recognized by distinct sets of T cells. These T cells are structurally characterized by the surface expression of CD4 or CD8. Whereas $CD4^+$ T cells recognize antigen presented by class II MHC, $CD8^+$ T cells recognize antigen presented by class I.

The specificity of CD4 or CD8 T cells for class II or I MHC results from several effects. The class II MHC molecule's β_2 domain contains a binding site for CD4, and the class I MHC molecule's α_2 and α_3 domain contain binding sites for CD8.[77, 78] Adhesion of CD4 or CD8 with class II or class I, respectively, increases the binding affinity of the T cell for the MHC expressing APC. Of more importance is that, after TCR stimulation, CD4 or CD8 associates with the TCR. By crosslinking TCR with

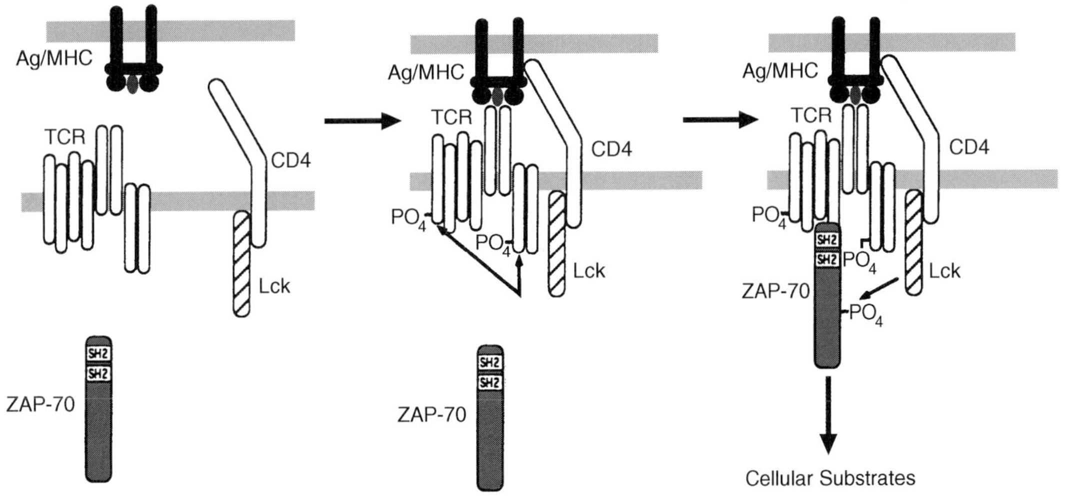

Figure 5–5. Model of TCR, Lck, and ζ-associated protein (ZAP)–70 interactions during antigen (Ag) recognition by a CD4+ T cell. The phosphorylation of tyrosine residues of the ITAMs within the ζ and CD3 chains has been simplified. MHC, major histocompatibility complex. (From Weiss A. T-cell antigen receptor signal transduction: a tale of tails and cytoplasmic protein kinases. Cell 1993; 73:211.)

MHC, it stabilizes the TCR-MHC interaction, thereby enhancing signaling through the TCR. CD4 and CD8 also have a more direct influence in activating T cells. The src-family tyrosine kinase lck is associated with the cytoplasmic tails of CD4 and CD8.[79, 80] After TCR stimulation, lck phosphorylates tyrosine residues in the cytoplasmic domains of the TCR CD3 and ζ chains. This phosphorylation is the first event in TCR signaling and triggers further downstream signaling (Fig. 5–5). The CD4 or CD8 molecules therefore usher lck into position near the TCR. Because CD4 or CD8 molecules act in concert with the TCR during antigen recognition, they are commonly referred to as co-receptors for the TCR.[77] Their presence enhances signaling through the TCR approximately 100-fold.[81]

Different Categories of Antigen Are Presented by Class I and Class II MHC

A second reason why class I and class II MHC are functionally distinct is that they present different categories of peptide antigens.[82–84] Whereas class I molecules present peptides synthesized within a cell, class II molecules present antigens derived primarily from exogenous sources. This difference in antigen source reflects a difference in the role of class I and class II MHC molecules: class I MHC reveals a cell's *intracellular* milieu; class II MHC reveals that which is *extracellular.* Class I and class II MHC molecules cannot intrinsically distinguish an antigen's source. Rather, cellular pathways that function to subserve the immune system provide for this difference in antigen type.

Peptide antigens destined for class I MHC molecules are produced largely by protein cleavage in a 700-kD multicatalytic protease complex termed the *proteasome*[85] (Fig. 5–6). Although the proteasome is cytosolic, peptides derived from cell surface, exocytosed, or endoplasmic reticulum (ER) and Golgi proteins may also be presented on class I MHC. Proteasomal degradation is important for these too. IFN-γ, produced in the course of an immune response, can enhance antigen presentation in part by increasing proteasome activity and the generation of small peptide fragments that can serve as class I ligands.[86] This occurs through the induction of the PA28 proteasome activator complex. Peptides derived from the proteasome are translocated into the ER by an adenosine triphosphate (ATP)–dependent peptide transporter, TAP1/2.[87] It is here that they encounter class I MHC.

MHC molecules contain leader sequences directing their transport into the ER during messenger RNA translation. The nascent class I MHC molecules require assistance in folding as they enter the ER. This is provided by resident ER proteins termed *chaperones.* Calnexin first associates with the class I heavy chain.[88] After association with β_{2m}, the class I heterodimer dissociates from calnexin and complexes with two other resident ER proteins, calreticulin and tapasin.[89] The MHC molecules at this point are devoid of peptide. The TAP1/2 heterodimer associates with the class I–calreticulin–tapasin complex.[90] TAP preferentially transports peptides of 8 to 12 amino acids, the appropriate size for binding class I molecules, from the cytosol to the ER.[91] Peptide binding releases the class I molecules, which then proceed to the cell surface.

Whereas the process of class I MHC folding and transit ensure its association with endogenously synthesized peptides, class II MHC transit and folding promote association with exogenously derived peptides[83] (Fig. 5–7). Like class I molecules, the two chains of class II MHC assemble in the ER with the assistance of chaperones.[92] However, they also associate with a third molecule, the invariant chain (Ii).[93] Ii contains a peptidic portion, CLIP, that binds to the groove of class II molecules. This prevents antigenic peptides present in the ER from filling this groove.[94] A separate domain of Ii mediates its trimerization. Nonamers of αβ class II-Ii complexes are then transported from the ER to the *trans*-Golgi network. Whereas class I molecules at this point continue onward

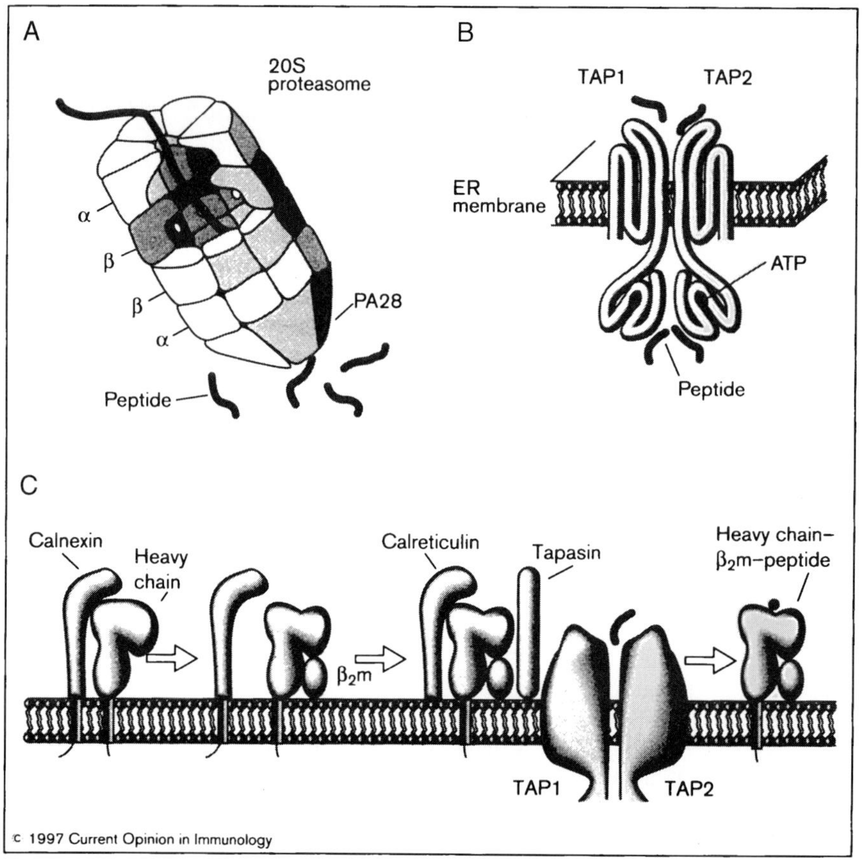

Figure 5–6. *A,* Schematic drawing of a cut-open 20S proteasome generating peptide fragments out of an unfolded polypeptide chain threaded into the narrow entry formed by an outer ring of α-type subunits. Cleavage occurs in the central cavity formed by two seven-membered rings of β-type subunits. A PA28 regulator complex is bound at the bottom of the cylinder. *B,* Hypothetical cross-section of a TAP1/TAP2 heterodimer embedded into the endoplasmic reticulum (ER) membrane. In the hydrophobic domains, 4 of the presumed 8 to 10 membrane-spanning segments (per TAP monomer) are shown. The adenosine triphosphate (ATP)–binding domains extend into the cytoplasm. *C,* Maturation of human class I molecules in the ER. Nascent class I heavy chains initially associate with calnexin. Upon binding of β_2m, the heterodimer dissociates form calnexin. A new complex containing class I heavy-chain, β_2m, calreticulin, tapasin, and TAP1/TAP2 is formed. After peptide loading, heavy-chain β_2m-peptide complexes are released to exit to the cell surface. (From Koopmann JO, Hammerling GJ, Momburg F. Generation, intracellular transport, and loading of peptides associated with MHC class I molecules. Curr Opin Immunol 1997; 9:81.)

to the cell surface, class II-Ii detours to the endocytic pathway.[95] Within the endocytic pathway, specialized compartment for antigen loading onto class II MHC exists in some cells. However, antigen may be loaded onto class II within multiple vesicular compartments,[96, 97] where class II MHC encounters peptide fragments from degraded extracellular proteins. Cathepsins cleave the invariant chain from the class II molecule, leaving the CLIP peptide behind.[98] A class II–like molecule, HLA-DM, next catalyzes the replacement of CLIP with antigenic peptide.[99] The class II–peptide complex finally is transported to the cell surface.

The antigens presented by class II molecules reflect the external environment because of the unique pathway for class II folding and migration to the cell surface. Within the endocytic compartment, class II molecules are bathed in a sea of exogenous antigens. These antigens may have been internalized by pinocytosis.[100] However, receptor-mediated internalization may be more important. Receptors that can bring antigens into the endocytic compartment include the BCR (sIg), the mannose receptor, and lectin-like receptors.[101, 102]

Cell-Specific Expression Patterns Differ for Class I and Class II MHC

A final manner in which class I and class II MHC molecules distinguish themselves is in their expression patterns. These patterns follow logically from the distinct presentation characteristics of class I and II molecules. Because class I molecules present endogenously derived peptides, they allow T cells to survey cells for the presence of internal abnormalities. Antigens derived from intracellular pathogens such as viruses and, in some cases, neoantigens formed as a result of malignant transformation can associate with class I MHC for presentation to $CD8^+$ T cells. Matured effector $CD8^+$ T cells recognizing these antigens can prevent spread of virus or malignancy by lysing affected target cells. It is therefore essential that all nucleated cells express MHC class I molecules.

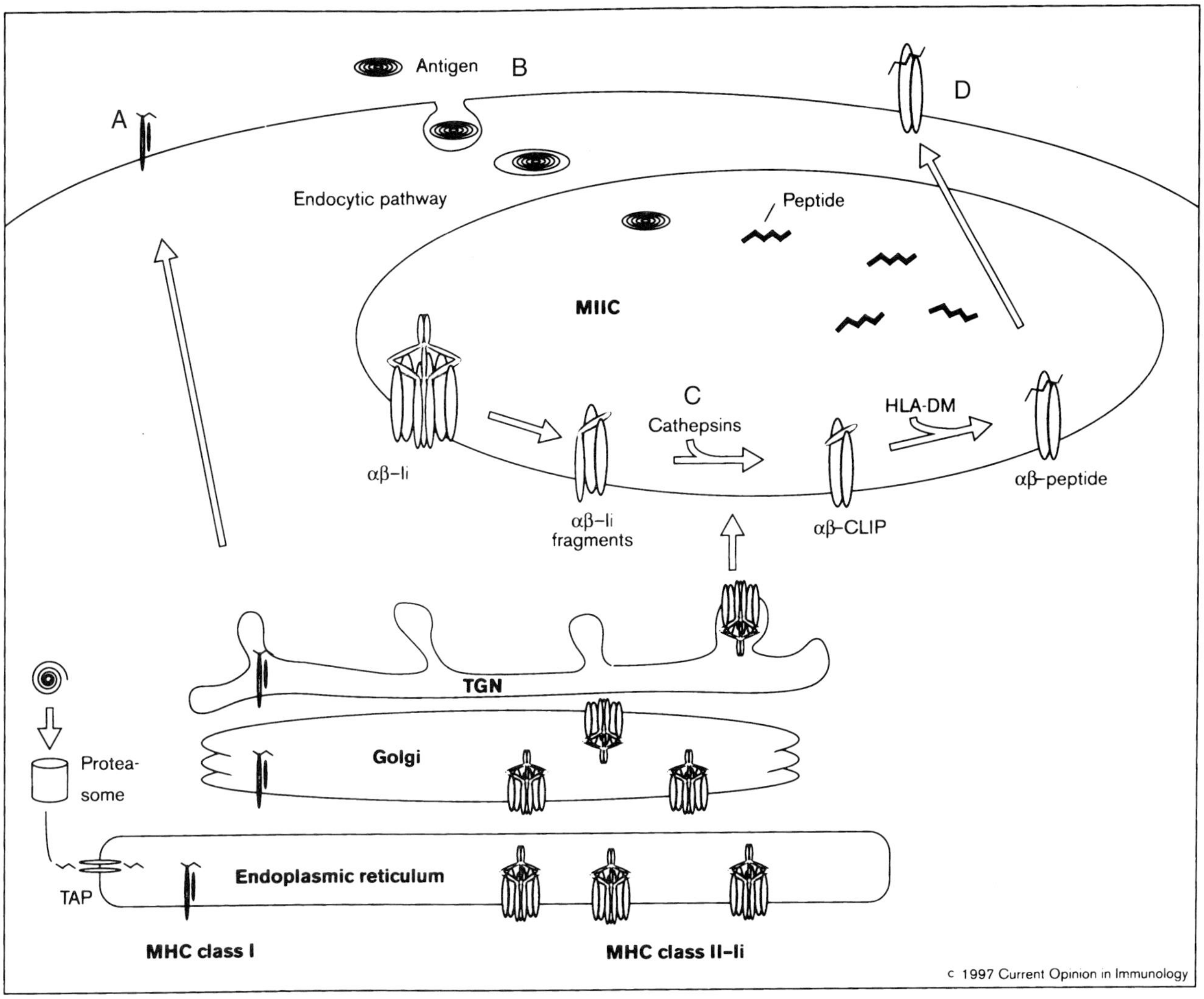

Figure 5–7. Intracellular pathways of major histocompatibility complex (MHC) class I and class II molecules. MHC class I molecules acquire antigenic peptides, generated by the proteasome, from the cytosol that are translocated into the endoplasmic reticulum by the TAP molecules (bottom of the figure). The MHC class I-peptide complex is transported through the Golgi complex directly to the cell surface for presentation to CD8⁺ T cells *(A)*. In contrast, MHC class II molecules acquire antigenic peptides derived from antigens that are internalized in the endocytic pathway *(B)*. MHC class II heterodimers associate in the endoplasmic reticulum (bottom of figure) with invariant chains to form nonameric αβ-Ii complexes. At the *trans*-Golgi network (TGN), these complexes are targeted to MHC class II compartments (MIIC) in the endocytic pathway as a result of targeting signals within the Ii cytoplasmic tail (not shown). There the MHC class II–associated Ii is degraded in distinct steps, at least partially by cathepsins *(C)*, leaving the CLIP peptide associated with the MHC class II peptide binding groove. CLIP can then be exchanged for antigenic peptides, and this exchange process is catalyzed by HLA-DM molecules. Peptide-loaded MHC class II complexes are then transported to the plasma membrane for presentation to CD4⁺ T cells *(D)*. TAP, transporter associated with antigen processing. (From Pieters J. MHC class II restricted antigen presentation. Curr Opin Immunol 1997; 9:91.)

Although viruses and tumors may attempt to cloak themselves by downregulating class I MHC, this strategy is not altogether effective. NK cells are preferentially activated by class I–deficient cells.[103, 104] Killer inhibitory receptors (KIRs) that bind class I molecules normally downregulate NK responses to class I MHC expressing cells. In the absence of class I MHC, cells are left susceptible to NK mediated lysis. NK cells are indeed found to be important in the control of viruses and some tumors. Nevertheless, some viruses still find it beneficial to downregulate class I MHC molecules. For example, cytomegalovirus destroys fledgling class I molecules in the ER, and herpes simplex virus blocks peptide translocation by the transporter for antigen processing (TAP).[105, 106]

In contrast to class I molecules, it is not necessary that all cells express class II MHC. Only select cells need scrutinize the extracellular environment. The cells that are dedicated to this task constitutively express class II MHC and are termed *professional APCs*. These consist of macrophages, dendritic cells, B cells, and some endothelial cells.[7, 9]

Professional APCs are unified in their ability to acquire antigens for presentation to CD4⁺ T cells. The means of this accumulation and the biology of the individual cell types differ, however. Although normally quiescent, macrophages are particularly potent phagocytic cells when activated by inflammatory stimuli such as lipopolysaccharide. They are capable of ingesting and digesting entire microorganisms, as well as internalizing antigens through cell surface receptors.

Dendritic cells constitutively macropinocytose extracellular fluid, concentrating extracellular antigens through their filter feeding behavior. Like macrophages, dendritic cells also express receptors for specific antigen types, including the mannose receptor and the low affinity receptor for immunoglobulin, crystallizable fragment γ receptor II (FcγRII). The long dendrites emanating from these cells are ideal for interacting with many cells and sampling the antigenic environment. Inflammatory stimuli induce their migration to lymphoid organs, where they are exceedingly potent activators of antigen-specific T cells.

B cells internalize antigen primarily through their BCR. Although B cells possess FcγRII, as do macrophages and dendritic cells, they express only a noninternalizing version, FcγRIIB1.[107] B cells therefore concentrate antigens specifically recognized by their own cell surface immunoglobulin. They present peptide fragments derived from these antigens to $CD4^+$ T cells, effectively informing them that the antigen to which they possess specific immunoglobulin is in the environment. The $CD4^+$ T cell, if appropriately activated, can then induce proliferation and differentiation of the antigen-specific B cell. When antigens are present in only minute quantities the ability to focus antigen with the BCR is important. Antigen concentrations too small to generate a significant density of antigen-MHC complexes on dendritic cells and macrophages may not be too low for presentation by antigen-specific B cells. However, the consequence of antigen presentation by B cells (and other APC) is not necessarily T cell activation. Indeed, B cells, particularly nonactivated B cells, have been shown to be extremely efficient inducers of T cell tolerance.[35, 108]

NONPEPTIDE ANTIGENS

Small peptides serve as the most general form of antigen presented to T lymphocytes. Peptide presentation, however, is not exclusive. Nonpeptides may be presented to T lymphocytes as well. The CD1 molecule is a nonpolymorphic transmembrane glycoprotein that is structurally similar to MHC.[109, 110] The key difference between CD1 and other MHC molecules is that CD1 contains a highly hydrophobic groove where other MHC molecules bind peptide. This groove is divided into two pockets, each of which binds a lipid arm of diacyl glycolipid molecules. CD1 seems particularly adept at binding and presenting the mycolic acids of mycobacteria.

Antigens of a second class do not even bind in the groove of the MHC molecule. Superantigens include a variety of proteins with binding sites for both the surface of MHC class II molecules and for the β chain of the TCR.[111, 112] These include bacterial products such as some staphylococcal enterotoxins and toxic shock syndrome toxin 1, as well as viral products. Each superantigen is specific for one or several TCR β chains. By directly crosslinking TCR with MHC, superantigens activate T cells independently of the TCR specificity and of the actual peptide bound in the MHC molecule's groove.

THE CONSEQUENCES OF ANTIGEN-MHC RECOGNITION

New approaches such as surface plasmon resonance, as well as an improved understanding of cell signaling pathways, have helped illuminate how TCRs respond to peptide-MHC complexes.[113–115] Studies of the binding of specific TCR for peptide-MHC reveal a low-affinity interaction, in the range of 5×10^{-4} to 10^{-7} mol/liter.[116–118] Dissociation rates are also rapid, at speeds of 10^{-2} to 10^{-1} seconds and even less. The interaction of TCR with peptide-MHC does not therefore result in the tight fit that occurs when immunoglobulin binds antigen. This observation does not imply that the TCR is indiscriminate in its binding. Unlike circulating antibody, the TCR is constrained by the two-dimensional surface of the plasma membrane. Furthermore, TCRs interact with MHC in the presence of additional cell-cell interactions, including those mediated by CD4 or CD8 as well as various adhesion molecules. These stabilize contact between the T cell and the APC, permitting the TCR to adequately examine the MHC-peptides presented by an APC. The T cell must be able to search rapidly among the hundreds of thousands of MHC molecules present on an APC for cognate antigen. In some studies, recognition of as few as 100 peptide-MHC specific complexes is sufficient to activate T cells.[119] However, this number undoubtedly varies with specific T cells, APCs, and antigens.

The consequences of TCR interaction with peptide-MHC are not uniform. Antigenic peptides can be roughly categorized into three classes: agonists, partial agonists, and antagonists.[120] When presented by a uniform population of APCs to a uniform population of T cells, these different types of peptides have different effects. Agonists fully activate T cells, and a stereotyped package of effector responses results. Partial agonists partially activate them, and some, but not all, of the consequences of full activation results; for instance, T cells may express interleukin (IL-2)–receptor, but fail to synthesize IL-2. Antagonists not only fail to activate T cells, but they prevent activation by simultaneously presented agonists. In some cases, they can induce a more prolonged state of T cell unresponsiveness termed *anergy.* (Note that this type of anergy is a cellular state and thus differs from the clinical use of the term *anergy,* meaning loss of T cell functional activity.)

The differences among agonists, partial agonists, and antagonists are subtle. Single amino acid changes may convert an agonist into a partial agonist or antagonist. Antagonists are associated with weaker TCR binding and increased TCR-MHC dissociation rates in comparison with agonists.[121–124] How this translates into distinct biological effects is not clear. One model, termed *kinetic proofreading,* postulates that the consequences of TCR engagement depend on the duration and fidelity of the interaction with MHC-peptide.[125, 126] Indeed, a large assembly of signaling molecules congregate at the point of T cell–APC contact. These include stimulatory as well as inhibitory proteins. Much like a snowball that starts an avalanche, subtle differences in affinity and duration of TCR contact with peptide-MHC may be sufficient to alter the balance of these components, leading either to cell activation or cell inhibition.

How TCR recognition of MHC translates into intracellular signaling is not understood. Two possibilities exist: allosteric changes in the TCR structure transmitted through the plasma membrane may induce cell activation, or crosslinking of multiple TCRs may stabilize a topological state capable of effectively signaling. Crosslinking seems to be important in cell activation through other receptors, such as the receptor for immunoglobulin E (IgE), FcεR. The fact that crosslinking antibodies bound to the TCR or the CD3 chains results in T cell stimulation suggests that receptor crosslinking is also important for the TCR.

Once a signal is transduced inside the T cell, the earliest detectable event is the phosphorylation of tyrosine residues on several proteins.[115] This phosphorylation is detectable within seconds of TCR engagement. The TCR-CD3 complex contains specific sites for tyrosine phosphorylation located within sequences called *immune tyrosine activation motifs* (ITAMs).[127] Each ITAM contains two tyrosine-X-X-leucine sequences, where X is an undefined amino acid. In a typical $\alpha\beta\gamma\delta\epsilon_2\zeta_2$ receptor, a total of 10 ITAMs are present, one in each of the CD3 chains and three in each of the ζ chains. Lck, which binds to CD4 or CD8, phosphorylates these ITAMs.[128] A second src family member, fyn, may play a similar role, but lck appears to be more important. Phosphorylation of the ζ chain attracts a second tyrosine kinase, ζ-associated protein (ZAP)–70. ZAP-70 is then activated by phosphorylation, possibly through lck or other src kinase–mediated activity, and a variety of downstream substrates are phosphorylated. In addition to its intrinsic kinase activity, ZAP-70 serves as a docking site for additional signaling molecules.[115]

Among the earliest of phosphorylation substrates arising from T cell activation is phosphatidylinositol phospholipase C-γ1 (PI-PLC-γ1).[129] Phosphorylation of PI-PLC-γ1, along with proteins that associate with it, both activates this enzyme and directs it to the plasma membrane. It then catalyzes the breakdown of phosphatidylinositol-4,5-bisphosphate into inositol 1,4,5-triphosphate (IP_3) and diacylglycerol (DAG). IP_3 mediates a rise in the cytoplasmic Ca^{2+} concentration by promoting release from intracellular stores. The Ca^{2+} complexes with the regulatory protein calmodulin. Ca^{2+}-calmodulin then activates several enzymes important for the activation of transcription factors. For example, members of the nuclear factor of activated T cells (NFAT) family of transcription factors are important in regulating transcription of IL-2, IL-4, and other cytokine genes. Ca^{2+}-calmodulin activates the serine-threonine specific protein phosphatase calcineurin. Calcineurin, in turn, dephosphorylates NFAT sequestered in the cell cytoplasm. This exposes a nuclear localization signal, directing NFAT to the nucleus, where it may regulate gene expression.

The DAG released as a result of PI-PLC-γ1 activity induces other signaling pathways through protein kinase C (PKC). PKC is a serine-threonine kinase capable of phosphorylating numerous substrates. Its relevance to T cell activation is demonstrated by the ability of pharmacological inducers of PKC to synergize with Ca^{2+} ionophores in activating T cells.

Although the PI-PLC-γ1–induced signaling pathways are essential to T cell activation, TCR signaling is not limited to them. The mitogen-activated protein (MAP) kinase pathways consist of cascades of serine-threonine kinases.[130] An MAP-kinase kinase kinase phosphorylates and activates an MAP-kinase kinase. This similarly activates an MAP kinase. These pathways are named after the identity of the MAP kinase. In T cell activation, the extracellular signal regulated kinase (ERK), c-Jun-N-terminal kinase (JNK), and p38 pathways are important in signaling. Within these individual pathways there may be several MAP kinases. Thus there are multiple ERK, JNK, and p38 family members. One example of the importance of these kinase cascades is in the induction of the transcription factor AP-1.[131] AP-1 is a heterodimer consisting of two proteins, Jun and Fos. Fos is regulated transcriptionally. Activated ERK-1 or other MAP kinases phosphorylate Elk-1, which in turn promotes Fos gene transcription. Jun is regulated by phosphorylation. Activated JNK phosphorylates Jun which is then translocated into the nucleus and associates with Fos to form AP-1. The AP-1 transcription factor can bind the enhancer region of several cytokine genes and can even bind other transcription factors, such as NFAT, promoting cytokine gene transcription.

Like PI-PLC-γ1, the MAP kinase pathways are coupled to the TCR by phosphorylation. Several steps must occur before the initiation of these pathways. Thus, for the ERK pathway, ZAP-70 phosphorylates an adaptor protein, possibly Grb-2, which activates a guanosine triphosphate/guanosine diphosphate (GTP/GDP) exchanger. This replaces the GDP on Ras with a GTP molecule, thereby activating it. Ras then binds to and activates the MAP-kinase kinase kinase.

T cell signaling pathways seem inordinately complex. However, the multiple intersecting pathways and the number of intermediates involved form a web of interactive strands. As the spider can sense minor perturbations at specific places in its web, the T cell can discriminate and amplify subtle changes that result from the occupation of even a small number of its TCR molecules. As discussed later, information from the TCR is integrated with that arising from a number of other signaling molecules. The T cell therefore uses its receptors to sense its environment, uses its signaling pathways as a brain to integrate the information, and then responds accordingly.

ADDITIONAL SIGNALING MOLECULES

Although the TCR is foremost in T cell signaling, a number of other molecules are important modifiers of T cell responses.[132] Some of these are listed in Table 5–1. The roles of CD4 and CD8 have already been discussed. As shown in the table, a number of signaling molecules are also adhesion molecules; hence T cells can adaptively

Table 5–1. T Cell Surface Accessory Molecules

Name	Synonyms	Biochemical Characteristics	Gene Family	Cellular Distribution	Ligand	Function in T Cells: Adhesion	Function in T Cells: Signal Transduction
CD4	T4 (human), L3T4 (mouse)	55-kD monomer	Ig	TCR α/β positive class II MHC–restricted T cells; macrophages	Class II MHC molecules	+	+
CD8	T8 (human), Lyt-2 (mouse)	α/α homodimer with 78-kD α chain or α/β heterodimer	Ig	TCR α/β positive class I MHC–restricted T cells	Class I MHC molecules	+	+
CD49CD29	VLA-4, VLA-5, VLA-6	α/β heterodimer	Integrin	Leukocytes, other cells	Matrix molecules, VCAM-1	+	+
CD11aCD18	LFA-1	α/β heterodimer with 180-kD α chain, 95-kD β chain	Integrin	All bone marrow–derived cells	ICAM-1, ICAM-2	+	+
CD28	Tp44	80- to 90-kD homodimer	Ig	All $CD4^+$ T cells; 50% $CD8^+$ T cells	B7-1, B7-2	–	+
CD2	T11, LFA-2, Leu-5, SRBC receptor	50-kD monomer	Ig	>90% mature human T cells, >70% human thymocytes	LFA-3	+	+
CD45R	T200; leukocyte common antigen; B220 (on B cells)	180- to 220-kD monomers; cytoplasmic tyrosine phosphatase domain		All immmature and mature leukocytes		–	+
CD40 ligand	gp39	Trimers of 39-kD chains	TNF	Activated T cells and mast cells	CD40	–	+
Fas ligand		Trimers of ~40-kD chains	TNF	Activated T cells	Fas (CD950)	–	+
CD5	T1, Leu-1 (humans), Lyt-1 (mice)	67-kD monomer		All T cells and thymocytes		–	+
Ly6		10- to 18-kD monomers; glycophospholipid membrane anchor		Immature and mature T and B cells; various other tissues		–	+
CD44	PgP-1	80- to 200-kD monomer; variably glycosylated, chondroitin sulfated	Cartilage link proteins	Thymocytes, T cells, granulocytes, macrophages, erythrocytes, fibroblasts	Collagen fibronectin, hyaluronate	+	?+
L-selectin	CD62L Mel-14 Lam-1	150-kD monomer	Selectin	B cell, T cells, monocytes, NK cells	Sialylated glycoproteins on high HEV	+	–

HEV, high endothelial venule; ICAM, intercellular adhesion molecule; Ig, immunoglobulin, LFA, leukocyte function–associated antigen; MHC, major histocompatibility complex; NK, natural killer; TCR, T cell receptor; TNF, tumor necrosis factor; VCAM, vascular cell adhesion molecule; VLA, very late activation.

respond to the cell that they are binding. For example, the CD11a/18 complex, a β_2 integrin called *leukocyte function–associated antigen-1* (LFA-1), binds intracellular adhesion molecule (ICAM)–1.[133] ICAM-1 is expressed on a variety of cells, including lymphocytes, endothelial, and epithelial cells. Cell-bound ICAM-1 can promote T cell activation because of its adhesive properties. However, soluble ICAM can also enhance the stimulation of T lymphocytes. Thus LFA-1 seems to function not only as an adhesion protein but also as a stimulatory receptor. Interestingly, much as LFA-1 signaling enhances T cell activation, activation through the TCR increases the avidity of LFA-1.[134, 135] This would be expected to stabilize the T cell–APC association when a T cell is stimulated by cognate antigen. Increased LFA-1 avidity likely results from changes in the molecule after phosphorylation of its cytoplasmic tail.

Another cell surface molecule enhances T cell activation through a distinct mechanism. CD45, or leukocyte common antigen, is a protein ubiquitously expressed on cells of myeloid or lymphoid origin.[136] Its cytoplasmic tail is a protein tyrosine phosphatase. The activity of the CD45 phosphatase may be considered in T cell signaling to be much like the gain on an amplifier. CD45 dephosphorylates a critical inhibitory residue on lck and other src family protein tyrosine kinases.[137, 138] When phosphorylated lck folds upon itself, its catalytic site is sterically blocked; conversely, lck dephosphorylation opens its confirmation, permitting activity. Because lck is a crucial initiator of T cell activation, the activity of CD45 helps establish the sensitivity of T cells to TCR signaling.

A number of isoforms of the CD45 molecule are found. Three of the exons (A, B, and C) are alternatively spliced, resulting in a total of eight possible variants. These variants are differentially expressed on different types of T cells. Thus T cells that have had prior antigen exposure and have differentiated into memory cells (discussed later) preferentially express CD45RO, whereas T cells that have not been exposed to cognate antigen (i.e. naive cells) preferentially express CD45RA. Although naive and memory T cells have significantly different sensitivities to antigen, the role of differences in CD45 isoforms is not clear. Differential interactions between the CD45 isoforms and T cell signaling molecules such as the TCR, CD4, and CD2 may be important in this regard.[139, 140]

The molecules just described assist in TCR-mediated signaling by enhancing the binding of T cell to APC and/or by enhancing the signal that the TCR transmits. Thus LFA-1 signaling, much like TCR signaling, results in calcium mobilization and increased PI-PLC-γ1 and PKC activity. However, there are some accessory signaling molecules that transmit signals distinct from those of the TCR, signals that are critical for T cell activation. These molecules are termed *costimulators.* CD28 is the best characterized costimulatory molecule on T cells.

COSTIMULATION IS A PREREQUISITE FOR T CELL ACTIVATION

In 1970 Bretscher and Cohn observed that immune responses to nonhematopoietic cells required the additional presence of hematopoietic cells.[141] They hypothesized that antigen by itself was insufficient to provoke immune responses and that additional costimulatory molecules are required. Lafferty and associates, who demonstrated the importance of hematopoietic cells in graft rejection, extended this hypothesis, asserting that T cell activation requires costimulation.[142] The nature of this costimulation was debated and soluble effector molecules, such as IL-1, were believed to be the most likely candidates for costimulation. However, Jenkins and Schwartz showed that cell surface molecules distinct from peptide-MHC were critical for the activation of some T cell clones.[143, 144] In a more impressive finding, they demonstrated that in the absence of these molecules, the T cells not only failed to respond to antigen—as measured by proliferation and cytokine production—but they also became refractory to restimulation. This state of antigen-induced unresponsiveness, as mentioned earlier, is termed *anergy.*

The search for the costimulatory factor led to many candidates, but CD28 appears preeminent.[145] CD28 is a glycoprotein in the immunoglobulin superfamily that serves as a receptor for two known ligands, CD80 (B7.1) and CD86 (B7.2). Binding of CD28 to its receptor augments T cell proliferation and cytokine secretion. It also protects T cells from activation-induced cell death by increasing expression of the antiapoptotic protein Bcl-x.[146] The importance of CD28 is apparent from mice in which CD28 is eliminated by homologous recombination.[147–150] T cell responses in such mice are abortive, and proliferative responses are not sustained. Responses to superantigens are weak. Whereas highly virulent viruses are capable of inducing a sufficient response for viral clearance, less virulent strains trigger inadequate responses. Therefore, CD28 is critical in sustaining immune responses. Whether it is indeed the only costimulatory molecule to do so is not clear. The activities of other costimulators may be sufficient to allow the parsimonious responses seen in the CD28-deficient mice.[132]

The importance of CD28/B7-mediated costimulation is also apparent from other studies. Expression of B7 in vitro can transform an APC that renders T cells anergic to one that activates them. Expression of B7 on specific tissues in vivo augments immunity and can even promote autoimmunity. For example, mice expressing a class II MHC molecule transgenically on their β-islet cells do not develop diabetes, although the islet cells become more adept at presenting islet-specific antigens to T cells. Likewise, mice expressing B7 transgenically on their islets do not become diabetic. In contrast, mice expressing both islet-specific class II molecules and B7 develop islet specific autoimmunity and diabetes.[151] Therefore, the presence of effective costimulation along with a sufficient dose of MHC-peptide is critical in defining a competent APC. Many types of cells, such as the β-islet cells in this example, can be transformed into effective APC through the expression of adequate levels of peptide-MHC accompanied with a costimulatory ligand.

Whereas CD28 is constitutively expressed on the majority of T cells, the B7 molecules are expressed on professional APCs only after activation. The induction kinetics and cell specificity of B7.1 and B7.2 differ.[152] Whether these two ligands also relay unique signals through CD28 is not known. Because B7 molecules are so important in transforming a T cell encounter with antigen that may be tolerance inducing or nonactivating into one resulting in active immunity, their regulation is critical. Upregulation of B7 is observed with activation of the innate immune system.[11] This may be important in linking the adaptive and innate immune systems, ensuring that immune responses are limited to situations in which a genuine threat exists.

Activated T cells can also induce the upregulation of B7 on APCs through cell-cell interactions. CD40 is expressed on professional APCs. Its ligand, CD154 (CD40L), is expressed on activated T cells. Ligation of CD40 with CD40L induces the upregulation of B7.[153, 154] The CD40-CD154 interaction also upregulates immune responses in other ways. For example, it increases CD58 (LFA-3) expression on dendritic cells and induces the synthesis of various cytokines and chemokines, including IL-8, macrophage inflammatory protein (MIP)–1α, tumor necrosis factor (TNF)–α, and IL-12. It is also required for macrophage nitric oxide synthesis and IL-12 production. Congenital absence of CD154 leads to impaired T cell–APC interactions. Hyper-IgM syndrome and impaired responses to a variety of pathogens are seen.

In addition to CD28, T cells express a second receptor for the B7 molecules, CTLA-4 (CD152).[155] CTLA-4 binds the B7 molecules with 10-fold higher affinity than does CD28.[156] Although it shares ligands with CD28, its function is quite different. Whereas CD28-deficient mice have limited T cell responses, CTLA-4 deficiency results in uncontrolled T cell activation.[157–159] Lymphoproliferation results in death within a month, with most T cells blastic and expressing various surface activation markers. When CTLA-4–deficient T cells are cultured in vitro, they spontaneously proliferate and produce a variety of cytokines. Whereas CD28 augments T cell responses, CTLA-4 restricts them. The kinetics of CTLA-4 expression follow logically from this presumed function. Unlike CD28, CTLA-4 is not normally expressed or is expressed at very low levels on the resting T cell surface. CTLA-4 expression is greatly enhanced, however, after T-cell activation. Thus a T cell that encounters antigen and costimulation will be activated, but the response will be limited by expression of CTLA-4. Stimulation of T cells through CTLA-4 indeed results in cell cycle arrest and inhibition of IL-2 production.[160]

The mechanism of CTLA-4 action remains uncertain. One possibility is that it serves as a competitive antagonist for CD28. Its higher avidity for the B7 molecules should allow it to outcompete CD28 for binding of costimulator. Indeed, the phenotype of mice deficient for both B7-1 and B7-2 is similar to that of CD28-deficient mice, which implies that the B7–CTLA-4 interaction contributes little beyond suppressing the B7-CD28 interaction.[161] In contrast, however, there is evidence that CTLA-4 can signal T cells. The cytoplasmic tail of CTLA-4 contains SH2 and SH3 domains.[162] These domains in other proteins have been found to bind signal transducing molecules. In CTLA-4–deficient mice, several TCR-associated tyrosine kinases are found to be constitutively activated through phosphorylation. Although not proof, this implies that CTLA-4 normally downmodulates the activities of these kinases. In support of this hypothesis, CTLA-4 is found to interact with the tyrosine phosphatase SHP-2.[163] This or other CTLA-4–protein associations could conceivably downregulate T cell signaling by dephosphorylating or otherwise inhibiting TCR-associated tyrosine kinases.

THYMIC MATURATION DETERMINES THE NAIVE T CELL REPERTOIRE

The challenge in developing the T cell repertoire differs from that in developing the B cell repertoire. Unlike B cells, T cells recognize only antigen presented by MHC molecules. Rearrangement of the V, D, and J components of the TCR occurs randomly and independently of the MHC. Although there may be a gross coevolution of TCR and MHC genes to ensure compatibility, this similarity does not guarantee that an individual's T cell repertoire will be able to interact well with the corresponding complement of MHC genes. In view of the polymorphism of the MHC locus, which involves particularly the region of the MHC molecule that interacts with the TCR, it is surprising that a functional repertoire of T cells develops at all. Indeed, it has been estimated that only 20% of randomly rearranged TCRs can recognize the MHC molecules of an individual.[164] Nonetheless, the immune system is much more efficient, because the repertoire of antigen-inexperienced, or antigen-naive, T cells is actively crafted during T cell development.

T cells develop in the thymus.[165] T cell precursors emigrate from the bone marrow to the thymus. The developmental progress of T cells in the thymus is most conveniently described by the expression of surface markers[166] (Fig. 5–8). The earliest T cell progenitors are $CD4^-$/dim$CD8^-TCR^-$.[167, 168] These constitute a small percentage of thymocytes. During this early state, the TCR β chain rearranges. If the rearrangement is productive, the β chain associates with an α chain surrogate, pTα, and this pair associates with the CD3 complex.[169] Although little pTα-β chain complex is found on the cell surface, it does transmit signals into the developing thymocyte. The developing thymocyte stops rearrangement of the second β chain allele (if this allele is in its germ line state). It upregulates CD4 and CD8, and it proliferates and expands. IL-7 is particularly important for blastogenesis in this early population of cells.[170, 171]

Next, the T cell begins rearranging its α chain genes. If a productively rearranged α chain capable of pairing with the β chain is formed, it replaces the pTα chain. Because timing of the shutdown of α chain rearrangement is not as rigid as that of the β chain, a portion of T cells develop without allelic exclusion of the α chain.[172] These cells may express two distinct functional TCRs on their surface if they can pair equivalently with the β chain. Although up to 30% of T cells have two productively rearranged α chain genes, most express only a single αβ heterodimer, because one α chain usually outcompetes the second chain in binding β chain.

Numerically, $CD4^+CD8^+$ thymocytes—either $pT\alpha^+$ that have not yet rearranged their α chain or $\alpha\beta^+$ that have successfully completed this rearrangement—constitute the bulk of thymocytes.[173] Whereas the pTα-β^+ receptor has no known ligand, $\alpha\beta^+$ T cells are capable

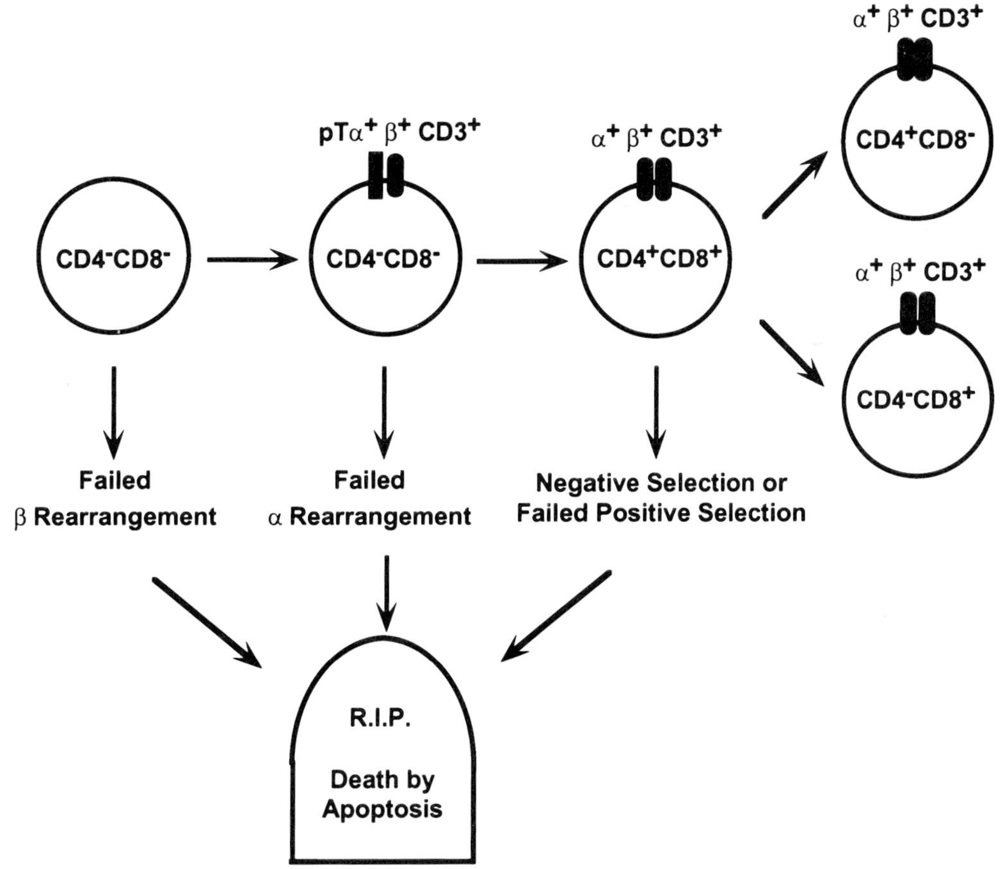

Figure 5–8. Schematic representation of the progression of thymocyte cell surface phenotypes during T cell development. The majority of thymocytes are $CD4^+CD8^+$; 5% or fewer are $CD4^-CD8^-$, and fewer than 20% are $CD4^+CD8^-$ or $CD4^-CD8^+$. These latter "single positive" cells exit the thymus and migrate to peripheral lymphoid organs.

of functional interactions with MHC. The level of TCR on $CD4^+CD8^+TCR\alpha\beta^+$ thymocytes is initially low, but with development the TCR increases to levels seen on mature T cells. The T cells also commit to lineage, down-regulating either CD4 or CD8. Thus $CD4^+CD8^-$ or $CD4^-CD8^+$ thymocytes with a surface phenotype identical to that of peripheral naive T cells develop. These cells exit the thymus to populate the peripheral lymphoid organs.

The majority of thymocytes undergo programmed cell death, or apoptosis, before they can fully mature. Fewer than 5% of developing thymocytes actually survive to exit the thymus.[58] This cell death does not reflect a lack of economy in T cell development. On the contrary, thymocytes must run a gantlet of selective forces to help ensure that only the cells most likely to contribute to a functional yet diverse repertoire are produced. Very few T cells react to any specific antigen-MHC complex. By eliminating T cells with specificities likely to be useless, thymic selection ensures that precursor frequencies do not become so low that a critical mass of T cells specific for a particular antigen cannot be found.

Two selective processes guide survival and death of developing thymocytes. The first, negative selection, acts to eliminate cells reactive to self antigens, serving to tolerize the immune system. If a developing thymocyte encounters cognate antigen, rather than being activated to proliferate and develop into an effector cell, it undergoes apoptosis.[174–178] Negative selection is extremely powerful. Conceptually, it can eliminate the bulk of self-reactive T cells. Antigens common to all cells in the body will be presented in the thymus, deleting reactive cells. Even antigens expressed outside the thymus may be presented within the thymus.

Hematopoietically derived APCs are particularly effective inducers of negative selection.[179, 180] These APCs may accumulate antigens throughout the body, load them onto their MHC class II molecules, and present them in the thymus. Antigens present in blood can also enter the thymus and there be loaded onto APCs.[181] Therefore, negative selection can theoretically be wholly responsible for tolerance among $CD4^+$ T cells, which recognize antigen presented by class II molecules. Whether antigens expressed outside the thymus can also be presented on class I molecules to tolerize the $CD8^+$ T cell lineage is less clear. Although the possible presentation of extracellular antigens by class I MHC has been described, the biological relevance of this observation is uncertain.[182, 183] Indeed, mice made transgenic with a variety of proteins expressed only outside the thymus fail to eliminate reactive $CD8^+$ T cells.[46, 184, 185] Nevertheless, the importance of $CD4^+$ T cell tolerance cannot be underestimated. Many $CD8^+$ T cell responses are not possible without help from $CD4^+$ T cells.[186, 187] Thus elimination of self-reactive $CD4^+$ T cells can prevent autoaggression by some $CD8^+$ T cells.

Although negative selection is the major mechanism for self-tolerance, it cannot account for the entirety of tolerance to self. Some antigens are expressed only after birth.[188, 189] T cells maturing before their expression may become autoaggressive. A small number of T cells have been observed to mature extrathymically.[190] These cells cannot profit from thymic deletion. Indeed, T cells specific for self antigens can be isolated even in the absence of autoimmune disease.[38–42] These cells circulate quiescently under normal circumstances. Clearly, thymic deletion is not acting to check their potential for autoaggression.

Although thymic deletion is the largest force ensuring self-tolerance, other mechanisms fill its loopholes. These mechanisms include anergy and ignorance, as well as active suppression by regulatory T cells.

The second selective force in T cell development is positive selection. Positive selection ensures that all T cells have the capability of interacting with an individual's complement of MHC molecules. The idea that T cells are developmentally selected to interact with self MHC molecules originated with studies in the late 1970s demonstrating that the reactivity of T cells from a mouse immunized with a random antigen on host MHC molecules was substantially greater than that for the same antigen presented on different MHC alleles.[191] For example, T cells from MHC A-type mice responded well to antigen X only when X was presented by A-type MHC, not B-type MHC. Conversely, T cells from MHC B-type mice responded well only to X presented by B-type MHC. Studies of mice made chimeric for either bone marrow or the thymus demonstrated that the thymic epithelium is the key cell type in imparting this recognition bias.

The generation of mice transgenic for a single rearranged TCR in the late 1980s permitted positive selection to be directly observed. Virtually all T cells in TCR transgenic mice express a single receptor. Studies with TCR transgenic animals demonstrated that each individual T cell must interact with a positively selecting ligand. In the absence of this interaction, the cell dies.[175, 192] Thus if the TCR used to make the TCR transgenic mice was derived from MHC A-type mice, MHC type A (or potentially a few other positively selecting MHC types) must be present developmentally in order for the thymocytes to progress from the $CD4^+CD8^+$ stage to the more mature $CD4^+CD8^-$ or $CD4^-CD8^+$ stages. In the absence of MHC type A, all thymocytes die before completing development.

It is paradoxical that some encounters of T cells with MHC lead to negative selection and cell death, whereas other encounters lead to positive selection and survival. The exclusive loading of single peptides onto MHC molecules in either in vitro organ culture systems or in vivo has allowed the study of how individual peptides may alternatively lead to negative versus positive selection.[124, 193–195] Three categories of peptides have been distinguished: peptides that have no effect, peptides that positively select, and peptides that negatively select. The selecting peptide–MHC complexes can be distinguished on the basis of their affinity for TCR: ligands with no effect have negligible affinities, positively selecting ligands have weak affinities, and negatively selecting ligands have high affinities. This system ensures that only T cells capable of interacting with, but not being activated by, self MHC with self peptides are allowed to mature. Among the T cells that are positively selected by a weak interaction with MHC and self-peptide are those capable of interacting with a slightly different ligand: foreign peptide presented by self MHC. Therefore, selection biases the T cell repertoire toward cells capable of recognizing foreign antigens.

Although it is possible that single peptide–MHC ligands positively select T cells, it seems more likely that multiple different peptide-MHC complexes, all with low affinity, mediate positive selection.[193] When mice are limited to expressing single MHC alleles containing single peptides, 20% to 50% of normal numbers of T cells still develop.[196–198] This suggests that many TCRs have weak affinity for and can be positively selected by any single ligand. It can be presumed that the corollary of this—namely that many MHC peptide ligands have a weak affinity for a randomly selected TCR—is also true. Because thousands of unique peptide-MHC complexes are present on any APC, it is likely that many low-affinity interactions, rather than a few of low to moderate affinity, induce positive selection in vivo.

MATURE T CELLS CAN BE CATEGORIZED INTO DISTINCT CLASSES ON THE BASIS OF PHENOTYPE AND FUNCTION

T cells are most readily categorized into broad groups according to the presence of CD4 or CD8 and the presence of αβ or γδ TCR. This phenotypic categorization reflects functional divisions. $CD4^+$ T cells recognize antigen acquired and presented by professional APC. After activation, $CD4^+$ T cells may acquire effector functions; however, much of their role is to verify that antigen is present and provide help to other effector cells, such as $CD8^+$ T cells or B cells. For this reason, the term *helper T cell*, although somewhat inaccurate, is sometimes used synonymously with $CD4^+$ T cell. The help may come in the form of secreted cytokines, such as IL-2 and IL-4, or cell surface molecules such as CD40L. $CD8^+$ T cells recognize antigens derived from intracellular sources. Although some regulatory roles have been ascribed to $CD8^+$ T cells, their primary function is to eliminate cells with undesirable intracellular antigens, such as virally or bacterially infected cells. Hence $CD8^+$ T cells are often inaccurately referred to as cytolytic T lymphocytes (CTL) or CTL precursors.

Although it is convenient to distinguish T cells on the basis of these phenotypic markers, significant functional differences exist among $CD4^+$ or among $CD8^+$ T cells. These differences are not necessarily flagged by the expression of unique cell surface markers. Functional discrimination of T cells has resulted from studies of the profile of effector functions that follow from stimulation of subsets of T cells.

The best characterized functional T cell subsets are the T helper–1 and T helper–2 (Th1 and Th2) subsets of

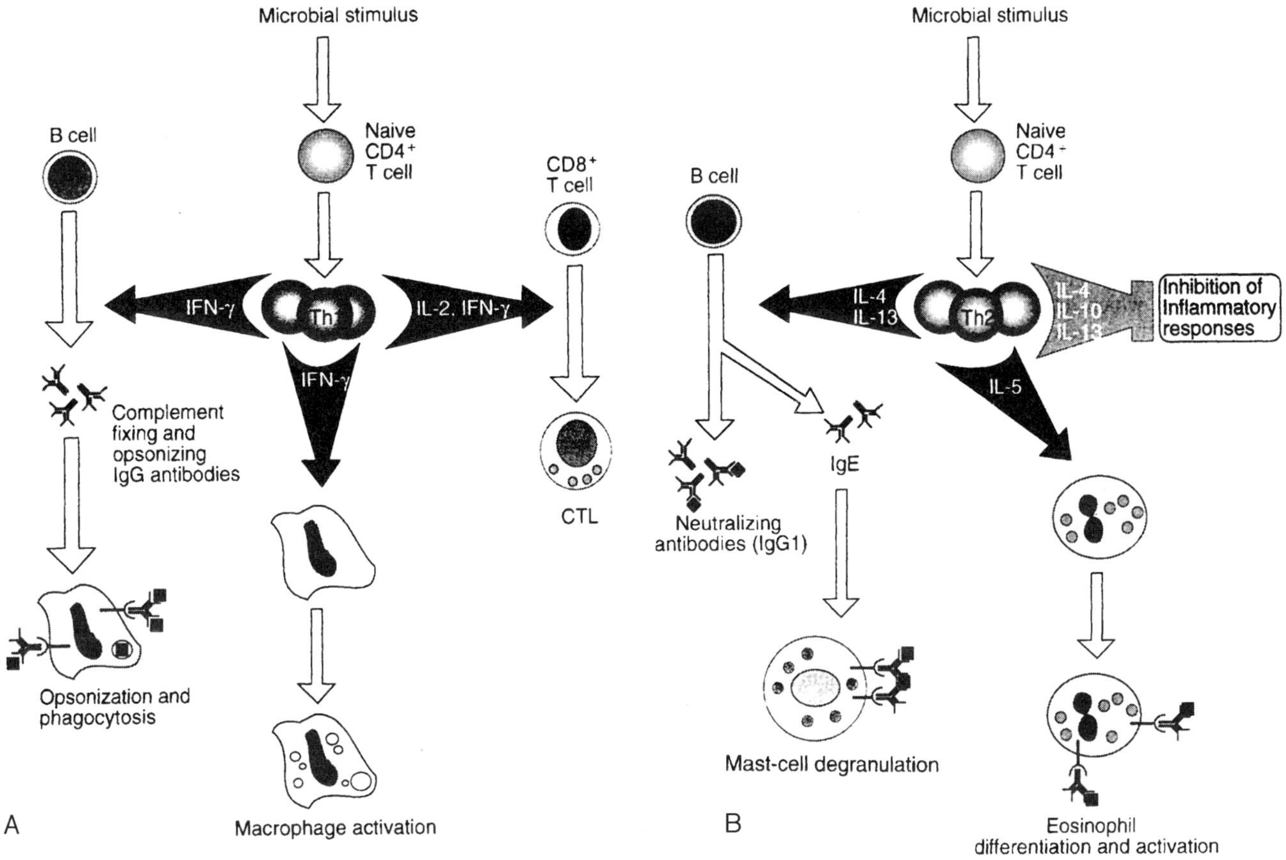

Figure 5–9. Effector function of Th1 and Th2 subsets of CD4+ helper T lymphocytes. Th1 cells *(A)* induce phagocyte and T cell mediated defense reactions against microbes; Th2 cells *(B)* induce immunoglobulin E (IgE)–dependent mast cell degranulation and eosinophil activation, two components of the immediate hypersensitivity response. CTL, cytolytic T lymphocytes. (From Abbas AK, Murphy KM, Sher A. Functional diversity of helper T lymphocytes. Nature 1996; 383:789.)

CD4+ T cells[199, 200] (Fig. 5–9). The distinction between Th1 and Th2 cells followed the recognition that specific immunity frequently involves patterned responses. One such response is delayed-type hypersensitivity (DTH).[9, 19] The DTH reaction is an inflammatory cell-mediated immune response ultimately resulting in the activation of macrophage. At the site of antigen introduction, initial T cell activation leads to endothelial cell activation, followed by neutrophil, monocyte, and lymphocyte recruitment and activation and by a loss of vascular integrity. The resulting leakage of fibrinogen and other plasma-derived macromolecules causes induration. Recruited monocytes transform into activated macrophages. These macrophages are highly competent at eliminating various intracellular pathogens, including bacteria and protozoa. They are efficient phagocytes, producing significant amounts of nitrous oxide and other activated oxygen species that can kill internalized organisms. They stimulate T cells by serving as APCs, which can promote the amplification of the immune response, as well as the development of CTL activity. CTL activity may result from the activation of CD8+ T cells. Some CD4+ T cells also possess a more limited cytolytic ability. Activated macrophages further produce multiple cytokines that promote inflammation. If the DTH response persists, stimulation of fibrous tissue synthesis by transforming growth factor (TGF)–β and other cytokines results in scarring at the site of inflammation and in granuloma formation. Although the primary effector cells in DTH are macrophage and not CD4+ T cells, T cells are required for DTH initiation.

A second example of a patterned response to pathogens is the humoral and allergic response mediated by B cell–derived antibodies. Like DTH, these responses are frequently dependent on CD4+ T cell activity. This immune pathway is frequently used in responses against extracellular pathogens such as helminths. Pathogen-specific antibodies can induce antibody-dependent cell-mediated cytotoxicity (ADCC) and the elimination of the offending organism.

Although both DTH and allergic responses rely on CD4+ T cells, the T cells are quite different. The cells that initiate DTH are Th1 cells; those that initiate the allergic/antibody reaction are Th2 cells. Both Th1 and Th2 cells derive from a common precursor.[201] These cells have the capacity to secrete a large array of cytokines upon stimulation, but with differentiation into Th1 or Th2 cells, the cytokine secretion patterns become more limited. Whereas Th1 cells secrete IL-2, IFN-γ, and TNF-β upon activation, Th2 cells secrete IL-4, IL-5, IL-6, and IL-13.[199, 202, 203] Cytokine secretion profiles of Th1 and Th2 cells explain their functional specialization. Each cytokine profile includes factors with several functions. Autocrine growth factors, such as IL-2 in Th1 cells or IL-4 in Th2 cells, promote expansion of antigen-specific T cells. Other cytokines promote effector functions. Thus IFN-γ and TNF-β activate macrophage and leukocytes for cytocidal activity. IFN-γ further promotes the formation of IgG isotypes that bind to high-affinity IgG receptors and complement, promoting opsonization or destruction of pathogenic organisms. IL-4, in contrast, is the major cytokine promoting immunoglobulin class switching to the IgE subset. IL-5 activates eosinophils, which are important in the elimination of some parasites.

More interesting from the standpoint of global immune regulation is that Th1 and Th2 cells produce cytokines that both promote their own and inhibit each other's development. Thus IFN-γ induces both IL-12 production by macrophages and expression of IL-12 receptor on T lymphocytes. IL-12 is the major cytokine known to promote differentiation of T cells along the Th1 pathway. IFN-γ also inhibits the generation of Th2 cells. Likewise, IL-4 promotes Th2 differentiation and inhibits Th1 differentiation. As a result, adaptive immune responses are not only amplified but also polarized. Either a Th1 or a Th2 response predominates. The net observed response, DTH versus allergic/antibody, reflects this polarization.

The events that support progression along a Th1 or Th2 pathway are not fully understood. Clearly, innate immune responses are important in defining pathogen type and thus in supporting either of these developmental responses. NK cells can secrete IFN-γ, and this may be important in initiating Th1 responses.[204] Likewise, a class of CD4$^+$ T cells that express the NK1.1 marker releases substantial amounts of IL-4 upon activation.[205] These cells seem to recognize a nonpolymorphic MHC molecule. Although they are potential initiators of Th2 development, their role in in vivo responses remains uncertain.

Biochemical changes involving transcription factor activities, and possibly chromatin accessibility associated with differentiation of Th1 and Th2 cells, promote their stability.[110] Differentiated Th1 and Th2 cells may be long-lived,[206, 207] and so restimulation with antigen can resurrect a Th1 response with production of IFN-γ, and residual Th2 cells can induce a Th2 response.

The polarization of T cell responses has important clinical consequences. Allograft acceptance is frequently associated with the development of a Th2 pattern of response, whereas Th1 responses result in graft rejection. A Th1 pattern has also been associated with some autoimmune states.[199] Furthermore, Th1 and Th2 responses relate to pathogen clearance. A humoral response to leprosy results in the progressive lepromatous pattern; a DTH response results in the localized tuberculoid pattern.

Th1 and Th2 are the best characterized functional subsets of T cells. However, these cells and their progenitors are not the only types of CD4$^+$ T cells. Studies of antigenic responses by gut-associated mucosal tissue have revealed two other types. One CD4$^+$ subset identified and termed *Th3 cells* produces TGF-β and variable levels of the Th2 cytokines IL-4 and IL-10.[208] These Th3 cells were shown to downmodulate experimentally induced autoimmune encephalomyelitis. A second subset that bears regulatory functions, T-regulatory-1 cells (Tr1), produce IL-10 (which is also produced by Th2 and some Th1 cells) but only a small amount of IL-2 and no IL-4.[209] The presence of regulatory cells such as the Th3 and Tr1 cells implies that downmodulation of immune responses is an active process involving networks of specific regulatory cells and not just the isolated reduction in the activity of specific effector cells.

Much as CD4$^+$ T cells are functionally divisible, CD8$^+$ effector cells can be separated into Tc1 and Tc2 subsets.[210] These subsets are analogous to Th1 and Th2 cells in regard to cytokine production. Although both Tc1 and Tc2 cells are cytolytic, whether there are differences in their cytolytic abilities is unclear.

The Th1/Th2 paradigm clearly demonstrates how effector responses coincide with the need to produce stereotyped biological responses. How these responses are regulated so as to clear pathogens effectively without harming the host is only now appreciated.

ACTIVATED T CELLS MAY DIE OR FORM MEMORY CELLS

Activated T cells proliferate in response to autocrine or paracrine cytokines, such as IL-2 and IL-4. However, as the initiating stimulus is cleared, there are two needs. First, the adaptive response must be downmodulated to prevent damage to the host. Second, the immune system must remember the insult. It must maintain an armamentarium of specific lymphocytes, available for quick response to recrudescent or recurrent disease. Downmodulation of T cell responses occurs in two ways. First, receptors such as CTLA-4 downregulate T cell activities. This activity, however, does not clear the large cohort of T cell clones expanded after antigen exposure. Indeed, in some experimental systems, a 100- to 5000-fold increase in antigen-specific T cells is observed.[211, 212] If all of such cells survived after multiple antigenic encounters, the immune system would become overloaded with them. Instead, the majority of activated T cells are eliminated shortly after an immune response through their apoptotic death in a process called *activation-induced cell death* (AICD).[213, 214] Both CD95 (fas) and its ligand are upregulated on T cells after activation. Engagement of CD95 by its ligand initiates a chain of events leading to nuclear breakdown, mitochondrial dysfunction, and DNA fragmentation. AICD occurs after the initial proliferative stage in immune responses. In cases in which stimuli are particularly strong, AICD may be so complete that tolerance results. This may be important in ensuring that immune responses to abundant antigens, such as autoantigens, do not become so pervasive that they severely harm the host. Indeed, the immune system selectively deploys the CD95 ligand in places where even small-scale T cell responses may be particularly onerous, such as in the eyes and the testes. Cells in these sites, called *immune privileged sites,* constitutively express CD95 ligand.[215] Interaction of this with CD95 downregulates incipient T cell responses.

Not all T cells die after most immune responses. Some enter a quiescent and yet readily triggerable state. These cells are termed *memory cells.*[212, 216] They are available should antigen resurface. Vaccines are effective because they can induce memory cell formation. Likewise, Rh hemolytic disease of the newborn, clotting factor sensitization, and some transfusion and allograft reactions are rapid and severe when preceded by the formation of memory cells.

Why some cells are destined to die after antigenic stimulation and others turn into long-lived memory cells is not known. Whereas some cellular proteins such as CD95 promote apoptotic death, others such as bcl-2 and bcl-xL are inhibitory.[217] One model is that the balance between pro-apoptotic and anti-apoptotic proteins most likely determines a cell's fate. Signals through some cytokine receptors, such as the IL-2R, or cell surface molecules, such as CD28, promote the accumulation of anti-apoptotic proteins. Other signals unleash pro-apoptotic forces. The environment of the T cell during its activation will thus determine whether it ultimately survives its encounter with cognate antigen. Other explanations of memory cell development, however, exist. For instance, it is possible that T cells do not all have equivalent potential to form memory cells; memory cells may form exclusively from a committed subset of T cells resistant to AICD.

Memory T cells are distinguished from their naive counterparts by surface immunophenotype.[216] After T cell activation, surface molecules are differentially regulated. For instance, expression of CD69, CD25, and CD30 may be induced early after activation. Changes in the expression of only a limited number of molecules persist and are found on memory cells. In mouse $CD4^+$ T cells, there is downregulation of CD62L and CD45RB in relation to naive cells and upregulation of CD44. In humans the most consistent difference is a downregulation of CD45RA and CD45RB and upregulation of CD45RO on memory cells. CD45RO memory T cells are difficult to find in the neonate but constitute the majority of T cells in the elderly.

In order for memory cells to be useful, they must be able to survive for long periods. Immunization with *Vaccinia,* for example, leads to an elevated precursor frequency of antigen-reactive T cells more than 30 years after exposure.[218] These cells are able to survive in the absence of exposure to pathogen. Whether they require regular antigen exposure, however, is less clear. Even after the elimination of pathogen, antigen stores can remain for extended periods. Indeed, follicular dendritic cells can retain antigen-antibody complexes for long periods of time and may serve as reservoirs for antigen.[219] Some studies show that memory T cells adoptively transferred into an antigenically inexperienced recipient are rapidly lost or revert to a naive phenotype,[150, 220, 221] which implies that memory requires persistent antigen presentation. Other studies do not confirm these findings.[222, 223] For instance, in vivo labeling studies analyzing cell turnover rates as a surrogate for antigenic stimulation are ambiguous as to whether persistence of antigen is required.

THE COORDINATED MOVEMENT OF ANTIGEN AND LYMPHOCYTES PERMITS ADAPTIVE IMMUNE RESPONSES

Adaptive immunity arises only within an anatomical system designed to filter out antigens and present them in a controlled manner to lymphocytes. The anatomy of the immune system is designed to focus antigen on critical sites where they may be presented to lymphocytes and where lymphocytes may mature. Three major locations serve as focal points for antigen concentration[7, 9, 224] (Fig. 5–10).

Lymph nodes are distributed throughout the body. Lymphocytes, primarily blood derived, enter lymph nodes through the high endothelial venules. They then segregate into distinct regions. The B cells move to follicles containing follicular dendritic cells specialized in presenting antigen. T cells stay within the surrounding paracortical regions. Lymph fluid derived from tissues is directed through conduits of lymphatic vessels and then percolates through these nodes. Antigens present within this fluid are retrieved by professional APC and presented to lymphocytes. Alternatively, tissue derived APCs can migrate through the lymph into the draining lymph nodes to present antigens. For instance, inflammation activates local dendritic cells, increasing their antigen uptake and

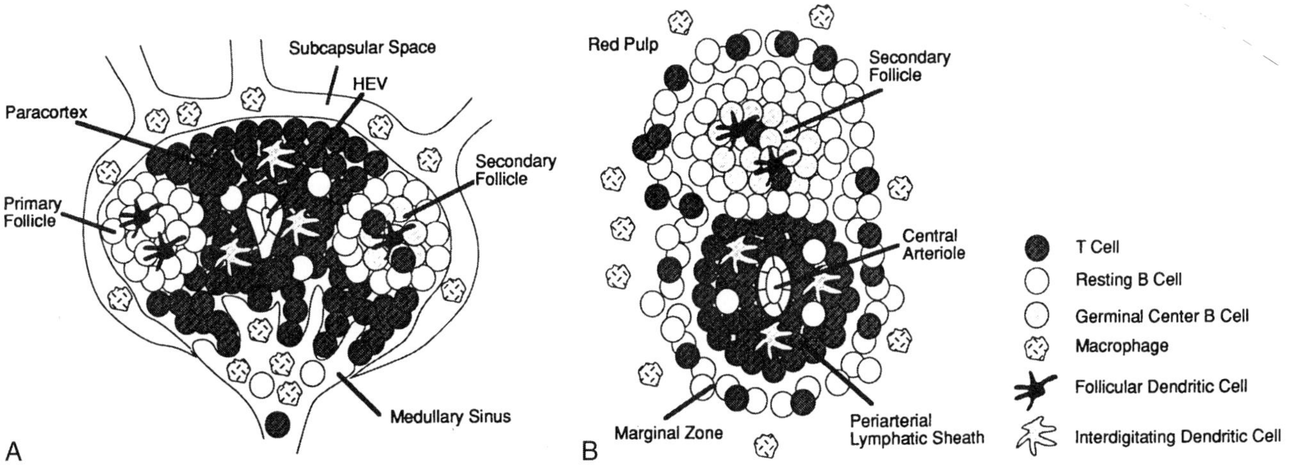

Figure 5–10. Schematic depiction of the structure of a lymph node *(A)* and an area of splenic white pulp *(B)*. The white pulp is seen as a transverse cross-section through one branch of a central arteriole. (From Mondino A, Khoruts A, Jenkins MK. The anatomy of T cell activation. Proc Natl Acad Sci U S A 1996; 93:2246.)

presentation capabilities and promoting their migration to local lymph nodes. These dendritic cells settle in the T cell zone of the lymph node, where circulating T cells can "survey" their antigenic holdings. In the absence of antigen encounter, T cells will remain for a short time—on the order of 1 day or less—before exiting through the efferent lymphatic vessels to eventually return to the circulation.

The structure and function of the mucosa-associated lymphatic tissue (MALT) are similar to those of the lymph node. However, unlike the lymph node, these sites can sample antigens from across epithelial surfaces. Peyer's patches embedded within the intestinal epithelium abut specialized epithelial cells, M cells, that transport antigens from the intestinal lumen, permitting continuous surveillance of epithelium-lined cavities. Lymphocytes enter MALT from the blood, much as they do lymph nodes, but the endothelial receptors that they use to guide them differ from those expressed by lymph node endothelium.

The spleen surveys antigens that have entered the circulation. Blood is continuously filtered by the spleen. Although the histological anatomy of the spleen differs from that of the lymph node, functional regions are analogous. Encircling small arterioles in the white pulp of the spleen are periarteriolar lymphatic sheaths (PALS), consisting primarily of T lymphocytes. Embedded within or adjacent to the T cell areas are B cell–rich follicles. Surrounding the PALS and follicles is a less dense sinusoidal region, the marginal zone. Naive T and B cells exit into the splenic parenchyma in these marginal zones and from there migrate into the PALS and follicles, respectively.

The design of all three of these lymphoid tissues coerces T and B cells to interact with each other and to interact with APCs. Although T and B cells are segregated as they migrate through lymphatic tissue to their respective anatomical zones, they are forced to interact, especially after an immunizing event. Activated B cells, whether present in the marginal zone or follicles, will redirect themselves to the T cell zones. It is here that antigen-specific T cells are activated by APCs. These T cells can provide necessary help to B cells, permitting their differentiation into antibody-secreting plasma cells or into memory B cells. The primed T and B cells move again to the follicles, where the B cells form germinal centers. In these sites, their receptors undergo mutation, termed *affinity maturation,* and B cells with increasing affinity for antigen are selected. The mature lymphocytes may terminally differentiate, turning into effector cells such as plasma cells or cytolytic or regulatory T cells before dying, or they may develop into long-lived memory cells.

Although the lymph nodes, MALT, and spleen are designed to foster the cell-cell contacts necessary to initiate adaptive immune responses, lymphocytes and lymphoid responses are not restricted to these sites. Lymphocytes may circulate through most organs in the body. Activated T cells will selectively home to sites of inflammation. Some lymphocytes selectively home to the skin or to the epithelial lining of the gut. Other cells may localize in the lungs, liver, or bone marrow. Within these different sites, structured lymphoid aggregates may form.

The tissue localization of lymphocytes is not random but results from their selective migratory patterns.[225] Much as T cells may be classified into Th1 and Th2 according to their cytokine profiles, T cells may also be categorized on the basis of their homing properties. T cell function and T cell localization are not independent. The immune response to an antigen entering from the gut is different from that of an antigen entering through the skin. Different types of lymphocytes selectively migrate to different tissues in order to accommodate specific immunological needs. An appropriate response to protein antigens encountered in the gut may be IgA production or immune tolerance, whereas DTH may be appropriate for the same antigen encountered in the subcutaneous space.

T cell homing results from a collaboration of various adhesion molecules and cytokines.[225, 226] Although the actual mechanics of differential lymphocyte migration are complicated, the general concept is not. The first stage of migration for a circulating T cell is recognition of receptors on vascular endothelium. Movement into the tissue space of organized lymphoid tissues, such as lymph nodes and Peyer's patches, occurs at high endothelial venules (HEV). These small venules are places where blood flow is most sluggish. Because the shear forces that the lymphocytes must overcome are minimized, they are the optimal sites for tissue entry.

Binding and transmigration of lymphocytes at HEV is divided into several steps (Fig. 5–11). First, in the contact step, the lymphocyte binds to the endothelium by using receptors present on their cell surface microvilli. For naive T cells entering Peyer's patches L-selectin (CD62L) is important in this regard. L-selectin binds fucosylated carbohydrates that are particularly rich on

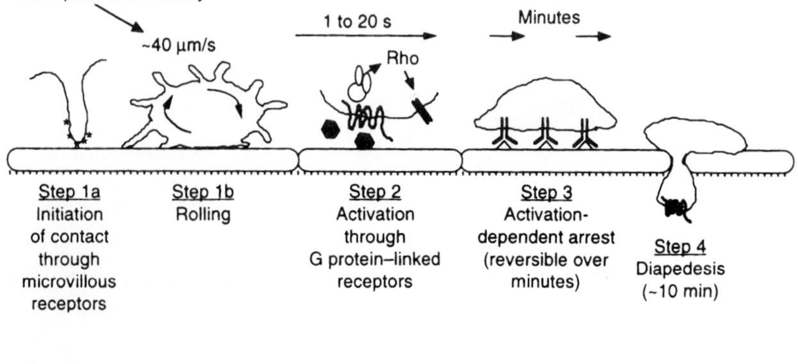

Figure 5–11. The multi-step model of lymphocyte-endothelial cell recognition and recruitment of lymphocytes from the blood. (From Butcher EC, Picker LJ. Lymphocyte homing and homeostasis. Science 1996; 272:63.)

HEV glycoproteins. This interaction slows the lymphocyte down approximately 100-fold, and the lymphocyte is observed to roll on the endothelium. In the absence of advancement to the next migratory step, the lymphocyte is released by proteases that cleave the L-selectin molecule from the T cell surface. Additional molecular interactions, such as that between the α_4 integrins and their receptors, can further slow rolling. Next, activation through G-protein coupled cell surface receptors mediates an activation-dependent arrest. Activation results in the enhanced binding of the α_4 and β_2 integrin family of receptors to the vascular endothelium. The signals causing this activation have not been fully elucidated. Chemokines may play an important, but not necessarily exclusive, role. The stable arrest of cells on the endothelium is followed by their diapedesis into the underlying tissue. Once inside the tissue, T cells further localize to specific sites. The molecular forces driving these migratory patterns are poorly characterized.

This scenario represents a general paradigm for lymphocyte trafficking. Individual tissues differ. Whereas the α_4 integrins are necessary to slow down the lymphocyte for β_2 integrin–mediated arrest on Peyer's patch HEVs, they are not required for lymph node HEVs. This difference possibly reflects the higher density of L-selectin ligands on the lymph node HEVs. Peyer's patches restrict entry to T lymphocytes expressing the α_4 integrin, whereas lymph nodes do not. Homing of memory T cells to the skin requires a distinct selectin, cutaneous lymphocyte-associated antigen (CLA), that binds E-selectin. Even with a small number of specific homing receptors, it is easy to see that a large number of migratory patterns are possible. Table 5–2 lists some cell surface molecules important in lymphocyte homing and migration.

Table 5–2. Lymphocyte Homing Receptors

	T Cell Homing Receptor	Endothelial Ligand
Homing of naive T cells to peripheral lymphoid organs	L-selectin	GlyCAM-1, CD34, MadCAM-1, others
Homing of T cells to mucosal tissues (e.g., Peyer's patches)	$\alpha_4\beta_7$ integrin CD44	MadCAM-1 Hyaluronate
Homing of memory T cells to inflamed skin	CLA-1	E-selectin
Homing of memory and effector T cells to sites of inflammation (general)	LFA-1 VLA-4 CD44	ICAM-1, ICAM-2 VCAM-1 Hyaluronate

GlyCAM, glycerol cellular adhesion molecule; MadCAM, mucosal addressin cellular adhesion molecule; CLA, cutaneous lymphocyte-associated antigen; LFA, leukocyte function–associated antigen; ICAM, intracellular adhesion molecule; VLA, very late antigen; VCAM, vascular cell adhesion molecule.

CONCLUSION

The immune system is designed to recognize and react to potential dangers to the host. It can do so largely because of the ability of T lymphocytes to interact with peptide fragments presented by MHC molecules. Any T cell interaction with peptide-MHC has three possible outcomes: tolerance, ignorance, and immunity. The resulting T cell response depends on many factors, including the physical properties of the antigen, the tissues and cell types that present the antigen, the prior activation state and type of T cell and APC, and the intercellular milieu of cytokines, stimulatory factors, and inhibitory factors during antigen presentation. The immunological self consists of host antigens presented so that they may potentially be perceived by the immune system. T cells are partially tolerized to this set of antigens. Deletion of self-specific T cells in the thymus eliminates the majority of self-reactive T cells before they are allowed to fully mature. Anergy, regulatory T cell interactions, and activated T cell death are all potential mechanisms for tolerizing self-reactive T cells that escape thymic deletion. Nevertheless, not all T cells specific for self are tolerant of self. Some circulate in a seemingly ignorant manner. Activation of these cells may produce autoimmunity.

Activation of T cells and the generation of an adaptive immune response occurs only in the presence of danger signals. These signals may be derived from pathogens themselves. Molecules such as lipopolysaccharide can activate the innate and adaptive immune systems. Danger signals initiating adaptive immunity may come from the innate immune system in the context of inflammation, or they may be derived from preactivated or memory T cells that have less stringent activation requirements than do their naive counterparts. Immunizing responses include antibody production, DTH, and cytolytic T cell activity. The nature of the response depends on the nature of the stimulus as well on its tissue location. Some sites, including the eyes and testes, constitutively express fasL, thereby downregulating incipient immune responses and preventing damage to these sensitive tissues. Lymphoid tissue, particularly the lymph nodes, spleen, and MALT, are constructed to focus antigen and foster immune responses. Activated T cells differentiate into effector or regulatory cell types that can be discriminated on the basis of functional differences, such as cytokine production. Once an antigen and the danger signals associated with it have been cleared, these T cells may die through apoptosis or may convert to long-lived memory cells. Memory cells maintain a state of readiness and can generate secondary responses to antigen that are more rapid and more resolute than are primary ones.

An understanding of T cell–mediated immunity is vital to a mechanistic understanding of transfusion medicine. T cells are required for the antibody production that mediates many transfusion reactions and alloimmunization states. They are the causative agents of transfusion-associated graft-versus-host disease. They are central to the immunomodulation caused by transfusion. They have also demonstrated increased promise as independent therapeutic agents for chronic myelogenous leukemia and other diseases. As an understanding of the role of the adaptive immune system in transfusion and disease increases, new approaches specifically designed to take advantage of this knowledge will become increasingly prominent in transfusion medicine.

REFERENCES

1. Silverstein AM. The history of immunology. *In* Paul WE (ed): Fundamental Immunology. New York: Raven Press, 1989.
2. Nossal GJV. Immunological tolerance. *In* Paul WE (ed): Fundamental Immunology. New York: Raven Press, 1989, p 571.
3. Billingham RE, Brent L, Medawar PB. Actively acquired tolerance of foreign cells. Nature 1953; 172:603–606.
4. Forsthuber T, Yip H, Lehmann P. Induction of Th1 and Th2 immunity in neonatal mice. Science 1996; 271:1728.
5. Ridge J, Fuchs E, Matzinger P. Neonatal tolerance revisited: turning on newborn T cells with dendritic cells. Science 1996; 271:1723.
6. Bendelac A, Fearon D. Innate immunity: innate pathways that control acquired immunity. Curr Opin Immunol 1997; 9:1.
7. Janeway CJ, Travers P. Immunobiology—the immune system in health and disease. Curr Biol 1997.
8. Male D, Cooke A, Owen M, et al. Advanced Immunology. London: Mosby–Year Book, 1996.
9. Abbas A, Lichtman A, Pober J. Cellular and Molecular Immunology. Philadelphia: WB Saunders, 1997.
10. Janeway JA Jr. The immune system evolved to discriminate infectious nonself from noninfectious self. Immunol Today 1992; 13:11.
11. Medzhitov R, Janeway CA Jr. Innate immunity: impact on the adaptive immune response. Curr Opin Immunol 1997; 9:4.
12. Lengyel P. Double stranded RNA and interferon action. J Interferon Res 1987; 7:511.
13. Honja T, Habu S. Origin of immune diversity: genetic variation and selection. Annu Rev Biochem 1985; 54:803.
14. Tse H, Schwarz R, Paul W. Cell-cell interactions in the T cell proliferative response. J Immunol 1980; 125:401.
15. Fischer M, Ma M, Goerg S, et al. Regulation of the B cell response to T dependent antigens by classical pathway complement. J Immunol 1996; 157:549.
16. Ahearn J, Fischer M, Croix D, et al. Disruption of the Cr2 locus results in a reduction of B-1a cells and in an impaired B cell response to T-dependent antigen. Immunity 1996; 4:251.
17. Croix D, Ahearn J, Rosengard A, et al. Antibody response to a T-dependent antigen requires B cell expression of complement receptors. J Exp Med 1996; 183:1857.
18. Berke G. The binding and lysis of target cells by cytotoxic lymphocytes. Annu Rev Immunol 1994; 12:735.
19. Mossman T, Coffman R. Th1 and Th2 cells: different patterns of lymphokine secretion lead to different functional properties. Annu Rev Immunol 1989; 7:145.
20. Parker D. T cell dependent B cell activation. Annu Rev Immunol 1993; 11:331.
21. Billingham RE, Silvers WK. Studies on tolerance of the Y chromosome antigen in mice. J Immunol 1960; 85:14.
22. Dresser DW, Mitchison NA. The mechanism of immunological paralysis. Adv Immunol 1968; 8:129.
23. Weigle WO. Immunological unresponsiveness. Adv Immunol 1973; 16:61.
24. Ildstad ST, Sachs DH. Reconstitution with syngeneic plus allogeneic or xenogeneic bone marrow leads to specific acceptance of allografts or xenografts. Nature 1984; 308:168.
25. Slavin S, Strober S, Fuks Z, Kaplan HS. Induction of specific transplantation tolerance using fractionated total lymphoid irradiation in adult mice: long term survival of allogeneic bone marrow and skin grafts. J Exp Med 1977; 146:34.
26. Eto M, Mayumi H, Tomita Y, et al. Intrathymic clonal deletion of Vb6+ T Cells in cyclophosphamide-induced tolerance to H-2 compatible, Mls-disparate antigens. J Exp Med 1990; 171:97.
27. Qin S, Cobbold S, Benjamin R, Waldmann R. Induction of classical transplantation tolerance in the adult. J Exp Med 1989; 169:779.
28. Isobe M, Yagita H, Okumara K, Ihara A. Specific acceptance of cardiac allograft after treatment with antibodies to ICAM-1 and LFA-1. Science 1992; 255:1125.
29. Ryan JJ, Gress RE, Hathcock KS, Hodes RJ. Recognition and response to alloantigens in vivo. J Immunol 1984; 133:2343.
30. Hori S, Sato S, Kitagawa S, et al. Tolerance induction of allo-class II H-2 antigen-reactive L3T4+ helper T cells and prolonged survival of the corresponding class II H-2 disparate skin graft. J Immunol 1989; 143:1447.
31. Sato S, Azuma T, Shimizu J, et al. Property of class I H-2 alloantigen-reactive Lyt-2+ helper T cell subset. J Immunol 1988; 141:721.
32. Sato S, Iwata H, Kitagawa S, et al. The lymphoid cell populations required for induction of tolerance of different subsets of alloantigen-reactive T cells. Transplantation 1991; 52:862.
33. Fink PJ, Shimonkevtz RP, Bevan MJ. Veto cells. Annu Rev Immunol 1988; 6:115.
34. Rammensee H-G, Bevan MJ. Mutual tolerization of histoincompatible lymphocytes. Eur J Immunol 1987; 17:893.
35. Eynon EE, Parker DC. Small B cells as antigen-presenting cells in the induction of tolerance to soluble protein antigens. J Exp Med 1992; 175:131.
36. Parker DC, Eynon EE. Antigen presentation in acquired immunological tolerance. FASEB J 1991; 5:2777.
37. Fuchs E, Matzinger P. B cells turn off virgin but not memory T cells. Science 1992; 258:1156.
38. Burns J, Littlefield K. Isolation of human lymphocyte cell lines reactive with whole human myelin. Ann N Y Acad Sci 1988; 540:367.
39. Hohfeld R, Conti-Tronconi B, Kalies I, et al. Genetic restriction of autoreactive acetylcholine receptor specific T lymphocytes in myasthenia gravis. J Immunol 1985; 135:2393.
40. Naquet P, Ellis J, Tibensky D, et al. T cell autoreactivity to insulin in diabetic and related nondiabetic individuals. J Immunol 1988; 140:2569.
41. Romball CG, Weigle WO. Transfer of experimental autoimmune thyroiditis with T cell clones. J Immunol 1987; 138:1092.
42. van der Veen RC, Trotter JL, Hickey WF, Kapp JA. The development and characterization of encephalitogenic cloned T cells specific for myelin proteolipid protein. J Neuroimmunol 1990; 26:139.
43. Holmdahl R, Andersson M, Goldschmidt TJ, et al. Type II collagen autoimmunity in animals and provocations leading to arthritis. Immunol Rev 1990; 118:193.
44. Lennon VA, Lindstrom JM, Seybold ME. Experimental autoimmune myasthenia gravis in mice: cellular and humoral immune responses. Ann N Y Acad Sci 1976; 274:283.
45. Zamvil SS, Steinman L. The T lymphocyte in experimental allergic encephalomyelitis. Annu Rev Immunol 1990; 8:579.
46. Ohashi PS, Oehen S, Buerki K, et al. Ablation of tolerance and induction of diabetes by virus infection in viral antigen transgenic mice. Cell 1991; 65:305.
47. Zinkernagel RM, Pircher HP, Ohashi P, et al. T and B cell tolerance and responses to viral antigens in transgenic mice: implications for the pathogenesis of autoimmune versus immunopathological disease. Immunol Rev 1991; 122:133.
48. Fowlkes B, Pardoll D. Molecular and cellular events in T cell development. Adv Immunol 1989; 44:207.
49. Toyonaga B, Mak T. Genes of the T-cell antigen receptor in normal and malignant T cells. Annu Rev Immunol 1987; 5:585.
50. Schatz D, Oettinger M, Baltimore D. The V(D)J recombination activating gene RAG-1. Cell 1989; 59:1035.
51. Oettinger M, Schatz D, Gorka C, Baltimore D. RAG-1 and RAG-2, adjacent genes that synergistically activate V(D)J recombination. Science 1990; 248:1517.
52. Rawsden D, Gent DV, Gellert M. Specificity in V(D)J recombination: new lessons from biochemistry and genetics. Curr Opin Immunol 1997; 9:114.
53. Stanhope-Baker P, Hudson K, Shaffer A, et al. Cell type specific chromatin structure determines the targeting of V(D)J recombinase activity. Cell 1996; 85:887.
54. Chothia C, Boswell DR, Lesk AM. The outline structure of the T-cell αβ receptor. EMBO J 1988; 7:3745.
55. Claverie JM, Prochnicka-Chalufour A, Bougueleret L. Implications of a Fab like structure for the T-cell receptor. Immunol Today 1989; 10:10.
56. Fields B, Mariuzzara R. Structure and function of the T cell receptor: insights from x-ray crystallography. Immunol Today 1996; 17:330.
57. Weiss A. T cell antigen receptor signal transduction: a tale of tails and cytoplasmic protein tyrosine kinases. Cell 1993; 73:209.
58. Sprent J. T lymphocytes and the thymus. *In* Paul W (ed): Fundamental Immunology. New York: Raven Press, 1989, pp 69–93.
59. Campbell R, Trowsdale J. Map of the human MHC. Immunol Today 1993; 14:349.
60. Bjorkman PJ, Saper MA, Samraoui B, et al. The foreign antigen binding site and T cell recognition regions of class I histocompatibility antigens. Nature 1987; 329:512.

61. Bjorkman PJ, Saper MA, Samraoui B, et al. Structure of the human class I histocompatability antigen, HLA-A2. Nature 1987; 329:506.
62. Davis MM, Bjorkman PJ. T-cell antigen receptor genes and T-cell recognition. Nature 1988; 334:395.
63. Fremont D, Hendrikson W, Marrack P, Kappler J. Structures of an MHC class II molecule with covalently bound single peptide. Science 1996; 272:1001.
64. Babbitt BP, Allen PM, Matsueda G, et al. Binding of immunogenic peptides to Ia histocompatibility molecules. Nature 1985; 317:359.
65. Jardetzky TS, Lane WS, Robinson RA, et al. Identification of self peptides bound to purified HLA-B27. Nature 1991; 353:326.
66. Rudensky AY, Preston-Hulbert P, Hong S-C, et al. Sequence analysis of peptides bound to MHC class II molecules. Nature 1991; 353:622.
67. Rudensky AY, Rath S, Preston-Hurlburt P, et al. On the complexity of self. Nature 1991; 353:660.
68. Townsend ARM, Rothbard J, Gotch FM, et al. The epitopes of influenza nucleoprotein recognized by cytotoxic T lymphocytes can be defined with short synthetic peptides. Cell 1986; 44:959.
69. Falk K, Rotzsche O, Stevanovic S, et al. Allele specific motifs revealed by sequencing of self peptides eluted from MHC molecules. Nature 1991; 351:290.
70. Hunt D, Henderson R, Shabanowitz J, et al. Characterization of peptides bound to the class I molecule HLA-A2.1 by mass spectrometry. Science 1992; 255:1261.
71. Fremont D, Stura E, Matsumara M, et al. Crystal structure of an H-2Kb-coalbumin peptide complex reveals the interplay of primary and secondary anchor positions in the major histocompatibility complex binding groove. Proc Natl Acad Sci U S A 1995; 92:2479.
72. Garboczi D, Ghosh P, Utz U, et al. Structure of the complex between human T cell receptor, viral peptide, and HLA-A2. Nature 1996; 384:134.
73. Garcia K, Degano M, Pease L, et al. Structural basis of plasticity in T cell receptor recognition of a self peptide-MHC antigen. Science 1998; 279:1166.
74. Parham P, Ohta T. Population biology of antigen presentation by MHC class I molecules. Science 1996; 272:67.
75. Burrows J, Burrows S, Poulsen L, et al. Unusually high frequency of Epstein-Barr virus genetic variants in Papua–New Guinea that can escape cytotoxic T cell recognition: implications for virus evolution. J Virol 1996; 70:2490.
76. Hill A, Elvin J, Willis A, et al. Molecular analysis of the association of B53 and resistance to severe malaria. Nature 1992; 360:434.
77. Janeway CJ. The T cell receptor as a multicomponent signaling machine. Annu Rev Immunol 1992; 10:645.
78. Sun J, Leahy D, Kavathas PB. Interaction between CD8 and major histocompatibility complex (MHC) class I mediated by multiple contact surfaces that include the α 2 and α 3 domains of MHC class I. J Exp Med 1995; 182:1275.
79. Rudd C, Trvillyan J, Dasgupta J, et al. The CD4 antigen is complexed in detergent lysates to a protein tyrosine kinase (pp58) from human T lymphocytes. Proc Natl Acad Sci U S A 1988; 85:5190.
80. Veillette A, Bookman M, Viorak E, Bolen J. The CD4 and CD8 T cell surface antigens are associated with the internal membrane tyrosine protein kinase p56lck. Cell 1988; 55:301.
81. Janeway CJ, Carding S, Jones B, et al. $CD4^+$ T cells: specificity and function. Immunol Rev 1988; 101:39.
82. Cresswell P, Howard J. Antigen recognition. Curr Opin Immunol 1997; 9:71.
83. Pieters J. MHC class II restricted antigen presentation. Curr Opin Immunol 1997; 9:89.
84. Koopman J, Hammerling G, Momburg F. Generation, intracellular transport and loading of peptides associated with MHC class I molecules. Curr Opin Immunol 1997; 9:80.
85. Groettrup M, Soza A, Kuckelkorn U, Kloetzel P. Peptide antigen production by the proteasome: complexity provides efficiency. Immunol Today 1996; 17:429.
86. Groettrup M, Soza A, Eggers M, et al. A role for the PA28 activator complex on the generation of class I binding antigenic peptides is demonstrated in vivo and in vitro. Nature 1996; 381:166.
87. Lehner P, Cresswell P. Processing and delivery of peptides presented by MHC class I molecules. Curr Opin Immunol 1996; 8:59.
88. Vassilakos A, Cohen-Doyle M, Peterson P, et al. The molecular chaperone calnexin facilitates folding and assembly of class I histocompatibility molecules. EMBO J 1996; 15:1495.
89. Sadasivan B, Lehner P, Ortmann B, et al. Roles for calreticulin and a novel glycoprotein, tapasin, in the interaction of class I MHC molecules with TAP. Immunity 1996; 5:103.
90. Ortmann B, Ansrolewicz M, Cresswell P. MHC class I/b2-microglobulin complexes associate with TAP transporters before peptide binding. Nature 1994; 368:864.
91. Koopman J, Post M, Neefjes J, et al. Translocation of long peptides by transporters associated with antigen processing (TAP). Eur J Immunol 1996; 26:1720.
92. Schaiff WT, Hruska KA Jr, McCourt DW, et al. HLA-DR associates with specific stress proteins and is retained in the endoplasmic reticulum in invariant chain negative cells. J Exp Med 1992; 176:657.
93. Cresswell P. Invariant chain structure and MHC class II function. Cell 1996; 84:505.
94. Ghosh P, Amaya M, Mellins E, Wiley D. The structure of an intermediate in class II MHC maturation: CLIP bound to HLA-DR3. Nature 1995; 378:457.
95. Bakke O, Doberstein B. MHC class II associated invariant chain contains a sorting signal for endosomal compartments. Cell 1990; 63:707.
96. Amigorena S, Drake J, Webster P, Mellman I. Transient accumulation of new MHC molecules in a novel endocytic compartment in B lymphocytes. Nature 1994; 369:113.
97. Castellino F, Germain R. Extensive trafficking of MHC class II invariant chain complexes in the endocytic pathway and appearance of peptide loaded class II in multiple compartments. Immunity 1995; 2:73.
98. Riese R, Wolf P, Bromme D, et al. Essential role for cathepsin S in the MHC class II associated invariant chain processing and peptide loading. Immunity 1996; 4:357.
99. Denzin L, Cresswell P. HLA-DM induces CLIP dissociation from MHC class II αβ dimers and facilitates peptide loading. Cell 1995; 82:155.
100. Sallusto F, Sella M, Danieli C, Lanzavecchia A. Dendritic cells use macropinocytosis and the mannose receptor to concentrate macromolecules in the major histocompatibility complex class II compartment: downregulation by cytokines and bacterial products. J Exp Med 1995; 182:389.
101. Bonnerot C, Lankar D, Hanau D, et al. Role of B cell receptor Ig A and B subunits in MHC class II-restricted antigen presentation. Immunity 1995; 3:335.
102. Lanzavecchia A. Mechanisms of antigen uptake for presentation. Curr Opin Immunol 1996; 8:348.
103. Moretta A, Moretta L. HLA class I specific inhibitory receptors. Curr Opin Immunol 1997; 9:694.
104. Hoglund P, Sundback J, Olsson-Alheim M, et al. Host MHC class I gene control of NK-cell specificity in the mouse. Immunol Rev 1997; 155:11.
105. Hill A, Jugovic P, York I, et al. Herpes simplex virus turns off the TAP to evade host immunity. Nature 1995; 375:411.
106. Hengel H, Flohr T, Hammerling G, et al. Human cytomegalovirus inhibits peptide translocation into the endoplasmic for MHC class I assembly. J Gen Virol 1996; 77:2287.
107. Amigorena S, Bonnerot C, Drake J, et al. Cytoplasmic domain heterogeneity and function of IgG Fc receptors in B lymphocytes. Science 1992; 265:1808.
108. Croft M, Joseph S, Miner K. Partial activation of naive CD4 T cells and tolerance induction in response to peptide presented by resting B cells. J Immunol 1997; 159:3257.
109. Maher J, Ronenberg M. The role of CD1 molecules in immune responses to infection. Curr Opin Immunol 1997; 9:456.
110. Zheng W, Flavell R. The transcription factor GATA-3 is necessary and sufficient for Th2 cytokine gene expression in CD4 T cells. Cell 1997; 89:587.
111. Choi Y, Herman A, DiGiusto D, et al. Residues of the variable region of the T-cell receptor beta chain that interact with the *S. aureus* toxin superantigens. Nature 1990; 346:471.
112. Fields B, Malchiodi E, Li H, et al. Crystal structure of a T cell receptor beta chain complexed with a superantigen. Nature 1996; 384:188.
113. Margulies D. Interactions of TCR with MHC-peptide complexes: a quantitative basis for mechanistic models. Curr Opin Immunol 1997; 9:390.
114. Margulies D, Plaskin D, Khilko S, Jelonek M. Interactions involving the T cell antigen receptor by surface plasmon resonance. Curr Opin Immunol 1996; 8:262.

115. Wange R, Samelson L. Complex complexes: signals at the TCR. Immunity 1996; 5:197.
116. Sykulev Y, Brunmark A, Jackson M, et al. Kinetics and affinity of reactions between an antigen-specific T cell receptor and peptide-MHC complexes. Immunity 1994; 1:15.
117. Matsui K, Boniface J, Steffner P, et al. Kinetics of T-cell receptor binding to peptide/I-Ek complexes: correlation of the dissociation rate with T-cell responsiveness. Proc Natl Acad Sci U S A 1994; 91:12862.
118. Matsui K, Boniface J, Reay P, et al. Low affinity interaction of peptide-MHC complexes with TCR. Science 1991; 254:1788.
119. Demotz S, Grey HM, Sette A. The minimal number of class II MHC-antigen complexes needed for T cell activation. Science 1990; 249:1028.
120. Sloan-Lanoister J, Allen P. Altered peptide ligand induced partial T cell activation: molecular mechanisms and role in T cell biology. Annu Rev Immunol 1996; 14:1.
121. Al-Ramadi B, Jelonek M, Boyd L, et al. Lack of strict correlation of functional sensitization with the apparent affinity of MHC-peptide complexes for the TCR. J Immunol 1995; 155:662.
122. Plaksin D, Polakova K, McPhie P, Margulies D. A three domain TCR is biologically active and specifically stains cell surface MHC-peptide complexes. J Immunol 1997; 158:2218.
123. Lyons D, Lieberman S, Hampl J, et al. A TCR binds to antagonist ligands with lower affinities and faster dissociation rates than to agonists. Immunity 1996; 5:53.
124. Alam S, Travers P, Wung J, et al. TCR affinity and thymocyte positive selection. Nature 1996; 381:616.
125. McKeithan T. Kinetic proofreading in T-cell receptor signal transduction. Proc Natl Acad Sci U S A 1995; 92:5042.
126. Rabinowitz J, Beeson C, Lyons DS, et al. Kinetic discrimination in T cell activation. Proc Natl Acad Sci U S A 1996; 93:1401.
127. Samelson L, Klausner R. Tyrosine kinases and tyrosine-based activation motifs. Current research on activation via the T cell antigen receptor. J Biol Chem 1992; 267:24913.
128. Iwashima M, Irving B, Oers NV, et al. Sequential interactions of the TCR with two distinct cytoplasmic tyrosine kinases. Science 1994; 263:1136.
129. Cantrell D. T cell antigen receptor signal transduction pathways. Annu Rev Immunol 1996; 14:259.
130. Robinson M, Cobb M. Mitogen-activated protein kinase pathways. Curr Opin Cell Biol 1997; 9:180.
131. Whitmarsh A, Davis R. Transcription factor AP-1 regulation by mitogen-activated protein kinase signal transduction pathways. J Mol Med 1996; 74:589.
132. Croft M, Dubey C. Accessory molecules and costimulation requirements for CD4 T cells. Crit Rev Immunol 1997; 17:89.
133. Binnerts M, Simmons D, Figdor C. Distinct binding of T lymphocytes to ICAM-1, -2, or -3 upon activation of LFA-1. Eur J Immunol 1994; 24:2155.
134. Dustin M, Springer T. T-cell receptor cross-linking transiently stimulates adhesiveness through LFA-1. Nature 1989; 341:619.
135. Dustin M. Two way signaling through the LFA-1 lymphocyte adhesion receptor. Bioessays 1990; 12:421.
136. Justement L. The role of CD45 in signal transduction. Adv Immunol 1997; 66:1.
137. Hurley T, Hyman R, Sefton B. Differential effects of the expression of the CD45 tyrosine protein phosphatase on the tyrosine phosphorylation of lck, fyn, and c-src tyrosine protein kinases. Mol Cell Biol 1993; 13:1651.
138. Sieh M, Bolen J, Weiss A. CD45 specifically modulates binding of lck to a phosphopeptide encompassing the negative regulatory tyrosine of lck. EMBO J 1993; 12:315.
139. Dianzani U, Luqman M, Rojo J, et al. Molecular associations on the T cell surface correlate with immunological memory. Eur J Immunol 1990; 20:2249.
140. Dianzani U, Redoglia V, Malavasi F, et al. Isoform-specific associations of CD45 with accessory molecules in human T lymphocytes. Eur J Immunol 1992; 22:365.
141. Bretscher P, Cohn M. A theory of self-nonself discrimination. Science 1970; 169:1042.
142. Lafferty KJ, Prowse SJ, Simeonovic CJ. Immunobiology of tissue transplantation: a return to the passenger leukocyte concept. Annu Rev Immunol 1983; 1:143.
143. Jenkins MK, Schwartz RH. Antigen presentation by chemically modified splenocytes induces antigen specific T cell unresponsiveness in vitro and in vivo. J Exp Med 1987; 165:302.
144. Jenkins MK. The role of cell division in the induction of clonal anergy. Immunol Today 1992; 13:69.
145. Chambers C, Allison J. Co-stimulation in T cell responses. Curr Opin Immunol 1997; 9:396.
146. Boise L, Noel P, Thompson C. CD28 and apoptosis. Curr Opin Immunol 1995; 7:620.
147. Green J, Noel P, Sperling A, et al. Absence of B7 dependent responses in CD28-deficient mice. Immunity 1994; 1:501.
148. Mittrucker H, Shahinian A, Bouchard D, et al. Induction of unresponsiveness and impaired T cell expansion by staphylococcal enterotoxin B in CD28 deficient mice. J Exp Med 1996; 183:2481.
149. Saha B, Harlan D, Lee K, June C, Abe R. Protection against lethal toxic shock by targeted disruption of the CD28 gene. J Exp Med 1996; 183:2675.
150. Kundig T, Shinian A, Kawai K, et al. Duration of TCR stimulation determines co-stimulatory requirement of T cells. Immunity 1996; 5:41.
151. Guerder S, Flavell R. The role of the T cell costimulator B7-1 in the induction and maintenance of tolerance to peripheral antigen. Immunity 1994; 1:155.
152. June C, Bluestone J, Nadler L, Thompson C. The B7 and CD28 receptor families. Immunol Today 1994; 15:321.
153. Grewal I, Borrow P, Pamer E, et al. The CD40-CD154 system in anti-infective host defense. Curr Opin Immunol 1997; 9:491.
154. Grewal I, Foellmer H, Grewal K, et al. Requirement for CD40 ligand in costimulation induction, T cell activation, and experimental allergic encephalomyelitis. Science 1996; 273:1864.
155. Thompson C, Allison J. The emerging role of CTLA-4 as an immune attenuator. Immunity 1997; 7:445.
156. van der Merwe P, Bodian D, Daenke S, et al. CD80 (B7-1) binds both CD28 and CTLA-4 with a low affinity and very fast kinetics. J Exp Med 1997; 185:393.
157. Krummel M, Allison J. CD28 and CTLA-4 have opposing effects on the response of T cells to stimulation. J Exp Med 1995; 182:459.
158. Waterhouse P, Penninger J, Timms E, et al. CTLA-4 deficiency causes lymphoproliferative disorder with early lethality. Science 1995; 270:985.
159. Tivol E, Borriello F, Schweitzer A, et al. Loss of CTLA-4 leads to massive lymphoproliferation and fatal multiorgan tissue destruction, revealing a critical negative regulatory role for CTLA-4. Immunity 1995; 3:541.
160. Krummel M, Allison J. CTLA-4 engagement inhibits IL-2 accumulation and cell cycle progression upon activation of resting T cells. J Exp Med 1996; 183:2533.
161. Borriello F, Sethna M, Boyd S, et al. B7-1 and B7-2 have overlapping, critical roles in immunoglobulin class switching and germinal center formation. Immunity 1997; 6:303.
162. Pawson T. Protein modules and signalling networks. Nature 1995; 373:573.
163. Marengere L, Waterhouse P, Duncan G, et al. Regulation of T cell receptor signaling by tyrosine phosphatase SYP association with CTLA-4. Science 1996; 272:1170.
164. Zerrahn J, Held W, Raulet D. The MHC reactivity of the T cell repertoire prior to positive and negative selection. Cell 1997; 88:627.
165. Kieslow P, von Boehmer H. Development and selection of T cells: facts and puzzles. Adv Immunol 1995; 58:87.
166. Boyd RL, Hugo P. Towards an integrated view of thymopoiesis. Immunol Today 1991; 12:71.
167. Fehling H, von Boehmer H. Early αβ T cell development in the thymus of normal and genetically altered mice. Curr Opin Immunol 1997; 9:263.
168. Wu L, Scollay R, Egerton M, et al. CD4 expressed on earliest T-lineage precursor cells in adult murine thymus. Nature 1991; 349:71.
169. von Boehmer H, Fehling H. Structure and function of the pre–T cell receptor. Annu Rev Immunol 1997; 15:433.
170. Von Freeden-Jeffry U, Vieira P, Lucian L, et al. Lymphopenia in interleukin 7 gene deleted mice identifies IL-7 as a nonredundant cytokine. J Exp Med 1995; 181:1519.
171. Cao X, Shores E, Hu-Li J, et al. Defective lymphoid development in mice lacking expression of the common cytokine receptor γ chain. Immunity 1995; 2:223.

172. Casanova J, Romero P, Widman C, et al. T cell receptor genes in a series of class I major histocompatibility complex–restricted cytolytic T lymphocyte clones specific for a *Plasmodium berghei* nonapeptide: implications for T cell allelic exclusion and antigen-specific repertoire. J Exp Med 1991; 174:1371.
173. Roehm N, Herron L, Cambier J, et al. The major histocompatibility complex–restricted antigen receptor on T cells: distribution on thymus and peripheral T cells. Cell 1984; 38:577.
174. Kappler JW, Roehm N, Marrack P. T cell tolerance by clonal elimination in the thymus. Cell 1987; 49:273.
175. Sha WC, Nelson CA, Newberry RD, et al. Positive and negative selection of an antigen receptor on T cells in transgenic mice. Nature 1988; 336:73.
176. Pircher H, Burki K, Lang R, et al. Tolerance induction in double specific T-cell receptor transgenic mice varies with antigen. Nature 1989; 342:559.
177. Smith CA, Williams GT, Kingston R, et al. Antibodies to CD3/T-cell receptor complex induce death by apoptosis in immature T cells in thymic cultures. Nature 1989; 337:181.
178. Murphy KM, Heimberger AB, Loh DY. Induction by antigen of intrathymic apoptosis of $CD4^+CD8^+$ TCRlo thymocytes in vivo. Science 1990; 250:1720.
179. Sprent J, Lo D, Gao E-K, Ron Y. T cell selection in the thymus. Immunol Rev 1988; 101:173.
180. Marrack P, Lo D, Brinster R, et al. The effect of thymus environment on T cell development and tolerance. Cell 1988; 53:627.
181. Lorenz RG, Allen PM. Thymic cortical epithelial cells can present self-antigens in vivo. Nature 1989; 337:560.
182. Gooding LR, Edwards CB. H-2 antigen requirements in the in vitro induction of SV40-specific cytotoxic T lymphocytes. J Immunol 1980; 124:1258.
183. Carbone F, Bevan MJ. Class I restricted processing and presentation of exogenous cell associated antigen in vivo. J Exp Med 1990; 171:377.
184. Geiger T, Gooding LR, Flavell RA. T-cell responsiveness to an oncogenic peripheral protein and spontaneous autoimmunity in transgenic mice. Proc Natl Acad Sci U S A 1992; 89:2985.
185. Geiger T, Soldavila G, Flavell R. T-cells are responsive to the simian virus 40 large tumor antigen transgenically expressed in pancreatic islets. J Immunol 1993; 151:7030.
186. Singer A, Munitz TI, Golding H, et al. Recognition requirements for the activation, differentiation, and function of T-helper cells specific for class I MHC alloantigens. Immunol Rev 1987; 98:143.
187. Guerder S, Matzinger P. Activation versus tolerance: a decision made by T helper cells. Cold Spring Harb Symp Quant Biol 1989; 54:799.
188. Dannecker G, Mecheri S, Hoffman MK. Induction of neonatal tolerance to the Mls-1a self-super-antigen. J Immunol 1991; 147:2833.
189. Haba S, Nisonoff A. Induction of tolerance to syngeneic IgE in neonatal mice. J Immunol 1991; 146:807.
190. Abromson-Leeman SR, Dorf ME. Extrathymic clonal deletion of self-reactive cells in athymic mice. J Immunol 1991; 147:1.
191. Fink P, Bevan M. H-2 antigens of the thymus determine lymphocyte specificity. J Exp Med 1978; 148:766.
192. Teh HS, Kisielow P, Scott B, et al. Thymic major histocompatibility complex antigens and the αβ T-cell receptor determine the CD4/CD8 phenotype of T cells. Nature 1988; 335:229.
193. Bevan M. In thymic selection peptide diversity gives and takes away. Immunity 1997; 7:175.
194. Jameson S, Hogquist K, Bevan M. Positive selection of thymocytes. Annu Rev Immunol 1995; 13:93.
195. Hu Q, Walker CB, Girao C, et al. Specific recognition of thymic self peptides induces the positive selection of cytotoxic T lymphocytes. Immunity 1997; 7:221.
196. Ignatowicz L, Rees W, Pacholczyk R, et al. T cells can be activated by peptides that are unrelated in sequence to their selecting peptide. Immunity 1997; 7:179.
197. Surh C, Lee D, Fung-Lung W, et al. Thymic selection by a single MHC/peptide ligand produces a semidiverse repertoire of $CD4^+$ T cells. Immunity 1997; 7:209.
198. Tourne S, Miyazaki T, Oxenius A, et al. Selection of a broad repertoire of $CD4^+$ T cells in H-2Ma$^{0/0}$ mice. Immunity 1997; 7:187.
199. Abbas A, Murphy M, Sher A. Functional diversity of helper T lymphocytes. Nature 1996; 383:787.
200. Constant S, Bottomly K. Induction of Th1 and Th2 responses: the alternative approaches. Annu Rev Immunol 1997; 15:297.
201. Seder R, Paul W. Acquisition of lymphokine producing phenotype by $CD4^+$ T cells. Annu Rev Immunol 1994; 12:635.
202. Cher D, Mossman T. Two types of murine helper T cell clone: II. Delayed type hypersensitivity is mediated by Th1 clones. J Immunol 1987; 138:3688.
203. Coffman R, Seymour B, Lebman D, et al. The role of helper T cell products in mouse B cell differentiation and isotype regulation. J Immunol 1988; 102:5.
204. Unanue E. Interrelationship among macrophages, natural killer cells and neutrophils in early stages of *Listeria* resistance. Curr Opin Immunol 1997; 9:35.
205. Yoshimoto T, Paul W. CD4pos, NK1.1pos T cells promptly produce interleukin 4 in response to in vivo challenge with anti-CD3. J Exp Med 1994; 179:1285.
206. Sornasse T, Larenas P, Davis K, et al. Differentiation and stability of T helper 1 and 2 cells derived from naive human neonatal $CD4^+$ T cells, analyzed at the single cell level. J Exp Med 1996; 184:473.
207. Perez V, Lederer J, Lichtman A, Abbas A. Stability of Th1 and Th2 populations. Int Immunol 1995; 7:869.
208. Chen Y, Kuchroo V, Inobe J, et al. Regulatory T cell clones induced by oral tolerance: suppression of autoimmune encephalomyelitis. Science 1994; 265:1237.
209. Groux H, Ogarra A, Bigler M, et al. A $CD4^+$ T-cell subset inhibits antigen specific T-cell responses and prevents colitis. Nature 1997; 389:737.
210. Carter L, Dutton R. Type 1 and type 2: a fundamental dichotomy for all T cell subsets. Curr Opin Immunol 1996; 8:336.
211. McHeyzer-Williams M, Davis M. Antigen specific development of primary and memory T cells in vivo. Science 1995; 268:106.
212. Ahmed R, Gray D. Immunologic memory and protective immunity: understanding their relation. Science 1996; 272:54.
213. Singer G, Abbas A. The fas antigen is involved in the peripheral but not thymic deletion of T lymphocytes in TCR transgenic mice. Immunity 1994; 1:415.
214. Nagata S, Golstein P. The Fas death factor. Science 1995; 267:1449.
215. Streilein J. Unraveling immune privilege. Science 1995; 270:1158.
216. Sprent J. Immunologic memory. Curr Opin Immunol 1997; 9:371.
217. Cory S. Regulation of lymphocyte by the bcl-2 gene family. Annu Rev Immunol 1995; 13:513.
218. Demkowicz W, Littaua R, Wang J, Ennis F. Human cytotoxic T cell memory: long lived responses to *Vaccinia* virus. J Virol 1996; 70:2627.
219. MacLennan I. Germinal centers. Annu Rev Immunol 1994; 12:117.
220. Gray D, Matzinger P. T cell memory is short lived in the absence of antigen. J Exp Med 1991; 174:969.
221. Oehen S, Waldner H, Kundig T, et al. Antivirally protective cytotoxic T cell memory to lymphocytic choriomeningitis virus is governed by persisting antigen. J Exp Med 1992; 176:1273.
222. Mullbacher A. The long term maintenance of cytotoxic T cell memory does not require persistence of antigen. J Exp Med 1994; 179:317.
223. Lau L, Jamieson B, Somamsundaram R, Ahmed R. Cytotoxic T cell memory without antigen. Nature 1994; 369:648.
224. Goodnow C. Chance encounters and organized rendezvous. Immunol Rev 1997; 156:5.
225. Butcher E, Picker L. Lymphocyte homing and homeostasis. Science 1996; 272:60.
226. Salmi M, Jalkanen S. How do lymphocytes know where to go? Current concepts and enigmas of lymphocyte homing. Adv Immunol 1997; 64:139.

CHAPTER 6

The Humoral Immune Response

Thomas F. Tedder
Yuan Zhuang
Michael McHeyzer-Williams

The humoral immune response has evolved as a mechanism to help protect vertebrates against infection by pathogenic microorganisms. The importance of this response is clearly demonstrated by the occurrence of humoral immunodeficiencies in which patients are susceptible to uncontrolled infections by a variety of pathogens, particularly pyogenic bacteria. Humoral responses are mediated by a distinct lineage of hematopoietic cells, termed *B lymphocytes.* The protective capacity of B lymphocytes results from their ability to produce antigen (Ag)-binding antibody (Ab) molecules, collectively called immunoglobulins (Igs). Abs are capable of binding specifically to foreign substances and targeting them for subsequent destruction and removal by various effector systems. They are a primary means of defense and are found in most body fluids.

ANTIBODY STRUCTURE

Early biochemical experiments examining the structure of Igs used proteolytic enzymes and reducing agents to dissect Ab molecules into fragments that could be independently analyzed. Digestion of Ig with papain generated two distinct fragments that together contained all of the recognized characteristics of the intact Ab molecule. The first fragment, termed *Fc* because it was readily crystallized, contained the portion of the molecule responsible for mediating effector functions (Fig. 6–1). The remaining fragment was named the *Fab* fragment because it retained Ag-binding activity. Fab and Fc fragments are generated at a stoichiometry of two and one per intact Ab molecule, respectively.

Monomeric Abs secreted during the course of an immune response are composed of four polypeptide chains: two identical heavy chains and two identical light chains held together by interchain and intrachain disulfide bonds (see Fig. 6–1). Carbohydrate makes up a substantial fraction of the total Ab mass (Table 6–1) and appears to be restricted almost exclusively to the heavy-chain constant regions. Although the function of carbohydrate on Abs is not completely understood, it may protect the hinge regions from proteolysis, regulate IgA and IgE synthesis and secretion, and aid in clearance of Ig by the liver.

Ab light chains are composed of two globular domains of approximately 110 amino acids each that have a characteristic structure termed an *Ig fold.* This structure consists of two disulfide-linked parallel β-pleated sheets that form a hydrophobic core between them. Light chains of two different isotypes (κ and λ) are present in humans and mice. Heavy chains are made up of four (or five in the case of IgM and IgE) of these globular domains. These domains serve as the prototype for evolutionarily related structural units found in a number of proteins that collectively comprise the Ig superfamily. Many members of the Ig superfamily mediate adhesive interactions of both immunological and nonimmunological cells through interaction of their Ig-like domains with specific ligands.[1]

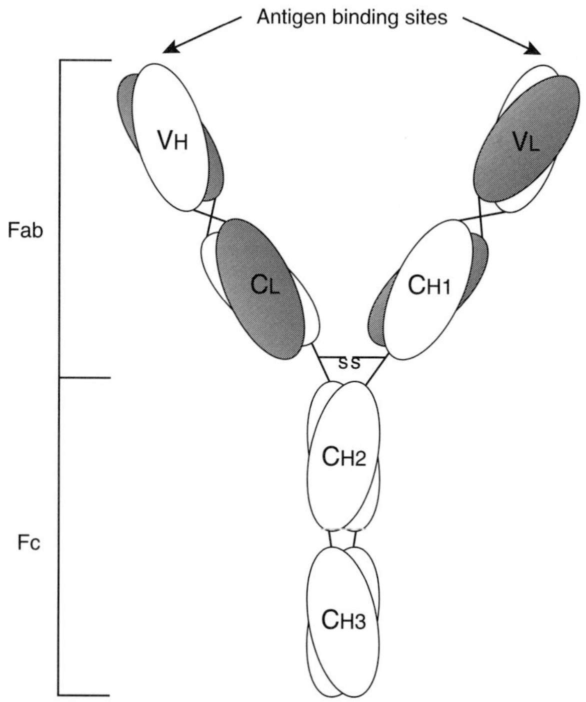

Figure 6–1. Structure of a prototypical, monomeric, secreted Ab molecule. Ovals represent Ig domains. Heavy chains are indicated by *white fill.* Light chains are indicated by *gray fill.* Polypeptide linkages between domains are indicated by *lines.* A single representative disulfide linkage between the hinge regions of the heavy chains is indicated; other interchain and intrachain disulfide bonds are not shown.

Table 6–1. Human Serum Immunoglobulins

	IgM	IgG				IgA	IgE
		IgG₁	IgG₂	IgG₃	IgG₄		
Molecular weight (kD)	950	150	150	150	150	160	190
Formula	10μ 10L 1J	2γ 2L	2γ 2L	2γ 2L	2γ 2L	4α 4L 1J	2ε 2L
Carbohydrate content	10%	<——— 2.5–4% ———>				10%	11.7%
% of total serum Ig	5–10%	~49%	~24%	~4%	~3%	5–15%	<1%
Half-life (days)	9–11	<——— 25–35 ———>				6–8	2–3

The amino-terminal globular domains of both the heavy- and light-chain proteins are diversified in amino acid sequence as a result of several genetic processes and are called variable domains V_H and V_L, respectively. This randomization is directly responsible for generating the diversity of Ab-binding specificities because V_H and V_L associate to form the Ag-combining site, a unique steric and electrostatic topology capable of interacting with Ag of complementary structure. The alterations in sequence are not randomly dispersed along the length of the V regions but are localized to three discrete regions on the polypeptide chains. These regions are called hypervariable or complementarity-determining regions. Hypervariable regions coincide with loops between the β strands of the Ig fold and lie in the Ag-binding cleft formed between the heavy and light chains. The less variable portions of the V domains, called the framework regions, coincide with the β strands themselves and provide the structure necessary to allow proper folding of the V region.

The remaining portions of each chain are identical between Abs of the same isotype and are therefore designated as constant regions C_H and C_L. The amino proximal C_H domain (C_H1) interacts with the C_L domain whereas the carboxyl-terminal C_H domains associate with their respective twin domains on the other heavy chain, forming the Fc portion of the molecule (see Fig. 6–1). A flexible hinge linking the Fc fragment to each of the two Fab fragments allows the bivalent molecule the freedom of motion necessary to interact with two antigenic determinants simultaneously. Because the variable and constant regions for both heavy and light chains are encoded by separate exons, it is possible for a given Ag-binding specificity to be linked to any one of several functionally distinct heavy-chain C regions. This occurs through a genetic process termed *class* or *isotype switching* (Fig. 6–2). The different heavy-chain isotypes, designated μ, δ, γ1, γ2, γ3, γ4, α1, α2, and ε in humans, induce distinct effector responses on Ag binding.

IgM is the first isotype secreted during the primary response and generally has a low affinity for Ag. The secreted form of IgM is pentameric (see Table 6–1) and can therefore bind multivalent Ags such as bacteria or viruses with high avidity. On binding to Ag, IgM can activate the classical complement cascade, resulting in complement-mediated lysis of IgM bound cells or in complement receptor–mediated phagocytosis of Ag/Ab complexes. IgG is the most common isotype expressed during secondary antigenic challenge and makes up approximately 80% of serum Ig. All four subtypes of IgG activate the complement cascade, although with variable efficiency. In addition, cell surface receptors for various IgG subclasses are expressed on macrophages, mast cells, polymorphonuclear cells, and lymphocytes. Binding of these receptors mediates a number of functions, including phagocytosis of Ag/Ab complexes, the release of inflammatory factors, and killing of the Ab-coated cells, a process termed *Ab-dependent cellular cytotoxicity.*[2] In addition, IgG is able to cross the maternal-fetal boundary because of the presence of IgG-specific Fc receptors on the placenta. IgA is uniquely localized to external secretions where it provides the first line of defense against pathogens at mucosal surfaces. This is due to its interaction with IgA receptors at the basolateral surface of epithelial cells of secretory organs that transport it to the apical surface where it is released. High-affinity receptors for IgE present on mast cells and basophils bind to soluble IgE in the serum, thus providing these cells with Ag-specific receptors. IgE binding of Ag results in cross-linking of these Fc receptors, activating the cell and inducing the release of potent inflammatory and chemoattractant mediators. Isotype switching thereby allows Abs with identical Ag-binding abilities to diversify their functions, including activation of complement, selective tissue localization, and the ability to stimulate different effector cells. Thus, the selection of B cells using alternative heavy chains adjusts humoral immune responses to suit the conditions of Ag encounter.

During the course of B cell development, Ab molecules first appear as cell surface–bound receptors before being found in the serum. This was demonstrated by injecting newborn mice with anti-μ Ab, which completely inhibited the development of mature B cells, leading to agammaglobulinemia.[3] Ag stimulation of the B cell induces alternative splicing of exons located at the 3′ end of the Ig messenger RNA, resulting in the production of a soluble form of the molecule. The membrane forms of all Abs are monomeric, as are the soluble forms of IgD, IgG, and IgE. IgM and IgA are secreted as multimers consisting of five and two Ab molecules, respectively, covalently associated by disulfide linkage to an accessory molecule called J chain. In addition, the secreted form of IgA is covalently associated with an additional polypeptide called secretory component, a cleavage fragment of the poly-Ig receptor that remains after transport of IgA across the epithelial layer.

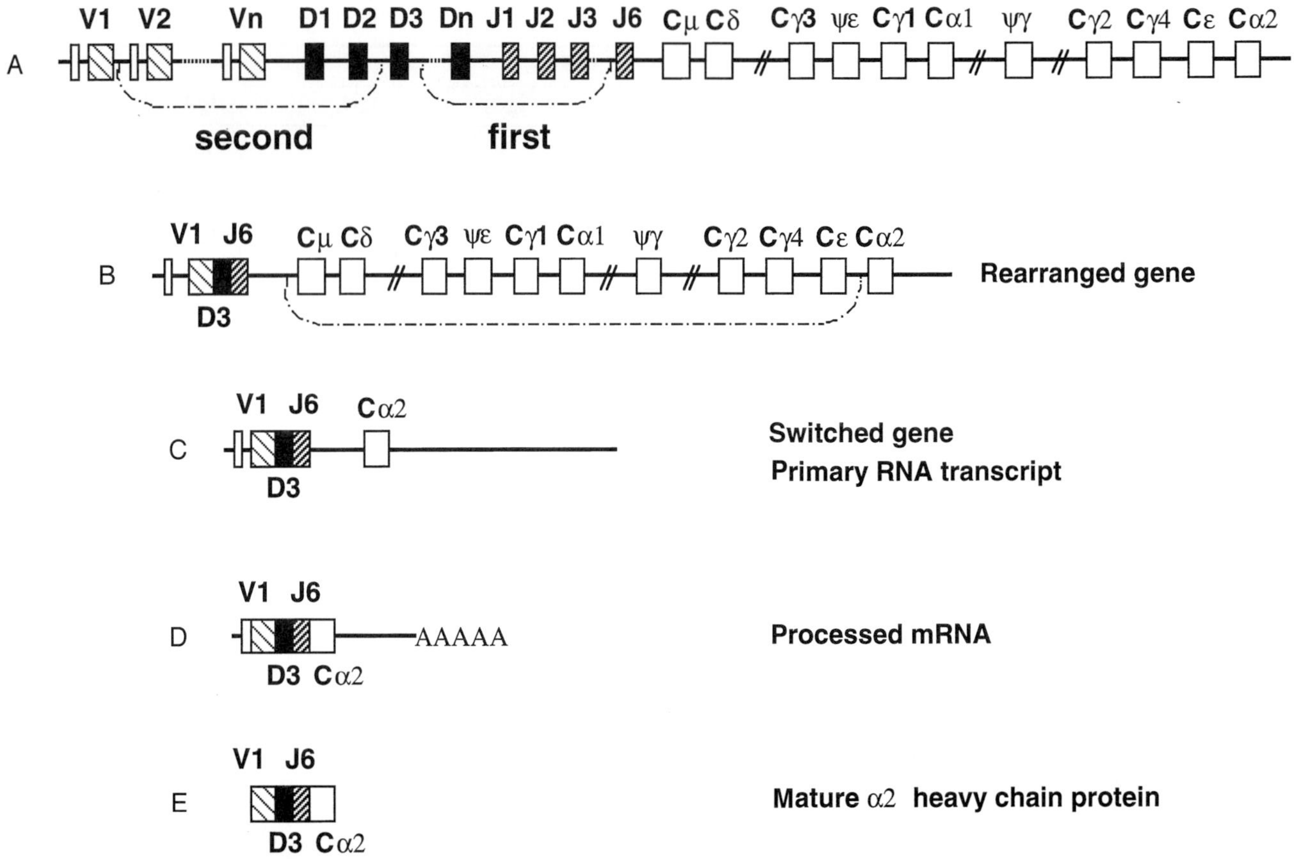

Figure 6–2. Rearrangements of the Ig heavy-chain locus. *A*, Germline configuration of the heavy-chain locus found in all non–B cells. Variable, diversity, joining, and constant elements are indicated and are numbered or designated according to isotype. Elements of indeterminate number are indicated by *n. Dotted lines* indicate regions with elements not shown. *Dashed lines* indicate rearrangements. Constant region pseudogenes are indicated by ψ. The rearranged form of the locus *(B)* is present in immature B cells and mature, IgM-secreting B cells. Specific conditions of Ag exposure induce class switching to IgA, resulting in the deletion of Cμ and the remainder of the intervening DNA *(C)*. RNA processing of the primary transcript results in the form depicted *(D)*, leading ultimately to the production of mature α2 heavy-chain proteins *(E)*.

Immunoglobulin Gene Rearrangements

The humoral immune system is capable of producing Abs against a seemingly limitless array of Ags, including synthetic chemical structures that do not occur naturally. The amount of genetic material necessary to encode such a large number of different Abs was initially calculated to be significantly greater than the total size of the genome. However, nucleic acid hybridization studies revealed that only a limited number of genes encode Ig proteins. Early "instructionists" resolved this paradox by proposing that Ag directed the appropriate folding of a multipotential precursor Ab molecule. However, amino acid sequence variability at the amino terminus of heavy and light chains indicated that the amino acid sequence of the Ag-combining site determined Ab specificity, suggesting genetic scrambling as a potential mechanism for generating Ab diversity.[4]

The gene rearrangement model for Ab diversification was confirmed when the structure of Ig genes was found to be altered in Ab-producing cells.[5] The genes that encode H and L chains are assembled using individual members of syntenic families of discrete exons through an ordered series of genetic rearrangements (see Fig. 6–2). Heavy chains are composed of V(ariable), D(iversity), J(oining), and C(onstant) segments (exons), whereas light chains contain only V, J, and C elements. D_H and J_H elements are the first to be rearranged, and V_H is then linked to the DJ_H unit. Rearrangements that generate a functional protein product are designated "productive" and result in the synthesis of μ protein, which is sequestered in the cytoplasm. Subsequently, rearrangements are sequentially initiated at the light-chain loci: V_κ to J_κ and finally, if no functional V_κ is produced, V_λ to J_λ. Interestingly, κ makes up 90% to 95% of the expressed pool of light chains in the adult mouse whereas in humans κ and λ are expressed at similar levels. This variation may relate to the stoichiometric ratio of functional V_κ and V_λ elements in each species. Once a particular heavy- or light-chain gene is successfully rearranged, the gene is expressed; and further rearrangements of the heavy- or light-chain genes, respectively, are suppressed, a process called *allelic exclusion.* B cells with nonproductive rearrangements of heavy chains or of both light chains are blocked from further development and eventually undergo apoptosis in the bone marrow.

Ig gene rearrangements are directed by conserved signal sequences located 3′ of V elements, 5′ of J elements, and both 3′ and 5′ of D elements. Rearrangement involves cleavage of the DNA at the signal sequences adjacent to the genetic elements to be juxtaposed. The ends of the intervening DNA are ligated together, forming a large circular extrachromosomal element, which is eventually degraded. During the process of recombination, junctional diversity is generated through the degradation, by one or a few nucleotides, of the free ends of genetic elements to be fused. In the heavy chain, the enzyme terminal deoxynucleotide transferase (TdT) adds short stretches of random nucleotides to the ends of segments after exonucleolytic degradation, further altering Ab sequences, a process termed *N region diversification.*[6]

Some of the proteins responsible for the rearrangement of Ig genes have been characterized. The recombination-activating genes, *RAG-1* and *RAG-2,* are expressed in primary lymphoid organs at the time when B and T lymphocytes are rearranging their Ag receptor genes.[7] Transfection of these two closely linked genes into murine fibroblasts confers the ability to recombine artificial substrates that mimic Ig gene elements.[8] The importance of *RAG-1* and *RAG-2* is clearly demonstrated by the complete absence of mature lymphocytes in mice that carry targeted mutations in either of these loci.[9, 10] There are additional components of the recombinase machinery because the defect in severe combined immunodeficiency (SCID) mice, which are severely impaired in their ability to rearrange Ig genes, maps to a different chromosome than *RAG-1* and *RAG-2.* Interestingly, the SCID defect resides in a general DNA repair activity rather than a VDJ recombination specific factor. Most cells isolated from SCID mice are defective in the repair of DNA damage induced by ultraviolet light or certain chemical treatments.[11]

Several mechanisms have evolved to diversify amino acid sequences within the Ab-combining site. For a given heavy or light chain any one of the multiple copies of each genetic element (V, D, or J) may be associated with any one of the copies of the other elements providing for heterogeneity through random assortment. In addition, any heavy chain may be associated with any light chain. Calculations based on estimated numbers for each element suggest that about 10^7 different Abs may be produced through combinational diversification. Additional mechanisms such as N-region diversification have arisen to expand the Ab repertoire even further, suggesting that this number is insufficient to ensure protection against all Ags that may be encountered.

Affinity maturation is an Ag-driven process in which Ig gene sequences are randomly altered, presumably through poor fidelity in Ig sequence replication during S phase of the cell cycle. B cells that develop an enhanced affinity for Ags because of fortuitous mutations continue to clonally expand in the presence of Ag whereas B cells with low-affinity receptors become diluted within the pool of B lymphocytes. Affinity maturation results from the accumulation of mutations within the variable regions of Ig that occur at a rate of approximately one base-pair mutation per V region per cell division. Alternatively, a *gene conversion* mechanism may be activated that allows short sequences of V region pseudogenes to be transposed onto the sequence of the Ag-reactive V region, thereby altering its sequence. A similar mechanism generates V region diversity in chickens.[12]

Isotype Switching

Ab Fc regions can be of several successive isotypes, allowing the Ag-binding V region to be associated with alternative heavy-chain sequences. Isotype switching appears to involve homologous recombination between conserved repetitive switch sequences located 5′ of all Ig heavy-chain sequences (except IgD). Subsequently, the intervening DNA is looped out and deleted (see Fig. 6–2), analogous to what occurs during Ig gene rearrangements.[13] Isotype switching does not alter the assembled variable regions of the Ig gene but juxtaposes a new heavy-chain constant region with the variable region. Isotype switching uses a mechanism different from that of VDJ recombination.[14, 15] The timing and patterns of isotype switching are strongly influenced by cytokines produced by T cells. In mice, for example, interleukin (IL)-4 stimulates isotype switching to IgG1 and IgE whereas tumor growth factor-β (TGF-β) stimulates switching to IgA.[16]

B CELL DEVELOPMENT

Surface Ig (sIg) Expression During B Cell Development

Successive stages of B cell development have been primarily characterized by alternative patterns of cell surface marker and Ig expression (Fig. 6–3). The first identifiable B lineage–restricted precursor, called the *pro–B cell,* has not yet begun to rearrange its Ig genes. Pro–B cells express HLA-D region gene products but few other B cell surface markers (Fig. 6–4). The next identifiable stage of differentiation is the *pre–B cell.*[17] Pre–B cells have rearranged their Ig heavy-chain genes and express μ heavy chains within the cytoplasm, although rearrangements of light-chain genes are not apparent.[18] Pre–B cells express several B lineage cell surface markers, including cluster of differentiation antigen 10 (CD10), CD19, and CD20.[19] Initially, pre–B cells were thought not to express μ heavy chains on the cell surface because co-association with light chains was required for surface heavy-chain expression. However, light chain–like proteins λ5 and V_{pre-B}, expressed exclusively in pre–B cells,[20–22] associate with heavy chains on the cell surface. This complex of heavy chains and "surrogate" light chains is believed to signal the presence of a functional heavy chain, resulting in allelic exclusion at the heavy-chain locus and the initiation of light-chain gene rearrangements. It is unclear whether a ligand exists on the bone marrow stromal cells for this complex or whether the presence of the complex on the surface is sufficient to mediate the observed effects.

Functional cell surface IgM (sIgM) is expressed after successful light-chain gene rearrangement. These "immature" B cells then move out of the bone marrow into the

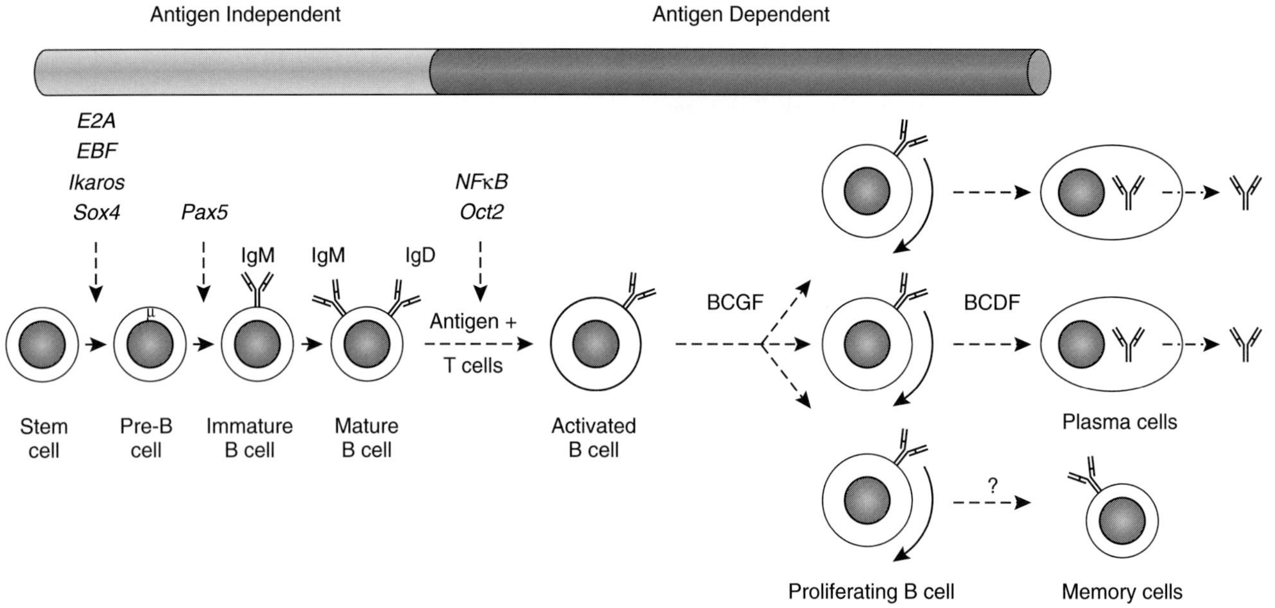

Figure 6–3. Stages and transcription factors of B lymphocyte development.

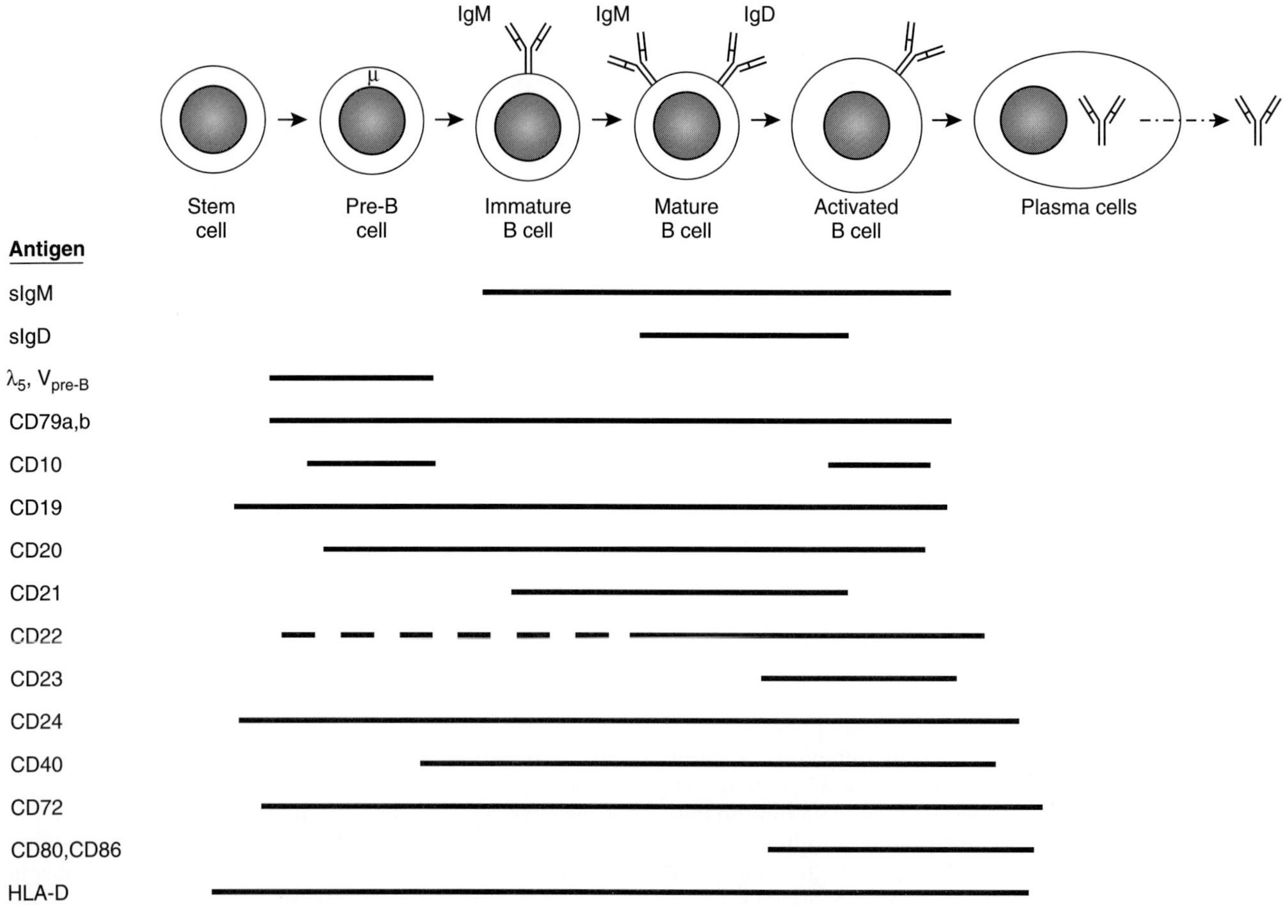

Figure 6–4. Cell surface Ag expression. The stages of expression of some B cell Ags are indicated by a *solid line.* Cytoplasmic but not surface expression is indicated by a *dashed line.*

periphery. Up to this point, B cell development proceeds without the necessity for foreign Ags. During this "Ag-independent" portion of development, crosslinking sIgM on immature B cells leads to cell death or to functional inactivation or "anergy" of the cell.[23] This may serve as a mechanism for eliminating self-reactive B cells. Surviving immature B cells subsequently coexpress both sIgM and sIgD and are considered "mature" B cells, which may be positively selected through interactions with Ags. Ag encounter is most likely to occur in secondary lymphoid organs because only about 2% of the total B cell population is found in the circulation. At this developmental stage, B cells respond to Ags either independently or with T cell help, proliferate and clonally expand, and can switch sIg isotypes. Most B cells appear to express sIgM before switching isotypes because IgG synthesis is suppressed as a result of treating animals with anti-IgM Ab, which inhibits the development of IgM^+ B cells.[3]

Expression of functional heavy- and light-chain genes is critical for progressive differentiation from pro–B cells to immature B cells. Gene targeting analysis in mice has shown that disruption of the μ heavy-chain gene blocks development at the pro–B cell stage and disruption of the light-chain gene blocks development at the pre–B cell stage. Sequential introduction of functional heavy- and light-chain genes into RAG2-deficient mice is sufficient to allow B cell development to proceed through the pro–B and pre–B stages, respectively. Finally, sustained cell surface Ag receptor expression is essential for mature B cells to survive in the periphery.[24] Presumably, sIg expression provides essential signals that instruct B cells during their different maturation steps, although the signals generated through sIg are not always equivalent.

B cell development is regulated by a complex interplay of external signals and internal differentiation programs. Although cell surface receptors such as the Ag receptor complex are important for cells to receive and interpret environmental signals, the final decision allowing a precursor cell to acquire more mature phenotypes is often made at the transcriptional level.[25] Gene targeting studies have demonstrated that the *E2A*, *EBF*, *Ikaros*, and *Sox4* gene products are transcription factors required for pro–B cell development. The Pax5 transcription factor is needed for pre–B cell development, whereas *NFκB* and *Oct2* gene products are involved in Ig gene transcription in mature B cells.[26] Further indicating the importance of these transcription factors during normal B cell development, alteration in the *E2A* gene induced by chromosomal translocations is a major cause of childhood lymphocytic leukemia.[27]

Pre–B cells and B cells are present at varied numbers in blood and lymphoid organs. B lineage cells represent approximately 7% of bone marrow nucleated cells, with $sIgM^+$ cells being about 2% of the cells. Although pre–B cells are rarely found outside the bone marrow, B cells represent 10% to 15% of circulating blood mononuclear cells, 35% to 50% of spleen cells, 25% to 30% of lymph node cells, and 40% of tonsil cells and are rarely found in the thymus (<1%). Among blood B cells, IgM is the predominant sIg isotype with concomitant expression of IgD (Table 6–2). Although IgD was first discovered in 1965, its role in the immune response is still poorly understood. IgD is localized mostly on the surface of B lymphocytes and is only present at low levels in serum. IgD may play a specialized role in the activation of B lymphocytes because it is only expressed at a discrete stage of differentiation by mature B cells. However, the exact nature of that role has yet to be fully discerned.

Table 6–2. Distribution of Human Blood B Cells Expressing Different Ig Isotypes*

Isotype	% of Newborn Blood	% of Adult Blood
IgM	18 (82% IgD^+)	9 (81% IgD^+)
IgD	15 (99% IgM^+)	7 (99% IgM^+)
IgG	6 (80% IgM^+ IgD^+)	3 (20% IgM^+ IgD^+)
IgA	1 (90% IgM^+ IgD^+)	1 (10% IgM^+ IgD^+)

*Values represent the approximate percentage of total mononuclear cells.[263]

Two developmental fates are available to a mature Ag-stimulated B lymphocyte; it may become an enlarged cycling cell called a *plasmablast*, or it may differentiate into a *memory cell*. Plasmablasts can be found in the circulation but represent only a few percent of B lineage cells. Interestingly, crosslinking of sIg on plasmablasts results in clonal abortion of those cells.[28] Thus, sIg can generate both positive and negative growth-modulating effects on B cells during different stages of development. The plasmablast terminally differentiates into a nondividing cell called a plasma cell that is highly specialized for the production of large quantities of Ab. The plasma cell is characterized by a well-developed Golgi apparatus, a large eccentric or "clock-face" nucleus, concentric laminae of endoplasmic reticulum, and high levels of cytoplasmic RNA—features all consistent with a tremendous protein synthetic capacity. These short-lived, noncirculating cells are capable of producing 2000 Ab molecules per second per cell. Plasma cell tumors were the first source of homogeneous myeloma proteins allowing the biochemical analysis of Ab structure.

Once B cells become activated and mature into plasmablasts, they are induced to complete their maturation in specific tissue sites. IgM-producing plasma cells are preferentially found in the spleen and lymph nodes. IgG-producing plasma cells are found in bone marrow, spleen, and lymph nodes. IgA-producing plasma cells are preferentially found in the gut- and bronchus-associated lymphoid tissue and mucosa. IgA is produced at the highest levels of all of the Ig isoforms but represents only a minor component of the serum. Most IgA is directed toward the gut and secretions where it leaves the body. IgE-producing plasma cells are found in the gut- and bronchus-associated lymphoid tissue and mesenteric lymph nodes. Factors in the microenvironment are likely to preferentially induce the expression and secretion of the different Ig isotypes.

Ontogeny of Development

Functionally distinct types of lymphocytes were initially identified in chickens, which possess a specialized organ called the bursa of Fabricius dedicated to the development of B cells.[29] Surgical removal of the bursa, an outcropping of the dorsal hindgut, from chicks before sIg+ cells begin to populate the periphery results in agammaglobulinemia and the absence of sIg+ cells and plasma cells in the adult. In mammals, no distinct organ is dedicated to B cell development. Rather, B cells are generated in hematopoietic tissues along with other blood cell types. B cells are produced in several successive locations within the embryo, first in placenta and embryonic blood, then in fetal liver and omentum, and finally in the spleen and bone marrow.

Pre–B cells are first detectable in the human fetus at approximately 8 weeks of gestation, and it is not until about 12 weeks that peripheralization of B cells occurs. In the human fetus, the liver is the principal hematopoietic organ from the 6th to the 22nd gestational week.[30] Stem cells generated in the yolk sac colonize the liver, where they proliferate and give rise to progenitor and precursor cells of the myeloid and lymphoid lineages. T cell precursors may develop in fetal liver in addition to B cell precursors. Within the fetal liver, no particular spatial relationship exists between the various hematopoietic cell lineages. Erythropoiesis and myleopoiesis occur in clusters around sinusoids and portal triad vessels, respectively, whereas lymphopoiesis occurs in a loosely scattered pattern without any sign of focal development. The fetal omentum is also a primary site of B cell development, and pre–B cells can be detected in the omentum and liver, but not spleen, as early as 8 weeks of gestation.[31] TdT+ cells have been detected in the fetal liver as early as 7 weeks of gestation and are believed to represent a stage of B cell development during which gene rearrangements occur.[6] At 12 weeks, the progenitor cells and B cells enter the circulation and populate the spleen where TdT+ B cell precursors are not found. This process is highly ordered and under the regulatory control of the hematopoietic inductive microenvironment. In the adult, B cell development is restricted to the bone marrow except with certain diseases or experimental treatments when the spleen may serve this function.

B lymphocytes derive from the same mesenchymal stem cells that give rise to T lymphocytes and all other blood leukocytes. Identifying and isolating hematopoietic stem cells is an active area of research because they will be clinically valuable for regenerating the immune system in immunodeficient patients. The existence of SCIDs in which B and T cells are deficient while the myeloid compartment remains unaffected suggests that there may be a further differentiated precursor cell restricted to lymphoid development. Additionally, precursor cells have been found that are capable of reconstituting the B and T cell compartments but not the myeloid compartment of irradiated recipients. Unfortunately, this lymphoid-restricted precursor remains elusive, owing to the absence of unique or distinctive cell surface Ags. Advances in the development of human bone marrow culture systems suggest that this goal is attainable.[32]

Progenitor cells in bone marrow colonize the proper environment, where they are guided to divide and differentiate by signals from proximal stromal cells that constitute the immediate microenvironment. The most immature B cell precursors in the adult are localized near the inner surface of the bone, where they divide most rapidly.[33] These cells migrate toward the center of the marrow as they mature, where they either die in situ of a lack of productive Ig gene rearrangements or migrate through the vascular endothelium of the venous sinuses to join the circulating lymphocyte pool. Immature B lymphocytes are rarely found in the circulation, indicating that their progression through this process is highly regulated and that a critical stage of maturation must be achieved before departing the bone marrow.

Much of the current understanding of early B cell maturation comes from studies using techniques previously developed for long-term culture of hematopoietic precursors and granulocytes that were adapted to promote selective growth of B lineage cells.[34] These cultures require a complex layer of stromal cells, including macrophages, endothelial cells, fat cells, adventitial reticular cells, and fibroblasts, as well as hematopoietic precursors and their more-differentiated progeny.[35] Bone marrow stromal cell lines have been generated to characterize the role of individual cell types in B cell development. These cloned stromal cell lines display significant variability in their ability to promote the growth and differentiation of B lineage cells and in the patterns of cytokines produced, including granulocyte, granulocyte-macrophage, and macrophage colony-forming factors, IL-6 and IL-7, TGF-β, and neuroleukin. IL-7 has the most dramatic effects on B cell hematopoiesis in that it promotes the outgrowth of B lineage cells in Whitlock-Witte cultures. However, it does not support their continued differentiation into mature B cells. Hematopoiesis is highly sensitive to inflammation and other stimuli, owing, in part, to the altered expression of hematopoietic growth factors by stromal cells in response to these external signals. Direct B cell/stromal cell interactions also play a critical role in proper B cell development, and the maintenance of early B lineage precursors is dependent on contact with the stromal layer.[36] Although long-term bone marrow cultures have proven extremely useful in characterizing the requirements for B lineage cell development, they nevertheless imperfectly mimic the in vivo situation. This is exemplified by the absence in bone marrow culture of a "quality control" mechanism normally active in vivo for the elimination of precursors with incorrectly rearranged Ig genes. Thus, these aberrant cells may make up a significant fraction of the B lineage population in vitro.

REGULATION OF B CELL FUNCTION

B lymphocytes respond to numerous stimuli that regulate development, negative selection in the bone marrow, activation, proliferation, the generation of humoral immune responses in the periphery, and the establishment and maintenance of tolerance, anergy, or memory. Each of these responses depends on the nature of the stimulus and the differentiation state of the B cell. Many of these responses are governed by the B cell Ag receptor (BCR) complex, which performs many highly specialized functions. For example, engagement of sIg by Ag triggers a signal transduction cascade that results in deletion or apoptosis of immature B cells yet activation and proliferation of mature B cells. The receptor complex is also

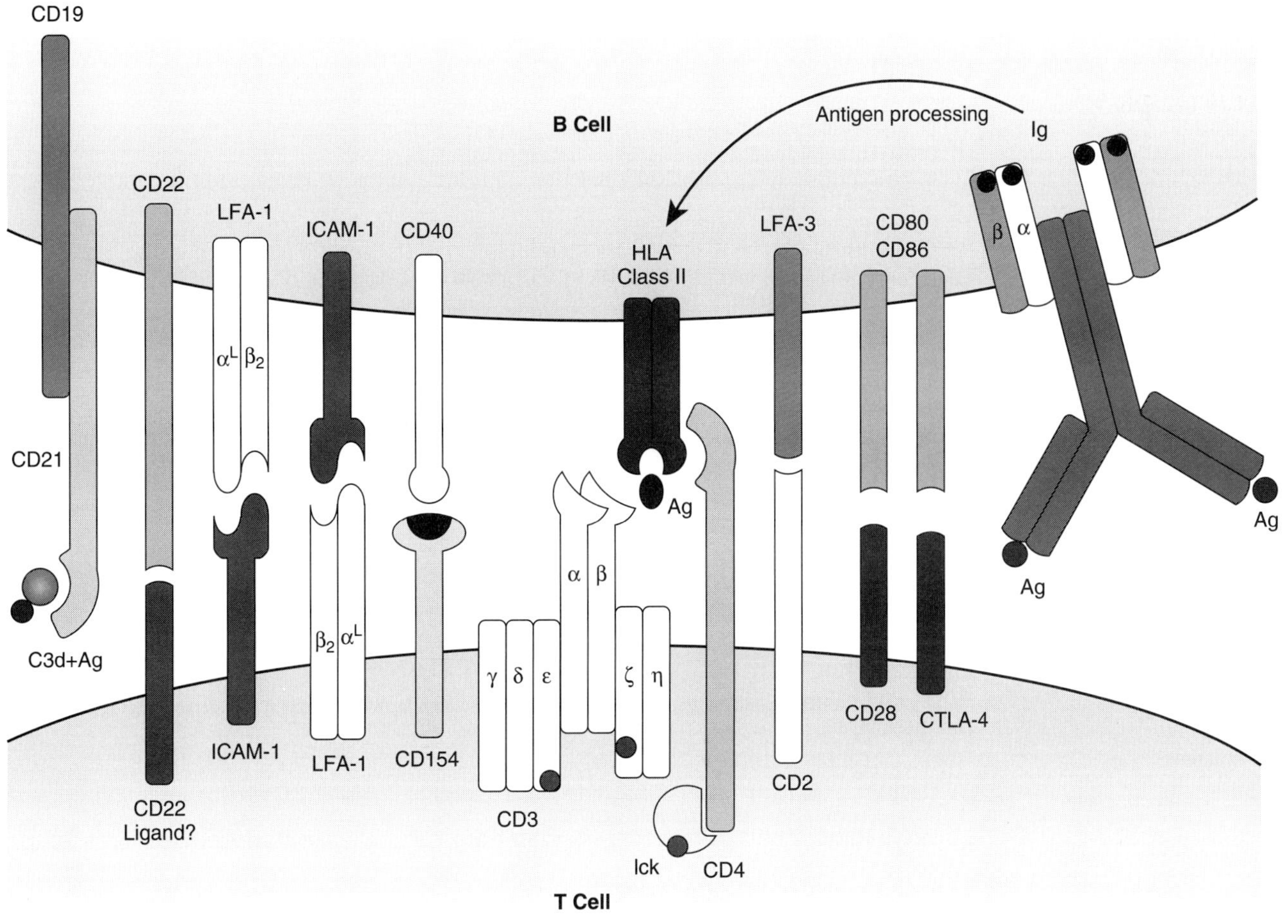

Figure 6–5. Cell surface molecules that facilitate T cell/B cell interactions.

required for the appropriate internalization and processing of Ag, which is then externalized in association with major histocompatibility complex (MHC) class II molecules for presentation to T cells (Fig. 6–5).[37] Expression of sIg also regulates B cell development by signaling the productive rearrangement of Ig genes.[38]

The outcome of the just-described developmental responses is determined in large part by signal transduction through the BCR complex.[39, 40] However, these signals are further regulated or "fine tuned" by an array of cytoplasmic signal transduction molecules that amplify or inhibit the outcome of BCR signaling during B cell development as well as during responses to self and foreign antigens (Table 6–3). Raising or lowering the thresholds required for transmembrane signals to initiate their downstream effects can also modulate the strength of transmembrane signals. Signaling through some cell surface molecules can also adjust signaling thresholds within B cells and thereby regulate how B cells sense and respond to their extracellular microenvironment.

BCR Signal Transduction

Cell surface IgM, IgD, and IgG have cytoplasmic domains of 3, 3, and 28 amino acids, respectively, and are believed to be incapable of transducing signals across the plasma membrane. Nonetheless, Ag binding by sIg leads to a series of intracellular events that are generated through a set of membrane proteins noncovalently associated with sIg, analogous to the CD3 components of the T cell Ag receptor complex.[41–43] Mouse sIgM is noncovalently associated with a disulfide-linked heterodimer composed of the 34-kD IgM-α (CD79a) and the 39-kD Ig-β (CD79b) signaling proteins. sIgD associates with a similar disulfide-linked heterodimer, although CD79a is replaced by a 35-kD protein that is also encoded by the *Cd79a* gene.[44] CD79a and CD79b are both membrane glycoproteins with single extracellular Ig-like domains.[45, 46] Ig-α and Ig-β isolated from B cells of various lymphoid organs and *Xid* mice show differences in molecular weight.[47] The function of this variability is unclear but may be the result of differential splicing of exons encoding the cytoplasmic domain in addition to differential post-translational processing of the proteins. CD79a may have other functions as well because most of the CD79a protein on mouse B cells is found as free monomer that can be transported to the cell surface without IgM.[48]

A similar molecular complex exists on human B cells, with two structurally distinct polypeptides of 47 kD and 37 kD co-precipitated with sIgM.[49] Human CD79a is B cell specific in expression, and it appears early in B cell differentiation, probably before expression of cytoplasmic μ chain, and persists until the plasma cell stage, where it

Table 6–3. B Cell Signaling Molecules

Function/Name	M_r (kD)	Comments
Surface Receptor		
CD79a	32	BCR-associated signaling component containing ITAM motifs
CD79b	37–39	BCR-associated signaling component containing ITAM motifs
CD19	95	Ig superfamily member complexed with CD81 and Leu-13; response regulator; associates with Fyn, Lyn, Vav, and PI-3 kinase
CD21	140	Complement receptor family, C3d receptor, associates with the CD19 complex
CD22	135	Ig superfamily adhesion receptor contains ITAMs and ITIMs; associates with SHP1, Lyn, Syk, and PI-3 kinase; association with SHP1 regulates CD19 and BCR signaling
Tyrosine Kinases		
Syk	72	Zap-70 related kinase; tandem SH2 domains that bind phosphorylated ITAMs
Lyn	53, 56	BCR-associated Src-family PTK
Blk	55	BCR-associated Src-family PTK
Lck	56	BCR-associated Src-family PTK
Fyn	59	BCR-associated Src-family PTK
Btk	77	Required for B cell development; mutated in X-linked Bruton's agammaglobulinemia; associates with Cbl adapter protein
Other Kinases		
PI-3 Kinase	85, 110	p110 subunit is catalytic, p85 subunit contains two SH2 domains, one SH3 domain, and proline-rich region; associated with Cbl, indirectly associated with BCR, associated with CD19
MAPK	42–44	Family of protein-serine/threonine kinases including ERK1 and 2; activated by MAPK kinases; leads to transcription factor phosphorylation and activation
JNK/SAPK	46, 54	Jun or stress-activated protein kinase; regulates transcription
Phospholipases		
PLCγ1,2	145	Contains two SH2 domains and one SH3 domain; activated by Syk; important for intracellular calcium mobilization
Phosphatases		
SHP1	65	Phosphotyrosine phosphatase; BCR-associated; also known as PTP1c, SHPTP1, HCP, and SHP; limits signal transduction; binds phosphorylated CD22
SHIP	145	SH2-containing inositol phosphatase; binds to FcγRIIb1, limits signal transduction by means of phosphatase activity or association with Shc
Adapter Proteins		
Shc	46, 52	Contains SH2, and phosphotyrosine-binding domains; binds Grb2, which in turn binds SOS; phosphorylation presumably leads to Ras activation.
Vav	95	Guanine-nucleotide exchange factor for Rac
Cbl	120	Ring finger and leucine zipper protein; contains proline-rich region; associates with PI-3 kinase and CD19 after BCR crosslinking

ITAM, immunoreceptor tyrosine-based activation motif; ITIM, immunoreceptor tyrosine-based inhibitory motif; PTK, protein tyrosine kinase; SH2, Src homology-2 domain; SH3, Src homology 3 domain.

is seen in the cytoplasm.[50] Expression of sIg is dependent on the presence of both CD79a and CD79b, and sIgM crosslinking stimulates tyrosine phosphorylation of these proteins.[51] Signal transmission after crosslinking CD79a also occurs in pre–B cell lines, even in the absence of significant sIgM, suggesting that CD79a may transmit signals for the pre–B cell Ag receptor complex as well.

In both mature and immature B cells, sIg crosslinking activates two major intracellular signaling pathways, protein tyrosine phosphorylation[52] and phosphoinositide hydrolysis.[53] Within seconds of sIgM or sIgD crosslinking, a small number of proteins become phosphorylated on tyrosine residues.[52, 54] Both CD79a and CD79b contain immunoreceptor tyrosine-based activation motifs (ITAMs) within their cytoplasmic domains that become phosphorylated after Ag binding by sIg.[55, 56] CD79 tyrosine phosphorylation facilitates the additional recruitment and activation of several Src-family protein tyrosine kinases (PTKs), including Lyn, Blk, Fyn, and lck, which further amplify CD79a and CD79b phosphorylation. Src-family PTK activity is also increased after sIg crosslinking.[57–59] Due to low-level kinase activity endogenous within primary B cells, tyrosines on some CD79a and CD79b proteins are phosphorylated, which results in the constitutive assembly of a preformed transducer complex organized by the B cell antigen receptor.[60] Phosphorylated CD79 ITAMs also serve as docking sites for the tandem Src homology 2 (SH2) domains of Syk, a Zap-70/Syk PTK family member. SH2 domains mediate recognition of proteins with specific phosphotyrosine-containing sequences. Syk recruited to CD79 becomes tyrosine phosphorylated by Src-family PTKs and thereby activated. Lyn is important for Syk activation because BCR crosslinking in Lyn-deficient B cells fails to induce Syk tyrosine phosphorylation.

After Syk and Src-family PTK activation, multiple cell surface receptors become rapidly tyrosine phosphorylated, including CD19 and CD22, which contain multiple SH2-docking sites. Crosslinking of sIgM also initiates a cascade of biochemical events that includes the tyrosine phosphorylation and activation of phospholipase Cγ1 and Cγ2 (PLC-γ) and phosphatidylinositol-3 (PI-3) kinase, the elevation of intracellular calcium ($[Ca^{2+}]_i$), and the translocation of protein kinase C (PKC) to the membrane.[61] There is also increased tyrosine phosphorylation of multiple downstream effector molecules, including Ras and the Vav and Shc adapter proteins. In addition, numerous phosphotyrosine phosphatases become activated, including SHP1 (an SH2-domain–containing phosphotyrosine phosphatase) and SH2-domain–containing inositol polyphosphate 5-phosphatase (SHIP). These molecules each contain one or more SH2 domains that facilitate their interactions either directly or indirectly with CD79a, CD79b, or other BCR-associated signaling molecules. Another phosphotyrosine phosphatase downstream of BCR signaling is CD45, a membrane spanning receptor of unknown specificity. Activation of Src-family PTKs after BCR ligation does not occur in CD45-deficient B cells.[62] CD45 is therefore likely to dephosphorylate a carboxyl-terminal tyrosine present in Src-family PTKs. Phosphorylation of this site is thought to downregulate Src-family PTK activity.

Tyrosine-phosphorylated PLC hydrolyzes phosphatidylinositol-(4,5)-bisphosphate (PIP_2) into two potent second messengers, diacylglycerol and inositol-(1,4,5)-trisphosphate (IP_3). IP_3 interacts with receptors on the endoplasmic reticulum, resulting in an efflux of Ca^{2+} from intracellular stores and increased $[Ca^{2+}]_i$ levels. Increased $[Ca^{2+}]_i$ results in the activation of a number of calcium-dependent proteins involved in propagating the stimulatory signal, such as calmodulin and calcineurin, which induce the nuclear localization of nuclear factor of activated T cells (NFAT). BCR crosslinking in Syk-deficient B cells does not lead to PLC-γ2 phosphorylation, which impairs $[Ca^{2+}]_i$ release.[63] Diacylglycerol activates PKC and several other members of the serine/threonine PKC family, which induces the subsequent translocation of PKC to the inner face of the plasma membrane. Activation of PKC leads to the activation and nuclear localization of transcription factors, including Fos, Jun, and NFκB.

BCR stimulation also induces activation of the guanosine triphosphate (GTP)-hydrolyzing enzyme Ras, although the precise mechanisms remain unknown. It is likely that the SH2-domain–containing adapter protein Shc contributes to Ras activation because Shc directly or indirectly associates with CD79 ITAM-binding proteins. Shc contains phosphotyrosine-binding domains in addition to its SH2 and SH3 domains. SH3 domains bind to proteins through proline-rich regions, whereas phosphotyrosine-binding domains mediate recognition of specific phosphotyrosine-containing sequences. Tyrosine phosphorylation of Shc results in the recruitment of another SH2/SH3-containing adapter molecule, growth factor–bound protein 2 (Grb2), and son of sevenless (SOS), a guanine nucleotide exchange factor. The Grb2/SOS protein complex catalyzes the activation of Ras through its binding of GTP. BCR crosslinking in Syk-deficient B cells fails to phosphorylate Shc, which likely impairs activation of the Ras signaling pathway. After BCR ligation, SHIP may complex with the Shc phosphotyrosine binding domain and thereby downregulate Ras activation.[64] SHIP activation may also block BCR-induced $[Ca^{2+}]_i$ responses by decreasing the availability of the major PLC-γ2 substrate, PIP_2.[65]

A downstream consequence of BCR-induced Ras activation is the activation of Raf-1, a serine/threonine-kinase, and activation of dual-specific (serine/threonine and tyrosine) kinases that subsequently trigger the mitogen-activated protein kinase (MAPK) cascade. The MAPK cascade includes extracellular signal-regulated mitogen-activated protein kinase (ERK), a serine/threonine kinase; Jun or stress-activated protein kinase (JNK/SAPK); and the kinase kinases (MEK, SEK, and MKK). MAPK activation leads to phosphorylation of a number of transcription factors, including Fos and Jun, thereby altering their DNA binding activity and downstream patterns of gene expression. The reconstitution of BCR signaling in a nonhematopoietic cell line suggests that activation of MAPK depends on the presence of Syk, which is consistent with the need for Syk to phosphorylate Shc and activate Ras.[66] Thus, a number of effector molecules are involved in translating BCR and other extracellular stimuli into nuclear events, which ultimately result in B cell proliferation and differentiation.

Cell Surface Regulators of Signal Transduction

Although sIg is central to the function of mature B cells, other surface molecules are also critical for normal development and regulation of B cell differentiation, activation, and proliferation (see Fig. 6–4). Signals generated through non-Ig receptors can also positively or negatively modulate the signals delivered through sIg. In this way, the anatomical location, local microenvironment, or milieu of localized "factors" can directly influence the outcome of a humoral response. The array and density of cell surface molecules expressed at any particular stage of B cell differentiation or on interacting T cells can have a directing influence as well.

Several cell surface receptors critically regulate BCR signaling (see Table 6–3). Included on this list is CD19, which forms a complex with the CD21 complement receptor on the surface of B cells.[67] CD22, a cell surface adhesion molecule, is also tightly coupled to intracellular signaling molecules and pathways that regulate BCR signaling.[68] As examples, these molecules include Lyn, Vav, and SHP1. The generation of knockout mice, or mice that overexpress these molecules, has demonstrated that these proteins regulate intracellular signaling thresholds and serve as "response regulators" or "threshold modulators" for dictating the magnitude of intracellular responses.[40] Thus, these molecules function as both positive and negative regulators, depending on the context in which function is being assessed.

An important consideration in B cell function is the delicate balance on which many of the key signaling molecules depend for function. Undoubtedly, competition between the binding elements of various regulatory proteins for limiting amounts of tyrosine-phosphorylated substrates or other docking sites occurs. Tipping the balance in favor of, or against, any interaction through regulatory cell surface molecules greatly influences the biological outcome of signaling. Thus, subtle changes in cell surface receptor density or the localized concentration of effector molecules within the cytoplasm of cells responding to external stimuli is likely to have amplified effects.

CD19

In addition to the sIg receptor complex, CD19 and CD21 are important signal transduction molecules that noncovalently associate to form a multimolecular complex on the cell surface.[69] CD19 is a member of the Ig superfamily.[70] It is uniquely expressed by B cells and follicular dendritic cells,[71] as is CD21 (CR2), a member of a family of complement receptors.[72] Two additional members of the CD19 complex are CD81, a broadly expressed member of the tetraspans protein family in which all members traverse the membrane four times,[73] and Leu-13, a broadly expressed protein.[74, 75] Thus, CD19, CD21, TAPA-1, and Leu-13 associate to form a signal transduction complex on B lymphocytes that is predominantly independent of the Ag receptor complex.

CD19 is a 95-kD protein expressed from the early stages of Ig heavy chain rearrangement until plasma cell differentiation.[19] CD19 has two extracellular Ig-like domains, a membrane-spanning domain, and a highly charged approximately 240 amino acid cytoplasmic tail containing localized regions of strong net negative charge.[70] Although the cytoplasmic domain of CD19 shares no significant amino acid sequence homology with other known proteins, this region is critical for CD19 function and is under significant evolutionary pressure for conservation of amino acid sequence. CD19 is generally a positive regulator of signaling because B cells are hyporesponsive in its absence and hyperresponsive when it is overexpressed.[76] CD19 expression regulates the activation of both kinases and tyrosine phosphatases that can have either positive or negative regulatory roles, depending on the assays or outcome employed. For example, BCR and CD19 crosslinking can deliver either potent mitogenic stimuli or inhibitory signals.[77–79] Crosslinking CD19 can inhibit $[Ca^{2+}]_i$ responses, and subsequent activation and proliferation that follow mitogen stimulation,[80] but can also induce tyrosine kinase activity,[80, 81] $[Ca^{2+}]_i$ release,[80] and internalization of the molecule.

The CD19 cytoplasmic domain contains nine well-conserved tyrosine residues, some of which are rapidly phosphorylated after BCR and/or CD19 ligation.[82] CD19 regulates BCR signaling by amplifying Src-family protein tyrosine kinase (PTK) activation[83] and mediating interactions between these PTKs and downstream effector molecules, including PI-3 kinase and Vav.[67] In the absence of CD19 expression, B cells from gene-targeted mice are hyporesponsive to transmembrane signals and generate modest immune responses.[84, 85] Uniquely, small increases in CD19 expression levels (20%–300%) in transgenic mice dramatically enhance B cell responses to transmembrane signals and predispose these mice to autoimmunity.[86–90] These observations suggest that CD19 expression and function are tightly regulated under normal circumstances.

Although a full understanding of CD19 function in vivo is not yet available, it appears that CD19 serves as a sensing mechanism for extracellular signals. An attractive hypothesis is that CD19 utilizes CD21 as a sensor to detect complement activation and alert B cells of inflammatory reactions.[76] Nonetheless, it is clear that CD19 is a major regulator of intracellular signal transduction thresholds.[67] Like in CD19-deficient mice, the *Btk*-deficient Xid mouse has lowered signaling thresholds and deficiencies in B cell function.[76, 91, 92] Mice deficient in the *Vav* proto-oncogene are also similarly affected.[93, 94] These and many other parallels suggest that CD19/CD21, *Vav*, and *Btk* regulate common or overlapping signaling pathways that also involve Src-family protein tyrosine kinase activity.

CD21

CD21 is the B cell receptor for the C3d,g fragment of complement[95] that also serves as the receptor for Epstein-Barr virus.[96] CD21 is first expressed by most B cells around the time of IgD expression and is lost after activation.[71] CD21 is a 145-kD protein that consists of 15 or 16 short consensus repeat units, each of 60 to 70 amino acids, followed by a transmembrane region and a 34 amino acid intracytoplasmic domain.[72] Although Ab binding to CD21 alone does not activate B cells, binding of CD21 by Ab or by crosslinked C3d,g can deliver a costimulatory signal to B cells suboptimally activated by phorbol myristate acetate (PMA), anti-IgM Ab, or T cell factors.[97] Crosslinking of IgM with CD21 also enhances the transient increase in intracellular $[Ca^{2+}]_i$ levels induced through IgM alone.[77] In vitro and in vivo, the simultaneous ligation of CD19/CD21 and membrane Ig lowers the threshold required for signaling through the Ag receptor, thereby promoting immune responses that are more effective.[98] Therefore, CD21 functional activity correlates with its co-association with CD19.

Recent in vivo studies demonstrate a direct role for CD21 in immune responses. In mice, CD21 is generated from a single gene that gives rise to a CD21/CD35 protein product.[99] Pretreatment of mice with a CD21/35 Ab blocks both T cell–dependent and T cell–independent immune responses and the generation of immunological memory.[100–102] The infusion of soluble recombinant mouse CD21 also blocks immune responses to T cell–dependent Ags in vivo.[103] Similar results are obtained with CD21/35-deficient mice.[104, 105] CD21/35-deficient mice have normal numbers of splenocytes and well-developed splenic follicles. The proliferative responses of B cells from CD21/35-deficient mice are normal, and serum Ig levels are generally within the normal range. However, CD21/35-deficient mice exhibit severe defects in their primary and secondary humoral responses to T cell–dependent Ags. IgM titers are moderately decreased whereas there is a dramatic impairment in IgG responses. The loss of CD21/35 expression results in a phenotype that is similar to, but much more subtle than, the phenotype of CD19-deficient mice.

The exact mechanism by which complement receptor deficiency affects the humoral immune response remains uncertain. The covalent coupling of C3 cleavage products onto Ags or immune complexes facilitates their clearance via the reticuloendothelial system and the localization of Ag onto B cells and follicular dendritic cells within germinal centers.[106, 107] Thereby, defective humoral immune responses in cases of complement deficiency may result from defective Ag localization and/or presentation within the follicular areas of the spleen. However, the defect in humoral immune responses in CD21/35-deficient mice appears to reside within the B cell compartment.[108] In one model explaining roles for the CD19 complex and C3 in B cell function, the association between CD19 and CD21 is envisioned to provide a mechanism for bridging the B cell Ag receptor complex with the CD19 complex through C3d-Ag.[109] A different model predicts that endogenous humoral C3d levels establish signaling thresholds for B cells in an Ag-independent manner through crosslinking the CD19 complex.[76] In this model, the CD19 complex would serve as a sensing mechanism for detecting activation of the innate immune system and adjust signaling thresholds accordingly. Complement activation during ongoing immune responses would heighten the humoral immune response by decreasing the signaling thresholds necessary for B cell activation. In the absence of infection or other immune stimulators, signaling thresholds would be modified to suppress humoral responses against weak self Ags.

CD22

CD22 is a 140-kD Ig-superfamily member, with an extracellular region of seven Ig-like domains that shares considerable homology with neural cell adhesion molecule, myelin-associated glycoprotein and carcinoembryonic Ag.[110, 111] Functional studies using COS cells transfected with CD22 complementary DNA indicate that it is an adhesion molecule involved in homotypical and heterotypical interactions with B and T cells, monocytes, and erythrocytes. The ligand for CD22 has not been specifically identified, but CD22 binds a broad variety of cell surface and soluble determinants bearing sialic acid.[112–114]

CD22 is uniquely expressed in the cytoplasm of progenitor B and pre–B cells, appears on the cell surface of mature B cells at the same time as IgD, and is lost upon activation.[115] In lymphoid tissues, CD22 is expressed at significant levels by follicular mantle and marginal zone B cells but only weakly by germinal center B cells. CD22 regulates B cell activation. The binding of CD22 Ab to B cells in vitro augments both $[Ca^{2+}]_i$ increases and proliferation induced after sIg crosslinking. The approximately 140 amino acid cytoplasmic domain of CD22 contains six tyrosines that are targets for rapid phosphorylation after surface Ig or CD22 ligation.[110, 116] The CD22 cytoplasmic domain uniquely contains ITAM and immunoreceptor tyrosine-based inhibition motif (ITIM) sequences, suggesting positive and negative signaling functions.[117, 118] Negative roles for CD22 in BCR signaling are proposed to be critical for normal B cell activation,[119–121] because tyrosine phosphorylated CD22 recruits SHP1, a potent intracellular phosphatase with inhibitory functions.[122–126] Consistent with a negative regulatory role for CD22, B cells from CD22-deficient mice display augmented $[Ca^{2+}]_i$ responses after BCR crosslinking and exhibit characteristics of chronic stimulation.[68, 127–130] By contrast, CD22 also associates with surface IgM and 1 positive × effector molecules.[117, 118, 125, 131, 132] This may explain why CD22-deficient mice generate reduced proliferative responses after BCR crosslinking.[127, 128] However, a major functional role for CD22 is the regulation of CD19 phosphorylation and function.[133] Nonetheless, it is clear that CD19 and CD22 serve as central signaling elements that are closely linked by tyrosine phosphorylation to multiple other signaling pathways and cell surface receptors, including the B cell antigen receptor.

CD5

A subpopulation of B cells express CD5, a marker found on nearly all T lymphocytes. Functional studies have suggested that CD5 B cells develop along a lineage distinct from that of conventional B cells.[134] However, considerable evidence now suggests that CD5$^+$ B cells represent a subpopulation of cells at a different stage of activation or differentiation than conventional B cells in response to different Ag receptor specificities.[135] This is likely because human B cells can be induced to express CD5 after treatment with phorbol esters[136] and crosslinking sIgM on newly emerging mouse B cells induces CD5 expression. CD5$^+$ B cells appear in the human fetal peritoneal and pleural cavities at 15 weeks of gestation; however, these cells are absent from the liver before 16 weeks and are rare in the bone marrow. During B cell development, 40% of the mature B cells found in the omentum and spleen are CD5$^+$, compared with only 20% in the liver.[31] In mouse, CD5 (Ly1$^+$) B cells are also generated in a compartment distinct from that of conventional B cells.

CD5$^+$ B cells differ from conventional B cells in their surface phenotype, tissue localization, and Ig repertoire. The most intriguing characteristic of CD5$^+$ B cells is their increased production of Ab with affinity for self Ag, including rheumatoid factor, and anti-DNA and anti–T cell reactivity.[137, 138] The overrepresentation of this specificity within CD5$^+$ B cells is clearly the result of Ag selection; however, the mechanism for the segregation of this Ab specificity and the nature of its function in vivo is unclear. Although there is an association between increased levels of CD5$^+$ B cells in certain autoimmune diseases such as rheumatoid arthritis, the exact role they play in the cause of autoimmune disease is unknown. One theory is that the amplification of CD5$^+$ B cell numbers reflects lowered B cell signaling thresholds, perhaps because of genetic alterations.[40] Alternatively, CD5 has been proposed to be an endogenous ligand selective for B cell surface Ig framework sequences.[139] In this context, CD5 would serve as a superantigen to sustain B cell activation and BCR signaling.

CD10

CD10, also known as CALLA for "common acute lymphoblastic leukemia Ag," is a 100-kD glycoprotein that is a member of a large family of cell surface proteases.[140] CD10 is primarily expressed during the early stages of pre–B cell development, by the majority of acute lymphoblastic leukemias, and by other lymphoid malignancies with an immature phenotype. Normal lymphoid progenitors that are either uncommitted or committed to only the earliest stages of B or T cell differentiation also express CD10, suggesting that the protein plays a role in the early stages of lymphoid ontogeny. However, CD10 is also expressed on granulocytes and nonhematopoietic cell types, including bronchial epithelial cells, cultured fibroblasts, renal proximal tubular epithelial cells, and certain solid tumor cell lines, indicating that its biological function is not restricted to lymphoid development. CD10 is a zinc metalloproteinase neutral endopeptidase 24.11. It cleaves peptide bonds on the amino side of hydrophobic amino acids and inactivates a variety of peptide hormones, including enkephalin, chemotactic peptide, substance P, atrial natriuretic factor, endothelin, oxytocin, neurotensin, bradykinin, angiotensin, and the bombesin-like peptides.[141] Although, the true function of CD10 on B cells remains unclear, the endopeptidase activity may serve to digest polypeptide factors present in the environment of maturing B lymphocytes, thereby altering their proliferation and differentiation.

CD20

CD20 was the first non-Ig differentiation Ag of human B cells to be identified by an mAb.[142] CD20 expression is B cell restricted, being found on early B cell precursors and all mature B cells but not plasma cells.[19] CD20 is a dominant phosphoprotein in activated B cells and B cell lines. It contains three extensive hydrophobic regions of sufficient length to pass through the membrane four times.[143] The long carboxyl- and amino-terminal ends of the molecule are located within the cytoplasm with only a minor portion of the molecule exposed to the extracellular environment. The transmembrane and cytoplasmic regions of both mouse and human CD20 are well conserved and may allow for interactions with the multiple proteins that are co-immunoprecipitated with CD20. Three isoforms of CD20—33 kD, 35 kD and 37 kD—result from differential phosphorylation of a single protein species at different serine and threonine residues within the cytoplasmic domain. CD20 shares a common chromosomal location, a similar overall structure, and a sequence homology with the β chain of the high-affinity IgE receptor found on mast cells.[144]

Ab binding to CD20 inhibits B cell entry into the $S/G2^{+}$ M stages of the cell cycle after mitogen stimulation and blocks differentiation.[145] In contrast, the binding of one Ab can induce B cell activation.[146] CD20 is not phosphorylated in resting B cells, but it becomes heavily phosphorylated after mitogen stimulation, providing further evidence that CD20 is involved in B cell activation and differentiation. In addition, Ab binding to CD20 generates a transmembrane signal that results in enhanced phosphorylation of the molecule. The presence of four membrane-spanning domains in CD20 is reminiscent of membrane transporters or ion channels. Indeed, CD20 has been found to be a component of a homo-oligomeric complex of perhaps four CD20 molecules that forms a Ca^{2+} channel critical for normal B cell function.[147]

Remarkably, anti-CD20 Ab treatment has evolved as a major therapy for non-Hodgkin's lymphoma.[148, 149] Anti-CD20 mAbs have been effectively employed for the immunotherapy of B cell lymphomas in multiple recent clinical trials in either unmodified form or conjugated to radionuclides.[150–154] A significant portion of the tumoricidal effect of anti-CD20 mAbs may be mediated by mechanisms independent of complement, antibody-dependent cellular cytotoxicity, or radioactive emissions.[155–157] Rather, we favor the notion that anti-CD20 Ab binding activates transmembrane Ca^{2+} channels that sustain elevated $[Ca^{2+}]_i$ levels that arrest the cells in cycle, which leads to their eventual apoptosis.[158]

CD23

CD23 is a low affinity receptor for IgE (FcεRII) that may have broad effects in immunoregulation.[159, 160] Differential splicing of a single gene results in an isoform of CD23 expressed by B cells (FcεRIIa) with a second form expressed by eosinophils, monocytes, and platelets (FcεRIIb).[161] CD23 is a 45-kD glycoprotein expressed on the surface of activated B cells that is a type II integral membrane protein (NH_2 terminus within the cell) with a carboxyl-terminal C-type lectin domain. A striking feature of CD23 is that it is cleaved into biologically active soluble fragments, some of which retain the ability to bind IgE and possess a variety of reported biological effects. Furthermore, soluble CD23 can be readily quantitated and isolated from biological fluids such as serum and urine.

CD24

CD24 is a pan–B cell marker expressed from the pro–B cell stage until plasma cell differentiation, which is also expressed by neutrophils.[162] CD24 is a single-chain sialoglycoprotein of 35 to 45 kD attached to the plasma membrane through a glycosyl polyphosphoinositol (GPI) anchor. Ab binding to CD24 negatively affects B cell differentiation but augments proliferation. It is not clear how CD24 transmits transmembrane signals; however, CD24 and other GPI-anchored cell surface molecules associate with protein tyrosine kinases, key regulators of cell activation, and signal transduction.[163] The CD24 complementary DNA encodes a remarkably small peptide of 31 to 35 amino acids with multiple sites for addition of N- and O-linked carbohydrates, suggesting that the bulk of the 35- to 45-kD molecule is carbohydrate.[164] Consistent with this, many of the CD24 Abs react with carbohydrate determinants present on CD24.

CD40

CD40 is a 50-kD glycoprotein expressed on most B cells that delivers a potent co-stimulatory signal for cell-cycle progression. CD40 is also expressed by activated macrophages, keratinocytes, follicular dendritic cells, bone marrow–derived dendritic cells, epithelial cells, and carcinoma cells. Quiescent B cells can be directly perturbed through CD40 to enlarge, aggregate, and acquire enhanced responsiveness to mitogenic triggering.[165] Moreover, CD40 Ab binding can act synergistically with other growth-promoting agents, such as IL-4, to sustain B cell proliferation.[166] CD40 ligation also prevents germinal center B cells from undergoing spontaneous apoptosis, thereby directing B cells toward plasma cell development on antigenic stimulation.[167]

CD40 is a member of the tumor necrosis factor (TNF)/nerve growth factor receptor family.[168] The CD40 ligand (CD154) is also a member of this receptor family, which is preferentially expressed by CD4+ T cells immediately after activation.[169] CD154 is also expressed by a number of other cell types, including dendritic cells. CD40 engagement by this ligand mediates B cell proliferation in the absence of a costimulus, as well as IgE production in the presence of IL-4. Thus, this receptor/ligand pair provides a rapid means of communication between B and T cells when they come into intimate contact after Ag recognition. A critical role for CD40/CD154 intercellular interactions during humoral immune responses is demonstrated in patients with X-linked hyper-IgM syndrome, who have defective CD154 genes.[170–172] These patients lack the ability to form germinal centers and undergo Ig isotype class switching from IgM to IgG, IgE, and IgA. Mice deficient in CD40 or CD154 expression exhibit a similar phenotype.[173, 174]

Among the earliest detectable signaling events after CD40 engagement are activation of Src-family protein tyrosine kinases (particularly Lyn), PI-3 kinase, and Ras.[175] CD40 ligation also activates two subfamilies of the stress-activated protein kinases, JNK/SAPKs and p38 MAPK, while inducing little or no activation of the more distantly related ERKs. Thus, CD40 plays a major role in the activation, proliferation, and differentiation of B lymphocytes.

CD72

CD72 is expressed at all stages of B cell differentiation except for the plasma cell stage and is identical to the mouse Lyb-2 differentiation Ag.[176] CD72 is an 80-kD glycoprotein composed of two disulfide-linked polypeptides of 39 and 43 kD that are derived from an identical protein precursor that is differentially proteolytically cleaved. CD72, like CD23, is a type II integral membrane protein that contains a carboxyl-terminal domain homologous with C-type animal lectins. Studies on mouse CD72 suggest that it participates in early B cell activation. With human B cells, CD72 Ab binding selectively augments certain activation pathways in tonsillar B cells. By itself CD72 Ab binding provides a weak stimulus to resting B cells, but it provides synergistic signals when added with immobilized anti-IgM Ab. Recent controversial studies suggest that CD72 serves as a counterreceptor for the CD5 differentiation Ag of T and B cells.[38]

Treatment of B cells with anti-CD72 Abs induces proliferation and augments B cell activation induced by BCR signaling.[177–181] Anti-CD72 mAbs also block BCR-mediated cell death of mature B cells.[182] CD72 also has an important role in B cell differentiation during responses to both thymic-independent and thymic-dependent Ags.[180, 183] Consistent with CD72 ligation modulating BCR signaling, the CD72 cytoplasmic domain contains an ITIM motif that recruits SHP-1 upon tyrosine phosphorylation.[184, 185] BCR ligation enhances CD72 phosphorylation and its recruitment of SHP-1, suggesting that CD72 may be a negative regulator of BCR signaling.

CD80

CD80, also called the B7-1 Ag, is a member of the Ig superfamily expressed on the surface of resting B cells after stimulation by crosslinking sIg or HLA-DR, by Epstein-Barr virus infection, or by exposure to IL-2 or IL-4.[186, 187] CD80 is expressed on some B cells 24 hours after activation, but maximal levels are apparent at 48 to 72 hours. In vivo, CD80 identifies a subpopulation of previously activated or primed B cells with accelerated responses to activation agents.[186] CD80 is also expressed on activated T cells,[188] monocytes in response to interferon (IFN)–γ,[189] dendritic cells,[190, 191] and human T lymphotropic virus type I–transformed T cells.[192] CD80 is a 50- to 60-kD glycoprotein composed of a V-type Ig-like domain, a C-type Ig-like domain, a transmembrane domain, and a short 16-amino acid cytoplasmic tail.[186, 193–195]

CD80 is a ligand for two structurally similar molecules expressed on T lymphocytes: CD28 and CTLA-4.[196–198] CD28 and CTLA-4 are important regulatory molecules for T cell activation.[199] Importantly, interactions between CD80 and its ligands (CD28/CTLA4) regulate immune responses. T cell Ag receptor signaling in the absence of CD80 costimulation results in the induction of Ag specific tolerance.[200] Binding of CD28 by Ab or by interactions with CD80 results in enhanced production of cytokines by activated T cells. B cell differentiation also involves interactions between CD28 on T cells and CD80 on activated B cells.[201] CTLA-4 is expressed at a lower level on the T cell surface than is CD28 but possesses a higher affinity for CD80.[198] B cells from mice lacking CD80 exhibit a 70% decrease in costimulation during alloantigen responses.[202] However, CD80-deficient mice have normal numbers of T cells and B cells, have normal levels of serum Ig, and respond normally to mitogens.

CD86

CD86, also called B7-2, is a second ligand for the CD28 and CTLA4 receptors on T cells.[203] CD86 is reactive with activated B cells, blood monocytes, large B cell lymphomas, CD30+ anaplastic large-cell lymphomas, and Reed-Sternberg cells of Hodgkin's disease.[204] This receptor appears 24 hours after B cell activation but induces IL-2 secretion and T cell proliferation.[205] Some T cells can also express CD86 after activation.[206] Among lymphoid tissues, CD86 is only weakly reactive with germinal center cells and is not present at detectable levels on other cells. CD86 is a single-chain 75- to 80-kD cell surface protein under reducing conditions.[204, 206] It belongs to the Ig superfamily and shares 26% amino acid sequence identity with CD80.[207]

Other Surface Molecules

Human leukocyte antigen class II Ags serve a critical role in the initiation of an immune response through their role as Ag-presenting molecules on the surface of B cells (see Fig. 6–5). Engagement of B lymphocyte class II region gene products with Ab also generates transmembrane signals. In addition, many other B cell–restricted and associated proteins are involved in regulating B cell development and proliferation. It is likely that many additional significant surface receptors have yet to be identified and functionally examined.

B Cell Growth and Differentiation Factors

Although cell surface receptors play a pivotal role in the regulation of immunological recognition, soluble factors and their receptors are also critical to the development of an immune response. All stages of lymphopoiesis are controlled by both agonistic and antagonist factors, as evidenced by the effects of soluble factors on in vitro cultures of B lineage precursors. Whereas stromal cell lines produce an array of cytokines, one of the most critical factors in early B cell growth is IL-7.[35] IL-7 does not appear to act on more mature B cells. IL-3 is also a potent growth stimulus for normal and leukemic B cell precursors, although no stromal cell lines have been found that express this cytokine. IL-4 also regulates the differentiation and proliferation of human precursor B cells and induces pre–B cells to mature into $sIgM^+$ B cells.[208] IL-5 may play an important role in the ontogeny of $CD5^+$ B cells. IL-1 induces expression of sIg on precursor B cells, but it is not clear whether this effect is direct or results from the induced release of other cytokines by stromal cells.

Cell cycle progression of mature B cells after antigen receptor ligation is dramatically augmented by soluble B cell growth factors derived primarily from helper T cells. This response is mediated by complex combinations of multiple cytokines, including IFN-γ, TNF, IL-1, IL-2, IL-4, IL-5, IL-6, IL-10, and others.[209, 210] Among its activities, IL-4 prepares resting B cells for optimal expansion in response to mitogenic stimuli and growth factors and induces the increased expression of multiple cell surface molecules that are central to B cell/T cell interactions. IFN-γ and IL-1 prime human B cells for accelerated entry into cell cycle,[211, 212] and the interferons enhance the proliferative response of human B cells. IL-2 serves as a growth factor for activated B cells. IL-5 is a late-acting B cell growth factor in mouse cells, whereas it does not augment the activation or proliferation of most human B cells. IL-10 is a potent growth and differentiation factor for activated human B cells.[213] In addition to the effects that these factors can induce alone, their combinations can also have dramatic synergistic or antagonistic effects.

Terminal differentiation of B cells is also regulated by soluble factors, presumably originating from helper T cells that initiate the differentiation cascade. These B cell differentiation factors can also have dramatic influence on the isotypes of secreted Ig as well. For example, the addition of IL-5 to cultures initiates IgM secretion and a switch to all Ig isotypes. IL-4 and IL-5, both alone and in combination, are capable of stimulating preferential production of IgE and some IgG subclasses. In addition, IFN-γ induces the production of different IgG subclasses. Induction of IgE synthesis can be significantly augmented by IL-4 and engagement of CD40. IL-10 and TGF-β cooperate to induce anti-CD40–activated B cells to secrete IgA. Although IL-6 mediates multiple functions on various cell types, it has dramatic effects on the proliferation of myeloma cells and late-stage activated B cells and is a potent differentiation factor.[214] Thus, in many instances, factors that affect early phases of the immune response have significant effects on the later stages as well.

PRIMARY IMMUNE RESPONSES

T Cell/Independent B Cell Differentiation

After Ag binding to sIg, a B cell can mount an immune response without T cell help. These T cell–independent responses can be initiated by bacterial products, such as lipopolysaccharide, that are potent polyclonal mitogens for mouse B lymphocytes. *Staphylococcus aureus* Cowan I is also a potent polyclonal activator of human B lymphocytes after interactions between protein A and sIg. Bacterial receptors for Ig that are distinct from protein A have also been identified on the surface of many other bacterial strains, including receptors specific for IgD. T cell–independent responses can also be initiated by polysaccharides that contain repeating antigenic units capable of binding to multiple sIg molecules simultaneously. Multivalent binding and subsequent crosslinking of sIg can provide a strong proliferative stimulus to resting B cells, which can result in the generation of a humoral response in vivo, usually restricted to the IgM subclass.

T Cell/Dependent B Cell Differentiation

Consistent with the critical role for T cells in the regulation of a normal immune response, most B cell responses are directed by interactions with helper T cells and their secreted factors. As indicated in Figure 6–5, T cell Ag receptor–mediated recognition of processed Ag/MHC class II complexes on the surface of B cells is the initiating event in the delivery of cognate help during T cell–dependent responses. The interaction of CD4 on T cells with MHC class II Ags on B cells is also essential for T cell activation, and Abs against either of these structures inhibit this. T cell/B cell interactions are also stabilized by the interaction of multiple adhesion receptors, including LFA-1 (CD11a)/ICAM-1 (CD54) and CD2/LFA-3 (CD58), and lymphocyte activation strengthens the adhesion between these co-receptors.[215] Abs directed against LFA-1 partially block T cell/B cell conjugate formation and subsequent B cell activation.[216, 217] Many adhesion molecules are capable of transmitting signals themselves, adding an additional layer of complexity to the B cell/T cell interaction paradigm.

Ag-activated B cells then clonally expand and differentiate in distinct microenvironments in vivo.[218, 219] These microenvironments are broadly divided into zones rich in T cells and zones rich in B cells. After appropriate T cell help, a cohort of Ag-specific B cells commits to plasma cell differentiation. These Ag-specific B cells expand in the T cell zones of secondary lymphoid organs and differentiate into short-lived plasma cells secreting IgM and downstream Ig isotypes.[219–223] Ag-binding cells in this non–germinal center (GC) pathway express high levels of syndecan (an integral membrane proteoglycan)[224, 225] and intermediate levels of B220 (the B cell isoform of CD45R) that helps distinguish Ab-secreting cells from either resting B cells or GC B cells.[226, 227] These Ag-specific plasma cells are best localized by immunohistochemistry with high levels of intracellular Ig,[219, 222, 223, 228] but they can also be isolated by flow cytometry and functionally characterized in vitro.[225–227] Mutational analysis of expressed V region genes after either microdissection or flow cytometry indicates that these non-GC plasma cells remain unmutated during early primary responses to Ag.

The Germinal Center Reaction

In response to Ag and T cell help, some of the Ag-activated B cells migrate into the B cell–rich follicular zones of secondary lymphoid organs. Clonal expansion in this microenvironment leads to the formation of GCs and a complex cycle of events referred to as the GC reaction. The GC reaction plays a pivotal role in specific immune responses to Ag.[218, 229, 230] The GC microenvironment serves to expand and diversify the repertoire of the early immune response to Ag and helps to select high-affinity variants for long-term maintenance of protective immunity.[226, 228, 231, 232] Oligoclonal expansion of Ag-specific B cells in the follicular regions of lymphoid organs is well described for a number of model systems.[228, 229, 232, 233] These rapidly dividing B cell blasts create secondary follicles that then give rise to the classical polarized GC reaction.[218, 221, 233] Dark zones within GCs house rapidly dividing centroblasts that continually give rise to noncycling centrocytes found within the light zone.[233] In the early phases of the GC cycle, selection proceeds without somatic diversification of the Ig receptor.[223, 226] During these first few days, Ag-specific clones expressing atypical V regions appear to be recruited and expanded in GCs but are rapidly selected against by unknown mechanisms.[223]

Maturation of the Antibody Response

Somatic hypermutation targets the rearranged V region genes of Ag-specific GC B cells with no regard to the final specificity of the variant clones produced.[234, 235] At some stage after diversification of the Ig receptor, selection takes place, presumably based on high-affinity Ag binding. The GC cycle also requires the purging of B cells with lowered Ag-binding capacity, as well as those acquiring self reactivity.[236–238] The infusion of a soluble deaggregated form of the immunizing protein Ag at the height of the GC reaction induces rapid cell death by apoptosis. This is thought to mimic the appearance of self-reactivity in the GC reaction. In addition, there is a heightened propensity of human GC B cells to undergo apoptosis in vitro.[167] In a recent series of studies, human tonsillar B differentiation has been staged with respect to expression of genes associated with apoptosis,[239] presence and extent of somatic hypermutation,[240] and the status of Ig isotype switch.[241] "Receptor editing" appears to be another means to diversify Ig genes during the GC reaction.[242] Exchanging the expressed light chain genes of self-reactive B cells by receptor editing was initially described in transgenic models of central tolerance as a means for avoiding clonal deletion. However, RAG-1 expression and V(D)J recombinase activity are now found in GC B cells and may serve to further diversify Ag-specific Ig receptors.[243, 244]

Microenvironments of Primary Immune Responses

Lymphocyte localization within the proper lymphoid tissues and microenvironment within each tissue is crucial to the development of appropriate humoral immune responses. The distribution of chemokines and their receptors regulates lymphocyte migration and helps organize tissue microenvironments in vivo. The BLR1/CXCR5 chemokine receptor not only controls B cell migration patterns to inguinal lymph nodes, Peyer's patches, and the spleen during homeostasis but also directs Ag-activated B cells to GC after priming with Ag.[245] BLC, a CXC chemokine expressed in lymphoid follicles, can selectively attract and activate B cells through BLR1/CXCR5.[246, 247] Three CC chemokines have also been implicated in the induction phase of B cell responses (ELC, SLC, and ABCD-1). ELC is expressed constitutively by dendritic cells of the T zones in lymph nodes and is chemotactic for T cells and activated B cells, signaling through the CCR7 receptor.[248, 249] SLC also signals through CCR7 and is expressed in high endothelial venules of lymph nodes and the T cell zones of spleen, lymph nodes, and Peyer's patches.[250, 251] SLC has a propensity for attracting resting T cells. ABCD-1, on the other hand, is produced by activated B cells and acts selectively on activated T cells.[252] These examples provide a glimpse of the molecular complexity that regulates the dynamic microenvironments of primary immune responses.

B CELL MEMORY

B cell memory is a systemic phenomenon most easily characterized by the high titer and affinity of the rapidly emerging Ab response that meets rechallenge with Ag.[253, 254] B cell memory develops in response to primary Ag challenge and can be divided broadly into four phases. The first phase involves the induction of B cell memory in the complex adaptive events that proceed in the GC reaction. The maintenance phase of B cell memory begins with the decline of this GC reaction about 3 weeks after initial priming. Third, "expression" of B cell memory refers to the typically rapid recall response that occurs on rechallenge with Ag. In the final phase, there must be some means for replenishment of the memory compartment after Ag recall. This last phase has received little attention experimentally. Retention of Ag in the immune system may be responsible for the maintenance of memory B cells.[255] This may be mediated by follicular dendritic cells present in germinal centers, which have the capacity to take up Ag in the form of immune complexes and retain it in an immunogenic form for many months.

The Memory B Cell Compartment

It is reasonable to consider all long-lived Ag-specific B cells that emerge from the GC reaction as memory B cells. According to this perspective, the phenomenon of B cell memory is regulated by a heterogeneous collection of cellular subtypes. Ig isotype expression offers one means of subdividing the memory B cell compartment. Expressing different Ig isotypes may indicate different cellular function. Similarly, localization and distinct migration patterns provide another way of subdividing the memory compartment. In the second schematic, memory B cells that preferentially circuit through particular regions (e.g., bone marrow, gut, lungs or skin) may express a unique physiology and serve different cellular functions. The last approach uses Ab secretion as the major defining characteristic. Therefore, one would consider long-lived Ab-secreting cells as belonging to the memory B cell compartment. There are also long-lived memory B cells that do not secrete Ab unless reexposed to Ag with cognate T cell help. In either case, a range of Ig isotypes could be expressed by both subtypes of memory B cells.

Long-Lived Plasma Cells

Ab production during acute infection is primarily an effector function. However, the continued production of Ag-specific Ab, often for the life of the animal, may be considered a long-term protective function. Recent studies highlight the longevity of Ag-specific plasma cells and provide a mechanism for prolonged humoral immunity that does not require cell turnover.[256, 257] Furthermore, adoptively transferred plasma cells continue to secrete Ab for extended periods in the absence of detectable Ag. The bone marrow houses the predominant long-lived plasma cell population. These bone marrow–homing plasma cells appear to be rapidly selected for high-affinity variants.[258] Furthermore, the average affinity of serum Ab continues to increase up to 120 days after primary immunization. This affinity increase continues long after the decline of the GC reaction in the spleen, indicating a phase of affinity-driven clonal competition without somatic diversification. The role of these cells in the maintenance of B cell memory and their relation to the quiescent memory B cell remain unclear.

Quiescent Memory B Cells

Typically, memory B cells are thought to be nonsecreting B cells that have affinity matured and are able to rapidly respond to secondary challenge with low doses of Ag. These cells are thought to express B220 (the B cell isoform of CD45R) and have switched Ig isotypes. There have been two studies of using CD27 expression to identify nonsecreting memory B cells in the spleen and peripheral blood of humans. The first study also uses expression of CD148 (a receptor protein tyrosine phosphatase) and marginal zone localization to identify memory B cells.[259] A large fraction of these cells express sIgM and sIgD with evidence of somatic hypermutation. The second study focused on $CD27^+IgM^+IgD^+$ cells, which comprise about 15% of peripheral blood B cell pool.[260] These cells also express somatically mutated V genes and are similar to IgM-only memory B cells that have been previously reported.[261] In human tonsils, CD38 expression increases with entry into the GC cycle. In the mouse, the opposite is true and CD38 is expressed highly on naive B cells and downregulates in the GC and on plasma cells.[262] Interestingly, expression of CD38 may increase on exit from the GC reaction and can be found on a subset of Ag-specific IgG_1 B cells late in the primary response.

CONCLUSIONS

The factors that coordinate the humoral branch of the immune response are complex, involving a programmed developmental pathway as well as regulatory interactions mediated through both cell surface and soluble receptors/factors. However, a thorough understanding of the biology of B cells will have broad applications for the treatment of agammaglobulinemias, autoimmunity, and other immunological disorders that affect this unique cell type. In addition, a molecular understanding of these cells may reveal why the majority of human leukemias and lymphomas derive from B lineage cells.

ACKNOWLEDGMENT

This work was supported by National Institutes of Health grants CA-81776 and CA-54464.

REFERENCES

1. Williams AF, Barclay AN. The immunoglobulin superfamily—domains for cell surface recognition. Annu Rev Immunol 1988; 88:381.
2. Unkeless JC, Scigliano E, Freedman V. Structure and function of human and murine receptors for IgG. Annu Rev Immunol 1988; 6:251.
3. Lawton AR, Asofsky R, Hylton MB, Cooper MD. Suppression of immunoglobulin class synthesis in mice: I. Effects of treatment with antibody to μ chain. J Exp Med 1972; 135:277.
4. Dreyer WJ, Bennett JC. The molecular basis of antibody formation. Proc Natl Acad Sci U S A 1965; 54:864.
5. Tonegawa S. Somatic generation of antibody diversity. Nature 1983; 302:575.
6. Desiderio SV, Yancopoulos GD, Paskind M, et al. Insertion of N regions into heavy-chain genes is correlated with expression of terminal deoxynucleotidyltransferase in B cells. Nature 1984; 311:752.
7. Oettinger MA, Schatz DG, Gorka C, Baltimore D. RAG-1 and RAG-2, adjacent genes that synergistically activate V(D)J recombination. Science 1990; 248:1517.
8. Schatz D, Baltimore D. Stable expression of immunoglobulin gene V(D)J recombinase activity by gene transfer into 3T3 fibroblasts. Cell 1988; 53:107.
9. Mombaerts P, Iacomini J, Johnson RS, et al. RAG-1 deficient mice have no mature B and T lymphocytes. Cell 1992; 68:869.
10. Shinkai Y, Rathbun G, Lam KP, et al. RAG-2 deficient mice lack mature lymphocytes owing to inability initiate V(D)J rearrangement. Cell 1992; 68:855.
11. Fulop GM, Phillips RA. The SCID mutation in mice causes a general defect in DNA repair. Nature 1990; 347:479.

12. Reynaud CA, Anquez V, Dahan A, Weill JC. A single rearrangement event generates most of the chicken immunoglobulin light chain diversity. Cell 1985; 40:283.
13. Kataoka T, Miyata T, Honjo T. Repetitive sequences in class switch recombination regions of immunoglobulin heavy chain genes. Cell 1981; 23:357.
14. Zheng B, Han S, Spanopoulou E, Kelsoe G. Immunoglobulin gene hypermutation in germinal centers is independent of the RAG-1 V(D)J recombinase. Immunol Rev 1998; 162:133.
15. Lansford R, Manis JP, Sonoda E, et al. Ig heavy chain class switching in Rag-deficient mice. Int Immunol 1998; 10:325.
16. Stavnezer J. Immunoglobulin class switching. Curr Opin Immunol 1996; 8:199.
17. Raff MC, Megson JJ, Cooper MD. Early production of intracellular IgM by lymphocyte precursors in mouse. Nature 1976; 259:224.
18. Maki R, Kearney J, Paige C, Tonegawa S. Immunoglobulin gene rearrangement in immature B cells. Science 1980; 209:1366.
19. Nadler LM, Korsmeyer SJ, Anderson KC, et al. B cell origin of non–T cell acute lymphoblastic leukemia: a model for discrete stages of neoplastic and normal pre–B cell differentiation. J Clin Invest 1984; 74:332.
20. Sakaguchi N, Melchers F. λ5, a new light-chain–related locus selectively expressed in pre–B lymphocytes. Nature 1986; 324:579.
21. Kudo A, Melchers F. A second gene, V_{preB} in the λ5 locus of the mouse, which appears to be selectively expressed in pre–B lymphocytes. EMBO J 1987; 6:2267.
22. Pillai S, Baltimore D. The omega and iota surrogate light chains. Curr Top Microbiol Immunol 1988; 137:136.
23. Cooper MD, Kearney JF, Gathings WE, Lawton AR. Effects of anti-Ig antibodies on the development and differentiation of B cells. Immunol Rev 1980; 52:29.
24. Lam KP, Kuhn R, Rajewsky K. In vivo ablation of surface immunoglobulin on mature B cells by inducible gene targeting results in rapid cell death. Cell 1997; 90:1073.
25. Henderson A, Calame K. Transcriptional regulation during B cell development. Annu Rev Immunol 1998; 16:163.
26. Clevers HC, Grosschedl R. Transcriptional control of lymphoid development: lessons from gene targeting. Immunol Today 1996; 17:336.
27. Korsmeyer SJ. Chromosomal translocations in lymphoid malignancies reveal novel proto-oncogenes. Annu Rev Immunol 1992; 10:785.
28. Maruyama S, Kubagawa H, Cooper MD. Activation of human B cells and inhibition of their terminal differentiation by monoclonal anti-μ antibodies. J Immunol 1985; 135:192.
29. Cooper MD, Peterson RDA, Good RA. Delineation of the thymic and bursal lymphoid systems in the chicken. Nature 1965; 205:143.
30. Cooper MD. Pre–B cells: normal and abnormal development. J Clin Immunol 1981; 1:81.
31. Solvason N, Kearney JF. The human fetal omentum: a site of B cell generation. J Exp Med 1992; 175:397.
32. Wolf ML, Buckley JA, Goldfarb A, et al. Development of a bone marrow culture for maintenance and growth of normal human B cell precursors. J Immunol 1991; 147:3324.
33. Jacobsen K, Osmond DG. Microenvironmental organization and stromal cell associations of B lymphocyte precursor cells in mouse bone marrow. Eur J Immunol 1990; 20:2395.
34. Whitlock CA, Witte ON. Long term culture of B lymphocytes and their precursors from murine bone marrow. Proc Natl Acad Sci U S A 1984; 79:3602.
35. Kincade PW, Lee G, Pietrangeli CE, et al. Cells and molecules that regulate B lymphopoiesis in bone marrow. Annu Rev Immunol 1989; 7:111.
36. Bentley SA. Close range cell:cell interaction required for stem cell maintenance in continuous bone marrow culture. Exp Hematol 1981; 9:308.
37. Lanzavecchia A. Antigen uptake and accumulation in antigen-specific B cells. Immunol Rev 1987; 99:39.
38. Rolink A, Melchers F. Molecular and cellular origins of B lymphocyte diversity. Cell 1991; 66:1081.
39. Goodnow CC. Balancing immunity and tolerance: deleting and tuning lymphocyte repertoires. Proc Natl Acad Sci U S A 1996; 93:2264.
40. Tedder TF. Response-regulators of B lymphocyte signaling thresholds provide a context for antigen receptor signal transduction. Semin Immunol 1998; 10:259.
41. O'Shea JJ, Johnston JA, Kehrl J, et al. Key molecules involved in receptor-mediated lymphocyte activation. Curr Protocols Immunol 1997:A.1J.
42. DeFranco AL. The complexity of signaling pathways activated by the BCR. Curr Opin Immunol 1997; 9:296.
43. Reth M, Wienands J. Initiation and processing of signals from the B cell antigen receptor. Annu Rev Immunol 1997; 15:453.
44. Hombach J, Lottspeich F, Reth M. Identification of the genes encoding the IgM-α components of the IgM antigen receptor complex by amino-terminal sequencing. Eur J Immunol 1990; 20:2795.
45. Sakaguchi N, Kashiwamura S, Kimoto M, et al. B lymphocyte lineage-restricted expression of mb-1, a gene with CD3-like structural properties. EMBO J 1988; 7:3457.
46. Hermanson GG, Eisenberg D, Kincade PW, Wall R. B29: a member of the immunoglobulin gene superfamily exclusively expressed on B-lineage cells. Proc Natl Acad Sci U S A 1988; 85:6890.
47. Chen J, Stall AM, Herzenberg LA, Herzenberg LA. Differences in glycoprotein complexes associated with IgM and IgD on normal murine B cells potentially enable transduction of different signals. EMBO J 1990; 9:2117.
48. Matsuo T, Kimoto M, Sakaguchi N. Direct identification of the putative surface IgM receptor–associated molecule encoded by murine B cell-specific mb-1 gene. J Immunol 1991; 146:1584.
49. van Noesel CJM, van Lier RAW, Cordell JL, et al. The membrane IgM-associated heterodimer on human B cells is a newly defined B-cell antigen that contains the protein product of the *mb-1* gene. J Immunol 1991; 146:3881.
50. Mason DY, Cordell JL, Tse AGD, et al. The IgM-associated protein mb-1 as a marker of normal and neoplastic B cells. J Immunol 1991; 147:2474.
51. Gold MR, Matsuuchi L, Kelly RB, DeFranco AL. Tyrosine phosphorylation of components of the B-cell antigen receptors following receptor crosslinking. Proc Natl Acad Sci U S A 1991; 88:3436.
52. Gold MR, Law DA, DeFranco AL. Stimulation of protein tyrosine phosphorylation by the B-lymphocyte antigen receptor. Nature 1990; 345:810.
53. Bijsterbosch MK, Meade CJ, Turner GA, Klaus GGB. B lymphocyte receptors and polyphosphoinositide degradation. Cell 1985; 41:999.
54. Lane PJL, McConnell FM, Schieven GL, et al. The role of class II molecules in human B cell activation: association with phosphatidylinositol turnover, protein tyrosine phosphorylation, and proliferation. J Immunol 1990; 144:3684.
55. Reth M. Antigen receptor tail clue. Nature 1989; 338:383.
56. Cambier JC. New nomenclature for the Reth motif (or ARH1/TAM/ARAM/YXXL). Immunol Today 1995; 16:110.
57. Yamanashi Y, Kakiuchi T, Mizuguchi J, et al. Association of B cell antigen receptor with protein tyrosine kinase Lyn. Science 1991; 251:192.
58. Dymecki SM, Niederhuber JE, Desiderio SV. Specific expression of a tyrosine kinase gene *blk,* in B lymphoid cells. Science 1989; 247:332.
59. Burkhardt AL, Brunswick M, Bolen JB, Mond JJ. Anti-immunoglobulin stimulation of B lymphocytes activates *src*-related protein-tyrosine kinases. Proc Natl Acad Sci U S A 1991; 88:7410.
60. Wienands J, Larbolette O, Reth M. Evidence for a preformed transducer complex organized by the B cell antigen receptor. Proc Natl Acad Sci U S A 1996; 93:7865.
61. Cambier JC, Ransom JT. Molecular mechanisms of transmembrane signaling in B lymphocytes. Ann Rev Immunol 1987; 5:175.
62. Trowbridge IS, Thomas ML. CD45: an emerging role as a protein tyrosine phosphatase required for lymphocyte activation and development. Annu Rev Immunol 1994; 12:85.
63. Nagai K, Takata M, Yamamura H, Kurosaki T. Tyrosine phosphorylation of Shc is mediated through Lyn and Syk in B cell receptor signaling. J Biol Chem 1995; 270:6824.
64. Tridandapani S, Kelley T, Cooney D, et al. Negative signaling in B cells: SHIP Grbs Shc. Immunol Today 1997; 18:424.
65. Scharenberg AM, Kinet J-P. The emerging field of receptor-mediated inhibitory signaling: SHP or SHIP? Cell 1996; 87:961.
66. Richards JD, Golds MR, Hourihane SL, et al. Reconstitution of B cell antigen receptor–induced signaling events in a nonlymphoid cell line by expression of the Syk protein-tyrosine kinase. J Biol Chem 1996; 271:6458.

67. Fujimoto M, Poe JC, Inaoki M, Tedder TF. CD19 regulates B lymphocyte responses to transmembrane signals. Semin Immunol 1998; 10:267.
68. Sato S, Tuscano JM, Inaoki M, Tedder TF. CD22 negatively and positively regulates signal transduction through the B lymphocyte antigen receptor. Semin Immunol 1998; 10:287.
69. Bradbury LE, Kansas GS, Levy S, et al. The CD19/CD21 signal transducing complex of human B lymphocytes includes the target of antiproliferative antibody-1 and Leu-13 molecules. J Immunol 1992; 149:2841.
70. Tedder TF, Isaacs CM. Isolation of cDNAs encoding the CD19 antigen of human and mouse B lymphocytes: a new member of the immunoglobulin superfamily. J Immunol 1989; 143:712.
71. Tedder TF, Clement LT, Cooper MD. Expression of C3d receptors during human B cell differentiation: immunofluorescence analysis with the HB-5 monoclonal antibody. J Immunol 1984; 133:678.
72. Moore MD, Cooper NR, Tack BF, Nemerow GR. Molecular cloning of the cDNA encoding the Epstein-Barr virus/C3d receptor (complement receptor type 2) of human B lymphocytes. Proc Natl Acad Sci U S A 1987; 84:9194.
73. Oren R, Takahashi S, Doss C, et al. TAPA-1, the target of an antiproliferative antibody, defines a new family of transmembrane proteins. Mol Cell Biol 1990; 10:4007.
74. Chen YX, Welte K, Gebhard DH, Evans RL. Induction of T cell aggregation by antibody to a 16-kd human leukocyte surface antigen. J Immunol 1984; 133:2496.
75. Deblandre GA, Marinx OP, Evans SS, et al. Expression cloning of an interferon-inducible 17-kDa membrane protein implicated in the control of cell growth. J Biol Chem 1995; 270:23860.
76. Tedder TF, Inaoki M, Sato S. The CD19/21 complex regulates signal transduction thresholds governing humoral immunity and autoimmunity. Immunity 1997; 6:107.
77. Carter RH, Spycher MO, Ng YC, et al. Synergistic interaction between complement receptor type 2 and membrane IgM on B lymphocytes. J Immunol 1988; 141:457.
78. Callard RE, Rigley KP, Smith SH, et al. CD19 regulation of human B cell responses: B cell proliferation and antibody secretion are inhibited or enhanced by ligation of the CD19 surface glycoprotein depending on the stimulating signal used. J Immunol 1992; 148:2983.
79. Rigley KP, Callard RE. Inhibition of B cell proliferation with CD19 monoclonal antibodies: CD19 antibodies do not interfere with early signalling events triggered by anti-IgM or IL-4. Eur J Immunol 1991; 21:535.
80. Pezzutto A, Dorken B, Rabinovitch PS, et al. CD19 monoclonal antibody HD37 inhibits anti-immunoglobulin–induced B cell activation and proliferation. J Immunol 1987; 138:2793.
81. Kansas GS, Tedder TF. Transmembrane signals generated through MHC class II, CD19, CD20, CD39, and CD40 antigens induce LFA-1–dependent and independent adhesion in human B cells through a tyrosine kinase–dependent pathway. J Immunol 1991; 147:4094.
82. Chalupny NJ, Kanner SB, Schieven GL, et al. Tyrosine phosphorylation of CD19 in pre–B and mature B cells. EMBO J 1993; 12:2691.
83. Fujimoto M, Poe JC, Jansen PJ, et al. CD19 amplifies B lymphocyte signal transduction by regulating Src-family protein tyrosine kinase activation. J Immunol 1999 (in press).
84. Engel P, Zhou L-J, Ord DC, et al. Abnormal B lymphocyte development, activation, and differentiation in mice that lack or overexpress the CD19 signal transduction molecule. Immunity 1995; 3:39.
85. Rickert RC, Rajewsky K, Roes J. Impairment of T-cell–dependent B-cell responses and B-1 cell development in CD19-deficient mice. Nature 1995; 376:352.
86. Zhou L-J, Smith HM, Waldschmidt TJ, et al. Tissue-specific expression of the human CD19 gene in transgenic mice inhibits antigen-independent B lymphocyte development. Mol Cell Biol 1994; 14:3884.
87. Sato S, Steeber DA, Tedder TF. The CD19 signal transduction molecule is a response regulator of B-lymphocyte differentiation. Proc Natl Acad Sci U S A 1995; 92:11558.
88. Sato S, Ono N, Steeber DA, et al. CD19 regulates B lymphocyte signaling thresholds critical for the development of B-1 lineage cells and autoimmunity. J Immunol 1996; 157:4371.
89. Sato S, Miller AS, Howard MC, Tedder TF. Regulation of B lymphocyte development and activation by the CD19/CD21/CD81/Leu 13 complex requires the cytoplasmic domain of CD19. J Immunol 1997; 159:3278.
90. Sato S, Steeber DA, Jansen PJ, Tedder TF. CD19 expression levels regulate B lymphocyte development: human CD19 restores normal function in mice lacking endogenous CD19. J Immunol 1997; 158:4662.
91. Hayakawa K, Hardy RR, Herzenberg LA. Peritoneal Ly-1 B cells: genetic control, autoantibody production, increased light chain expression. Eur J Immunol 1986; 16:450.
92. Khan WN, Alt FW, Gerstein RM, et al. Defective B cell development and function in Btk-deficient mice. Immunity 1995; 3:283.
93. Tarakhovsky A, Turner M, Shaal S, et al. Defective antigen receptor–mediated proliferation of B and T cells in the absence of *Vav.* Nature 1995; 374:467.
94. Zhang R, Alt FW, Davidson L, et al. Defective signalling through the T- and B-cell antigen receptors in lymphoid cells lacking the vav proto-oncogene. Nature 1995; 374:470.
95. Iida K, Nadler L, Nussenzweig V. Identification of the membrane receptor for the complement fragment C3d by means of a monoclonal antibody. J Exp Med 1983; 158:1021.
96. Fingeroth JD, Weiss JJ, Tedder TF, et al. The Epstein-Barr virus receptor of human B lymphocytes is the C3d receptor (CR2). Proc Natl Acad Sci U S A 1984; 81:4510.
97. Bohnsack JF, Cooper NR. CR2 ligands modulate human B cell activation. J Immunol 1988; 141:2569.
98. Dempsey PW, Allison MED, Akkaraju S, et al. C3d of complement as a molecular adjuvant: bridging innate and acquired immunity. Science 1996; 271:348.
99. Carroll MC. CD21/CD35 in B cell activation. Semin Immunol 1998; 10:279.
100. Heyman B, Wiersma EJ, Kinoshita T. In vivo inhibition of the antibody response to a complement receptor–specific monoclonal antibody. J Exp Med 1990; 172:665.
101. Wiersma E, Kinoshita T, Heyman B. Inhibition of immunological memory and T-independent humoral responses by monoclonal antibodies specific for murine complement receptors. Eur J Immunol 1991; 21:2501.
102. Gustavsson S, Kinoshita T, Heyman B. Antibodies to murine complement receptor 1 and 2 can inhibit the antibody response in vivo without inhibiting T helper cell induction. J Immunol 1995; 154:6524.
103. Hebell T, Ahearn JM, Fearon DT. Suppression of the immune response by a soluble complement receptor of B lymphocytes. Science 1991; 254:102.
104. Ahearn JM, Fischer MB, Croix D, et al. Disruption of the Cr2 locus results in a reduction in B-1a cells and in an impaired B cell response to T-dependent antigen. Immunity 1996; 4:251.
105. Molina H, Holers VM, Li B, et al. Markedly impaired humoral immune response in mice deficient in complement receptors 1 and 2. Proc Natl Acad Sci U S A 1996; 93:3357.
106. Papamichail M, Gutierrez C, Embling P, et al. Complement dependence of localization of aggregated IgG in germinal centers. Scand J Immunol 1975; 4:343.
107. Klaus GG, Humphrey JH. The generation of memory cells: I. The role of C3 in the generation of B memory cells. Immunology 1977; 33:31.
108. Croix DA, Ahearn JM, Rosengard AM, et al. Antibody response to a T-dependent antigen requires B cell expression of complement receptors. J Exp Med 1996; 183:1857.
109. van Noesel CJM, Lankester AC, van Lier RAW. Dual antigen recognition by B cells. Immunol Today 1993; 14:8.
110. Wilson GL, Fox CH, Fauci AS, Kehrl JH. cDNA cloning of the B cell membrane protein CD22: a mediator of B-B cell interactions. J Exp Med 1991; 173:137.
111. Tedder TF, Tuscano J, Sato S, Kehrl JH. CD22, a B lymphocyte–specific adhesion molecule that regulates antigen receptor signaling. Annu Rev Immunol 1997; 15:481.
112. Engel P, Nojima Y, Rothstein D, et al. The same epitope on CD22 of B lymphocytes mediates the adhesion of erythrocytes, T and B lymphocytes, neutrophils and monocytes. J Immunol 1993; 150:4719.
113. Kelm S, Pelz A, Schauer R, et al. Sialoadhesin, myelin-associated glycoprotein and CD22 define a new family of sialic acid–

dependent adhesion molecules of the immunoglobulin superfamily. Curr Biol 1994; 4:965.
114. Engel P, Wagner N, Miller A, Tedder TF. Identification of the ligand binding domains of CD22, a member of the immunoglobulin superfamily that uniquely binds a sialic acid–dependent ligand. J Exp Med 1995; 181:1581.
115. Dörken B, Moldenhauer G, Pezzutto A, et al. HD39 (B3), a B lineage–restricted antigen whose cell surface expression is limited to resting and activated human B lymphocytes. J Immunol 1986; 136:4470.
116. Schulte RJ, Campbell M-A, Fischer WH, Sefton BM. Tyrosine phosphorylation of CD22 during B cell activation. Science 1992; 258:1001.
117. Leprince C, Draves KE, Geahlen RL, et al. CD22 associates with the human surface IgM-B cell antigen receptor complex. Proc Natl Acad Sci U S A 1993; 90:3236.
118. Peaker CJG, Neuberger MS. Association of CD22 with the B cell antigen receptor. Eur J Immunol 1993; 23:1358.
119. Smith KGC, Tarlinton DM, Doody GM, et al. Inhibition of the B cell by CD22: a requirement for Lyn. J Exp Med 1998; 187:807.
120. Cornall RJ, Cyster JG, Hibbs ML, et al. Polygenic autoimmune traits: Lyn, CD22, and SHP-1 are limiting elements of a biochemical pathway regulating BCR signaling and selection. Immunity 1998; 8:497.
121. DeFranco AL, Chan VWF, Lowell CA. Positive and negative roles of the tyrosine kinase Lyn in B cell function. Semin Immunol 1998; 10:299.
122. Doody GM, Justement LB, Delibrias CC, et al. A role in B cell activation for CD22 and the protein tyrosine phosphatase SHP. Science 1995; 269:242.
123. Lankester AC, van Schijndel GM, van Lier RA. Hematopoietic cell phosphatase is recruited to CD22 following B cell antigen receptor ligation. J Biol Chem 1995; 270:20305.
124. Campbell MA, Klinman NR. Phosphotyrosine-dependent association between CD22 and protein tyrosine phosphatase 1C. Eur J Immunol 1995; 25:1573.
125. Law C-L, Sidorenko SP, Chandran KA, et al. CD22 associates with protein tyrosine phosphatase 1C, Syk, and phospholipase C-γ1 upon B cell activation. J Exp Med 1996; 183:547.
126. Blasiolo J, Paust S, Thomas ML. Definition of the sites of interaction between the protein tyrosine phosphatase SHP-1 and CD22. J Biol Chem 1999; 274:2303.
127. Sato S, Miller AS, Inaoki M, et al. CD22 is both a positive and negative regulator of B lymphocyte antigen receptor signal transduction: altered signaling in CD22-deficient mice. Immunity 1996; 5:551.
128. Otipoby KL, Andersson KB, Draves KE, et al. CD22 regulates thymus-independent responses and the lifespan of B cells. Nature 1996; 384:634.
129. O'Keefe TL, Williams GT, Davies SL, Neuberger MS. Hyperresponsive B cells in CD22-deficient mice. Science 1996; 274:798.
130. Nitschke L, Carsetti R, Ocker B, et al. CD22 is a negative regulator of B-cell receptor signalling. Curr Biol 1997; 7:133.
131. Tuscano J, Engel P, Tedder TF, Kehrl JH. Engagement of the adhesion receptor CD22 triggers a potent stimulatory signal for B cells and blocking CD22/CD22L interactions impairs T-cell proliferation. Blood 1996; 87:4723.
132. Tuscano JM, Engel P, Tedder TF, et al. Involvement of p72syk kinase, p53/56lyn kinase and phosphatidylinositol-3 kinase in signal transduction via the human B lymphocyte antigen CD22. Eur J Immunol 1996; 26:1246.
133. Fujimoto M, Bradney AP, Poe JC, et al. CD22 functions downstream of CD19 regulation during B lymphocyte activation. (Submitted for publication.)
134. Hardy RR, Carmack CE, Li YS, Hayakawa K. Distinctive developmental origins and specificities of murine CD5$^+$ B cells. Immunol Rev 1994; 137:91.
135. Haughton G, Arnold LW, Whitmore AC, Clarke SH. B-1 cells are made, not born. Immunol Today 1993; 14:84.
136. Freedman AS, Freeman G, Whitman J, et al. Expression and regulation of CD5 on in vitro activated human B cells. Eur J Immunol 1989; 19:849.
137. Casali P, Burastero SE, Nakamura M, et al. Human lymphocytes making rheumatoid factor and antibody to ssDNA belong to Leu-1$^+$ B-cell subset. Science 1987; 236:77.
138. Hardy RR, Hayakawa K, Shimizu M, et al. Rheumatoid factor secretion from human Leu-1 B cells. Science 1987; 236:81.
139. Pospisil R, Mage RG. CD5 and other superantigens as "ticklers" of the B-cell receptor. Immunol Today 1998; 19:106.
140. LeBien TW, McCormack RT. The common acute lymphoblastic leukemia antigen (CD10)$^-$: emancipation from a functional enigma. Blood 1989; 73:625.
141. LeTarte M, Vera S, Tran R, et al. Common acute lymphoblastic leukemia antigen is identical to neutral endopeptidase. J Exp Med 1988; 168:1247.
142. Stashenko P, Nadler LM, Hardy R, Schlossman SF. Characterization of a human B lymphocyte–specific antigen. J Immunol 1980; 125:1678.
143. Tedder TF, Streuli M, Schlossman SF, Saito H. Isolation and structure of a cDNA encoding the B1 (CD20) cell-surface antigen of human B lymphocytes. Proc Natl Acad Sci U S A 1988; 85:208.
144. Hupp K, Siwarski D, Mock BA, Kinet J-P. Gene mapping of the three subunits of the high affinity FcR for IgE to mouse chromosomes 1 and 19. J Immunol 1989; 143:3787.
145. Tedder TF, Boyd AW, Freedman AS, et al. The B cell surface molecule B1 is functionally linked with B cell activation and differentiation. J Immunol 1985; 135:973.
146. Clark EA, Shu G, Ledbetter JA. Role of the Bp35 cell surface polypeptide in human B-cell activation. Proc Natl Acad Sci U S A 1985; 82:1766.
147. Ord DC, Elelhoff S, Dushkin H, et al. CD19 maps to a region of conservation between human chromosome 16 and mouse chromosome 7. Immunogenetics 1994; 39:322.
148. Shan D, Ledbetter JA, Press OW. Apoptosis of malignant human B cells by ligation of CD20 with monoclonal antibodies. Blood 1998; 91:1644.
149. Demidem A, Lam T, Alas S, et al. Chimeric anti-CD20 antibody (IDEC-C2B8) monoclonal antibody sensitizes a B cell lymphoma cell line to cell killing by cytotoxic drugs. Cancer Biother Radiopharmaceuticals 1997; 12:177.
150. Press OW, Eary JF, Appelbaum FR, et al. Radio-labeled antibody therapy of B-cell lymphoma with autologous bone marrow support. N Engl J Med 1993; 329:1219.
151. Press OW, Eary JF, Appelbaum FR, et al. Phase II trial of 131-1-B1 (anti-CD20) antibody therapy with autologous stem cell transplantation for relapsed B cell lymphomas. Lancet 1995; 346:336.
152. Kaminski MS, Zasadny KR, Francis IR, et al. Radioimmunotherapy of B-cell lymphoma with [^{131}I]anti-B1 (anti-CD20) antibody. N Engl J Med 1993; 329:459.
153. Kaminski MS, Zasadny KR, Francis IR, et al. Iodine-131-anti-B1 radioimmunotherapy for B-cell lymphoma. J Clin Oncol 1996; 14:1974.
154. Maloney DG, Grillo-Lopez AJ, White CA, et al. IDEC-C2B8 (Rituximab) anti-CD20 monoclonal antibody therapy in patients with relapsed low-grade non-Hodgkin's lymphoma. Blood 1997; 90:2188.
155. Reff ME, Carner K, Chambers KS, et al. Depletion of B cells in vivo by a chimeric mouse human monoclonal antibody to CD20. Blood 1994; 83:435.
156. Press OW, Appelbaum F, Ledbetter JA, et al. Monoclonal antibody 1F5 (anti-CD20) serotherapy of human B cell lymphomas. Blood 1987; 69:584.
157. Buchsbaum DJ, Wahl RL, Normolle DP, Kaminski MS. Therapy with unlabeled and 131-I–labeled pan–B-cell monoclonal antibodies in nude mice bearing Raji Burkitt's lymphoma xenografts. Cancer Res 1992; 52:6476.
158. Tedder TF, Engel P. CD20: a regulator of cell-cycle progression of B lymphocytes. Immunol Today 1994; 15:450.
159. Gordon J, Flores-Romo L, Cairns JA, et al. CD23: a multi-functional receptor/lymphokine? Immunol Today 1989; 10:153.
160. Kikutani H, Inui S, Sato R, et al. Molecular structure of human lymphocyte receptor for immunoglobulin E. Cell 1986; 47:657.
161. Yokota A, Kikutani H, Tanaka T, et al. Two species of human Fc epsilon receptor II (Fc epsilon RII/CD23): tissue-specific and IL-4-specific regulation of gene expression. Cell 1988; 55:611.
162. Abramson CS, Kersey JH, LeBien TW. A monoclonal antibody (BA-1) reactive with cells of human B lymphocyte lineage. J Immunol 1981; 126:83.
163. Stefanova I, Horejsi V, Ansotegui IJ, et al. GPI-anchored cell-surface molecules complexed to protein tyrosine kinases. Science 1991; 254:1016.

164. Kay R, Rosten PM, Humphries RK. CD24, a signal transducer modulating B cell activation responses, is a very short peptide with a glycosyl phosphatidylinositol membrane anchor. J Immunol 1991; 147:1412.
165. Gordon J, Millsum MJ, Guy GR, Ledbetter JA. Resting B lymphocytes can be triggered directly through the CDw40 (Bp50) antigen. J Immunol 1988; 140:1425.
166. Banchereau J, Rousset F. Growing human B lymphocytes in the CD40 system. Nature 1991; 353:678.
167. Liu Y-J, Hoshua DE, Willimas GT, et al. Mechanism of antigen-driven selection in germinal centres. Nature 1989; 342:929.
168. Stamenkovic I, Clark EA, Seed B. A B-lymphocyte activation molecule related to the nerve growth factor receptor and induced by cytokines in carcinomas. EMBO J 1989; 8:1403.
169. Armitage RJ, Fanslow WC, Strockbine L, et al. Molecular and biological characterization of a murine ligand for CD40. Nature 1992; 357:80.
170. Korthauer U, Graf D, Mages HW, et al. Defective expression of T-cell CD40 ligand causes X-linked immunodeficiency with hyper-IgM. Nature 1993; 361:539.
171. Allen RC, Armitage RJ, Conley ME, et al. CD40 ligand gene defects responsible for X-linked hyper-IgM syndrome. Science 1993; 259:990.
172. DiSanto JP, Bonnefoy JY, Gauchat JF, et al. CD40 ligand mutations in X-linked immunodeficiency with hyper-IgM. Nature 1993; 361:541.
173. Kawabe T, Naka T, Yoshida K, et al. The immune responses in the CD40-deficient mice: impaired immunoglobulin class switching and germinal center formation. Immunity 1994; 1:167.
174. Xu J, Foy TM, Laman JD, et al. Mice deficient for the CD40 ligand. Immunity 1994; 1:423.
175. Craxton A, Shu G, Graves JD, et al. p38 MAPK is required for CD40-induced gene expression and proliferation in B lymphocytes. J Immunol 1998; 161:3225.
176. von Hoegen I, Nakayama E, Parnes JR. Identification of a human protein homologous to the mouse Lyb-2 B cell differentiation antigen and sequence of the corresponding cDNA. J Immunol 1990; 144:4870.
177. Subbarao B, Mosier DE. Activation of B lymphocytes by monovalent anti-Lyb-2 antibodies. J Exp Med 1984; 159:1796.
178. Subbarao B, Mosier DE. Lyb antigens and their role in B lymphocyte activation. Immunol Rev 1982; 69:81.
179. Yakura H, Kawabata I, Ashida T, et al. A role for Lyb-2 in B cell activation mediated by a B cell stimulatory factor. J Immunol 1986; 137:1475.
180. Kamal M, Katira A, Gordon J. Stimulation of B lymphocytes via CD72 (human Lyb-2). Eur J Immunol 1991; 21:1419.
181. Muthusamy N, Baluyut AR, Subbarao B. Differential regulation of surface Ig- and Lyb-2-mediated B cell activation by cyclic AMP: I. Evidence for alternative regulation of signaling through two different receptors linked to phosphatidylinositol hydrolysis in murine B cells. J Immuno 1991; 147:2483.
182. Nomura T, Han H, Howard MC, et al. Antigen receptor–mediated B cell death is blocked by signaling via CD72 or treatment with dextran sulfate and is defective in autoimmunity-prone mice. Int Immunol 1996; 8:867.
183. Snow EC, Mond JJ, Subbarao B. Enhancement by monoclonal anti-Lyb2 antibody of antigen-specific B lymphocyte expansion stimulated by TNP-Ficoll and T lymphocyte–derived factors. J Immunol 1986; 137:1793.
184. Adachi T, Flaswinkel H, Yakura H, et al. The B cell surface protein CD72 recruits the tyrosine phosphatase SHP1 upon tyrosine phosphorylation. J Immunol 1998; 160:4662.
185. Wu Y, Nadler MJS, Brennan LA, et al. The B-cell transmembrane protein CD72 binds to and is an in vivo substrate of the protein tyrosine phosphatase SHP-1. Curr Biol 1998; 8:1009.
186. Freedman AS, Freeman G, Horowitz JC, et al. B7, a B cell-restricted antigen that identifies preactivated B cells. J Immunol 1987; 139:3260.
187. Koulova L, Clark EA, Shu G, Dupont B. The CD28 ligand B7/BB1 provides a costimulatory signal for alloactivation of CD4+ T cells. J Exp Med 1991; 173:759.
188. Sansom DM, Hall ND. B7/BB1, the ligand for CD28, is expressed on repeatedly activated human T cells in vitro. Eur J Immunol 1993; 23:295.
189. Freedman AS, Freeman GJ, Rhynhart K, Nadler LM. Selective induction of B7/BB-1 on interferon-γ stimulated monocytes: a potential mechanism for amplification of T cell activation through the CD28 pathway. Cell Immunol 1991; 137:429.
190. Young JW, Koulova L, Soergei SA, et al. The B7/BB1 antigen provides one of several costimulatory signals for the activation of CD4+ T lymphocytes by human blood dendritic cells in vitro. J Clin Invest 1992; 90:229.
191. Hart DNJ, Starling GC, Calder VL, Fernando NS. B7/BB1 is a leukocyte differentiation antigen on human dendritic cells induced by activation. Immunology 1993; 79:616.
192. Valle A, Yssel GH, Bonnefoy J-Y, et al. mAb 104, a new monoclonal antibody, recognizes the B7 antigen that is expressed on activated B cells and HTLV-1-transformed T cells. Immunol 1990; 69:531.
193. Freeman GJ, Freedman AS, Segil JM, et al. B7, a new member of the Ig superfamily with unique expression on activated and neoplastic B cells. J Immunol 1989; 143:2714.
194. Freeman GJ, Gray GS, Gimmi CD, et al. Structure, expression, and T cell costimulatory activity of the murine homologue of the human B lymphocyte activation antigen B7. J Exp Med 1991; 174:625.
195. Reiser H, Freeman GJ, Razi-Wolf Z, et al. Murine B7 antigen provides an efficient costimulatory signal for activation of murine T lymphocytes via the T-cell receptor/CD3 complex. Proc Natl Acad Sci U S A 1992; 89:271.
196. Hathcock KS, Laszlo G, Dickler HB, et al. Identification of an alternative CTLA-4 ligand costimulatory for T cell activation. Science 1993; 262:905.
197. Linsley PS, Clark EA, Ledbetter JA. T-cell antigen CD28 mediates adhesion with B cells by interacting with activation antigen B7/BB-1. Proc Natl Acad Sci U S A 1990; 87:5031.
198. Linsley PS, Brady W, Urnes M, et al. CTLA-4 is a second receptor for the B cell activation antigen B7. J Exp Med 1991; 174:561.
199. Hathcock KS, Hodes RJ. Role of the CD28-B7 costimulatory pathways in T cell–dependent B cell responses. Adv Immunol 1996; 62:131.
200. Schwartz RH. Costimulation of T lymphocytes: the role of CD28, CTLA-4, and B7/BB1 in interleukin-2 production and immunotherapy. Cell 1992; 71:1065.
201. Damle NK, Linsley PS, Ledbetter JA. Direct helper T cell–induced B cell differentiation involves interaction between T cell antigen CD28 and B cell activation antigen B7. Eur J Immunol 1991; 21:1277.
202. Freeman GJ, Borriello F, Hodes RJ, et al. Uncovering of functional alternative CTLA-4 counter-receptor in B7-deficient mice. Science 1993; 262:907.
203. Engel P, Gribben JG, Freeman GG, et al. The B7-2 (B70) costimulatory molecule expressed by monocytes and activated B lymphocytes is the CD86 differentiation antigen. Blood 1994; 84:1402.
204. Nozawa Y, Wachi E, Tominaga K, et al. A novel monoclonal antibody (FUN-1) identifies an activation antigen in cells of the B-cell lineage and Reed-Sternberg cells. J Pathol 1993; 169:309.
205. Boussiotis VA, Freeman GJ, Gribben JG, et al. Activated human B lymphocytes express three CTLA4 counter-receptors which costimulate T cell activation. Proc Natl Acad Sci U S A 1993; 90:11059.
206. Engel P, Wagner N, Zhou L-J, Tedder TF. CD86 Workshop report. *In* Schlossman SF, Boumsell L, Gilks W, et al. (eds): Leukocyte Typing V, vol 1. Oxford, UK: Oxford University Press, 1994, pp 703–705.
207. Freeman GJ, Gribben JG, Boussiotis VA, et al. Cloning of B7-2: a CTLA-4 counter-receptor that costimulates human T cell proliferation. Science 1993; 262:909.
208. Hofman FM, Brock M, Taylor CR, Lyons B. IL-4 regulated differentiation and proliferation of human precursor B cells. J Immunol 1988; 141:1185.
209. Miyajima A, Miyatake S, Schreurs J, et al. Coordinate regulation of immune and inflammatory responses by T cell–derived lymphokines. FASEB J 1988; 2:2462.
210. Banchereau J, Rousset F. Functions of interleukin-4 on human B lymphocytes. Immunol Res 1991; 10:423.
211. Boyd AW, Tedder TF, Griffin JD, et al. Pre-exposure of resting B cells to interferon-gamma enhances their proliferative response to subsequent activation signals. Cell Immunol 1987; 106:355.
212. Freedman AS, Freeman G, Whitman J, et al. Pre-exposure of

human B cells to recombinant IL-1 enhances subsequent proliferation. J Immunol 1988; 141:3398.
213. Rousset F, Garcia E, Defrance T, et al. Interleukin 10 is a potent growth and differentiation factor for activated human B lymphocytes. Proc Natl Acad Sci U S A 1992; 89:1890.
214. Akira S, Hirano T, Taga T, Kishimoto T. Biology of multifunctional cytokines: IL 6 and related molecules (IL 1 and TNF). FASEB J 1990; 4:2860.
215. Springer TA. Traffic signals on endothelium for lymphocyte recirculation and leukocyte emigration. Annu Rev Physiol 1995; 57:827.
216. Tedder TF, Schmidt R, Rudd CE, et al. Function of the LFA-1 and T4 molecules in the direct activation of resting human B lymphocytes by T lymphocytes. Eur J Immunol 1986; 16:1539.
217. Fischer A, Durandy A, Sterkers G, Griscelli C. Role of the LFA-1 molecule in cellular interactions required for antibody production in humans. J Immunol 1986; 136:3198.
218. MacLennan ICM, Gray D. Antigen-driven selection of virgin and memory B cells. Immunol Rev 1986; 91:61.
219. Jacob R, Kassir R, Kelsoe G. In situ studies of the primary immune response to (4-hydroxy-3-nitrophenyl)acetyl: I. The architecture and dynamics of responding cell populations. J Exp Med 1991; 173:1165.
220. Ho F, Lortan JE, MacLennan IC, Khan M. Distinct short-lived and long-lived antibody-producing cell populations. Eur J Immunol 1986; 16:1297.
221. MacLennan ICM, Liu YJ, Oldfield S, et al. The evolution of B-cell clones. Curr Top Microbiol Immunol 1990; 159:37.
222. Jacob J, Kelsoe G. In situ studies of the primary immune response to (4-hydroxy-3-nitrophenyl)acetyl: II. A common clonal origin for periarteriolar lymphoid sheath–associated foci and germinal centers. J Exp Med 1992; 176:679.
223. Jacob J, Przylepa J, Miller C, Kelsoe G. In situ studies of the primary immune response to (4-hydroxy-3-nitrophenyl)acetyl: III. The kinetics of V-region mutation and selection in germinal center B cells. J Exp Med 1993; 178:1293.
224. Sanderson RD, Lalor P, Bernfield M. B lymphocytes express and lose syndecan at specific stages of differentiation. Cell Reg 1989; 1:27.
225. Lalor PA, Nossal GJV, Sanderson RD, McHeyzer-Williams MG. Functional and molecular characterization of single, (4-hydroxy-3-nitropheny)acetyl (NP)-specific, $I_8G_1^+$ B cells from antibody-secreting and memory B cell pathways in the C57BL/6 immune response to NP. Eur J Immunol 1992; 22:3001.
226. McHeyzer-Williams MG, McLean MJ, Lalor PA, Nossal GJV. Antigen-driven B cell differentiation in vivo. J Exp Med 1993; 178:295.
227. Smith KG, Hewitson TD, Nossal GJV, Tarlinton DM. The phenotype and fate of the antibody-forming cells of the splenic foci. Eur J Immunol 1996; 26:444.
228. Jacob J, Kelsoe G, Rajewsky K, Weiss U. Intraclonal generation of antibody mutants in germinal centres. Nature 1991; 354:389.
229. Coico RF, Bhogal BS, Thorbecke GJ. Relationship of germinal centers in lymphoid tissue to immunologic memory: VI. Transfer of B cell memory with lymph node cells fractionated according to their receptors for peanut agglutinin. J Immunol 1983; 131:2254.
230. Rajewsky K. Clonal selection and learning in the antibody system. Nature 1996; 381:751.
231. Berek C, Berger A, Apel M. Maturation of the immune response in germinal centers. Cell 1991; 67:1121.
232. Ziegner M, Steinhauser G, Berek C. Development of antibody diversity in single germinal centers: selective expansion of high-affinity variants. Eur J Immunol 1994; 24:2393.
233. Liu YJ, Zhang J, Lane PJ, et al. Sites of specific B cell activation in primary and secondary responses to T cell–dependent and T cell–independent antigens. Eur J Immunol 1991; 21:2951.
234. Betz AG, Rada C, Pannell R, et al. Passenger transgenes reveal intrinsic specificity of the antibody hypermutation mechanism: clustering, polarity, and specific hot spots. Proc Natl Acad Sci U S A 1993; 90:2385.
235. Yelamos J, Klix N, Goyenechea B, et al. Targeting of non-Ig sequences in place of the V segment by somatic hypermutation. Nature 1995; 376:225.
236. Shokat KM, Goodnow CC. Antigen-induced B-cell death and elimination during germinal-centre immune responses. Nature 1995; 375:334.
237. Pulendran B, Kannourakis G, Nouri S, et al. Soluble antigen can cause enhanced apoptosis of germinal-centre B cells. Nature 1995; 375:331.
238. Han S, Zheng B, Dal Porto J, Kelsoe G. In situ studies of the primary immune response to (4-hydroxy-3-nitrophenyl)acetyl: IV. Affinity-dependent, antigen-driven B cell apoptosis in germinal centers as a mechanism for maintaining self-tolerance. J Exp Med 1995; 182:1635.
239. Martinez-Valdez H, Guret C, de Bouteiller O, et al. Human germinal center B cells express the apoptosis-inducing genes *Fas, c-myc, P53,* and *Bax* but not the survival gene *bcl-2.* J Exp Med 1996; 183:971.
240. Pascual V, Liu YJ, Magalski A, et al. Analysis of somatic mutation in five B cell subsets of human tonsil. J Exp Med 1994; 180:329.
241. Liu YJ, Malisan F, de Bouteiller O, et al. Within germinal centers, isotype switching of immunoglobulin genes occurs after the onset of somatic mutation. Immunity 1996; 4:241.
242. Kelsoe G. V(D)J hypermutation and receptor revision: coloring outside the lines. 1999 (in press).
243. Han S, Dillon SR, Zheng B, et al. V(D)J recombinase activity in a subset of germinal center B lymphocytes. Science 1997; 278:301.
244. Papavasiliou F, Casellas R, Suh H, et al. V(D)J recombination in mature B cells: a mechanism for altering antibody responses. Science 1997; 278:298.
245. Forster R, Mattis AE, Kremmer E, et al. A putative chemokine receptor, BLR1, directs B cell migration to defined lymphoid organs and specific anatomic compartments of the spleen. Cell 1996; 87:1037.
246. Gunn MD, Ngo VN, Ansel KM, et al. A B-cell-homing chemokine made in lymphoid follicles activates Burkitt's lymphoma receptor-1. Nature 1998; 391:799.
247. Legler DF, Loetscher M, Roos RS, et al. B cell–attracting chemokine 1, a human CXC chemokine expressed in lymphoid tissues, selectively attracts B lymphocytes via BLR1/CXCR5. J Exp Med 1998; 187:655.
248. Ngo VN, Tang HL, Cyster JG. Epstein-Barr virus-induced molecule 1 ligand chemokine is expressed by dendritic cells in lymphoid tissues and strongly attracts naive T cells and activated B cells. J Exp Med 1998; 188:181.
249. Yoshida R, Nagira M, Imai T, et al. EBII-ligand chemokine (ELC) attracts a broad spectrum of lymphocytes: activated T cells strongly up-regulate CCR7 and efficiently migrate toward ELC. Int Immunol 1998; 10:901.
250. Gunn MD, Tangemann K, Tam C, et al. A chemokine expressed in lymphoid high endothelial venules promotes the adhesion and chemotaxis of naive T lymphocytes. Proc Natl Acad Sci U S A 1998; 95:258.
251. Willimann K, Legler DF, Loetscher M, et al. The chemokine SLC is expressed in T cell areas of lymph nodes and mucosal lymphoid tissues and attracts activated T cells via CCR7. Eur J Immunol 1998; 28:2025.
252. Schaniel C, Pardali E, Sallusto F, et al. Activated murine B lymphocytes and dendritic cells produce a novel CC chemokine which acts selectively on activated T cells. J Exp Med 1998; 188:451.
253. Ahmed R, Gray D. Immunological memory and protective immunity: understanding their relation. Science 1996; 272:54.
254. Przylepa J, Himes C, Kelsoe G. Lymphocyte development and selection in germinal centers. Curr Top Microbiol Immunol 1998; 229:85.
255. Gray D. B cell memory is short lived in the absence of antigen. Nature 1988; 336:70.
256. Slifka MK, Ahmed R. Long-lived plasma cells: a mechanism for maintaining persistent antibody production. Curr Opin Immunol 1998; 10:252.
257. Slifka MK, Antia R, Whitmire JK, Ahmed R. Humoral immunity due to long-lived plasma cells. Immunity 1998; 8:363.
258. Smith KG, Light A, Nossal GJV, Tarlinton DM. The extent of affinity maturation differs between the memory and antibody-forming compartments in the primary immune response. EMBO J 1997; 16:2996.
259. Tangye SG, Liu YJ, Aversa G, et al. Identification of functional human splenic memory B cells by expression of CD148 and CD27. J Exp Med 1988; 188:1691.
260. Klein U, Rajewsky K, Kuppers R. Human immunoglobulin (Ig)M^+ IgD^+ peripheral blood B cells expressing the CD27 cell surface antigen carry somatically mutated variable region genes: CD27 as

a general marker for somatically mutated (memory) B cells. J Exp Med 1998; 188:1679.
261. Klein U, Kuppers R, Rajewsky K. Evidence for a large compartment of IgM-expressing memory B cells in humans. Blood 1997; 89:1288.
262. Ridderstad A, Tarlinton DM. Kinetics of establishing the memory B cell population as revealed by CD38 expression. J Immunol 1998; 160:4688.
263. Gathings WE, Lawton AR, Cooper MD. Immunofluorescent studies of the development of pre-B cells, B lymphocytes and immunoglobulin isotype diversity in humans. Eur J Immunol 1977; 7:804.

CHAPTER 7
Complement

Dana V. Devine

The existence of the complement system has great impact on the practice of transfusion medicine. In its normal immune activities, complement functions to kill pathogens, mediate inflammation, maintain the solubility of immune complexes, and opsonize particles for phagocytosis. However, complement can also mediate pathogenic processes, including anaphylaxis, intravascular hemolysis of transfused blood cells, and activation of platelets.

The group of proteins known to constitute the complement system was first recognized in the 1880s as the labile bactericidal activity in serum.[1] Paul Ehrlich coined the term for the phenomenon by proposing a model of antibody-mediated cytotoxicity in which a serum factor "complements" the bactericidal activity of antibody. A detailed understanding of the biochemistry of the complement system required the development of techniques that would permit the isolation of individual complement proteins; this technology finally appeared in the 1960s. With the explosion of research activity in the complement field in the 1970s came the recognition that this system was much more complex than had been imagined. This complexity is amply demonstrated by the fact that at least 25 complement proteins are involved in the activation and regulation of that activity known to Ehrlich simply as "complement."

The understanding of the complement system is made easier by setting a proper context. Like coagulation, the complement system is an activated enzyme cascade. In such cascades, proteins normally circulate in an inactive form, the zymogen. When the pathway is initiated, the first protein in the sequence is converted from a zymogen to an activated enzyme, which acts on the next protein zymogen in the cascade. Such pathways are amplifying, because each enzyme molecule generated can act on multiple substrate molecules. Activated enzyme pathways are also characterized by the presence of regulatory proteins, both humoral and cellular, that prevent the activated enzymes from converting all available substrate.

The nuances of the complement system have long struck fear into the hearts of basic scientist and clinician alike. Clinical aspects of complement biology in the pathophysiology of disease have been reviewed by Morgan.[2] This chapter describes the central role of complement in many physiological processes, including those associated with the use of blood components.

Table 7–1. Activators of the Classical Pathway

IgG_1 and IgG_3; IgG_2 weakly
IgM
C-reactive protein
Mannose-binding lectin
Some negatively charged surfaces
Crystalline cholesterol

Ig, immunoglobulin.

BASIC BIOCHEMISTRY OF THE COMPLEMENT SYSTEM

Classical Pathway Activation

Activation of the complement system occurs via two pathways; with the activation of C3 (the third component of complement), these pathways join to form a common pathway that completes the cascade (Fig. 7–1). The primary function of both pathways is the generation of enzyme complexes that activate C3 by cleaving it to C3b. The antibody-mediated activation of complement occurs by the *classical pathway,* so called because it was the first pathway recognized. Activators of the classical pathway include not only antibody molecules but also several non-immunoglobulin proteins (Table 7–1). Only immunoglobulins (Igs) of the M and G isotypes activate complement by the classical pathway. In humans, immunoglobulins G_3 and G_1 are strong complement activators, but IgG_2 is a poor activator, and IgG_4 does not activate complement. These differences result from variation in the ability of the different IgG subclasses to bind the first component of complement, C1. The ability of an antibody to activate complement with the accompanying opsonization and perhaps lysis of the cell parallels the opsonic potential of the IgGs themselves. The varying risk of phagocytic destruction by crystallizable fragment (Fc) receptor–mediated recognition of IgG is an important feature in distinguishing clinically significant antibodies from those with less destructive potential.

C1 is a multisubunit complex that contains the initial antibody-binding subunits, C1q, as well as two types of zymogen subunits, C1r and C1s, that acquire serine protease activity upon activation of the complex. Each molecule of C1 contains six C1q subunits, and two each of the C1r and C1s subunits. The fixation of a C1 molecule to the surface of the cell by the C1q subunits requires a minimum of one molecule of IgM or at least two molecules of IgG for efficient activation. C1q itself contains six identical subunits composed of a triple helical region with homology to collagen and a globular domain at the

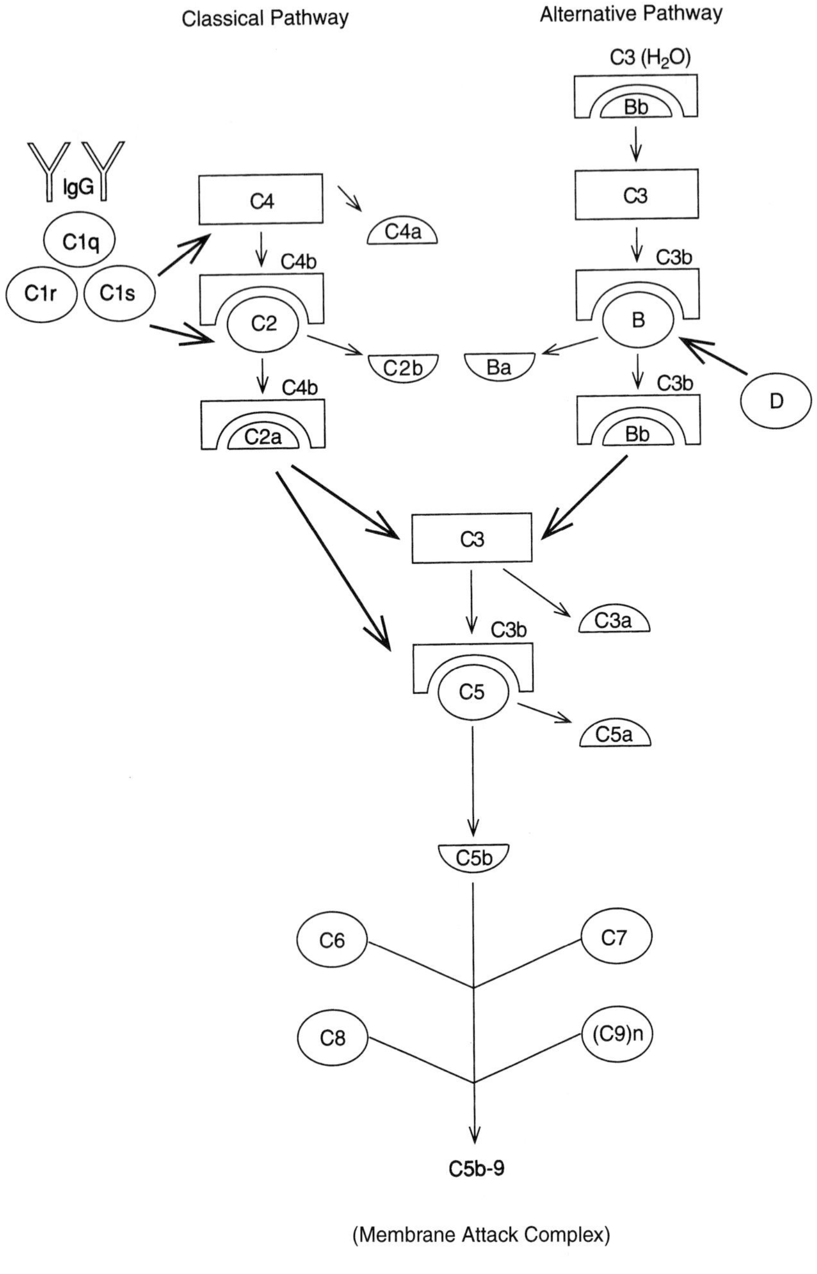

Figure 7–1. The activation pathway of complement. The activation of complement may proceed by the classical pathway or the alternative pathway. Inactive (zymogen) forms of complement proteins are cleaved by activated proteins that have serine protease activity *(heavy arrows)*. Once cleaved, a substrate acquires enzymic activity and acts on the next substrate in the pathway. The membrane attack complex forms by the assembly of the individual components in an enzyme-independent manner.

distal end. The proximal end of C1q is associated with the other subunits of the C1 complex, C1r and C1s, in a calcium-dependent manner. Two of the six C1q subunits must be bound by antibody to effect activation. Although a single molecule of IgM is capable of activating complement, it must be bound to antigen, where it assumes a staple-shaped conformation. Fluid-phase or planar IgM does not activate complement, inasmuch as the C1q-binding sites are exposed only in the staple form.[3]

Once two subunits of C1q are bound to antibody, the molecular conformation changes, in that the angle between the subunits is greatly reduced; the resulting stress on the molecule facilitates the autocatalysis of the C1r subunits.[4] Upon autoactivation, C1r acquires serine protease activity, which is directed against the C1s subunits. Once C1s is cleaved by activated C1r, it also acquires serine protease activity. This activated C1 complex is the initiation complex of the classical pathway.

Although the majority of classical pathway activation is antibody mediated, antibody-independent activation of the classical pathway has been described in several situations (see Table 7–1). Such activation may involve the direct binding of C1q to a surface, or it may be mediated by other plasma proteins, such as C-reactive protein or mannose-binding protein. Activated C1s has the next two proteins in the pathway, C4 and C2, as its substrates. The C4 molecule is cleaved by C1s to C4a and C4b. Some of the C4b molecules bind covalently to the cell surface through a reactive thiolester bond that is exposed when the C4a fragment is removed; most C4b molecules are inactivated by hydrolysis and never bind to a cell surface. In a magnesium-dependent reaction, a C2 molecule binds to a molecule of C4b; the C2 is then also cleaved by C1s. This cleavage results in the generation of the active serine protease, C2a, which remains associated with C4b. Clearly, the cleavage of both C4 and C2 by the same molecule of C1s is sensitive to the local geometry; deposition of the C4b molecule far from the activated C1 molecule results in the termination of the activation pathway.

The bimolecular complex, C4b2a, is the C3-converting complex of the classical pathway. The cleavage of C3 by C4b2a results in the formation of two fragments, C3a and C3b. C3b, like C4b, contains a reactive thiolester bond that enables it to bind covalently to the cell surface. The intramolecular thiolester present within C3 is formed by a transacylation reaction between the thiol group of Cys^{988} and the gamma amide group of Gln^{991}.[5] The exposure of this reactive center results in the interaction with cell surface moieties through the formation of an ester or an amide bond.

As indicated earlier, the activation of the classical pathway does not require immunoglobulin. The most recent developments in complement biochemistry have included an appreciation for the role of molecules of the pentraxin and lectin families in the activation of complement. Pentraxins, a family of molecules named for their cyclic pentameric subunit structure, include two proteins that have been implicated in complement activation: C-reactive protein (CRP) and serum amyloid P.[6–8] Both proteins bind C1q, thereby initiating the classical pathway without a requirement for antibody.

The carbohydrate-binding properties of plant-derived lectins are well known in the field of blood banking, in which they are useful phenotyping reagents. Lectins are also found in mammals. One of the C-type animal lectins, mannose-binding lectin (MBL), has been reported to mediate complement activation.[9] The hexameric form of MBL is structurally similar to C1q and will bind the $C1r_2s_2$ complex. MBL is found complexed to a serine protease, MBL-associated protease (MASP). Complement activation may be mediated by either $C1r_2s_2$ or perhaps by the direct action of MASP. Although the relative biological significance of the pentraxin and lectin pathways is not fully understood, both CRP and MBL are acute-phase reactants and may reach significant serum concentration during infection or inflammation.

Alternative Pathway Activation

A different C3-converting complex is generated by the activation of the *alternative pathway of complement.* The term *alternative* arises from the fact that this mechanism of C3 cleavage was discovered many decades after the classical pathway. It should in no way be considered a secondary pathway of complement activation, because it is the only pathway of complement that can respond to microorganisms in the absence of specific antibody. It is, therefore, a front-line host defense. Activators of the alternative pathway include a broad spectrum of substances, from renal dialysis membranes to immune complexes to microorganisms (Table 7–2). The initial step in the activation of the alternative pathway is the generation

Table 7–2. Activators of the Alternative Pathway

Some dialysis membranes, especially cuprophane
Desialated erythrocytes
Surfaces that promote the binding of factor B
IgA complexes
Protein aggregates
Microbial pathogens
Tumor cells

IgA, immunoglobulin A.

of a partially activated molecule of C3, which has been described as "C3b-like."[10] This molecule is presumably generated by the low-grade, spontaneous hydrolysis of C3 that occurs in the body and is not the result of the presence of the activator substance per se. $C3(H_2O)$ has the important characteristic of being able to interact in the fluid phase with the complement protein factor B in a magnesium-dependent manner. Once factor B has associated with $C3(H_2O)$, it is cleaved by factor D, a circulating serine protease that has specificity for factor B bound to $C3(H_2O)$. This cleavage results in the formation of two fragments, Ba and Bb. The Bb fragment has serine protease activity and remains associated with $C3(H_2O)$. The bimolecular complex $C3(H_2O)Bb$ has C3 as its substrate. The $C3(H_2O)Bb$ complex cleaves C3 in the same way as C4b2a, and the resulting C3b molecules can bind covalently to the cell surface. If C3b binds to an activator surface, factor B associates with it and is cleaved by factor D. This results in the formation of an alternative-pathway C3-converting complex on the surface of the activator. Because this complex has C3 as its substrate, it produces a feedback amplification loop for the deposition of C3b onto the activator.

The binding of a C3b molecule in the immediate vicinity of a C4b2a or C3bBb enzyme complex produces a trimolecular complex that is capable of cleaving C5. The C3b molecule has a binding site for C5; if the geometry is appropriate, C5 is presented to the enzyme complex, where it is cleaved by C2a or Bb serine proteases. The cleavage produces the fragments C5a and C5b. Although there is a great deal of homology among C3, C4, and C5, there is no reactive thiolester in the C5 molecule. Therefore, the cleavage of C5 does not generate a fragment capable of binding covalently to a cell surface. The C5b molecule remains briefly associated with C3b before its association with the terminal proteins of the complement pathway.

Formation of the Membrane Attack Complex

Membrane attack complex of complement refers to the association of the complement proteins C5, C6, C7, C8, and C9 to form a potentially cytolytic complex. When C5 is activated in either the classical or alternative pathway, the resulting C5b molecule contains binding sites for the next components in the pathway. This part of the complement pathway is still a cascade, but the activation of a component results in the exposure of binding sites for other terminal complement proteins rather than in the acquisition of enzymatic activity. C5b, but not C5, contains a binding site for C6, which becomes bound while the C5b molecule is associated with its C3b tether. The C5b6 complex may be released from C3b, or it may remain anchored until it binds a molecule of C7. Once C7 is attached, the trimolecular complex undergoes a transition in which the normal hydrophilic character of the individual members of the complex is lost and a transient hydrophobic character is acquired. At this time, C5b-7 may associate with a membrane through the hydrophobic region; if it fails to interact with a membrane, the complex inactivates by self-aggregation or by interaction with the inhibitors described later.

Once C5b-7 is membrane associated, a binding site for C8 is exposed in C5b. The binding of C8 causes the complex to insert more deeply into the membrane. C9 binds to C8 and undergoes significant conformational changes. Not only does it acquire considerable hydrophobic character, pushing the membrane attack complex deeper into the membrane, but it gains affinity for other molecules of C9, which polymerize into the complex. Electron-microscopic studies suggest that the $C5b\text{-}9_{(n)}$ complex resembles a hollow cylinder. This cylinder is formed by the polymerized C9 molecules, which number between 12 and 18 in each complex. The C5b-8 is thought to play little active role in the structure of the cylindrical pore; it is, however, the essential catalyst for the pore's formation. The biochemical characteristics of the complement proteins are given in Table 7–3.

The Regulation of Complement Activation

Plasma Proteins

As discussed previously, the activation of the complement system is expressed as the activation of several enzymes of the serine protease group. As with any zymogen-to-enzyme conversion, there must be a way of regulating the activity of the enzyme, or else it will cleave all available substrate molecules. With the complement proteins, this regulation is achieved by multiple mechanisms. The geometric arrangement of the proteins is the simplest of these, inasmuch as several of the key enzymes function only when surface associated. The continuing activation of the complement pathway is highly dependent on the spatial arrangement of the enzyme and substrate molecules. For example, a C2 molecule associated with a C4b molecule that has been deposited more than 60 nm from the activated C1 will not be activated. Also, the enzymatic proteins of complement all occur in multisubunit or multimolecular complexes, each of which has a divalent cation requirement. The reduction of divalent cation concentration, as well as the inherent dissociation constant of the protein-protein interaction, means that the complement enzyme complexes simply fall apart.

An important way in which the body controls complement activation is through the action of specific protein inhibitors of the complement proteins. These proteins are of two sorts: plasma proteins and cellular membrane proteins (Table 7–4). Cells that are constantly exposed to the plasma milieu have evolved their own defense mechanisms against complement activation. Selective pressure to evolve defense proteins is present because the complement system does not distinguish between "good" and "bad" targets. A variety of proteins that are involved in complement regulation on cell surfaces have been described.[11]

The plasma proteins that inhibit complement work at all steps of complement activation. The only known inhibitor of activated C1 is the C1 inhibitor protein, which

Table 7–3. Characteristics of the Proteins of Complement

Pathway	Protein	Molecular Weight (kDa)	Structure	Average Serum Concentration (mg/mL)
Activation complex classical pathway	C1q	Subunit A: 27 Subunit B: 27 Subunit C: 24 Complex: 465	6 each of subunits A, B, and C	80
	C1r	83	If full complex, C1q + 2 C1r + 2 C1; if no C1q, then 2 C1r + 2 C1s	50
	C1s	83		50
	C4	Subunit a: 97 Subunit b: 75 Subunit c: 33 Complex: 205	One each of subunits a, b, and c synthesized from a single precursor	600
Activation complex alternative pathway	Factor B	92	Single chain	210
	Factor D	24	Single chain	<2
Common pathway	C3	Subunit a: 110 Subunit b: 75 Complex: 185	One each of subunits a and b synthesized from a single precursor	1,300
	C5	Subunit a: 115 Subunit b: 75 Complex: 190	One each of subunits a and b synthesized from a single precursor	70
	C6	120	Single chain	65
	C7	110	Single chain	56
	C8	Subunit a: 64 Subunit b: 64 Subunit c: 22 Complex: 150	One each of subunits a, b, and c	55
	C9	70	Single chain	60

Table 7–4. Characteristics of the Complement Regulatory Proteins

Pathway	Protein	Molecular Weight (kDa)	Structure	Average Serum Concentration (mg/mL)
Activation complex classical pathway	C1 inhibitor	110	Single chain	200
	C4BP	Subunit: 70 Complex: 500	Complex of 7 subunits	250
	Factor I	Subunit a: 50 Subunit b: 38 Complex: 80	One each of subunits a and b	35
	Decay-accelerating factor (DAF)	70	Single chain; phosphatidylinositol membrane anchor	N/A
	Membrane cofactor protein (MCP)	45–70	Single chain	N/A
Activation complex alternative pathway	Factor H	150	Single chain	500
	CR1	160–250	Single chain	N/A
Terminal complex	S-protein (vitronectin)	83	Single chain	500
	Sp-40,40	Subunit: 40 Complex: 75	Two subunits in complex	50
	CD59	20	Single chain; phosphatidylinositol membrane anchor	N/A

N/A, not applicable.

is also an inhibitor of kallikrein, plasmin, factor XIa, and factor XIIa. C1 inhibitor inactivates C1 by binding to the active sites of the C1r and C1s subunits with very high affinity; this binding has been suggested to be covalent. Because the C1 complex is composed of two subunits each of C1r and C1s, the inactivation of the complex requires the binding of two molecules of C1 inhibitor. Inhibition of enzymatic activity of C1 by C1 inhibitor does not modulate the ability of the C1q subunits to bind either to immunoglobulin or to specific cellular receptors for C1q.

The critical role of C1 inhibitor in the control of the complement pathway can be illustrated by the disease hereditary angioedema (HAE).[12] Approximately 80% of patients with type I HAE are shown, by both immunological and functional assays, to have less than 50% normal levels of C1 inhibitor. The remaining 20% of patients have a normal level of a dysfunctional protein. Patients with both types of HAE are subjected to periodic attacks of acute edema that may be life-threatening if there is laryngeal involvement. HAE attacks are thought to arise from minor trauma that produces localized complement activation. The ineffective regulation of C1, caused by the depletion of C1 inhibitor, results in the generation of activation peptides that induce edema. Although the exact nature of the mediators is yet to be determined, both kinin and bradykinin are candidate molecules. The levels of C2 and C4 in patients suffering HAE attacks are greatly reduced, which reflects the requirement for rapid inactivation of activated C1 to prevent substrate depletion. A similar clinical picture also arises in patients who have acquired angioedema (AAE) as a result of the presence of an autoantibody reactive with C1 inhibitor. These antibodies can cause accelerated clearance of C1 inhibitor or may functionally interfere with the protein.

The other plasma proteins that regulate the classical pathway all act on the C4b2a complex. Two plasma proteins that bind C4b have been described. C4-binding protein (C4BP) is a multisubunit protein that circulates complexed with protein S of the coagulation system.[13] Bound protein S does not affect the complement inhibitory activity of C4BP. C4BP accelerates the decay of the C4b2a complex, as well as acting as a cofactor for the degradation of C4b by factor I. The other C4-binding plasma protein is a sialoglycoprotein called SGP 120.[14] This molecule copurifies with C2 during C4b-sepharose affinity chromatography. It apparently is a competitive inhibitor for the C2-binding site on C4b. The precise biological role of SGP 120 remains to be determined.

The plasma proteins that regulate the alternative pathway are molecules that are either inhibitory or stabilizing for the C3bBb complex. As described previously, the alternative pathway begins in the fluid phase. It is the fate of the C3b molecules deposited on the surface that distinguishes an activator from a nonactivator. The major plasma protein that regulates complement activation is factor H. The interplay between factor B and factor H, in their competition for C3b, actually determines whether a surface is "activating." On some surfaces, the binding of factor B is promoted over the binding of factor H; these surfaces are said to be activators of the alternative pathway because the C3bBb complex readily forms. If the binding of factor H is favored, the surface does not activate complement. Factor H has cofactor activity for factor I, the C3b inactivator. Factor I is a circulating serine protease that has C4b and C3b as its substrates. The degradation of C3b by factor I results in the formation of biologically important fragments of C3 that interact with specific cellular receptors.

Although the plasma regulatory proteins just described act to downregulate the activation of complement, one protein of the alternative pathway, properdin, modulates the activity of the pathway by stabilizing the C3bBb complex. Properdin circulates in an inactive form, which becomes activated upon association with C3b. Although properdin apparently binds to a site on C3b, the binding affinity increases considerably if C3b is complexed to Bb.[15]

The terminal complex of complement is regulated by two plasma proteins: vitronectin and clusterin (or SP40,40). Vitronectin, the major plasma regulator of the membrane attack complex, was initially called *S-protein* by investigators in the complement field; current literature may still use this designation. This molecule is not the same as protein S of the coagulation system. Vitronectin regulates the membrane attack complex at the C5b-7 stage. When C5b-7 is formed, several molecules of vitronectin bind to the hydrophobic regions of the complex, increasing its water solubility. Inactivated C5b-7, known as SC5b-7, is capable of binding C8 and C9, but C9 polymerization is blocked. SP40,40 was described as an inhibitor of membrane attack complex, which appears to act at the C5-6 level.[16, 17] The protein is a disulfide-linked heterodimer; each subunit has a molecular weight of approximately 40 kDa. SP40,40 co-localizes with vitronectin and membrane attack complexes in tissue sections. There is some in vitro evidence to suggest that SP40,40 may be complexed in plasma with vitronectin. SP40,40 most likely shares identity with the protein clusterin, a cell-agglutinating protein that circulates in plasma complexed to apolipoprotein A-I.[18] The relative functions of this molecule in complement regulation, cholesterol transport, and cell-cell interaction remain to be determined.

Cell Membrane Proteins

Cells that come into contact with activated complement have evolved additional mechanisms to protect themselves from opsonization or cytolysis. One such adaptation is to evolve proteins that inactivate complement at the membrane surface. The analysis of such proteins has been the focus of much of the activity in complement biology since their discovery in the early 1980s.

The first such molecule described was *decay-accelerating factor* (DAF), which was discovered simultaneously by two groups.[19, 20] As its name suggests, DAF functions by accelerating the decay of the C3bBb or C4b2a enzyme complexes. In the alternative pathway, DAF binds to C3b, thereby disrupting the C3bBb complex. The mode of action of DAF on C4b2a is not completely clear; published studies have demonstrated the binding of DAF to both C2a and C4b.[21, 22] DAF is expressed on a wide variety of tissues other than blood cells, including endothelial cells and kidney glomerular epithelial cells. The number of molecules of DAF per cell varics from 10^3 to 10^4, depending on the cell type; in addition, DAF expression in some cells can be modulated in response to mitogens and cytokines.[23] DAF has no cofactor activity for factor I inactivation of either C3b or C4b.

Membrane cofactor protein (MCP) is an integral membrane protein that regulates the C3bBb and C4b2a complexes by binding to C3b or C4b and acting as a cofactor for factor I inactivation.[24] The molecule has no decay-accelerating activity. MCP acts only on C3b and C4b bound to the cell that contains the MCP; that is, it acts to regulate complement only at a very local level. The affinity of MCP for C3b is much greater than for C4b; hence its cofactor function is greater for C3b inactivation.

The third membrane protein capable of regulating complement activation at the C3 step is the complement receptor CR1 (CD35). The ligand for this receptor is C3b or C4b that is present on an exogenous cell—that is, not on the cell that bears the CR1 molecule. CR1 is an integral membrane protein with a wide tissue distribution; as discussed later, it is crucially important in the clearance of C3b-containing immune complexes from the circulation.

The plethora of proteins that have been identified as regulators of the C3/C5-converting enzymes seems at first to suggest redundancy in the complement system. However, these proteins, both plasma and membrane, act in concert to regulate complement activation in all situations in which it may arise. In the fluid phase of plasma, C4-binding protein, SGP 120, and factor I control the activation of the classical pathway; factor H and factor I control the alternative pathway. The membrane proteins DAF and MCP regulate the activation of complement on autologous cell surfaces, whereas CR1 acts to regulate exogenous complement activation, particularly in immune complexes. The evolution of proteins to specifically control all activation scenarios prevents the negative physiological sequelae of unregulated complement enzymes.

Two membrane proteins that regulate the membrane attack complex of complement by preventing the complete assembly of $C5b\text{-}9_{(n)}$ have been described.[25, 26] These proteins are important in controlling the formation of membrane attack complex on cells that bear C5-converting enzyme complexes. They are also essential for protecting the cell from "reactive lysis" or "bystander lysis," whereby the cell picks up C5b-7 from the surrounding medium even though it may not bear the C5-converting enzymes that generated the C5b-7 complex. C8-binding protein, also known as homologous restriction factor, is a 65-kDa protein first identified in the red blood cell membrane. It binds to C8 and prohibits the polymerization of C9 into the membrane attack complex. This protein has the characteristic of homologous restriction; that is, human C8-binding protein works best on human membrane attack complex and less efficiently or not at all with complement proteins from other species. Such species selectivity has been noted for other proteins in the complement pathway. In 1988 and 1989, four separate groups found another membrane protein that regulates the activity of the membrane attack complex.[27–30] This molecule, now known as CD59, was also called 1F5 antigen, P-18, MEM-43, homologous restriction factor 20, H-19, membrane inhibitor of reactive lysis (MIRL), and MAC inhibitory factor. CD59 contains binding sites for C8 and C9 and thus appears to regulate at both C5b-8 and C5b-9.[31, 32]

The regulatory proteins DAF, CD59, and C8-binding protein all belong to an unusual group of proteins that are attached to the cell membrane by a phosphatidylinositol anchor, rather than by cytoplasmic and transmembrane stretches of amino acids.[33] This anchor structure, which is synthesized in the endoplasmic reticulum, involves the attachment of a protein moiety to the phospholipid through a series of carbohydrate residues. Abnormalities in genes encoding enzymes responsible for the addition of carbohydrates to the anchor structure are associated with the development of the acquired myelodysplastic condition paroxysmal nocturnal hemoglobinuria (PNH).[33] Gene defects in PNH are clustered in the so-called PIG-A gene, a putative glycosyltransferase with specificity for *N*-acetylglucosamine; abnormalities often result in the complete lack of protein product. The defects in PIG-A gene in PNH are expressed phenotypically as the complete or near-complete absence of phosphatidylinositol-anchored proteins from the cell membrane. The lack of CD55, CD59, and C8-binding protein from PNH cells is associated with accelerated complement-mediated intravascular hemolysis and gives rise to the hemoglobinuria that is a hallmark of the disease.

Two sets of observations in other conditions suggest that it is the deficiency of membrane attack complex regulatory proteins that is responsible for the hemolytic anemia of PNH. First, it was determined by two groups of investigators that erythrocytes lacking the blood group antigens of the Cromer complex (the Inab phenotype) are deficient in DAF, the molecule that carries the Cromer antigen system.[34, 35] Affected persons demonstrate no intravascular hemolysis. The second observation is a description of one patient who has a genetic deficiency of CD59.[36] This condition is associated, in this patient, with a mild hemolytic anemia and cerebrovascular thrombosis; thrombosis is the major cause of mortality in PNH. Together, these observations suggest that the regulators of the terminal complex are the most important in protecting cells from destruction by complement. The relative importance of CD59 and C8-binding protein in vivo remains to be determined.

These factors—molecular geometry, complex instability, and regulatory proteins—contribute to marked inefficiency of the complement system. Circulating erythrocytes from a patient with cold agglutinin disease can carry over 100,000 molecules of C3 per cell; normal erythrocytes can defend themselves against as many as 20,000 membrane attack complexes. Even given the inherent inefficiency of complement, the presence of multiple regulatory mechanisms at each step of the complement pathway attests to the importance of regulating the activity of this system.

The Ontogeny and Phylogeny of Complement Proteins

The application of molecular biology to the complement system has demonstrated heretofore unidentified relationships among the proteins of complement. Many structural homologies exist within the complement system. As might be expected, structure and function are closely aligned in the complement proteins (Table 7–5). Four distinct "families" of complement proteins can be identified. The first of these is the serine protease family, which contains C1r, C1s, C2, factor B, factor D, and factor I. These proteins are related to the well-studied serine proteases trypsin and chymotrypsin. All of these proteins contain a 25-kDa protease domain at the carboxyl terminus of the protein. Because 25 kDa is the approximate molecular weight of factor D, this activator of factor B can be considered the quintessential serine protease. C1r and C1s are identical in size and contain very similar molecular features, including a set of 60–amino acid short consensus repeats (SCRs) and a type III cysteine-rich domain similar to that in epidermal growth factor. The genes encoding these two proteins are closely linked on chromosome 12 and presumably arose by gene duplication.

Table 7–5. Structural/Functional Homologies Within the Complement System

Proteins	Homology
C1r, C1s	Serine proteases with similar subunit structure Genes linked
C2, factor B	Similar size, activation Highly homologous by structure Linked in major histocompatibility complex locus
C3, C4, C5	Activation by cleavage from α chain C3 and C4 contain reactive thiolester Amino acid sequences show >20% overall identity
C6, C7, C8, C9	Share overall homology to one another ranging from 16% to 33% C6 and C7 share greatest homology All undergo amphipathic conversion to acquire membrane-binding character
CR1, CR2, factor H, DAF, MCP, C4-binding protein	All function to regulate complement activation All have multiple (60–70)–amino acid short consensus repeats

DAF, delay-accelerating factor; MCP, membrane cofactor protein.

As indicated previously, the serine proteases of the early classical and alternative pathways are both C3/C5-converting enzymes. In addition to this functional similarity, C2 and factor B have considerable structural homology. They are similarly sized proteins composed of a single polypeptide chain; they contain similar SCRs, similar serine protease domains (shared by all serine proteases), and a region shared only by these two. The genes for both C2 and factor B lie in the class III region of the major histocompatibility complex (MHC) on chromosome 6, a region that also contains the genes for C4.

C3, C4, and C5 are highly homologous proteins. As discussed, each protein is activated by the cleavage of a small "a" fragment from the α chain of the native molecule. C3 and C4 share the feature of the reactive thiolester bond in the α chain; this bond is lacking in C5. All three proteins are synthesized as single "proproteins" that undergo modification before release into the plasma to generate the two chains of C3 and C5 and the three chains of C4. Interestingly, despite the high degree of overall homology of amino acids in these proteins (about 25%), the genes for the three proteins are located on three different chromosomes: the C3 gene is on chromosome 19; the C4 genes are in the MHC on chromosome 6; and the C5 gene is on chromosome 9. Although both C3 and C5 are encoded by single genes, two genes encode C4. These genes, known as C4A and C4B, give rise to the isotypic variants of the C4 protein. On the basis of the structure of C3-like proteins in other organisms, it has been postulated that C3 arose first and C4 and C5 arose later as gene duplication products.

The terminal complement proteins (C6 to C9) also exhibit a considerable degree of homology. Each of the terminal proteins exhibits an overall amino acid homology of 18% to 33% with the other proteins. If an analysis is made considering conservative substitutions, the homology increases to more than 50%. The predominant characteristic of the terminal complement proteins is the presence of cysteine-rich regions. From the amino-terminus and with the nomenclature of Morgan,[2] the four types of cysteine-rich domains are known as type I, type II, type III, and the SCR (Fig. 7–2). The terminal complement proteins all contain type I cysteine-rich domains of approximately 60 amino acids, as well as other cysteine-rich domains of approximately 40 amino acids that share sequence homology to those in the low-density lipoprotein (LDL) receptor (types II and III). These cysteine-rich domains, which greatly contribute to the tertiary structure of the protein, are clearly important for function. The SCRs are present in at least 12 of the complement proteins, and 8 proteins contain the other types of cysteine-rich domains. C6, C7, and C9 are single-polypeptide chains encoded by single genes; C8 is composed of three polypeptide chains, each of which is encoded by its own gene. The C8 α and β proteins are highly homologous, but the C8 gamma chain shows no homology to any complement protein; it shows homology to α_1-microglobulin.

The proteins involved in the regulation of complement activation are also structurally related. In addition, the genes encoding the proteins that modulate C3 and C4 activation are grouped in one region of the long arm of chromosome 6 known as the *regulators of complement activation* (RCA) cluster.[37] The RCA group includes factor H, C4-binding protein, DAF, membrane cofactor protein, and the complement receptors CR1 and CR2. These proteins contain a variable number of SCRs of 60 to 70 amino acids. The chromosomal assignments of the complement proteins are given in Table 7–6.

Molecular biology has also proved invaluable in the identification of polymorphisms of complement proteins that had previously been noted as variants in electrophoretic mobility or antigenicity. Polymorphisms have been described for most of the complement proteins.[38, 39] Some of the complement protein polymorphisms are associated with a loss or decrease of complement activity. Others demonstrate some degree of disease association; however, no disease associations have been established for any polymorphisms of the terminal complex proteins.

THE PHYSIOLOGICAL RESPONSE TO COMPLEMENT ACTIVATION

Anaphylatoxins

The cleavage of C3, C4, or C5 by the enzyme complexes of the alternative or classical pathways results in the formation of two fragments. The fate of the C3b, C4b, and C5b fragments was discussed previously. The other fragments, C3a, C4a, and C5a, are known as the *anaphylatoxic fragments of complement.* These very small fragments of complement can produce a very large and potentially life-threatening physiological response. The C3bBb and C4b2a enzyme complexes recognize an Arg-X-sequence near the amino terminus of C3, C4, and C5. Cleavage of this bond results in the formation of a small N-terminal peptide of 77 amino acids for C3a and C4a and a small N-terminal peptide of 74 amino acids for C5a, each with a C-terminal arginine residue.

Although these peptides are very similar in structure, their potency in mediating cellular responses varies considerably. C5a is the most potent of the complement-derived anaphylatoxins, and C3a is the least potent. These complement fragments exert their anaphylatoxic effects by interacting with specific cellular receptors present on the surface of mast cells and basophils. The occupation

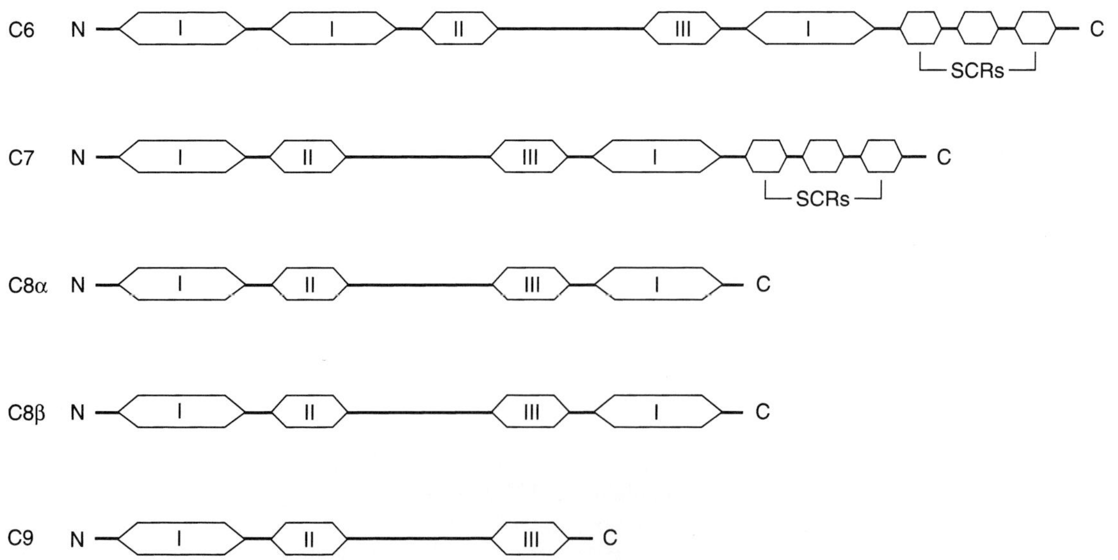

Figure 7–2. The domain structure of the terminal complex proteins. This figure illustrates the relative homologies among the proteins of the membrane attack complex. The highly homologous regions are found within cysteine-rich domains types I, II, and III (according to Morgan[2]). In addition, C6 and C7 contain cysteine-rich short consensus repeats (SCRs).

Table 7–6. Chromosomal Assignments of the Complement Proteins

Protein(s)	Chromosomal Assignment
C1q	A and B chains on 1; C chain unassigned
C1r/C1s	Closely linked on 12
C2, C4A, C4B	In MHC locus on 6
C1 inhibitor, CD59	11
C4-binding protein, factor H, CR1, CR2, MCP, DAF	In RCA cluster on 1
Factor B	In MHC locus on 6
Factor D	Unassigned
Factor I	4
Properdin	X
C3	19
C5	9
C6/C7	Closely linked on 5
C8	α and β chains on 1; γ chain on 9
C9	5

MCP, membrane cofactor protein; DAF, delay-accelerating factor; MHC, major histocompatibility complex; RCA, regulators of complement activation.

of the receptor triggers the release of histamine and serotonin from intracellular granules. These two soluble factors cause contraction of smooth muscle cells and increased vascular permeability of blood vessels. Neutrophils, monocytes, macrophages, and platelets also bind anaphylatoxic fragments of complement; the occupation of these receptors activates the cell and, in the case of neutrophils, induces chemotaxis toward the site of complement activation.

Although the anaphylatoxic fragments of C3, C4, and C5 are potent biological response modifiers, they are rapidly inactivated in plasma by the action of a pair of carboxypeptidases. The best known, serum carboxypeptidase N, removes the C-terminal arginine residue from the peptide. Another enzyme, carboxypeptidase R, has been identified as the primary inactivator of kinin as well as anaphylatoxin peptides.[40] Unlike carboxypeptidase N, carboxypeptidase R is itself rapidly inactivated under normal purification conditions. After removal of the arginine, the peptide acquires the designation "des arg." C3a and C4a are rapidly and completely inactivated by the two carboxypeptidases; C5a is somewhat more resistant to inactivation. In addition, neutrophils can still respond to C5a des arg, albeit with some 10^3 weaker affinity; the removal of arginine from C3a and C4a results in complete loss of biological activity.

The relative resistance to carboxypeptidases and retention of bioactivity make C5a the most physiologically important of the anaphylactic complement peptides. Generation of C5a causes many of the effects seen in inflammation that are mediated by neutrophils. After activation by the binding of C5a into specific receptors, neutrophils bind to the capillary endothelium and migrate through the vessel wall, after the concentration gradient of the C5a. Once they are in contact with the higher concentrations of C5a present at the site of complement activation, neutrophils release granule contents and reactive metabolites, including lysozyme, reactive oxygen species, and eicosanoids. Although this is part of the normal mechanism of response to tissue injury or infection, the generation of large amounts of C5a or its presence in inappropriate locations can cause significant damage to uninvolved tissues.

Other Complement Activation Peptides

Other peptides generated during the course of complement activation have been identified as inducing cell activation or chemotaxis. Factor Ba, the peptide cleaved from factor B by factor D, is a weak chemotactic factor. The cleavage products of factor B, Ba and Bb, have been reported to inhibit and stimulate B cell proliferation, respectively. Peptides with function similar to those of C3a and C5a can be generated by the action of non-complement enzymes, particularly plasmin, on C3 and C5. These C3a-like and C5a-like peptides may play a significant role in the activation of both platelets and white cells under existing blood storage protocols. The use of negatively charged leukoreduction filters may significantly affect the levels of various contact activation peptides in blood products.[41] In general, negatively charged artificial membrane surfaces promote complement activation; however, some types of filters appear to remove C3a that is generated during processing and storage.[42]

The membrane attack complex itself causes significant activation in a wide variety of cell types. Because most studies of the C5b-9 complex have focused on its lytic effect on erythrocytes, the functional effect on nucleated cells and platelets has lately gained appreciation. Although there are some reports in the literature that C5b-7 has chemotactic activity for neutrophils, it is the fully formed C5b-9 that has the greatest effect on these cells. In comparison with erythrocytes, nucleated cells are very resistant to C5b-9 lysis. In response to C5b-9, nucleated cells and platelets coalesce the C5b-9 complexes and bud them off in vesicles of plasma membrane. In nucleated cells, especially neutrophils, this process is accompanied by the activation of the cell and the release of enzymes, leukotrienes, prostaglandins, thromboxanes, and reactive oxygen metabolites from the cell.[43]

Platelets interact with the activated proteins of the complement system at several levels.[44] Specific platelet receptors for C1q have been identified.[45–47] Although the precise role of C1q receptors remains to be determined, one such receptor has been reported to play a role in phagocytosis in other cell types.[48] The exposure of human platelets to C3a alters the response to physiological agonists but does not induce platelet aggregation. The effect of C5a on human platelets has not been investigated. Membrane attack complex can also affect platelet function.[49] C5b-9 can induce the formation of platelet membrane vesicles (or "microparticles"), increase the procoagulant activity of the platelet, and cause some degree of arachidonic acid generation.[50] Studies of the effects of C5b-9 on platelets have been carried out in purified protein systems; the significance of these observations for the whole plasma system remains to be determined. The platelet may modify the effects of activated complement fragments through the action of its surface regulatory proteins, DAF, MCP, C8-binding protein, and CD59.

Platelets also contain internal pools of vitronectin, which may contribute to the local modulation of complement. The significant effects of activated complement fragments on the physiological processes of platelets must be considered in the setting of platelet concentrate storage. Complement is activated under storage conditions,[51] with or without prestorage leukoreduction. Activated complement fragments as well as C5b-9 may contribute to the platelet storage lesion.[52]

EFFECTS OF COMPLEMENT ACTIVATION ON CELL SURVIVAL

Cytotoxic Effects

In the transfusion medicine setting, the effects of complement activation are graphically illustrated by the acute intravascular transfusion reaction. The generation of C3a and C5a produces bronchospasm and hypotension. C5a can also stimulate the production of interleukin-1 from macrophages, thereby causing fever.[53] The recruitment of large numbers of neutrophils to the lung by C5a generation produces ventilation-perfusion abnormalities. Two other hallmarks of the acute intravascular transfusion reaction, hemoglobinemia and hemoglobinuria, result from the activation of complement on the red cell surface in sufficient amounts to overwhelm the cellular and plasma control proteins, thereby lysing the cell. The generation of activated complement proteins affects more than red cell survival. The activation of cells with the concomitant release of enzymes contributes to the activation of the coagulation system, as does the action of complement proteins on coagulation substrates and endothelial cells. In vitro studies suggest that these processes may trigger the disseminated intravascular coagulation seen in severe cases of hemolytic transfusion reaction. Evidence for the direct cytolysis of platelets or granulocytes during transfusion is not abundant, perhaps because of the difficulty in constructing study design. However, complement activation may be directly linked to platelet destruction in the setting of paroxysmal nocturnal hemoglobinuria, sepsis, and thrombotic thrombocytopenic purpura/hemolytic uremia syndrome. Each of these conditions is associated with complement activation and platelet dysfunction. The complement-mediated destruction of antibody-coated platelets can be experimentally induced. Antibody to the Pl^{A1} antigen (HPA-1) fixes sufficient complement to lyse target platelets.[54] In vitro platelet lysis can also be induced by cold agglutinin anti-I antibodies[55]; antibodies of this specificity have been proposed to mediate the thrombocytopenia associated with Epstein-Barr virus infection.

Opsonic Effects

The opsonic effects of complement activation result in the accelerated clearance of particles or cells that bear C3 as well as IgG. Although complement activation is the primary mechanism of cell destruction in the acute hemolytic transfusion reaction, the extravascular destruction of erythrocytes does not have the absolute requirement of complement activation. The primary clearance mechanism is through the phagocyte Fc receptor with recognition of the IgG present on the cell surface. Opsonization of cells by complement, rather than through lysis, means that the cell has been able to regulate complement effectively in order to prevent the assembly of cytolytic membrane attack complexes. This regulation may reflect the titer, avidity, affinity, or thermal amplitude of the antibody in its interaction with the cell target.

In addition, as described previously, only IgG_1 and IgG_3 are efficient complement activators. The presence of C3b (or its degradation products) on the cell target in addition to antibody accelerates the clearance by the reticuloendothelial system. If a macrophage is already activated, it will bind and ingest cells that bear only C3b. Normal, resting macrophages require that IgG is also present on the erythrocyte surface. This experimental result is supported by the in vivo observation that the erythrocytes of patients with cold agglutinin disease circulate through the spleen bearing C3b but no IgG and are not sequestered. That is not to say that C3 has no in vivo role in clearance. Bacteria coated with C3 only are efficiently phagocytized by macrophages, resting or activated, even in the absence of IgG. Macrophages in the liver (Kupffer cells) are capable of clearing erythrocytes coated with C3b only. In addition, persons who are genetically deficient in one of the components of the early classical pathway are unable to bind C3 to anti–D-coated erythrocytes; those target cells are cleared from the circulation much more slowly than in persons with intact complement systems.[56]

The opsonic and cytotoxic effects of complement are important in the ex vivo setting of blood storage. Many types of bacteria that have been implicated in transfusion-mediated sepsis are either lysed or opsonized by the complement proteins in the blood unit. These bacteria are then engulfed by phagocytes also present in the bag. The removal of phagocytes by leukodepletion within 24 hours of collection results in the removal of contaminating bacteria as well. Leukodepletion more than 24 hours after collection may fail to sterilize the unit, because white cell breakdown may result in the release of viable bacteria from phagolysosomes.

The Role of Complement Receptors in Cell Clearance and in Maintenance of the Immune Response

The removal of complement-coated target cells is mediated by specific receptors for C3 and its activation and degradation fragments. As previously discussed, the activation of C3 produces two fragments, C3a, the anaphylatoxin, and C3b, which is covalently bound to the cell surface. In the presence of factor H, MCP, or the complement receptor CR1, C3b is rapidly cleaved by factor I to an inactivated form, C3bi (Fig. 7–3). This cleavage is estimated to occur in vivo within 5 minutes of the generation of C3b. Inactivated C3b undergoes another, slower interaction with factor I that results in a second cleavage on the opposite side of the thiolester bond from the initial cleavage. This second cleavage occurs within 30 minutes of generation of C3b and results in the generation of the

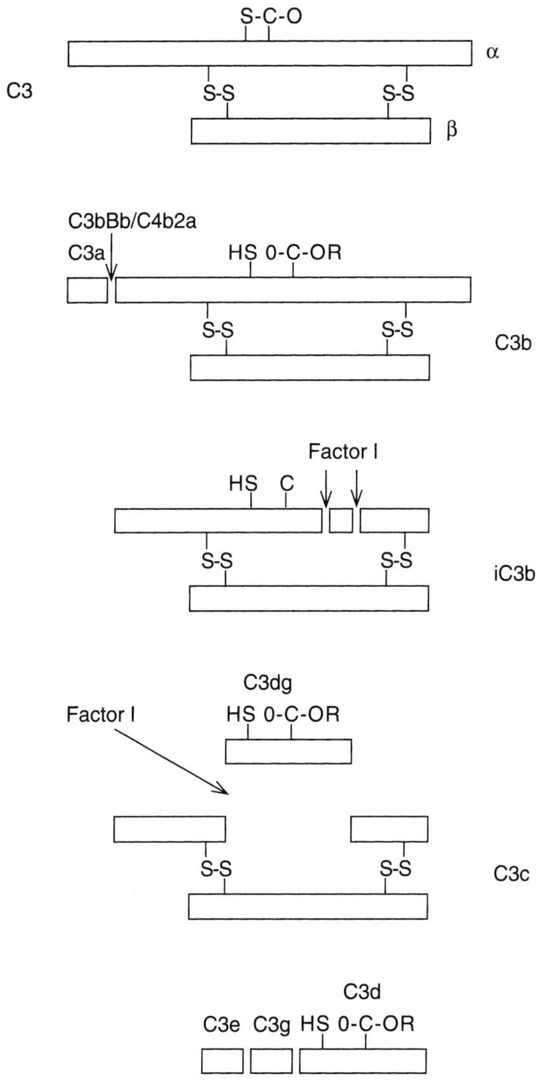

Figure 7–3. Degradation fragments of C3. Native C3 is cleaved by C4b2a or C3bBb, resulting in the exposure of a reactive thiolester in the α chain of C3 and the generation of two fragments, C3a and C3b. C3b is inactivated by factor I in the presence of factor H or CR1 to iC3b, which remains bound to the surface by the thiolester. A further cleavage by factor I on the other side of the covalent bond from the first cleavage results in the release of the C3c fragment; the C3dg fragment remains surface bound. In vitro, the C3dg fragment may be further degraded to C3d, C3f, and C3g. The C3d fragment, a terminal breakdown product of C3, remains covalently bound to the surface.

C3c fragment, which is no longer tethered to the cell, and the C3dg fragment, which contains the thiolester bond and remains bound to the cell surface. Under laboratory conditions, the C3dg fragment can be further cleaved by trypsin to leave the C3d fragment on the cell surface; the frequency of generation of this fragment in vivo is uncertain.

Several complement receptors have been identified to date. They have overlapping cell distribution (Table 7–7). The specificity of these receptors for individual fragments of C3 is reflected in the biological response to receptor occupation. The central function of the complement receptor CR1 is clearance of immune complexes from the circulation through its interaction with C3b contained in the complex.[57] The bulk of the total CR1 in the circulation is present on red cells, as they provide the greatest mass of cells in the peripheral blood. The erythrocyte is therefore essential in transporting immune complexes from the plasma to the resident macrophages in the spleen.

The further processing of C3b to iC3b enables the complement fragment to interact with the complement receptor CR3, also known as CD11b/CD18. This receptor, with its distribution on monocytes, macrophages, and neutrophils, plays a major role in immune-mediated phagocytosis. CR3 belongs to a family of related receptor molecules that have the β chain CD18. The pairing of the CD11a α chain to CD18 defines the leukocyte function antigen-1 (LFA-1), which is important in mediating killing by T lymphocytes. CD18 may also pair with the α chain CD11c, forming the complex known as p150,95. This molecule has been unofficially designated CR4 in recognition of its binding affinity for iC3b.

The importance of the complement receptors CR3 and CR4 is indicated by the severity of the deficiency state in which patients have defective phagocytic function and are susceptible to recurrent infections.[58] The degradation of iC3b by factor I produces C3dg, the principal ligand for the receptor CR2. The expression of CR2 is restricted to B lymphocytes, on which the binding of C3dg triggers B cell activation and proliferation. In addition to its role as a C3dg-binding protein, CR2 is the cellular receptor through which the Epstein-Barr virus gains entry to B lymphocytes. The identification and characterization of the complement receptors has led to the development of new therapeutic modalities. For example, a recombinant CR1 has been engineered with the transmembrane region missing. This molecule retains the complement-regulatory ability of CR1 but is soluble in plasma. In animal models, this protein, sCR1, has proved efficacious in reducing the complement activation seen during thrombolytic therapy.[59]

Fragments of C3 are important in maintaining the immune response.[60] Animals with an experimental depletion of C3 fail to mount a normal IgG response to secondary immunization. This observation suggests that C3 is important in the development of immunological memory, but such a role for C3 has not been confirmed in humans.

LABORATORY ANALYSIS OF COMPLEMENT

Measurement of Cell-Associated Complement

The methods available for the measurement of cell-associated immunoglobulins are readily adaptable to the detection of cell-bound complement. Traditionally, the presence of cell-associated C3b and its cleavage products is *detected* by means of an aggregating anti-C3d antibody (C3 Coombs' test). The presence of small amounts of C4d antigen on the erythrocyte is identified in the blood bank as the Chido-Rodgers blood group antigen system. The antigenic difference is actually determined by the C4A and C4B alleles, with Rodgers specificity found in

Table 7–7. Structure and Distribution of Complement Receptors

Receptor	Molecular Structure	Cellular Distribution
C1q	65 kDa, single chain	Platelets, monocytes, macrophages, B lymphocytes, endothelial cells
C3a	Unknown	Mast cells, monocytes, macrophages, neutrophils, basophils, T cells
C5a	45 kDa, single chain	Monocytes, macrophages, neutrophils, mast cells
CR1 (CD35)	Four allotypes ranging from 160 to 250 kDa	Erythrocytes, monocytes, neutrophils, B lymphocytes
CR2 (CD21)	145 kDa, single chain	B cells, follicular dendritic cells
CR3 (CD11b/CD18)	Two chains, 165 kDa and 95 kDa	Neutrophils, monocytes, macrophages, follicular dendritic cells, natural killer cells
CD11c/CD18 (CR4)*	Two chains, of 150 kDa and 95 kDa	Neutrophils, monocytes, macrophages, natural killer cells
(CR5)*	Unknown	Neutrophils, platelets

*CR designations are unofficial.

the C4A isotypes and Chido specificity found in the C4B isotypes. Techniques developed to measure cell-associated immunoglobulin can all be adapted to measure cell-bound complement, especially C3. These methods include fluorescence flow cytometry, radioimmunoassay, and enzyme-linked immunosorbent assay (ELISA).[61, 62] In addition, the development of monoclonal antibodies that can distinguish among the various fragments of C3 may prove useful in laboratory diagnosis.

Measurement of Complement Activation

Until the mid-1980s, there were no readily accessible tests of complement activation. The activation of complement was implied by a decrease in the level of an individual component, most often C4, in a clinical setting in which activation was suspected. Although this approach may be of some utility in the outpatient setting, it is of little use in the investigation of very sick patients, especially those receiving blood products. The problem with this diagnostic approach is twofold. First, reduction in the C4 level can occur from decreased synthesis of the protein in the liver rather than from consumption. Second, because of the presence of null genes for C4, the normal range for C4 is very wide; a person with a C4 level that usually is at the high end of the normal range may activate more than 50% of C4 before the measured level exceeds the normal range. Only laboratories with specialized complement expertise had methods permitting the detection of activation peptides of complement, generally by gel electrophoresis techniques or by radioimmunoassay of small complement fragments remaining in solution after precipitation of native protein and large fragments.

With the advent of monoclonal antibody technology, antibodies have been made that are capable of recognizing neoantigens expressed in the activation peptides of complement. These antibodies have been used in the formulation of commercial ELISA kits. ELISA tests that detect the activation peptides of either the classical (C4d) or alternative (factor Bb) pathway or both (C3a, C5a, iC3b, and C5b-9) are currently available. In addition, descriptions of many other monoclonal antibody-based activation peptide assays can now be found in the literature. These activation-dependent assays enable the definite differentiation between the patients with complement activation and those with decreased production of complement proteins.

In summary, the burgeoning of research activity on the complement system has produced a clearer understanding of the biochemistry of these important proteins. This knowledge has led to the development of better diagnostic tools, as well as to the invention of therapeutic modalities to control unwanted complement activation.

REFERENCES

1. Ross GD. Immunobiology of the Complement System. Orlando, FL: Academic Press, 1986, pp 1–19.
2. Morgan BP. Complement: Clinical Aspects and Relevance to Disease. New York: Academic Press, 1990.
3. Sim RB, Reid KBM. C1: molecular interactions with activating systems. Immunol Today 1991; 12:307.
4. Perkins SJ, Nealis AS. Solution structure of human and mouse immunoglobulin M by synchrotron X-ray scattering and molecular graphics modelling. J Mol Biol 1991; 221:1345.
5. Levine RP, Dodds AW. The thiolester bond of C3. Curr Top Microbiol Immunol 1989; 153:73.
6. Szalai AJ, Briles DE, Volanakis JE. Role of complement in C-reactive protein-mediated protection of mice from *Streptococcus pneumoniae.* Infect Immunol 1996; 64:4850.
7. Bristow CL, Boackle RJ. Evidence for the binding of human serum amyloid P component to C1q and Fab. Mol Immunol 1986; 23:1045.
8. Pepys MB, Blatz ML. Acute phase proteins with special reference to C-reactive protein and related proteins (pentraxins) and serum amyloid A protein. Adv Immunol 1983; 34:141.
9. Lu JH, Thiel S, Wiedemann H, et al. Binding of the pentamer/hexamer forms of mannan-binding protein to zymosan activates the proenzyme C1rC1s2 complex of the classical pathway of complement, without involvement of C1q. J Immunol 1990; 144:2287.
10. Lachmann PJ, Hughes-Jones NC. Initiation of complement activation. Springer Semin Immunopathol 1984; 7:143.
11. Devine DV. The regulation of complement on cell surfaces. Trans Med Rev 1991; 5:123.
12. Donaldson VH, Bissler JJ. C1 inhibitors and their genes: an update. J Clin Lab Med 1992; 119:330.
13. Hillarp A, Dahlback B. The protein S–binding site localized to the central core of C4b-binding protein. J Biol Chem 1987; 262:11300.
14. Hammer CH, Jacobs RM, Frank MM. Isolation and characterization of a novel plasma protein which binds to activated C4 of the classical complement pathway. J Biol Chem 1989; 264:2283.
15. Farries TC, Lachmann PJ, Harrison RA. Analysis of the interaction between properdin and factor B, components of the alternative pathway C3 convertase of complement. Biochem J 1988; 253:667.
16. Murphy BF, Kirszbaum L, Walker ID, et al. SP-40,40, a newly identified normal human serum protein found in the SC5b-9 complex of complement and in the immune deposits in glomerulonephritis. J Clin Invest 1988; 81:1858.
17. Choi NH, Mazda T, Tomita M. A serum protein SP40,40 modulates the formation of membrane attack complex of complement on erythrocytes. Mol Immunol 1989; 26:835.
18. Jenne DE, Lowin B, Peitsch MC, et al. Clusterin (complement lysis inhibitor) forms a high density lipoprotein complex with apolipoprotein A-I in human plasma. J Biol Chem 1991; 266:11030.

19. Nicholson-Weller A, Burge J, Fearon DT, et al. Isolation of a human erythrocyte membrane glycoprotein with decay accelerating activity for C3 convertases of the complement system. J Immunol 1982; 129:184.
20. Medof ME, Kinoshita T, Nussenzweig V. Inhibition of complement activation on the surface of cells after incorporation of decay-accelerating factor (DAF) into their membranes. J Exp Med 1984; 160:1558.
21. Pangburn MK. Differences between the binding sites of the complement regulatory proteins DAF, CR1, and factor H on C3 convertases. J Immunol 1986; 136:2216.
22. Kinoshita T, Medof ME, Nussenzweig V. Endogenous association of decay-accelerating factor (DAF) with C4b and C3b on cell membranes. J Immunol 1986; 136:3390.
23. Berger M, Medof ME. Increased expression of complement decay accelerating factor during activation of human neutrophils. J Clin Invest 1987; 79:214.
24. Seya T, Atkinson JP. Functional properties of membrane cofactor protein of complement. Biochem J 1989; 264:581.
25. Schoermark S, Rauterberg, EW, Shin ML, et al. Homologous species restriction in lysis of human erythrocytes: a membrane-derived protein with C8-binding capacity functions as an inhibitor. J Immunol 1986; 136:1772.
26. Zalman LS, Wood LM, Muller-Eberhard JH. Isolation of a human erythrocyte membrane protein capable of inhibiting expression of homologous complement transmembrane channels. Proc Nat Acad Sci U S A 1986; 82:7711.
27. Holguin MH, Frederick LR, Bernshaw NJ, et al. Isolation and characterization of a membrane protein from normal human erythrocytes that inhibits reactive lysis of the erythrocytes of paroxysmal nocturnal hemoglobinuria. J Clin Invest 1989; 84:7.
28. Sugita Y, Nakamo Y, Tomita M. Isolation from human erythrocytes of a new membrane protein which inhibits the formation of complement transmembrane channels. J Biochem (Tokyo) 1988; 104:633.
29. Okada N, Harada R, Fujita T, et al. Monoclonal antibodies capable of causing hemolysis of neuraminidase-treated human erythrocytes by homologous complement. J Immunol 1989; 143:2262.
30. Stefanova I, Hilgert I, Kirstofova H, et al. Characterization of a broadly expressed human leukocyte antigen MEM-43 anchored in membrane through phosphatidylinositol. Mol Immunol 1989; 26:153.
31. Lockert DH, Kaufman KM, Chang CP, et al. Identity of the segment of human complement C8 recognized by complement regulatory protein CD59. J Biol Chem 1995; 270:19723.
32. Husler T, Lockert DH, Kaufman KM, et al. Chimeras of human complement C9 reveal the site recognized by complement regulatory protein CD59. J Biol Chem 1995; 270:3483.
33. Rosse WF. Paroxysmal nocturnal hemoglobinuria as a molecular disease. Medicine 1997; 76:63.
34. Telen MJ, Green AM. The Inab phenotype: characterization of the membrane protein and complement regulatory defect. Blood 1989; 74:437.
35. Merry AH, Rawlinson VI, Uchikawa M, et al. Studies on the sensitivity to complement-mediated lysis of erythrocytes (Inab phenotype) with a deficiency of DAF (decay accelerating factor). Br J Haematol 1989; 73:248.
36. Yamashina M, Ueda E, Kinoshita T, et al. Inherited complete deficiency of 20-kilodalton homologous restriction factor (CD59) as a cause of paroxysmal nocturnal hemoglobinuria. N Engl J Med 1990; 323:1184.
37. Farries TC, Atkinson JP. Evolution of the complement system. Immunol Today 1991; 12:295.
38. Marcus D, Alper CA. Methods for allotyping complement proteins. *In* Manual of Clinical Immunology. Washington, DC: American Society for Microbiology, 1986, pp 185–196.
39. Winkelstein JA, Colten HR. Genetically determined disorders of the complement system. *In* The Metabolic Basis of Disease. St. Louis: McGraw-Hill, 1987, pp 2711–2737.
40. Campbell W, Okada H. An arginine specific carboxypeptidase generated in blood during coagulation or inflammation which is unrelated to carboxypeptidase N or its subunits. Biochem Biophys Res Comm 1989; 162:933.
41. Shiba M, Tadokoro K, Sawanobori M, et al. Activation of the contact system by filtration of platelet concentrates with a negatively charged white cell–removal filter and measurement of venous blood bradykinin level in patients who received filtered platelets. Transfusion 1997; 37:457.
42. Snyder EL, Mechanic S, Baril L, et al. Removal of soluble biologic response modifiers (complement and chemokines) by a bedside white cell–reduction filter. Transfusion 1996; 36:707.
43. Morgan BP. Complement membrane attack on nucleated cells: resistance, recovery and non-lethal effects. Biochem J 1989; 264:1.
44. Devine DV. The effects of complement activation on platelets. Curr Top Microbiol Immunol 1992; 178:101.
45. Peerschke EIB, Ghebrehiwet B. Human blood platelets possess specific binding sites for C1q. J Immunol 1987; 138:1537.
46. Nepomuceno RR, Henschen-Edman AH, Burgess WH, et al. cDNA cloning and primary structure analysis of C1qR(P), the human C1q/MBL/SPA receptor that mediates enhanced phagocytosis in vitro. Immunity 1997; 6:119.
47. Nepomuceno RR, Tenner AJ. C1qRP, the C1q receptor that enhances phagocytosis, is detected specifically in human cells of myeloid lineage, endothelial cells, and platelets. J Immunol 1998; 160:1929.
48. Butko P, Nicholson-Weller A, Wessels MR. Role of complement and complement receptor C1qR in the antibody-independent killing of group B streptococcus. Adv Exp Med Biol 1997; 418:941.
49. Sims PJ, Wiedmer T. The response of human platelets to activated components of the complement system. Immunol Today 1991; 12:338.
50. Wiedmer T, Esmon CT, Sims PJ. Complement proteins C5b–9 stimulate procoagulant activity through platelet prothrombinase. Blood 1986; 68:875.
51. Bode AP, Miller DT, Newman SL, et al. Plasmin activity and complement activation during storage of citrated platelet concentrates. J Lab Clin Med 1989; 113:94.
52. Gyongyossy-issa MIC, McLeod E, Devine DV. Complement activation in platelet concentrates is surface-dependent and modulated by the platelets. J Lab Clin Med 1994; 123:859.
53. Dalmasso AP. Complement in the pathophysiology and diagnosis of human disease. CRC Crit Rev Clin Lab Sci 1986; 24:123.
54. Cines DB, Schreiber RD. Effect of anti-$P1^{A1}$ antibody on human platelets: I. The role of complement. Blood 1979; 53:567.
55. Dixon RH, Rosse WF. Mechanisms of complement-mediated activation of human blood platelets in vitro: comparison of normal and paroxysmal nocturnal hemoglobinuria platelets. J Clin Invest 1977; 59:360.
56. Schreiber AD. An experimental model of immune hemolytic anemia. Ann Intern Med 1977; 87:211.
57. Schifferli JA, Ng YC, Peters DK. The role of complement and its receptor in the elimination of immune complexes. N Engl J Med 1986; 315:488.
58. Anderson DC, Springer TA. Leukocyte adhesion deficiency: an inherited defect in the MAC-1, LFA-1, and p150,95 glycoproteins. Annu Rev Med 1987; 38:175.
59. Weisman HF, Bartow T, Leppo MK, et al. Soluble complement receptor type 1: in vivo inhibitor of complement suppressing post-ischemic myocardial inflammation and necrosis. Science 1990; 249:146.
60. Erdei A, Fust G, Gergely J. The role of C3 in the immune response. Immunol Today 1991; 12:332.
61. Garraty G. The significance of IgG on the red cell surface. Trans Med Rev 1987; 1:47.
62. Schwartz KA. Platelet antibody: review of detection methods. Am J Hematol 1988; 29:106.

CHAPTER 8

Transfusion Genetics

Geoff Daniels
Emanuel Hackel

DEVELOPMENT OF THE MENDELIAN THEORY OF INHERITANCE

The year 1900 was indeed a propitious one for the science of transfusion medicine. It was the year of the landmark, although serendipitous, discovery by Landsteiner[1, 2] of the basis for normal antigenic variations in human blood. Moreover, it was the year of the discovery, independently by three investigators (DeVries,[3] Correns,[4] and von Tschermak[5]), of what Mendel[6] had published 35 years earlier, thereby inaugurating the modern science of genetics. Landsteiner and his colleagues[2, 7] appreciated the implications of his findings for transfusion as well as for forensic medicine. Nonetheless, 10 more years passed before von Dungern and Hirszfeld[8] could establish unequivocally that the ABO blood groups were inherited according to mendelian principles, as had been suggested by Epstein and Ottenberg[9] in 1908. Even though they demonstrated inheritance, von Dungern and Hirszfeld were not able to deduce the exact manner by which it occurred. Analysis by Bernstein[10, 11] more than 12 years later elucidated the three-allele explanation for inheritance of blood groups.

During the early years of the investigation of blood groups, a comparable extension of mendelian principles developed from the work of many investigators studying many different species. However, except for ABO blood groups, very little of this work concerned humans. A notable exception was the study of the human metabolic disorder, alkaptonuria, in which Garrod[12] identified a pattern of inheritance expected for a mendelian recessive trait. A few years later, Bateson[13] described several human inherited traits. Although he anticipated the finding of more of them, he apparently had serious doubts as late as 1909 as to the widespread applicability of mendelian principles to normal variations in human populations.[14] By that time, Garrod[15] had identified still more of what he called *inborn errors of metabolism,* all inherited as mendelian recessive traits. Human biochemical genetics was thus initiated, although relatively few people realized it then.

It was a time of great activity in the field of genetics. There was strong interest in using mendelian principles to improve the breeding stock of commercially important species. Certainly, breeders of both plant and animal species had adopted a number of practices before the rediscovery of Mendel's work, but these were neither uniformly nor consistently successful. The application of mendelian principles did indeed resolve a number of problems, but not until 1908 were the basic principles of population genetics clearly and unequivocally enunciated by Hardy[16] and Weinberg.[17] Although there is no evidence of any communication between them, they independently presented the concept of gene frequency in a population as a governing characteristic of genotype and phenotype frequencies. Castle[18] earlier had presented the concept of equilibrium—that is, unchanging frequencies of genotypes—in a randomly mating population not subject to selection. It remained for Hardy, a mathematician, and Weinberg, a biologist and physician, to set down the rules and mathematical model for what is now called the *Hardy-Weinberg equilibrium.*

Although it took a quarter of a century for the general details of the union between blood groups and genetics to be worked out, developments thereafter proceeded at a more rapid pace. Not long after Bernstein's[10, 11] explanation of ABO inheritance, Landsteiner and Levine[19–22] used antibodies made in rabbits to discover the MN and P systems, which were independent of the ABO system. The pattern of inheritance that they found was precisely that expected from classical mendelian genetics. Subsequently, many more systems were uncovered, which in all cases were shown to be inherited according to mendelian principles.

Gregor Mendel was an Augustinian monk in the Czech city of Brno who taught mathematics at the monastery school. (During his life the city was known as Brünn and was in the Austro-Hungarian Empire.) Much of what is known today in genetics is traceable to him and his experiments on garden peas (*Pisum sativum*). His formulation of a theory to explain his experimental results may well have been successful as a result of his mathematical acumen. Scientists have speculated for years as to why Mendel's work was overlooked for 35 years; there are many hypotheses but no real answers. Even today, in the era of molecular genetics, the fundamental basis for the transmission of characters from one generation to the next is, with minor modification, as Mendel explained it.

The importance of the numerical relationship introduced by Mendel cannot be overemphasized. Using the mathematical relationships implied by his theory, Mendel was able to explain the results of his experiments. An essential factor in his theory was the particulate nature of factors transmitted from one generation to the next.

(Mendel never used the term *gene;* that was introduced much later.) How he first conceived the idea of particulate factors of inheritance remains unclear. Chromosomes had not yet been discovered, and he made no mention of any other specific objects or structures in body cells or gametes. It is clear from his paper, however, that Mendel imagined a distinct unchanging entity or particle to be present in all cells. He attributed two of these (per trait) to each body (somatic) cell, but only one to each gamete.

Mendel carried out a large number of matings between garden pea plants. He chose several traits for consideration, and these formed the basis for his conclusions. When individuals from pure strains were mated, he observed that the "hybrids" (F_1 heterozygotes) showed one or the other of the parental types:

> These characters which are transmitted entire, or almost unchanged in the hybridization, and therefore in themselves constitute the characters of the hybrid, are termed the *dominant,* and those which become latent in the process *recessive.* The expression "recessive" has been chosen because the characters thereby designated withdraw or entirely disappear in the hybrids, but nevertheless reappear unchanged in their progeny. . . .
>
> It was furthermore shown by the whole of the experiments that it is perfectly immaterial whether the dominant character belongs to the seed-bearer or to the pollen-parent; the form of the hybrid remains identical in both cases.[6]

In mating the hybrids (F_1 individuals) to obtain an F_2 generation, Mendel did nothing new. However, in counting the different kinds of individuals in F_2, he must have had some theory in mind. For this, his training as a mathematician yields an important clue to his thinking. The very act of bringing in the concept of a numerical relationship among the F_2 individuals was a revolutionary one at the time and clearly indicates a conceptual scheme (or theory.)[23]

"If now the results of the whole of the experiments be brought together, there is found, as between the number of forms with the dominant and recessive characters, an average ratio of 2.98 to 1, or 3 to 1."[6] This conclusion was based on his observations of more than 20,000 F_2 examples.

Commenting upon Mendel's work in 1936, Fisher[24] found that the data were too close to expectation to have arisen by chance. Bennett[25] summarized the situation as follows (quotations are from Fisher[24]): "To account for the rather sensational evidence that 'the data of most, if not all, of the experiments have been falsified so as to agree closely with Mendel's expectations,' Fisher suggested that Mendel was possibly deceived by an assistant 'who knew too well what was expected.' " The controversy has long since subsided and currently receives little if any attention. Even in this era of molecular genetics, Mendel's theory, with its subsequent modifications, remains the touchstone of classical genetics.

In addition to the numerical relationships, Mendel had to know that the dominant individuals among his subjects were of two different types. As he described the situation,

> The dominant character can have here a *double signification*—[namely] that of a parental character [homozygote], or a hybrid-character [heterozygote]. In which of the two significations it appears in each separate case can only be determined by the following generation. As a parental character [homozygote] it must pass over unchanged to the whole of the offspring; as a hybrid character [heterozygote], on the other hand, it must maintain the same behavior as in the first generation [F_2].[6]

(Mendel was concerned primarily with the nature of the offspring of hybrids, so he referred to the F_2 as the "first" generation.)

For the critical determination of the genotypes of the F_2 individuals, Mendel conducted the necessary experimental matings, the results of which he described as follows:

> Those forms which in the first generation [F_2] exhibit the recessive character do not further vary in the second generation [F_3] as regards this character; they remain constant in their offspring.
>
> It is otherwise with those which possess the dominant character in the first generation [bred from the hybrids]. Of those, *two*-thirds yield offspring which display the dominant and recessive characters in the proportion of 3 to 1, and thereby show exactly the same ratio as the hybrid form, while only *one*-third remains with the dominant character constant.[6]

Here he was able to show clearly that among the F_2 individuals exhibiting the dominant phenotype, there were two distinct genotypes occurring in a ratio of 2 heterozygotes to 1 homozygote. This could happen only if the factors were particulate and unchanging, as opposed to the notion of an infinitely divisible fluid. Mendel summarized this portion of the work as follows:

> The ratio of 3 to 1, in accordance with which the distribution of the dominant and recessive characters results in the first generation [F_2], resolves itself therefore in all experiments into the ratio of 2:1:1 if the dominant character be differentiated according to its significance as a hybrid-character [heterozygote] or as a parental one [homozygote]. Since the members of the first generation [F_2] spring directly from the seed of hybrids [F_1], *it is now clear that the hybrids form seeds having one or the other of the two differentiating characters, and of these one half develop again the hybrid form, while the other half yield plants which remain constant and receive the dominant or the recessive characters [respectively] in equal numbers.*[6]

Without naming specifically the hereditary factors to which he referred, Mendel nevertheless had postulated a pattern for their behavior. Only by assuming the activity of these imagined particles could his factual observations be explained.

This is a classic illustration of the role of theory in science. Theories not only enable investigators to explain otherwise unexplainable observations; they also yield many deductions from which researchers can draw working hypotheses that can be tested empirically. These tests, if they confirm the hypotheses, lend further support to the theory. So it was in the case of Mendel's experiments. His results, obtained empirically, supported the hypotheses deduced from his conceptual scheme. Since then, there have been countless modifications and improvements, but the mendelian theory regarding the transmission of characters from one generation to the next remains a sine qua non for the study of genetics. Of course, the "imagined particle" need no longer be imagined; first chromosomes and then DNA and its elaborate behavior readily fit with what had been postulated for genes. There have been other accommodations as well to account for concepts such as linkage, crossing over, penetrance, and mutation. But the modifications made over the years have not detracted from the value, and indeed the elegance, of what Mendel presented in 1865.[23]

Reduced to its simplest form, Mendel's theory may best be summarized by these postulates:

1. There are particles governing hereditary traits that are passed from one generation to the next.
2. Each individual contains two such particles for each trait; these, however, segregate at gamete formation, with only one of each pair going to a single gamete. (This is the *law of segregation.*)
3. An individual containing two unlike particles for a given trait may show the effect of only one of these. (This is the concept of *dominance.*) The dominant or recessive nature of the particles does not affect their transmission to the next generation.
4. The assortment of a pair of these particles is independent of the other pairs. (This is the *law of independent assortment.*) Thus the presence of the particles in a single gamete results from random distribution of the particles contained in the individual.
5. The results of matings are describable in terms of mathematical probability.

REFINEMENTS OF MENDEL'S THEORY

During the years 1865 to 1900, there were a number of technical developments that should have contributed to the acceptability of the mendelian theory. Among them were those that led to the discovery of chromosomes and their observed behavior, which was very similar to that proposed by Mendel for his imagined particles. During somatic cell division, the cell nucleus divides by mitosis, ensuring each new cell the same number and same kinds of chromosomes as the original cell. During gametogenesis, however, meiosis occurs. This reduction division results in only one of each pair of homologous chromosomes in any given gamete. Together, both these findings provide a mechanism for what Mendel had postulated.

By 1900, the world was more prepared for mendelian theory. Three investigators[3–5] had published their findings, giving Mendel full credit for his earlier theory, and Garrod,[12, 15] publishing as early as 1902, made full use of mendelian theory. Fisher[24] commented that "Mendel's contemporaries may be blamed for failing to recognize his discovery, perhaps through resting too great a confidence on comprehensive compilations."

Mendel's genetic mechanism, universally applicable as it was, required some modification to conform with subsequent findings. The similarity between the postulated behavior of Mendel's particles during segregation and the observed behavior of chromosomes during meiosis was so great that chromosomes soon came to be regarded as the carriers of the particles. It was during this time that Johannsen[26] introduced the term *gene,* which was at once almost universally adopted. Mendel's factors or particles at last had a name. It soon became apparent that there were far more genes than chromosomes, and thus there had to be many genes on a given chromosome.

Genes for different traits, when carried on the same chromosome, may *not* follow the law of independent assortment. Because the chromosome is the unit of transmission to gametes (and thus to the zygote and to the offspring), genes on the same chromosome are transmitted together. The gametes of heterozygotes are therefore not random; they contain genes in the same combinations as they were received from the parents. In 1910, this explanation was offered by Morgan,[27] who hypothesized that some genes were apparently transmitted together because they were on the same chromosome. He called this *linkage.* If a given chromosome contains a number of genes, all of these are assorted to the gametes together, not independently. Mendel, in considering the results of his experiments, based his conclusion regarding multifactorial crosses only on traits governed by unlinked genes that assorted independently.

Morgan's concept of linkage had to be incorporated into Mendel's basic theory because it explained the exceptions to independent assortment and aided considerably in understanding the gene-chromosome relationship. Initially at Columbia University and later at the California Institute of Technology, Morgan worked with *Drosophila,* for which hundreds of traits were known but only four pairs of chromosomes were observed. A one-to-one relationship between genes and chromosomes was therefore impossible. However, if the assumption were made that genes are *in* or *on* chromosomes, then it was possible for relatively few chromosomes to carry all the genes postulated. Because the chromosomes are the units independently assorted, it follows that genes on the same chromosome are *not* independently assorted.

Theories are sometimes still new when exceptions to them are noted. Morgan and other investigators found a number of instances in which it was not possible to explain empirical data on the basis of the old (Mendel) or the new (Mendel-Morgan) principle of independent assortment. Morgan attributed the lack of expected mendelian ratios in some of his experiments to linkage. However, when dealing with large numbers, he sometimes found that his results were close to what he expected on the basis of linkage but not precisely so. Among the offspring there were individuals whose phenotypes could not be explained on the basis of either independent assortment or linkage. This may be illustrated by a hypothetical example:

Consider the following mating in which *A* and *a* are genes for one trait, and *B* and *b* are genes for a different trait:

$$AABB \times aabb$$

$$\downarrow$$

$$AaBb$$

Situation 1: No linkage; therefore, independent assortment occurs, and the heterozygote, *AaBb,* produces four kinds of gametes in equal numbers, resulting in four genotypic combinations in equal numbers, as shown:

$$AaBb \times aabb$$

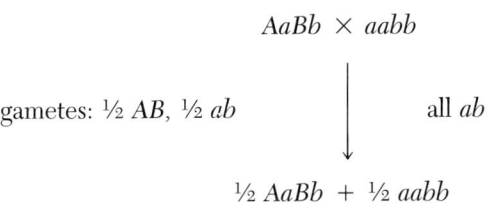

gametes: ¼ *AB*, ¼ *Ab*, ¼ *aB*, ¼ *ab* ↓ all *ab*

$$\tfrac{1}{4}\,AaBB + \tfrac{1}{4}\,Aabb + \tfrac{1}{4}\,aaBb + \tfrac{1}{4}\,aabb$$

Situation 2: Linkage; therefore, independent assortment does not occur, and the heterozygote produces only two kinds of gametes in equal numbers. The gene combinations in the gametes depend on the combinations in the parents of the heterozygote; in this example, *A* and *B* came from one parent and *a* and *b* from the other. Therefore, in this case, only two kinds of offspring are expected from the mating shown:

$$AaBb \times aabb$$

gametes: ½ *AB*, ½ *ab* ↓ all *ab*

$$\tfrac{1}{2}\,AaBb + \tfrac{1}{2}\,aabb$$

Situation 3: However, what Morgan and his associates observed was the following:

$$AaBb \times aabb$$

↓

$$x\%\ AaBb + y\%\ Aabb + y\%\ aaBb + x\%\ aabb$$
$$(2x + 2y = 100\%)$$

It is apparent that if x = y, the results are exactly the same as those obtained in the nonlinked case (situation 1), in which independent assortment occurs. In such a case, it is impossible to recognize linkage. On the other hand, if y = 0, only the results of linkage are found, as described in situation 2. Morgan and colleagues, to account for their actual observations (situation 3), assumed that the genes were arranged in a linear order on the chromosomes and that occasionally these chromosomes exchanged parts, causing new combinations of heretofore linked genes. This phenomenon, called *crossing-over* or *recombination,* occurred in the hypothetical example in the formation of 2y% of the gametes of the heterozygous parent. (Crossing-over in homozygotes is obviously not detectable.)

Observations of chromosomes during meiosis showed that homologous chromosomes are entwined for a time preceding division. Sometimes, during this entwining process, breaks occur in the chromosome, resulting in an exchange of parts. This exchange of chromosome parts causes the production of progeny that have combinations of genes opposite to those expected from linkage. It must be realized that many primordial germ cells undergo meiosis at a given time. In only a certain percentage of these does chromosome breakage and exchange occur between gene locations (loci; singular, locus) under consideration, causing crossing-over of genes. This crossing-over, however, has been found to occur with regular frequency between any two genes. By reasoning that genes existing closer together in the linear arrangement on the chromosome would have fewer crossovers and genes farther apart would show more crossing-over, it has been possible to infer the relative distances between the various genes on a chromosome. The percentage of crossing-over between two linked genes therefore represents the relative distance between them. For example, if crossing-over between the *A-a* and *B-b* loci occurs 5% of the time, these genes are presumed to be five units apart on the chromosomes; if 20% of crossovers are detected, these loci are said to be 20 units apart. The unit of relative distance on the chromosome is the *centimorgan,* which equals 1% of crossing-over.

Linkage has been universally applied whenever genes appear to be on the same chromosome. However, what about the situation in which such gene loci are 50 or more units apart? On the basis of crossover percentage, such loci would give no evidence of linkage, and yet, they are on the same chromosome. Renwick[28] proposed that the term *synteny* be used for all genes on the same chromosome, including those too far apart for the crossover percentage to interfere with apparently independent assortment ratios. That they were on the same chromosome would be established from their relationship to other genes on the chromosome. Thus linkage is a special kind of synteny and the term would be used only to denote a sufficiently close proximity on the chromosome so that the absence of independent assortment is clearly detectable.

The crossover percentages obtained from linkage studies made it possible to infer the relative distances between loci, which in turn allowed construction of a chromosome map showing the relative positions of the loci along the length of a given chromosome. Additional techniques have been developed for such studies: when used in combination with the classic (crossover) method, these techniques have permitted a great increase in the rate at which gene loci are positioned relative to one another. Cytological techniques, based on observed changes in staining and banding patterns due to insertions and deletions and chromosomal breakage, provide much useful information. Hybrid cell lines, somatic cell tissue cultures, base pair sequencing of DNA and RNA, restriction fragment length polymorphisms, and in situ hybridization, among others, all have important functions in determining the order of loci (and thus the genes) on the chromosome. This mapping is the goal of the Human Genome Project. On January 20, 1999, Online Mendelian Inheritance in Man (www.ncbi.nlm.nih.gov/Omim/) listed 6981 established human gene loci: 6561 autosomal, 357 X-linked, 26 Y-linked, and 37 mitochondrial.

Although the expanding knowledge of human genetics includes the blood group systems, and although the mechanisms of their inheritance and immunology are better understood than ever before, most blood groups continue to follow the "WYGTG-YMTA" (pronounced "wig-tig yimta" or "wiggy-tiggy yimta") system of immu-

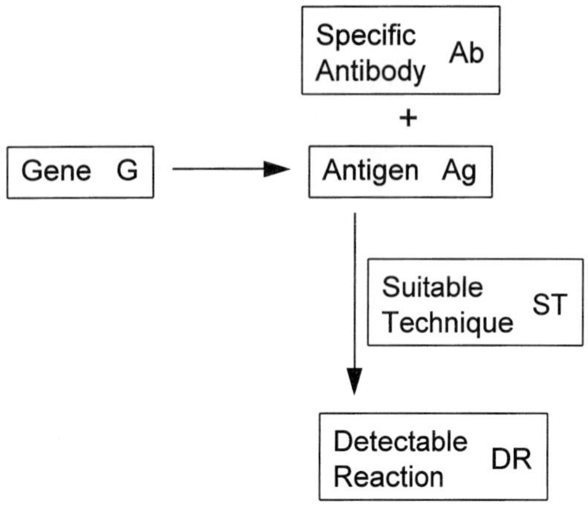

Figure 8–1. A schematic portrayal of a gene-antigen-antibody relationship: The "WYGTG-YMTA" hypothesis.

nogenetics. A simple mnemonic for this system is "*W*hen *y*ou've *g*ot *t*he *g*ene, *y*ou *m*ake *t*he *a*ntigen." Figure 8–1 is a schematic diagram of this system.

Initially the existence of genes, antigens, and antibodies had to be imagined, but this is no longer the case. The ever more refined probing of their molecular depths provides consistent and workable elucidation of what they really are and, indeed, that they really exist.

If in the course of testing, a detectable reaction (DR) is obtained, the usual conclusion is that antigen (Ag) is present and that it is due to the presence of the gene (G). Easily overlooked is the required presence of antibody (Ab) and a suitable technique (ST), without either of which, DR cannot be obtained even in the presence of Ag and G. In view of all the elements of this system, it becomes easy to reason that a DR means that Ag, and therefore G, are present.

A problem arises when, with Ab and ST present, DR is not obtained when G presumably must be present. Yet, in terms of the system, G must be considered absent unless the situation is one shown in Figure 8–2. In this instance, not only must G be present to obtain Ag (and DR), but a second gene (G′) must also be present; two different genes are required for the antigen to be produced in this case.

In the example shown in Figure 8–2, the second gene (G′) functions to make a precursor (P), on which the original gene (G) can act. There are other possible patterns of action for G′. It may be a regulator for G, or it may be the functional allele to an inhibitor that has a negative effect on G. Indeed, it may be that a series of genes, G′, G″,..., G_n, is required to make a series of products that act on the original G to make the necessary Ag to produce DR. As discussed later, further analyses of blood groups, particularly by molecular methods, have shown that many such complexities occur.

The classical approach to genetics is rooted in the study of inherited characters. These characters, such as eye color, the height of a plant, or the presence or absence of a disease, may be easily recognized or measured, but the underlying genetics may be extremely complex involving interactions between genes at a number of different loci. A biochemical assay, in which the polypeptide gene product is analyzed, quantitatively or qualitatively, can be interpreted more directly in terms of single genes. The discovery in the 1950s that the genetic code resides in the DNA, and the subsequent deciphering of that code, opened the study of a molecular approach to genetics.[29, 30] Genetic variation may now be scrutinized by determining the sequences of individual genes or their messenger RNA transcripts.

APPLICATIONS OF GENETICS TO HUMAN BLOOD GROUPS

An understanding of the relationship between genes and antigens has been extremely fruitful for dealing with problems in transfusion medicine. Race and Sanger,[31] for example, used knowledge from classical genetics in the consideration of transfusion and other related immunological problems. The concepts of classical genetics are still widely in use, but to these must be added the more recent input from biochemistry and molecular genetics. For most of the remainder of this chapter, human red cell antigens are used as examples.

In 1900 Landsteiner[1, 2] identified two antigens, A and B, and these were later recognized to represent alleles at a single locus.[8–11] There are now 268 blood group antigens recognized by the International Society of Blood Transfusion, and some of these antigens have variant forms. Most of the blood group antigens are classified into 25 genetically defined systems, each containing one or more antigens encoded by a single gene or, in the case of the MNS, Rh, and Chido-Rodgers systems, by two or three very closely linked homologous genes.[32–34] The chromosomal locations of all these genes have now been determined. Each system is genetically discrete. Some genes representing different systems are syntenic (e.g., *KEL*, *YT*, and *CO* on chromosome 7) and some are even linked, but there is always a measurable recombination rate between them (e.g., *LU* and *LW* are approximately 5 centimorgans apart on chromosome 19). Genes representing all but 4 of the 25 systems have been cloned, and in most cases, the molecular bases of the polymorphisms have

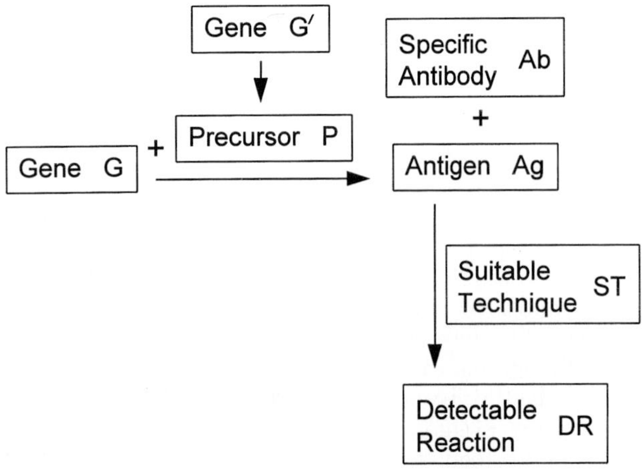

Figure 8–2. A modification of Figure 8–1 to accommodate expansion of the gene-antigen-antibody relationship.

been elucidated.[35] The majority of polymorphisms result from one or more missense mutations, single nucleotide base changes that alter the encoded amino acid. The amino acid substitutions usually occur within the red cell surface protein, but in the ABO system, for example, the amino acid substitutions alter the specificity of a glycosyltransferase that catalyzes the biosynthesis of the carbohydrate chains of membrane glycoproteins and glycolipids. In addition, other genetic mechanisms account for blood group polymorphism, including single nucleotide deletions, deletion of a whole gene, and exchange of genetic material between closely linked homologous genes.

Often a blood group phenotype may be predicted from the DNA sequence of the encoding gene, but it is important to remember that an antigen is defined by an antibody, or at least by an immune response, not by a nucleotide sequence. As discussed later, blood groups can be accurately determined only by analyzing the red cell surface, because there are many, often unpredicted factors that can prevent the expected reflection of a DNA sequence at the cell surface.

The ABO System

ABO, the most important blood group system from the transfusion standpoint, is a suitable vehicle for considering the changing "styles" in genetics. It is still essentially explicable in terms of mendelian classical genetics; indeed, those fundamental concepts are all that is needed for a simple but nonetheless satisfactory explanation.[10, 11] Add to this the many twists and nuances developed over the years,[31, 32] and classical gene action, though modified, still suffices as an explanation. The work of many investigators on the biochemical nature of the ABO antigens and the transferases that make (or do not make) the antigens has added immeasurably to the understanding of the system and its genetics.[36–39] Most recently comes the work of the molecular geneticists. They have stripped away the mystique of the ABO genes, permitting a thorough examination of what goes on inside.

ABO, the first blood group system discovered, was not only one of the first human characters shown to be inherited in a mendelian manner but was also the first blood group to enter the biochemical era of human genetics. The immunodominant oligosaccharides of A- and B-active structures, however, were originally determined not from red cell membrane–borne antigens but from soluble antigens in body fluids.[36–39] Clausen and Hakomori[40] introduced the term *histo-blood group* for ABO, H, and related antigens when they emphasized that these structures constitute major allogeneic antigens of most epithelial cell types and that these antigens appear earlier in evolution in ectodermal and endodermal tissue than in mesenchymal hematopoietic tissues and cells.

The products of the *A* and *B* alleles of the *ABO* gene are glycosyltransferases that catalyze the transfer of *N*-acetylgalactosamine and galactose, respectively, to a precursor oligosaccharide chain called H. In people with group O blood types, the *A* and *B* allele–specified glycosyltransferases are not present and H remains unmodified. H, the precursor of A and B, is synthesized by a glycosyltransferase produced by a gene independent of *ABO*. Thus the genetic control of the ABO antigens can be considered in terms of the model in Figure 8–2, in which gene *G* represents an *A* or *B* allele of the *ABO* gene and gene *G′* represents an active allele of the *H* gene. This model provided an explanation for the rare Bombay phenotype, initially reported by Bhende and colleagues[41] in 1952, in which persons with *A* or *B* genes had no A, B, or H antigen on their red cells or in their secretions. By the early 1930s, Putkonen[42] had already noticed that a proportion of people with type A, B, or AB red cells had no A or B antigen in their body fluids. This inability to secrete ABH antigen was found to be inherited in a mendelian manner, genetically independent of *ABO*.[43] When, in rare individuals, red cells were found with the Bombay phenotype but secretions contained normal quantities of A, B, and H antigens (according to their ABO genotype), tissue-specific regulatory genes active on the *H* gene (gene *G′* in Fig. 8–2) were postulated to explain these discordances between red cell and secretory phenotype.[39, 44] Then in the 1980s, Oriol and his colleagues[45] proposed an alternative thesis, in which two genes control the biosynthesis of H antigen, one active in the ectoderm and mesoderm and responsible for H on red cells, the other active in the endoderm and responsible for H in exocrine secretions. Two fucosyltransferase genes, both on chromosome 19, have subsequently been identified and cloned.[46, 47] These genes, called *FUT1* and *FUT2*, are responsible for biosynthesis of H antigen on red cells and in secretions, respectively. A variety of rare inactivating mutations has been identified in *FUT1* to account for the absence of ABH antigen on red cells in Bombay and related phenotypes,[48, 49] and several mutations in *FUT2* for the absence of ABH antigen from secretions in the nonsecretor phenotype.[47, 50–53]

The *ABO* gene contains seven exons, of which exons 6 and 7 constitute 77% of the coding sequence.[54] *ABO* is unusual in that two alleles at the same locus produce transferase enzymes with different substrate specificities: GDP-*N*-acetylgalactosamine and GDP-galactose are the donor substrates for the *A* and *B* gene products, respectively. The *A* and *B* genes differ by a number of nucleotide base substitutions, four of which, all in exon 7, result in amino acid substitutions, two of which appear to be responsible for determining whether the gene product has *N*-acetylgalactosaminyltransferase (A) or galactosyltransferase (B) activity.[55, 56] There are three common *O* alleles. O^1, the most common, has the same sequence as an *A* allele, apart from a single nucleotide deletion in exon 6 that disrupts the nucleotide-triplet code.[55] The resultant shift in the reading frame changes the code to that of a completely different sequence of amino acids and introduces a premature translation stop codon. Any gene product would be very truncated and lack the catalytic site. A variant O^1 allele (O^{1v}) has the same nucleotide deletion but has a number of other, irrelevant changes in the sequence.[57] The O^2 allele does not have the nucleotide deletion, but it does have a missense mutation that converts the important glycine residue of A-transferase to arginine, presumably inactivating the gene product.[58]

Before the introduction of more sophisticated techniques, such as human leukocyte antigen (HLA) testing and then genetic fingerprinting, blood groups were considered reliable markers for paternity testing, because they followed the basic rules of mendelian inheritance. Suzuki and associates[59] described a paternity case in which the mother had a group B blood type, the child group A, and the putative father group O: an apparent first-order exclusion of paternity. However, many other polymorphic markers failed to support this exclusion. Sequencing of the *ABO* genes of the family showed that the child had an *ABO* gene consisting partly of a *B* gene and partly of an O^1 gene. This hybrid gene had probably arisen in the germline of the mother as a result of crossing-over during meiosis (Fig. 8–3). O^1 and *A* alleles have identical sequences apart from a single nucleotide deletion in exon 6 that prevents the production of an enzymatically active product. In the *B-O* hybrid gene, exon 6 (and, presumably exons 1 to 5) is derived from a *B* allele and therefore does not have the inactivating single nucleotide deletion. This means that the gene product would be enzymatically active, but exons 1 to 6 have no effect on the specificity of the enzyme product, so B-transferase activity would not be expected. Exon 7, which contains the sequence that determines transferase specificity, was derived from an O^1 allele. As exon 7 of an O^1 allele has an identical sequence to that of an *A* allele, the product of this *B-O* hybrid gene has A-transferase activity and the child had group A red cells, despite the fact that neither parent had an *A* gene. Such genetic events may

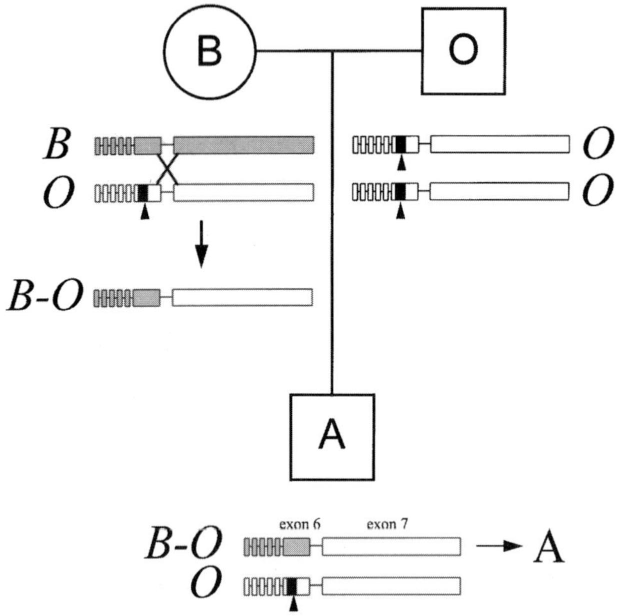

Figure 8–3. Paternity case with a mother with group B blood type, putative father with group O blood type, and child with group A blood type, showing likely crossover event in germline of mother between *B* and *O* alleles to produce an A-transferase–active *B-O* fusion gene.[59] The *large X* represents the site of recombination; the *black triangle* represents the site of nucleotide deletion in *O* allele; *open boxes* represent exons derived from an *O* gene; *shaded boxes* represent exons derived from a *B* allele. Exon 7 derived from an *O* gene has an identical sequence to that derived from an *A* gene.

be considered to be rare, yet Suzuki and associates[59] estimate that similar recombinant alleles occur with a frequency of about 1% in the Japanese population.

The Rh System

Rh is the most complex of the blood group systems, with a total of at least 45 antigens.[32] The complexities of the system began to be appreciated in the early 1940s, and classical genetic analysis of serological data led to two contrasting philosophies: (1) that of Fisher and Race,[60] who considered that the Rh antigens are controlled by three closely linked genes, one producing C or c, one producing D or no D, and one producing E or e; and (2) that of Wiener, who believed that there was only one Rh gene with multiple alleles, each capable of producing multiple antigenic determinants (reviewed by Wiener and Wexler[61]). Many years later, based on a wealth of additional serological information, Tippett[62] proposed that there are two Rh genes, one producing D or no D antigen, the other producing the Cc and Ee antigens. Resolution of this puzzle had to await the cloning of the Rh genes. In 1990 Chérif-Zahar and colleagues[63] and Avent and associates[64] cloned a gene encoding Cc and Ee antigens, and a second gene, encoding D antigen, was cloned by Le Van Kim and coworkers[65] in 1992. Thus it appears that there are two Rh genes, called *RHCE* and *RHD*, as predicted by Tippett.[62] This is not totally at variance with the proposals of Fisher and Race, as Race and Sanger[66] wrote in 1958:

> The existence of three sites where Mendelian inheritance can go on seems unassailable, and to argue whether the three sites are to be placed within or without the boundary of one gene appears particularly unprofitable at the present time when no one seems to know what the boundaries of a gene are.

From the frequencies of the eight possible gene complexes or haplotypes producing D or d (absence of D), C or c, and E or e antigens, Fisher[67] devised a hypothesis that the less frequent haplotypes *(Dce, dcE, dCe, DCE)* were created by crossover events involving two of the more common haplotypes *(Dce, dce, DcE)* and that the very rare haplotype *(dCE)* arose from a crossover event that involved a common haplotype and one of the less common haplotypes. Fisher[67] then extrapolated his theory to postulate that the *Cc* gene lies between *D* and *Ee (D-Cc-Ee)*. This elegant piece of logic, however, has not survived the molecular era: the *C/c* polymorphism is controlled by nucleotide substitutions within exons 1 and 2 of *RHCE* and the *E/e* polymorphism by a nucleotide substitution within exon 5 of *RHCE*, so *C/c* is 5′ of *E/e*; yet a yeast artificial chromosome clone containing the whole of *RHD* and all of *RHCE* except its 5′ end revealed that *RHCE* lies 5′ of *RHD (Cc-Ee-D)* (Fig. 8–4).[68]

After the identification of anti-c and anti-e, the antibodies antithetical to anti-C and anti-E, it was considered only a matter of time before anti-d would be discovered. It took a further 45 years and the application of molecular genetics research to explain why anti-d was never found. Colin and colleagues[69] reported that D-negative people are homozygous for a deletion of *RHD* and, therefore,

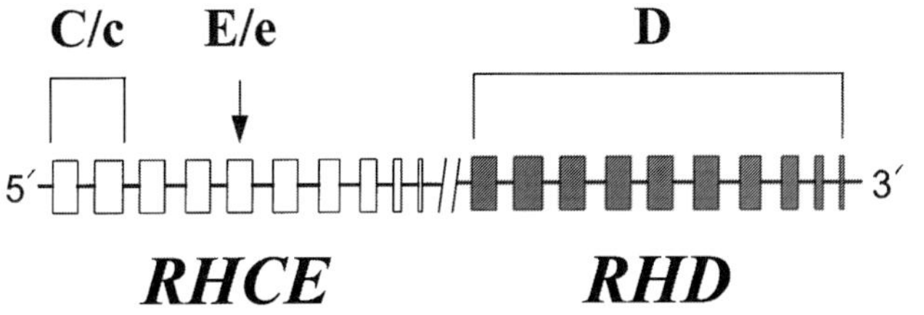

Figure 8–4. Genomic organization of the Rh genes *RHCE* and *RHD*, each comprising 10 exons of coding sequence. The *C/c* polymorphism is associated with four amino acid substitutions encoded by exons 1 and 2 of *RHCE;* the *E/e* polymorphism is associated with an amino acid substitution encoded by exon 5 of *RHCE;* and the numerous D epitopes are encoded by various regions of *RHD.*

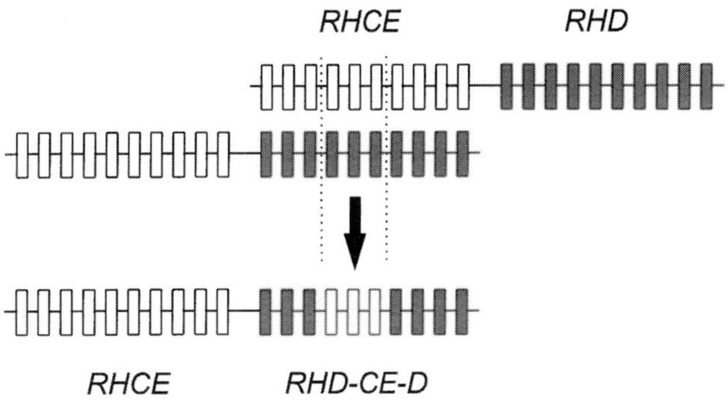

Figure 8–5. Diagrammatic representation of misalignment at meiosis between *RHCE* and *RHD* and recombination, either by double crossover or gene conversion, to produce an *RHD-CE-D* fusion gene.

have no D polypeptide. This explains why D is so immunogenic. Most blood group polymorphisms arise from a single amino acid change within a cell surface protein, and for antibody to be produced, an immune response must be mounted against a relatively trivial change on the protein. D-negative people, however, lack the whole D polypeptide, so an anti-D immune response is mounted against the whole protein, and anti-D serum may contain antibody molecules directed at multiple epitopes on the whole extracellular region of the D protein.

The serological and classical genetic approach to Rh revealed a blood group system that was exceedingly complex. Molecular genetics has provided at least three explanations for this level of complexity.[35, 70–72]

The first of these involves recombination between *RHD* and *RHCE*. These two genes are highly homologous, and it is likely that mispairing at meiosis may occur in rare instances, in which *RHD* pairs with *RHCE*. If recombination then occurs—as a result of one or more crossover events or as a result of another mechanism called gene conversion in which a segment of one gene may be replaced by the equivalent segment of its homologue—the result is a fusion of gene that encodes a hybrid protein consisting partly of D protein and partly of CcEe protein. For example, there are rare phenotypes in which the red cells lack some D epitopes. Despite being D-positive, people with these phenotypes may make antibodies to the D epitopes they lack, antibodies that generally behave as anti-D. Most of these partial D phenotypes result from *RHD-CE-D* hybrid genes, *RHD* genes in which an internal segment has been replaced by an equivalent segment from an *RHCE* gene. For example, D^{VI}, one of the most common partial D antigens, is produced by an *RHD* gene in which the fourth, fifth, and sixth of the 10 exons are replaced by the equivalent exons from an *RHCE* gene (Fig. 8–5).[73]

Second, analysis of the amino acid sequences of the Rh polypeptides to predict their hydrophobic and hydrophilic domains suggested that they cross the red cell membrane 12 times, with the N- and C-termini inside the cytosol and six loops at the exterior of the cell (Fig. 8–6).[64, 74] Rh antigens are not simply linear chains of amino acids; they are very dependent on the shape of the molecule and may also involve interactions between different extracellular domains. Minor changes in the amino acid sequence, such as a single amino acid change, even within a membrane-spanning domain, may cause conformational changes that create new antigens and affect the expression of existing ones.

Third, Rh proteins exist in the red cell membrane not in isolation but as part of a complex involving several, genetically unrelated proteins. Of these, the most important with regard to Rh antigen expression is the Rh-associated glycoprotein (RhAG, often referred to as Rh50). RhAG is a glycoprotein with sequence and conformational similarities to the Rh polypeptides but is encoded by a gene on chromosome 6,[75] whereas the Rh loci are on chromosome 1. Rh_{null} and Rh_{mod} are rare phenotypes in which all Rh antigens either are totally absent or are expressed only weakly. It has been known from family evidence for many years that these phenotypes result from homozygosity for rare alleles at one or more loci genetically independent of the Rh locus.[76, 77] Sequencing of *RHAG* gene transcripts revealed inactivating mutations in Rh_{null} persons and a missense mutation, encoding a single amino acid substitution, in an Rh_{mod} person.[78] It therefore appears that absence of RhAG from the red cell prevents expression of Rh antigens, and that changes

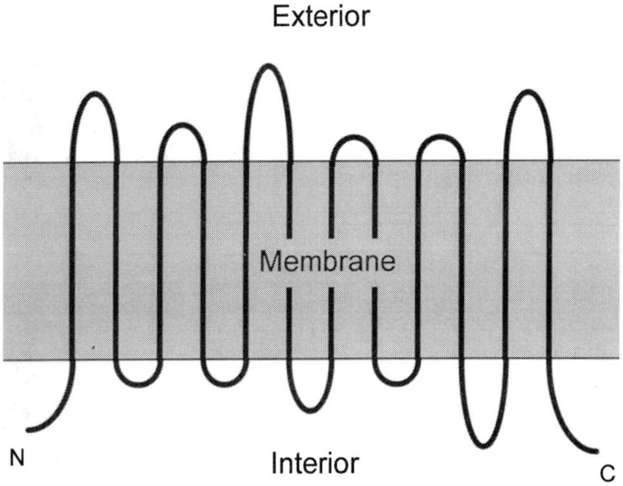

Figure 8–6. Diagram of probable conformation of Rh polypeptides in the red cell membrane, showing 12 membrane-spanning domains, cytosolic termini, and six extracellular loops.

in the amino acid sequence of RhAG may have other, less profound effects on Rh phenotypes.

The prevalence of hemolytic disease of the newborn (HDN) caused by anti-D antibody has been greatly reduced by anti-D immunoglobulin prophylaxis; however, some D-negative women do still produce anti-D antibody, and when they are pregnant, it is valuable to know the D phenotype of their fetus. If the fetus is D-positive, management of the potential HDN can be planned; if the fetus is D-negative, there is no need for further concern. Appreciation of the molecular backgrounds to the D phenotypes has made it possible to predict fetal D type from fetal DNA, obtained by amniocentesis. Several techniques that involve the polymerase chain reaction (PCR) with primers that amplify different regions of *RHD* have been developed to reveal whether a fetus possesses an *RHD* gene.[79] It is important that more than one region of *RHD* is amplified in any test, in order to avoid obtaining negative results with partial D phenotypes, in which part of the *RHD* gene is absent (see Fig. 8–5). A new complication, however, has arisen. The precept that D-negative people lack *RHD* was based on tests on DNA from people of European origin. Two thirds of D-negative black Africans, however, have an apparently intact *RHD* gene.[80] These Africans are genuinely D-negative and can produce anti-D antibody, and the reason why their *RHD* gene is not expressed at the red cell surface is not known. All PCR-based tests devised so far for predicting D phenotype are therefore unsuitable for use on black populations or on any population that contains a significant proportion of people of African origin.

Functional and Evolutionary Aspects of Blood Groups

The classical genetic approach to studying blood groups revealed a great deal about their inheritance but almost nothing about their function. Molecular analysis of blood group genes, however, has made it possible to predict the functions of many blood group antigens, either by analogy with other molecules of similar structure or by showing that certain blood groups are located on proteins of known function. The functions of some blood group antigens are known: the Cromer and Knops antigens are the complement regulatory glycoproteins decay-accelerating factor (CD55) and complement receptor type 1 (CD35); the Diego antigen is the red cell anion exchanger (band 3); the Kidd antigen is an urea transporter; the Colton antigen is a water transporter (aquaporin 1); and the Duffy glycoprotein is a chemokine receptor. The functions of some blood group antigens can be speculated upon because of their homology with structures of known function. For example, the Lutheran and LW glycoproteins are members of the immunoglobulin superfamily of receptors and adhesion molecules, the Rh polypeptides show homology with ammonium transporters, and the Kell glycoprotein resembles a family of endopeptidases.[81, 82]

Most blood group systems include null phenotypes in which the blood group protein, and hence all the antigens of that system, are absent from the red cells.[32] In many cases, inactivating mutations within the blood group gene have been identified, and so the gene product must be absent from all tissues, not just the red cells. However, people with these null phenotypes generally appear healthy. Despite the apparent important functions of some blood group antigens, either on red cells or in other tissues, most are redundant, inasmuch as other structures are able to carry out those functions in their absence.

Almost nothing is known regarding the function and evolutionary significance of blood group polymorphism. In any polymorphism, one of the alleles must have a selective advantage in order to achieve a frequency of more than 1% in a large population, but what that advantage is or was is not known. It is now apparent that glycoproteins and glycolipids carrying blood group activity, either on red cells or in other tissues, are exploited by pathogenic microorganisms as receptors for attachment to the cells and subsequent entry.[83] It is therefore probable that pathogens have played the major part in the evolution of blood group polymorphisms. There may be mutations in blood group genes that do not adversely affect the function of the membrane glycoprotein or glycolipid but render it less suitable as a receptor for a parasite. This might have nothing to do with red cells; the target for the parasite may be other cells that carry the protein. The mutant form would then have a selective advantage and establish itself as a polymorphism. Subsequently, the selective advantage could disappear, either because the parasite evolves to be able utilize the alternative form of the membrane structure or because the parasite is no longer present to infect the host. This is purely speculative, but it does provide one possible explanation for the existence of blood group polymorphism.

Two examples in which a selective advantage of a blood group polymorphism is apparent involve different forms of malaria. Merozoites of *Plasmodium vivax*, a parasite common and widespread in Africa that causes benign tertian malaria, utilize the Duffy glycoprotein, a red cell chemokine receptor, to gain access to the red cells.[84] In people of European and Asian origin, the Duffy glycoprotein is almost universally present and carries the Fy^a/Fy^b blood group polymorphism. In people of African origin, a third allele, *Fy*, that produces neither Fy^a nor Fy^b is very common. Homozygosity for *Fy* is responsible for the Fy(a−b−) red cell phenotype and absence of Duffy glycoprotein from the red cells. The Fy^a/Fy^b polymorphism is a single nucleotide change encoding an amino acid substitution within the coding region of the Duffy gene. The *Fy* allele results from a T→C change in the promoter region of the Duffy gene, upstream of the translation-initiating methionine codon.[85] This mutation prevents binding of the erythroid specific GATA-1 transcription factor and prevents expression of the gene in erythroid tissue, although the Duffy glycoprotein is present in endothelial cells of postcapillary venules. Africans homozygous for *Fy* have the selective advantage of being resistant to *P. vivax* malaria, without the potential disadvantage that may result from the absence of a functional Duffy chemokine receptor in their postcapillary venules. In some regions of Africa the frequency of Fy(a−b−) approaches 100%.

Plasmodium falciparum causes a far more severe form of malaria that is responsible for an estimated 2 million deaths per year, mostly in Africa.[86] In *P. falciparum* infection, parasites are sequestered from the peripheral circulation during the second half of their intraerythrocytic cycle, and infected red cells adhere to postcapillary venular endothelium. Mortality from this type of malaria may be related to the distribution of sequestered parasites in the body. Red cells infected with certain strains of *P. falciparum* bind other, infected or noninfected, red cells (rosetting). The process of rosetting probably involves an interaction between a parasite-derived lectin-like protein on the infected red cell surface and receptors naturally present on the surface of red cells. One of these receptors appears to be complement receptor type 1 (CR1 or CD35), the glycoprotein that carries the Knops blood group polymorphisms.[87] A correlation was found between low levels of CR1 and reduced rosetting. Absence of the Knops blood group antigen Sl^a (KN4) reduced binding of the red cells to the parasite-derived lectin-like protein and possibly reduced the pathogenicity of the parasite in individuals with Sl(a−) phenotype.[87] Sl(a−) has a frequency of 40% to 50% in African Americans, in comparison with 1% to 2% in white Americans,[32] which suggests a selective advantage for the Sl(a−) phenotype in Africa.

Current and Future Applications of Genetics to Transfusion Medicine

Although it has always been important to understand the inheritance of blood groups, classical genetics has never played a direct role in transfusion medicine. Molecular genetics, on the other hand, is making a continuously increasing impact on the application of blood transfusion, as it is with virtually every branch of medicine.

Prediction of fetal red cell phenotypes by PCR-based methods, as described in the Rh section earlier, is already provided as a service in some countries. Methods are now developed for predicting most red cell antigens that may be involved in HDN; Rh D and K are the most frequently requested. Currently, tests are usually performed on DNA derived from amniocytes, obtained by amniocentesis. It would be extremely beneficial if less invasive methods were developed, and the most likely source of fetal material is the very small numbers of fetal erythroblasts in maternal peripheral blood. One way to overcome problems posed by the extremely small numbers of these cells may be to isolate messenger RNA, because each cell would contain only one or two copies of the pertinent gene but many copies of its messenger RNA transcript.[88] The introduction of less invasive methods would make fetal phenotyping more routine and may even be used to determine fetal Rh D phenotype before it is decided whether to give prenatal Rh immunoglobulin to Rh D-negative pregnant women.[79]

It is unlikely that molecular methods will regularly be used for red cell antigen phenotyping when red cells are available; serological techniques for directly determining the presence of antigens on red cells are far easier, cheaper, and more accurate. This is not, however, always the case for identifying cell surface polymorphisms on other blood cells. PCR-based methods are used routinely for predicting cell surface antigen phenotypes on platelets[89] and granulocytes,[90] mainly in investigations into neonatal alloimmune thrombocytopenia and neutropenia, respectively. In an attempt to provide matched allografts, HLA-DR tissue typing is now usually carried out on DNA by PCR-based methods, and similar methods are also being introduced for HLA class I testing.[91, 92] Most PCR-based typing of leukocytes is carried out with sequence-specific primers.

One aspect of red cell serology in which recombinant DNA technology may prove valuable is the production of blood group antigens by transfecting suitable cultured cells with complementary DNA encoding the antigen. These recombinant antigens could then prove valuable in the identification of antibodies to red cell surface antigens. So far, the application of soluble recombinant CR1 and delay-accelerating factor for identifying Knops system and Cromer system antibodies, respectively, has been reported.[93, 94] Eventually it may be possible to produce a panel of recombinant antigens for identifying most blood group antibodies; however, some antigens, such as those of the Rh system, which are conformational and are lost when isolated from the membrane, will provide a challenge.

Production of immunohematological reagents was revolutionized in the 1980s by monoclonal antibody technology. Future developments for in vitro synthesis of antibodies will come from recombinant DNA technology. The most commonly used techniques involve phage-display, in which PCR-amplified complementary DNA derived from B cell heavy chain and light chain gene segments are packaged in phage particles, which express encoded immunoglobulin Fab (fragment antigen binding) or Fv (fragment variable) fragments at their surfaces.[95] These phage particles can be selected by binding them, through the expressed Fab or Fv fragments, to an appropriate, immobilized, antigen. Selected phage can then be expanded in *Escherichia coli* organisms and eventually expressed as small soluble antibody-like antigen-binding molecules. It may also be possible to improve these "antibodies" by in vitro mutagenesis of the immunoglobulin DNA. So far, no reagent for use in transfusion practice has been produced by these methods, but recombinant technology will certainly play an important role in future immunohematological testing, diagnosis, and therapy.

Amplification assays for the detection of microbial genomes in donor blood and pooled plasma are rapidly being introduced into transfusion practice.[96, 97] The main purpose of these assays is to enhance, rather than replace, currently used serological assays, in an attempt to detect viruses during the "window" period of infection when they are not detectable by serological tests. Assays, usually involving PCR but occasionally involving other amplification techniques such as the ligase chain reaction, are used to detect nucleic acid derived from human immunodeficiency virus, hepatitis B and C viruses, human T cell leukemia/lymphoma virus, cytomegalovirus, various bacteria, and parasites responsible for malaria and Chagas' disease. Multiplex assays are being introduced to reduce the number of amplifications required.

The changing concept of the gene has been accompanied by comparable conceptual changes throughout biology. Genetics, as a diagnostic tool or as a basis for disease prevention, and increasingly as a means for treatment (directly or indirectly), is becoming more and more intricately involved in medicine. Gene therapy is the correction of a disease by genetic manipulation. Gene therapy has not yet lived up to its initial promise, but it could still be the way forward for treating a large range of inherited and acquired diseases.[98, 99] Many gene therapy protocols involve the ex vivo manipulation of cells: removal of cells from the patient, transduction of those cells with an appropriate recombinant gene, and return of the transduced cells to the patient. Much of the expertise required for ex vivo gene therapy is similar to that demanded for blood transfusion, particularly the reliable handling of donor cells. Blood banks therefore should expect to play a part in ex vivo gene therapy, should it ever become a routine medical procedure.

REFERENCES

1. Landsteiner K. Zur kenntnis der antifermentativen, lytischen und agglutinierenden wirkungen des blutserums und der lymphe. Zentralbl Bakt 1900; 27:357.
2. Landsteiner K. Über agglutinationserscheinungen normalen menschlichen blutes. Wien Klin Wschr 1901; 14:1132.
3. DeVries H. Sur la loi de disjonction des hybrides. CR Acad Sci 1900; 130:845.
4. Correns C. G. Mendel's regel über das verhalten der nachkommenschaft der rassenbastarde. Deutsch Bot Ges Berlin 1900; 18:158.
5. von Tschermak E. Über kunstliche kreuzung bei *Pisum sativum*. Deutsch Bot Ges Berlin 1900; 18:232.
6. Mendel GJ. Versche über pflanzenhybriden. Verh Naturf Ver Brünn 1865;4:3–47.
7. von Decastello A, Sturli A. Über die isoagglutinine im serum gesunder und kranker menschen. Münch Med Wschr 1902; 26:1090.
8. von Dungern E, Hirszfeld L. Über gruppenspezifische strukturen des Blutes III. Z Immun Forsch 1911; 8:526–62.
9. Epstein AA, Ottenberg R. Simple method of performing serum reactions. Proc N Y Pathol Soc 1908; 8:117.
10. Bernstein F. Ergebnisse einer biostatischen zusammenfassenden betrachtung über die erblichen blutstrukturen des menschen. Klin Wschr 1924; 3:1495.
11. Bernstein F. Zusammenfassende betrachtungen über die erblichen blutstrukturen des menschen. Z Indukt Abstamm Vererb Lehre 1925; 37:237.
12. Garrod AE. The incidence of alkaptonuria: a study in chemical individuality. Lancet 1902; 2:1616.
13. Bateson W. An address on mendelian heredity and its applications to man. Brain 1906; 29:157.
14. Bateson W. Mendel's Principles of Heredity. Cambridge, UK: Cambridge University Press, 1909, p 205.
15. Garrod AE. The Croonian Lectures on Inborn Errors of Metabolism. Lancet 1908; 2:1.
16. Hardy GH. Mendelian proportions in a mixed population. Science 1908; 28:49.
17. Weinberg W. Über den nachweis der vererbung beim menschen. Jahreshefte d Vereins f vaterl Naturkinde in Württ. 1908; 64:369. [Cited in Stern C. The Hardy Weinberg law. Science 1943; 97:137.]
18. Castle WE. The laws of heredity of Galton and Mendel, and some laws governing race improvement by selection. Proc Am Acad Arts Sci 1903; 39:223.
19. Landsteiner K, Levine P. A new agglutinable factor differentiating individual human bloods. Proc Soc Exp Biol N Y 1927; 24:600.
20. Landsteiner K, Levine P. Further observations on individual differences of human blood. Proc Soc Exp Biol N Y 1927; 24:941.
21. Landsteiner K, Levine P. On individual differences in human blood. J Exp Med 1928; 47:757.
22. Landsteiner K, Levine P. On the inheritance of agglutinogens of human blood demonstrable by immune agglutinins. J Exp Med 1928; 48:731.
23. Hackel E. Basic genetic concepts for blood bankers. *In* Wilson JK (ed): Genetics for Blood Bankers. Washington, DC: American Association of Blood Banks, 1980, pp 1–17.
24. Fisher RA. Has Mendel's work been rediscovered? Ann Sci 1936; 1:115.
25. Bennett JH (ed). Mendel's Experiments in Plant Hybridization [Reprint]. Edinburgh: Oliver & Boyd, 1965, p 29.
26. Johannsen W. Über erblichkeit in populationen und in reinen linien. Jena, 1903.
27. Morgan TH. Sex limited inheritance in *Drosophila*. Science 1910; 32:120.
28. Renwick JH. The mapping of human chromosomes. Annu Rev Genet 1971; 5:81.
29. Watson JD, Crick FHC. Genetical implications of the structure of deoxyribonucleic acid. Nature 1953; 171:964.
30. Crick FHC. The genetic code: III. Sci Am 1966; 215(4):55.
31. Race RR, Sanger R. Blood Groups in Man, 6th ed. Oxford, UK: Blackwell, 1975.
32. Daniels GL. Human Blood Groups. Oxford, UK: Blackwell Science, 1995.
33. Daniels GL, Anstee DJ, Cartron JP, et al. Blood group terminology 1995. ISBT Working Party on Terminology for Red Cell Surface Antigens. Vox Sang 1995; 69:265.
34. Daniels GL, Anstee DJ, Cartron JP, et al. Terminology for red cell surface antigens. Oslo report. Vox Sang, in press.
35. Avent ND. Human erythrocyte antigen expression: its molecular bases. Br J Biomed Sci 1997; 54:16.
36. Morgan WTJ. A contribution to human biochemical genetics: the chemical basis of blood group specificity (the Croonian Lecture). Proc R Soc Lond B 1960; 151:308.
37. Watkins WM. Blood-group substances. Science 1966; 152:172.
38. Kabat EA. Blood Group Substances: Their Chemistry and Immunochemistry. New York: Academic Press, 1956.
39. Watkins WM. Biochemistry and genetics of the ABO, Lewis, and P blood group systems. Adv Hum Genet 1980; 10:1.
40. Clausen H, Hakomori S. ABH and related histo-blood group antigens; immunochemical differences in carrier isotypes and their distribution. Vox Sang 1989; 56:1.
41. Bhende YM, Deshpande CK, Bhatia HM, et al. A 'new' blood-group character related to the ABO system. Lancet 1952; 1:903.
42. Putkonen T. Uber die gruppenspezifischen Eigenschaften Verschiedener Korperflussigkeiten. Acta Soc Med Fenn Duodecim Ser A 1930; 14:113.
43. Schiff F, Sasaki H. Der Ausscheidungstypus, ein auf serologischem Wege nachweisbares Mendelndes Merkmal. Klin Woch 1932; 11:1426.
44. Solomon JM, Waggoner R, Leyshon WC. A quantitative immunogenetic study of gene suppression involving A_1 and H antigens of the erythrocyte without affecting secreted blood group substances. The ABH phenotypes $A^h{}_m$ and $O^h{}_m$. Blood 1965; 25:470.
45. Oriol R, Danilovs J, Hawkins BR. A new genetic model proposing that the *Se* gene is a structural gene closely linked to the *H* gene. Amer J Hum Genet 1981; 33:421.
46. Larsen RD, Ernst LK, Nair RP, et al. Molecular cloning, sequence, and expression of a human GDP-L-fucose:β-D-galactoside 2-α-L-fucosyltransferase cDNA that can form the H blood group antigen. Proc Natl Acad Sci U S A 1990; 87:6674.
47. Kelly RJ, Rouquier S, Giorgi D, et al. Sequence and expression of a candidate for the human *Secretor* blood group α(1,2)fucosyltransferase gene (*FUT2*). Homozygosity for an enzyme-inactivating nonsense mutation commonly correlates with the non-secretor phenotype. J Biol Chem 1995; 270:4640.
48. Kaneko M, Nidhihara S, Shinya N, et al. Wide variety of point mutations in the *H* gene of Bombay and para-Bombay individuals that inactivate H enzyme. Blood 1997; 90:839.
49. Wagner FF, Flegel WA. Polymorphism of the *h* allele and the population frequency of sporadic nonfunctional alleles. Transfusion 1997; 37:284.
50. Yu L-C, Broadberry RE, Yang Y-H, et al. Heterogeneity of the human *Secretor* α(1,2)fucosyltransferase gene among Lewis(a+b–) non-secretors. Biochem Biophys Res Comm 1996; 222:390.
51. Koda Y, Soejima M, Liu Y, et al. Molecular basis for secretor type

α(1,2)-fucosyltransferase gene deficiency in a Japanese population: a fusion gene generated by unequal crossover responsible for the enzyme deficiency. Am J Hum Genet 1996; 59:343.
52. Kudo T, Iwasaki H, Nishihara S, et al. Molecular genetic analysis of the human Lewis histo-blood group system. II Secretor gene inactivation by a novel single missense mutation A385T in Japanese nonsecretor individuals. J Biol Chem 1996; 271:9830.
53. Henry S, Mollicone R, Lowe JB, et al. A second nonsecretor allele of the blood group α(1,2)fucosyltransferase gene (FUT2). Vox Sang 1996; 70:21.
54. Bennett EP, Steffensen R, Clausen H, et al. Genomic cloning of the human histo-blood group ABO locus. Biochem Biophys Res Comm 1995; 206:318.
55. Yamamoto F, Clausen H, White T, et al. Molecular genetic basis of the histo-blood group ABO system. Nature 1990; 345:229.
56. Yamamoto F. Molecular genetics of the ABO histo-blood group system. Vox Sang 1995; 69:1.
57. Olsson ML, Chester MA. Frequent occurrence of a variant O^1 gene at the blood group ABO locus. Vox Sang 1996; 70:26.
58. Yamamoto F, McNeill PD, Yamamoto M, et al. Molecular genetic analysis of the ABO blood group system: 4. Another type of *O* allele. Vox Sang 1993; 64:175.
59. Suzuki K, Iwata M, Tsuji H, et al. A de novo recombination in the ABO blood group gene and evidence for the occurrence of recombination products. Hum Genet 1997; 99:454.
60. Fisher RA. [Cited by Race RR.] An 'incomplete' antibody in human serum. Nature 1944; 153:771.
61. Wiener AS, Wexler IB. An Rh-Hr Syllabus, 2nd ed. New York: Grune & Stratton, 1963.
62. Tippett P. A speculative model for the Rh blood groups. Ann Hum Genet 1986; 50:241.
63. Chérif-Zahar B, Bloy C, Le Van Kim C, et al. Molecular cloning and protein structure of a human blood group Rh polypeptide. Proc Natl Acad Sci U S A 1990; 87:6243.
64. Avent ND, Ridgwell K, Tanner JA, et al. cDNA cloning of a 30 kDa erythrocyte membrane protein associated with Rh (Rhesus) blood-group-antigen expression. Biochem J 1990; 271:821.
65. Le Van Kim C, Mouro I, Chérif-Zahar B, et al. Molecular cloning and primary structure of the human blood group RhD polypeptide. Proc Natl Acad Sci U S A 1992; 89:10925.
66. Race RR, Sanger R. Blood Groups in Man, 3rd ed. Oxford, UK: Blackwell Scientific, 1958, p 123.
67. Fisher R. Population genetics. Proc R Soc Lond B 1953; 141:510.
68. Carritt B, Kemp TJ, Poulter M. Evolution of the human RH (rhesus) blood group genes: a 50 year old prediction (partially) fulfilled. Hum Mol Genet 1997; 6:843.
69. Colin Y, Chérif-Zahar B, Le Van Kim C, et al. Genetic basis of the RhD-positive and RhD-negative blood group polymorphism as determined by Southern analysis. Blood 1991; 78:2747.
70. Cartron J-P, Agre P. RH blood groups and Rh-deficiency syndrome. *In* Cartron J-P, Rouger P (eds): Blood Cell Biochemistry, vol 6. New York: Plenum Press, 1995, pp 189–225.
71. Huang C-H. Molecular insights into the Rh protein family and associated antigens. Curr Opin Hematol 1997; 4:94.
72. Sonneborn H-H, Voak D (eds). A review of 50 years of the Rh blood group system. Biotest Bull 1997; 5:389.
73. Mouro I, Le Van Kim C, Rouillac C, et al. Rearrangements of the blood group RhD gene associated with the D^{VI} category phenotype. Blood 1994; 83:1129.
74. Avent ND, Butcher SK, Liu W, et al. Localization of the C termini of the Rh (Rhesus) polypeptides to the cytoplasmic face of the human erythrocyte membrane. J Biol Chem 1992; 267:15134.
75. Ridgwell K, Spurr NK, Laguda B, et al. Isolation of cDNA clones for a 50 kDa glycoprotein of the human erythrocyte membrane associated with Rh (Rhesus) blood-group antigen expression. Biochem J 1992; 287:223.
76. Levine P, Celano MJ, Falkowski F, et al. A second example of −/− or Rh_{null} blood. Transfusion 1965; 5:492.
77. Chown B, Lewis M, Kaita H, et al. An unlinked modifier of Rh blood groups: effects when heterozygous and when homozygous. Am J Hum Genet 1972; 24:623.
78. Cherif-Zahar B, Raynal V, Gane P, et al. Candidate gene acting as a suppressor of the *RH* locus in most cases of Rh-deficiency. Nature Genet 1996; 12:168.
79. Avent ND. Prenatal determination of fetal Rh status using the PCR. Biotest Bull 1997; 5:429.
80. Daniels G, Green C, Smart E. Differences between RhD-negative Africans and RhD-negative Europeans. Lancet 1997; 350:862.
81. Anstee DJ, Cartron J-P. Toward an understanding of the red cell surface. *In* Garratty G (ed): Applications of Molecular Biology to Blood Transfusion Medicine. Bethesda, MD: American Association of Blood Banks, 1997, pp 17–49.
82. Daniels G. Functional aspects of red cell antigens. Blood Rev, in press.
83. Moulds JM, Nowicki S, Moulds JJ, et al. Human blood groups: incidental receptors for viruses and bacteria. Transfusion 1996; 36:362.
84. Hadley TJ, Peiper SC. From malaria to chemokine receptor: the emerging physiologic role of the Duffy blood group antigen. Blood 1997; 89:3077.
85. Tournamille C, Le Van Kim C, Gane P, et al. Molecular basis and PCR-DNA typing of the Fya/fyb blood group polymorphism. Hum Genet 1995; 95:407.
86. Targett G. The value of death. Malaria research—an audit of international activity. Immunol News 1997; April:76.
87. Rowe JA, Moulds JM, Newbold CI, et al. *P. falciparum* rosetting mediated by a parasite-variant erythrocyte membrane protein and complement-receptor 1. Nature 1997; 388:292.
88. Hamlington J, Cunningham J, Mason G, et al. Prenatal detection of Rhesus D genotype. Lancet 1997; 349:540.
89. Newman PJ, McFarland JG, Aster RH. The alloimmune thrombocytopenias. *In* Loscalzo J, Schafer AI (eds): Thrombosis and Hemorrhage, 2nd ed. Baltimore: Williams & Wilkins, 1998.
90. Bux J, Stein EL, Santoso S, et al. NA gene frequencies in the German population, determined by polymerase chain reaction with sequence-specific primers. Transfusion 1995; 35:54.
91. Bunce M, O'Neill CM, Barnardo MCNM, et al. Phototyping: comprehensive DNA typing for HLA-A, B, C, DRB3, DRB4, DRB5 & DQB1 by PCR with 144 primer mixes utilizing sequence-specific primers (PCR-SSP). Tissue Antigens 1995; 46:355.
92. Wassmuth R. Molecular analysis of HLA polymorphism and relevance for transplantation. Biotest Bull 1997; 5:539.
93. Moulds JM, Rowe KE. Neutralization of Knops system antibodies using soluble complement receptor 1. Transfusion 1996; 36:517.
94. Daniels GL, Green CA, Powell RM, et al. Hemagglutination-inhibition of Cromer blood group antibodies with soluble recombinant decay-accelerating factor. Transfusion 1998; 38:332.
95. Siegel DL. New approaches for monoclonal antibody function. *In* Garratty G (ed): Applications of Molecular Biology to Blood Transfusion Medicine. Bethesda, MD: American Association of Blood Banks, 1997, pp 73–102.
96. Busch MP, Stramer SL, Kleinmann SH. Evolving applications of nucleic acid amplification assays for prevention of virus transmission by blood components and derivatives. *In* Garratty G (ed): Applications of Molecular Biology to Blood Transfusion Medicine. Bethesda, MD: American Association of Blood Banks, 1997, pp 123–175.
97. Barbara JAJ. Molecular biology: applications in transfusion microbiology. Education Programme of the 26th Congress of the International Society of Haematology, Singapore, 1996, pp 151–156.
98. Anderson WF. Human gene therapy. Science 1992; 256:808.
99. Kay MA, Liu D, Hoogerbrugge PM. Gene therapy. Proc Natl Acad Sci U S A 1997; 94:12744.

SECTION

III Red Cells

CHAPTER 9

Red Cell Metabolism

Ernest Beutler

GENERAL CONSIDERATIONS

The mammalian red blood cell leaves the marrow as a reticulocyte and retains the capacity to circulate and to carry oxygen and carbon dioxide for about 120 days. Although it has lost its nucleus by the time it is discharged from the marrow, it retains the enzymes necessary to carry out the complex metabolic reactions that help it remain viable and maintain its hemoglobin so that it can perform its important functions. Although it was once thought that the final event that led to loss of red cell viability was probably the gradual attrition of its enzymatic machinery,[1–4] we still do not know what signals the demise of the erythrocyte.[5–7] Of the various proposals that have been advanced, the most attractive is that exposure of phosphatidyl serine on the outer leaflet of the erythrocyte membrane is an important aging signal,[8] but this signal does not seem to play a role in the storage lesion.[9]

A metabolically active erythrocyte survives in the circulation at 37°C for 4 months, but a cell that has been removed from its normal environment for storage at 4°C unfortunately does not go into a state of suspended animation. Although cold-stored red cells do not continue to age, they eventually lose their capacity to circulate. How long red cells can be stored before they are no longer suitable for transfusion depends on the medium in which they are suspended and how well it serves their metabolic needs. Thus an understanding of red cell metabolism has been important in the development of media to maintain the viability and function of cold-stored erythrocytes.

ENERGY METABOLISM[10–12]

Glycolysis

During its circulation the erythrocyte must continually carry out certain energy-requiring processes to perform its functions. The reduced form of nicotinamide adenine dinucleotide (NADH) must be generated to maintain the iron of hemoglobin in the reduced, divalent form. Adenosine triphosphate (ATP) is needed to power the sodium–potassium–adenosine triphosphatase (Na^+, K^+-ATPase) that, through its pumping action, maintains high intracellular potassium and low sodium concentrations in the face of low plasma potassium and high plasma sodium. ATP powers other membrane pumps, including one that extrudes calcium from the interior of the cell,[13] another that transports magnesium,[14] and still others that transport oxidized glutathione[15] and glutathione conjugates.[16, 17] ATP is required for the synthesis of glutathione[18] and phosphoribosyl pyrophosphate (PRPP),[19, 20] essential for the production of adenosine monophosphate (AMP) by the erythrocyte. ATP is also needed to sustain membrane structure, possibly by phosphorylating critical sites in membrane proteins.[21–24]

The physiological substrate for energy metabolism of the human erythrocyte is glucose. Glucose does not merely diffuse into the erythrocyte. It is carried into the cell by a saturable, temperature-sensitive glucose transporter, Gluc 1. This transporter has been thought to be associated with membrane band 3[25, 26] or membrane band 4.5.[27, 28] Although transport is not energy dependent, it is thought to be modulated by ATP.[29–31] The red cells of many mammals lose their permeability to glucose as the mammal matures; adult pig erythrocytes, for example, are almost totally impermeable to glucose,[32] and some other source of energy must be present, likely inosine.[33] However, human red cells are so permeable to glucose that even at cold temperatures, glucose transport is not a limiting factor for glycolysis.

The pathway of glucose metabolism by the red cell is illustrated in Figure 9–1. Utilization of glucose requires its phosphorylation by ATP first in the hexokinase reaction and then, after isomerization to fructose-6-phosphate, in the phosphofructokinase (PFK) reaction. There are, in fact, two kinases. One of these, PFK-2, phosphorylates fructose-6-phosphate at the 2-position, forming fructose-2,6-diphosphate,[34] an important regulatory compound. The other, PFK-1,[35] phosphorylates fructose-6-phosphate at the 1-position, forming fructose-1,6-diphosphate, an intermediate in the glycolytic pathway. This fructose diphosphate ester is cleaved by aldolase into trioses, which are metabolized ultimately to pyruvic and/or lactic acid. The glycolytic pathway branches because 1,3-diphosphoglycerate (1,3-DPG) can serve as a substrate for either

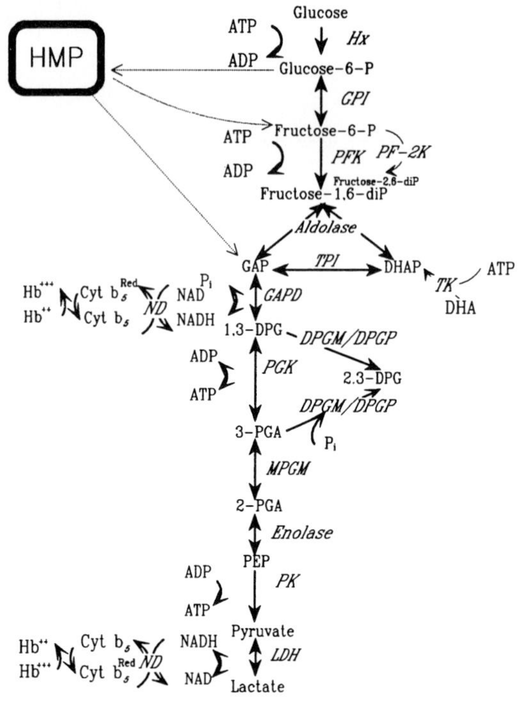

Figure 9–1. The glycolytic pathway of red cell metabolism. Enzymes are shown in italics. Hx, hexokinase; GPI, glucose phosphate isomerase; PFK, phosphofructokinase; PF-2K, fructose-6-phosphate, 2-kinase; GAP, D-glyceraldehyde-3-P; TPI, triose phosphate isomerase; DHA, dihydroxyacetone; DHAP, dihydroxyacetone phosphate; GAPD, glyceraldehyde phosphate dehydrogenase; 1,3-DPG, 1,3-diphosphoglyceric acid; DPGM, diphosphoglyceromutase; DPGP, diphosphoglycerophosphatase; PGK, phosphoglycerate kinase; 2,3-DPG, 2,3-diphosphoglyceric acid; 3-PGA, 3-phosphoglyceric acid; MPGM, monophosphoglyceromutase; 2-PGA, 2-phosphoglyceric acid; PEP, phospho(enol)pyruvate; PK, pyruvate kinase; LDH, lactate dehydrogenase.

of two competing reactions: the phosphoglycerate kinase reaction, which phosphorylates adenosine diphosphate (ADP) to ATP, and the diphosphoglycerate mutase reaction, which forms 2,3-diphosphoglycerate (2,3-DPG). The latter compound is particularly important in the erythrocyte because it serves as a modulator of the oxygen affinity of hemoglobin.[36–38] The final acid products of glucose catabolism, lactic acid and pyruvic acid, are transported through the membrane[39, 40] and carried away from the circulating red cell by the plasma, but in a closed storage system these acids are responsible for the progressive fall in pH that occurs during storage.

Although glucose is the physiological substrate for the reactions of glycolysis, certain other sugars can also be used by the red cells. Fructose is efficiently phosphorylated by hexokinase,[41] and the fructose-6-phosphate formed is a normal glycolytic intermediate. Mannose is phosphorylated to mannose-6-phosphate, which mannose phosphate isomerase can convert to fructose-6-phosphate.[42] The activity of the latter enzyme is relatively low, so that mannose utilization is not nearly as efficient as glucose use.[43] The metabolism of galactose is even less efficient.[42]

Dihydroxyacetone (DHA) is phosphorylated to dihydroxyacetone phosphate (DHAP) by triokinase,[44] and it has the capability of maintaining ATP and 2,3-DPG levels in stored erythrocytes.[45–49] Under proper conditions, red cells are permeable to phospho(enol)pyruvate (PEP).[50] The PEP that gains entry into the erythrocyte can be metabolized to pyruvate, phosphorylating ADP to ATP. Accordingly, it has been used as a means of rejuvenating stored cells.[51, 52] However, because of the low pH required for penetration of PEP through the membrane, it is not effective as a substitute for glucose when added at the beginning of storage.[53]

Hexosemonophosphate Shunt

Normally, most of the glucose metabolized by erythrocytes is broken down to pyruvic acid and lactic acid by way of the glycolytic pathway (see Fig. 9–1), but the hexosemonophosphate (HMP) shunt (Fig. 9–2) is also used, particularly under conditions of oxidative stress. In this pathway, glucose undergoes oxidative decarboxylation to pentose. After several enzymatically catalyzed rearrangements, sugars rejoin the glycolytic pathway as fructose-6-phosphate and glyceraldehyde-3-phosphate.

The first step of the HMP shunt is catalyzed by glucose-6-phosphate dehydrogenase (G6PD). The unimpeded activity of this enzyme is about 10 times as high as that of the hexokinase reaction, and G6PD could readily metabolize all the glucose-6-phosphate formed by the erythrocyte. However, the enzyme is markedly inhibited by reduced nicotinamide adenine dinucleotide phosphate (NADPH),[54, 55] and the level of NADP in red cells is too low to support its maximal rate of activity. The very high NADPH-to-NADP ratio of normal red cells[56] therefore markedly limits metabolism by way of the HMP shunt. However, when NADPH is oxidized to NADP, G6PD inhibition is relieved and glucose-6-phosphate is oxidized. This process serves to regenerate the NADPH that may be needed to protect the cell against oxidative insult, largely by regenerating reduced glutathione (GSH) from oxidized glutathione (GSSG).

The HMP shunt serves another useful physiological role in the metabolism of erythrocytes. Pentose in the form of PRPP[57] is required for the synthesis of adenine nucleotides from adenine base in the adenine phosphoribosyltransferase (APRT) reaction (see later discussion). The ribose-5-phosphate needed for the synthesis of PRPP is one of the intermediates of the HMP shunt (see Fig. 9–2).

In the context of red cell storage, the reactions of the HMP shunt are also vital in the utilization of inosine as a source of high-energy phosphate. Ribose-1-phosphate formed by the purine nucleoside phosphorylase (PNP) reaction is isomerized to ribose-5-phosphate, a normal intermediate in the pathway, and is ultimately converted to the products of the HMP shunt, fructose-6-phosphate and glyceraldehyde-3-phosphate. The inorganic phosphate esterified to pentose in the PNP reaction ultimately becomes the source of high-energy phosphate to form ATP. Thus this pathway is a way of creating high-energy

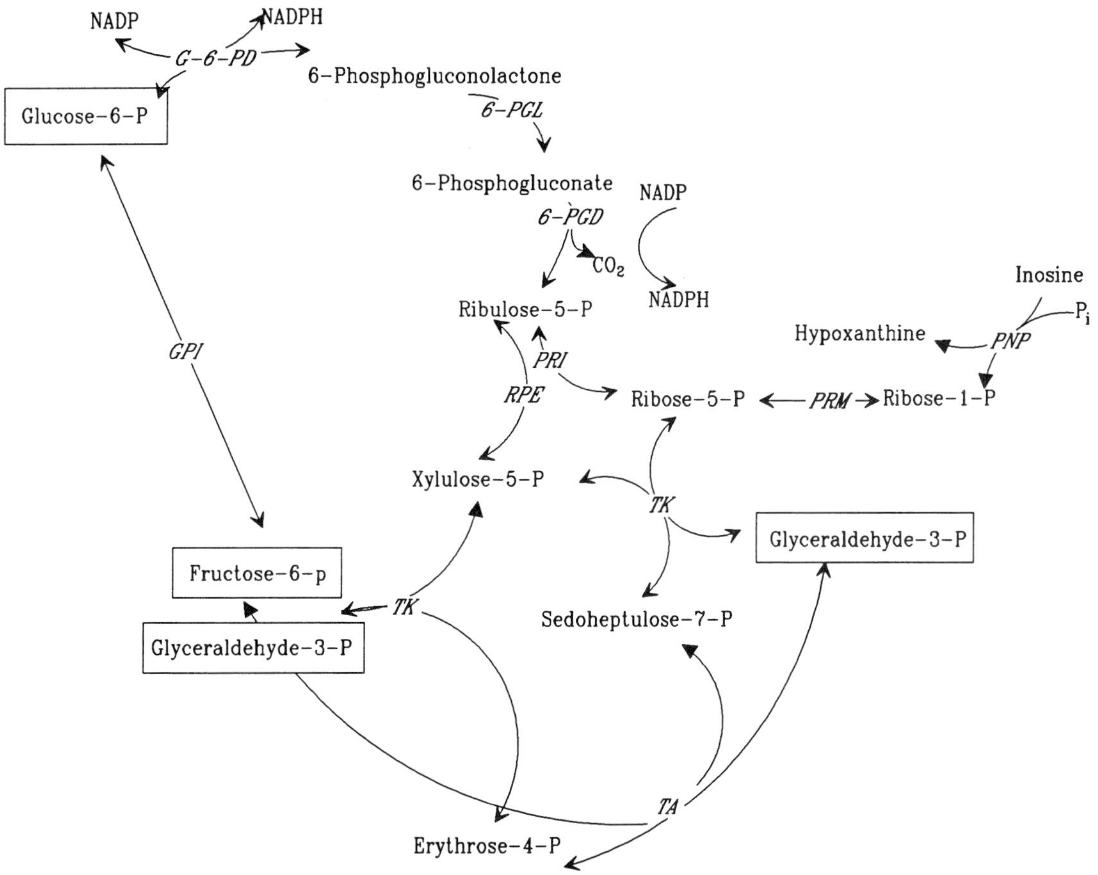

Figure 9–2. The hexosemonophosphate pathway (HMP). Enzymes are shown in italics. G-6-PD, glucose-6-phosphate dehydrogenase; 6-PGL, 6-phosphogluconolactonase; 6-PGD, 6-phosphogluconate dehydrogenase; GPI, glucose phosphate isomerase; PRI, phosphoribose isomerase; PNP, purine nucleoside phosphorylase; RPE, ribulosephosphate 3-epimerase; PRM, phosphoribomutase; TK, transketolase; TA, transaldolase.

phosphate bonds without the expenditure of ATP, a mechanism that has been used to salvage red cells that have lost their ATP during storage.

Nucleotide Metabolism

Adenine nucleotides are essential to red cell metabolism. A guanine nucleotide pool is present as well and probably plays an important role.[58–60]

Phosphorylation of Adenine Nucleotides. AMP is phosphorylated to ADP by ATP through the action of the enzyme adenylate kinase (AK). ADP, in turn, is phosphorylated to ATP in the phosphoglycerate kinase (PGK) and pyruvate kinase (PK) reactions. The AK reaction is readily reversible so that two molecules of ADP can react to form one of AMP and one of ATP. Thus the two terminal phosphates of ATP are in a continuous state of exchange while the phosphate attached to the ribose is firmly fixed.

Deamination of Adenine Nucleotides. The red cell continually deaminates the adenine moiety to inosine in the adenosine deaminase and AMP-deaminase reactions. Of these enzymes, it is probably AMP-deaminase that plays the most important regulatory role. Hereditary deficiency of this enzyme causes an increase in red cell ATP levels.[61, 62] Further evidence comes from the fact that as red cells age in vivo, the level of ATP rises because the activity of red cell ATP-deaminase falls with red cell senescence,[63–65] contrary to earlier suggestions that red cell ATP levels decline during aging.[66–68]

Incorporation of Adenine into the Adenine Nucleotide Pool. Although it cannot synthesize adenine to replace that which has been deaminated, the erythrocyte maintains the capacity to incorporate preformed adenine into the adenine nucleotide pool. The main mechanism for performing this function appears to be the APRT reaction, in which adenine and PRPP react to form AMP.[69] The source of preformed adenine used by the erythrocyte is probably the liver, and it may obtain sufficient amounts of adenine as it passes through this organ for its needs. A second mechanism for the incorporation of adenine moiety into erythrocyte nucleotide pool is the adenosine kinase reaction, which phosphorylates the nucleoside adenosine to AMP.[70]

Guanine Nucleotides. Erythrocytes contain guanine nucleotides as well as adenine nucleotides, although at a considerably lower concentration.[71, 72] The role of these nucleotides is less well established than the role of adenine nucleotides. Guanosine triphosphatase (GTPase) activity has been demonstrated to be present in human erythrocytes,[73] and guanosine triphosphate (GTP) can substitute for ATP in a number of kinase reactions.[74, 75]

GTP inhibits transglutaminase activity.[76] GTP-binding proteins have been found in erythrocytes.[58, 60, 77]

RED CELLS IN LIQUID STORAGE

History of Liquid Storage

Introduction of Sodium Citrate–Glucose Preservatives. Although the first blood transfusions were administered centuries ago—a hazardous undertaking before the recognition of blood groups less than 100 years ago—the storage of blood for transfusion has a much shorter history. Rous and Turner[78, 79] found that glucose retarded in vitro hemolysis of stored cells. O. H. Robertson, a young Canadian medical officer later to achieve fame in the field of infectious diseases, transfused stored erythrocytes on the battlefields of France during World War I.[80] The cells had been preserved for as long as 27 days in large volumes of glucose-citrate solutions. At the time and under the circumstances, there was no way of determining whether the blood transfusions were efficacious, but several of his patients survived.

Acid Citrate–Glucose Solutions. Between World War I and World War II, progress was made in studying the physiology of red blood cells. Particularly notable was the development by Ashby of an ingenious differential agglutination method for the study of survival of red cells in the circulation.[81] However, trisodium citrate–glucose solutions remained the mainstay of blood preservation. Solutions of glucose and citrate had to be autoclaved separately because the glucose caramelized in the presence of the alkaline citrate. Loutit and Mollison,[82, 83] attempting to overcome this inconvenience, devised an acidified citrate medium, acid-citrate-dextrose (ACD), that could be autoclaved as a single solution and actually improved red cell preservation, as measured by differential agglutination. This solution and minor modifications, one of which was citrate-phosphate-dextrose (CPD),[84] became the mainstay of blood transfusion practice for a third of a century and are still in extensive use today.

Biochemical and Physiological Studies. The biochemistry and physiology of stored red cells have been explored in detail. In a remarkably prescient paper, Rapoport[85] studied the physical and biochemical properties of erythrocytes stored in different media. A few years later, Finch and colleagues, using modern tracer techniques, explored the fate of stored cells.[86–92] Noting the correlation between ATP loss and decline in viability of reinfused erythrocytes, they attempted to repair this manifestation of the storage lesion by adding adenosine to storage media.[88, 89] When they found that adenosine tended to cause hypotension in recipients, they turned to inosine as a possible energy source to replenish the ATP of stored erythrocytes.[86, 87] Promising results were obtained and a large national study was undertaken, but the findings were disappointing.[93] In retrospect, it appears that some of the early inosine solutions might have been contaminated with adenine.[94] Indeed, in 1962 Nakao and colleagues[95] demonstrated that the addition of inosine and adenine had a pronounced effect on restoring the ATP levels of stored red cells. The use of inosine was undesirable because it could serve as a precursor of uric acid formation in the recipient, and Simon showed that the addition of adenine at the beginning of storage greatly improved not only the ATP levels but also the viability of the reinfused, stored red cells.[96, 97]

Appreciation of the Role of 2,3-DPG. The fact that 2,3-DPG was rapidly lost from red cells stored in ACD or CPD solutions, with or without added adenine, was well known but generally ignored, because it appeared to have no effect on the viability of the stored erythrocytes. Indeed, Valtis and Kennedy[98] had shown that the oxygen dissociation curve of stored erythrocytes was abnormal, but without a rationale for this isolated finding, its significance was not appreciated. However, when Benesch and Benesch[99] and Chanutin and Curnish[100] independently recognized that 2,3-DPG interacted with hemoglobin to cause a right shift in the oxygen dissociation curve, it was appreciated that red cells that had been stored for even 1 week in ACD or 2 weeks in CPD might show excellent viability, but that their oxygen delivery properties were far from optimal. Even though it was soon shown that the 2,3-DPG level returned to normal within about 24 hours,[101, 102] the development of media that preserved red cell 2,3-DPG throughout the storage period became an important goal.

Development of Artificial Storage Media for Erythrocytes. The desire to develop storage media to improve preservation of red cell 2,3-DPG, as well as the increased use of red cell concentrates and other blood fractions, stimulated the introduction of artificial storage media in 1971.[103, 104] One of the early solutions that was developed, bicarbonate-adenine-glucose-phosphate-mannitol (BAGPM),[105–108] maintained normal 2,3-DPG levels and excellent viability for 6 to 7 weeks. Several years later, Högman and associates introduced another artificial preservative, saline-adenine-glucose (SAG),[109] which maintains viability but not 2,3-DPG levels. The addition of mannitol[110] decreased the marked hemolysis that was observed with SAG. Subsequently modified formulas such as SAGM,[111–113] Adsol,[114–117] and Nutricel[118] have been widely used in the past few years.

Changes Occurring During Red Cell Storage: The Storage Lesion

During storage in conventional storage media such as ACD, ACD-adenine, CPD, CPD-adenine, or Adsol, the 2,3-DPG level, the ATP level, and the potassium content of the red cells decline.[104, 119, 120] The pH of the suspension falls as the lactate and pyruvate levels rise.[119] The ammonia concentration increases as AMP is deaminated and the level of red cell sodium increases.[121] Vesicles of membrane and hemoglobin accumulate,[122] and there is frank hemolysis of stored cells. However, the volume of red cells remains constant throughout storage.[117] When stored red cells are reinfused, some of the cells are rapidly removed from the circulation within the first 24 hours. Those cells that survive the first postinfusion day have a normal lifespan. The cells that fail to survive are designated *nonviable*, whereas those that do survive are *viable*.[90–92] When less than 70% of the erythrocytes are viable, the red cells are generally considered to be unsatisfactory for transfusion.

The changes that occur during storage of red cells at 4°C and that presumably lead to loss of viability after reinfusion are collectively known as the *storage lesion*. Because there is some correlation between loss of ATP during storage and the percentage of cells that are viable, ATP levels have often been used as a surrogate marker for viability measurements.[123–125] In reality, the correlation between ATP levels and viability is poor,[105, 126–128] and the precise factors that determine the viability of stored erythrocytes are still not understood.

Many efforts have been made to identify other factors that may correlate with loss of viability. The suggestion that increased annexin V binding to erythrocytes (a measure of exposed phosphotidyl serine) during storage could be used to assess the quality of stored red cells[129] could not be confirmed.[9, 130] Increased binding of anti–band 3 immunoglobulin G (IgG) antibody to stored cells has been reported.[131] Considerable attention has been paid to the possibility that oxidative damage is an important component of the storage lesion,[132–134] but its role has not been clearly defined.

Measurement of Erythrocyte Viability

It has been generally recognized since the early studies of Finch and colleagues that transfused erythrocytes that survive the first 24 hours after reinfusion have an essentially normal lifespan. It is the loss of nonviable cells in the first hours after transfusion that increases with storage time and makes it necessary to discard blood after 21 days in ACD solution and 42 days in Adsol. Estimation of the percentage of cells that are still viable is thus essential in the evaluation of any new preservative; there is currently no substitute for making this measurement directly.

To measure the viability of stored erythrocytes, it is necessary to label the stored cells, infuse them into a normal human subject, and calculate, from a second sample, the percentage of the originally infused cells that are still present in the circulation after 24 hours. The classical means of identifying the transfused cells is the use of an immunological difference between the cells of the donor and those of the recipient, as originally done with the ABO group by Ashby.[81] This method has been used, even relatively recently,[135, 136] but is suitable only for measuring viability of stored red cells in patients who need transfusions. Because the evaluation of red cells stored in preservatives is ordinarily carried out by reinfusing autologous blood into normal donors, it is usually necessary to label the cells with a radioisotopic tag, although nonradioactive isotopes may also be used.[137–140] Chromium-51 is most frequently employed, because the binding of chromate to the red cell is relatively firm and it is technically easy to count. Although other tags such as carbon-14 cyanate[141] or biotin[142] might serve as well, the large body of experience with the use of ^{51}Cr has made it the most frequently used tag.

It is not enough, however, to know how many tagged cells have been infused. The volume through which they are distributed must also be determined, so that the number remaining can be calculated from a blood sample drawn 24 hours after infusion. The most commonly used method for determining this distribution space, the red cell mass, is to draw samples frequently after the infusion of the labeled cells and to back-extrapolate to the time of infusion.[128, 143, 144] This approach has been criticized because it assumes that the loss of cells is exponential even during the first few minutes after infusion, when mixing is incomplete and no measurements can be made. It has been suggested that an independent measurement of the red cell volume be made instead, with the use of iodine-131 albumin.[145, 146] This is an indirect measurement of the red cell mass, because it is plasma volume that is actually estimated. The latter is then converted to an estimate of the red cell mass by means of an empirical conversion factor.[145, 147] Recent studies suggest that such measurements may be sufficiently reliable for clinical purposes.[148]

Fortunately, another method for accurate measurement of red cell mass has become available. Red cells labeled with technetium-99m are stable for 20 to 30 minutes, which is long enough to permit dilution of labeled red cells to be measured accurately.[149] This technique can be used to measure viability of stored cells, labeling the stored cells with ^{51}Cr and the subject's own freshly drawn cells with ^{99m}Tc. This method has made it possible to demonstrate that the classical back-extrapolation method overestimates viability by less than 4%,[144] which suggests its suitability for routine use (Fig. 9–3). For more exact results, the combined ^{51}Cr-^{99m}Tc method can be used; its validity has been confirmed in a number of studies.[150, 151]

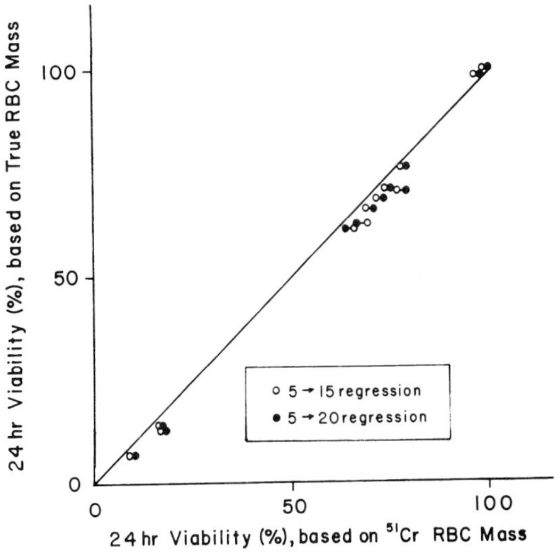

Figure 9–3. A comparison of estimation of the viability of stored red cells based on back extrapolation of ^{51}Cr-labeled red cells (abscissa) and on measurement of the red cell mass with ^{99m}Tc ("True RBC Mass") (ordinate). Separate values are shown for back extrapolation for 5 to 15 minutes *(hollow circles)* and 5 to 20 minutes *(solid circles)*. The former measurement is more reliable, because the 20-minute point tends to deviate from linearity. (From Beutler E, West C. Measurement of the viability of stored red cells by the single isotope technique using ^{51}Cr. Analysis of validity. Transfusion 1984; 24:100.)

Additives

ACD, the prototype of the first generation of modern preservatives, maintained viability of at least 70% of stored red cells for 21 days.[135] 2,3-DPG is virtually entirely depleted within 1 week.[119, 152] A number of modifications in ACD solutions have been made in an attempt to improve the storage of red cells.

Phosphate. The first major attempt to modify ACD consisted of slightly raising its pH and adding a small amount of phosphate ion. The resultant solution, CPD, was initially claimed to support viability of red cells for 28 rather than 21 days,[153] but this was not uniformly found to be the case.[135] What was clear, although its importance was not appreciated at first, is that CPD maintains higher 2,3-DPG levels than ACD because of its higher pH.[119]

Much higher levels of phosphates in CPD solution have also been studied.[154, 155] Inorganic phosphate strongly stimulates glycolysis in erythrocytes by relieving the inhibition of hexokinase by glucose-6-phosphate and possibly by stimulating the glyceraldehyde phosphate dehydrogenase reaction.[156] As a result, both ATP and 2,3-DPG levels are enhanced by high phosphate levels in the preservative. To a considerable extent, however, the addition of excess phosphate is self-defeating, because the increased rate of glycolysis results in a more rapid generation of lactic acid and fall in pH. Even when ATP levels were enhanced, no improvement in viability was noted.[127]

Inosine. When inosine is added to storage media, it is cleaved in the presence of phosphate by nucleoside phosphorylase to yield ribose-1-phosphate and hypoxanthine (see Fig. 9–2). The ribose-1-phosphate ultimately enters the glycolytic pathway and serves as a source of phosphate for the phosphorylation of ADP to ATP.[86, 87] Unfortunately, upon reinfusion, the hypoxanthine is converted to uric acid, and a marked rise in the level of plasma urate is observed.[157] Moreover, the loss of adenine moiety from the red cells by deamination cannot be corrected by inosine; adenosine can be converted to inosine, but the reverse reaction does not occur. Thus when purified inosine was used as an additive to ACD solution, no improvement in viability was noted.[93, 94]

Adenine. Adenine has proved to be a much more valuable additive than inosine. Effective at only one tenth or less the concentration of inosine, it can restore the adenine nucleotide pool through the action of APRT.[97] Its effectiveness in improving the viability of red cells was demonstrated first with inosine[95] but subsequently simply by its addition to the ACD preservative at the beginning of storage.[96] The remarkable effect of adenine in prolonging the storage life of blood has been confirmed by numerous investigators over the past 30 years.[126, 158–162]

Guanine Nucleosides. Limited studies of the effect of guanine nucleosides have been carried out.[157, 163–167] There is some suggestion that the addition of guanosine may improve viability of stored cells beyond the level that can be achieved with adenine.[157] The mechanism of such an effect is not altogether clear, although red cells do have active guanine nucleotide metabolism,[167] GTPase activity,[73] and, as shown recently by a number of investigators, GTP-binding membrane proteins.[58–60, 77]

Dihydroxyacetone. DHA improves maintenance of 2,3-DPG by stored red cells[46, 48, 49, 168, 169] but is metabolized too slowly to be useful as a rejuvenation solution.[46] The pH optimum of phosphorylation of DHA by triokinase, the limiting step in its metabolism, is much more favorable than the pH optimum of phosphorylation of glucose by hexokinase.[44] The toxicity of DHA appears to be extremely low. High concentrations can be intravenously infused directly into rabbits.[44, 46] Although it was introduced more than two decades ago, little attention has been paid to this potentially valuable additive. Part of the reason for this may be that DHA is unstable in CPD solution, probably because of the presence of phosphate. However, in slightly acidic water, DHA is very stable, and it could be readily incorporated into a preservative system by placing it in a separate pouch.

Ascorbate and Oxalate. In 1972 my colleagues and I discovered that the addition of ascorbic acid to ACD or CPD preservative media appeared to exert a profound effect on the preservation of 2,3-DPG in stored blood,[106, 170, 171] but we were unable to elucidate the mechanism of this effect. Synergism with DHA was demonstrated.[45] Subsequently, the ascorbate derivatives dehydroascorbate and ascorbate-2-phosphate were alleged to raise 2,3-DPG levels.[123, 124, 172] The mysterious effect of ascorbate was clarified when industry attempted to develop a commercial system by using highly purified ascorbate. It was found that ascorbate had no effect but that the oxalate that contaminated ascorbate profoundly affected red cell 2,3-DPG levels during storage,[173] apparently by inhibiting the PK reaction.[174] The toxic effect of oxalate[175]—the development of urolithiasis—limits its applicability as a blood preservation additive.

Addition of glyoxylate and ethyl oxaloacetate to CPD-adenine also increases 2,3-DPG levels of stored red cells.[176] These compounds can be metabolized to oxalate, which probably explains their effect.

Pyruvate. Pyruvate is known to stimulate red cell glycolysis by oxidizing NADH to NAD, thus facilitating the glyceraldehyde phosphate dehydrogenase reaction. The addition of pyruvate to blood storage media improves preservation of both ATP and 2,3-DPG.[177] The effect of pyruvate is relatively modest. Moreover, pyruvate solutions tend to be unstable, so the use of pyruvate-based media has not been implemented.

Xanthones. Xanthone compound BW A827C [2-ethoxy-6-(5-tetrazolyl)xanthone], known to influence the oxygen dissociation curve by direct interaction with hemoglobin, was tested for its effect on stored red cells. Surprisingly, it caused a right shift in the oxygen dissociation curve not only by directly affecting hemoglobin but also by increasing red cell 2,3-DPG levels.[178] A closely related xanthone compound, BW A440C [2-(2-hydroxyethoxy)-6-(1-*H*-tetrazole-5-yl)xanthen-9-one], was found to have a similar effect.[179] These results have been confirmed, and it has been demonstrated that at low concentrations, BW A440C inhibits PK and diphosphoglycerate phosphatase.[180] Inhibition of either of these enzymes leads to an increase in 2,3-DPG levels; thus the effect of xanthone compounds can be readily explained by their impact on the metabolic flow in stored erythrocytes. Although the effect exerted by this class of compounds is interesting, it is unlikely that these substances, which do not occur normally in the body, will be useful as additives to preservative solutions.

Phthalates. Di-2-ethylhexylphthalate (DEHP) is a component of the polyvinyl chloride plastic films that are used as blood containers. Phthalates have been a necessary part of the formulation, in that they provide suitable physical properties to the plastic film. These hydrophobic compounds are leached from the film into stored blood. The fate of the phthalate upon infusion into the recipient is uncertain, but it has been suggested that it may have significant toxic properties.[181–184] To avoid the use of phthalates, formulations without this type of plasticizer have been tested. Surprisingly, it was found that in vitro and in vivo hemolysis of red cells was greatly accelerated in the absence of phthalate.

Thus, although not an additive in the true sense of the word, phthalates may play an important role in maintaining the physical integrity of stored red blood cells[185–188] and even their viability after reinfusion.[189] A different plasticizer[112] appears to maintain the integrity of the stored red cells and is readily metabolized upon reinfusion. The mechanism by which phthalates or other plasticizers prevent in vitro hemolysis is not well understood.

Other Additives. Because PK deficiency is characterized by an increase in red cell 2,3-DPG levels, and inhibitors of PK such as oxalate or xanthones increase 2,3-DPG during storage (see earlier), it seems reasonable that other inhibitors of this enzyme might be useful as additives to storage solutions. Alanine is such a compound and appears to have a positive effect on 2,3-DPG levels during blood storage.[53, 176, 190, 191] L-Phenylalanyl-L-alanine has a similar effect, probably being hydrolyzed to L-alanine.[176] However, the effect of alanine is modest, and no major studies of its possible usefulness have been undertaken.

The ammonium ion appears to have a striking effect on the preservation of red cell ATP levels. It was shown to have such an effect in 1981 by Debski,[192] and interest in its possible role was sparked by storage of red cells in a hypotonic medium containing high concentrations of phosphate, ammonium ion, low sodium, and low pH.[193]

Artificial Storage Media

Artificial storage media are added to red cell concentrates prepared from whole blood collected in ACD storage media. The use of half-strength CPD (0.5 CPD) as the collection medium appears to have some advantage, in that 2,3-DPG levels are better maintained while the whole blood is held before concentration of the cells and their resuspension in the artificial medium.[194] Currently used solutions have in common the inclusion of sodium chloride to provide iso-osmolarity, adenine to maintain adenine nucleotide levels, glucose as a source of energy, and mannitol to prevent in vitro hemolysis. We originally proposed the use of mannitol in such solutions because we thought that this impermeable solute would provide the osmotic support for erythrocytes needed when plasma proteins and citrate are removed. However, the effect of mannitol on red cell volume during storage is modest, suggesting some other mechanism of action.[117] The inclusion of citrate in such solutions[161, 195, 196] may be useful, because this polyanion increases intracellular pH through the Donnan membrane equilibrium.[197]

Experimental media containing high concentrations of phosphate and ammonium ion and a low sodium content have been found to have remarkable effects on red cell ADP levels.[193] When the effects of the various components were dissected systematically, it became apparent that the most important component of this solution was ammonium,[198–200] although, as had been shown much earlier, high phosphate concentrations also stimulate ATP levels in stored cells. It is well known that ammonium ion releases phosphofructokinase from inhibition by its substrate, ATP, and thus serves to stimulate glycolysis.[198] One such experimental additive solution designated EAS-2 maintained viability at 79.5% ± 7.1% at 9 weeks of storage.[201] Studies have also been performed with other additives designed to cause cell swelling and generate ammonia[202] and with L-carnitine.[203]

The flexibility of components of artificial storage media greatly exceeds that of preservatives in which whole blood or red cells are stored. The bicarbonate ion is an ideal buffer for red cells because it is nontoxic and its acid product carbonic acid can be lost from the preservative solution by diffusion through the plastic film of a container.[105] Alternatively, it can be absorbed by an internal calcium hydroxide pack.[107] One of the earliest artificial media was BAGPM. This medium maintains viability and 2,3-DPG levels for over 6 weeks, but it has never been used, partly because of difficulties in the manufacturing of bicarbonate-containing solutions.

Rejuvenation Solutions

Red cells that have been stored in conventional media for several weeks may be metabolically rejuvenated by raising the pH[204] and by adding substrate such as inosine. One such effective rejuvenating solution is phosphate-inosine-glucose-pyruvate-adenine (PIGPA).[205] PEP has also been used for this purpose.[52, 206] Although incubation with such solutions can undoubtedly improve the metabolic integrity of long-stored erythrocytes, the economic benefits of rejuvenation are dubious, and such solutions are not currently in wide use except for autologous cells or cells with unusual phenotypes.

Effect of Irradiation

In the context of providing red cell transfusion therapy to severely immunosuppressed individuals, it is necessary to irradiate the cells with gamma rays to render lymphocytes nonviable and thus prevent graft-versus-host disease. It appears that treatment with 30 cGy results in some increase of in vitro hemolysis,[207, 208] but reported data regarding the effect on post-transfusion viability are contradictory: one study reported a substantial decrease in red cell viability,[207] while no effect was found in another.[208]

Future Prospects

The trend toward fractionation of blood has continued for over two decades, and red blood cells are now typically separated and administered as a component. It is logical to store these red cells in a suspending medium especially designed to prolong their survival and maintain their functional properties. Artificial preservatives currently in use fall far short of the ideal because they do not maintain 2,3-DPG levels. A solution that does maintain both viability and 2,3-DPG levels (BAGPM) exists, but advances in manufacturing techniques are needed to implement this solution. Selective addition of supplementary compounds to stored cells would be greatly facilitated by the development of inexpensive sterile docking devices. These systems would allow separate addition of components that may not be compatible with the basic storage medium.

With increasing concern over the risk of infection from transfusion, technologies for extensive washing of stored red cells before infusion are being developed. Such technologies broaden the types of compounds that can be added to red cells during storage. For example, although the hypoxanthine formed from inosine during storage presents a hazard to the patient because of its metabolism to uric acid, inosine-containing media would be safe if the cells were washed before reinfusion. Similarly, oxalate, which has a potent effect on 2,3-DPG levels, could be added to red cells during storage if it were removed by washing before reinfusion.

Attempts to add antiviral agents to red cell suspensions pose a new challenge. In reality, screening for viruses has become so efficient that the infection rate from transfusion of red cells is extremely low. This fact makes ironic the intense effort being undertaken in many quarters to develop virucidal techniques that can be applied to erythrocytes. Many of the agents being studied are foreign substances, and it is doubtful that they will pass a risk-benefit analysis, because the risk is now so low. Indeed, the main argument for the development of virucidal techniques is the prevention of transmission of infectious agents that might appear in the blood supply in the future.

Because detergents that disrupt viral envelopes disrupt red cell membranes as well, the search for substances that can be used in whole blood as opposed to plasma has been difficult. Moreover, because some infectious agents, such as the human immunodeficiency virus, may be located intracellularly in contaminating lymphocytes and monocytes, sterilization of the plasma surrounding the red cells is not sufficient. Trials have been carried out on photoreactive agents such as aluminum phthalocyanine tetrasulfanes and related compounds,[209–212] benzoporphyrin derivatives,[213] and methylene blue and related dyes,[214–215] but no practical means of red cell sterilization is yet at hand.

There seems little doubt that additional effort and the development of the necessary technology will make red cell transfusion even safer and more effective than it is today.

REFERENCES

1. Chapman RG, Schaumburg L. Glycolysis and glycolytic enzyme activity of aging red cells in man. Changes in hexokinase, aldolase, glyceraldehyde-3-phosphate dehydrogenase, pyruvate kinase and glutamic-oxalacetic transaminase. Br J Haematol 1967; 13:665.
2. Brewer GJ, Powell RD. Hexokinase activity as a function of age of the human erythrocyte. Nature 1963; 199:704.
3. Löhr GW, Waller HD. Zellstoffwechsel und Zellalterung. Klin Wochenschr 1959; 37:833.
4. Allison AC, Burn GP. Enzyme activity as a function of age in the human erythrocyte. Br J Haematol 1955; 1:291.
5. Beutler E. Isolation of the aged. Blood Cells 1988; 14:1.
6. Beutler E. The relationship of red cell enzymes to red cell life-span. Blood Cells 1988; 14:69.
7. Suzuki T, Dale GL. Senescent erythrocytes: isolation of in vivo aged cells and their biochemical characteristics. Proc Natl Acad Sci U S A 1988; 85:1647.
8. Connor J, Pak CC, Schroit AJ. Exposure of phosphatidylserine in the outer leaflet of human red blood cells. Relationship to cell density, cell age, and clearance by mononuclear cells. J Biol Chem 1994; 269:2399.
9. Boas E, Forman L, Beutler E. Phosphatidyl serine exposure and red cell viability in red cell ageing, storage, and in hemolytic anemia. Blood 1997; 90(Suppl 1):272a.
10. Beutler E. Energy metabolism and maintenance of erythrocytes. *In* Williams WJ, Beutler E, Erslev AJ, Lichtman MA (eds): Hematology, 4th ed. New York: McGraw-Hill, 1990, pp 355–368.
11. Beutler E. Red cell enzyme defects. Hematol Pathol 1990; 4:103.
12. Valentine WN, Tanaka KR, Paglia DE. Hemolytic anemias and erythrocyte enzymopathies. Ann Intern Med 1985; 103:245.
13. Benaim G, De Meis L. Activation of the purified erythrocyte plasma membrane Ca^{2+}-ATPase by organic solvents. FEBS Lett 1989; 244:484.
14. Morrot G, Zachowski A, Devaux PF. Partial purification and characterization of the human erythrocyte Mg^{2+}-ATPase. FEBS Lett 1990; 266:29.
15. Kondo T, Kawakami Y, Taniguchi N, Beutler E. Glutathione disulfide–stimulated Mg^{2+}-ATPase of human erythrocyte membranes. Proc Natl Acad Sci U S A 1987; 84:7373.
16. Sharma R, Gupta S, Ahmad H, et al. Stimulation of a human erythrocyte membrane ATPase by glutathione conjugates. Toxicol Appl Pharmacol 1990; 104:421.
17. Sharma R, Gupta S, Singh SV, et al. Purification and characterization of dinitrophenylglutathione ATPase of human erythrocytes and its expression in other tissues. Biochem Biophys Res Commun 1990; 171:155.
18. Beutler E, Dale GL. Erythrocyte glutathione: function and metabolism. *In* Dolphin D, Poulson R, Avramovic O (eds): Glutathione: Chemical, Biochemical, and Medical Aspects. New York: John Wiley and Sons, 1989, pp 291–317.
19. Yip LC, Roome S, Balis ME. In vitro and in vivo age-related modification of human erythrocyte phosphoribosyl pyrophosphate synthetase. Biochemistry 1978; 17:3286.
20. Becker MA, Meyer LJ, Huisman W, et al. Human erythrocyte phosphoribosylpyrophosphate synthetase. J Biol Chem 1977; 252:3911.
21. Wei T, Tao M. Human erythrocyte casein kinase II: characterization and phosphorylation of membrane cytoskeletal proteins. Arch Biochem Biophys 1993; 307:206.
22. Wright L, Chen S, Roufogalis BD. Regulation of the activity and phosphorylation of the plasma membrane Ca^{2}-ATPase by protein kinase C in intact human erythrocytes. Arch Biochem Biophys 1993; 306:277.
23. Norris ER, Howard TA, Marcus SJ, Ware RE. Structural and functional analysis of the PIG-A protein that is mutated in paroxysmal nocturnal hemoglobinuria. Blood Cells Mol Dis 1997; 23:350.
24. Xu W, Beutler E. An exonic polymorphism in the human glucose phosphate isomerase (GPI) gene. Blood Cells Mol Dis 1997; 23:377.
25. Langdon RG, Holman VP. Immunological evidence that band 3 is the major glucose transporter of the human erythrocyte membrane. Biochim Biophys Acta 1988; 945:23.
26. Shelton RL, Langdon RG. Reconstitution of glucose transport using human erythrocyte band 3. Biochim Biophys Acta 1983; 733:25.
27. Kondo T, Beutler E. Developmental changes in glucose transport of guinea pig erythrocytes. J Clin Invest 1980; 65:1.
28. Kahlenberg A, Zala CA. Reconstitution of D-glucose transport in vesicles composed of lipids and intrinsic protein (zone 4.5) of the erythrocyte membrane. J Supramol Struct 1977; 7:287.

29. Jacquez JA. Modulation of glucose transport in human red blood cells by ATP. Biochim Biophys Acta 1983; 727:367.
30. Carruthers A. ATP regulation of the human red cell sugar transporter. J Biochem 1986; 261:11028.
31. May JM. Effects of ATP depletion on the mechanism of hexose transport in intact human erythrocytes. FEBS Lett 1988; 241:188.
32. Kim HD, McManus TJ. Studies on the energy metabolism of pig red cells: I. The limiting role of membrane permeability in glycolysis. Biochim Biophys Acta 1971; 230:1.
33. Verma IM, Somia N. Gene therapy—promises, problems and prospects. Nature 1997; 389:239.
34. Fujii S, Matsuda M, Okuya S, et al. Fructose-6-phosphate, 2-kinase activity in human erythrocytes. Blood 1987; 70:1211.
35. Vora S. Isozymes of phosphofructokinase. *In* Rattazzi MC, Scandalios JG, Whitt GS (eds): Isozymes: Current Topics in Biological and Medical Research. New York: AR Liss, 1982, pp 119–167.
36. Duhm J, Gerlach E. On the mechanisms of the hypoxia-induced increase of 2,3-diphosphoglycerate in erythrocytes. Studies on rat erythrocytes in vivo and on human erythrocytes in vitro. Pflugers Arch 1971; 326:254.
37. Rorth M. Hemoglobin interactions and red cell metabolism. Semin Haematol 1972; 5:7.
38. Sasaki R, Ikura K, Narita H, et al. 2,3-Bisphosphoglycerate in erythroid cells. TIBS Rev 1982; 7:140.
39. De Bruijne AW, Vreeburg H, Van Steveninck J. Kinetic analysis of L-lactate transport in human erythrocytes via the monocarboxylate-specific carrier system. Biochim Biophys Acta 1983; 732:562.
40. Halestrap AP. Transport of pyruvate and lactate into human erythrocytes. Biochem J 1976; 156:193.
41. Moses SW, Bashan N. Fructose metabolism in the human red blood cell. Isr J Med Sci 1974; 10:707.
42. Beutler E, Duron O. Studies of blood preservation. The relative capacities of hexoses, hexitols and ethanol to maintain red cell ATP levels during storage. Transfusion 1966; 6:537.
43. Beutler E, Teeple L. Mannose metabolism in the human erythrocyte. J Clin Invest 1969; 48:461.
44. Beutler E, Guinto E. Dihydroxyacetone metabolism by human erythrocytes: demonstration of triokinase activity and its characterization. Blood 1973; 41:559.
45. Wood L, Beutler E. The effect of ascorbate and dihydroxyacetone on the 2,3-diphosphoglycerate and ATP levels of stored human red cells. Transfusion 1974; 14:272.
46. Beutler E, Guinto E. The metabolism of dihydroxyacetone by intact erythrocytes. J Lab Clin Med 1973; 82:534.
47. Laborit H. Concerning the use of dihydroxyacetone as a new substrate in blood preservation mediums. Agressologie 1972; 13:243.
48. Brake JM, Deindoerfer FH. Preservation of red blood cell 2,3-diphosphoglycerate in stored blood containing dihydroxyacetone. Transfusion 1973; 13:84.
49. Dawson RB. Blood preservation using metabolic regulators and nutrients: XXI. Further studies on pyruvate and DHA (dihydroxyacetone). Transfusion 1976; 16:446.
50. Hamasaki N, Hardjono IS, Minakami S. Transport of phosphoenolpyruvate through the erythrocyte membrane. Biochem J 1978; 170:39.
51. Hamasaki N, Ideguchi H, Ikehara Y. Regeneration of 2,3-bisphosphoglycerate and ATP in stored erythrocytes by phosphoenolpyruvate: a new preservative for blood storage. Transfusion 1981; 21:391.
52. Matsuyama H, Niklasson F, de Verdier CH, Högman CF. Phosphoenolpyruvate in the rejuvenation of stored red cells in SAGM medium: optimal conditions and the indirect effect of methemoglobin formation. Transfusion 1989; 29:614.
53. Matsuyama H, Ericson ÅA, Högman CF, et al. Lack of success with a combination of alanine and phosphoenolpyruvate as an additive for liquid storage of red cells at 4°C. Transfusion 1990; 30:339.
54. Luzzatto L. Regulation of the activity of glucose-6-phosphate dehydrogenase by NADP+ and NADPH. Biochim Biophys Acta 1967; 146:18.
55. Yoshida A. Hemolytic anemia and G-6-PD deficiency. Science 1973; 179:532.
56. Kirkman HN, Gaetani GD, Clemons EH, Mareni C. Red cell $NADP^+$ and NADPH in glucose-6-phosphate dehydrogenase deficiency. J Clin Invest 1975; 55:875.
57. Fox IH, Kelley WN. Phosphoribosylpyrophosphate in man: biochemical and clinical significance. Ann Intern Med 1971; 74:424.
58. Damonte G, Morelli A, Piu M, et al. "In situ" characterization of guanine nucleotide-binding properties of erythrocyte membranes. Biochem Biophys Res Commun 1989; 159:41.
59. Bergamini CM. GTP modulates calcium binding and cation-induced conformational changes in erythrocyte transglutaminase. FEBS Lett 1988; 239:255.
60. Ikeda K, Kikuchi A, Takai Y. Small molecular weight GTP-binding proteins in human erythrocyte ghosts. Biochem Biophys Res Commun 1988; 156:889.
61. Ogasawara N, Goto H, Yamada Y, Hasegawa I. Deficiency of erythrocyte type isozyme of AMP deaminase in human. Adv Exp Med Biol 1986; 195:123.
62. Ogasawara N, Goto H, Yamada Y, et al. Deficiency of AMP deaminase in erythrocytes. Hum Genet 1987; 75:15.
63. Dale GL, Norenberg SL, Suzuki T, Forman L. Altered adenine nucleotide metabolism in senescent erythrocytes from the rabbit. Prog Clin Biol Res 1989; 319:259.
64. Paglia DE, Valentine WN, Nakatani M, Brockway RA. AMP deaminase as a cell-age marker in transient erythroblastopenia of childhood and its role in the adenylate economy of erythrocytes. Blood 1989; 74:2161.
65. Dale GL, Norenberg SL. Time-dependent loss of adenosine 5′-monophosphate deaminase activity may explain elevated adenosine 5′-triphosphate levels in senescent erythrocytes. Blood 1989; 74:2157.
66. Brok F, Ramot B, Zwang E, Danon D. Enzyme activities in human red blood cells of different age groups. Isr J Med Sci 1966; 2:291.
67. Bartosz G, Grzelinska E, Wagner J. Aging of the erythrocyte: XIV. ATP content does decrease. Experientia 1982; 38:575.
68. Magnani M, Stocchi V, Dacha M, Fornaini G. Rabbit red blood cell hexokinase. Evidences for an ATP-dependent decay during cell maturation. Mol Cell Biochem 1984; 61:83.
69. Srivastava SK, Beutler E. Purification and kinetic studies of adenine phosphoribosyltransferase from human erythrocytes. Arch Biochem Biophys 1971; 142:426.
70. Meyskens FL, Williams HE. Adenosine metabolism in human erythrocytes. Biochim Biophys Acta 1971; 240:170.
71. Sidi Y, Gelvan I, Brosh S, et al. Guanine nucleotide metabolism in red blood cells: the metabolic basis for GTP depletion in HGPRT and PNP deficiency. Adv Exp Med Biol 1990; 253A:67.
72. Bishop C, Rankine D, Talbott JH. The nucleotides in normal human blood. J Biol Chem 1959; 234:1233.
73. Beutler E, Kuhl W. Guanosine triphosphatase activity in human erythrocyte membranes. Biochim Biophys Acta 1980; 601:372.
74. Hosey MM, Tao M. Selective phosphorylation of erythrocyte membrane proteins by the solubilized membrane protein kinases. Biochemistry 1977; 16:4578.
75. Lee CS, O'Sullivan WJ. Properties and mechanism of human erythrocyte phosphoglycerate kinase. J Biol Chem 1975; 250:1275.
76. Bergamini CM, Signorini M, Poltronieri L. Inhibition of erythrocyte transglutaminase by GTP. Biochim Biophys Acta 1987; 916:149.
77. Carty DJ, Iyengar R. A 43 kDa form of the GTP-binding protein G_{i3} in human erythrocytes. FEBS Lett 1990; 262:101.
78. Rous P, Turner JR. The preservation of living red blood cells in vitro: I. Methods of preservation. J Exp Med 1916; 23:219.
79. Rous P, Turner JR. The preservation of living red blood cells in vitro: II. The transfusion of kept cells. J Exp Med 1916; 23:239.
80. Robertson OH. Transfusion with preserved red blood cells. BMJ 1918; 1:691.
81. Ashby W. The determination of the length of life of transfused blood corpuscles in man. J Exp Med 1919; 29:267.
82. Loutit JF, Mollison PL, Young IM, Lucas EJ. Citric acid–sodium citrate–glucose mixtures for blood storage. Q J Exp Physiol 1943; 32:183.
83. Loutit JF, Mollison PL. Advantages of a disodium-citrate-glucose mixture as a blood preservative. BMJ 1943; 2:744.
84. Gibson JG, Rees SB, McManus TJ, Scheitlin WA II. A citrate-phosphate-dextrose solution for the preservation of human blood. Am J Clin Pathol 1957; 28:569.
85. Rapoport S. Dimensional, osmotic, and chemical changes of erythrocytes in stored blood: I. Blood preserved in sodium citrate, neutral, and acid citrate-glucose (ACD) mixtures. J Clin Invest 1947; 26:591.

86. Gabrio BW, Finch CA, Huennekens FM. Erythrocyte preservation: a topic in molecular biochemistry. Blood 1956; 11:103.
87. Gabrio BW, Donohue DM, Huennekens FM, Finch CA. Erythrocyte preservation: VII. Acid-citrate-dextrose-inosine (ACDI) as a preservative for blood during storage at 4 degrees C. J Clin Invest 1956; 35:657.
88. Donohue DM, Finch CA, Gabrio BW. Erythrocyte preservation: VI. The storage of blood with purine nucleosides. J Clin Invest 1956; 35:562.
89. Gabrio BW, Donohue DM, Finch CA. Erythrocyte preservation: V. Relationship between chemical changes and viability of stored blood treated with adenosine. J Clin Invest 1956; 34:1509.
90. Gabrio BW, Stevens AR, Finch CA. Erythrocyte preservation: III. The reversibility of the storage lesion. J Clin Invest 1954; 33:252.
91. Gabrio BW, Stevens AR, Finch CA. Erythrocyte preservation: II. A study of extra-erythrocyte factors in the storage of blood in acid-citrate-dextrose. J Clin Invest 1954; 33:247.
92. Gabrio BW, Finch CA. Erythrocyte preservation: I. The relation of the storage lesion to in vivo erythrocyte senescence. J Clin Invest 1954; 33:242.
93. Lange RD, Crosby WH, Donohue DM, et al. Effect of inosine on red cell preservation. J Clin Invest 1958; 37:1485.
94. Finch CA. Adenine-supplemented blood. Vox Sang 1985; 48:319.
95. Nakao K, Wada T, Kamiyama T, et al. A direct relationship between adenosine triphosphate-level and in vivo viability of erythrocytes. Nature 1962; 194:877.
96. Simon ER. Red cell preservation: further studies with adenine. Blood 1962; 20:485.
97. Sugita Y, Simon ER. The mechanism of action of adenine in red cell preservation. J Clin Invest 1965; 44:629.
98. Valtis DJ, Kennedy AC. Defective gas-transport function of stored red blood-cells. Lancet 1954; 1:119.
99. Benesch R, Benesch RE. The effect of organic phosphates from the human erythrocyte on the allosteric properties of hemoglobin. Biochem Biophys Res Commun 1967; 26:162.
100. Chanutin A, Curnish RR. Effect of organic and inorganic phosphates on the oxygen equilibrium of human erythrocytes. Arch Biochem Biophys 1967; 121:96.
101. Beutler E, Wood L. The in vivo regeneration of red cell 2,3-diphosphoglyceric acid (DPG) after transfusion of stored blood. J Lab Clin Med 1969; 74:300.
102. Valeri CR, Hirsch NM. Restoration in vivo of erythrocyte adenosine triphosphate, 2,3-diphosphoglycerate, potassium ion, and sodium ion concentrations following the transfusion of acid-citrate-dextrose-stored human red blood cells. J Lab Clin Med 1969; 73:722.
103. Beutler E, Wood LA. Preservation of red cell 2,3-DPG in modified ACD solution and in experimental artificial storage media. Vox Sang 1971; 20:403.
104. Wood L, Beutler E. Storage of erythrocytes in artificial media. Transfusion 1971; 11:123.
105. Beutler E, Wood LA. Preservation of red cell 2,3-DPG and viability in bicarbonate-containing medium: the effect of blood-bag permeability. J Lab Clin Med 1972; 80:723.
106. Beutler E. Viability, function, and rejuvenation of liquid-stored red cells. *In* Chaplin HJ, Jaffe ER, Lenfant C, Valeri CR (eds): Preservation of Red Blood Cells. Washington, DC: National Academy of Sciences, 1973, pp 195–214.
107. Bensinger TA, Chillar R, Beutler E. Prolonged maintenance of 2,3-DPG in liquid storage: use of an internal CO_2 trap to stabilize pH. J Lab Clin Med 1977; 89:498.
108. Chillar RK, Bensinger TA, Beutler E. Maintenance of low screen filtration pressure in blood stored in a new liquid medium: BAGPM. J Lab Clin Med 1977; 89:504.
109. Högman CF, Hedlund K, Zetterstroem H. Clinical usefulness of red cells preserved in protein-poor mediums. N Engl J Med 1978; 299:1377.
110. Beutler E. Red cell suspensions. N Engl J Med 1979; 300:984.
111. Högman CF, Åkerblom O, Hedlund K, et al. Red cell suspensions in SAGM medium. Vox Sang 1983; 45:217.
112. Högman CF, Eriksson L, Ericson ÅA, Reppucci AJ. Storage of saline-adenine-glucose-mannitol–suspended red cells in a new plastic container: polyvinylchloride plasticized with butyryl-n-trihexyl-citrate. Transfusion 1991; 31:26.
113. Högman CF. Additive system approach in blood transfusion: birth of the SAG and Sagman systems. Vox Sang 1986; 51:339.
114. Valeri CR, Pivacek LE, Palter M, et al. A clinical experience with Adsol preserved erythrocytes. Surg Gynecol Obstet 1988; 166:33.
115. Moroff G, Holme S, Keegan T, Heaton A. Storage of Adsol-preserved red cells at 2.5 and 5.5°C: comparable retention of in vitro properties. Vox Sang 1990; 59:136.
116. Heaton A, Miripol J, Aster R, et al. Use of Adsol preservation solution for prolonged storage of low viscosity AS-1 red blood cells. Br J Haematol 1984; 57:467.
117. Beutler E, Kuhl W. Volume control of erythrocytes during storage: the role of mannitol. Transfusion 1988; 28:353.
118. Simon TL, Marcus CS, Myhre BA, Nelson EJ. Effects of AS-3 nutrient-additive solution on 42 and 49 days of storage of red cells. Transfusion 1987; 27:178.
119. Beutler E, Meul A, Wood LA. Depletion and regeneration of 2,3-diphosphoglyceric acid in stored red blood cells. Transfusion 1969; 9:109.
120. Beutler E. Preservation of liquid red cells. *In* Rossi EC, Simon TL, Moss GS (eds): Principles of Transfusion Medicine. Baltimore: Williams & Wilkins, 1990, pp 47–56.
121. Bontemps F, Van Den Berghe G, Hers HG. Pathways of adenine nucleotide catabolism in erythrocytes. J Clin Invest 1986; 77:824.
122. Greenwalt TJ, Zehner Sostok C, Dumaswala UJ. Studies in red blood cell preservation: 2. Comparison of vesicle formation, morphology, and membrane lipids during storage in AS-1 and CPDA-1. Vox Sang 1990; 58:90.
123. Moore GL, Marks DH, Carmen RA, et al. Ascorbate-2-phosphate in red cell preservation. Clinical trials and active components. Transfusion 1988; 28:221.
124. Moore GL, Ledford ME, Brummell MR. Improved red cell storage using optional additive systems (OAS) containing adenine, glucose and ascorbate-2-phosphate. Transfusion 1981; 21:723.
125. De Mendonca M, Appel M, Bidault J, et al. Maintenance of 2,3-DPG and ATP levels in blood stored for 30 days at a constant pH obtained by variation of CO_2. Vox Sang 1978; 35:184.
126. Åkerblom O, Kreuger A. Studies on citrate-phosphate-dextrose (CPD) blood supplemented with adenine. Vox Sang 1975; 29:90.
127. Wood L, Beutler E. The viability of human blood stored in phosphate adenine media. Transfusion 1967; 7:401.
128. Dern RJ, Brewer GJ, Wiorkowski JJ. Studies on the preservation of human blood: II. The relationship of erythrocyte adenosine triphosphate levels and other in vitro measures to red cell storageability. J Lab Clin Med 1967; 69:968.
129. Sestier C, Sabolovic D, Geldwerth D, et al. Use of annexin V-ferrofluid to enumerate erythrocytes damaged in various pathologies or during storage in vitro. C R Acad Sci III 1995; 318:1141.
130. Geldwerth D, Kuypers FA, Butikofer P, et al. Transbilayer mobility and distribution of red cell phospholipids during storage. J Clin Invest 1993; 92:308.
131. Ando K, Beppu M, Kikugawa K, Hamasaki N. Increased susceptibility of stored erythrocytes to anti–band 3 IgG autoantibody binding. Biochim Biophys Acta 1993; 1178:127.
132. Knight JA, Searles DA, Clayton FC. The effect of desferrioxamine on stored erythrocytes: lipid peroxidation, deformability, and morphology. Ann Clin Lab Sci 1996; 26:283.
133. Knight JA, Voorhees RP, Martin L, Anstall H. Lipid peroxidation in stored red cells. Transfusion 1992; 32:354.
134. Knight JA, Blaylock RC, Searles DA. The effect of vitamins C and E on lipid peroxidation in stored erythrocytes. Ann Clin Lab Sci 1993; 23:51.
135. Valeri CR, Szymanski IO, Zaroulis CG. 24-Hour survival of ACD- and CPD-stored red cells: 1. Evaluation of nonwashed and washed stored red cells. Vox Sang 1972; 22:289.
136. Szymanski IO, Valeri CR. Clinical evaluation of concentrated red cells. N Engl J Med 1969; 280:281.
137. Sioufi HA, Button LN, Jacobson MS, Kevy SV. Nonradioactive chromium technique for red cell labeling. Vox Sang 1990; 58:204.
138. Dever M, Smith JE, Hausler DW. A new approach for measuring the erythrocyte life span with a nonradioisotope. Clin Chim Acta 1989; 181:337.
139. Heaton WAL, Hanbury CM, Keegan TE, et al. Studies with nonradioisotopic sodium chromate: I. Development of a technique for measuring red cell volume. Transfusion 1989; 29:696.
140. Drysdale HC, Emerson PM, Holmes A. An improved method for the measurement of red cell survival using non-radioactive chromium. J Clin Pathol 1979; 32:655.

141. Eschbach JW, Korn D, Finch CA. ^{14}C cyanate as a tag for red cell survival in normal and uremic man. J Lab Clin Med 1977; 89:823.
142. Suzuki T, Dale GL. Biotinylated erythrocytes: in vivo survival and in vitro recovery. Blood 1987; 70:791.
143. Dern RJ. Studies on the preservation of human blood: III. The posttransfusion survival of stored and damaged erythrocytes in healthy donors and patients with severe trauma. J Lab Clin Med 1968; 71:254.
144. Beutler E, West C. Measurement of the viability of stored red cells by the single-isotope technique using 51-Cr: analysis of validity. Transfusion 1984; 24:100.
145. Button LN, Gibson JG II, Walter CW. Simultaneous determination of the volume of red cells and plasma for survival studies of stored blood. Transfusion 1965; 5:143.
146. Valeri CR. Measurement of viable Adsol-preserved human red cells. N Engl J Med 1985; 612:377.
147. Valeri CR, Cooper AG, Pivacek LE. Limitations of measuring blood volume with iodinated I 125 serum albumin. Arch Intern Med 1973; 132:534.
148. Fairbanks VF, Klee GG, Wiseman GA, et al. Measurement of blood volume and red cell mass: re-examination of ^{51}Cr and ^{125}I methods. Blood Cells Mol Dis 1996; 22:169.
149. Jones J, Mollison PL. A simple and efficient method of labelling red cells with 99m Tc for determination of red cell volume. Br J Haematol 1978; 38:141.
150. Heaton A, Keegan T, Hartman P, et al. Evaluation of single and double red cell label methods to measure red cell volume and post-transfusion recoveries of Terumo SAGM red cells [Abstract]. *In* Proceedings of the 20th Congress of the International Society of Blood Transfusion, 1988, p 283A.
151. Heaton WAL, Keegan T, Holme S, Momoda G. Evaluation of ^{99m}technetium/^{51}chromium post-transfusion recovery of red cells stored in saline, adenine, glucose, mannitol for 42 days. Vox Sang 1989; 57:37.
152. Chanutin A. Effect of storage of blood in ACD–adenine–inorganic phosphate plus nucleosides on metabolic intermediates of human red cells. Transfusion 1967; 7:409.
153. Gibson JG, Gregory CB, Button LN. Citrate-phosphate-dextrose solution for preservation of human blood: a further report. Transfusion 1961; 1:280.
154. Beutler E, Duron O. The preservation of red cell ATP: the effect of phosphate. Transfusion 1966; 6:124.
155. Dawson RB. Blood storage: XXII. Improvement in red blood cell 2,3-DPG levels at six weeks by 20 mM PO4 in CPD-adenine-inosine. Transfusion 1976; 16:450.
156. Rose IA, Warms JVB, O'Connell EL. Role of inorganic phosphate in stimulating the glucose utilization of human red blood cells. Biochem Biophys Res Commun 1964; 15:33.
157. Seidl S. Survival studies on the effect of the addition of adenine and different combinations of nucleosides in red cell preservation. Bibl Haematol 1971; 38:190.
158. Herve P, Lamy B, Peters A, et al. Preservation of human erythrocytes in the liquid state: biological results with a new medium. Vox Sang 1980; 39:195.
159. Messeter L, Ugander L, Monti M, et al. CPD-adenine as a blood preservative—studies in vitro and in vivo. Transfusion 1977; 17:210.
160. Zuck TF, Bensinger TA, Peck CC, et al. The in vivo survival of red blood cells stored in modified CPD with adenine: report of a multi-institutional cooperative effort. Transfusion 1977; 17:374.
161. Lovric VA, Prince B, Bryant J. Packed red cell transfusions—improved survival, quality and storage. Vox Sang 1977; 33:346.
162. Simon ER. Adenine in blood banking. Transfusion 1977; 17:317.
163. Strauss D, Raderecht HJ. Zum Einfluss von Adenin und Guanosin auf die Überlebensrate von Erythrozyten nach Lagerung bei Temperaturen zwischen 4 degrees C und 25 degrees C. Folia Haematol (Leipz) 1974; 101:232.
164. Stigge V, Lun A, Ziemer S, et al. Weitere Optimierung der ACD-AG-Konservierungsloesung fuer Blut. Folia Haematol (Leipz) 1974; 101:256.
165. Lun A, Stigge V, Ziemer S, et al. Weitere Optimierung der ACD-AG-Konservierungsloesung fuer Blut III. Mitteilung: Verbesserung der Sauerstofftransportfunktion von Erythrozyten in Sorbit-xylit-pyruvat-lösungen mit erhöhtem pH. Folia Haematol (Leipz) 1975; 102:335.
166. Stigge V, Seidel B. Verhalten von Adeninnukleotiden im Konservenblut mit Adenin und Guanosinzusatzen. Acta Biol Med Ger 1977; 36:549.
167. de Verdier CH, Strauss D, Ericson A, et al. Purine metabolism of erythrocytes preserved in adenine, adenine-inosine, and adenine-guanosine supplemented media. Transfusion 1981; 21:397.
168. Brake JM, Deindoerfer FH. The effect of dihydroxyacetone on the 2,3-diphosphoglycerate (2,3-DPG) level of stored blood. *In* Proceedings of the 13th Congress of the International Society of Blood Transfusion, 1972, p 60.
169. Moore GL, Ledford ME, Brummell MR. Red cell ATP and 2,3-diphosphoglycerate concentrations as a function of dihydroxyacetone supplementation of CPD adenine. Vox Sang 1981; 41:11.
170. Beutler E. The maintenance of red cell function during liquid storage. *In* Schmidt PJ (ed): Progress in Transfusion and Transplantation. Chicago: American Association of Blood Banks, 1972, pp 285–297.
171. Wood LA, Beutler E. The effect of ascorbate on the maintenance of 2,3-diphosphoglycerate (2,3-DPG) in stored red cells. Br J Haematol 1973; 25:611.
172. Dawson RB, Hershey RT, Myers CS, Eaton JW. Blood preservation: XLIV. 2,3-DPG maintenance by dehydroascorbate better than D-ascorbic acid. Transfusion 1980; 20:321.
173. Kandler R, Grode G, Symbol R, Hickey G. Oxalate is the active component that produces increased 2,3-DPG in ascorbate stored red cells. Transfusion 1986; 26:563.
174. Beutler E, Forman L, West C. Effect of oxalate and malonate on red cell metabolism. Blood 1987; 70:1389.
175. Laerum E, Aarseth S. Urolithiasis in railroad shopmen in relation to oxalic acid exposure at work. Scand J Work Environ Health 1985; 11:97.
176. Vora S, West C, Beutler E. The effect of additives on red cell 2,3-DPG levels in CPDA preservatives. Transfusion 1989; 29:226.
177. Paniker NV, Beutler E. Pyruvate effect in maintenance of ATP and 2,3-DPG of stored blood. J Lab Clin Med 1971; 78:472.
178. Hyde RM, Paterson RA, Livingstone DJ, et al. Modification of the haemoglobin oxygen dissociation curve in whole blood by a compound with dual action. Lancet 1984; 2:15.
179. Paterson RA, Dawson J, Hyde RM, et al. Xanthone additives for blood storage which maintains its potential for oxygen delivery: I. 2-hydroxyethoxy- and 2-ethoxy-6-(5-tetrazoyl) xanthones in citrate-phosphate-dextrose-adenine (CPDA-1) blood. Transfusion 1988; 28:34.
180. Beutler E, Forman L, West C, Gelbart T. The mechanism of improved maintenance of 2,3-diphosphoglycerate in stored blood by the xanthone compound BW A440C. Biochem Pharmacol 1988; 37:1057.
181. Rock G, Labow RS, Franklin C, et al. Hypotension and cardiac arrest in rats after infusion of mono(2-ethylhexyl) phthalate (MEHP), a contaminant of stored blood. N Engl J Med 1987; 316:1218.
182. Rock G, Tocchi M, Ganz PR, Tackaberry ES. Incorporation of plasticizer into red cells during storage. Transfusion 1984; 24:493.
183. Collins JA. Massive blood transfusion. Clin Haematol 1976; 5:201.
184. Jaeger RJ, Rubin RJ. Migration of a phthalate ester plasticizer from polyvinyl chloride blood bags into stored human blood and its localization in human tissues. N Engl J Med 1972; 287:1114.
185. Estep TN, Pedersen RA, Miller TJ, Stupar KR. Characterization of erythrocyte quality during the refrigerated storage of whole blood containing di-(2-ethylhexyl)phthalate. Blood 1984; 64:1270.
186. Rock G, Tocchi M, Ganz PR, Tackaberry ES. Incorporation of plasticizer into red cells during storage. Transfusion 1984; 24:493.
187. Horowitz B, Stryker MH, Waldman AA, et al. Stabilization of red blood cells by the plasticizer, diethylhexylphthalate. Vox Sang 1985; 48:150.
188. Stern IJ, Carmen RA. Hemolysis in stored blood: stabilizing effect of phthalate plasticizer. *In* Proceedings of the 16th Congress of the International Society of Hematology, 1980, p 151.
189. AuBuchon JP, Estep TN, Davey RJ. The effect of the plasticizer di-2-ethylhexyl phthalate on the survival of stored RBCs. Blood 1988; 71:448.
190. Dawson RB, Ottinger WE, Chiu WM, et al. Control of red cell 2,3-DPG levels in vitro and a proposal for in vivo control in response to hypoxia and metabolic demand. Prog Clin Biol Res 1985; 195:349.

191. Vora S. Metabolic manipulation of key glycolytic enzymes: a novel proposal for the maintenance of red cell 2,3-DPG and ATP levels during storage. Biomed Biochim Acta 1987; 46:285.
192. Debski B. The influence of the ammonium ion and adenosine on glucose metabolism in preserved human erythrocytes. Acta Physiol Pol 1981; 32:73.
193. Meryman HT, Hornblower ML, Syring RL. Prolonged storage of red cells at 4 degrees C. Transfusion 1986; 26:500.
194. Högman CF, Eriksson L, Gong J, et al. Half-strength citrate CPD combined with a new additive solution for improved storage of red blood cells suitable for clinical use. Vox Sang 1993; 65:271.
195. Stewart IM, Chapman BE, Kirk K, et al. Intracellular pH in stored erythrocytes. Refinement and further characterisation of the 31P-NMR methylphosphonate procedure. Biochim Biophys Acta 1986; 885:23.
196. Farrugia A, Douglas S, James J, Whyte G. Red cell and platelet concentrates from blood collected into half-strength citrate anticoagulant: improved maintenance of red cell 2,3-diphosphoglycerate in half-citrate red cells. Vox Sang 1992; 63:31.
197. Poyart CF, Bursaux E, Freminet A. Citrate and the Donnan equilibrium in human blood p507.4 or p507.2. Biomedicine 1973; 19:52.
198. Kay A, Beutler E. The effect of ammonium, phosphate, potassium, and hypotonicity on stored red blood cells. Transfusion 1992; 32:37.
199. Greenwalt TJ, McGuinness CG, Dumaswala UJ, Carter HW. Studies in red blood cell preservation: 3. A phosphate-ammonium-adenine additive solution. Vox Sang 1990; 58:94.
200. Dumaswala UJ, Oreskovic RT, Petrosky TL, Greenwalt TJ. Studies in red blood cell preservation: 5. Determining the limiting concentrations of NH_4Cl and Na_2HPO_4 needed to maintain red blood cell ATP during storage. Vox Sang 1992; 62:136.
201. Greenwalt TJ, Dumaswala UJ, Dhingra N, et al. Studies in red blood cell preservation: 7. In vivo and in vitro studies with a modified phosphate-ammonium additive solution. Vox Sang 1993; 65:87.
202. Dumaswala UJ, Rugg N, Greenwalt TJ. Studies in red blood cell preservation: 9. The role of glutamine in red cell preservation. Vox Sang 1994; 67:255.
203. Greenwalt TJ. Recent developments in the long-term preservation of red blood cells. Curr Opin Hematol 1997; 4:431.
204. Beutler E, Duron O. Effect of pH on preservation of red cell ATP. Transfusion 1965; 5:17.
205. Valeri CR, Zaroulis CG. Rejuvenation and freezing of outdated stored human red cells. N Engl J Med 1972; 287:1307.
206. Hamasaki N, Hirota C, Ideguchi H, Ikehara Y. Regeneration of 2,3-bisphosphoglycerate and ATP of stored erythrocytes by phosphoenolpyruvate; a new preservative for blood storage. Prog Clin Biol Res 1981; 55:577.
207. Davey RJ, McCoy NC, Yu M, et al. The effect of prestorage irradiation on posttransfusion red cell survival. Transfusion 1992; 32:525.
208. Mintz PD, Anderson G. Effect of gamma irradiation on the in vivo recovery of stored red blood cells. Ann Clin Lab Sci 1993; 23:216.
209. Horowitz B, Rywkin S, Margolis-Nunno H, et al. Inactivation of viruses in red cell and platelet concentrates with aluminum phthalocyanine (AlPc) sulfonates. Blood Cells 1992; 18:141; discussion 150.
210. Margolis-Nunno H, Ben-Hur E, Gottlieb P, Robinson R, Oetjen J, Horowitz B. Inactivation by phthalocyanine photosensitization of multiple forms of human immunodeficiency virus in red cell concentrates. Transfusion 1996; 36:743.
211. Ben-Hur E, Barshtein G, Chen S, Yedgar S. Photodynamic treatment of red blood cell concentrates for virus inactivation enhances red blood cell aggregation: protection with antioxidants. Photochem Photobiol 1997; 66:509.
212. Moor AC, Lagerberg JW, Tijssen K, et al. In vitro fluence rate effects in photodynamic reactions with AlPcS4 as sensitizer. Photochem Photobiol 1997; 66:860.
213. North J, Neyndorff H, King D, Levy JG. Viral inactivation in blood and red cell concentrates with benzoporphyrin derivative. Blood Cells 1992; 18:129.
214. Wagner SJ, Storry JR, Mallory DA, et al. Red cell alterations associated with virucidal methylene blue phototreatment. Transfusion 1993; 33:30.
215. Wagner SJ, Robinette D, Storry J, et al. Differential sensitivities of viruses in red cell suspensions to methylene blue photosensitization. Transfusion 1994; 34:521.

CHAPTER 10
Red Cell Antigens

Marilyn J. Telen

Blood group antigens are portions of blood cell surface molecules that are recognized by antibodies. Such antigens may reside on a variety of structures, including proteins, polysaccharides, glycoproteins, glycolipids, and lipoproteins. Antibodies themselves are capable of spanning a region of only 5 to 10 amino acids or three to five glycosidic units. Thus, blood group antigens can often be characterized as small differences in largely nonpolymorphic molecules.

Since the description of the ABO antigens in 1901 by Karl Landsteiner, the practice of blood transfusion has led to the serological identification of hundreds of individual blood group antigens. Many of these antigens are related to one another by arising from polymorphisms of the same parent molecule and thus together form blood group systems. Within these systems, some antigens may exist as different epitopes on the same molecule or multimolecular complex, whereas others may be expressed as the products of allelic genes. It speaks well for the perspicacity of many hard-working serologists that many such relationships were determined on the basis of serological investigations of unusual phenotypes and the families of such individuals long before the genetic bases of these antigens were defined.

A list of well-recognized antigens that can be put into blood group systems is presented in Table 10–1. Biochemical and molecular genetic investigations have now clarified many of the relationships among antigens and have allowed classification of heretofore poorly understood antigens into blood group systems. In this chapter, the current understanding of the biochemical and genetic basis of the major and some minor blood group antigen systems is discussed.

POLYSACCHARIDE BLOOD GROUP ANTIGENS

The ABO Blood Group System

Until recognition of the ABO antigen system and the fact that essentially all individuals have isoagglutinins for A and/or B antigens if they themselves lack these antigens, blood transfusion was an extremely dangerous practice. However, in this century, we have been able to understand the biochemical basis for the A, B, and H antigens and to identify the gene structures leading to expression of the major ABO phenotypes.

Antigen specificity in this blood group system resides in oligosaccharide structures, which are the products of several glycosyltransferases that act sequentially on a substrate (Fig. 10–1).[1, 2] The substrate, or backbone, to which these sugars are added is called paragloboside. Paragloboside is a tetrasaccharide whose terminal residue is a galactose attached via a β(1–3) or β(1–4) linkage to produce type 1 or type 2 paragloboside, respectively. Type 1 paragloboside chains are found in secreted antigens, whereas type 2 chains are indigenous to red cells. The H gene *(FUT1)* encodes a fucosyltransferase that attaches a fucose via an α(1–2) linkage to the terminal galactose of type 2 chains. The *Se* (Secretor) gene *(FUT2)* encodes a fucosyltransferase that acts similarly on type 1 paragloboside chains. Individuals whose paragloboside molecules have no sugars added, other than fucose by the H transferase, are denoted blood group type O and express the H antigen. Rarely, the H fucosyltransferase may be absent, resulting in the hh, or Bombay, phenotype. In group A or B individuals, another glycosyltransferase acts to add an additional "immunodominant" sugar to the galactose. The *A* gene encodes a transferase that adds N-acetylgalactosamine via an α(1–3) bond, whereas the *B* gene encodes an enzyme that adds galactose by means of a similar bond. Individuals who do not express the H transferase cannot express the A and B antigens.

Table 10–1. Well-Recognized Blood Group Antigen Systems

	Name of System	Symbol
Polysaccharide Blood Groups	Hh	H
	ABO	ABO
	Lewis	Le
	Ii	I
	P	P
Protein Blood Groups	Rh	Rh
	MNS	MNSs
	Kell	K
	Lutheran	Lu
	Kidd	Jk
	Duffy	Fy
	Gerbich	Ge
	Cromer	Cr
	Diego	Di
	Cartwright	Yt
	Xg	Xg
	Scianna	Sc
	Dombrock	Do
	LW	LW
	Colton	Co
	Chido/Rodgers	Ch/Rg
	XK	Kx
	Knops/McCoy	Kn
	Indian	In

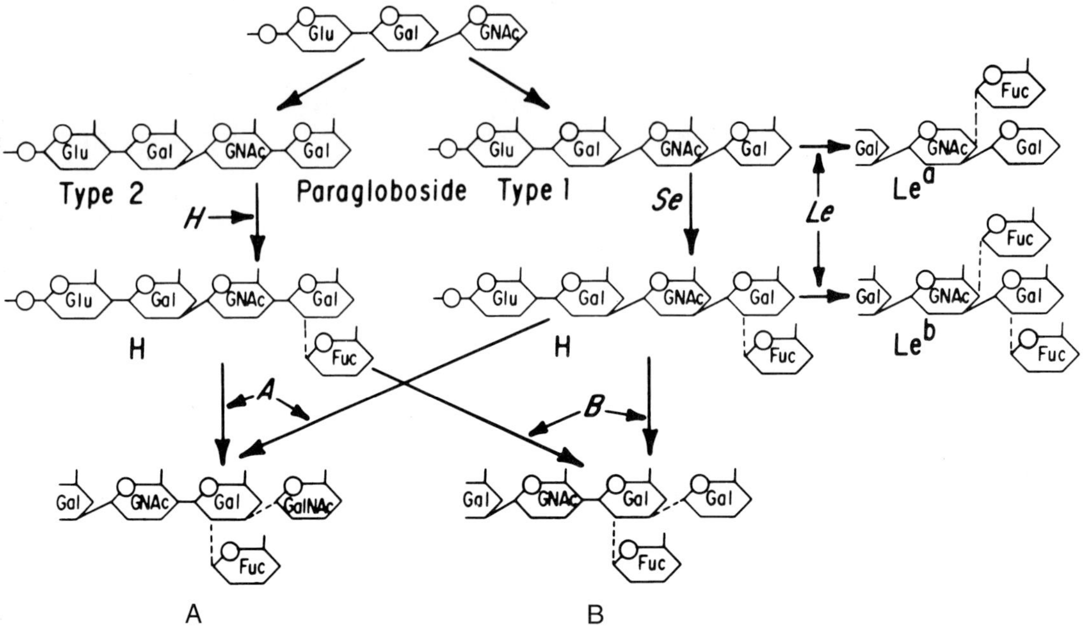

Figure 10–1. Formation of the H, A, B, and Lewis antigens. Glu, glucose; GNAc, N-acetylglucosamine; Gal, galactose; GalNAc, N-acetylgalactosamine; Fuc, fucose. Interrupted lines indicate α-glycosidic linkages, and β-linkages are indicated by solid lines. Antigens are indicated by normal type, genes by italic type. (From Rosse WF, Telen MJ. The biochemistry of the antigens of the red blood cell membrane. *In* Agre P, Parker JC [eds]: Red Blood Cell Membranes: Structure, Function, Clinical Implications. New York: Marcel Dekker, 1989, p 301. Reprinted courtesy of Marcel Dekker, Inc.)

The Genetic Basis of ABO Antigens

The *ABO* gene locus has been localized to chromosome 9q34.[3, 4] In 1990, Yamamoto and colleagues[5, 6] reported the isolation and then cloning of a complementary DNA (cDNA) encoding the human blood group A transferase. The encoded protein of 353 amino acids contained a short N-terminal domain, a single hydrophobic transmembrane domain, and a large C-terminal domain most likely containing the active catalytic site. This cDNA sequence was not extensively homologous to the cDNA sequence for human H fucosyltransferase, described by Larsen and associates[7] the same year.

Further work by Yamamoto's group[8] elucidated the genetic basis of the common ABO antigen phenotypes by describing the differences among the allelic group A, group O, and group B cDNAs. Comparison of the cDNAs for the A and B (and silent O) transferases demonstrates well how relatively small changes at the genetic level can give rise to markedly different phenotypes (Fig. 10–2).[8] When the cDNA of group O individuals was compared with that of group A individuals, only one difference was found: a single base deletion was present near the N-terminus, resulting in a shift of the reading frame and generation of a stop codon after amino acid 116. This common *O* allele is denoted as O^1. A variant of the O^1 allele (O^{1var}) occurs in about 40% of *O* alleles and has at least seven point mutations as compared with the original O^1 allele.[9] In addition, the O^2 allele contains nucleotides typical of the B gene at position 526 and of the A gene at position 703.[10, 11]

The cDNAs for the A and B transferases differ from each other at seven nucleotides, producing amino acid sequence differences only at residues 176, 235, 266, and 268.[8] Of these, at least the last three have been shown, through transfection and expression of mutant constructs, to influence the sugar specificity of the product transferase; the last two amino acid positions, which are situated close to each other, are most important in determin-

```
        10         20         30         40         50
MAEVLRTLAG KPKCHALRPM ILFLIMLVLV LFGYGVLSPR SLMPGSLERG      A
********** ********** ********** ********** **********      B
********** ********** ********** ********** **********      O

        60         70         80         90        100
FCMAVREPDH LQRVSLPRMV YPQPKVLTPCRKDVLVVTPWL APIVWEGTFN      A
********** ********** ********************* **********      B
********** ********** *****************PLGW LPLSGRAHST      O

       110        120        130        140        150
IDILNEQFRL QNTTIGLTVF AIKKYVAFLK LFLETAEKHF MVGHRVHYYV      A
********** ********** ********** ********** **********      B
STSSTSSSGS RTPPLG-                                          O

       160        170        180        190        200
FTDQLAAVPR VTLGTGRQLS VLEVRAYKRW QDVSMRRMEM ISDFCERRFL      A
********** ********** ****G***** ********** **********      B

       210        220        230        240        250
SEVDYLVCVD VDMEFRDHVG VEILTPLFGT LHPGFYGSSR EAFTYERRPQ      A
********** ********** ********** ***S****** **********      B

       260        270        280        290        300
SQAYIPKDEG DFYYLGGFFG GSVQEVQRLT RACHQAMMVD QANGIEAVWH      A
********** ****M*A*** ********** ********** **********      B

       310        320        330        340        350
DESHLNKYLL RHKPTKVLSP EYLWDQQLLG WPAVLRKLRF TAVPKNHQAV      A
********** ********** ********** ********** **********      B

       360
RNP-                                                        A
****                                                        B
```

Figure 10–2. Amino acid sequences of the A, B, and "O" transferases, represented in one-letter code. *, amino acid identical to that in the A transferase; -, stop codon. The product of the O gene differs from that of the A and B genes starting at amino acid 87 because of a single base pair deletion and resultant frame shift. The A and B transferases differ by four amino acids. (Adapted from Yamamoto F-I, Clausen H, White T, et al. Molecular genetic basis of the histo-blood group ABO system. Nature 1990; 345:229.)

ing substrate specificity of the glycosyltransferase.[9] Thus, the A and B transferases are homologous proteins that differ from each other by only four amino acids; their substrate specificities depend largely on variation of two amino acids at positions 266 and 268.

Additional *A* and *B* alleles also have been identified. The A^2 allele (the A^1 allele encodes for the A transferase) has a single base deletion in the carboxy end, resulting in a frame shift.[12] The A^2 transferase possesses an extra domain; when the A^2 transferase is expressed as a recombinant protein in HeLa cells, there is decreased A transferase activity.

Another variant allele produces the so-called cis-AB phenotype, in which family studies show that expression of the A and B antigens are inherited by subsequent generations via a single chromosome. The cis-AB phenotype results from a point mutation in a single allele. The *cis-AB* allele differs from the *B* allele in only three instead of four positions.[13, 14] This gene encodes a transferase that is capable of adding either galactose or N-acetylgalactosamine to fucosylated paragloboside.

Another variant phenotype, the B(A) phenotype, has been characterized as expressing both B antigen as well as very small amounts of A antigen, with both antigens apparently resulting from a gene on a single chromosome, as in the cis-AB phenotype. In at least one individual, this phenotype results from an *AB* allele that encodes two amino acids characteristic of the A transferase and two typical of the B transferase.[15]

The Bombay and para-Bombay phenotypes result from variant H alleles. Individuals with these rare phenotypes fail to express erythrocyte H antigen, owing to a lack of activity of *FUT1*-encoded α(1,2)-fucosyltransferase. The Bombay phenotype also lacks any *FUT2*-encoded α(1,2)-fucosyltransferase activity (a product of the *Se* gene, see later). Koda and colleagues[16] studied individuals with the Bombay phenotype and discovered a single mutation in the *FUT1* gene leading to inactivity of the *FUT1*-encoded α(1,2)-fucosyltransferase. In these same individuals, there was a gene deletion of *FUT2*.

Other Polysaccharide Antigens

Polysaccharide antigens other than A and B are relatively rarely of clinical significance in transfusion medicine. Some polysaccharide blood group antigens reside on glycoproteins, whereas others are borne for the most part by glycolipids. The Lewis (Le), P, and Ii systems constitute the other polysaccharide human blood groups.

Lewis Blood Group System

Lewis antigens reside on glycosphingolipids that are absorbed onto red cells from plasma.[17] Lewis antigens result from the action of two genes, *Le* and *Se* (see Fig. 10–1). The *Le* gene, now renamed *FUT3*, is located on chromosome 19p13.3 and encodes an α(1–3/1–4)-fucosyltransferase that adds a fucose to the penultimate N-acetylglucosamine of type 1 paragloboside.[18] The so-called *le* allele, which appears not to encode an active transferase, has now been shown to arise from a variety of *FUT3* gene mutations that result in inactive or unstable enzymes.[19, 20]

The *Se* gene, now identified as *FUT2*, also resides on chromosome 19p13.3 but at a locus separate from that of *FUT3;* it produces an α(1–2)-fucosyltransferase that acts on type 1 paragloboside; this enzyme adds a fucose to the terminal sugar of type 1 paragloboside.[21] There appears also to be a pseudogene highly homologous to *FUT2* about 35 kb away from it. The "null" allele for *Se* is denoted *se;* like the *le* allele, the *se* allele can arise from a number of different mutations, leading to failure to produce a functional transferase. When only the penultimate sugar of the paragloboside is fucosylated, owing to presence of an *Le* allele but not an *Se* allele, the Le^a antigen is produced. When the products of both the *Le* and *Se* genes are present, the Le^b antigen is produced. In some Asian populations, the Le(a+b+) phenotype occurs due to a weakly active FUT2 enzyme.[22] Alloantibodies to the Le antigens are relatively common, cold-reacting IgM antibodies that rarely cause clinically evident problems.

The Ii Blood Group System

The I and i antigens, unlike the Le antigens, do not represent the products of allelic genes. Instead, they are developmentally determined structures that reside on type 2 paragloboside linked to proteins or lipids. The i antigen may simplistically be thought of as consisting of a chain of repeated galactose-N-acetylglucosamine units,[23] whereas the I antigen is composed of a branching structure containing these similar units.[24, 25] Although both fetal and adult red cells express both I and i antigens, fetal cells express relatively more i and less I, whereas adult cells express more I and less i. Rarely, an adult may fail to exhibit normal expression of I (the adult i phenotype) and produce anti-I; this antibody is sometimes referred to as allo-anti-I, but careful studies can show that such individuals express small amounts of I and thus produce an autoantibody rather than alloantibody. Such anti-I may be, but is not uniformly, clinically significant.

Two genes encoding β-1,6-N-acetylglucosaminyltransferases have been found on chromosome 9q21. One, *C2GnT,* is able to catalyze the addition of N-acetylglucosamine β1→6 to galactose β1→3N-acetylgalactosamine, whereas the homologous *IGnT* is also an acetylglucosaminyltransferase and is, moreover, capable of producing I antigen in transfected cells. However, it is not known whether the i phenotype is associated with mutations in the *IgnT* gene.[26, 27]

Although antibodies to the I and i antigens are usually naturally occurring, cold-reacting IgM antibodies of little clinical import, certain infectious diseases (especially infectious mononucleosis and *Mycoplasma* infections) may be associated with high-titer, high-thermal amplitude hemolytic antibodies, and hemolytic anti-i has also been associated with lymphomas. Finally, cold agglutinin disease, most often found in the elderly, is a hemolytic syndrome caused by production of a monoclonal or oligoclonal cold-reacting antibody, usually anti-I.

The P Blood Group System

The P antigen system consists of a number of antigens produced by interacting glycosyltransferases that may be the products of two or more genes.[17] The antigens of the P system are P, P_1, P^k, and Luke (LKE). Commonly, red cells express both P and P_1 (75% of the population) or P but not P_1 (25%). Rarely, cells may express no P antigens or only P^k. Absence of all P system antigens, sometimes referred to as the Tj(a−) phenotype, results in the development of a broadly reactive antibody, anti-Tj^a, which is associated with an increased risk of spontaneous abortions.[28]

Biochemically, P antigens are constructed from ceramide dihexoside. P^k results from addition of an additional galactose to form ceramide trihexoside. The P antigen, also called globoside, results from addition of N-acetylgalactosamine to ceramide trihexoside. P_1, on the other hand, results from addition of galactose to paragloboside, which is derived from ceramide dihexoside by a different set of glycosyltransferase reactions than globoside. The structure of the Luke antigen may be that of the so-called embryonic antigen SSEA-4, which appears to result from addition of galactose and then sialic acid to globoside.

Clinically, the P blood group is also important because the P antigen serves as the receptor for B19 parvovirus, the causative agent of fifth disease, as well as infectious erythroblastopenia. Individuals who fail to express the P antigen are not infected by parvovirus B19 and do not develop antibodies to it.[29, 30] The P antigen is also the target of so-called Donath-Landsteiner cold-reacting IgG autoantibodies, the cause of paroxysmal cold hemoglobinuria.[31]

BLOOD GROUP ANTIGENS ON TRANSMEMBRANE PROTEINS

The Rh Blood Group System

After the ABO system, the Rh blood group system is the most important human blood group system in clinical transfusion medicine. Antibodies to antigens in this system make up far more than half the alloantibodies made by recipients of ABO type-specific blood products, as well as by mothers of infants affected by hemolytic disease of the newborn. In addition, Rh antigen structures appear to be frequent targets of autoantibodies found in autoimmune hemolytic anemia and drug-induced hemolytic anemia. The extreme antigenicity of the Rh structures, however, is thus far not explained by what we know about the structure of Rh proteins. However, the basis of the serological complexity of the Rh blood group system, which contains over 40 antigens, is slowly being elucidated.

The Rh Antigens

The first Rh antigen was described when a woman received a postpartum blood transfusion from her husband and had an immediate and severe transfusion reaction.[32] The name Rhesus was derived from the fact that this woman's antibody appeared to have the same specificity as an antibody made by rabbits to rhesus monkey cells, although later investigations proved that the rabbit antibody actually had specificity for the antigen now called LW (Landsteiner-Weiner). Not long after identification of anti-Rh, it became clear that the Rh system contained many antigenic variants.

Present understanding of the Rh system defines three major Rh epitopes: the Rh_o or D antigen may be present or absent, giving rise to the Rh-positive (D+) or Rh-negative (D−, sometimes written d) phenotype. (No antigen antithetical to D has been described.) In addition, most red cells express the C and/or c and E and/or e antigens. The D antigen is encoded by the *D* gene on chromosome 1p34.3-1p36.13. The C/c and E/e antigens are encoded by a second gene *(CE)* within the *RH* locus; recombination between the *D* and *CE* genes does not frequently occur. Because the genetic material encoding C/c and E/e is so tightly linked to that controlling D/(d), the *RH* locus is considered a single gene complex for gene frequency calculations. The frequency of the various combinations is listed in Table 10–2.

The Rh system also encompasses a large number of rare antigens and phenotypes. Occasionally, an individual's phenotype may be cD, with no E or e antigens expressed. Unusual individuals may also have the D− − phenotype, with expression of the D antigen but no C/c or E/e antigens. Still other individuals may have cells that express what appear to be weakened or rare variants of D, C/c, or E/e antigens. When there is a weakened D antigen but normal expression of C/c and E/e, the phenotype has been denoted D^u. Some D variants, as well as C/c and E/e variants, may be found in conjunction with antibody to the normal corresponding antigen and have been referred to as "mosaics"; this nomenclature, although it preceded understanding of these antigens on a molecular level, has proven to be apt, as is explained below.

Individuals whose red cells lack all Rh antigens (the Rh_{null} phenotype) have also been identified. Lack of all Rh antigens has been shown by serological studies to occur from either an abnormality linked to the *RH* locus ("amorph" type) or to a gene not linked to the *RH* locus ("regulator" type). Rh_{null} red cells may also lack non-Rh antigens and have multiple cell membrane abnormalities, attesting to the probable physiological importance of Rh structures in the membrane.[33–35] Both types of Rh_{null} red

Table 10–2. Differences in Frequency of Rh Gene Complexes in Different Populations

Gene Complex	Frequency: White Population	Frequency: African-American Population
DCe	0.40	0.17
dce	0.39	0.26
DcE	0.16	0.11
Dce	0.02	0.44
dCe	0.01	0.02
dcE	0.01	0.01
DCE	0.001	0.001
dCE	<0.001	<0.001

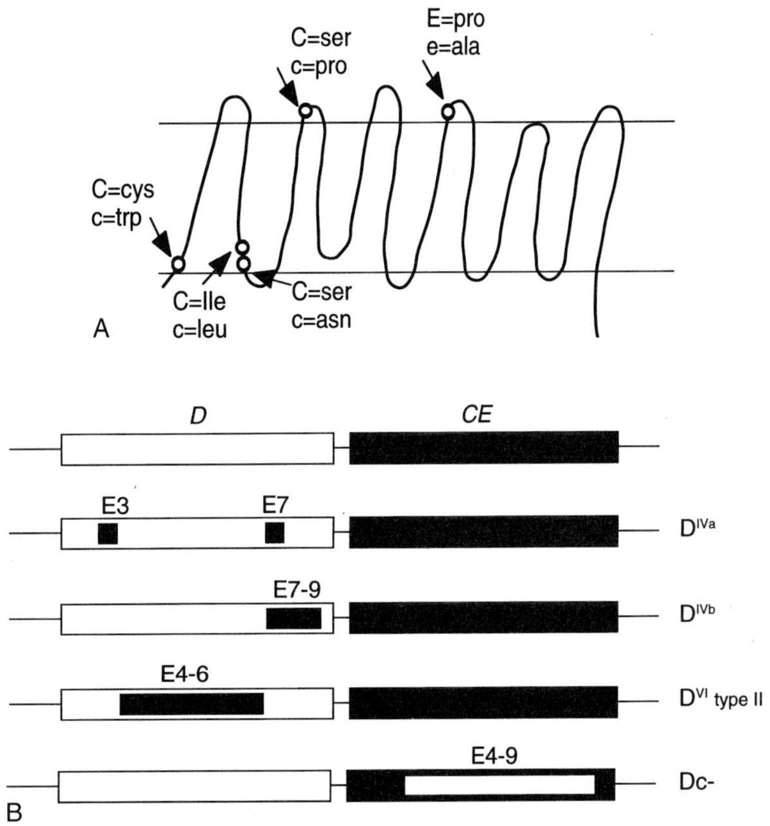

Figure 10–3. *A,* Schematic representation of an RhCE protein with 12 membrane-spanning domains and both the N- and C-termini in the cytosol. Points of sequence divergence associated with expression of the E/e and C/c antigens are shown. *B,* Schematic representation of the molecular genetic basis of some Rh system variants. Boxed areas in white represent genetic material derived from the *RHD* gene, whereas shaded areas represent genetic material derived from the *RHCE* gene. E, exon.

cells are stomatocytic and have shortened in vivo survival, leading to a variable degree of chronic hemolytic anemia. Rh_{null} cells have multiple biochemical abnormalities, including elevated ATPase activity, reduced cation and water content, reduced membrane stability, and abnormal phospholipid distribution.

Rh Biochemistry and Genetics

Investigators have now been successful in elucidating this serological maze with biochemical and genetic techniques. In 1982, several groups used immunoprecipitation techniques to show that anti-D, anti-c, and anti-E reacted specifically with proteins of 28 to 33 kD.[36, 37] Shortly thereafter, investigators began to discover how unusual the Rh protein was. First, even though it is a membrane-spanning protein, the Rh protein contains no detectable carbohydrate.[38] Second, the Rh protein contains exposed tyrosine that can be radiolabeled on intact cells but it has thus far been impervious to cleavage by proteases.[39] The Rh protein is also very poorly soluble. This characteristic may be partly dependent on Rh protein/cytoskeleton interactions, although such interactions have been only indirectly demonstrated.[40, 41] Finally, the Rh protein is one of the major red cell fatty-acylated proteins. The fatty acylation appears to be reversible and to occur by means of constant exchange of free palmitate for palmitate esterified onto cysteine residues within the Rh polypeptide.[42]

Several groups of investigators independently isolated Rh protein, and two groups published a cDNA sequence later shown to encode one polymorphic form of the RHCE polypeptide.[43, 44] The open reading frame of this cDNA encodes a peptide of 417 amino acids (the first of which, methionine, is absent from the mature protein). More than 30% of the amino acid residues are hydrophobic, and the peptide most likely has 12 transmembrane domains (Fig. 10–3A), with both termini in the cytosol. Somewhat later, three groups of investigators published the cDNA sequence encoding the RhD protein.[45–47] The D protein has the same number of amino acids as the CE protein and is 92% identical. The difference between the cDNA encoding an Rh protein expressing the E antigen and one expressing the e antigen is a single amino acid, whereas the C and c polypeptides differ by four amino acids, only one of which, however, is predicted to be in the extracellular domain (see Fig. 10–3A).[48]

Colin and colleagues[49] were the first to suggest that there are only two *RH* genes, one for D, and the other for Cc/Ee. Using exon-specific probes corresponding to the originally described *RHCE* cDNA, they showed that these DNA fragments hybridized to two DNA restriction fragments in DNA from Rh-positive individuals but to only one fragment in DNA from Rh-negative individuals. In whites, the majority of D-negative individuals lack *RHD* genes; however, it is now clear that at least some D-negative individuals have at least some part of the D gene.[50] This fact has become important to efforts to use molecular genetic techniques to determine if fetuses are at risk for Rh hemolytic disease of the newborn; to be accurate, it is necessary to examine at least three different regions of the *RHD* gene before declaring a fetus RhD positive or RhD negative.[51]

The high degree of homology between the *D* and *CE* genes has led to a number of crossing-over and gene conversion events, giving rise to a relatively large number of variant genes that contain some material derived from the *D* gene and some derived from the *CE* gene (see Fig. 10–3*B*). At least 13 variant *D* genes give rise to so-called partial D antigens (previously called D mosaics). In some, only one or two exons are derived from the *CE* gene, whereas the R^{oHar} phenotype arises from expression of a gene that is predominantly *CE* in derivation but whose fifth exon is that of a normal *D* gene.[52–55]

Whereas the Rh proteins are nonglycosylated, there is also a glycosylated protein that is structurally similar to the Rh proteins.[56] The protein, called Rh glycoprotein, is encoded by a gene on chromosome 6 and is known to carry ABH antigens. Much evidence suggests that Rh glycoprotein expression is necessary for expression of the RhD and RhCE proteins at the cell surface and that the Rh proteins and glycoprotein form a complex in the membrane, perhaps composed of two Rh proteins and two Rh glycoproteins. Thus far, most examples of the Rh_{null} phenotype appear to be due to structural defects in the gene encoding the Rh glycoprotein.[57]

Rh_{null} cells fail to express not only Rh antigens but also LW and glycophorin B antigens; Duffy antigen expression is also altered in these cells. Work of many researchers has contributed to the theory of a multiprotein Rh membrane complex, in which the Rh proteins themselves play a key role. Other members of this complex may be the Rh-related glycoprotein, as well as glycophorin B and the Duffy proteins.

Functionally, the Rh protein remains uncharacterized. Its structure is reminiscent of a transporter protein, and it has significant homology to a family of nonmammalian NH^+ transporters.[58]

In summary, although the Rh antigens are clinically among the most important of the protein antigens, and our extensive serological knowledge of these antigens and phenotypes has recently been complemented by biochemical and genetic understanding of the bases for expression of antigens in this system, the apparently important physiological role of the Rh proteins remains to be understood.

Landsteiner-Weiner (LW) Antigens

The LW antigens are more strongly expressed on D+ than on D− red cells and are absent from Rh_{null} cells. For this reason, the first-identified human anti-D was mistakenly thought to recognize the same antigen identified by heterologous antibody to rhesus monkey red cells. However, LW is now known to be the true "Rhesus" antigen, and the *LW* locus has been localized to chromosome 19p13-cen and is thus independent of Rh on chromosome 1. Since its discovery, the LW antigen has also been "subdivided" into LW^a and LW^b, and varying terminology exists for LW variants. LW antigens reside on glycoproteins of 37 to 47 kD.[59] The cDNA encoding the LW protein predicts a protein with a single transmembrane domain and two extracellular Ig-like domains.[60] LW protein is about 30% homologous to ICAM-1, ICAM-2, and ICAM-3, which are intercellular adhesion molecules. This similarity has prompted investigators to search for an adhesive function for LW, and LW does appear capable of mediating integrin-dependent leukocyte adhesion.[61] It is not known whether LW's adhesive capability is important during such events as erythroid maturation.

The MNSs Blood Group Antigens on Glycophorins A and B

Glycophorins A and B are highly glycosylated, high copy number, integral membrane proteins. Approximately 0.5 to 1 × 10^6 copies of glycophorin A (GPA) are expressed per red cell, but glycophorin B (GPB) is expressed in much lower amounts (0.8–3 × 10^5 copies per red cell).[62] Initially recognized as the major proteins in red cell membranes to stain with periodic acid–Schiff (PAS) (85% and 10% of total PAS-positive proteins, respectively), GPA and GPB have since been found to be highly related proteins encoded on chromosome 4q28-q31 by genes that undoubtedly arose by gene duplication.[62]

Biochemistry of MNSs

GPA carries the M or N blood group antigen at its N-terminus. These blood group antigens depend on a pair of polymorphisms in the first and fifth amino acids of GPA,[63] as shown below:

Amino acid:	1	2	3	4	5	6	7	8
M type:	Ser	Ser	Thr	Thr	Gly	Val	Ala	Met....
N type:	Leu	Ser	Thr	Thr	Glu	Val	Ala	Met....

However, most human antibodies to the M and N antigens fail to recognize their antigens unless the amino acids at positions 2 through 4 are properly O-glycosylated.

GPB is a highly homologous protein whose N-terminus is the same as the N-terminal 26 amino acids of N-type GPA.[62] However, no peptide corresponding to amino acids 27 through 55 of GPA is present in GPB. The rest of the extracellular portion of GPB, as well as its transmembrane domain, are also quite homologous to GPA, but GPB lacks amino acids corresponding to the cytoplasmic tail of GPA. In addition, GPB is polymorphic at amino acid 29, where a methionine gives rise to the S antigen, and threonine at this site forms the s antigen.[64]

Null Phenotypes

Since the original description of the MNSs antigens, a number of null and variant phenotypes have been described. Persons whose cells lack GPA but express GPB are designated En(a−).[65–67] Antibodies made by such persons, however, may recognize a variety of epitopes on GPA, and not all En(a−) cells lack all such epitopes. The antigens recognized by anti-En^a sera are generally classified into three types (see reference 68) (Fig. 10–4): En^aTS denotes an antigen removed by trypsin treatment of intact red cells, thus presumably N-terminal to the trypsin cleavage sites at amino acids 30 and 39. En^aTS, therefore, must reside between residues 26 and 39, because anti-En^aTS is glycophorin A specific and does not recognize the N-terminal 26 amino acids common to both

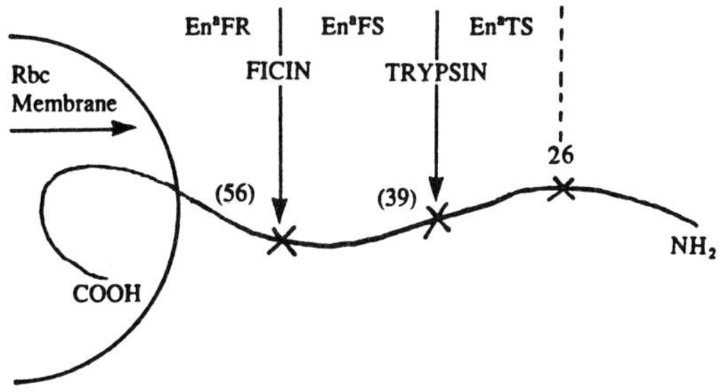

Figure 10–4. Diagrammatic representation of En^a antigens of glycophorin A. On intact cells, trypsin cleaves at residues 30 and 39, whereas ficin is believed to cleave the protein at residue 56. The protein enters the membrane at residue 70. Therefore, three broad epitopes can be defined by their resistance to trypsin and ficin degradation: En^{a}TS resides in the part of the trypsin-cleavable peptide not homologous to glycophorin B (between residues 26 and 39); En^{a}FS resides between the trypsin and ficin cleavage sites; and En^{a}FR resides between the ficin cleavage site and the point at which the protein enters the membrane. Human antisera corresponding to all three epitopes have been described. (Adapted from Issitt PD. Applied Blood Group Serology, 3rd ed. Miami: Montgomery Scientific, 1985, p 357.)

glycophorins A and B. En^{a}TR, on the other hand, refers to epitopes not affected by trypsin treatment; however, En^{a}TR is also by definition ficin (and papain) sensitive and thus must involve residues between the trypsin cleavage site at residue 39 and the ficin cleavage site at residue 56. Finally, En^{a}FR denotes ficin-resistant, glycophorin A–specific epitopes involving residues between the ficin cleavage site and the membrane, or residues C-terminal to amino acid 56 and N-terminal to amino acid 70.

There is also a glycophorin B–negative phenotype, termed S−s−, or sometimes S−s−U−. The S−s− phenotype is found in about 1 in 80 to 425 black persons, depending on the antiserum used for typing. The red cells of most U− persons lack glycophorin B when examined biochemically.[69] However, some S−s− cells carry small amounts of glycophorin B, and the abnormality of the GPB in these cells is not determined. The U antigen, however, appears to be glycophorin B dependent but perhaps not totally determined by glycophorin B alone; it may depend on the association of glycophorin B with another membrane constituent, possibly an Rh protein.[70]

Finally, there is a glycophorin A- and B-negative phenotype. The gene responsible for this phenotype is *Mk*, and totally GPA- and GPB-negative individuals are homozygous for this gene. Initial evidence suggests that the MkMk phenotype represents deletion of most of the GPA and GPB genes.[71]

Variants of Glycophorins A and B

In addition to various En(a−) and S−s−U− phenotypes, a number of variant glycophorins have been described. The glycophorin A and B genes are highly homologous (in both their exons and introns) and are situated quite close to each other, similarly to the *RHD* and *RHCE* genes. A third gene, sometimes denoted the glycophorin E gene, is also situated close by on chromosome 4.[72]

Unequal crossing-over, as well as gene conversion events, have been shown to produce a large number of variant and hybrid glycophorins. The serological literature refers to these molecules as Miltenberger (Mi) variants, although this nomenclature is now decreasing in popularity. Many of these molecules have been studied on the biochemical and genetic levels, and antibodies to some of them have been defined with the use of synthetic inhibitory peptides.[73–77] Brief characterization of some of these variants is given in Table 10–3. Red cells with certain molecules, such as the Miltenberger V (MiV) type, which contains the N-terminal portion of GPA attached to the C-terminal portion of GPB, have also served as means to

Table 10–3. Variants of Glycophorins A and B

Name	Description
MiI	Substitution of a methionine for threonine at residue #28 interferes with attachment of the N-linked oligosaccharide at position 26, leading to a GPA with lower than normal molecular weight on SDS-PAGE. This may have arisen from a gene conversion event involving the glycophorin B pseudoexon. This protein bears the Vw antigen.
MiII	Substitution of a lysine for threonine at residue #28 interferes with attachment of the N-linked oligosaccharide at position 26, leading to a GPA with lower than normal molecular weight on SDS-PAGE. This may have arisen from a gene conversion event involving the glycophorin B pseudoexon. This protein bears the Hut antigen.
MiIII	An abnormal GPB-type protein in which the glycophorin B pseudoexon corresponding to amino acids 27 through 48 of glycophorin A is expressed, along with amino acids 49–57 of glycophorin A, resulting in an abnormal glycophorin B only moderately smaller than normal glycophorin A. This protein bears the Mur antigen.
MiIV	An abnormal GPB-type protein similar to MiIII in molecular weight; exact structure unreported.
MiV	A GPA-GPB hybrid in which the glycophorin A segment forms the N-terminal domain and the glycophorin B segment forms the C-terminal domain. Most of the extracellular protein corresponds to glycophorin A, but the molecular weight is intermediate between glycophorins A and B.
MiVI	An abnormal GPB-like protein similar to MiIII, except that a threonine is substituted for arginine at residue #49.
MiVII	An abnormal protein that differs from glycophorin A at residues #49 and #52 (threonine for arginine and serine for tyrosine, respectively); proposed to result from a GPA-GPB-GPA hybrid gene structure.
MiVIII	An abnormal GPA with substitution of threonine for arginine at residue #49, proposed to result from a GPA-GPB-GPA hybrid gene structure.
MiIX	A GPA-like protein with residues 35–41 replaced by glycophorin B. The N-terminus and C-terminus appear normal. This protein carries the Mur antigen.
MiX	An abnormal GPB-type protein produced by gene conversion, in which a short insert of GPA DNA sequence causes expression of the GPB pseudoexon.
Dantu	An abnormal protein composed of the N-terminal domain of glycophorin B and the C-terminal domain of glycophorin A.
St^a	This phenotype has been shown to arise from multiple, different, unequal crossing-over events. Several St(a+) phenotypes are due to glycophorin A–glycophorin B hybrid proteins, whereas others arise from complex gene conversion events or simple mutations.

investigate the importance of various domains of the GPA structure.

Physiological Roles of the Major Glycophorins

Glycophorins A and B appear to have significant interactions with other membrane structures. Glycophorin A appears to interact with components of the cytoskeleton, most probably protein 4.1.[78] In addition, glycophorin A apparently interacts with band 3, and this interaction is required for expression of the Wright (Wr) antigens.[79] In transfected mammalian cells, expression of recombinant GPA facilitates expression of recombinant band 3.[80] However, in human red cells lacking GPA, expression of band 3 is at normal levels, although the function of band 3 as an anion transporter is slightly altered.[81]

Glycophorin B may interact with the Rh complex. Serological evidence of such an interaction comes from studies of Rh_{null} phenotypes. Many Rh_{null} cells fail to express glycophorin B antigens. In addition, an antibody to an antigen named Duclos appears to depend on glycophorin B expression and yet also to coprecipitate the Rh protein.[70]

Glycophorins A and B provide most of the negative charge of the red cell surface, owing to the large amount of sialic acid they bear. However, En(a−), S−s−U−, and MkMk cells are morphologically and functionally normal.

The Gerbich Antigens on Glycophorins C and D

Glycophorins C and D together constitute the other major sialoglycoproteins of human erythrocytes, although they constitute by weight only 4% and 1% of erythrocyte membrane sialoglycoproteins, respectively. Initially named glycophorins because they share many of the characteristics of GPA and GPB, glycophorins C and D are the product of a single gene unrelated to the genes encoding GPA and GPB. Furthermore, unlike the other glycophorins, GPC and GPD have been shown to be structurally important to the red cell membrane.[82] Finally, GPC and GPD, unlike GPA and GPB, appear to be more widely expressed; an alternately spliced isoform of GPC is expressed in lymphoid cells.[83]

The Gerbich Blood Group Antigens

Glycophorin C is encoded by four exons, the second and third of which are highly homologous to each other.[62] Glycophorin D arises from the same gene via an alternate transcription initiation site within exon 2 (Fig. 10–5).[84] The Gerbich blood group antigens have been shown to reside on GPC and GPD (see Fig. 10–5). This family of antigens has three high-frequency antigens, denoted Ge2, Ge3, and Ge4, as well as a number of low-frequency antigens. The Ge3 epitope lies within the protein domain encoded by exon 3 and is thus shared by glycophorins C and D. However, the Ge2 epitope is unique to glycophorin D and depends on the N-terminus of that protein;

```
Normal Glycophorin C:

   exon 1             exon 2                  exon 3           exon 4

MWSTRSPNSTAWPLSL/EPDPGMASASTTMHTTTIA/EPDPGMSGWPDGRMETSTPTIMDIVVIA/GVIAAV...
                                                 -------------
                                                      Ge3

Normal Glycophorin D:

                      exon 2                  exon 3           exon 4

                    MASASTTMHTTTIA/EPDPGMSGWPDGRMETSTPTIMDIVVIA/GVIAAV...
                    --------                     -------------
                      Ge2                             Ge3

Ge:-2,3 (Yus Type):

   exon 1                exon 3              exon 4

MWSTRSPNSTAWPLSL/EPDPGMSGWPDGRMETSTPTIMDIVVIA/GVIAAVAIV...
                     -------------
                          Ge3

Ge:-2,-3 (Ge type):

   exon 1             exon 2      exon 4

MWSTRSPNSTAWPLSL/EPDPGMASASTTMHTTTIA/GVIAAVAIV...
```

Figure 10–5. Normal and variant glycophorin C/D proteins. Normal glycophorin C is encoded by four exons and carries the Ge3 antigen in a domain encoded by exon 3. Glycophorin D is similar to glycophorin C, except that the material encoded by exon 1 and the 5′ end of exon 2 is missing; an alternative start site (AUG) in exon 2 is used. Glycophorin D bears the Ge2 antigen near its N-terminus. A Ge:-2,3 or Ge:-2,-3 variant protein arises when exon 2 or exon 3, respectively, has been lost because of unequal crossing-over.

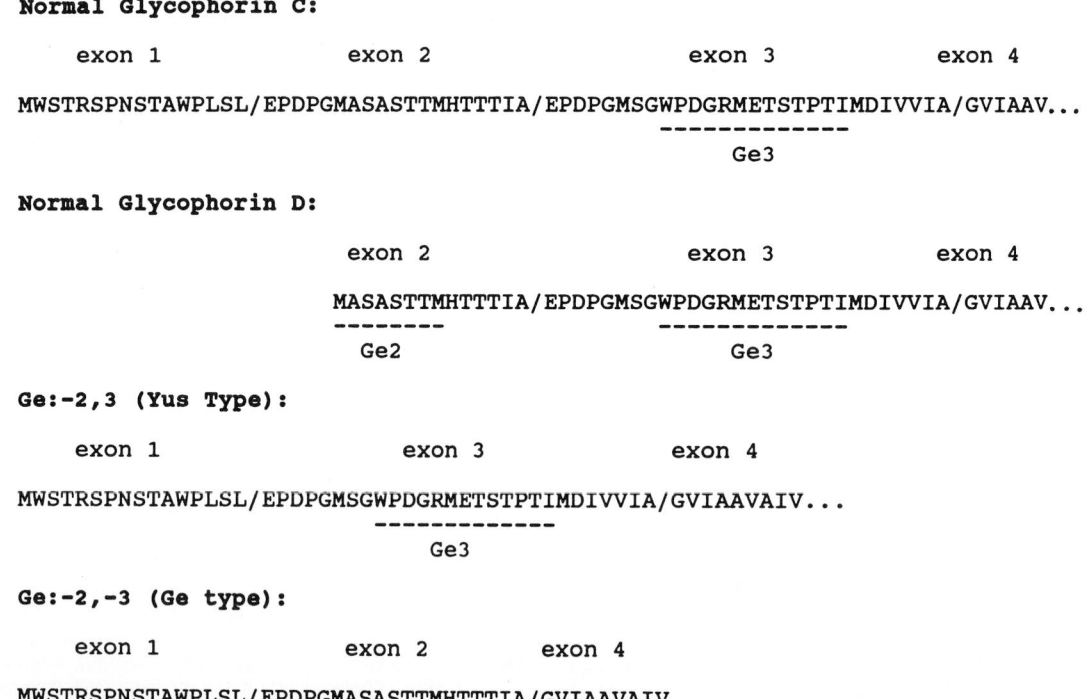

although the same sequence is expressed by GPC, the fact that it does not comprise the N-terminus of GPC apparently accounts for its lack of antigen activity on GPC. Ge4 is near the N-terminus of GPC and therefore is not present on GPD.[85]

Variants of Glycophorins C and D

The rare variants of GPC and GPD arise from somewhat different mechanisms from those giving rise to GPA and GPB variants. Some arise from unequal crossing over involving the homologous exons 2 and 3.[86–88] Thus, the Ge:-2,-3 phenotype arises when exon 3 has been lost during unequal crossing-over, whereas the Ge:-2,3 (Yus) phenotype arises from loss of exon 2 (see Fig. 10–5). Both mutations give rise to protein that does not express Ge2 but does express Ge4. The reciprocal result of this type of unequal crossing over has also been described: The Ls(a+) phenotype results from duplication of exon 3, giving rise to a larger than normal GPC and a novel amino acid sequence at the exon 3-exon 3 boundary. Anti-Ls^a antisera react with a synthetic peptide corresponding to this novel amino acid sequence.[89]

Finally, several low-incidence Gerbich antigens arise from point mutations. In the Webb (Wb+) phenotype, a smaller than normal GPC is expressed. The lower molecular weight of this protein is due to a point mutation that causes loss of the normally N-glycosylated asparagine (residue 8) and substitution of a presumably O-glycosylated serine.[90] In the Dh(a+) phenotype, the Dh^a antigen is expressed by GPC but not GPD. Consistent with expression only on glycophorin C, this antigen appears to correlate with a point mutation substituting phenylalanine for leucine at amino acid residue 14 of glycophorin C.[91]

Perhaps the most interesting variant phenotype in the Gerbich system is the Leach phenotype, in which no glycophorin C or D is expressed.[92] These cells are elliptocytic, and people with this phenotype have laboratory evidence of low-grade hemolysis. The first investigation of such an individual demonstrated a deletion of exons 3 and 4 of the glycophorin C gene.[87] Investigation of three other instances of this phenotype has confirmed this abnormality to be the most common cause of the phenotype, although one example of a small complex mutation involving deletion of one base has also been shown to be responsible for a similar phenotype.[93]

The Kell Antigens

The Kell blood group system is one of the larger and more clinically important of the protein blood group systems. It comprises three well-defined sets of antithetical antigens as well as a number of high-frequency and low-frequency antigens more rarely encountered in transfusion medicine. The more commonly encountered antigens are listed in Table 10–4. Anti-K is one of the most commonly encountered, clinically significant alloantibodies made by transfusion recipients; it is also a significant cause of mild to moderately severe hemolytic disease of the newborn. About 0.2% of whites (and fewer black persons) are k-negative. When this phenotype occurs, anti-k can be a severe obstacle to transfusion because of the rarity of k-negative donors.

Table 10–4. Commonly Encountered Antithetical Pairs of Kell System Antigens

Traditional Symbol and Name	Alphanumeric Symbol	Frequency
K (Kell)	K1	Low
k (Cellano)	K2	High
Kp^a (Penney)	K3	Low
Kp^b (Rautenberg)	K4	High
Js^a (Sutter)	K6	Low
Js^b (Matthews)	K7	High

Unusual Kell Phenotypes

Although the Kell system antigens listed in Table 10–4 account for most of the clinical alloimmune problems caused by Kell antigens, some of the more interesting phenomena involve the rarest Kell phenotypes. A Kell$_{null}$ phenotype, in which no Kell antigens are expressed, has been described.[94] This phenotype appears to result from presence of two amorphic Kell genes and thus is inherited as a recessive characteristic. Red cells from individuals with this K$_0$ phenotype are morphologically and functionally normal. However, these cells overexpress an antigen denoted Kx. Although originally it was proposed that the *XK* gene encoded the precursor for Kell antigens, this theory has now been proven false, and the Kx protein—the product of the *XK* gene—has now been shown to be structurally unrelated to the Kell protein.

Biochemistry and Genetics of the Kell Antigens

The Kell blood group system was mapped to chromosome 7 owing to linkage to the prolactin-inducible protein locus.[95] Numerous antisera to various Kell antigens have been shown to identify the same 93-kD red cell membrane protein in immunoprecipitation experiments.[96–98] Cloning of the Kell protein cDNA has shown that the Kell protein consists of 732 amino acids, oriented with its C-terminus extracellular and its N-terminus in the cytoplasm; only one membrane-spanning domain is present (Fig. 10–6).[99] The Kell protein appears to belong to the family of proteins that are zinc-binding neutral endopeptidases; this family of proteins includes the common acute lymphocytic leukemia antigen (CALLA). Evidence suggests that the Kell protein is an active enzyme capable of cleaving big endothelin, a precursor of endothelin-1, as well as other vasoactive peptides.[100] The various non-antithetical Kell antigens have now been shown to represent different epitopes on a single protein[101–103] (see Fig. 10–6).

In early investigations of the biochemistry of Kell antigens, a 34-kD protein was also reported to be coprecipitated by antisera to Kell antigens by at least two groups of investigators.[96, 98] A protein of approximately the same molecular weight was isolated by immunoprecipitation with human anti-Kx,[104] suggesting that the Kell

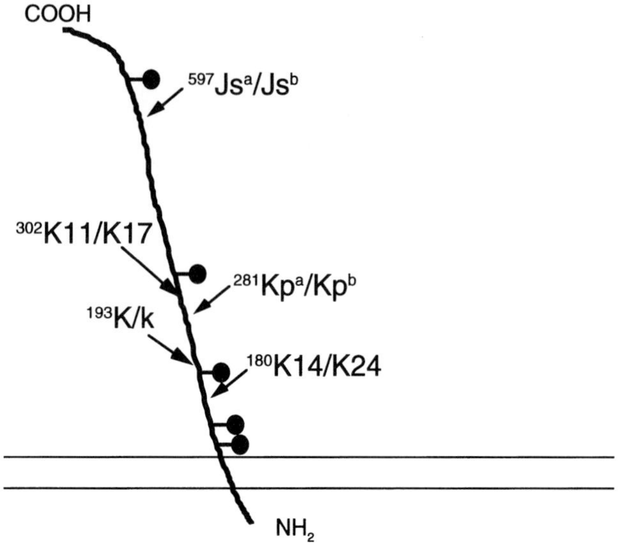

Figure 10–6. Schematic diagram of the Kell protein, including the sites of the various antithetical antigens whose structures are known.

and Kx proteins might be associated with each other in the membrane. It is interesting to speculate that Kx protein might be required for normal expression of Kell protein because of such an interaction, thus explaining why absence of Kx protein leads to poor expression of Kell antigens. Cloning of the cDNA encoding the Kx protein has demonstrated that Kx is a multipass membrane protein with structural but not sequence homology to a family of neurotransmitter transport proteins.[105] Although the function of Kx has not been demonstrated, mutations in the *XK* gene that prevent Kx expression or alter the Xk protein are associated with neuroacanthocytosis, a progressive neurological disorder.[106] The Kx antigen is encoded by the *XK* gene on the X chromosome, as shown by the fact that it has been found missing in various syndromes involving deletions or alterations of that gene, including X-linked chronic granulomatous disease and Duchenne's muscular dystrophy.[107, 108] The Kx-negative phenotype, also called the McLeod phenotype, totally lacks the Kx antigen but does express inherited Kell system antigens weakly. In addition, unlike K_0 red cells, McLeod red cells are morphologically and functionally abnormal[109, 110]; absence of Kx protein is associated with acanthocytosis and concomitant mild hemolysis that is not usually clinically significant. The acanthocytosis is correctable in vitro by incubation with dimyristoyl phosphatidylserine or chlorpromazine.[111]

Kidd System Antigens

The Kidd system antigens are clinically important antigens that also furnish insight into the normal physiology of red cells. The genes for the two Kidd antigens—Jk^a and Jk^b—occur with nearly equal frequency in the white population, although Jk^a appears to be a better immunogen than Jk^b. Antibodies to these antigens are notorious for causing severe delayed transfusion reactions, which may include intravascular hemolysis and even transient renal failure. Unfortunately, antibodies to Jk^a and Jk^b appear to be more short-lived and harder to detect than many other blood group antisera.

A hereditary Jk(a−b−) phenotype has been described and appears most common in Asia, although its frequency is still less than 1 in 10,000 in Japan. Although no clinical syndrome is associated with this phenotype, in vitro studies have shown that Jk(a−b−) red cells are resistant to lysis by 2M urea.[112, 113] More extensive experiments have further shown that Jk(a−b−) cells are deficient in urea transport, thus implying that the Kidd protein constitutes a urea transport mechanism.[114]

The gene that encodes the Kidd protein has now been identified. It is located on chromosome 18q11-q12, and its product has now been shown to be a urea transport protein.[115] The molecular basis of the Jk^a/Jk^b polymorphism has also been shown to be a single amino acid substitution, like so many other blood group antigen polymorphisms.[116]

Duffy Antigens

The Duffy blood group system is of interest both for its importance in alloimmunization and for the putative role of the Duffy protein as a receptor for malarial parasites. The two major antigens in this system—Fy^a and Fy^b—occur with only slightly unequal frequency in the white population. However, they are both low-frequency antigens in the black population: Two thirds of African-Americans and 90% of West African blacks are Fy(a−b−). The *FY* locus is located on the long arm of chromosome 1.

Although Fy antibodies are not uncommon, Duffy antigens are relatively poor immunogens. Anti-Fy^a is more commonly encountered than anti-Fy^b. The Fy3 antigen is expressed whenever Fy^a or Fy^b is present, and the antigen Fy4 is poorly understood at present. Fy5 is an antigen expressed by all Fy(a+) or Fy(b+) red cells; Fy5 is absent from Fy(a−b−) and Rh_{null} red cells. A biochemical or genetic basis for this interaction between the Duffy and Rh systems is not understood.

Biochemical characterization of a Duffy antigen was initially accomplished by Western blotting with anti-Fy^a,[117] and further work has suggested that the antigenic Duffy protein exists as part of a protein complex.[118] The 35- to 46-kD proteins reactive with Fy antisera appear to aggregate and generate higher-molecular-weight components, perhaps as do glycophorins A and B. The anti-Fy^a–reactive protein is a glycoprotein bearing both N-linked and O-linked oligosaccharide. After deglycosylation, the Fy protein has a molecular weight of only 26 kD.[119] The Fy protein has now been shown to be part of the chemokine receptor family, and Fy protein itself can act as a receptor for a number of chemokines, including interleukin-8.[120] Fy protein expression is not limited to erythroid cells,[121] and whether endothelial Fy protein plays a role in leukocyte migration out of vessels into tissues is under investigation. Interestingly, the Fy(a−b−) phenotype of African origin is not a true "null" phenotype. In this phenotype, Fy antigens are not expressed on red cells, owing to a mutation in the GATA site of the *FY* promoter, interrupting expression in these cells[122]; however, this mutation, thus far always associated with a *FY*B* gene, does not interrupt expression outside the bone marrow.

The relationship between Duffy antigens and malaria is an interesting one. Good evidence exists showing that *Plasmodium vivax,* the causative agent of malaria in Asia, and *Plasmodium knowlesi,* a cause of malaria in monkeys, cannot invade Fy(a−b−) erythrocytes,[123] although the parasites can attach to Fy(a−b−) cells. Moreover, antibodies to Fy^a or Fy^b can prevent invasion of antigen-positive cells by *P. vivax* or *P. knowlesi.*[124] However, the West African malarial parasite *Plasmodium falciparum* can both attach to and invade Fy(a−b−) red cells.

Colton Antigens

Antibodies to the Colton (Co) antigens are rarely encountered. More than 99% of people have Co(a+) red cells, whereas 8% to 9% have Co(b+) cells. However, when produced as a result of transfusion or pregnancy, antibodies to these antigens can accelerate destruction of transfused red cells in vivo.

Although it was theorized for many years that erythrocytes expressed a specialized protein that facilitated passage of water through the plasma membrane, this protein eluded detection until the 1990s. The major water channel of erythrocytes is now known as aquaporin-1 (AQP-1) and has become the founding member of a family of such proteins expressed in mammalian cells.[125] AQP-1 is a channel-forming integral membrane protein that accounts for more than 2% of the total membrane protein of the red cell. It is believed to occur in the membrane as a tetramer, with one molecule in the tetramer carrying ABH determinants on a complex polysaccharide. Soon after identification of the AQP-1 protein and mapping of its gene to chromosome 7p14,[126] the connection was made to the Colton antigens, which reside on AQP-1.[127] Some leukemias and myelodysplasias are associated with monosomy 7 and manifest with weak expression of Colton antigens. However, the Co(a−b−) phenotype, which results from a variety of mutations in the *AQP-1* gene, is not associated with significantly abnormal red cells,[128] nor does it cause significantly abnormal renal function, despite the fact that AQP-1 is the major water channel in normal kidney cells.

Diego and Wright Antigens

The Diego and Wright antigens reside on the major erythrocyte membrane protein known as band 3 or the anion channel (also called the anion exchanger-1 [AE-1]). Although not originally understood to be related, these antigens now clearly represent polymorphisms at different sites of the large band 3 protein. The incidence of Di^a antigen is highly variable from one geographic location to another; most people who express Di^a are of Mongolian origin. Among whites, more than 99.9% are both Di(b+) and Wr(b+). There is also a relatively long list of rare band 3 polymorphisms associated with low-frequency blood group antigens. Although several antibodies to band 3 antigens have been reported to cause hemolytic disease of the newborn, few have been reported to cause hemolysis in a delayed transfusion reaction setting.

Band 3 structure is now well understood, because the cDNA has been cloned, and the molecular bases for many of its antigens have been defined.[129, 130] The structural basis of the Wright antigens is particularly interesting, because it had been observed for many years that normal expression of glycophorin A was necessary for Wr^b expression, although at least one individual was identified as being Wr(a+b−) in the presence of normal glycophorin A. Ultimately, biochemical and molecular genetic evidence led to the conclusion that the Wr^b antigen is dependent on an interaction between glycophorin A and band 3.[81, 131] Band 3 also interacts with the cytoskeletal protein ankyrin, and alterations in the cytoplasmic domain of band 3 are associated with hereditary spherocytosis and southeast Asian ovalocytosis.[132–135]

Antigens Regulated by *In(Lu)*

The Lutheran blood group system antigens are rarely clinically important, although other aspects of these antigens are fascinating. Historically, the alleles encoding Lu^a and Lu^b at the Lutheran locus, along with the two alleles at the *Se (Secretor)* locus, were used to demonstrate autosomal linkage in humans for the first time.[136] This same *LU-SE* linkage was later used to document a sex-related variation in the frequency of crossing-over in humans.[137] Since these early studies, the *LU* locus has been localized to chromosome 19 and has been shown to be closely linked to a number of other loci, including *C3, LDLR, LW,* and *APOC2.*[138]

The Lutheran Blood Group System

After the Rh and Kell systems, the Lutheran blood group system encompasses one of the largest groups of antigens. Four antithetical pairs of antigens are now recognized (Table 10–5). In total, 16 Lutheran or para-Lutheran antigens have been defined. Those designated Lutheran antigens have been clearly shown to be linked to expression of other Lutheran antigens. The term *para-Lutheran* is used for antigens suppressed by the Lutheran regula-

Table 10–5. Antithetical Antigen Pairs in the Lutheran Blood Group System

Traditional Symbol or Name	Alphanumeric Symbol	Frequency
Lu^a	Lu1	Low
Lu^b	Lu2	High
Mull	Lu9	Low
Jan	Lu6	High
Hof	Lu14	Low
Taylor	Lu8	High
Au^a	Lu18	High
Au^b	Lu19	Low

tory gene *In(Lu)* but not unequivocally linked to the Lutheran locus. In general, antibodies to Lutheran antigens rarely cause accelerated red cell destruction; and when they do so, the pace of hemolysis is usually relatively slow. Lutheran antigens are also poorly developed on fetal red cells, which may contribute to the rarity of hemolytic disease of the newborn due to Lutheran antibodies.

Biochemistry and Function of Lutheran Antigens

The Lu^a and Lu^b antigens, as well as several other Lutheran antigens, have all been shown to be carried by two proteins of approximately 78 and 85 kD, respectively[139, 140]; these two proteins are encoded by a single cDNA and differ from each other only in their cytoplasmic tails, as a result of alternative mRNA splicing.[141–143] The bases for the antigenic differences between antithetical antigens such as Lu^a/Lu^b and Au^a/Au^b are single variations in amino acid sequence.[144,145]

The Lutheran protein is an immunoglobulin superfamily protein, as are many receptors and adhesion molecules. The Lutheran protein has now been shown to act as a laminin receptor.[146] Although minimally or not active on normal red cells, Lutheran protein expressed on red cells of individuals with sickle cell anemia avidly mediates adhesion to laminin.[146, 147] Moreover, Lutheran appears to be overexpressed by such erythrocytes.[147]

Lu(a−b−) Phenotypes (Table 10–6) and the *In(Lu)* Gene

The expression of Lutheran antigens can be suppressed by the presence of a single copy of the *In(Lu)* gene, a rare gene that nevertheless may occur in as many as 1 in 3,000 persons.[148] The *In(Lu)* gene was first described as a cause of the Lu(a−b−) phenotype,[149] which was soon shown to be due to an autosomal dominant gene.[150] In addition to reducing the expression of Lutheran antigens to levels undetectable by normal serological methods, *In(Lu)* affects the expression of antigens genetically and biochemically unrelated to Lutheran antigens. These include the polysaccharide antigens P1 and i,[150] the protein antigens In^a/In^b[151]—which reside on the CD44 protein,[152–154] and the AnWj antigen, to which *Haemophilus influenzae* is known to bind.[155, 156] Although the product of the *In(Lu)* gene is unknown, as is the mechanism whereby *In(Lu)* has such profound effects on the expression of unrelated genes, it is unusual if not unique among blood group system–related genes for its dominant inhibitory role.

The *In(Lu)* gene is the most common but not the only cause of the Lu(a−b−) phenotype. A recessive Lu(a−b−) phenotype has been reported,[157] and one family with an X-linked Lu(a−b−) phenotype has also been described.[158] In the *In(Lu)* Lu(a−b−) phenotype, small amounts of inherited Lutheran antigens can be demonstrated to be expressed by sensitive serological techniques, such as absorption and elution. The X-linked recessive Lu(a−b−) phenotype is similar, except that non-Lutheran antigens, such as those on CD44 and the AnWj antigen, are not diminished. However, in the recessive Lu(a−b−) phenotype, only Lutheran antigens are affected.

Interestingly, among the various Lu(a−b−) phenotypes, only *In(Lu)* Lu(a−b−) red cells have been reported to be morphologically abnormal; they have both mild morphological abnormalities and abnormal cation homeostasis.[159] In vivo, however, *In(Lu)* red cells are not associated with hemolytic syndromes. Also, because the *In(Lu)* gene apparently has relatively erythroid-specific effects, CD44 expression on leukocytes appears normal or near normal.[160]

The CD44-In^a/In^b Protein

As noted previously, the In^a/In^b antigens reside on CD44, an 80 kD protein with wide tissue distribution. First described on red cells as *In(Lu)*-related p80,[160, 161] this protein is now known to be present on a wide variety of cells, including lymphocytes, neutrophils, monocytes, fibroblasts, and epithelial cells. The protein is also found in human serum. Its importance as a lymphocyte surface marker and its involvement in lymphocyte homing has led to extensive work on this protein by investigators interested in immune processes. The protein has received the lymphocyte differentiation antigen designation CD44.

The effect of the *In(Lu)* gene on erythrocyte CD44 expression, as on Lu antigen expression, is profound. Red cells from persons with the *In(Lu)* gene bind five times less monoclonal antibody to CD44 than do cells from normal individuals. The cDNA for CD44 has been cloned.[162, 163] The 341-amino acid protein encoded by this cDNA is highly N- and O-glycosylated and, in some tissues, also bears chondroitin sulfate. Variant cDNAs that appear to arise from use of exons not found in the originally described cDNAs are also expressed in some tissues. The In^a and In^b antigens were assigned to CD44 on the basis of biochemical studies.[152, 153] Although many monoclonal antibodies to CD44 exist, none has yet been shown to recognize the same epitope(s) as human sera to In^a/In^b.

The CD44 protein is known to be a hyaluronan receptor and to function as a lymphocyte homing receptor.[164–166] Transfection of CD44 cDNA into nonadherent cell lines confers an adherent phenotype.[167] CD44 may also have a role in immune processes requiring cell/cell

Table 10–6. Lutheran-Negative Phenotypes

Inheritance and Genotype	Phenotype	Absorbs and Elutes Anti-Lu^b?	Expression of Other Antigens
Recessive, *lulu*	Lu (a− b−)	No or little	Unaffected
Dominant, *In(Lu)*	Lu (a− b−)	Yes	Reduced P_1, i, AnWj, and CD44 (In^b)
X-linked recessive, *XS2*	Lu (a− b−)	Yes	AnWj and CD44 (In^b) unaffected

Table 10–7. Cromer Blood Group System

High-frequency antigens (antithetical low-frequency antigens listed in parentheses)	Cr^a Tc^a (Tc^b, Tc^c) Dr^a Es^a WES^b (WES^a) UMC IFC
Variant phenotypes	
Dr(a−)	Absence of Dr^a antigen and decreased expression of DAF (and other Cromer antigens)
Inab	Absence of all Cromer antigens; no detectable DAF
Paroxysmal nocturnal hemoglobinuria	Clonal deficiency of all GPI-linked proteins leads to weakened or absent expression of all Cromer antigens

interaction.[168, 169] Although direct testing of these functions in *In(Lu)* individuals has not been reported, the phenotype has not been associated with immune dysfunction. CD44 also cooperates with VLA-4 as a fibronectin receptor of early erythroid progenitors.[170]

Knops/McCoy Antigens

The Knops/McCoy antigens, reported by one group also to be downregulated by the *In(Lu)* gene,[171] have now been localized to the erythrocyte C3b/C4b complement receptor (CR1, or CD35), along with the Swain-Langley and York antigens.[172, 173] CR1 expression on erythroid cells is known to vary considerably from donor to donor and to be correlated to a restriction fragment length polymorphism detectable with some CR1 DNA probes.[174] Thus, it is not entirely clear whether *In(Lu)* truly has an effect on CR1 expression, because studies implicating *In(Lu)* in regulating Knops/McCoy expression did not control for the CR1-regulatory genotype.

ANTIGENS ON PHOSPHATIDYLINOSITOL-LINKED PROTEINS

During the 1980s, it became clear that a number of cell surface membrane proteins belonged to a unique class of proteins that did not attach to membranes by insertion of one or more hydrophobic peptide segments. Instead, such proteins consisted of a peptide domain attached to the cell surface by means of a phosphatidylinositol glycan anchor.[175] The biochemistry of these anchors was first worked out in trypanosomes and later in mammals.[176] The peptide is linked by means of ethanolamine to a tetrasaccharide, which is in turn attached to an inositol. The inositol is then attached via a phosphate group to two anchoring fatty acids; a third fatty acid may frequently be directly attached to the inositol in erythrocytes.[177, 178]

During the late 1980s and early 1990s, failure to express proteins of this class was shown to be the crucial defect in the acquired stem cell disorder paroxysmal nocturnal hemoglobinuria.[179] Two phosphatidylinositol-linked GPI-linked erythrocyte proteins have complement regulatory function: decay-accelerating factor (DAF, CD55) and membrane inhibitor of reactive lysis (MIRL, CD59, protectin). Lack of these proteins, but especially of CD59, accounts for the hemolysis that is the cardinal feature of paroxysmal nocturnal hemoglobinuria. It is likely that lack of one or more GPI-linked proteins in platelets also accounts for the tendency to thrombosis in this disease.

Cromer Antigens and Decay-Accelerating Factor

The first blood group antigens shown to reside on a GPI-linked protein were the Cromer antigens (Table 10–7).[180] Antigens of this system constitute epitopes on DAF (Fig. 10–7), and the null phenotype in this system—Inab—fails to express DAF on all circulating blood cells.[180, 181] The existence of the Inab phenotype, in fact, led to confirmation that DAF is not the major defense against autologous complement, because Inab red cells have only a mild in vitro complement regulatory defect and Inab individuals do not have hemolytic anemia.[182] Nevertheless, work on the Cromer antigens has led to interesting observations regarding blood group antigen expression.

The Dr(a−) phenotype is one in which the Cromer antigen Dr^a is lacking and all other Cromer antigens are only weakly expressed. The point mutation responsible for the antigenic difference between Dr(a+) and Dr(a−) red cells has been defined, and transfected cells expressing wild-type and mutant DAF cDNA have been used to demonstrate that such allele-specific transfectants can be used serologically.[183] In addition, the Dr(a−) phenotype, like the Inab phenotype, expresses other GPI-linked proteins and antigens normally. Thus, the decrease in DAF expression in the Dr(a−) phenotype is due to a defect intrinsic to the DAF gene. This defect has now been

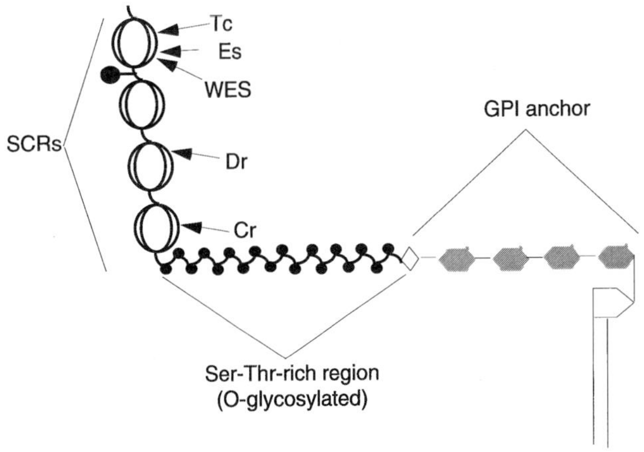

Figure 10–7. Schematic representation of the GPI-anchored protein decay-accelerating factor and localization of several blood group antigen epitopes. Decay-accelerating factor contains four short consensus repeats (SCRs) and a highly O-glycosylated region rich in serine (Ser) and threonine (Thr). The C-terminus is attached to the phosphatidylinositol-glycan anchor, from which two fatty acids insert into the membrane lipid bilayer.

shown to be a missplicing event involving the same exon that contains the point mutation responsible for the antigenic phenotype.[184]

Other Antigens on GPI-Linked Proteins

Other red cell proteins known to be GPI linked include acetylcholinesterase, lymphocyte function-associated antigen-3, and nicotinamide adenine dinucleotide glycohydrylase. In addition, blood group antigens that appear to reside on GPI-linked proteins include not only Cromer antigens but also Holley/Gregory (Hy/Gy^a), JMH, Cartwright (Yt^a/Yt^b), and Dombrock (Do^a/Do^b).[185] The Hy/Gy^a and JMH antigens appear to reside on proteins of 47 to 58 kD and 76 kD, respectively.[186–188] The Cartwright antigens have now been shown to reside on erythrocyte acetylcholinesterase.[189–191] Erythrocyte acetylcholinesterase differs from that found in other tissues, owing to alternate splicing and use of an erythrocyte-specific exon; it is this latter exon that encodes the amino acids necessary for attachment of the phosphatidylinositol anchor unique to erythrocyte acetylcholinesterase.[192] JMH antigens reside on a protein also identified as the leukocyte surface molecule CD108;[193] its function is thought to be adhesion, although its ligand has not been identified. Dombrock antigens appear to reside on the same protein as do the Hy and Gy^a antigens.[187, 194]

CONCLUSION

Our knowledge of the biochemical and genetic basis of blood group antigens has grown exponentially over the past decade. In addition to defining, at the molecular level, the targets recognized by human antibodies, investigators have elucidated the genetic mechanisms responsible for many of the unusual phenotypes recognized in the course of pre- and post-transfusion serological testing. Perhaps even more interesting has been the wealth of information gained about functionally important red cell membrane proteins during these investigations. It is now evident that the existence of blood group antigens, and the antibodies to them, provides a valuable tool for investigating important molecules expressed both by red cells as well other tissues.

REFERENCES

1. Hakomori S-I. Blood group ABH and Ii antigens of human erythrocytes: chemistry, polymorphism, and their developmental change. Semin Hematol 1981; 18:39.
2. Watkins WM. The glycosyltransferase products of the A, B, H, and Le genes and their relationship to the structure of the blood group antigens. *In* Mohn JF, Plunkett RW, Cunningham RK, Lambert RM (eds): Human Blood Groups. Basel: S Karger, 1976, pp 134–142.
3. Yamamoto F, McNeill PD, Hakomori S. Genomic organization of human histo-blood group ABO genes. Glycobiology 1995; 5:51.
4. Olsson ML, Chester MA. Frequent occurrence of a variant *O^1* allele at the blood group *ABO* locus. Vox Sang 1996; 70:26.
5. Clausen H, White T, Takio K, et al. Isolation to homogeneity and partial characterization of a histo-blood group A defined Fucα1–2Galα1–3-N-acetylgalactosaminyltransferase from human lung tissue. J Biol Chem 1990; 265:1139.
6. Yamamoto F-I, Marken J, Tsuji T, et al. Cloning and characterization of DNA complementary to human UDP-GalNAc: Fucα1–2Galα1–3GalNAc transferase (histo-blood group A transferase) mRNA. J Biol Chem 1990; 265:1146.
7. Larsen RD, Ernst LK, Nair RP, Lowe JB. Molecular cloning, sequence, and expression of a human GDP-L-fucose:β-D-galactoside 2-α-L-fucosyltransferase cDNA that can form the H blood group antigen. Proc Natl Acad Sci U S A 1990; 87:6674.
8. Yamamoto F-I, Clausen H, White T, et al: Molecular genetic basis of the histo-blood group ABO system. Nature 1990; 345:229.
9. Yamamoto F-I, Hakomori S-I. Sugar-nucleotide donor specificity of histo-blood group A and B transferase is based on amino acid substitutions. J Biol Chem 1990; 265:19257.
10. Yamamoto F, McNeill PD, Yamamoto M, et al. Molecular genetic analysis of the ABO blood group system: 4. Another type of *O* allele. Vox Sang 1993; 64:175.
11. Grunnet N, Steffenson R, Bennett EP, Clausen H. Evaluation of histo-blood group ABO genotyping in a Danish population: frequency of a novel *O* allele defined as *O^2*. Vox Sang 1994; 67:210.
12. Yamamoto F, McNeill PD, Hakamori S. Human histo-blood group A^2 transferase coded by *A^2* allele, one of the A subtypes, is characterized by a single base deletion in the coding sequence, which results in an additional domain at the carboxy terminal. Biochem Biophys Res Commun 1992; 187:366.
13. Yamamoto F, McNeill PD, Kominato Y, et al. Molecular genetic analysis of the ABO blood group system: 2. *cis-AB* alleles. Vox Sang 1993; 64:120.
14. Fukumori Y, Ohnoki S, Yoshimura K, et al. Rapid detection of the *cis-AB* allele consisting of a chimera of normal *A* and *B* alleles by PCR-RFLPs. Transfus Med 1996; 6:337.
15. Yamamoto F, McNeill PD, Yamamoto M, et al. Molecular genetic analysis of the ABO blood group system: 3. *A(X)* and *B(A)* alleles. Vox Sang 1993; 64:171.
16. Koda Y, Soejima M, Johnson PH, et al. Missense mutation of *FUT1* and deletion of *FUT2* are responsible for Indian Bombay phenotype of ABO blood group system. Biochem Biophys Res Commun 1997; 238:21.
17. Rosse WF. Immunohematology: Basic Concepts and Clinical Applications. Boston: Blackwell Scientific, 1990, pp 198–202.
18. Kukoowska-Latallo JF, Larsen RD, Nair RP, et al. A cloned human cDNA determines expression of a mouse stage-specific embryonic antigen and the Lewis blood group α(1,3/1,4)fucosyltransferase. Genes Dev 1990; 4:1288.
19. Koda Y, Kimura H, Mekada E. Analysis of fucosyltransferase genes from the human gastric mucosa of Lewis-positive and -negative individuals. Blood 1993; 82:2915.
20. Mollicone R, Reguigne I, Kelly RJ, et al. Molecular basis for Lewis α(1,3/1,4)-fucosyltransferase gene deficiency *(FUT3)* found in Lewis-negative Indonesian pedigrees. J Biol Chem 1994; 269:20987.
21. Kelly RJ, Rouquier S, Giorgi D, et al. Sequence and expression of a candidate for the human Secretor blood group α(1,2)fucosyltransferase gene *(FUT2)*. J Biol Chem 1995; 270:4640.
22. Koda Y, Soejima M, Liu Y, et al. Molecular basis for secretor type α(1,2)-fucosyltransferase gene deficiency in a Japanese population: a fusion gene generated by unequal crossover responsible for the enzyme deficiency. Am J Hum Genet 1996; 59:343.
23. Niemann H, Watanabe K, Hakomori S-I, et al. Blood groups i and I activities of lacto-N-norhexosylceramide and its analogues: the structural requirements for i specificities. Biochem Biophys Res Commun 1978; 81:1286.
24. Watanabe K, Hakomori S-I, Childs RA, Feizi T. Characterization of a blood group I active ganglioside: structural requirements for the I and i specificities. J Biol Chem 1979; 254:3221.
25. Watanabe K, Laine RA, Hakomori S-I. On neutral fucoglycolipids having long, branched carbohydrate chains: H-active and I-active glycosphingolipids of human erythrocyte membranes. Biochemistry 1975; 14:2725.
26. Roelcke D. Serology, biochemistry, and pathology of antigens defined by cold agglutinins. *In* Blood Cell Biochemistry, vol 6. New York: Plenum, 1995, pp 117–152.
27. Bierhuizen MFA, Mattei MG, Fukuda M. Expression of the developmental I antigen by a cloned human cDNA encoding a member

of a β-1, 6-N-acetylglucosaminyltransferase gene family. Genes Dev 1993; 7:468.
28. Levine P, Koch E. The rare human isoagglutinin anti-Tj[a] and habitual abortion. Science 1954; 120:239.
29. Brown KE, Anderson SM, Young NS. Erythrocyte P antigen: cellular receptor for B19 parvovirus. Science 1993; 262:114.
30. Brown KE, Hibbs JR, Gallinella G, et al. Resistance to B19 parvovirus infection due to lack of virus receptor (erythrocyte P antigen). N Engl J Med 1994; 330:1192.
31. Schwarting GA, Kundu SK, Marcus DM. Reaction of antibodies that cause paroxysmal cold hemoglobinuria (PCH) with globoside and Forssman glycosphingolipids. Blood 1979; 53:186.
32. Levine P, Stetson RE. An unusual case of intragroup agglutination. JAMA 1939; 113:126.
33. Sturgeon P. Hematological observations on the anemia associated with blood type Rh_{null}. Blood 1970; 36:310.
34. Lauf PK, Joiner CH. Increased potassium transport and ouabain binding in human Rh_{null} red blood cells. Blood 1976; 48:457.
35. Kuypers F, van Linde-Sibenius-Trip M, Roelofsen B, et al. Rh_{null} human erythrocytes have an abnormal membrane phospholipid organization. Biochem J 1984; 221:931.
36. Gahmberg CG. Molecular identification of the human Rh_0(D) antigen. FEBS Lett 1982; 140:93.
37. Moore S, Woodrow CF, McClelland DBL. Isolation of membrane components associated with human red cell antigens Rh(D), (C), (E) and Fy(a). Nature 1982; 285:529.
38. Gahmberg CG. Molecular characterization of the human red cell Rh_0(D) antigen. EMBO J 1982; 2:223.
39. Agre P, Saboori AM, Asimos A, Smith BL. Purification and partial characterization of the Mr 30,000 integral membrane protein associated with the erythrocyte Rh(D) antigen. J Biol Chem 1987; 262:17497.
40. Gahmberg CG, Karhi KK. Association of Rh_0(D) polypeptides with the membrane skeleton in Rh_0(D)-positive human red cells. J Immunol 1984; 133:334.
41. Ridgwell K, Tanner MJA, Anstee DJ. The Rhesus (D) polypeptide is linked to the human erythrocyte cytoskeleton. FEBS Lett 1984; 174:7.
42. de Vetten MP, Agre P. The Rh polypeptide is a major fatty-acid acylated erythrocyte membrane protein. J Biol Chem 1988; 263:18193.
43. Cherif-Zahar B, Bloy C, Le Van Kim C, et al. Molecular cloning and protein structure of a human blood group Rh polypeptide. Proc Natl Acad Sci U S A 1990; 87:6243.
44. Avent ND, Ridgwell K, Tanner MJA, Anstee DJ. cDNA cloning of a 30 kDa erythrocyte membrane protein associated with Rh (Rhesus) blood group antigen expression. Biochem J 1990; 271:821.
45. Le Van Kim C, Mouro I, Cherif-Zahar B, et al. Molecular cloning and primary structure of the human blood group RhD polypeptide. Proc Natl Acad Sci U S A 1992; 89:10925.
46. Arce MA, Thompson ES, Wagner S, et al. Molecular cloning of RhD cDNA derived from a gene present in RhD-positive, but not RhD-negative individuals. Blood 1993; 82:651
47. Kajii E, Umenishi F, Iwamoto S, et al. Isolation of a new cDNA clone encoding an Rh polypeptide associated with the Rh blood group system. Hum Genet 1993; 91:157.
48. Mouro I, Colin Y, Cherif-Zahar B, et al. Molecular genetic basis of the human Rhesus blood group system. Nat Genet 1993; 5:62.
49. Colin Y, Cherif-Zahar B, Le Van Kim C, et al. Genetic basis of the RhD-positive and RhD-negative blood group polymorphism as determined by Southern analysis. Blood 1991; 78:2747.
50. Hyland CA, Wolter LC, Saul A. Three unrelated Rh D gene polymorphisms identified among blood donors with Rhesus CCee (r′r′) phenotypes. Blood 1994; 84:321.
51. Gassner C, Schmarda A, Kilga-Nogler S, et al. RHD/CE typing by polymerase chain reaction using sequence-specific primers. Transfusion 1997; 37:1020.
52. Daniels G, Lomas-Francis C, Wallace M, Tippett P. Epitopes of Rh D: serology and molecular genetics. *In* Silberstein LE, (ed): Molecular and Functional Aspects of Blood Group Antigens. Bethesda, MD: American Association of Blood Banks, 1995, pp 193–228.
53. Rouillac C, Colin Y, Hughes-Jones NC, et al. Transcript analysis of D category phenotypes predicts hybrid Rh D-CE-D proteins associated with alteration of D epitopes. Blood 1995; 85:2937.
54. Mouro I, Le Van Kim C, Rouillac C, et al. Rearrangements of the blood group RhD gene associated with the DVI category phenotype. Blood 1995; 83:1129.
55. Cherif-Zahar B, Raynal V, D'Ambrosio AM, et al. Molecular analysis of the structure and expression of the RH locus in individuals with D–, Dc-, and DCw-gene complexes. Blood 1994; 84:4354.
56. Ridgwell K, Spurr NK, Laguda B, et al: Isolation of cDNA clones for a 50 kDa glycoprotein of the human erythrocyte membrane associated with Rh (rhesus)-blood-group antigen expression. Biochem J 1992; 287:223.
57. Cherif-Zahar B, Raynal V, Gane P, et al. Candidate gene acting as a suppressor of the *RH* locus in most cases of Rh-deficiency. Nat Genet 1996; 12:168.
58. Marini AM, Urrestarazu A, Beauwens R, Andre B. The Rj (Rhesus) blood group polypeptides are related to NH_4^+ transporters. Trends Biochem Sci 1997; 22:460.
59. Mallinson G, Martin PG, Anstee DJ. Identification and partial characterization of the human erythrocyte membrane component(s) which express the antigens of the LW blood group system. Biochem J 1986; 234:649.
60. Bailly P, Hermand P, Callebaut I, et al. The LW blood group glycoprotein is homologous to intercellular adhesion molecules. Proc Natl Acad Sci U S A. 1994; 91:5306.
61. Bailly P, Tontti E, Hermand P, et al. The red cell LW blood group protein is an intercellular adhesion molecule which binds to CD11/CD18 leukocyte integrins. Eur J Immunol 1995; 25:3316.
62. Cartron J-P, Colin Y, Kudo S, Fukuda M. Molecular genetics of human erythrocyte sialoglycoproteins, glycophorins A, B, C, and D. *In* Harris JR (ed): Blood Cell Biochemistry 1: Erythroid Cells. London: Plenum Press, 1990, pp 299–335.
63. Dahr W, Uhlenbruck G, Janssen E, Schmalisch R. Different N-terminal amino acids in the M,N glycoprotein from MM and NN erythrocytes. Hum Genet 1977; 35:335.
64. Dahr W, Beyreuther K, Steinbach H, et al. Structure of the Ss blood group antigens: II. A methionine/threonine polymorphism with the N-terminal sequence of Ss glycoprotein. Hoppe-Seyler's Z Physiol Chem 1980; 361:895.
65. Darnborough J, Dunsford I, Wallace J. The Ena antigen and antibod: a genetical modification of human red cells affecting their blood grouping reactions. Vox Sang 1969; 17:241.
66. Furuhjelm U, Myllyla G, Nevanlinna HR, et al. The red cell phenotype En(a−) and anti-Ena: serological and physicochemical aspects. Vox Sang 1969; 17:256.
67. Furuhjelm U, Nevanlinna HR, Pirkola A. A second Finnish En(a−) propositus wuth anti-Ena. Vox Sang 1973; 24:545.
68. Issitt PD, Anstee DJ. Applied Blood Group Serology, 4th ed. Miami: Montgomery Scientific, 1998, pp 501–507.
69. Dahr W, Uhlenbruck G, Issitt PD. SDS-polyacrylamide gel electrophoretic analysis of the membrane glycoproteins from S-s-U-erythrocytes. J Immunogenet 1975; 2:249.
70. Mallinson G, Anstee DJ, Avent ND, et al. Murine monoclonal antibody MB-2D10 recognizes Rh-related glycoproteins in the human red cell membrane. Transfusion 1990; 30:222.
71. Rahuel C, London J, Vignal A, et al. Alteration of the genes for glycophorin A and B in glycophorin-A–deficient individuals. Eur J Biochem 1988; 177:605.
72. Vignal A, Rahuel C, London J, et al. A novel gene member of the human glycophorin A and B gene family: molecular cloning and expression. Eur J Biochem 1990; 191:619.
73. Huang C-H, Blumenfeld OO. Characterization of a genomic hybrid specifying the human erythrocyte antigen Dantu: Dantu gene is duplicated and linked to a delta glycophorin gene deletion. Proc Natl Acad Sci U S A 1988; 85:9640.
74. Vignal A, Rahuel C, El Maliki B, et al. Molecular analysis of glycophorin A and B gene structure and expression in homozygous Miltenberger class V (Mi.V) human erythrocytes. Eur J Biochem 1989; 184:337.
75. Huang C-H, Blumenfeld OO. Molecular genetics of human erythrocyte MiIII and MiVI glycophorins: use of a pseudoexon in construction of two delta-alpha-delta hybrid genes resulting in antigenic diversification. J Biol Chem 1991; 266:7248.
76. Huang C-H, Blumenfeld OO. Multiple origins of the human glycophorin St[a] gene: identification of hot spots for independent unequal homologous recombinations. J Biol Chem 1991; 266:23306.
77. Johe KK, Vengelen-Tyler V, Leger R, Blumenfeld OO. Synthetic

peptides homologous to human glycophorins of the Miltenberger complex of variants of MNSs blood group system specify the epitopes for Hil, SJL, Hop, and Mur antisera. Blood 1991; 78:2456.
78. Chasis JA, Mohandas N, Shohet SB. Erythrocyte membrane rigidity induced by glycophorin A-ligand interaction: evidence for a ligand-induced association between glycophorin A and skeletal proteins. J Clin Invest 1985; 75:1919.
79. Telen MJ, Chasis JA. Relationship of the human erythrocyte Wr^b antigen to an interaction between glycophorin A and band 3. Blood 1990; 76:842.
80. Groves JD, Tanner MJ. The effects of glycophorin A on the expression of the human red cell anion transporter (band 3) in *Xenopus* oocytes. J Membr Biol 1994; 140:81.
81. Bruce LJ, Groves JD, Okubo Y, et al. Altered band 3 structure and function in glycophorin A- and B-deficient (MkMk) red blood cells. Blood 1994; 84:916.
82. Reid ME, Chasis JA, Mohandas N. Identification of a functional role for human erythrocyte sialoglycoproteins beta and gamma. Blood 1987; 69:1068.
83. Le Van Kim C, Mitjavila M-T, Clerget M, et al. An ubiquitous isoform of glycophorin C is produced by alternative splicing. Nucl Acids Res 1990; 18:3076.
84. El Maliki B, Blanchard D, Dahr W, et al. Structural homology between glycophorins C and D of human erythrocytes. Eur J Biochem 1989; 183:639.
85. Poole J, Reid ME, Banks J, et al. Serological and immunochemical specificity of a human autoanti-Gerbich-like antibody. Vox Sang 1990; 58:287.
86. Le Van Kim C, Colin Y, Blanchard D, et al. Gerbich blood group deficiency of the Ge:-1,-2,-3 and Ge:-1,-2,3 types: immunochemical study and genomic analysis with cDNA probes. Eur J Biochem 1987; 165:571.
87. High S, Tanner MJA, MacDonald EB, Anstee DJ. Rearrangements of the red-cell membrane glycophorin C (sialoglycoprotein b) gene: a further study of alterations in the glycophorin C gene. Biochem J 1989; 262:47.
88. Colin Y, Le Van Kim C, Tsapis A, et al. Human erythrocyte glycophorin C: gene structure and rearrangement in genetic variants. J Biol Chem 1989; 264:3773.
89. King M-J, Reid ME, Avent ND, et al. Molecular characterization of the low incidence antigen, Lsa. Blood 1991; 78(suppl):387a.
90. Telen MJ, Le Van Kim C, Guizzo ML, et al. Erythrocyte Webb-type glycophorin C variant lacks N-glycosylation due to an asparagine to serine substitution. Am J Hematol 1991; 37:51.
91. King M-J, Avent ND, Mallinson G, Reid ME. The Dh^a blood group antigen is the result of a single amino acid substitution (leucine—phenylalanine) at the N-terminus of glycophorin C. Blood 1991; 78(suppl):177a.
92. Daniels GL, Shaw M-A, Judson PA, et al. A family demonstrating inheritance of the Leach phenotype: a Gerbich-negative phenotype associated with elliptocytosis. Vox Sang 1986; 50:117.
93. Telen MJ, Le Van Kim M, Chung A, et al. Molecular basis for elliptocytosis associated with glycophorin C and D deficiency in the Leach phenotype. Blood 1991; 78:1603.
94. Chown B, Lewis M, Kaita H. A "new" Kell blood group phenotype. Nature 1957; 180:711.
95. Zelinski T, Coghlan G, Myal Y, et al. Genetic linkage between the Kell blood group system and prolactin-inducible protein loci: provisional assignment of KEL to chromosome 7. Ann Hum Genet 1991; 55:137.
96. Redman CM, Marsh WL, Mueller KA, et al. Isolation of Kell-active protein from the red cell membrane. Transfusion 1984; 24:176.
97. Redman CM, Avellino G, Pfeffer SR, et al. Kell blood group antigens are part of a 93,000 dalton red cell membrane protein. J Biol Chem 1986; 261:9521.
98. Jaber A, Blanchard D, Goossens D, et al. Characterization of the blood group Kell (K1) antigen with a human monoclonal antibody. Blood 1989; 73:1597.
99. Lee S, Zambas ED, Marsh LW, Redman CM. Molecular cloning and primary structure of Kell blood group protein. Proc Natl Acad Sci U S A 1991; 88:6353.
100. Lee S, Lin MH, Farmar JG, et al. Kell blood group protein proteolytically cleaves vasoactive peptides. Blood 1998; 92(suppl 1):4a.
101. Lee S, Wu X, Reid M, et al. Molecular basis of the Kell (K1) phenotype. Blood 1995; 85:912.
102. Lee S, Wu X, Reid M, Redman C. Molecular basis of the K:6,-7 [Js(a+b−)] phenotype in the Kell blood group system. Transfusion 1995; 35:822.
103. Lee S, Wu X, Son S, et al. Point mutations characterize *KEL10,* the *KEL3, KEL4,* and *KEL21* alleles, and the *KEL17* and *KEL11* alleles. Transfusion 1996; 36:490.
104. Redman CM, Marsh WL, Scarborough A, et al. Biochemical studies on McLeod phenotype red cells and isolation of the Kx antigen. Br J Haematol 1988; 68:131.
105. Ho M, Chelly J, Carter N, et al. Isolation of the gene for McLeod syndrome that encodes a novel membrane transport protein. Cell 1994; 77:869.
106. Witt TN, Danek A, Reiter M, et al. McLeod syndrome: a distinct form of neuroacanthocytosis: Report of two cases and literature review with emphasis on neuromuscular manifestations. J Neurol 1992; 239:302.
107. Bertelson CJ, Pogo AO, Chaudhuri A, et al. Localization of the McLeod locus *(Xk)* within *XP21* by deletion analysis. Am J Hum Genet 1988; 42:703.
108. Frey D, Maechler M, Seger R, et al. Gene deletion in a patient with chronic granulomatous disease and McLeod syndrome: fine mapping of the *Xk* gene locus. Blood 1988; 71:252.
109. Kuypers FA, Van Linke-Sibenius Trip M, Roelofsen B, et al. The phospholipid organization in the membranes of McLeod and Leach phenotype erythrocytes. FEBS Lett 1985; 184:20.
110. Wimer BM, Marsh WL, Taswell HF, Galey WR. Haematological changes associated with the McLeod phenotype of the Kell blood group system. Br J Haematol 1977; 36:219.
111. Redman CM, Huima T, Robbins E, et al. Effect of phosphatidylserine on the shape of McLeod red cell acanthocytes. Blood 1989; 74:1826.
112. Heaton DC, McLoughlin K. Jk(a−b−) red blood cells resist urea lysis. Transfusion 1982; 22:70.
113. Edwards-Moulds J, Kasschau MR. The effect of 2 Molar urea on Jk(a−b−) red cells. Vox Sang 1988; 55:181.
114. Frohlich O, Macey RI, Edwards-Moulds J, et al. Urea transport deficiency in Jk(a−b−) erythrocytes. Am J Physiol 1991; 260:778.
115. Olives B, Neau P, Bailly P, et al. Cloning and functional expression of a urea transporter from human bone marrow cells. J Biol Chem 1994; 269:31649.
116. Olives B, Merriman M, Bailly P, et al. The molecular basis of the Kidd blood group polymorphism and its lack of association with type I diabetes susceptibility. Hum Mol Genet 1997; 6:1017.
117. Hadley TJ, David P, McGinniss MH, Miller LH. Identification of an erythrocyte component carrying the Duffy blood group Fy^a antigen. Science 1984; 223:597.
118. Chaudhuri A, Zbrzezna V, Johnson C, et al. Purification and characterization of an erythrocyte membrane protein complex carrying Duffy blood group antigenicity: possible receptor for *Plasmodium vivax* and *Plasmodium knowlesi* malaria parasite. J Biol Chem 1989; 254:13770.
119. Tanner MJA, Anstee DJ, Mallinson G, et al. Effect of endoglycosidase F-peptidyl N-glycosidase F preparations on the surface of the human erythrocyte. Carbohydr Res 1988; 178:203.
120. Horuk R, Chitnis CE, Darbonne WC, et al. A receptor for the malarial parasite *Plasmodium vivax:* the erythrocyte chemokine receptor. Science 1993; 261:1182.
121. Hadley TJ, Lu Zh, Wasniowska K, et al. Postcapillary venule epithelial cells in kidney express a multispecific chemokine receptor that is structurally and functionally identical to the erythrocyte isoform, which is the Duffy blood group antigen. J Clin Invest 1994; 94:985.
122. Tournamille C, Colin Y, Cartron JP, Le Van Kim C. Disruption of a GATA motif in the Duffy gene promoter abolishes erythroid gene expression in Duffy-negative individuals. Nat Genet 1995; 10:224.
123. Miller LH, Mason SJ, Dvorak JA, et al. Erythrocyte receptors for *(Plasmodium knowlesi)* malaria. Science 1975; 189:561.
124. Mason SJ, Miller LH, Shiroishi T, et al. The Duffy blood group determinants: their role in the susceptibility of human and animal erythrocytes to *Plasmodium knowlesi* malaria. Br J Haematol 1977; 36:327.
125. Preston GM, Agre P. Isolation of the cDNA for erythrocyte integral membrane protein of 28 kilodaltons: member of an ancient channel family. Proc Natl Acad Sci U S A 1991; 88:11110.

126. Moon C, Preston GM, Griffin C, et al. The human aquaporin-CHIP gene: structure, organization, and chromosomal localization. J Biol Chem 1993; 268:15772.
127. Smith BL, Preston GM, Spring F, et al. Human red cell aquaporin CHIP: I. Molecular characterization of ABH and Colton blood group antigens. J Clin Invest 1994; 94:1043.
128. Preston GM, Smith BL, Zeidel NI, et al. Mutations in aquaporin-1 in phenotypically normal humans without functional CHIP water channels. Science 1994; 265:1585.
129. Tanner MJA, Martin PG, High S. The complete amino acid sequence of the human erythrocyte membrane anion-transport protein deduced from the cDNA sequence. Biochem J 1988; 256:703.
130. Lux SE, John KM, Kopito RR, Lodish HF. Cloning and characterization of band 3, the human erythrocyte anion-exchange protein (AE1). Proc Natl Acad Sci USA 1989; 86:9089.
131. Telen MJ, Chasis JA. Relationship of the human erythrocyte Wr^b antigen to an interaction between glycophorin A and band 3. Blood 1990; 76:842.
132. Jarolim P, Rubin HL, Liu SC, et al. Duplication of 10 nucleotides in the erythroid band 3 (AE1) gene in a kindred with hereditary spherocytosis and band 3 protein deficiency (band 3^{PRAGUE}). J Clin Invest 1994; 93:121.
133. Dhermy D, Galand C, Bournier O, et al. Heterogeneous band 3 deficiency in hereditary spherocytosis related to different band 3 gene defects. Br J Haematol 1997; 98:32.
134. Jarolim P, Palek J, Amato D, et al. Deletion in erythrocyte band 3 gene in malaria resistant Southeast Asian ovalocytosis. Proc Natl Acad Sci U S A 1991; 88:11022.
135. Tanner MJA, Bruce L, Martin PG, et al. Melanesian hereditary ovalocytes have a deletion in red cell band 3. Blood 1991; 78:2785.
136. Mohr J. A Study of Linkage in Man. Copenhagen: Munksgaard, 1954.
137. Cook PJL. The Lutheran-Secretor recombination fraction in man: a possible sex difference. Ann Hum Genet 1965; 28:393.
138. Lewis M, Kaita H, Coghlan G, et al. The chromosome 19 linkage group LDLR, C3, LW, APOC2, Lu, Se in man. Ann Hum Genet 1988; 52:137.
139. Parsons SF, Mallinson G, Judson PA, et al. Evidence that the Lu^b blood group antigen is located on red cell membrane glycoproteins of 85 and 78 kD. Transfusion 1987; 27:61.
140. Daniels G, Khalid G. Identification, by immunoblotting, of the structures carrying Lutheran and para-Lutheran blood group antigens. Vox Sang 1989; 57:137.
141. Campbell IG, Foulkes WD, Senger G, et al. Molecular cloning of the B-CAM cell surface glycoprotein of epithelial cancers: a novel member of the immunoglobulin superfamily. Cancer Res 1994; 54:5761.
142. Parsons SF, Mallinson G, Holmes CH, et al. The Lutheran blood group glycoprotein, another member of the immunoglobulin superfamily, is widely expressed in human tissues and is developmentally regulated in human liver. Proc Natl Acad Sci U S A 1995; 92:5496.
143. Rahuel C, Le Van Kim C, Mattei MG, et al. A unique gene encodes spliceoforms of the B-cell adhesion molecule cell surface glycoprotein of epithelial cancer and of the Lutheran blood group glycoprotein. Blood 1996; 88:1865.
144. El Nemer W, Rahuel C, Colin Y, et al. Organization of the human LU gene and molecular basis of the Lu(a)/Lu(b) blood group polymorphism. Blood 1997; 89:4608.
145. Parsons SF, Mallinson G, Daniels GL, et al. Use of domain-deletion mutants to locate Lutheran blood group antigens to each of the five immunoglobulin superfamily domains of the Lutheran glycoprotein: elucidation of the molecular basis of the Lu(a)/Lu(b) and the Au(a)/Au(b) polymorphisms. Blood 1997; 89:4219.
146. Udani M, Zen Q, Cottman M, et al. Basal cell adhesion molecule/Lutheran protein: the receptor critical for sickle cell adhesion to laminin. J Clin Invest 1998; 101:2550.
147. Zen JQ, Cottman M, Truskey G, et al. Critical factors in basal cell adhesion molecule/Lutheran-mediated adhesion to laminin. J Biol Chem 1999; 274:728.
148. Shaw MA, Leak MR, Daniels GL, Tippett P. The rare Lutheran blood group phenotype Lu(a−b−): a genetic study. Ann Hum Genet 1984; 48:229.
149. Crawford MN, Greenwalt TG, Sasaki T, et al. The phenotype Lu(a−b−) together with unconventional Kidd groups in one family. Transfusion 1961; 1:228.
150. Taliano V, Guevin R-M, Tippett P. The genetics of a dominant inhibitor of the Lutheran antigens. Vox Sang 1973; 24:42.
151. Ferguson DJ, Gaal HD. Some observations on the In^b antigen and evidence that anti-In^b causes accelerated destruction of radiolabeled red cells. Transfusion 1988; 28:479.
152. Spring FA, Dalchau R, Daniels GL, et al. The In^a and In^b blood group antigens are located on a glycoprotein of 80,000 MW (the CDw44 glycoprotein) whose expression is influenced by the In(Lu) gene. Immunology 1988; 64:37.
153. Telen MJ, Ferguson DJ. Relationship of In^b antigen to other antigens on In(Lu)-related p80. Vox Sang 1990; 58:118.
154. Telen MJ, Udani M, Washington MK, et al. A blood group–related polymorphism of CD44 abolishes a hyaluronan-binding consensus sequence without preventing hyaluronan binding. J Biol Chem 1996; 271:7147.
155. Poole J, Giles CM. Observations on the Anton antigen and antibody. Vox Sang 1982; 43:220.
156. Gilsdorf JR, Judd WJ, Cinat M. Relationship of *Hemophilus influenzae* type b pilus structure and adherence to human erythrocytes. Infect Immun 1989; 57:3259.
157. Brown F, Simpson S, Cornwall S, et al. The recessive Lu(a−b−) phenotype: a family study. Vox Sang 1974; 26:259.
158. Norman PC, Tippett P, Beal RW. An Lu(a−b−) phenotype caused by an X-linked recessive gene. Vox Sang 1986; 51:49.
159. Udden MM, Umeda M, Hirano Y, Marcus DM. New abnormalities in the morphology, cell surface receptors, and electrolyte metabolism of *In(Lu)* erythrocytes. Blood 1987; 69:52.
160. Telen MJ, Eisenbarth GS, Haynes BF. Human erythrocyte antigens; regulation of a novel red cell surface antigen by the inhibitor Lutheran *In(Lu)* gene. J Clin Invest 1983; 71:1978.
161. Telen MJ, Palker TJ, Haynes BF. Human erythrocyte antigens: II. The *In(Lu)* gene regulates expression of an antigen residing on an 80-kilodalton protein of human erythrocytes. Blood 1984; 64:599.
162. Stamenkovic I, Amiot M, Pesandro JM, Seed B. A lymphocyte molecule implicated in lymphocyte homing is a member of the cartilage link protein family. Cell 1989; 56:1057.
163. Goldstein LA, Zhou DF, Picker LJ, et al. A human lymphocyte homing receptor, the Hermes antigen, is related to cartilage proteoglycan core and link proteins. Cell 1989; 56:1063.
164. Aruffo A, Stemankovic I, Melnick M, et al. CD44 is the principal cell surface receptor for hyaluronidate. Cell 1990; 61:1303.
165. Jalkanen ST, Bargatze RF, Herron LR, Butcher EC. A lymphoid cell surface glycoprotein involved in endothelial cell recognition and lymphocyte homing in man. Eur J Immunol 1986; 16:1195.
166. Berg EL, Goldstein LA, Jutila MA, et al. Homing receptors and vascular addressins: cell adhesion molecules that direct lymphocyte traffic. Immunol Rev 1988; 108:5.
167. St John T, Meyer J, Idzerda R, Gallatin WM. Expression of CD44 confers a new adhesive phenotype on transfected cells. Cell 1990; 60:45.
168. Hale LP, Singer KH, Haynes BF. CD44 antibody against In(Lu)-related p80, lymphocyte homing receptor molecule inhibits the binding of human erythrocytes to T cells. J Immunol 1990; 143:3944.
169. Haynes BF, Telen MJ, Hale LP, Denning SM. CD44: a molecule involved in leukocyte adherence and T-cell activation. Immunol Today 1989; 10:423.
170. Verfaillie CM, Benis A, Iida J, et al. Adhesion of committed human hematopoietic progenitors to synthetic peptides from the C-terminal heparin-binding domain of fibronectin: cooperation between the integrin alpha 4 beta 1 and the CD44 adhesion receptor. Blood 1994; 84:1802.
171. Daniels GL, Shaw MA, Lomas CG, et al. The effect of *In(Lu)* on some high incidence antigens. Transfusion 1986; 26:171.
172. Rao N, Ferguson DJ, Lee S-F, Telen MJ. Identification of human erythrocyte blood group antigens on the C3b/C4b receptor. J Immunol 1991; 146:3502.
173. Moulds JM, Nickells MW, Moulds JJ, et al. The C3b/C4b receptor is recognized by the Knops, McCoy, Swain-Langley, and York blood group antisera. J Exp Med 1991; 173:1159.
174. Wilson JG, Murphy EE, Wong WW, et al. Identification of a restriction fragment length polymorphism by a CR1 cDNA that correlates with the number of CR1 on erythrocytes. J Exp Med 1986; 164:50.
175. Low MG. Glycosyl-phosphatidylinositol: a versatile anchor for cell surface proteins. FASEB J 1989; 3:1600.

176. Low MG. Biochemistry of the glycosyl-phosphatidylinositol membrane protein anchor. Biochem J 1987; 244:1.
177. Roberts WL, Kim BH, Rosenberry TL. Differences in the glycolipid membrane anchors of bovine and human erythrocyte acetylcholinesterases. Proc Natl Acad Sci U S A 1987; 84:7817.
178. Roberts WL, Santikarn S, Reinhold VN, Rosenberry TL. Structural characterization of the glycoinositol phospholipid membrane anchor of human erythrocyte acetylcholinesterase by fast atom bombardment mass spectrometry. J Biol Chem 1988; 263:18776.
179. Rosse WF. Phosphatidylinositol-linked proteins and paroxysmal nocturnal hemoglobinuria. Blood 1990; 75:1595.
180. Telen MJ, Hall SE, Green AM, et al. Identification of human erythrocyte blood group antigens on decay accelerating factor (DAF) and identification of an erythrocyte phenotype negative for DAF. J Exp Med 1988; 167:1993.
181. Spring FA, Judson PA, Daniels GL, et al. A human cell-surface glycoprotein that carries Cromer-related blood group antigens on erythrocytes and is also expressed on leucocytes and platelets. Immunology 1987; 62:307.
182. Telen MJ, Green AM. The Inab phenotype: characterization of the membrane protein and complement regulatory defect. Blood 1989; 74:437.
183. Lublin DM, Thompson ES, Green AM, et al. Dr(a−) polymorphism of decay accelerating factor: biochemical, functional, and molecular characterization and production of allele-specific transfectants. J Clin Invest 1991; 87:1945.
184. Lublin DM, Mallinson G, Poole J, et al. Molecular basis of reduced or absent expression of decay-accelerating factor in Cromer blood group phenotypes. Blood. 94; 84:1276.
185. Telen MJ, Rosse WF, Parker CJ, et al. Evidence that several high frequency blood group antigens reside on phosphatidylinositol-linked erythrocyte membrane proteins. Blood 1990; 75:1404.
186. Spring FA, Reid ME. Evidence that the human blood group antigens Gy^a and Hy are carried on a novel glycosylphosphatidylinositol-linked erythrocyte membrane glycoprotein. Vox Sang 1991; 60:53.
187. Rao N, Udani M, et al. Investigations using a novel monoclonal antibody to the glycosylphosphatidylinositol-anchored protein that carries Gregory, Holley, and Dombrock blood group antigens. Transfusion 1995:35:459.
188. Bobolis KA, Moulds JJ, Telen MJ. Isolation of the JMH antigen on a novel phosphatidylinositol-linked human membrane protein. Blood 1992; 79:1574.
189. Spring FA, Gardner B, Anstee DJ. Evidence that the antigens of the Yt blood group system are located on human erythrocyte acetylcholinesterase. Blood 1992; 80:2136.
190. Rao N, Whitsett CF, Oxendine SM, Telen MJ. Human erythrocyte acetylcholinesterase bears the Yta blood group antigen and is reduced or absent in the Yt(a−b−) phenotype. Blood 1993; 81:815.
191. Bartels CF, Zelinski T, Lockridge O. Mutation at codon 322 in the human acetylcholinesterase *(ACHE)* gene accounts for YT blood group polymorphism. Am J Hum Genet 1993; 52:928.
192. Li Y, Camp S, Rachinsky TL, et al. Gene structure of mammalian acetylcholinesterase: alternative exons dictate tissue-specific expression. J Biol Chem 1991; 266:23083.
193. Mudad R, Rao N, Angelisova P, et al. Evidence that CDw108 membrane protein bears the JMH blood group antigen. Transfusion 1995; 35:566.
194. Banks JA, Hemming N, Poole J. Evidence that the Gya, Hy and Joa antigens belong to the Dombrock blood group system. Vox Sang 1995; 68:177.

SECTION

IV Granulocytes

CHAPTER 11

Granulocyte Storage and Metabolism

Thomas A. Lane

This chapter reviews aspects of the structure and metabolism of granulocytes that are relevant to granulocyte transfusion and the storage of granulocyte concentrates before transfusion. The scientific bases of the granulocyte storage techniques and procedures commonly used to provide functional granulocytes to patients are demonstrated. Although transfusion of granulocyte concentrates is infrequently indicated, it may nonetheless be helpful to selected patients, and the advent of improved methods to harvest granulocytes by treatment of donors with granulocyte colony stimulating factor (G-CSF) has led to increasing interest in the therapeutic use of granulocytes. Consequently, it is important for blood banks to provide granulocyte concentrates with optimal function and the lowest possible potential for adverse effects. For the purpose of this chapter, the term *granulocyte* refers only to the mature (circulating) neutrophilic polymorphonuclear leukocyte (PMN) unless otherwise specified.

THE PHYSIOLOGICAL ROLE OF GRANULOCYTES

The primary physiological function of granulocytes is to kill microbes that penetrate the initial lines of host defense (e.g., skin, mucous membranes) or that escape normal clearance mechanisms (e.g., respiratory, gastrointestinal, and genitourinary mechanisms; spleen and liver). The importance to host defense of sufficient numbers of circulating granulocytes has long been appreciated by clinicians who care either for patients who have agranulocytosis[1] or for patients who have severe, prolonged leukopenia as a result of cancer chemotherapy.[2] Patients with severe neutropenia suffer from repeated infections and commonly die from them. In addition to the requirement for a minimum number in the circulation, granulocytes must function properly in order to prevent infection. Thus a wide variety of disorders of granulocyte function, both congenital and acquired, have been associated with decreased host resistance to infection.[3–5] The clinical features and microbial etiology of infections encountered by persons who have deficient numbers or defective function of granulocytes are to some extent characteristic. These patients commonly suffer from infections in the skin, soft tissues, sinopulmonary tract, and blood stream, and the infections are most commonly caused by high-grade bacterial and fungal pathogens, such as *Staphylococcus, Klebsiella, Serratia, Pseudomonas, Candida,* and *Aspergillus* species and *Escherichia coli.*[3–5]

GRANULOCYTE CONCENTRATE TRANSFUSION

The development of technological methods designed to collect large numbers of normal granulocytes for transfusion evolved from a need to support the antimicrobial defenses of patients who had been rendered severely neutropenic by leukemia therapy.[6] The leading cause of death in such patients was infection with bacteria, partly because optimal antibiotic therapy was sometimes ineffective in infected patients who were severely neutropenic ($<500 \times 10^9$ leukocytes/L).[6, 7] In view of this problem, investigators collected and transfused granulocytes in an effort to augment the patients' antimicrobial defenses. A series of controlled clinical studies of granulocyte transfusion therapy was performed with these goals in mind. Although most of the early studies of granulocyte transfusion demonstrated efficacy with regard to both survival of patients and clearance of infection, later studies achieved less favorable results.[8–14] The variation in success demonstrated by the later studies may have resulted from a variety of factors, including variability in patient selection, the low dose of granulocytes transfused (increments in granulocyte counts were rarely achieved, even for brief periods), improvements in supportive therapy (including antimicrobial therapy), and shorter duration of severe neutropenia because of improvements in chemotherapy.[7, 15–20] The advent of therapy with growth factors to prevent or shorten the duration of chemotherapy-induced severe neutropenia,[21–23] the high cost and limited availability of granulocyte transfusions, and the adverse effects of granulocyte transfusion (e.g., alloimmunization to human leukocyte antigens [HLAs], cytomegalovirus transmission, and possible pulmonary reactions)[24–26] have reduced the use of granulocyte transfusion.[15–20] Nevertheless, granulocyte transfusion is still considered beneficial for selected patients.[16, 20, 26]

The current clinical settings in which granulocyte transfusion is employed include bacterial or fungal infections that are accompanied by severe neutropenia and are unresponsive to optimal antimicrobial therapy. Ideally, the patient has a good chance of marrow recovery if he or she can survive the current infection.[16, 18, 26] The use of granulocyte transfusions is most common in patients who are undergoing leukemia induction therapy or bone marrow transplantation,[15, 17, 20, 26] in neonates who are septic and have bone marrow failure,[27–30] and in patients who have certain granulocyte dysfunction syndromes (e.g., chronic granulomatous disease).[17, 18] A discussion of these important issues relating to the indications for granulocyte transfusion, compatibility testing, and granulocyte collection techniques is beyond the scope of this chapter, but these topics have been reviewed elsewhere.[7, 15–18, 20, 26, 27, 30] This chapter focuses on the effects of short-term storage on the function of granulocytes and on the efforts designed to improve upon the available methods of granulocyte storage. The term *granulocyte concentrate,* which is widely used in the literature, refers essentially to blood neutrophils (PMNs), the most numerous of the circulating granulocytes.

GRANULOCYTE STORAGE

The importance of granulocyte storage technology, and therefore its investigation, stems from two sources. First, even though granulocytes for transfusion are collected on an as-needed basis, it is nevertheless inevitable that granulocyte concentrates are stored before infusion. Because a major goal in granulocyte transfusion therapy is to provide an adequate number of granulocytes with optimal function, some studies have focused on the effects of short-term liquid storage both on the survival of granulocytes during storage and on granulocyte function. Other studies have focused on the mechanisms of the adverse effects of blood bank storage on granulocytes. Together, these investigations have provided the scientific basis of the current guidelines for storage of granulocyte concentrates. As a result of these studies, it is clear that granulocyte concentrates for transfusion cannot be banked as are red cells and platelets, but must be collected when needed and transfused as soon as possible. Finally, as evidenced by reviews on the subject, optimal methods of granulocyte storage are still important to investigators of granulocyte function, who may find it necessary to ship patient samples from one location to another.[31–33]

OVERVIEW OF GRANULOCYTE FUNCTION

In order to prevent or combat bacterial or fungal infection, granulocytes must be capable of performing three critical cellular functions (Table 11–1 and Fig. 11–1): (1) circulating in blood, (2) adhering to and migrating from capillaries toward loci of infection (chemotaxis), and then (3) killing invading microbes.[3–5] Each of these cellular functions in turn depends on the maintenance of certain subcellular structures or on the execution of critical intracellular biochemical or physical mechanisms.

Table 11–1. Critical Functions of Granulocytes

Circulation
Deformability
Membrane nonadherence/repulsion (?)
Migration (Chemotaxis)
Margination (adherence augmentation)
Chemotaxin receptor binding
Stimulus-response coupling
Mechanical translocation
Microbial Killing
Energy metabolism
Phagocytosis
Oxygen radical generation
Degranulation (nonoxidative mechanisms)

Circulation

In order for granulocytes to circulate, they must be sufficiently deformable to pass through small capillaries, and they must remain in a relatively low adherence (unactivated) state. Because granulocytes normally have a very short circulation time in blood—approximately 6 hours—there is little or no time for any metabolic, functional, or structural abnormality caused by storage (the so-called storage lesion) to be corrected after transfusion.[34, 35] This is greatly in contrast to transfusion of red cells, which circulate long enough for some of the metabolic disturbances induced by storage to be corrected.

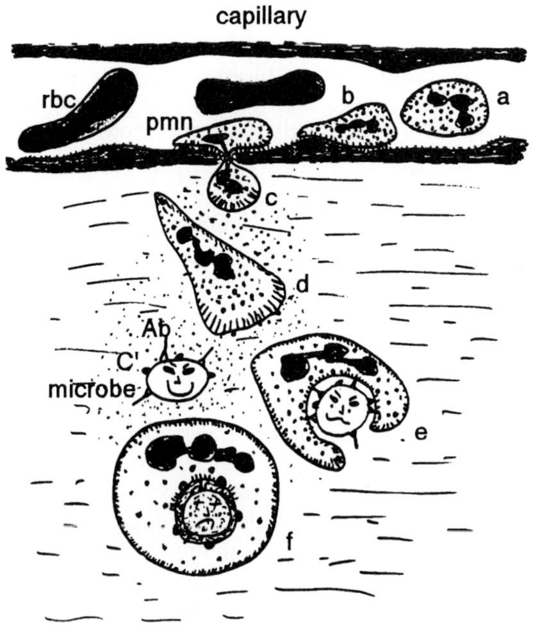

Figure 11–1. In order for granulocytes (pmn) to function properly they must be available in sufficient numbers and must circulate in the bloodstream (a); adhere to postcapillary endothelium that has been activated by inflammatory mediators (b); squeeze through the capillary walls between endothelial cells (c); migrate vectorially toward a gradient of one or more chemotactic factors (chemotaxis); engulf microbes (microbe) that have been opsonized by antibody (Ab) and complement (C) (e); and kill the invading microbes (f).

Migration

Exit of granulocytes from the blood stream and entry into the tissues *(diapedesis)* depends on augmentation of adherence, adequate function of chemotaxin receptors, integration of the chemotactic response into a vectorially accurate path of migration, and an intact mechanical response. In the normal circulation, granulocytes that have traversed capillaries adhere for a brief time to the endothelium of postcapillary venules and then are swept into the moving stream of blood.[36] In response to localized inflammation, granulocyte adherence to the postcapillary vasculature in the inflamed site is prolonged and enhanced by two events, both of which depend on the local generation of a variety of inflammatory mediators.

First, the leukocyte adherence properties of the postcapillary endothelial cells are increased near the inflamed tissue site.[37] This increase in adherence is caused by the activation of endothelial cells by such agents as interleukin-1, tumor necrosis factor, interferon-γ, and bacterial lipopolysaccharide, which are generated locally.[37, 38] The activation of endothelial cells by these substances is associated with increased endothelial cell membrane display of specific leukocyte adherence molecules,[37–46] increasing granulocyte adherence to postcapillary endothelium. Second, some of the same cytokines (tumor necrosis factor, interleukin-1) and other inflammatory mediators, including complement, bacteria-derived chemotactic factors, and nonchemotactic bacterial products, also directly activate granulocytes.[47–49] This results in augmentation of the adherence function of existing granulocyte membrane adherence molecules, such as leukocyte function–associated antigen-1 (LFA-1), as well as increased display of additional granulocyte membrane adherence molecules.[47–52] Specific classes of granulocyte and endothelial cell adhesion receptors initially result in increased rolling adhesion of neutrophils to postcapillary endothelial cells, followed by firm adhesion and ultimately transmigration of granulocytes through postcapillary endothelial cells[50–52] (Table 11–2). In the setting of endothelial cell activation, and even in the absence of a chemotactic gradient, granulocytes may migrate between endothelial cells and into the subendothelial space.[53]

Once the granulocytes arrive in the subendothelial space, they are exposed to the chemical gradient of chemotactic factors. Chemotaxis toward a locus of microbes is initiated by chemotaxin binding to specific granulocyte membrane receptors.[54–56] A large number of potential chemotactic factors generated by inflammation, including complement component fragment C5a, bacterial factors, interleukin-8 (IL-8), and other cell-derived factors such as leukotrienes, augment the response.[53, 57, 58] Chemotaxin receptor binding also initiates an activation response.[47, 49–52, 54] This series of events, which results in vectorial migration up the chemical gradient of chemotactic factor, is referred to collectively as *stimulus-response coupling.*[59] Stimulus-response coupling in granulocytes is incompletely understood, but effective granulocyte function requires the activation of cellular mechanisms that give rise to an increase in intracellular calcium[60, 61] and the generation of leukotriene B_4 (LTB_4).[62] This highly integrated function ultimately leads to orientation of the granulocyte toward the chemical gradient of chemotaxin.[59]

Mechanical translocation of the granulocyte, the final event in the process of chemotaxis, depends on a supply of intracellular adenosine triphosphate (ATP) and an intact cytoskeleton. The continued expression of chemotaxin receptors and adherence molecules is also required, because granulocytes migrate by extending pseudopodia forward between cells, then retracting the remainder of the cell toward the leading edge of the cell (as opposed to swimming).[54–56] Once at the locus of inflammation, granulocytes are discouraged from further migration by high concentrations of the same chemotactic factors that initiated migration. This process, referred to as *deactivation,* results partly from downregulation (decreased expression) of membrane chemotaxin receptors and increased granulocyte adherence properties.[47, 58]

Table 11–2. Adhesion Molecules and Transendothelial Migration of Granulocytes

Granulocyte Adhesion Molecule	Endothelial Cell Counter Receptor
Augmented Rolling Ahesion	
L-selectin (CD62L)	CD34 and others
PSGL-1/SLe^x	P selectin (CD62P)
ESL-1/SLe^x	E selectin (CD62-E)
Firm Adhesion	
LFA-1 (integrin α_L β_2; CD11a/CD18)	ICAM-1 (CD54), ICAM-2
Mac-1 (integrin α_M β_2; CD11b/CD18)	ICAM-1 (CD54), fibrinogen
Endothelial Transmigration	
IAP (CD47)	unknown
Integrin-α_V β_3?	PECAM (CD31)
PECAM (CD31)?	Integrin-α_V β_3

PSGL-1, P selectin glycoprotein ligand-1; Sle^x, sialyl Lewis X carbohydrate; ESL-1, E selectin ligand-1; LFA-1, leukocyte function–associated antigen-1; Mac-1, macrophage-1; ICAM, intracellular adhesion molecule; IAP, integrin–associated protein; PECAM, platelet endothelial cell adhesion molecule.

Microbial Killing

Microbial killing is initiated by phagocytosis of the invading organism. Phagocytosis is facilitated by the binding of antibody and complement to the organism. The coated organism then binds via these molecules to granulocyte receptors for immunoglobulin G (IgG) and complement. Binding is followed by mechanical translocation of the granulocyte membrane around the microorganism, enveloping the microorganism and forming a phagosome after resealing of the membranes surrounding the invagination.[3] During formation of the phagosome, yet another series of activation events results in the fusion of lysosomal granules with the phagosome, which at this stage is called a phagolysosome. The discharge of cytotoxic granule contents into the phagolysosome is followed by the generation of additional cytotoxic metabolites within the phagolysosome.

To accomplish their microbicidal function, granulocytes nonselectively employ a variety of mechanisms to kill either attached or ingested organisms, depending on the type of microbe (Table 11–3).[3–5] Microbicidal mechanisms may be broadly divided into oxygen-dependent and

Table 11–3. Microbicidal Mechanisms of Granulocytes*

Formation of superoxide anion	$NADPH + 2O_2$	$\xrightarrow{\text{NADPH oxidase}}$	$NADP^+ + 2O_2^- + H^+$	(A)
Formation of hydrogen peroxide	$2O_2^- + 2H^+$	$\xrightarrow{\text{Superoxide dismutase}}$	$O_2 + H_2O_2$	(B)
Formation of hydroxyl radical	$O_2^- + H_2O_2$	$\xrightarrow{\text{(Fe2+; Haber-Weiss)}}$	$O_2 + OH^- + OH\cdot$	(C)
Formation of hypochlorous acid	$H_2O_2 + Cl^- + H^+$	$\xrightarrow{\text{Myeloperoxidase}}$	$HOCl + H_2O$	(D)

Oxygen-Independent Mechanisms

Primary granule contents	Specific granule contents
Lysozyme	Lysozyme
Defensins	Lactoferrin
Azurocidin	
BPI	Miscellaneous
Cathepsin G	Acidification
Elastase	
Collagenase	

NADPH, reduced nicotinamide-adenine dinucleotide phosphate; BPI, bactericidal permeability-increasing factor.

*Oxygen-dependent mechanisms require conversion of molecular oxygen to superoxide anion (O_2^-) by NADPH oxidase (equation A). In the presence of hydrogen ion, superoxide dismutase generates hydrogen peroxide from O_2^- (equation B). Hydroxyl radical ($OH\cdot$) is formed by the spontaneous reaction of O_2^- with H_2O_2 in the presence of trace amounts of iron (equation C). Hypochlorous acid (HOCl) is generated from H_2O_2 by myeloperoxidase, in the presence of chloride (equation D).

oxygen-independent categories.[63, 64] Oxidative microbicidal mechanisms are initiated by both phagocytosis and chemical inflammatory stimuli.[47, 54, 65] They depend on the assembly and activation (on the outer leaflet of the granulocyte membrane) of a multimolecular reduced nicotinamide-adenine dinucleotide phosphate (NADPH) oxidase that, in the dormant state, consists of both cytosolic and membrane components.[66] Activation events result in the assembly of the full multimolecular complex on the membrane. This fully active NADPH oxidase uses molecular oxygen as a substrate for the generation of superoxide anion (equation A in Table 11–3) adjacent to the outer leaflet of the membrane. Superoxide anion is itself cytotoxic, but more importantly, it serves as a precursor to other, even more toxic oxygen radicals. One of the most important, hypochlorous acid (HOCl, approximately equivalent to household bleach), is synthesized as a result of degranulation and the release of myeloperoxidase into the phagolysosome (equation D in Table 11–3). Others, such as hydroxyl radical and hydrogen peroxide, are generated by cytosolic enzymes, and to some extent spontaneously (equations B and C in Table 11–3).

Nonoxidative microbicidal mechanisms are initiated by degranulation of lysosomal contents.[67] Lysozyme, lactoferrin, granulocyte defensins, bactericidal permeability-increasing factor (BPI), serprocidins (cathepsin G, azurocidin/CAP37), elastase, and phospholipases are released into the phagolysosome, along with hydrogen ion.[67, 68] These factors act upon selective groups of microorganisms, either in a microbicidal manner or by impairing their ability to divide.

Subcellular Mechanisms

More detailed discussions of the subcellular mechanisms underlying the granulocyte functions—circulation, migration, and microbial killing—may be found in reviews.[3–5, 43, 59, 63, 64, 66, 67] All the individual steps constituting normal granulocyte activation physiology must function properly, and in the correct sequence, for granulocytes to find and kill microbes successfully.

Any test of granulocyte function that ascertains that an individual granulocyte structure (e.g., chemotaxin receptors), enzyme activity (e.g., phospholipase), or subcellular mechanism (e.g., agonist-stimulated calcium flux) is intact under experimental conditions does not ensure the adequacy of the critical cellular function that is dependent on it (e.g., chemotaxis). Each of the critical granulocyte functions is highly integrated with and dependent on several subcellular mechanisms. Thus the degree of maintenance of any critical granulocyte function can be ascertained only by studying the function itself. Awareness of this caveat is an important prerequisite for valid evaluation and interpretation of the literature regarding granulocyte storage. The "viability" of granulocytes (more properly referred to as membrane integrity) as ascertained in an experiment by supravital dye exclusion thus does not predict that the chemotactic response of the cells will be normal or even present. The literature on granulocyte storage reveals that granulocyte "survival" frequently refers only to the ability of the membrane to exclude a supravital dye. Thus the reader must recall that such "viable" cells may be incapable of any relevant function. A corollary is that the most straightforward and economical experimental approach to the evaluation of a new method or technique for granulocyte storage will first address the effect of the technique on the three critical granulocyte functions listed in Table 11–1.

TESTS USED TO EVALUATE GRANULOCYTE FUNCTION

Granulocyte function studies can be divided into two broad categories: tests that provide important information regarding functions critical to the ability of the cells to perform in vivo (see Table 11–1) and tests that address the subcellular mechanisms on which the critical functions depend.[3, 55, 63, 64] The best test of the function of transfused granulocytes is in their ability to facilitate the cure of a documented infection in the host, ideally in the setting of a well-designed, well-controlled clinical trial. However, clinical trials are costly, time consuming, labor intensive, and difficult to control and may show benefit only under ideal conditions.[15, 16] It is therefore not surprising that there have been no clinical trials of granulocyte transfusion that directly address the efficacy of granulocyte storage as an experimental question.

In order to circumvent the difficulties associated with performance of clinical trials, investigators of granulocyte storage have employed a variety of surrogate techniques to ascertain the function of stored granulocytes, with the overall goal of predicting their function after transfusion. These techniques include tests of granulocyte function both in vivo and in vitro after varying periods of storage. The clinical relevance of these granulocyte functions is demonstrated by clear associations between increased susceptibility of infection and severe granulocyte function defects in patients who have congenital granulocyte disorders[3–5] or severe neutropenia.[69] Techniques used to harvest granulocytes for function testing may influence their behavior; consequently, great care must be taken to avoid artifacts in the collection of granulocytes before testing.[70, 71] Likewise, for studies of granulocyte storage, it is important for the investigator to know how similar the experimental conditions are to conditions used in practice. For example, some investigations of granulocyte storage employ extensively manipulated cells that are stored (or "cultured") in plastic tubes, sometimes at 37°C. This type of experimental design introduces artifacts that severely limit the value of the results toward the purpose of predicting the utility of storage (in plastic bags at 22°C–24°C) of granulocyte concentrates collected for clinical transfusion purposes.[72]

Circulation Kinetics

The ability of granulocytes to circulate in the blood stream is measured through isotopic labeling techniques and is reported as the percentage of recovery and the half-disappearance time, or T/2, of the transfused cells.[73] Studies that employ a strong gamma ray–emitting radionuclide, such as indium-111, may also provide information regarding the distribution of the transfused granulocytes and their migration into inflammatory loci.[74] Investigations employing isotopically labeled granulocytes for transfusion have provided extremely useful information regarding the localization of stored granulocytes and the effects of recipient alloimmunization to HLAs.[75] In view of the extraordinarily large numbers of granulocytes transfused when the donor has been treated with G-CSF, it has become possible to use the granulocyte count itself to assess the circulation of transfused granulocytes.[16] This advance should also facilitate the investigation of the kinetics of stored granulocytes.

To date, the kinetics of stored granulocytes have been studied only by isotopic methods, but granulocyte kinetics may be modified by the possible effects of the labeling process on granulocyte function. Thus a subpopulation of stored fragile granulocytes may be lost or destroyed during the labeling procedure, leaving the more normal cells for injection and analysis. The average functional integrity of the entire population of granulocytes might thus be overestimated. There is also the counterbalancing possibility that the labeling process may select out partially damaged cells.[73, 74] These general criticisms apply to nearly all studies of granulocyte function; consequently, investigators must have proper controls and must assess the extent to which their assay systems introduce artifact.

Adherence and Chemotaxis

In vitro tests of granulocyte adherence may employ artificial substrates, extracellular matrix, or cultured endothelial cells and may or may not include serum proteins.[76–78] Although adherence of granulocytes to artificial surfaces may be convenient, the use of endothelial cells to measure the adherence function of granulocytes is the preferred substrate, because endothelial cells provide a clinically relevant substrate and express adhesion molecules, such as endothelial-leukocyte adhesion molecule-1 (ELAM-1) and intercellular adhesion molecule-1 (ICAM-1).[76, 79] Granulocytes from patients with leukocyte adhesion deficiency (LAD) may not always yield the same results on artificial substrates as on endothelium.[80] Once an adhesion defect has been identified functionally, it would be appropriate to ascertain which, if any, of the known neutrophil membrane adhesion molecules is responsible for the change, through the use of flow cytometry and other techniques.[50–52]

In vitro tests of granulocyte motility and chemotaxis generally employ one of two techniques: the Boyden chamber filter-migration technique and techniques that use migration of granulocytes under an agarose gel.[81] Some investigators argue that the Boyden chamber method is more sensitive and more likely to identify clinically relevant abnormalities; the agarose technique has the advantage of allowing direct visualization of migrating cells and locomotion analysis of individual cells.[82] Some of the subcellular mechanisms that support granulocyte chemotaxis can be measured directly. Granulocyte membrane chemotaxin receptor numbers and function are measured through the use of labeled probes,[83, 84] and the process of stimulus-response coupling may be measured by a variety of techniques, including chemotaxin-induced alterations in calcium flux, cyclic nucleotide levels, and the generation of LTB_4.[59] The specific roles of some of the metabolic steps and paths proposed to be involved in stimulus-response coupling are controversial, and these steps may vary, depending on the cell function of interest.[59, 61, 85] Certain aspects of mechanical and cytoskeletal mechanisms underlying granulocyte functions can be measured by electron microscopy and biochemical assays of the state of actin within the cell.[86]

Phagocytosis and Microbial Killing

Phagocytosis may be measured by a variety of techniques, but those that employ visual analysis of particle uptake are only semiquantitative, in comparison with spectrophotometric and isotopic techniques, which have objective end points.[87] The chief subcellular mechanisms supporting phagocytic function can be assessed by measuring immunoglobulin, complement, and adhesion receptors, specific stimulus-response coupling pathways and actin-myosin function.[59, 61, 85, 86] Measurement of granulocyte microbicidal activity by classical, colony-forming unit techniques is a difficult, labor-intensive task, and numerous variations to make it simpler and more quantitative have been described.[55, 63, 64, 71, 88] A variety of microbes may be used, including gram-positive (usually *Staphylococcus aureus*), gram-negative (usually *E. coli*), and fungal (most often *Candida albicans*).

Subcellular mechanisms supporting microbial killing can be evaluated by several techniques. The specific technique employed in such tests should be tailored to the microbe of interest, on the basis of the results of microbicidal assays.[55, 71] Microbicidal activity, especially toward catalase-positive microbes,[64] depends largely on superoxide anion generation by NADPH oxidase and enzymatic conversion of superoxide into oxygen radicals. The state of mechanisms that facilitate oxygen radical–dependent killing can be easily assessed by a variety of simple quantitative techniques: For example, superoxide anion generation with cytochrome c reduction; the quantitative nitroblue tetrazolium (NBT) test; or the more accurate dihydrorhodamine 123 fluorescence assay; and quantitative assays of myeloperoxidase activity.[64] Visual assays of NBT and myeloperoxidase staining provide information on the fraction of granulocytes capable of generating superoxide or containing peroxide, but they are not quantitative. Also, the chemiluminescence assay is of limited use because what it measures is not clear and because it is only semiquantitative.[89]

In addition to oxidative microbicidal mechanisms, granulocytes have a number of nonoxidative mechanisms.[3, 63, 67] Because most of the oxygen-independent killing mechanisms employ the contents of granulocyte primary and specific granules, these mechanisms are crucially dependent on the integrity of the granules and their fusion with the phagosome at the appropriate time (referred to as *degranulation*). The overall function of degranulation is usually measured by employing a maximal nonspecific stimulus (e.g., phorbol ester) in conjunction with a marker for primary granules (e.g., β-glucuronidase or peroxidase), specific granules (e.g., lactoferrin or vitamin B_{12}–binding protein), and a marker for cell lysis (e.g., lactate dehydrogenase). Both total granulocyte content of the marker to be assessed and the extent of its discharge during granulocyte activation are measured.[3] In addition, individual microbicidal agents can be measured (e.g., cathepsin G, BPI, and defensins).[67] With use of specific probes, it is also possible to measure alteration of phagolysosomal pH during phagocytosis.[68]

Summary

The preceding description is not an all-inclusive list of the tests of granulocyte function. It is focused, however, on the chief subcellular mechanisms upon which critical granulocyte functions depend. The types of studies reviewed have been employed by investigators both to assess granulocyte function in persons suspected of having granulocyte dysfunction syndromes and to determine granulocyte function abnormalities induced by storage. Although the choice of function test to be employed depends on specific goals, several principles are constant: to access not only subcellular mechanisms but also critical granulocyte functions; to employ sufficient controls; to perform sufficient preliminary experiments; to ascertain the reliability and sensitivity of the assays used; and to determine their comparability with previously used techniques. Finally, if abnormalities of granulocyte function are identified, it is important to assess their relevance.

RELATIONSHIP BETWEEN GRANULOCYTE FUNCTION AND SUSCEPTIBILITY TO INFECTION

Circulation Kinetics

Like most other physiological functions, granulocyte-dependent microbicidal function has considerable reserve capacity. The significance of minor alterations in the number of circulating granulocytes per microliter or in granulocyte functions is questionable. The point at which a quantitative abnormality of granulocyte function is clinically relevant is not always clear. The most relevant single measure of granulocyte function is prevention of infection. In this regard, a clear concentration-dependent relationship between the number of circulating neutrophils and the likelihood of bacterial infection in patients has been reported. In a classic study, Bodey and colleagues[69] demonstrated a progressive increase in the risk of infection as the granulocyte count fell below 500×10^9 PMNs/L (Fig. 11–2). A quantitative relationship between the other critical granulocyte functions (adhesion, chemotaxis, and microbial killing) and susceptibility to infection is more difficult to ascertain. Information regarding this issue must be based on studies of patients who have granulocyte function defects. A variety of granulocyte function defects have been reported, and many of these are clearly associated with increased susceptibility to infection.[3–5]

Adhesion and Chemotaxis

Considering the reported clinical disorders associated with abnormalities of granulocyte chemotaxis, it is worthwhile to remember that both in vitro and in vivo assays of granulocyte motility demonstrate wide variability in the chemotactic response. Substantial variability in the chemotaxis of granulocytes from normal persons is an inherent, consistent weakness of all techniques used to evaluate granulocyte migration.[81] In most patients who have been reported to have increased susceptibility to infection in association with a chemotactic defect, extremely low levels of granulocyte chemotaxis were observed.[82, 88] Indeed, it is largely on the basis of the severity (and repeatability) of the granulocyte defect in specific patients that the chemotactic abnormalities have

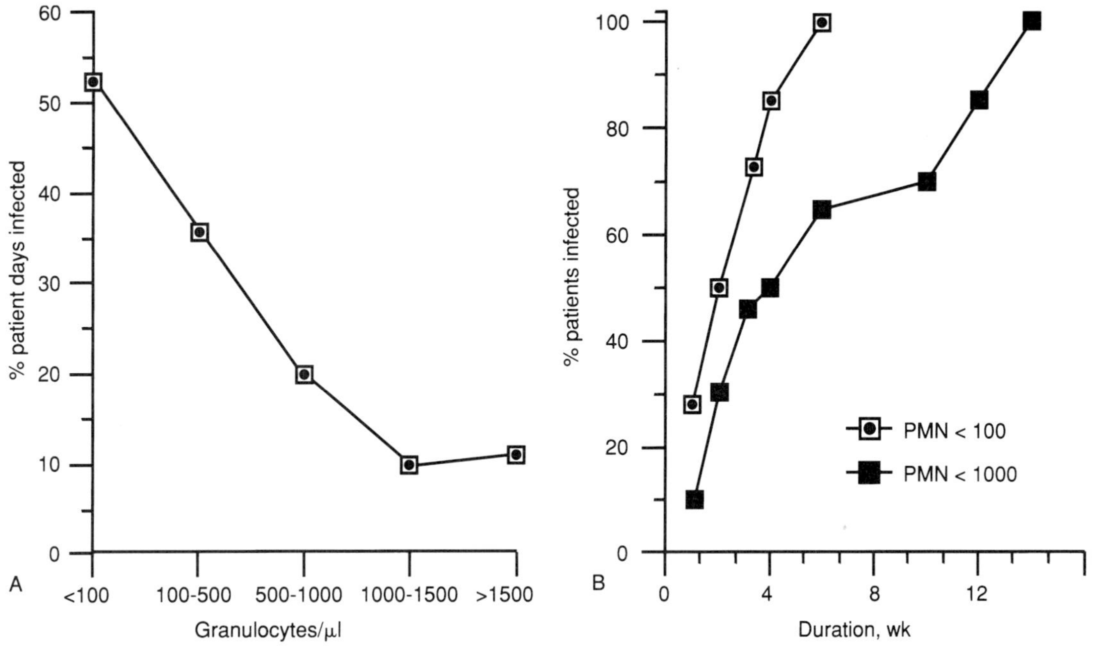

Figure 11–2. *A,* Relationship between granulocyte count and risk of infection: the granulocyte count in cells per microliter (or cells × 10^9/L) versus the percentage of patient days spent with the documented infection. *B,* Relationship between the duration of granulocytopenia in weeks and the percentage of patients infected. PMN < 100 refers to an absolute granulocyte count of less than 100 per microliter (less than 100 × 10^9/L) and PMN < 1000 refers to an absolute granulocyte count of less than 1000 per microliter (less than 100 × 10^9/L). (Modified from Bodey GP, Buckley M, Sathe YS, et al. Quantitative relationships between circulating leukocytes and infection in patients with acute leukemia. Ann Intern Med 1966; 64:328.)

been judged to be clinically relevant. In other reports describing patients who had increased susceptibility to infection in association with (and presumably because of) mild defects in granulocyte chemotaxis, the actual role of the granulocyte defect is more difficult to assess.[3–5] Clinical studies do not provide a clear guideline as to the degree of in vitro abnormality in chemotaxis that is required before increased susceptibility to infection is manifested. Moreover, the degree of abnormality in granulocyte function that would render a person susceptible to infection would be expected to vary among people, inasmuch as a multitude of host factors besides chemotaxis play a role in infection susceptibility. However, some general conclusions may be drawn from the available literature.

Several reports have described patients with congenital leukocyte adhesion deficiency (LAD).[63, 76–79, 90] LAD-1 occurs with a frequency of about 1 per 1,000,000 persons and results from a mutation in the gene on chromosome 21q22.3 that encodes the common β_2 leukocyte integrin subunit (CD18).[3] Another defect in leukocyte adhesion that has been reported in a few patients, LAD-2, is associated with normal integrins, and its genetic basis is unknown.[3] Patients with LAD-1 suffer from recurrent infections, and their granulocytes have complete or near-complete deficiency of membrane adherence receptors of the integrin class (CD18/11a; CD18/11b; CD18/11c). In addition, granulocytes from persons with LAD-1 fail to upregulate (increase the expression of) adherence receptors upon chemotaxin binding and have abnormal chemotaxis, but they mediate normal bacterial killing.[90] Obligate heterozygotes for LAD-1 have normal granulocyte function. One report classified patients who had symptomatic LAD-1 into two groups on the basis of clinical severity[91]: those who had severe, symptomatic disease had absence of skin window migration of granulocytes and an in vitro chemotactic response that was 25% to 35% of normal (according to a modified Boyden chamber assay), whereas patients who had only moderate symptoms had delayed and diminished skin window migration and an in vitro chemotactic response that was 30% to 70% that of healthy controls.[91]

These findings suggest not only that the skin window technique measures a clinically relevant granulocyte function but also that moderate to marked alterations in the in vitro chemotactic response, as measured by the modified Boyden chamber assay, may also be clinically relevant. However, it should be noted that LAD-1 is also associated with a diminution in phagocytosis of opsonized particles; hence abnormalities in this function, along with chemotaxis, may also contribute to infection susceptibility. The conclusion that partial diminution in the in vitro chemotactic response, as well as total absence of the response, may be clinically relevant is supported by experiments in animals showing that diminution in the early exudation of granulocytes after an infectious challenge significantly influences the eventual outcome of the infection.[92]

Microbial Killing

The best-studied group of patients who have recurrent infections and defective bacterial killing by granulocytes have X-linked severe chronic granulomatous disease

(CGD). CGD occurs with a frequency of about 5 per 1,000,000 persons and consists of three autosomal recessive variants and one X-linked variant. Each variant is associated with a defect in one of the subunits of the phagocyte NADPH oxidase that is responsible for generation of superoxide anion. Granulocytes from such patients share common laboratory features, including almost no capacity to generate superoxide anion, in association with severely defective killing of catalase-positive bacteria (less than 10% of the value in healthy controls).[64, 89] On the other hand, a wide spectrum of intermediate defects in NADPH oxidase–dependent function, ranging from 10% to 90% of normal, are observed in obligate carriers who are asymptomatic.[89] Female carriers who, owing to nonrandom inactivation of X chromosomes, have less than 10% of the normal oxidative burst function, may be only mildly symptomatic. In these people, in vitro assays of superoxide generation and microbicidal function are poor predictors of host susceptibility to infection unless the results are severely abnormal.[89, 93] These findings also suggest that, in contrast to chemotaxis, granulocytes have a much greater reserve capacity for superoxide anion generation and microbicidal function. This conclusion is supported by the fact that patients with myeloperoxidase deficiency and whose granulocytes therefore cannot generate relevant toxic oxygen radicals beyond superoxide anion have significant abnormalities in the rate of microbial killing as measured in vitro but are nevertheless essentially asymptomatic.[64, 94] Together, these studies indicate that mild or moderate, isolated deficiencies of respiratory burst activity and microbicidal function are unlikely to be clinically relevant.

Summary

Investigations of granulocyte storage have been hampered for the following reasons: tests of granulocyte function show a wide range of variability; even in normal persons, there is no known simple, consistent, quantitative relationship between the degree of abnormality of many granulocyte functions and clinical susceptibility to infection; and at least some granulocyte functions appear to have a great deal of reserve capacity (e.g., respiratory burst and microbicidal activity). On the basis of the information available, however, it seems reasonable to conclude that storage-induced alterations in granulocytes that result in more than 50% reduction in chemotactic function of the cells are likely to be clinically relevant. The relevance of defects in respiratory burst activity and microbicidal function is more difficult to ascertain. It is unclear to what extent statistically significant but intermediate-level abnormalities detected in tests of these functions of stored granulocytes (e.g., 50% of control levels) are clinically relevant, because granulocyte microbicidal function may be reduced by 50% to 75% in asymptomatic people.[89, 93] Moreover, it would appear that isolated defects of respiratory burst activity associated with more than 50% of the normal enzyme activity are unlikely to be relevant. This conclusion must be balanced against the fact that stored granulocytes may have multiple functional abnormalities. Thus a given level of abnormality in the relatively small dose of granulocyte concentrate that is to be given to a patient may be more consequential than a similar degree of abnormality in a noninfected patient who has normal numbers of granulocytes.[7]

LIQUID STORAGE OF GRANULOCYTES

Effect of Donor Treatment and Collection Technique on Granulocyte Function

Early investigations of granulocyte transfusion therapy employed two competing techniques for granulocyte harvesting from normal donors: filtration leukapheresis (FL) and centrifugation leukapheresis (CL).

FL was a technically simple procedure with the ability to collect large numbers of granulocytes, but it was associated with occasional donor and recipient reactions and poor granulocyte function.[95, 96] Granulocytes collected by FL had morphological abnormalities, defective microbicidal activity, increased adherence, and poor in vivo recovery and survival, and they migrated poorly into inflamed loci.[97, 98] Three times as many FL-collected PMNs as CL-collected granulocytes were required to protect septicemic dogs.[99] American Association of Blood Banks (AABB) standards no longer refer to FL as a method for granulocyte collection.[103a]

Collection of granulocytes by CL exploits differences in cell density between granulocytes and other blood cells.[100] In order to enhance granulocyte yields, most pheresis programs premedicate donors with steroids and employ red cell–sedimenting agents, such as hydroxyethyl starch.[101] The physical forces involved in CL are considered gentle in comparison with the shear forces required to damage granulocytes.[102, 103] In contrast to PMNs collected by FL, granulocytes harvested by CL have normal microbicidal activity and chemotaxis and normal circulation kinetics.[103] For these reasons, FL has been supplanted by CL in the harvesting of granulocytes for transfusion. AABB standards call for at least 75% of the products to contain at least 1×10^{10} granulocytes.[103a] The use of injections of G-CSF to increase the level of circulating granulocytes in normal donors increases the yield of PMNs collected by leukapheresis by three- to five-fold in comparison with steroids alone and has also improved the survival, function, and possibly, the storage characteristics of the harvested PMN.[16]

General Comments on Granulocyte Storage

Granulocytes share several physiological attributes with red cells and platelets that influence their storage shelf life. All are end-stage cells (cell fragments in the case of platelets), with no capacity for self-renewal and very little for protein synthesis. Their capacity for repair of structural elements or enzymes that may be damaged during collection or storage is limited. Like platelets, but not red cells, granulocytes also have a very short in vivo life span (approximately 6 hours), which diminishes to minutes after activation.[34] The activation of granulocytes is to be avoided during storage because it results in degranulation, energy expenditure, and increased adherence.[47, 54] Activated granulocytes also have sharply diminished in vivo survival in association with sequestration in the reticuloendothelial system.[104] Unlike platelets, which are sufficiently small to pass through capillaries without deformation, granulocytes must deform as they squeeze through capillary networks during every circulation; consequently, even partial or limited degrees of activation are likely to result in a diminished life span. Studies indicate that certain granulocyte "priming" agents (e.g., G-CSF or interferon-γ, neither of which directly causes cell activation but does enhance activation caused by other stimuli), may protect granulocyte functions during ex vivo storage.[16]

Another feature unique to granulocytes is the fact that activation also leads to generation or release of their entire microbicidal armamentarium.[3, 61, 63, 64] This may result not only in autotoxicity but also in damage to nearby cells, further limiting the number of functional granulocytes during storage.[105] Important goals in granulocyte storage are to limit granulocyte metabolism (as with storage of red cells), to prevent activation, and to preserve the vital biochemical pathways and structural elements necessary for successful in vivo function. Finally, unlike red cells or platelets, which fulfill their purpose in a relatively passive way, granulocytes must respond to a variety of biological signals, integrate a complex series of biochemical mechanisms, and then undergo a sequential series of functional changes in order to carry out their physiological role. Hence, a defect in any one of several different complex systems can render granulocytes nonfunctional.

Storage-Induced Alterations in Granulocytes

Granulocyte concentrate is best stored in plastic bags with autologous plasma and citrate anticoagulant, unagitated, and at room temperature. Nonetheless, significant impairment in granulocyte function occurs within 24 hours from the time of collection, and storage beyond 24 hours is accompanied by increasingly severe alterations (Table 11–4).[103] The earliest critical granulocyte function to deteriorate is chemotaxis. In vitro experiments indicate that chemotaxis and random migration are abnormal in granulocytes from some units stored for 24 hours and that chemotaxis is even more impaired after 48 hours of storage.[106–109] These findings are supported by the results of in vivo experiments with labeled granulocytes in humans, which show that normal post-transfusion granulocyte recovery, circulation, and migration into inflammatory loci are maintained for at least 8 hours after granulocyte storage at room temperature; however, after 24 hours of storage, there are decreases in both post-transfusion recovery and migration into inflammatory loci.[110] Microbial killing by granulocytes is normal after 24 hours of storage, but thereafter diminishes.[106–109, 111] The number of granulocytes present in granulocyte concentrates is relatively stable during storage, decreasing by less than 15% after 48 hours.[106–109, 111]

The clinical relevance of the moderate impairment in chemotaxis after 24 hours of storage is uncertain because there has been no direct study in humans or animals of the efficacy of stored granulocytes after 24-hour storage. The degree of abnormality found in granulocytes from some units,[107] however, is similar to that noted in patients with granulocyte dysfunction syndromes and increased susceptibility to infection. The more severe decrease in chemotaxis after 48-hour storage is very likely to be clinically relevant. The extent of abnormality in granulocyte microbicidal activity after 48-hour storage would be of little clinical relevance in a person with a normal granulocyte count; it is more likely to be important in a patient who is being supported by granulocyte transfusion.[7] Granulocytes that are collected from donors stimulated with G-CSF may be somewhat resistant to the changes in these functions, but this has not been the subject of systematic investigation.

Experimental Modification of Storage Conditions

In view of the apparently short shelf life of granulocyte concentrates, several investigators have made attempts to improve the function of these concentrates after storage. Most investigators have used surrogate, in vitro models to examine the effects of storage on granulocyte function.[109] Attempts to improve the storage of granulocytes have focused on methods to augment their ability to migrate. Measurement of granulocyte migration in vivo cannot be used to perform extensive tests on stored granulocytes; consequently, tests of chemotactic function in vitro are commonly used as surrogate tests for in vivo localiza-

Table 11–4. Effect of Room Temperature Storage on Granulocyte Function

Function	Duration of Storage*		Reference(s)
	24 Hours	48 Hours	
In Vivo			
Recovery (%)	50	—	110
Survival (T/2)	100	—	110
In Vitro			
Recovery (%)	88–99	86–96	106, 109, 134
Chemotaxis level (%)	80–99	45–86	106, 107, 134
Microbial killing level (%)	94–100	71–97	106, 107, 109

T/2, half-disappearance time.
*Percentage of control (fresh) granulocytes.

tion.[109] The validity of chemotaxis as a surrogate test is based on the observations that (1) chemotaxis is the most labile of granulocyte functions measured in vitro after storage[103] and (2) the in vivo survival of stored granulocytes appears to become abnormal after a shorter duration of storage than that required to result in abnormal in vitro tests of granulocyte chemotaxis. Thus any abnormality in chemotactic function in vitro is very likely to be associated with diminished circulation kinetics and limited granulocyte efficacy.[110]

Anticoagulant/Preservative

The standard anticoagulant and preservative solutions (e.g., citrate, citrate-phosphate-dextrose, citrate-phosphate-dextrose-adenine) appear to be interchangeable with regard to maintenance of chemotaxis and other granulocyte functions after 24 hours of storage, but storage of granulocytes in heparin preserves chemotaxis less than does storage in citrate anticoagulants.[112, 113] There is an extracellular protein requirement for the liquid preservation of granulocytes, because granulocytes stored in the absence of protein have a marked chemotaxis defect.[108] The protein in the storage medium need not be plasma, inasmuch as chemotaxis in granulocytes stored in synthetic media supplemented with albumin is equal to that in cells stored in autologous plasma.[108] Supplementation of the citrate preservative with additional buffer may be beneficial if the granulocyte count in the unit exceeds 5×10^{10}/L, which occurs commonly with the use of some CL techniques.[114] In this setting, there is a marked decrease in the pH of the suspending plasma after 24 hours, in association with an equally marked decrease in granulocyte chemotaxis. Addition of extra buffer to the granulocyte concentrate has been reported to prevent the decreases in both pH and chemotaxis.[115] A specific study of the effect of pH on granulocyte preservation also identified an optimal range of 7.0 to 7.5 for maintenance of chemotaxis.[98]

Temperature

The optimal temperature for granulocyte storage has been studied extensively. Storage temperature has practical implications, because some blood centers employ units of whole blood stored at 4°C for the subsequent production of "buffy coat" preparations to be given to septic, neutropenic neonates.[116] In addition, storage of blood at 4°C has the theoretical advantage of slowing down metabolic processes and thereby maintaining cell function. An animal study of in vivo granulocyte post-transfusion kinetics and localization demonstrated near-normal recovery and survival of granulocytes stored at either 4°C or room temperature for up to 24 hours. The study suggested that after 24 hours of storage, granulocytes preserved at 4°C were superior with regard to both post-transfusion recovery and migration into an inflammatory locus.[117] A subsequent study in humans that employed only 4°C storage showed marked decreases in the recovery (30% to 66% of control levels), survival (36% to 50% of control levels), and skin chamber migration (25% of control levels) of granulocytes stored for 24 hours.[118] However, in the only study of in vivo granulocyte post-transfusion kinetics and localization in humans in which storage temperatures were compared, granulocyte storage at 4°C for only 8 hours was associated with significantly diminished post-infusion recovery (33% of control levels) and migration into skin chambers (17% of control levels).[110] In contrast, the recovery and skin chamber migration (93% and 50% of control levels, respectively) of granulocytes stored at room temperature for 8 hours were significantly better than those stored at 4°C and not significantly different from the corresponding values for unstored granulocytes.[110] In this study, after 24 hours there was still an advantage to room temperature storage, but the differences were less marked.

The effect of storage temperature on granulocyte function in vitro has also been studied. Because chemotaxis is the most labile function during storage, several studies have focused on it. In two comparative studies, granulocytes stored at 4°C for 24 hours had diminished in vitro chemotaxis in comparison with those stored at room temperature, and the differences were accentuated after 48 hours.[106, 107] In another report, even brief (1.5-hour) exposure to 4°C storage impaired granulocyte migration.[70] These reports were supported by studies using only 4°C storage, which showed a significant decrease in chemotactic response after 9 hours.[116] There were no significant differences between granulocytes stored at the two temperatures with regard to changes in cell number, phagocytosis, and generation of superoxide anion.[106, 107] However, one study reported an advantage for granulocytes stored at 4°C with regard to bacterial killing.[107] The pathogenesis of the adverse effects of 4°C storage on chemotaxis are unclear, but alterations in the granulocyte cytoskeleton and in adherence properties have been reported.[119] Finally, storage of granulocytes at 37°C appears to accelerate deterioration in their function.[106]

Agitation

Agitation of granulocyte concentrates by end-over-end rotation has been reported to result in extensive hemolysis of contaminating red cells, with diminution in chemotaxis and microbicidal activity of granulocytes.[106] A study employing horizontal agitation also confirmed hemolysis but reported no change in microbicidal activity and a striking improvement in the maintenance of chemotaxis.[120] To date, there has been no direct comparison of the two agitation methods by the same investigator. In studies comparing types of storage containers, the plasticizer used in some bags was reported to adversely affect granulocyte function.[121, 122] Prestorage irradiation of granulocyte units is apparently not harmful to post-storage granulocyte functions.[123–125]

Growth Factors and Other Conditions

Storage of PMNs in the presence of interferon-γ G-CSF, and granulocyte-macrophage colony-stimulating factor (GM-CSF) has been reported to delay some of the storage-associated alterations in a variety of PMN functions, including membrane integrity, adherence, chemotaxis, superoxide generation, and microbial killing. Collection of granulocytes from G-CSF–treated donors has also been reported to result in improved ex vivo adhesion and oxidative metabolism.[126–132] However, because all the aforementioned ex vivo studies were performed on granulocytes that had been extensively manipulated (e.g., density gradient separation, hypotonic lysis of red cells, multiple washing steps) and cultured in plastic containers at either 4°C[126] or 37°C[127–132] (not 22°C to 24°C, as is current practice), it is not clear to what extent the results of these studies will apply to granulocytes harvested by apheresis techniques and stored at room temperature in a closed bag system. For example, one study in which granulocytes were isolated and stored as noted reported severe defects in chemotaxis after 20 hours (20% of control)[131] that were far in excess of those reported for granulocytes harvested and stored under blood bank conditions (70% to 80% of control amounts),[106–109] and the defects were only partially prevented by incorporation of G-CSF and interferon in the culture medium. In contrast, a study carried out under conditions similar to that employed by blood banks failed to confirm an effect of GM-CSF on preservation of granulocyte function during storage.[133] Thus although it is not clear that these studies will translate into prolonged storage for granulocytes, this area represents the most provocative and promising work on the preservation of granulocytes for transfusion.

The presence of red cells in the granulocyte concentrate has no apparent adverse effect.[134] A variety of agents have been investigated as potential preservatives of granulocyte function. Addition of adenine to the storage medium appears to offer no advantages in preservation of granulocyte function.[113] As noted previously, supplemental buffer may prevent rapid loss of chemotaxis function in granulocyte concentrates with high cell counts.[115] A systematic investigation of several potential granulocyte preservatives suggested that a number of agents, including glucose, ATP, ascorbic acid, vitamin E, NADPH, amikacin, and ampicillin, all improved maintenance of one or more granulocyte functions.[135] Kannan and associates[136] suggested improved survival of murine neutrophils cultured in the presence of nerve growth factor, but granulocyte "viability" was assessed only by trypan blue dye exclusion.[136] It has also been reported that a modified low-molecular-weight gelatin may improve the "viability" and bactericidal capacity of granulocytes stored at 4°C for 1 week, but granulocyte recovery was only 63%, and no intermediate time points or alternative storage temperatures were reported.[137]

Summary and Current Recommendations

Current AABB standards call for granulocyte concentrate to be stored at room temperature and transfused as soon as practicable but within 24 hours from the time of collection.[103a] The functional efficacy of granulocyte concentrates is best reflected by their ability to combat infection in vivo. No studies employing this standard have been reported for stored granulocytes, but studies employing the next best standard—the ability of stored granulocytes to migrate to an infected site—have suggested that granulocyte concentrates can be stored in autologous citrate-anticoagulated plasma, unagitated, at room temperature for up to 8 hours. If the collection bag contains granulocytes in a concentration in excess of 5×10^{10}/L, it appears wise to transfuse the cells as soon as possible or to add plasma or buffer. It is not clear whether granulocytes from donors treated with G-CSF will have improved ex vivo storage characteristics, but care must be taken to ensure that the PMN concentrations in leukapheresis bags from G-CSF–treated donors are not so high that their metabolism causes excessive accumulation of hydrogen ion.[115]

PATHOGENESIS OF STORAGE-INDUCED GRANULOCYTE DYSFUNCTION

Because empirical attempts to improve granulocyte storage have been largely unsuccessful, investigators have endeavored to elucidate the pathogenesis of storage-induced granulocyte dysfunction. The rationale for these studies has generally been that a better understanding of the storage lesion would suggest specific strategies for improving the storage life of granulocytes.

Circulation Kinetics

No studies have directly addressed the pathogenesis of the abnormal kinetics of transfused granulocytes. The alteration in adherence properties of granulocytes stored at 4°C to 6°C may be responsible for the rapid pulmonary sequestration noted in cells stored at this temperature.[117, 118] It is not clear whether the increase in adherence properties of such cells results from an alteration or from an increase in expression of granulocyte adherence molecules.

Chemotaxis

A variety of abnormalities may be responsible for the chemotactic defect in stored granulocytes (see Table 11–1). Defects in mechanical translocation appear to be unlikely candidates, because granulocytes that have severe chemotactic defects after storage have intact phagocytic mechanisms.[106–109] As noted earlier, growth factors that prevent apoptosis have been reported to improve somewhat upon the chemotactic function of granulocytes stored at 37°C.[131] Other investigation has focused on granulocyte chemotaxin receptor function, energy metabolism, adherence properties, and stimulus-response coupling.

Receptors

Storage diminishes the chemotactic ability of the entire population of granulocytes, as opposed to a small minority of rapidly migrating cells.[107, 132] The fractional subpopulation of cells that migrate slowly is also increased with storage.[138] Both the speed of random migration and the maximal velocity of chemotactic migration are decreased.[107] In addition, the percentage of cells that do not orient in a chemotactic gradient enlarges after storage.[138] The finding that the concentration of an experimentally used chemotaxin (F-Met-Leu-Phe, or FMLP) required to stimulate half-maximal migration (ED50) is increased after storage[139] suggests an abnormality in the number or function of granulocyte FMLP receptors. A decrease in the mean FMLP receptor affinity has been reported after storage.[140] This decrease is apparently caused by an increase in the number of low-affinity FMLP receptors.[83, 140] A defect in FMLP receptor upregulation after exposure to FMLP was also reported.[140] These defects in granulocyte chemotaxin receptor function would be expected to result in an increase in the concentration of FMLP required to stimulate ED50, as has been reported.[139, 140] The effect of granulocyte storage on other chemotaxin receptors (e.g., C5a and LTB_4) has not been characterized.

Energy Metabolism, Cell Concentration, and pH

The chemotactic defect in stored granulocytes does not result exclusively from alterations in FMLP receptor affinity. Stored granulocytes also have diminished random migration (which is presumably independent of chemotaxin receptors), decreased maximal migration,[107] and diminished migration toward chemotaxins other than FMLP.[107, 108] These findings suggest a global abnormality in the ability of stored granulocytes to translocate.

Energy is required for chemotaxis,[141] and a relationship between the diminished ATP and defective chemotaxis in stored granulocytes has been reported in cells stored at 4°C.[142] In contrast to granulocytes stored at 4°C, granulocytes stored at 22°C to 24°C at a cell concentration less than 5 × 10^{10}/L maintained ATP both at rest and during exposure to chemotaxins. Defective maintenance of ATP levels was noted only during a phagocytic challenge.[114] Because granulocytes obtain ATP from glycolysis of ambient glucose or intracellular glycogen,[143] an abnormality in either glycolysis or glycogenolysis was suggested. Subsequent studies showed a normal glycolytic pathway and normal glycogen content in stored granulocytes[144] but a mild abnormality in glycogenolysis.[145]

Increases in both intracellular pyruvate and intracellular lactate during room-temperature storage of granulocytes have also been reported,[146] but the mechanism for these increases is unclear. These abnormalities are not considered severe enough, by themselves, to account for the chemotactic defect in stored granulocytes.[145] In the same studies, strong inverse correlations were noted between the concentration of granulocytes in the stored units and intracellular granulocyte ATP concentration, extracellular glucose concentrations, resting granulocyte glucose use, and suspending medium pH after storage.[114] A role for platelets in glucose use during granulocyte storage was also noted.[135, 147] The excessive depletion of ATP in granulocyte concentrates with high cell numbers may be prevented, the glucose use increased, and the pH of the medium maintained by addition of buffer but not by supplemental glucose.[114] An additional study showed that maintenance of the suspending medium pH (with additional buffer) in granulocyte concentrates with high cell numbers was also associated with maintenance of the chemotactic function of stored granulocytes.[115] These studies led to the recommendation that storage of granulocyte concentrates with cell numbers greater than 5 × 10^{10}/L should not be attempted in the absence of additional buffer.[115]

The precise role of ATP depletion in the chemotaxis impairment of stored granulocytes was not directly addressed by the studies just described. Depletion of ATP to levels far below those observed in stored granulocytes was not associated with a decrease in the chemotactic function of the cells.[148] It was concluded that granulocytes either require only a very low concentration of intracellular ATP to maintain chemotactic function or employ an alternative source of energy for chemotaxis.[148] This study indicated that decrements in ATP are unlikely to be related to chemotactic dysfunction after storage, but supported the conclusion that alterations in the pH of the suspending medium for stored granulocytes may be causally related to chemotactic dysfunction.[115, 148]

Stimulus-Response Coupling

Generation of LTB_4 is considered the chief intracellular (post–receptor-binding) mediator of chemotactic signal amplification.[59] One study suggested such an intracellular abnormality in the ability of stored granulocytes to translate chemotactic signals into effective migration, because stored granulocytes had diminished ability to generate LTB_4 after exposure to a chemotaxin.[149] This defect resulted from more than one abnormality in the enzymatic path responsible for LTB_4 generation, inasmuch as generation of other leukotrienes was also affected.[149] Because supplementation of the stored cells with exogenous LTB_4 during chemotaxis did not improve their function,[149] the overall role of the abnormality in LTB_4 generation remains uncertain.

Adherence

It has been reported that granulocytes stored at 22°C to 24°C develop increased adherence to both endothelial monolayers, to extracellular matrix, and to artificial surfaces.[119] One study reported accentuated increases in endothelial cell adhesion in granulocytes stored at 6°C in bags.[150] In one report in which granulocytes were extensively manipulated, cells stored in dishes at 37°C had decreased baseline and agonist-stimulated adherence to plastic.[128] In contrast, the ability of granulocytes to increase adherence in response to chemotaxins was unaltered by storage at room temperature in a closed-bag system.[150] The mechanism responsible for increased adherence, especially with storage at 4°C, is unclear, but altered expression of granulocyte adherence receptors seems a likely possibility.[79, 80] It is therefore somewhat paradoxical that one study in which isolated granulocytes were stored at 4°C in plastic dishes reported no change in the number of CD11b (Mac-1) or CD11c leukocyte integrin adhesion molecules, but a decrease in CD11a (LFA-1).[126] In contrast, another study in which granulocytes were stored at room temperature in a closed-bag system reported a significant increase in the CD11b

(Mac-1) integrin adherence molecule.[151] The latter study is most consistent with previous adherence data, but unfortunately, neither of the studies on adherence molecules included concomitant measurement of granulocyte adhesion to relevant substrates, such as endothelial cells. Agents that inhibit apoptosis have been reported to be associated with either maintenance or somewhat increased expression of CD11b,[126, 128] and in one study they maintained adherence function.[128] As with changes in adherence, the chemotaxin-induced aggregation of granulocytes was increased in cells stored at 6°C.[150] Interestingly, fresh granulocytes and those stored at 22°C to 24°C had very little spontaneous aggregation, but cells stored at 6°C had a marked tendency to aggregate spontaneously upon rewarming in physiological buffer.[150] The altered relationship between spontaneous and chemotaxin-induced aggregation in granulocytes stored at 6°C, which results in a decreased aggregation index after storage,[150] is presumably responsible for a previously reported decrease in chemotaxin-induced granulocyte aggregation with storage.[116]

Summary

Chemotaxis has received the most investigative attention of any granulocyte function during storage, because it is the most labile function of granulocytes. Although apoptosis appears to be a major candidate mechanism for defective function of granulocytes stored at 37°C, there appears to be no single unifying mechanism responsible for the altered chemotactic function of granulocytes stored at 22°C to 24°C, because a variety of abnormalities has been identified in the structure and function of these cells. Although none of the reported abnormalities may be individually sufficient to account for the extent of chemotactic dysfunction, the combined effects of all of the abnormalities may have adverse effects. As a result of these investigations, it may be concluded that chemotaxis is best preserved in granulocytes stored at room temperature in autologous plasma. If granulocytes are present in excess of 5×10^{10}/L, which is now routinely possible through the pretreatment of donors with G-CSF, either the cells should not be stored or buffer should be added. Questions still remain as to the effect of agitation on and the best storage bag for post-storage granulocyte function.[120, 121]

Microbial Killing

Microbial killing and microbicidal mechanisms in granulocytes, including phagocytosis, degranulation, proteolytic activity, lysosomal content, and generation of oxygen radicals, appear to be intact after 24 hours of storage either in refrigeration or at room temperature[106–109, 152]; consequently, these functions have received far less study than chemotaxis. By 48 hours after collection, some investigators noted up to a 30% decrease in microbial killing.[107–109] The significance of this finding, as an isolated event, is questionable in view of the substantial reserve capacity for microbial killing. As previously noted, extensively manipulated granulocytes stored at 37°C for less than 24 hours have markedly decreased function, in association with apoptosis, and this can be partially prevented by agents that inhibit apoptosis.[128, 130]

CRYOPRESERVATION OF GRANULOCYTES

Cryopreservation of red cells has overcome the problems associated with the long-term preservation of these blood elements; consequently, cryopreservation appears to be a rational approach to the storage of granulocytes. Unfortunately, the investigation of cryopreservation of granulocytes has been largely disappointing. Critical granulocyte functions either have not been studied or were severely decreased after cryopreservation and subsequent thawing.[153] A major problem has been the tendency of cryopreserved granulocytes to aggregate after thawing, possibly as a result of loss of surface constituents.[154] Although one study demonstrated the feasibility of cryopreserving anucleate granulocyte cytoplasts, the motility of the thawed cytoplasts was not evaluated quantitatively, and their microbicidal activity was diminished.[155] Cryopreservation of granulocytes thus remains a subject of laboratory investigation only.

MOLECULAR MECHANISMS OF GRANULOCYTE DYSFUNCTION DURING STORAGE

Circulating granulocytes are short-lived cells, with a vascular half-life of 6 hours and a tissue phase of 2 to 4 days.[34] Studies have suggested that granulocytes, like other end-stage cells, undergo a process of apoptosis, or programmed cell death, during storage, and this may be responsible for some or all of the structural and functional changes that occur during storage. In one report, granulocyte aging at 37°C in vitro and in vivo was associated with typical morphological changes indicative of apoptosis and with the recognition and ingestion of aging cells by macrophages.[156] This hypothesis is supported by reports that hematopoietic growth factors both inhibit apoptosis and prolong effective storage of granulocytes stored at 37°C.[128–130] It seems reasonable that inhibition of apoptosis may also be responsible for the prolonged in vivo circulation kinetics of PMNs harvested from donors treated with G-CSF.[157, 158] However, apoptosis may not explain the shortened in vivo survival or functional abnormalities of morphologically intact granulocytes that are stored at 22°C to 24°C. Thus although apoptosis may partially explain diminished ex vivo granulocyte function after storage, several additional possibilities appear also worthy of consideration.

Protein degradation is a constant event in living cells[159] and is thought to play a role in limiting preservation of other cell types.[160] Granulocytes have only limited capacity to regenerate proteins, so spontaneous protein degradation may play a key role in the limited shelf life of these cells. For example, degradation of glycolytic enzymes would explain altered ATP generation in these cells; likewise, an alteration in plasma membrane proteins might be responsible for increased adherence. Abnormalities in other proteins offer potential explanations for essentially all of the functional derangements that accompany storage. In addition to spontaneous protein degradation, proteolysis may play a role in granulocyte aging, because granulocytes contain a formidable array of proteolytic enzymes capable of degrading most proteins.[3] To date, there is only indirect evidence of proteolysis in granulocyte dysfunction with storage. Cytosolic fractions from disrupted granulocytes impair the chemotaxis[152] and chemotaxin receptor binding of intact cells,[161] but inclusion of a proteolysis inhibitor with granulocytes during storage only minimally prevents the decrease in chemotaxis that accompanied storage.[152] The overall role of protein degradation in storage-induced granulocyte dysfunction is thus unclear.

Various additional mechanisms have been proposed to explain the deterioration in granulocyte function that is associated with their storage.[162, 163] Granulocyte activation, resulting in the generation of the full oxidative and nonoxidative potential for toxicity, is one possible mechanism. Two reports assessed the spontaneous generation of oxygen radicals and spontaneous degranulation by granulocytes during storage.[144, 152] No evidence of a significant degree of activation was found in either study, but the recent finding of increased adhesiveness after granulocyte storage[151] is consistent with activation.[47] More sensitive techniques for ascertaining activation are now available[104] but have not been studied in stored granulocytes. At cold temperatures, there may be irreversible disruption of microtubules[119] and increased cell water as a result of inhibition of ion pumps.[115, 164] Loss of glycolytic enzymes appears to play a minor role in storage-induced dysfunction.[144] Alterations in hydrogen ion concentration that accompany storage of granulocytes in high cell numbers may irreversibly impair cell function independently of their effect on ATP synthesis, but the mechanism of this effect is unclear.[115, 148] Currently, there is no unifying theory sufficient to encompass all of the structural and functional alterations in granulocytes that accompany their storage.

FUTURE DIRECTIONS

The current understanding of the storage of granulocytes for transfusion leaves several key questions unanswered. From a practical standpoint, perhaps the most compelling question is the relationship between storage-induced alterations in granulocyte function and the clinical efficacy of the cells as measured by their ability to combat infection in vivo. This question seems unlikely to be addressed in humans: an animal model of neutropenia and infection is required. The information derived from such a study would serve as a basis for investigating the validity of surrogate tests, such as in vivo localization and in vitro chemotaxis, as predictors of the in vivo efficacy of stored human granulocytes. Such studies would also provide quantitative guidelines necessary for the evaluation of the relevance of alterations in surrogate functions that are induced by storage or are present in congenital or acquired granulocyte dysfunction syndromes. An additional, still unanswered question that can be studied in humans is the relationship between storage-induced alterations in granulocyte localization in in vivo and in vitro chemotaxis studies.

The effect of donor treatment with G-CSF on granulocyte function during storage is another compelling and readily answerable question, in view of the increasing use of this cytokine to collect the cells in large numbers. The provocative research on G-CSF and other agents, such as interferon-γ, that inhibit apoptosis should be performed on granulocytes collected and stored under blood bank conditions, because it seems possible that such agents might permit more prolonged storage or shipment of granulocytes.

A variety of additional practical questions relating to granulocyte storage remain to be studied, including the effect of short periods of cold exposure (e.g., less than 6 hours) followed by room-temperature storage on granulocyte function. The influence of storage containers and agitation may not be as clear-cut as once thought, and systematic investigation of the requirements of the storage medium requires additional investigation. Finally, although several studies have identified apoptosis as a major pathobiological event in granulocytes stored at 37°C, additional investigation is necessary to determine the extent to which apoptosis accounts for granulocyte dysfunction stored in cold at 22°C to 24°C. To researchers who have dedicated years to the investigation of these fragile cells, the possibility of prolonging the ex vivo (and in vivo) survival of granulocytes through the use of G-CSF or other relatively nontoxic agents is indeed an exciting prospect.

REFERENCES

1. Roberts SR, Kracke SS. Agranulocytosis. Ann Intern Med 1931; 5:40.
2. Hersh EM, Bodey GP, Nies BA, Freireich EJ. Causes of death in acute leukemia. JAMA 1965; 193:99.
3. Malech HL, Nauseef WM. Primary inherited defects in neutrophil function: etiology and treatment. Semin Hematol 1997; 34:279.
4. Matzner Y. Acquired neutrophil dysfunction and diseases with an inflammatory component. Semin Hematol 1997; 34:291.
5. Yang KD, Hill HR. Neutrophil function disorders: pathophysiology, prevention, and therapy. J Pediatr 1991; 119:343.
6. Herzig GP, Graw RG. Granulocyte transfusions for bacterial infections. Prog Hematol 1975; 9:207.
7. Schiffer CA. Granulocyte transfusion therapy. Cancer Treat Rep 1983; 67:113.
8. Graw RG Jr, Herzig G, Perry S, Henderson ES. Normal granulocyte transfusion therapy. Treatment of septicemia due to gram-negative bacteria. N Engl J Med 1972; 287:367.
9. Higby DJ, Yates JW, Henderson ES, Holland JF. Filtration leukapheresis for granulocyte transfusion therapy. Clinical and laboratory studies. N Engl J Med 1975; 292:761.
10. Fortuny E, Bloomfield CD, Hadlock DC, et al. Granulocyte transfusion: a controlled study in patients with acute nonlymphocytic leukemia. Transfusion 1975; 15:548.
11. Herzig RH, Herzig GP, Graw RG Jr, et al. Successful granulocyte transfusion therapy for gram-negative septicemia. N Engl J Med 1977; 296:701.
12. Alavi JB, Rott RK, Djerassi I, et al. A randomized clinical trial of granulocyte transfusions for infection in acute leukemia. N Engl J Med 1977; 296:706.
13. Vogler WR, Winton EF. A controlled study of the efficacy of granulocyte transfusions in patients with neutropenia. Am J Med 1977; 63:548.
14. Winston DJ, Ho WG, Gale RP. Therapeutic granulocyte transfusions for documented infections. A controlled trial in ninety-five

infectious granulocytopenic episodes. Ann Intern Med 1982; 97:509.
15. Strauss RG. Therapeutic granulocyte transfusions in 1993. Blood 1993; 81:1675.
16. Dale DC, Liles WC, Price TH. Renewed interest in granulocyte transfusion therapy. Br J Haematol 1997; 98:497.
17. Schiffer CA. Supportive care: issues in the use of blood products and treatment of infection. Semin Oncol 1987; 14:454.
18. Klein HG, Strauss RG. Granulocyte transfusion therapy. Semin Hematol 1996; 33:359.
19. Love LJ, Schimpff SC, Schiffer CA, et al. Improved prognosis for granulocytopenic patients with gram-negative bacteremia. Am J Med 1980; 68:643.
20. Lazarus HM. Granulocyte transfusions: have we learned anything? J Lab Clin Med 1990; 115:271.
21. Klingeman HG. Use of granulocyte-macrophage colony stimulating factor (GM-CSF) to support intensive chemotherapy. Prog Clin Biol Res 1990; 354B:211.
22. Gutterman J, Vadhan-Raj S, Logothetis C, et al. Effects of granulocyte-macrophage colony-stimulating factor in iatrogenic myelosuppression, bone marrow failure, and regulation of host defense. Semin Hematol 1990; 27:15.
23. Reuf C, Coleman DL. Granulocyte-macrophage colony-stimulating factor: pleiotropic cytokine with potential clinical usefulness. Rev Infect Dis 1990; 12:41.
24. Winston DJ, Ho WG, Howell CL, et al. Cytomegalovirus infection associated with leukocyte transfusions. Ann Intern Med 1980; 93:671.
25. Dutcher JP, Kendall J, Norris D, et al: Granulocyte transfusion therapy and amphotericin B: adverse reactions? Am J Hematol 1989; 31:102.
26. Herzig RH. The negative aspects of granulocyte transfusions. Cancer Invest 1989; 7:589.
27. Cairo MS, Worcester CC, Rucker RW, et al. Randomized trial of granulocyte transfusions versus intravenous immune globulin therapy for neutropenia and sepsis. J Pediatr 1992; 120:281.
28. Strauss RG. Current status of granulocyte transfusions to treat neonatal sepsis. J Clin Apheresis 1989; 5:25.
29. Berger M. Complement deficiency and neutrophil dysfunction as risk factors for bacterial infection in newborns and the role of granulocyte transfusion in therapy. Rev Infect Dis 1990; 12:S401.
30. Hill HR. Granulocyte transfusions in neonates. Pediatr Rev 1991; 12(10):298.
31. Rosiek A, Konecka G, Daszynski J, Furman J. Studies of the possibility of preservation of leukocyte concentrates. Acta Haematol Pol 1989; 20:42.
32. Lane TA. Granulocyte storage. Transfus Med Rev 1990; 4:23.
33. Verstraeten L, Marchand-Arvier M, Schooneman F, Vigneron C. Storage of granulocytes. Ann Biol Clin (Paris) 1991; 49:161.
34. Cronkhite EP, Fliedner TM. Granulocytopoiesis. N Engl J Med 1964; 270:1347.
35. Cronkhite EP. Analytical review of structure and regulation of hemopoiesis. Blood Cells 1988; 14:313.
36. Schmid-Schonbein GW, Engler RL. Perspectives of leukocyte activation in the microcirculation. Biorheology 1990; 27:859.
37. Cotran RS. New roles for the endothelium in inflammation and immunity. Am J Pathol 1987; 129:407.
38. Yong K, Khwaja A. Leucocyte cellular adhesion molecules. Blood Rev 1990; 4:211.
39. Rothlein R, Dustin ML, Marlin SD, Springer TA. A human intercellular adhesion molecule (ICAM-1) distinct from LFA-1. J Immunol 1986; 137:1270.
40. Springer TA. Adhesion receptors of the immune system. Nature 1990; 346:425.
41. Bevilacqua MP, Stengelin S, Gimbrone MA, Seed B. Endothelial leukocyte adhesion molecule-1: an inducible receptor for neutrophils related to complement regulatory proteins and lectins. Science 1989; 243:1160.
42. McEver RP. GMP-140: a receptor for neutrophils and monocytes on activated platelets and endothelium. J Cellular Biochem 1991; 45:156.
43. Gahmberg CG, Nortamo P, Kantor C, et al. The pivotal role of the Leu-CAM and ICAM molecules in human leukocyte adhesion. Cell Diff Dev 1990; 32:239.
44. Munro JM, Pober JS, Cotran RS. Recruitment of neutrophils in the local endotoxin response: association with de novo endothelial expression of endothelial leukocyte adhesion molecule-1. Lab Invest 1991; 64:295.
45. Kuijpers TW, Hakkert BC, Hoogerwerf M, et al. Role of endothelial leukocyte adhesion molecule-1 and platelet-activating factor in neutrophil adherence to IL-1–prestimulated endothelial cells. Endothelial leukocyte adhesion molecule-1–mediated CD18 activation. J Immunol 1991; 147:1369.
46. Luscinskas FW, Cybulsky MI, Kiely JM, et al. Cytokine-activated human endothelial monolayers support enhanced neutrophil transmigration via a mechanism involving both endothelial-leukocyte adhesion molecule-1 and intercellular adhesion molecule-1. J Immunol 1991; 146:1617.
47. Smith CW, Hollers JC, Patrick RA, et al. Motility and adhesiveness in human neutrophils: effects of chemotactic factors. J Clin Invest 1979; 64:221.
48. Kapp A, Zeck-Kapp G. Activation of the oxidative metabolism in human polymorphonuclear neutrophilic granulocytes: the role of immuno-modulating cytokines. J Invest Dermatol 1990; 95:94S.
49. Sklar LA, Omann GM. Kinetics and amplification in neutrophil activation and adaptation. Semin Cell Biol 1990; 1:115.
50. Springer TS. Traffic signals for lymphocyte recirculation and leukocyte emigration: the multistep paradigm. Cell 1994; 76:301.
51. Brown E. Neutrophil adhesion and the therapy of inflammation. Semin Hematol 1997; 34:319.
52. Celi A, Lorenzet R, Furie B, Furie B. Platelet–leukocyte–endothelial cell interaction on the blood vessel. Semin Hematol 1997; 34:327.
53. Smith WB, Gamble JR, Clark-Lewis I, Vadas MA. Interleukin-8 induces neutrophil transendothelial migration. Immunology 1991; 72:65.
54. Baggaiolini M, Kernen P, Deranleau DA, Dewald B. Control of motility, exocytosis and the respiratory burst in human neutrophils. Biochem Soc Trans 1991; 19:55.
55. Virella G. Diagnostic evaluation of phagocytic function. Immunol Serol 1990; 50:323.
56. Wilkinson PC. How do leucocytes perceive chemical gradients? FEMS Microbiol Immunol 1990; 2(5–6):303.
57. Kunkel SL, Standiford T, Kasahara K, Strieter RM. Interleukin-8 (IL-8): the major neutrophil chemotactic factor in the lung. Exp Lung Res 1991; 17:17.
58. Cassimeris L, Zigmond SH. Chemoattractant stimulation of polymorphonuclear leucocyte locomotion. Semin Cell Biol 1990; 1:125.
59. Snyderman R, Jhing RJ. Phagocytic cells: stimulus-response coupling mechanisms. *In* Gallin JI, Goldstein IM, Snyderman R (eds.): Inflammation: Basic Principles and Clinical Correlates. New York: Raven Press, 1988, p 309.
60. Krause KH, Campbell KP, Welsh MJ, Lew DP. The calcium signal and neutrophil activation. Clin Biochem 1990; 23:159.
61. Lew DP. Receptor signalling and intracellular calcium in neutrophil activation. Eur J Clin Invest 1989; 19:338.
62. Goldman G, Welbourn R, Valeri CR, et al. Thromboxane A_2 induces leukotriene B_4 synthesis that in turn mediates neutrophil diapedesis via CD18 activation. Microvasc Res 1991; 41:367.
63. Curnutte JT. Phagocytic defects I: abnormalities outside of the respiratory burst. Hematol Oncol Clin North Am 1988; 2:185.
64. Lehrer RI, Ganz T, Selsted ME, et al. Neutrophils and host defense. Ann Intern Med 1988; 109:127.
65. Aida Y, Pabst MJ. Neutrophil responses to lipopolysaccharide. Effect of adherence on triggering and priming of the respiratory burst. J Immunol 1991; 146:1271.
66. Smith RM, Curnutte JT. Molecular basis of chronic granulomatous disease. Blood 1991; 77:673.
67. Ganz T, Weiss J. Antimicrobial peptides of phagocytes and epithelia. Semin Hematol 1997; 34:343.
68. Cech P, Lehrer RI. Phagolysosomal pH of human neutrophils. Blood 1984; 63:88.
69. Bodey GP, Buckley M, Sathe YS, et al. Quantitative relationships between circulating leukocytes and infection in patients with acute leukemia. Ann Intern Med 1966; 64:328.
70. Glasser L, Fiederlein RL. The effect of various cell separation procedures on assays of neutrophil function. A critical appraisal. Am J Clin Pathol 1990; 93:662.
71. Haynes AP, Fletcher J. Neutrophil function tests. Baillières Clin Haematol 1990; 3:871.

72. Glasser L. Effect of storage on normal neutrophils collected by discontinuous-flow centrifugation leukapheresis. Blood 1977; 50:1145.
73. Peters AM: Granulocyte kinetics and methods of evaluating cell performance. Nucl Med Comm 1988; 9:687.
74. Peters AM, Saverymuttu SH. The value of indium-labelled leucocytes in clinical practice. Blood Rev 1987; 1:65.
75. Dutcher JP, Schiffer CA, Johnston GS, et al. Alloimmunization prevents the migration of transfused indium-111–labeled granulocytes to sites of infection. Blood 1983; 62:354.
76. Springer TS, Anderson DC. Leukocyte Adhesion Molecules: Structure, Function, and Regulation. New York: Springer-Verlag, 1988.
77. Crowley CA, Curnutte JT, Rosin RE, et al. An inherited abnormality of neutrophil adhesion: its genetic transmission and its association with a missing protein. N Engl J Med 1980; 302:1163.
78. Patarroyo M. Leukocyte adhesion in host defense and tissue injury. Clin Immunol Immunopathol 1991; 60:333.
79. Springer TA, Dustin ML, Kishimoto TK, et al. The lymphocyte function-associated LFA-1, CD2, and LFA-3 molecules: cell adhesion receptors of the immune system. Annu Rev Immunol 1987; 5:223.
80. Harlan JM, Killen PD, Senecal FM, et al. The role of neutrophil membrane glycoprotein GP-150 in neutrophil adherence to endothelium in vitro. Blood 1985; 66:167.
81. Gallin JI, Quie PG. Leukocyte Chemotaxis: Methods, Physiology, and Clinical Implications. New York: Raven Press, 1977.
82. Brown CC, Gallin JI. Chemotactic disorders. Hematol Oncol Clin North Am 1988; 2:61.
83. Snyderman R. Regulatory mechanisms of a chemoattractant receptor on leukocytes. Fed Proc 1984; 43:2743.
84. Chenoweth DE, Hugli TE. Demonstration of specific C5a receptor on intact human polymorphonuclear leukocytes. Proc Natl Acad Sci U S A 1978; 75:3943.
85. Brown GE, Reed EB, Lanser ME. Neutrophil CR3 expression and specific granule exocytosis are controlled by different signal transduction pathways. J Immunol 1991; 147:965.
86. Omann GM, Allen RA, Bokoch GM, et al. Signal transduction and cytoskeletal activation in the neutrophil. Physiol Rev 1987; 67:285.
87. Stossel TP, Mason RJ, Hartwig J, et al. Quantitative studies of phagocytosis by polymorphonuclear leukocytes: use of emulsions to measure the initial rate of phagocytosis. J Clin Invest 1972; 51:615.
88. Axtell RA. Evaluation of the patient with a possible phagocytic disorder. Hematol Oncol Clin North Am 1988; 2:1.
89. Curnutte JT, Babior BM. Chronic granulomatous disease. Adv Hum Genet 1987; 16:229.
90. Todd RF, Freyer DR. The CD11/CD18 leukocyte glycoprotein deficiency. Hematol Oncol Clin North Am 1988; 2:13.
91. Anderson DC, Schmalstieg FC, Finegold MJ, et al. The severe and moderate phenotypes of heritable Mac-1, LFA-1 deficiency: their quantitative definition and relation to leukocyte dysfunction and clinical features. J Infect Dis 1985; 152:668.
92. Miles AA, Miles EM, Burke J. The value and duration of defence reactions of the skin to the primary lodgement of bacteria. Br J Exp Pathol 1957; 38:79.
93. Curnutte JT, Berkow RL, Roberts RL, et al. Chronic granulomatous disease due to a defect in the cytosolic factor required for nicotinamide adenine dinucleotide phosphate oxidase activation. J Clin Invest 1988; 81:606.
94. Nauseef WM. Myeloperoxidase deficiency. Hematol Oncol Clin North Am 1988; 2:135.
95. Djerassi I, Kim JS, Suvansri U, et al. Continuous flow filtration leukapheresis. Transfusion 1972; 12:75.
96. Goldman JM, Heim L, Wright DG. Filtration leukaphresis: review and reevaluation. Exp Hematol 1979; 7:1.
97. Glasser L. Functional considerations of granulocyte concentrates used for clinical transfusions. Transfusion 1979; 19:1.
98. McCullough J. Liquid preservation of granulocytes. Transfusion 1980; 20:129.
99. Appelbaum FR, Bowles CA, Makuch RW, Deisseroth AB. Granulocyte transfusion therapy of experimental *Pseudomonas* septicemia: study of cell dose and collection technique. Blood 1978; 52:323.
100. Freireich EJ, Judson G, Levin RH. Separation and collection of leukocytes. Cancer Res 1965; 25:1516.
101. Strauss RG, Hester JP, Vogler WR, et al. A multicenter trial to document the efficacy and safety of a rapidly excreted analog of hydroxyethyl starch for leukapheresis with a note on steroid stimulation of granulocyte donors. Transfusion 1986; 26:258.
102. Dewitz TS, Hung TC, Martin RR, McIntire LV. Mechanical trauma in leukocytes. J Lab Clin Med 1977; 90:728.
103. Glasser L, Lane TA, McCullough J, Price TH. Neutrophil concentrates: functional considerations, storage, and quality control. J Clin Apheresis 1983; 1:179.
103a. Klein HG (ed.). Standards for Blood Banks and Transfusion Services, 18th ed. Bethesda, MD: American Association of Blood Banks, 1997.
104. Araout MA, Hakim RM, Todd RF, et al. Increased expression of an adhesion-promoting surface glycoprotein in the granulocytopenia of hemodialysis. N Engl J Med 1985; 312:457.
105. Jackson JH, Cochrane CG. Leukocyte-induced tissue injury. Hematol Oncol Clin North Am 1988; 2:317.
106. McCullough J, Weiblen BJ, Peterson PK, Quie PG. Effect of temperature on granulocyte preservation. Blood 1978; 52:301.
107. Lane TA, Windle BE. Granulocyte concentrate preservation: effect of temperature. Blood 1979; 54:216.
108. Glasser L, Fiederlein RL, Huestis DW. Liquid preservation of human neutrophils stored in synthetic media at 22°C: Controlled observations on storage variables. Blood 1985; 66:267.
109. Lane TA, Windle BE. A model for the study of granulocyte concentrate preservation. Transfusion 1980; 20:559.
110. McCullough J, Weiblen BJ, Fine D. Effects of storage of granulocytes on their fate in vivo. Transfusion 1983; 23:20.
111. McCullough J, Yunis EJ, Benson SJ, Quie PG. Effect of blood bank storage on leukocyte function. Lancet 1969; 2:1333.
112. McCullough J, Weiblen BJ, Quie PG. Chemotactic activity of human granulocytes preserved in various anticoagulants. J Lab Clin Med 1974; 84:902.
113. Strauss RG, Crouch J. Preservation of neutrophils in CPD-adenine. Transfusion 1981; 21:354.
114. Lane TA, Lamkin GE. Defective energy metabolism in stored granulocytes. Transfusion 1982; 22:368.
115. Lane TA, Lamkin GE. Hydrogen ion maintenance improves the chemotaxis of stored granulocytes. Transfusion 1984; 24:231.
116. Eastlund T, Charbonneau T, Britten A. Changes in neutrophil aggregation and chemotaxis response during 18-hour cold storage. Transfusion 1984; 24:513.
117. Price TH, Dale DC. Neutrophil preservation: the effect of short term storage on in vivo kinetics. J Clin Invest 1977; 59:475.
118. Price TH, Dale DC. Blood kinetics and in vivo chemotaxis of transfused neutrophils: effect of collection method, donor corticosteroid treatment, and short term storage. Blood 1979; 54:977.
119. Palm SL, Furcht LT, McCullough J. Effects of temperature and duration of storage on granulocyte adhesion, spreading and ultrastructure. Lab Invest 1981; 45:82.
120. Miyamoto M, Sasakawa S. Studies on granulocyte preservation: III. Effect of agitation on granulocyte concentrates. Transfusion 1987; 27:165.
121. Miyamoto M, Sasakawa S: Effects of plasticizers and plastic bags on granulocyte function during storage. Vox Sang 1987; 53:19.
122. Miyamoto M, Sasakawa S. Effects of autoclave sterilization on the physical properties of storage bags and granulocyte function. Vox Sang 1988; 54:74.
123. Patrone F, Dallegre F, Brema F, Sacchetti C. In vitro function of chronic myelocytic leukemia granulocytes. Effects of irradiation and storage. Tumori 1979; 65:27.
124. Wolber RA, Duque RE, Robinson JP, Oberman HA. Oxidative product formation in irradiated neutrophils: a flow cytometric analysis. Transfusion 1987; 27:167.
125. Eastlund DT, Charbonneau TT. Superoxide generation and cytotactic response of irradiated neutrophils. Transfusion 1988; 28:368.
126. Murea S, Fruehauf S, Zeller WJ, Haas R. Granulocytes harvested following G-CSF–enhanced leukocyte recovery retain their functional capacity during in vitro culture for 72 hours. J Hematother 1996; 5:351.
127. Begley CG, Lopez AF, Nicola NA, et al. Purified colony-stimulating factors enhance the survival of human neutrophils and eosinophils in vitro: a rapid and sensitive microassay for colony-stimulating factors. Blood 1986; 68:162.
128. Klebanoff SJ, Olszowski S, Van Voorhis WC, et al. Effects of gamma-interferon on human neutrophils: protection from deterioration on storage. Blood 1992; 80(1):225.

129. Colotta F, Re F, Polentarutti N, et al: Modulation of granulocyte survival and programmed cell death by cytokines and bacterial products. Blood 1992; 80(8):2012.
130. Brach MA, de Vos S, Gruss HJ, Herrmann F. Prolongation of survival of human polymorphonuclear neutrophils by granulocyte-macrophage colony-stimulating factor is caused by inhibition of programmed cell death. Blood 1992; 80:2920.
131. Rex JH, Bhalla SC, Cohen DM, et al. Protection of human polymorphonuclear leukocyte function from the deleterious effects of isolation, irradiation, and storage by interferon-gamma and granulocyte colony-stimulating factor. Transfusion 1995; 35(7):605.
132. Cohen DM, Bhalla SC, Anaissie EJ, et al. Effects of in vitro and in vivo cytokine treatment, leucapheresis and irradiation on the function of human neutrophils: implications for white blood cell transfusion therapy. Clin Lab Haematol 1997; 19:39.
133. Garley D, Clay M, McCullough J. The effects of recombinant granulocyte-macrophage colony stimulating factor (rGM-CSF) on 48-hour granulocyte storage [Abstract]. Transfusion 1987; 27:537.
134. Glasser L, Fiederlein RL. The effect of platelets and red cells on granulocytes stored at 22°C. Transfusion 1984; 24:310.
135. Verstraeten L, Marchand-Arvier M, Schooneman F, Vigneron C. Experimental study of a model for granulocyte storage. Ann Biol Clin 1991; 49:155.
136. Kannan Y, Ushio H, Koyama H, et al. 2.5S nerve growth factor enhances survival, phagocytosis, and superoxide production of murine neutrophils. Blood 1991; 77:1320.
137. Babior BM, Berkman E. Granulocyte storage. Lancet 1990; 335:50.
138. Burton JL, Bank HL, Law P. Kinematic analysis of chemotaxis of fresh and stored neutrophils. Ann Clin Lab Sci 1987; 17:398.
139. Lane TA, Windle BE. Decreased affinity for a chemotactic factor in stored granulocytes. Transfusion 1981; 21:450.
140. Lane TA, Lamkin GE. Chemotaxin receptor cycling in fresh and stored granulocytes. Transfusion 1988; 28:362.
141. Caruthers BM. Leukocyte motility II. Can J Physiol Pharmacol 1967; 45:269.
142. McCullough J, Weiblen BJ. The relationship of granulocyte ATP to chemotactic response during storage. Transfusion 1979; 19:764.
143. Klebanoff SJ, Clark RA. The Neutrophil: Function and Clinical Disorders. New York: North-Holland, 1978.
144. Lane TA, Beutler E, West C, et al: Glycolytic enzymes of stored granulocytes. Transfusion 1984; 24:153.
145. Lane TA, Lamkin GE: Glycogen metabolism of stored granulocytes. Transfusion 1985; 25:246.
146. Paul JL, Abbouyi AE, Roch-Arveiller M, et al. Effects of storage on the pyruvate-lactate system and random migration of human granulocytes. Vox Sang 1987; 52:24.
147. Glasser L, Fiederlein RL, Huestis DW. Granulocyte concentrates: glucose concentrations and glucose utilization during storage at 22°C. Transfusion 1985; 25:68.
148. Lane TA, Lamkin GE. A reassessment of the energy requirements for neutrophil migration: adenosine triphosphate depletion enhances chemotaxis. Blood 1984; 64:986.
149. Lane TA, Lamkin GE. Stimulus-response coupling in fresh and stored granulocytes. Transfusion 1988; 28:243.
150. Lane TA, Lamkin GE. Adherence of fresh and stored granulocytes to endothelial cells: effect of storage temperature. Transfusion 1988; 28:237.
151. Wikman A, Lundahl J, Fernvik E, Shanwell A. Altered expression of adhesion molecules L-selectin and Mac-1 on granulocytes during storage. Transfusion 1994; 34:167.
152. Lane TA, Lamkin GE. Effect of storage on degranulation by human neutrophils. Transfusion 1985; 25:155.
153. Frim J, Mazur P. Approaches to the cryopreservation of human granulocytes. Cryobiology 1980; 17:282.
154. Hill RS, Norris-Jones R, Still B, et al. Surface charge and hydrophobic properties of fresh and cryopreserved blood phagocytes as determined by partition in two-phase aqueous polymer systems. Am J Hematol 1986; 21:249.
155. Malawista SE, VanBlaricom G, Breitenstein MG. Cryopreservable neutrophil surrogates. J Clin Invest 1989; 83:728.
156. Savill JS, Wyllie AH, Henson JE, et al. Macrophage phagocytosis of aging neutrophils in inflammation: programmed cell death in the neutrophil leads to its recognition by macrophages. J Clin Invest 1989; 83:865.
157. Bensinger WI, Price TH, Dale DC, et al. The effects of daily recombinant human granulocyte colony-stimulating-factor administration on normal granulocyte donors undergoing leukapheresis. Blood 1993; 81:1883.
158. Caspar CB, Seger RA, Burger J, Gmur J. Effective stimulation of donors for granulocyte transfusions with recombinant methionyl granulocyte colony-stimulating factor. Blood 1993; 81:2866.
159. Pontremoli S, Mellone E. Extralysosomal protein degradation. Annu Rev Biochem 1986; 55:455.
160. Snyder EL, Horne WC, Napychank P, et al. Calcium-dependent proteolysis of actin during storage of platelet concentrates. Blood 1989; 73:1380.
161. Lane TA, Lamkin GE, Windle BE. Phagocytosis-induced modulation of human neutrophil chemotaxis receptors. Blood 1981; 58:228.
162. Lane T. The effect of storage on granulocyte function. Adv Biosci 1987; 66:97.
163. Glasser L. The molecular pathobiology of stored neutrophils. Plasma Ther Transfus Technol 1988; 9:295.
164. Contreras TJ, Hunt SM, Lionetti FJ, et al. Preservation of human granulocytes. III. Liquid preservation studied by electronic sizing. Transfusion 1978; 18:46.

CHAPTER 12

Granulocyte Immunology

Mary E. Clay
David F. Stroncek

Granulocyte immunology had its beginning in the late 19th century, when Elie Metchnikoff introduced his *Phagocytic Theory of Immunity* to Russian colleagues at the Odessa Congress in 1883.[1] However, Metchnikoff could only speculate at that time on how phagocytic cells participate in the processes of immunity and inflammation and provide defense against infection. Since then, much has been learned about granulopoiesis and the morphology and cellular physiology of granulocytes, as well as about the process of granulocyte stimulation by foreign materials and the consequences of those interactions (i.e., chemotaxis, phagocytosis, degranulation, and intracellular killing of bacteria). In addition, researchers have identified granulocyte membrane and cytoplasmic antigens that are both granulocyte-restricted and granulocyte-nonrestricted in their tissue and cell line distribution. Furthermore, alloantibodies and autoantibodies to these granulocyte antigens have been shown to play a key role in the pathophysiological processes of several clinical disorders, including autoimmune neutropenia, alloimmune neonatal neutropenia, febrile and pulmonary transfusion reactions, Wegener's granulomatosis, and leukocyte adhesion molecule deficiencies.

GRANULOCYTE ANTIGEN SYSTEMS

Clinically significant granulocyte antigens were originally defined from human allosera through studies of alloimmune neonatal neutropenia (ANN), autoimmune neutropenia, and transfusion reactions. Monoclonal antibodies that define granulocyte antigen epitopes associated with disease states have since been described.

Granulocyte-Specific Antigens Defined by Human Allosera

Lalezari and associates[2] first reported the existence of granulocyte-specific antigens that are found only on neutrophils, eosinophils, and basophils, in 1960. Characterization of antigens on basophils and eosinophils is difficult; therefore, most antigens on neutrophils have not been tested to determine whether they occur only on neutrophils or on all granulocytes.

Nomenclature

Lalezari and associates proposed the nomenclature now used for the majority of these antigens: N, for neutrophil-specific antigen; a capital letter designating the locus of the gene controlling the production of the antigen; and a number designating a specific allele at that locus (e.g., NA1, NA2). A standardized system of nomenclature of neutrophil-specific antigens, such as has been developed for human leukocyte antigens (HLA)[3] and platelet antigens,[4] is needed.

Antigen Specificities

To date, antigens that define genes at eight different loci (Table 12–1) have been reported. Allelic antigens have been described at three of these loci. These antigens and their gene frequencies have shown ethnic differences in American, Dutch, Japanese, and French population studies.[5–10] Although very little is known about the expression of granulocyte-specific antigens during myelopoiesis, there is evidence to suggest that they are absent on primitive myeloid precursor cells,[11] that their expression correlates with granulocyte differentiation and maturation,[12, 13] and that they are fully expressed at birth (in full-term infants).[14]

NA

NA1 was the first granulocyte-specific antigen described in 1960 by Lalezari and associates.[2] It was defined by an antibody from the serum of a woman who gave birth to an infant with transient ANN. Lalezari and Radel[15] subsequently found an antigen that appeared to be antithetical to NA1. Population studies supported the concept that NA2 was produced by allelic genes at the NA locus. The NA antigens are truly "neutrophil-specific," inasmuch as they occur on neutrophils but not on eosinophils or basophils.[2, 16] The NA antigen system has been located on the crystallizable fragment (Fc) γ receptor IIIb (FcγRIIIb)[17, 18] and has been the subject of extensive studies in biochemical and molecular biology. The Fc receptors on granulocytes are summarized in Table 12–2. FcγRIIIb is expressed on all segmented neutrophils, about half of neutrophilic metamyelocytes, and about 10% of neutrophilic myelocytes.[19]

NA Biochemistry. Granulocyte-specific antigens NA1 and NA2 are located on the granulocyte FcγRIIIb.[17, 18] The molecular weight of granulocyte FcγRIIIb has been found to be variable, and the differences in molecular weight are associated with the NA

Table 12–1. Granulocyte Antigen Identified by Human Alloantibodies: Antigen and Gene Frequencies in Four Populations*

		Antigen Frequency (%)				Gene Frequency			
Locus	**Antigen**	**American[5, 6]**	**Dutch[7, 8]**	**Japanese[9]**	**French[10]**	**American[5, 6]**	**Dutch[7, 8]**	**Japanese[9]**	**French[10]**
NA	NA1	46	54	88	55	0.37	0.32	0.65	0.32
	NA2	88	93	51	88	0.63	0.68	0.30	0.65
	NA null				*nd*				0.03
NB	NB1	97	92	88	87	0.83	0.72	0.66	
	NB2	32	31			0.17	0.17		
NC	NC1	91	96	70		0.72	0.80	0.46	
ND	ND1		98				0.88		
NE	NE1		23				0.12		
5	5a		33				0.18		
	5b		97				0.82		
9	9a	58	63			0.35	0.39		
MART	MART	99				0.91			

*Superscript numbers in column headings indicate chapter references.
nd, not determined.

antigen phenotype.[17, 18] FcγRIIIb has a molecular weight of 50 to 60 kD on NA1-positive granulocytes, 58 to 80 kD on NA2-positive granulocytes, and 50 to 80 kD on heterozygous cells. Granulocyte FcγRIIIb has been found to be a glycoprotein. Although carbohydrate side chains can be attached to proteins through O-linkages or N-linkages, granulocyte FcγRIIIb has only N-linked carbohydrate side chains. Much of the difference in molecular weight between the NA1 phenotype and the NA2 phenotype is attributable to the amount of carbohydrate present on each molecule. When N-linked carbohydrate chains are removed enzymatically from NA1 FcγRIIIb, the apparent molecular weight of the protein portion of the molecule is 29 kD. After removal of the N-linked carbohydrates from NA2 FcγRIIIb, the molecular weight of the remaining protein is 33 kD. FcγRIIIb from granulocytes that express NA1 and NA2 contains both the 29-kD and 33-kD proteins.

Although many blood cell membrane glycoproteins have both extracellular transmembrane and intracellular domains, granulocyte FcγRIIIb does not. It belongs to the glycosyl phosphatidylinositol (GPI) group of glycoproteins,[18] which are attached to plasma membranes through a lipid anchor. The C-terminus of these glycoproteins is typically attached covalently through a glycan to a phosphatidylinositol molecule, and the 1,2-diacylglycerol moiety of the phosphatidylinositol molecule is embedded in the lipid bilayer of the plasma membrane.[20] The GPI linkage allows the anchored glycoprotein to be highly mobile.[20] GPI-linked glycoproteins can be enzymatically cleaved from cells through the use of phosphatidylinositol-specific phospholipase C. Some GPI-linked glycoproteins are released when cells are stimulated. Granulocyte FcγRIIIb antigen is rapidly released from plasma membranes when granulocytes are stimulated with the chemotaxin F-Met-Leu-Phe (FMLP).[21] Soluble FcγRIIIb and NA1 and NA2 antigens have been found in plasma.[22] FcγRIIIb released from granulocytes has been found to be the source of the soluble glycoproteins.[22]

NA Molecular Biology. The gene encoding granulocyte FcγRIIIb is located on chromosome 1. The sequence of the genes encoding both the NA1 and NA2 FcγRIIIb molecules has been mapped.[23, 24] Both proteins contain 233 amino acids, and the protein sequences of the two molecules differ at only four amino acids (Table 12–3).[23–26] However, NA2 FcγRIIIb has six potential N-linked glycosylation sites, and NA1 FcγRIIIb has only four.[23] Interestingly, monoclonal antibody CLB gran 11, which is specific for NA1 antigen, recognizes an epitope specified by amino acids Val 176 and Ser 203. Because amino acids

Table 12–2. Crystallizable Fragment (Fc) Receptors on Human Granulocytes

Types	Ligand	Affinity	Molecular Weight (kD × 10^{-3})	Sites per Cell (× 10^{-3})	Expression
FcγRI	Monomeric IgG	High	72	Monocytes: 20	Monocytes, granulocytes*
FcγRII	Complexed IgG	Low	40	Granulocytes: 31 Monocytes: 36 B lymphocytes: 38 Platelets: 1.2	Granulocytes, monocytes, platelets, B lymphocytes, some T lymphocytes, some endothelial cells, and epithelial cells
FcγRIII	Complexed IgG	Low	50–80	Granulocytes: 100–200	Granulocytes, monocytes, large granular lymphocytes, natural killer lymphocytes, T lymphocytes
FcαR	IgA		50–70		Granulocytes

Adapted from Lalezari P. Leukocyte antigens and antibodies. *In* Hoffman R, Benz EJ, Shettil SJ, et al (eds): Hematology: Basic Principles and Practice. New York: Churchill Livingstone, 1991, pp 1566–1572.
*Inducible by interferon-γ.
IgG, immunoglobulin G; IgA, immunoglobulin A.

Table 12–3. Comparison of the Amino Acid Sequences of Neutrophils NA1 and NA2 FcγRIIIb and Natural Killer Cell FcγRIIIa

Amino Acid Number	FcγRIIIb		FcγRIIIa: Natural Killer Cell
	Neutrophil NA1	Neutrophil NA2	
Allele-Specific Differences			
36	Arg	Ser	Arg
65	Asn	Ser*	Ser*
82	Asp	Asn*	Asp
106	Val	Ile	Ile
Cell Type–Specific Differences			
147	Asp	Asp	Gly
158	His	His	Tyr
176	Val	Val	Phe
203	233	233	254
Total Number of Amino Acids	233	233	254

Data from references 23 to 26.
*Creates additional *N*-glycosylation sites at Asn63 and Asn85.
FcγRIII, crystallizable fragment γ receptor III.

Val 176 and Ser 203 are the same on NA1 FcγRIIIb and NA2 FcγRIIIb, it has been hypothesized that the amino acid changes at amino acids 30, 65, 82, 106, 122, and 151 associated with NA2 may result in a masking of the NA1 epitope at amino acids Val 176 and Ser 203.[23]

Differences in granulocyte NA phenotypes can be determined by restriction fragment length polymorphisms (RFLP).[23] When DNA from peripheral blood mononuclear cells was digested with restriction enzyme Taq 1 and analyzed by DNA hybridization with an *FcγRIIIB* probe, a 6.6-kilobase fragment was detected on cells obtained from patients whose granulocytes expressed NA1. This 6.6-kilobase fragment was absent from DNA obtained from persons who were homozygous for NA2. NA1 and NA2 forms of *FcγRIIIB* can also be distinguished through the use of sequence specific primers and restriction enzymes.[27, 28]

FcγRIII is also expressed on natural killer lymphocytes, but its structure is different from that of granulocyte FcγRIIIb, and it is denoted as FcγRIIIa. NA antigens are not expressed by natural killer cells. Furthermore, FcγRIIIa is not GPI-anchored.[23] The gene encoding FcγRIIIa has also been identified. The major difference between the granulocyte and natural killer cell genes is that the natural killer cell gene, *FcγRIIIA*, encodes 21 additional C-terminal amino acids.[23] The termination codon, which is TGA in the granulocyte gene, *FcγRIIIB*, is CGA (arginine) in the natural killer gene. There are few other amino acid differences between the natural killer FcγRIIIa and the granulocyte FcγRIIIb protein (see Table 12–3).[23]

The NA polymorphisms of FcγRIIIb may affect granulocyte function slightly. For example, NA2-positive granulocytes have been found to have slightly decreased phagocytosis of opsonized red cells in comparison with NA1-positive granulocytes.[29]

NA Variants and NA Null. Although the biallelic relationship between NA1 and NA2 has historically been noted in the families and populations initially studied, occasional exceptions have been noted[30, 31]; there may therefore be a silent or third allele at this locus.[9, 32] Of further interest has been the finding of several persons—patients and healthy blood donors—whose granulocytes were typed as "NA-null" with both human anti-NA sera and anti-NA monoclonal antibodies.[10] Subsequent studies demonstrated that the lack of both NA antigens was due to the absence of FcγRIIIb on granulocytes from these persons, which confirmed that they were NA-null.[33–35]

A polymorphism of FcγRlllb, SH, has been described. Antibodies to SH were detected by granulocyte agglutination and granulocyte immunofluorescence assays in four cases of ANN.[36] The antibodies were found to react with FcγRIIIb but were not specific for NA1 or NA2. SH is expressed on neutrophils from 5% of white people. The nucleotide sequence of the SH allele was found to differ from the NA1 and NA2 forms of *FcγRIIIB* at base 266, where a change from cytosine to adenosine was present. This resulted in an amino acid substitution of alanine to aspartate at amino acid 78. Three people with this polymorphism have been found to have duplicate FcγRIIIB genes and, as a result, have at least three FcγRIIIB genes.[37]

NB

The NB1 antigen, described by Lalezari and associates in 1971,[38] was also discovered during the investigation of a case of ANN. The NB1 antithetical allelic antigen (NB2) was concurrently described in 1982 from two patients: one experiencing a febrile transfusion reaction[39] and one with ANN.[40] In addition, Lalezari and associates[40] suggested that NB2 is identical to another granulocyte antigen known for many years as 9a. This association was also confirmed in the Red Cross Granulocyte Serology laboratory; however, the initial examination of this tissue, based on samples from a large number of donors that were examined with granulocyte agglutination, seemed to disprove the hypothesis. When the donors were retyped by means of the granulocyte immunofluorescence assay and flow cytometry, the data were found to be consistent with the hypothesis that NB2 is the same as the 9a antigen.

Unfortunately, what has not been confirmed is the

allelic association between the antigens detected by the currently available NB1 and NB2 human allosera. In prospective testing of 157 donors between 1988 and 1990, Kline and coworkers found gene frequencies of .79 for NB1 and .37 for NB2. The NB2 gene frequency was double that originally reported[6] (see Table 12–1) and reflected the variability in the pattern of serological reactivity that Kline and coworkers observed with the four NB2 antisera thus far identified. Furthermore, detection of the NB1 antigen requires agglutination and immunofluorescence techniques,[41] whereas the NB2 antigen as currently described is usually detectable only by agglutination.[42] Together, these observations suggest that the currently described NB2 antisera may not define an antigen that is the antithetical allele of NB1. These antigen systems, including 9a, and their respective allosera therefore need to be thoroughly reexamined.

NB1 antigen appears to be more than just a single epitope. Two murine monoclonal antibodies specific for NB1 react with different epitopes.[43] The epitope recognized by one of the monoclonal antibodies, 7D8, was also recognized by two NB1-specific alloantibodies, but a third alloantibody recognized a different epitope.[43]

NB1 antigen is unique in that it is expressed by subpopulations of granulocytes. The size of the antigen-positive subpopulation varies from 0% to 100%, but the average size of the NB1-positive population is 55% of neutrophils from adults.[19] When the size of the NB1-positive population is less than 45%, the NB1 antigen is often not detected by alloantisera in the granulocyte agglutination assay.[44]

A comparison of the size of the NB1-positive cell population with two different monoclonal antibodies also suggests that polymorphism of the NB1 antigen may exist. The size of the NB1-positive cell population was measured in 25 white patients and was the same with both antibodies in 23 people but differed in 2,[19] which suggests that at least two different forms of NB1 antigen exist.[43]

There is no difference in the expression of NB1 in adults and children, but NB1 expression is increased on neutrophils from umbilical cord blood. The average size of the NB1-positive neutrophil population in umbilical cord blood was 91%.[19] NB1 is also expressed on neutrophil precursors and on similar proportions of myelocytes, metamyelocytes, and segmented neutrophils.[19] The expression of NB1 is reduced in patients with chronic myelogenous leukemia. The average NB1-positive neutrophil population was only 29% in eight such patients studied and less than 10% in three patients.[19]

The expression of NB1 increases slightly when neutrophils are stimulated in vitro. NB1 expression is also increased in people who are given granulocyte colony-stimulating factor (G-CSF).[45]

NB Biochemistry. The biochemical structure of NB1 antigen, but not of NB2, has been determined. NB1 antigen is located on a 58- to 64-kD plasma membrane glycoprotein.[46–48] Like FcγRIIIb, the NB1 molecule is linked to the granulocyte membrane via a GPI anchor.[47, 48] The expression of NB1 antigen is increased on stimulated granulocytes, but NB1 antigen is not released from granulocyte surfaces, nor is it found in plasma.[46, 48] The NB1 glycoprotein contains N-linked, but not O-linked, carbohydrate side chains.[46, 48] The 58- to 64-kD molecule and the NB1 antigen have also been located on membranes of specific or secondary granules.[46, 48] The gene encoding this glycoprotein has not been identified, and the role of the molecule in granulocyte function is uncertain.

Alloantibodies to NB1 antigen were used in immunoblotting and immunoprecipitating assays to identify the 58- to 64-kD glycoprotein.[47] Although NB2 antibodies were also tested in immunoblotting and immunoprecipitation, the molecule on which NB2 is located has not yet been identified.[47] Studies with monoclonal antibodies and rabbit polyclonal antibodies to NB1 suggest that NB1 and NB2 differ markedly. Two NB1-specific rabbit polyclonal antibodies immunoblotted the 58- to 64-kD NB1 molecule but did not immunoblot any protein on NB1-negative cells.[49] Unfortunately, the NB1 protein has yet to be sequenced, and the gene has not been cloned. Once the gene expressing NB1 antigen is sequenced, a better understanding of NB polymorphisms will follow.

NC

A single antigen at the NC locus was defined in 1970 by the serum of a woman whose infant had ANN.[50] This serum also contained very strong HLA antibodies, which can yield misleading results and therefore must be completely removed by absorption techniques before such a serum is used as a typing reagent.

NC1 has been shown to have a very strong association with the NA2 antigen.[51–53] Schacter and colleagues[54] reported that the genes segregate independently in black people but are apparently identical in white people. Such a racial segregation pattern would be unprecedented and requires confirmation. Kline and coworkers' studies of the association between NA2 and NC1 showed discrepancies in only 3 of 281 predominantly white blood donors.[55] All three discrepant donors were typed as NA2-positive and NC1-negative. The cells of these donors failed to absorb anti-NC1, which led us to conclude that the donors truly lacked the NC1 antigen. Thus Kline and coworkers believe that these two specificities are difficult to differentiate but not identical. It is possible either that the NA2 and NC1 antigens are the products of two closely linked genes, except when a rare allele is present, or that the NA2 antigen is a precursor for the production of the NC1 antigen.[56]

ND

ND1 was described in 1978 by Verheugt and coworkers,[57] who used serum of two patients with autoimmune neutropenia. Family studies established that this new specificity was not related to the NA, NB, NC, or 9a loci. The ND1 antigen was called neutrophil-specific, although the results of cell line distribution studies were not reported. The antigen was present on 98.5% of neutrophils from 67 donors, and the gene frequency was 0.88, assuming a biallelic system.

NE

NE1 was defined in 1979 with the serum of a child with chronic benign neutropenia.[58] The preliminary population analysis showed no correlation between this antigen and NA1, NA2, NB1, NC1, or 9a. Its incidence in the Dutch population (based on testing 48 donors) was 28%, which corresponded to a gene frequency of 0.12. Because this gene frequency hinted that NE1 might be the antigen produced by the allele of ND1, several family studies were done. Two people were found whose granulocytes lacked both the ND1 and the NE1 antigens, which indicates that the antigens are not simply alleles.[59] Absorption tests showed that the NE1 antigen is present on granulocytes but not on lymphocytes, monocytes, platelets, or erythrocytes.

Granulocyte-Associated Antigens Identified by Human Allosera

In addition to granulocyte-specific antigens, granulocytes also have numerous membrane antigens that are expressed on other cell lines and tissues.[60] These systemic antigens are of interest because (1) they provide information about myeloid ontogeny and intercellular relationships, (2) they may play a role in transfusion therapy and immune-related granulocyte dysfunction, and (3) they are of use for ensuring correct interpretation of serological test results.

The 5 Antigen System

The human group 5 antigen system, first described in 1964,[8] has two known alleles (5a and 5b) that segregate independently of the HLA system.[62] These antigens are expressed on granulocytes, lymphocytes, platelets, kidney cells, spleen cells, placenta cells, and endothelial cells, but not on erythrocytes.[8] Cytogenetic studies have suggested that group 5 antigens are the product of genes located on chromosome 4.[63]

Although the biological role for this system has not been established, some clinical associations have been noted. While studying the group 5 antigens in patients receiving bone marrow grafts, Warren and colleagues[64] observed a striking association between the incidence of 5a and acute lymphocytic leukemia. The presence of the 5a antigen is also associated with a reduced level of natural killer cell function.[65] One case of febrile transfusion reaction associated with anti-5b has been described,[66] and immunization to the 5b antigen occurs frequently during pregnancy.[67] A case of transfusion-related acute lung injury (TRALI) has been associated with transfusion of plasma containing anti-5b.[68] This antibody was subsequently used to study the pathophysiological processes of TRALI.[69]

The 9 Antigen System

The 9a antigen, reported by van Rood and associates in 1965,[70] was defined by an antibody in the serum of a multiparous woman. Although there was no evidence that any of her children had developed neonatal neutropenia, anti-9a has been associated with one reported case of ANN[71] and shown to be granulocyte-specific.[72]

As previously discussed, 9a has been suggested to be identical to NB2 and therefore allelic to NB1. However, studies by Jager and co-workers[73] could not confirm that 9a and NB1 are alleles. These researchers found that human monocyte antigen–1 (HMA-1) and 9a appear to be identical, although the antibodies by which they are recognized react in different test systems.[73] Absorption studies indicated that 9a was present on granulocytes, monocytes, and B cells, but not on T cells or erythrocytes. To date, nothing is known about the biochemical properties or clinical relevance of 9a.

MART

The MART antigen was defined by antibody in the sera of three multiparous blood donors who had never received transfusions.[74] MART was found on granulocytes, monocytes, and lymphocytes, but not on platelets or erythrocytes. The antigen was shown to have autosomal dominant inheritance with a high phenotypic frequency (99.1% of white blood donors) and has no relation to known granulocyte, HLA, or red blood cell antigens. MART has been located on the α M chain (CD11b) of the C3bi receptor (CR3).[75] The detection of this alloantigen on a leukocyte cell adhesion molecule (Leu-CAM) illustrates its antigenic polymorphisms.[75] The significance of the antibody in mediating blood cell destruction is not known, because none of the infants of the three multiparous women with anti-MART showed evidence of ANN.

A second polymorphism of the β2 integrins, Ond, has been described. A male patient with aplastic anemia who had undergone numerous transfusions became alloimmunized to Ond. Ond was found to be expressed on the αL integrin unit (CD11a).[75]

HLA

HLA class I antigens (HLA-A and HLA-B) can be demonstrated on the surface of granulocytes by a variety of techniques, including absorption and elution,[76, 77] agglutination,[78] and immunofluorescence.[79] Conversely, routine serological methods have failed to detect the presence of class II HLA antigens on granulocyte membranes.[80, 81] Class I antigens appear to be present in smaller quantities on granulocytes than on lymphocytes,[76] and the fact that chloroquine removes HLA-A and HLA-B antigens from granulocytes without effect on cell-specific antigens may indicate that they are passively adsorbed onto granulocytes.[82] In addition, most of the easily detectable class I HLA antigens are also removed during preparation of neutroplasts,[83] which are granulocytes with the nuclei and most of the cytoplasmic granules removed by centrifugation.

The presence of HLA antigens on the surface of granulocytes is of practical importance from two standpoints. First, HLA antigens and antibodies can contribute to misleading results in serological investigations aimed at the detection of granulocyte-specific antigens and antibodies.[84] Second, HLA antigens must be considered when granulocyte transfusions are being provided for HLA-alloimmunized patients.[85, 86]

ABH

The search for evidence of ABH antigens on granulocytes illustrates the role that test materials and methods play in the analysis of results.[87] Studies demonstrating ABH antigens on granulocytes were performed primarily with absorption and elution techniques before 1969, when the technology for the preparation of purified granulocyte suspensions was not well established.[88–90] Therefore, the presence of blood cells other than granulocytes in these preparations may have led to erroneous conclusions. Subsequent attempts, performed with pure granulocyte suspensions, have been unable to demonstrate ABH antigens on granulocytes. A variety of techniques have been used, including agglutination,[91] avidin-biotin complex (ABC) immunoassay,[92] immunoperoxidase staining,[93] anti-A lectin studies with bone marrow precursor cells,[94] cytotoxicity,[91, 95] iodine-125–labeled staphylococcal protein A binding,[92] immunofluorescence microscopy and flow cytometry,[93, 96] immunoradiometry,[91] opsonization,[95] and rosette formation.[95] The only possible indication of ABH on granulocytes has been a report in which a microfilter plate radioimmunoassay was used; however, only plasma containing high-titer (1:512) anti-A or anti-B reacted with ABO-mismatched granulocytes.[97] Although the results of in vitro studies have been controversial, McCullough and associates[98] were unable to show any effect of anti-A and anti-B on in vivo survival of indium-111–labeled granulocytes or on their localization at the site of infection.[98] This is very strong evidence suggesting that there are no integral A and B antigens on granulocyte membranes, inasmuch as anti-A, anti-B, and anti-A,B are very efficient at destroying transfused incompatible cells.

Unclassified Granulocyte Antigens Identified by Human Allosera

Granulocyte antibodies that fail to demonstrate specificity for the granulocyte antigens classified to date are frequently detected serologically. Limited resources and reagents usually preclude further studies; thus the identification of new granulocyte antigens has been a very slow process. Although the number of investigations in this field has remained fairly constant over time, efforts are being made to establish organized activities that would permit systematic comparison and investigation of the multitude of antigens observed in the different laboratories. The first International Granulocyte Serology Workshop was conducted in 1989 in the United Kingdom,[99] and a second workshop was held in 1997.[100] Five reported, well-described antibodies appear to be defining new granulocyte antigens.

CN1

A granulocyte-specific antibody with specificity for an antigen more prevalent among American blacks was identified in the serum of a primipara who had never received transfusions and whose child had neonatal neutropenia.[101] The antigen, tentatively designated CN1 (Charleston 1), was found to be present in 31% of American black donors and in 1.5% of white blood donors tested.[102] Family studies suggested that the antigen was inherited in an autosomal dominant manner.

KEN

Serum from a mother of a child with severe ANN was found to contain a granulocyte-specific antibody, previously designated KEN, that reacted with all normal granulocytes tested.[33] Analysis of maternal granulocytes revealed that they lacked FcγRIIIb, the protein that expresses the NA locus antigens.[36] Autosomal recessive inheritance of this blank NA condition (resulting in an NA-null phenotype) was demonstrated through family studies, in which weakened KEN reactivity was used as a marker for the carrier state. The exact specificity of KEN is currently unknown. Subsequent studies evaluating the frequency of the NA-null phenotype in a donor population have detected a few persons with discordant NA (NA1, NA2) and KEN phenotypes,[103] which thus suggests the presence of additional low-frequency NA alleles or the need to better characterize the specificity of the KEN antibody.

LAN and LEA

Two cases of ANN in Australian aborigines suggest the existence of a new granulocyte antigen.[104] The maternal antibodies (designated LAN and LEA) reacted with more than 99% of the white blood donors tested; antibody reactivity was restricted to mature granulocytes (metamyelocytes, band, and segmented cells). Although both sera appeared to recognize the same antigen, this observation could not be confirmed.

SL

During Stroncek and associates' evaluation of a case of ANN, serum from the mother was found to contain a granulocyte antibody that appeared to identify a new granulocyte antigen, currently designated SL.[105] When the maternal serum was tested against a panel of granulocytes from 69 donors of known phenotype, reactivity was seen with 46 (67%) of the panel cells. Antibody activity was observed only with immunofluorescence and not with agglutination techniques. Preliminary family studies suggested that the antigen was inherited in an autosomal dominant manner. Further studies are needed to elucidate the serology, genetics, and biochemical nature of this antigen.

Granulocyte Cytoplasmic Antigens

Granulocyte cytoplasmic antigens were initially observed in the early 1960s and 1970s, during the study of selected patient sera for granulocyte-specific antinuclear factors.[106, 107] It was the work of the Dutch and Swedish scientists in the 1980s, however, that established an association between antibodies to neutrophil cytoplasmic components and active Wegener's granulomatosis and that ignited scientific interest in granulocyte subcellular antigens.[108, 109] These antibodies, now called *antineutrophil cytoplasmic autoantibodies* (ANCA), have been shown to be present in most patients with systemic necrotizing vasculitis.[110] The spectrum of ANCA-associated diseases includes renally limited disease (e.g., idiopathic crescentic glomerulonephritis), polyarteritis nodosa, Wegener's granulomatosis, and Churg-Strauss syndrome, in addition to clinicopathological syndromes that are more difficult to classify.[110] ANCA are serological markers for this spectrum of vascular inflammatory diseases and thus have proved useful for the diagnosis of systemic vasculitis and the estimation of disease activity.[111] The accelerating interest in this area of autoimmunity has been fostered through three international ANCA workshops that have focused on better elucidation of (1) ANCA detection, (2) ANCA antigen specificity, (3) disease specificity, (4) working nomenclature classification schemes, and (5) the pathogenic potential of ANCA.[112–114]

ANCA Antigen Specificity

Significant progress has been made since the 1980s in the identification of the antigens recognized by ANCA. The two major ANCA antigens are proteinase 3 (PR3) (a 29-kD diisopropylfluorophosphate-binding serine protease)[115–122] and myeloperoxidase (MPO),[122–124] both of which reside in neutrophil primary (azurophilic or alpha) granules.[122, 125] After neutrophil activation, PR3 and MPO are translocated to the cell surface and thus are able to interact with ANCA.[122]

A few other granulocyte cytoplasmic antigens with ANCA specificity have been identified. These include CAP 57 (an antimicrobial cationic protein contained in a subpopulation of neutrophil primary granules),[126, 127] human leukocyte elastase (located in the primary granules),[122, 128] lactoferrin (the only known ANCA antigen contained in the secondary granules),[122, 129–131] cathepsin G (a 25-kD neutral protease in the primary granules),[122, 132] and eosinophil peroxidase.[122, 132] Furthermore, from the results of the third international ANCA workshop in 1990, it is clear that additional antigen specificities remain to be identified, because numerous sera submitted for evaluation at the workshop contained antibodies to undefined granulocyte cytoplasmic antigens.

ANCA Antigen Classification

Through the use of indirect immunofluorescence microscopy with ethanol-fixed granulocytes as substrate, two major categories of ANCA have been established: one with a cytoplasmic staining pattern (C-ANCA) and one with a perinuclear staining pattern (P-ANCA).[133] Although the majority of C-ANCA have PR3 specificity and the majority of P-ANCA have MPO specificity,[133] additional C-ANCA and P-ANCA specificities have been identified across the spectrum of ANCA-associated diseases (Table 12–4).[122] P-ANCA are more commonly found in patients with renally limited disease, whereas C-ANCA are much more common in patients with biopsy-confirmed Wegener's granulomatosis.[114]

Table 12–4. Antigen Specificity of Antineutrophil Cytoplasmic Autoantibodies (ANCA)

ANCA Categories*	Antigen Specificity
C-ANCA	Proteinase 3 CAP57
P-ANCA	Myeloperoxidase Human leukocyte elastase
Homogeneous non–C-ANCA	Cathepsin G

From Lesavre P. Antineutrophil cytoplasmic autoantibodies antigen specificity. Am J Kidney Dis 1991; 18:159.

*ANCA categories established by indirect immunofluorescence microscopy with ethanol-fixed granulocytes as substrate.

C-ANCA, antineutrophil cytoplasmic autoantibodies with cytoplasmic staining pattern; P-ANCA, antineutrophil cytoplasmic autoantibodies with perinuclear staining pattern.

Granulocyte Antigens Identified by Monoclonal Antibodies

Numerous monoclonal antibodies have been produced that identify human granulocyte antigens. Some of these monoclonal antibodies detect antigens unique to granulocytes, and other reagents define antigens that are common to granulocytes, other cells, and tissues. Although many of these determinants appear to be differentiation markers, some represent epitopes on functionally significant membrane proteins: CR3, C3bi, Fc receptor for immunoglobulin G (IgG), and the lymphocyte function-associated antigen (LFA), which function as leukocyte adhesion molecules. The antigens listed in Table 12–5 represent granulocyte antigens of current interest and investigation that have been identified with monoclonal antibodies.[60] The clusters of differentiation (CD), as defined by the Fourth International Workshop and Conference on Human Leukocyte Differentiation Antigens,[134] are shown along with some basic information about their functional and biochemical characteristics. Only six of the many granulocyte monoclonal antibodies thus far reported have shown specificity for the polyclonal serologically defined granulocyte antigens, and these antibodies appear to be directed against the NA1, NA2, and NB1 antigens; against NA1, CLB-gran 11,[17] M3G8,[135, 136] and B73.1[137, 138]; against NA2, GRM1[137, 138]; and against NB1, 1B5,[139] and 7D8.[43]

Granulocyte Subpopulations and the Heterogeneous Expression of Granulocyte Antigens

Granulocyte subpopulations have been defined on the basis of physical properties, function, and antigen expression. With counterflow centrifugal elutriation, populations of granulocytes of different size have been isolated.[140] The function of these granulocytes was tested, and the volume of the granulocytes correlated directly with the quantity of superoxide anion produced in response to stimulation with FMLP and phorbol myristate acetate (PMA). Other groups have isolated granulocyte subpopulations on the basis of cell density and have found that cells with lower density have decreased FMLP-induced chemotaxis.[141]

Table 12–5. Representative Granulocyte Antigens Identified with Murine Monoclonal Antibodies

Antibody/Antigen Cluster Designation (CD)	Recognized Membrane Antigen	Molecular Weight (kD)	Function	Ligand
CD10	Common acute lymphoblastic leukemia antigen–1	gp 100	Neutral endopeptidase (enkephalinase)	—
CD11a	α L chain of LFA-1	gp 180	Integrin receptor Leukocyte-leukocyte adhesion Leukocyte–endothelial cell adhesion	ICAM-1; ICAM-2
CD11b	α M chain of complement (C3) receptor (CR3) (Mac-1, Mo1)*	gp 165	Integrin receptor Cell-cell adhesion (polymorphonuclear leukocyte–endothelial cell adhesion) Phagocytosis Complement binding	C3bi (proteolytic fragment of complement 3b) Fibrinogen Coagulation factor X Endotoxin
CD11c	α X chain of complement (C4) receptor 4 (CR4) (gp 150, 95)	gp 150	Integrin receptor Complement binding	C3bi
CD15	X-hapten (3-fucosy-N-acetyllactosamine, Lewis X)	gp 50, 68, 110, 180	Possible ligand for selectins	—
CD16	FcγRIII	gp 50–65	Low-affinity Fc receptor for complexed IgG (i.e., immune complexes) Main receptor for antibody-dependent cell-mediated cytotoxicity Crosslinked antibodies can activate cytotoxicity, cytokine production, and receptor expression	IgG (complexed)
CD18	β chain of LFA-1, CR3, CR4	gp 95	Same as for CD11a, CD11b, and CD11c functions	Same as for CD11a, CD11b, and CD11c ligands
CD29	β chain of VLA-6 (α6 β1)	gp 120–150	Laminin receptor	Laminin
CD31	PECAM-1	gp 130–140	Cell-cell adhesion Immunoglobulin gene superfamily adhesion molecule	
CDw32	FcγRII	gp 40	Low-affinity Fc receptor for aggregated IgG Cell activation molecule	IgG (aggregated)
CD44	Homing cell adhesion molecule (Hermes antigen)	gp 80–95	Cell-cell adhesion Homing receptor	Endothelial cell mucosal addressin Type I collagen Type VI collagen
CD45	Leukocyte common antigen (T200)	gp 180, 190, 205, 220	Signal transduction molecule Tyrosine phosphatase	—
CD49f	α chain of VLA-6 (α6β1)	gp 120	Laminin receptor	Laminin
CD55	Decay-accelerating factor	gp 70	Complement regulation	Complement proteins 3b and 4b
CD62L	LEC-CAM adhesion protein, $gp\text{-}100^{MEL\text{-}14}$	gp 100	Initial adhesion of granulocytes to endothelial cells adjacent to inflammation	Endothelial cell carbohydrate
CD64	FcγRI	gp 75	High-affinity Fc receptor for IgG Transduces activation signals	IgG (monomeric)
CD groups have not been assigned for the following monoclonal antibodies: CLB-gran 11, M3G8, B73.1,† GRM1†	NA1	gp 45–60	Unknown; located on neutrophil FcγRIII (CD16)	—
	NA2	gp 60–75	Unknown; located on neutrophil FcγRIIIb (CD16)	—
1B5	NB1	gp 58–64	Unknown	—

Compiled from data in references 134 to 139.

*Mac-1/Mo1 are monoclonal antibodies that initially identified the CD11b molecule; this antigen is often referred to as Mac-1 or Mo1.

†These monoclonal antibodies are neither granulocyte-specific nor absolutely NA allotype–specific.[135–138]

LFA-1, leukocyte function antigen–1; ICAM, intracellular adhesion molecule; FcγRIII, crystallizable fragment γ receptor III; IgG, immunoglobulin G; VLA-6, very late antigen–6; PECAM-1, platelet endothelial cell adhesion molecule–1; LEC-CAM, lectin–epidermal growth factor–complement–cell adhesion molecule.

Granulocyte subpopulations have also been identified by function. For example, when granulocytes are stimulated by FMLP or PMA, 40% to 83% undergo respiratory burst, as measured by reduction of nitroblue tetrazolium (NBT) or single-cell chemiluminescence.[142, 143] After stimulation with PMA, all granulocytes undergo depolarization, but when granulocytes are stimulated with FMLP, only 40% to 65% are depolarized.[143, 144] Granulocytes have also been separated on the basis of their ability to form rosettes with opsonized red cells. Approximately 50% to 80% of granulocytes form rosettes with IgG-coated red cells,[145–147] and approximately 40% of granulocytes form rosettes with immunoglobulin A (IgA)–coated red cells. When granulocytes that form rosettes with IgG-coated red cells were compared with those that do not form rosettes, no difference in receptors for C4b, C3b, C3d, or C3bi could be detected.[148] Other studies have shown that lactoferrin from granulocytes that did form rosettes inhibited granulocyte-macrophage colony-stimulating activity, whereas lactoferrin from granulocytes that did not form rosettes did not similarly inhibit this activity.[149] Finally, subpopulations of granulocytes have been isolated on the basis of their ability to migrate: fewer than 50% of granulocytes migrate in response to the C5a or FMLP.[149]

Although most granulocyte antigens are expressed on all granulocytes, some antigens are detected only on subpopulations of cells. Antigens found to be expressed heterogeneously on granulocytes include 31D8,[150] common acute lymphoblastic leukemia antigen (CALLA) (CD10),[151] 4D1,[139] 1B5,[139] 7D8,[43] and NB1.[48] 31D8 monoclonal antibody reacts strongly with approximately 85% of granulocytes, weakly with 15%, and not at all with fewer than 1%.[150, 151] Granulocytes with reduced expression of 31D8 show reductions in chemotaxis[150] and production of oxygen species in response to C5a and FMLP.[150, 152] The population of granulocytes that react with 31D8 has been found to be reduced in neonates,[153] in patients with chronic myelogenous leukemia,[154] in victims of blunt trauma,[155] and in healthy volunteers given endotoxin or steroids.[156] The expression of 31D8 increases on myeloid cells as they mature to polymorphonuclear cells; the population of peripheral blood granulocytes that react weakly with 31D8 may therefore represent functionally immature granulocytes.[157] CALLA (CD10), a neural endopeptidase, is expressed on approximately 95% of granulocytes. The antigen-negative cell population has enhanced response to C5a.[151]

Monoclonal antibodies 1B5 and 7D8 and human alloantibody NB1 recognize the same granulocyte antigen epitope.[43, 48] Interestingly, the size of the NB1 and 1B5 antigen population varies markedly among individuals (0% to 100% of granulocytes reactive).[43, 48, 49]

GRANULOCYTE ANTIBODIES

Detection Methods

Many methods are available to detect granulocyte antibodies (Table 12–6)[158–186]; however, correlations with clinical situations are not well established.[187] Because most of the assays are complicated and require the use of fresh test cells, there have been few studies comparing the value of different assays in detecting clinical problems. In addition, the composition of the test cell suspension—such as unseparated leukocytes versus isolated granulocyte suspensions—may lead to different results.

Table 12–6. Granulocyte Antibody Detection Methods

General Phenomenon	Specific Technique	Major Reference(s)
Agglutination of granulocytes	Agglutination	2, 158
	Macroscopic*	159, 160
	Microscopic*	161–163
	Microcapillary	
Antibody coating of granulocytes	Cytotoxicity	164–167
	Complement mediated	168, 169
	Dye (eosin) exclusion	
	Fluorochromasia	
	Cell mediated	7, 170, 171
	ADLG	
	Immunofluorescence	172–174
	Macroscopic*	175, 174
	Microscopic*	42
	Flow cytometry*	
	ABC immunoassay	177, 178
	ELISA	97, 179, 180, 181, 182
	Radioimmunoassay	
	Staphylococcal protein A	
	MAIGA	183
Alteration of granulocyte function	Opsonic assay	184–186

*Assays most commonly used to detect antibodies directed against the granulocyte antigens shown in Table 12–1.

ADLG, antibody-dependent, lymphocyte-mediated granulocyte cytotoxicity; ABC, avidin-biotin complex; ELISA, enzyme-linked immunosorbent assay; MAIGA, monoclonal antibody immunization of granulocyte antigens.

The current, well-described, classified granulocyte antigens shown in Table 12–1 have been detected primarily by granulocyte agglutination and granulocyte immunofluorescence (GIF).[42] Other serological methods, such as granulocytotoxicity and antibody-dependent cell-mediated cytotoxicity (ADCC) assays, do not produce reaction patterns showing the same granulocyte antigen specificities.[187] In studies using some of these other assay systems, sera that appear to define other systems of granulocyte antigens have been identified.[80, 168, 188, 189]

Granulocyte antibodies can be grouped, on the basis of the behavior of the antibodies, as those causing (1) direct agglutination of cells, (2) coating of cells with antibody and/or complement, and (3) alteration of granulocyte function (see Table 12–6).

Agglutination tests are the most traditional detection methods, but they are subject to problems with reproducibility and stringent test cell preparation and incubation time/temperature parameters. They should be conducted with a pure granulocyte suspension in test tubes, microtiter trays, or capillary tubes (see Table 12–6). Coating of granulocytes can be detected by a variety of methods, including cytotoxicity, immunofluorescence, ABC immunoassay, enzyme-linked immunosorbent assay (ELISA), radioimmunoassay, staphylococcal protein A, and monoclonal antibody immobilization of granulocyte antigen (MAIGA) assay (see Table 12–6). The advantage of the MAIGA assay is that it can distinguish antibodies directed to specific antigens even when HLA or several granulocyte-specific antibodies are present. A fundamentally different approach to detecting this class of granulocyte antibodies is based on their opsonic property.[184, 185] In the opsonic assay, indicator phagocytes such as rabbit macrophages are incubated with antibody-coated granulocytes, and metabolic changes associated with phagocytosis are measured in the indicator cells.

Complement fixation by granulocyte antibodies is usually detected in a granulocytotoxicity assay similar to the HLA lymphocytotoxicity assay (see Table 12–6). Treatment of cells with enzyme or cytochalasin B has been used to enhance granulocytotoxin reactivity. The method that appears most valuable involves double fluorochromasia.[188] Although a few studies have been done with antibody-dependent lymphocyte-mediated granulocytotoxicity,[7, 170, 171] this technique has not been developed into a widely used assay for granulocyte serology studies.

Detection of Antineutrophil Cytoplasmic Autoantibodies

Methods of detecting ANCA include indirect immunofluorescence,[190–192] ELISA,[115, 117, 193–196] radioimmunoassay,[197] Western blotting,[115] and immunoprecipitation.[115]

Indirect immunofluorescence with alcohol-fixed granulocytes was established, at the first international ANCA workshop in 1988, as the reference method for ANCA detection.[191] With this technique, two main ANCA fluorescence staining patterns are observed: (1) a cytoplasmic pattern (C-ANCA), in which granular staining is seen in the cytoplasm and often accentuated at the center of the cell between the nuclear segments, and (2) a perinuclear pattern (P-ANCA), which produces peripheral or diffuse nuclear staining.

Because some of the antigens that give rise to the C-ANCA and P-ANCA patterns are localized in the primary granules, researchers were initially puzzled as to how these antigens could produce two different ANCA patterns. It is now known that the P-ANCA pattern is a fixation artifact, inasmuch as the granule membranes are disrupted and basic proteins (positively charged) are redistributed to the negatively charged nucleus.[111] If fixation is in formaldehyde, which prevents the migration of proteins, it is impossible to distinguish between C-ANCA and P-ANCA patterns. In addition, properly prepared substrate slides are essential for differentiating among C-ANCA, P-ANCA, and the pattern of granulocyte-specific antinuclear antibodies.[133] When Cytospin-prepared slides were compared with air-dried slides for the identification of ANCA in 19 patients with Wegener's granulomatosis, the slides prepared with the Cytospin substrate were superior in differentiating among the three patterns of antibody reactivity.[198] The detection of ANCA with the indirect immunofluorescence technique also requires that the secondary antibody used in the assay be reactive with all immunoglobulin classes, because ANCA can be of different isotypes.[133]

The qualitative nature of the assay and the problems with interpretation of the immunofluorescence patterns established the need for antigen-specific solid-phase assays. Although numerous enzyme immunoassay and radioimmunoassay methods have been developed,[111] variations in the nature of the antigen preparation used as substrate and the specificity and label of the secondary antibody make it difficult to compare the assays. For example, the substrates may consist of whole cell extracts, granule extracts, or purified proteins; the secondary label may be anti-immunoglobulin or may be immunoglobulin class specific. Therefore, it is clear that as additional ANCA antigen specificities are detected, there will be a concomitant need for standardized solid-phase methods for detecting and/or measuring ANCA.

As expected, the solid-phase assays are more sensitive and less subjective than immunofluorescence. Some studies indicate that the correlation between disease activity and antibody titer is better in ELISA than in immunofluorescence.[111] Nonetheless, circulating levels of ANCA usually but not always parallel disease activity in individual patients.[193] Depending on the antigen substrate used in the solid-phase assays, indirect immunofluorescence microscopy may help detect patients with ANCA specificities for new antigens. It has been observed that approximately 80% to 90% of samples that are positive by indirect immunofluorescence are positive in ELISA and that 90% of samples that are positive in ELISA are positive in immunofluorescence.[111] The use of granulocyte primary granule extracts versus whole cell extracts as ELISA substrates for the detection of PR3-ANCA demonstrates a 20-fold increase in the response of the assay that used granule extract substrate, with a specificity greater than 95% and a sensitivity of 80% to 90%.[111]

The majority of ANCA-positive sera is monospecific for a single ANCA antigen,[122] and affected patients usually have either C-ANCA or P-ANCA but not both.[133] Therefore, until purified and standardized substrate antigens and/or reagents for solid-phase assays are more available, many laboratories will continue to screen for ANCA initially by using immunofluorescence and then use ELISA for confirmation of antigen specificity.[111]

Serological Characteristics

Granulocyte agglutinins are usually IgG, although mixtures of IgG, immunoglobulin M (IgM), and IgA have been reported.[12] This is in contrast to red cell serology, in which antibodies that cause direct agglutination are usually IgM. This difference may be explained by the occurrence of two kinds of granulocyte agglutination: an active process dependent on Fc-mediated antibody binding caused by IgG antibodies[199] and a separate process caused by IgM antibodies that is comparable to true agglutination.[12, 51]

Granulocyte cytotoxins are usually IgM[12, 186] but are occasionally IgG.[188] IgG is the active component of serum that facilitates lymphocyte-mediated granulocytotoxicity. Although IgM and IgG complement–activating antibodies have been detected in patients with ANN,[12, 200] autoimmune neutropenia,[187, 201, 202] and febrile[12] and pulmonary[203] transfusion reactions, many IgG antibodies are not detectable by granulocyte cytotoxicity.[12, 187, 200, 202] In these clinical situations, granulocyte antibodies are detected and identified with the granulocyte agglutination and immunofluorescence assays.[68, 201–207]

Immunochemical Characteristics

Very few studies have related the immunochemical nature of granulocyte antibodies to their serological reactivities and clinical effects. In a small study, Verheugt and coworkers[12] did not find any relationship between the immunoglobulin class or IgG subclass and the clinical effect of granulocyte-specific antibodies in patients with alloimmune or autoimmune neutropenia or febrile transfusion reactions or in patients receiving platelet or granulocyte transfusions except for the expected IgG antibodies associated with ANN. In contrast to the lack of association between immunoglobulin classes and clinical conditions, the immunochemical properties of the granulocyte antibodies were strongly related to their serological behavior: IgM antibodies were best detected by cytotoxicity and immunofluorescence assays, whereas IgG antibodies were optimally reactive in the agglutination and immunofluorescence assays.[12] Higher sensitivity of granulocyte immunofluorescence for the detection of granulocyte antibodies, especially in patients with autoimmune neutropenia, has also been reported by other investigators.[202, 207]

Subsequent immunochemical studies of granulocyte antibodies from a total of 66 infants with autoimmune neutropenia by three different groups of investigators[202, 207, 208] demonstrated the predominant role of IgG in this clinical disorder: serum from 48 infants (73%) had only IgG antibodies; serum from 14 (21%) had IgG and IgM antibodies; serum from 1 (1.5%) had IgG and IgA antibodies; serum from 2 (3%) had only IgM antibodies; and serum from 1 (1.5%) had IgM and IgA antibodies. Immunoglobulin subclass examinations were performed with 30 of the serum samples that contained IgG antibodies. IgG_1 and IgG_3 subclass granulocyte antibodies were demonstrable in 30 and 23 cases, respectively.[202] Similarly, IgG_1 and IgG_3 subclass antibodies have been detected in specimens from 18 patients with ANN.[200] Serum from one patient also contained IgA antibodies, and serum from another contained IgM antibodies.

In Vivo Effects

The specific in vivo effects of different leukocyte antibodies or in vitro tests that correlate with immune granulocyte destruction and adverse transfusion effects remain undefined. One major problem has been the lack of a satisfactory method of studying the in vivo fate of a single injection of a granulocyte suspension to determine the effect of antibodies present. However, the development of technology that involves the use of granulocytes labeled with radioisotope indium-111 allows measurement of both the intravascular and extravascular fate of injected granulocytes. Thus studies similar to those conducted in red cell serology are possible. Specifically, the fate of transfused granulocytes in patients with different kinds of leukocyte antibodies can establish the clinical sequelae of the individual antibodies.

Dutcher and colleagues[85] reported that indium-111–labeled granulocytes localized at sites of infection in all of 20 nonimmunized patients but in only 3 of 14 infected patients who also had lymphocytotoxic (HLA) antibody. In later studies,[86] these investigators showed that alloimmunization significantly increased pulmonary retention of indium-111–labeled granulocytes for 30 minutes after injection. Because most of the patients had both lymphocytotoxic and leukoagglutinating antibodies, the role of the antibodies detected in different assays could not be established.

McCullough and associates showed that granulocyte-agglutinating antibodies, alone and in combination with other leukocyte antibodies, were associated with decreased intravascular recovery of incompatible granulocytes.[98, 209] Although antibody identified by granulocytotoxicity, lymphocytotoxicity, GIF, or antibody-dependent lymphocyte-mediated granulocytotoxicity assays demonstrated similar effects, one patient whose serum reacted in GIF and other assays but not in granulocyte agglutination had decreased intravascular granulocyte recovery.

The ability of granulocytes to migrate to a site of inflammation may be more important than their survival in the intravascular space. In McCullough and associates' studies, granulocytes failed to localize at known sites of inflammation in three patients, and abnormal sequestration of transfused granulocytes was noted in the lungs of two patients.[98, 209] These patients had antibodies that were detected by both agglutination and immunofluorescence assays, which suggested that such antibodies either caused abnormal localization or accelerated intravascular clearance of transfused cells. Neither granulocytotoxic and lymphocytotoxic antibodies nor those causing lymphocyte-mediated granulocytotoxicity were associated with reduced intravascular recovery, failure of granulocytes to localize at a site of infection, or abnormal pulmonary sequestration.

Studies to date have not established which antigen systems are involved in interference with the in vivo fate of granulocytes. Granulocyte agglutination detects granulocyte-specific and some HLA antigens, and immunofluorescence detects both granulocyte-specific and HLA antigens, whereas lymphocytotoxicity identifies only HLA antigens. McCullough and associates' data indicate that granulocytes that are incompatible in a lymphocytotoxicity (HLA) crossmatch circulate normally, migrate to a site of infection normally, and are not abnormally sequestered in the lungs. In contrast, studies by Dutcher and colleagues[85, 86] suggested clinical sequelae mediated by lymphocytotoxic antibodies. Chow and associates[210] reported that immunofluorescence was more predictive of the in vivo fate of granulocytes in dogs than was agglutination or lymphocytotoxicity. Dahlke and coworkers[211] examined the correlation between alloimmunization and recovery from gram-negative sepsis in 25 patients receiving granulocyte transfusions and also demonstrated the clinical role of antibodies detected by immunofluorescence. Agglutination and immunofluorescence may be the best in vitro predictors of the in vivo fate of granulocytes.

ROLE OF GRANULOCYTE ANTIGENS IN INTERCELLULAR INTERACTIONS

Integrins

Several membrane structures are involved in granulocyte adhesion to cells and surfaces (Table 12–7). The most widely studied granulocyte adhesion molecules belong to the integrin and selectin families of adhesion proteins. The integrins are a group of cell membrane glycoproteins with two subunits, α and β, that are noncovalently associated.[212–215] Eleven α subunits and six β subunits have been described.[212] The α chain contains a calcium-binding region, and the β chain contains four cysteine-rich repeats. The extracellular domains of the α and β subunits contain the ligand-binding region. The cytoplasmic portion of the β subunits contains regions capable of binding to cytoskeletal actin.[213]

Three types of integrin molecules have been well characterized on granulocytes.[216] All three have the same β unit (β2, CD18) but different α subunits. LFA-1 (CD11a/CD18) is located on lymphocytes, monocytes, and granulocytes and contains the α L subunit (CD11a). The α L subunit is 177 kD, and the β2 subunit is 95 kD. LFA-1 is important in cell-to-cell adhesion, especially in granulocyte adhesion to endothelial cells. LFA-1 binds to two different counterreceptors on endothelial cells: intercellular cell adhesion molecule (ICAM)–1 (CD54), and ICAM-2.[217] Both ICAM-1 and ICAM-2 belong to the immunoglobulin gene superfamily of adhesion receptors. ICAM-1 is located on all hematopoietic cells, epithelial cells, and endothelial cells; moreover, the expression of ICAM-1 on endothelial cells is increased after stimulation with γ interferon, tumor necrosis factor (TNF), and interleukin-1.[217] The induction of expression of ICAM-1 is controlled at the complementary DNA level, and maximal expression on endothelial cells occurs approximately 24 hours after stimulation.[218] ICAM-2 is also located on endothelial cells, but its expression is not induced by mediators of inflammation.[217]

Another granulocyte integrin molecule, CR3, is the receptor for complement component C3bi.[213, 215] CR3 is made up of the α M subunit of 165 kD and a β2 subunit of 95 kD and is designated CD11b/CD18. In addition to binding complement, this receptor also binds fibrinogen, coagulation factor X, and endotoxin. Several monoclonal antibodies, including Mac-1, OKM-1, Mo-1, and Leu-15, recognize CR3. The CR3 receptor is located on granulocytes, monocytes, and natural killer cells. This receptor is involved in phagocytosis, complement binding, and cell-to-cell adhesion. The expression of CR3 is increased on the surface of granulocytes and monocytes that have been stimulated with the chemoattractant FMLP.

The third granulocyte integrin is p150, 95, which has a 150-kD α X subunit and a 95-kD β2 subunit.[213, 215] Integrin p150, 95 is located on granulocytes and monocytes. Little is known of the function of this molecule, but it does bind CB3i. The expression of p150, 95 is also increased on the surface of granulocytes and monocytes that have been stimulated with FMLP.

Polymorphisms of LFA-1 and CR3 have been described. Granulocyte alloantigen Ond is located on the α L subunit of LFA-1, and alloantigen MART is located on the α M subunit of CR3.[75] The biochemical changes in these molecules that result in the polymorphisms are not known, nor is it known whether these polymorphisms are important to granulocyte function.

The β2 family of granulocyte integrins function in the adhesion of granulocytes to endothelium and extracellular matrix, granulocyte aggregation, and phagocytosis of microbes. The granulocyte β2 integrins have a role in the interaction of granulocytes with extracellular matrix proteins. When plated on surfaces coated with extracellular matrix proteins fibronectin, laminin, vitronectin, or thrombospondin and cultured with TNF, granulocytes release greater amounts of hydrogen peroxide than do

Table 12–7. Granulocyte Adhesion Molecules

Integrin	Name	Molecular Weight (kD)	CD
CD11/CD18 (Leu-CAM; β2 Integrins)			
LFA-1 complex	α subunit: α L	177	CD11a
	β subunit: β2	95	CD18
CR3 complex	α subunit: α M	165	CD11b
CR4 complex (p150, 95)	α subunit: α X	150	CD11c
β1 Integrin			
VLA-6 complex	α subunit: α 6	120	CD49f
	β subunit: β1	120–150	CD29
Other	**Class**	**Molecular Weight (kD)**	**CD**
PECAM-1	Immunoglobulin superfamily	130–140	CD31
LAM-1	Selectin	90–100	Not determined
H-CAM (Hermes antigen)	Proteoglycan	80–95	CD44

Data from references 112, 230, and 241.

VLA-6, very late antigen–6; PECAM-1, platelet endothelial cell adhesion molecule–1; LAM-1, leukocyte adhesion molecule–1; H-CAM, homing cell adhesion molecule.

cells adherent to other surfaces.[219] This increased hydrogen peroxide production is blocked by antibodies specific for β2 and does not occur in patients with congenital deficiency of CD11/CD18. Granulocyte binding to microbes can occur through the CR3, LFA-1, and p150, 95 receptors even if complement and IgG are not bound to the microbes.[215]

Antibodies specific for granulocyte β2 integrins block several granulocyte functions. Monoclonal antibodies specific for CD18 and some specific for CD11b have been shown to block the following in vitro actions of granulocytes: adhesion to endothelial cells, spreading on surfaces, aggregation, and phagocytosis of zymosan particles.[220, 221] Also, in animal models, antibodies specific for CD18 block the extravasation and migration of granulocytes into sites of inflammation.[221] Monoclonal antibodies to CD11b/CD18 prevent reperfusion injury in animal models of ischemic intestines, myocardial infarction, and hemorrhagic shock.[218]

The stimulation of granulocytes not only results in the increased expression of β2 integrins but also changes the function of β2 integrins.[218] On resting granulocytes, the α chain is phosphorylated, but the β chain is not. When granulocytes are stimulated with FMLP or PMA, transient phosphorylation of the β chain results. This phosphorylation may enhance function by altering either the binding of CD11/CD18 to various ligands or its interaction with cytoskeletal elements.[218]

In addition to the β2 family, other integrins have been located on granulocytes. Granulocytes adhere to surfaces coated with the endothelial cell basement membrane protein laminin.[222] Although granulocyte adhesion to laminin is mediated partly by β2 integrins, monoclonal antibodies to CD18[213] do not completely block the adherence of stimulated granulocytes to laminin,[222] which suggests that another laminin receptor is located on granulocytes. The integrin very late antigen–6 (VLA-6) ($\alpha_5\beta_1$), also known as platelet glycoprotein complex Ic/IIa, which mediates the adherence of platelets to laminin, has also been located on granulocytes.[223] Another granulocyte integrin that does not belong to the β2 family has been described. This integrin is made up of a 130- to 140-kD unit and a 110-kD unit.[224] Binding of fibronectin, fibrinogen, vitronectin, von Willebrand's factor, and type IV collagen to this receptor enhances IgG-mediated granulocyte phagocytosis. The function of this integrin is inactivated by myeloperoxidase-dependent oxidants produced by granulocytes,[224] but it has not been further characterized.

Selectins

The selectin adhesion receptors are important in the interaction of circulating blood cells to vascular endothelium. All selectins have a common structure, consisting of an N-terminus lectin-binding domain, an epidermal growth factor (EGF)–like domain, and a varying number of short repeat motifs that are similar to those in complement regulatory proteins. The ligands for these selectins are carbohydrates.

One selectin, mouse leukocyte homing receptor for high endothelial venules–14 (MEL-14), is involved in the adhesion of murine lymphocytes to high endothelial venules (HEV) and has been described as a peripheral lymph node–endothelial homing receptor.[225] MEL-14 antigen is expressed on murine granulocytes and participates in granulocyte–endothelial cell interactions.[226] The selectin that mediates the binding of human lymphocytes to high endothelial venules of peripheral lymph nodes has been identified. This molecule is called the leukocyte adhesion molecule–1 (LAM-1, TQ1, Leu-8, CD62L).[227, 228] The selectin LAM-1 is expressed on human granulocytes as a 90- to 100-kD glycoprotein.[229, 230] Granulocyte expression of LAM-1 is first upregulated and then downregulated when granulocytes are treated with PMA; with chemotactic factors C5a, FMLP, and leukotriene B4; and with granulocyte-macrophage colony-stimulating factor and TNF.[229–231]

Two other selectins contribute to granulocyte-endothelial binding, but these selectins are located on endothelial cells. The two endothelial cell selectins, granule-membrane protein–140 (GMP-140, platelet activation–dependent granule external membrane [PADGEM], CD62P)[232] and endothelial cell–leukocyte adhesion molecule–1 (ELAM-1, CD62E),[233] recognize carbohydrates on granulocytes. GMP-140 is expressed in the α granules of platelets and in Weibel-Palade bodies of endothelial cells.[234] Endothelial cell surfaces express GMP-140 after they are stimulated with inflammatory agents or thrombotic agents.[235] The granulocyte ligands for GMP-140 are sialylated, fucosylated lactosaminoglycans, including sialyl Lewis X.[235] The selectin ELAM-1 is also expressed on the endothelial cells that have been stimulated with cytokines.[233] The granulocyte ligand for ELAM-1 is sialyl Lewis X antigen.[236] Although both GMP-140 and ELAM-1 are expressed on stimulated endothelial cells, the timing of their expressions differs. GMP-140 can be recruited from granules within minutes, but the maximal expression of ELAM-1 occurs after several hours.[233]

OTHER ADHESION MOLECULES LOCATED ON GRANULOCYTES

Another antigen expressed on granulocytes is CD44, which has been found to be involved in the binding of human lymphocytes to venous endothelium.[237, 238] At one time it was thought that this molecule could be a selectin homologous to the murine leukocyte selectin MEL-14; however, the structure of lymphocyte CD44 has been identified and is not that of a selectin. The N-terminus of the molecule has strong sequence homology to cartilage proteoglycan and link proteins.[239, 240] This 80- to 95-kD antigen is highly glycosylated,[213] but its exact structure and role in granulocyte function have not yet been determined.

Platelet-endothelial cell adhesion molecule–1 (PECAM-1, CD31) is a 130-kD glycoprotein that belongs to the immunoglobulin gene superfamily.[241] It likely plays a role in the binding of platelets to endothelium.[213] PECAM-1 is also found on granulocytes, but its role in granulocyte function is not certain.[241]

Adhesion of Granulocytes to Endothelium

The initiating event in a granulocyte-mediated inflammatory reaction in vivo is the rolling of granulocytes along endothelium. At first, only a few cells roll along the vessel wall, but the number of adherent cells gradually increases and their velocity decreases. Eventually, the movement of the granulocytes stops, and cells begin to flatten against the vessel wall. Granulocytes then migrate between endothelial cells and into the extravascular space. Several studies suggest that the initial rolling of granulocytes along endothelium is mediated by both granulocyte and endothelial cell selectins but that the later migration of granulocytes through endothelial cells depends on granulocyte β2 integrins.[234, 242]

A possible model of the mechanisms for the interactions between granulocytes and endothelial cells is shown in Figure 12–1. The initiating event may be the production of cytokines at the site of inflammation. Cytokines induce the expression of ICAM-1 and selectins GMP-140 and ELAM-1 on endothelial cells. The upregulated endothelial cell selectins GMP-140 and ELAM-1 bind to granulocyte ligands and mediate the rolling of unstimulated granulocytes on endothelial cells in vitro. Granulocyte selectin LAM-1 also contributes to the rolling of neutrophils, and neutrophil LAM-1 and endothelial cell ELAM-1 may interact with each other as receptor and counterreceptor.[243]

After granulocytes become stimulated with chemoattractants, their binding to endothelial cells becomes dependent on integrins LFA-1 and CR3. The slow, selectin-mediated rolling may permit granulocytes to react with chemotactic factors present at the inflammatory site. After the granulocytes are stimulated by the chemoattractants, the expression of CR3 and integrin p150, 95 increases, but the expression of neutrophil selectin LAM-1 transiently increases and then decreases. The upregulated integrins react with their endothelial cell ligands ICAM-2 and ICAM-1, which also have been upregulated. The resulting cell-to-cell interactions cause the granulocyte rolling to slow and stop. Granulocytes then begin to migrate between endothelial cells and extravasate.

Granulocytes stimulated with chemotactic factors have been found to aggregate, and the granulocyte-to-granulocyte adhesion likely helps recruit more granulocytes into sites of inflammation. Moreover, integrins also play an important role in granulocyte aggregation because in vitro granulocyte aggregation is blocked by antibodies

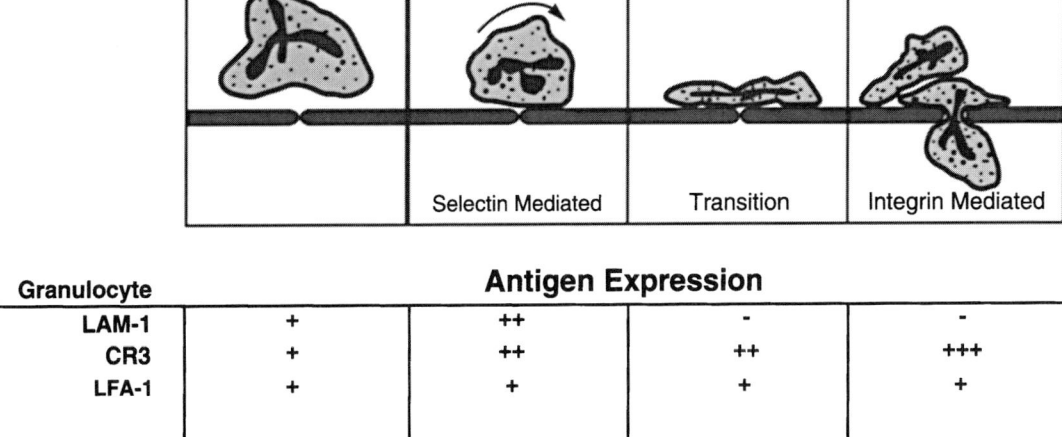

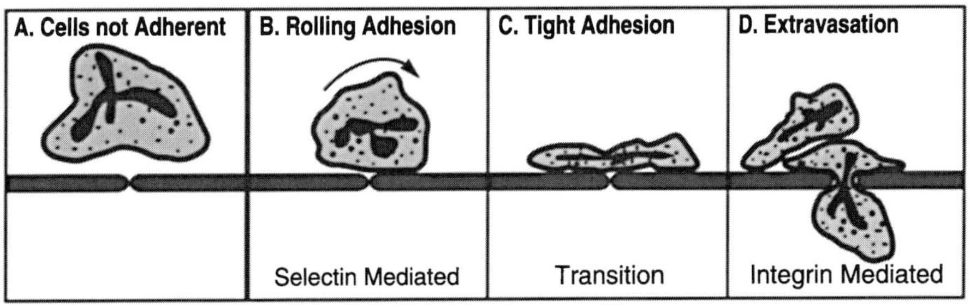

Antigen Expression

Granulocyte	A	B	C	D
LAM-1	+	++	-	-
CR3	+	++	++	+++
LFA-1	+	+	+	+
Endothelial Cell				
ICAM-1	-	+	+	+
ICAM-2	+	+	+	+
GMP-140	-	+	+	+
ELAM-1	-	+	+	+

Figure 12–1. A model of the interactions of granulocyte and endothelial cell antigens at sites of inflammation. *A*, When no inflammation is present, few granulocytes are adherent to endothelial cells. Granulocytes express LAM-1, CR3, and LFA-1. Endothelial cells express only ICAM-2. *B*, As inflammation develops, cytokines produced at the inflammatory site stimulate endothelial cells, whose expression of ICAM-1 and selectins ELAM-1 and GMP-140 is increased. Granulocyte selectin LAM-1 and the endothelial cell selectins mediate the first associations between neutrophils and endothelial cells. The result is the slow rolling of granulocytes along the vessel wall. *C*, As granulocytes roll along the endothelium, they are exposed to high concentrations of chemoattractants produced at the site of inflammation, and they are stimulated. The stimulated granulocytes lose the selectin LAM-1, but the expression of integrins LFA-1 and CR3 is upregulated. Granulocyte antigens CR3 and LFA-1 bind to cell molecules ICAM-2 and ICAM-1, which also has been upregulated. As a result, granulocyte rolling slows and finally stops. Granulocytes begin to spread on endothelium. *D*, Granulocytes migrate through the endothelium and extravasate through a CR3-dependent process. Additional granulocytes are recruited to the site of inflammation via aggregation. This granulocyte-to-granulocyte binding of stimulated cells depends on CR3. LAM-1, leukocyte adhesion molecule–1; LFA-1, lymphocyte function–associated antigen–1; ICAM, intercellular cell adhesion molecule; ELAM-1, endothelial cell–leukocyte adhesion molecule–1; GMP-140, granule-membrane protein–140. The number of + signs indicates the degree of antigen expression.

to β2 integrins.[221] Platelets may also contribute to the binding of granulocytes to vessel walls.[244] After tissue injury, platelets bind to the exposed endothelium. Such platelets become stimulated and express GMP-140, which then binds granulocytes.[245]

ROLE OF GRANULOCYTE ANTIGENS AND ANTIBODIES IN HUMAN DISEASES

Alloimmune Neonatal Neutropenia

Like hemolytic disease of the newborn and alloimmune neonatal thrombocytopenia, alloimmunization to granulocyte-specific antigens can occur during pregnancy. The maternal IgG can then cross the placenta and result in neonatal neutropenia. Such ANN can occur during a first pregnancy, and its clinical course is quite variable. Although some children have no infections, others may have cutaneous infections, respiratory tract infections, or bacteremias. These infections are usually mild, but fatalities have been reported in 5% of cases.[246] The neutropenia usually resolves in 2 to 8 weeks without treatment. Intravenous immunoglobulin treatment resulted in transient improvement in granulocyte counts in one neonate.[247]

Antibodies to granulocyte-specific antigens NA1,[16, 248, 249] NA2,[13] NB1,[38] and NC1[50] have been reported to cause neonatal alloimmune neutropenia; antibodies to NA1, NA2, and NB1 are most commonly involved.[200] Antibodies to FcγRIIIb (CD16) have been produced by several mothers who lack NA antigens and have also caused neonatal neutropenia.[33, 34–36] The reported incidence of ANN was 2 per 1000 births,[250] accounting for 1.5% of admissions to neonatal special care units.[250] The reported incidence of alloimmunization to granulocyte antibodies during pregnancies has varied markedly, from 0.17%[251] to 2%[248] of primigravida and multiparous women. Sera from 29 of 147 women at week 34 of their second or subsequent pregnancies contained antibodies to granulocytes, and the presence of the granulocyte antibodies in maternal serum was associated with decreased granulocyte counts in umbilical cord blood.[252]

Autoimmune Neutropenia of Infancy

Neutropenia mediated by autoantibodies has been well described in children (Table 12–8).[30, 202, 207, 253–255] Typically, the autoimmune neutropenia of children begins at 8 months of age, but children between 1 and 36 months of age can be affected.[207, 253, 255] One patient, who was 4 months old when the diagnosis was made, was documented to have had neutropenia beginning at age 3 weeks.[202] A second patient who was 33 days of age at the time of diagnosis had had a normal neutrophil count in the first week after birth.[255] Most studies found that neutrophil counts recover spontaneously by the age of 5 years,[207] with a median of 13 to 20 months of neutropenia.[202, 207, 253, 255] Slightly more females than males are affected.[207]

In most cases, children have severe neutropenia, with neutrophil counts less than 500 cells/μL; occasionally, however, patients may have neutrophil counts over 1000 cells/μL.[202, 253] Monocytosis has been reported to occur in up to 38% of patients.[202] Bone marrow biopsies in infected patients usually show normal to hypercellular marrow with a decreased number of mature granulocytes. Febrile episodes and infections, including bacterial skin infections, otitis media, respiratory tract infections, and urinary tract infections, are common. Life-threatening complications are rare. In some cases, patients treated with corticosteroids show either no or only temporary improvement.[207] Lalezari and colleagues[207, 256] reported that intravenous immunoglobulin resulted in transient recovery of neutrophil counts, lasting up to 9 days, in seven of eight patients; two patients had complete remission. Although the remissions were transient, at least one child showed response to a second treatment.[207]

Table 12–8. Autoimmune Neutropenia of Infancy: Summary of Three Studies

Statistic	Lalezari et al.[207]	Bux et al.[202]	Bux et al.[255]
Number of patients	121	76	240
% Female	59.5	*NA*	54
Age at diagnosis (months)			
Median	8	12	*NA*
Range	3–30	4–30	1–36
Follow-up period	Up to 12 years	6–36 months	*NA*
Number recovering	81	4	30
Age at recovery (months)			
Median	30	*NA*	*NA*
Range	6–60	*NA*	*NA*
Time to recovery (months)			
Median	20	18	17
Range	15–54	9–26	1–38
Granulocyte antibody detected (% of patients)	88.5	*NA*	100
Anti-NA1 detected (% of patients)	8	41	31
Anti-NA2 detected (% of patients)	2	None	3

NA, data not available.

Bux and colleagues treated 7 patients with corticosteroids, 20 with high-dose intravenous IgG (IVIG), and 8 with G-CSF.[255] Half the patients responded to IVIG, but their neutrophil counts remained elevated for only 1 week. All the patients responded to G-CSF and 75% to corticosteroids, and their neutrophil counts remained elevated as long as the drugs were given.

Kuijpers and colleagues used G-CSF to successfully treat an 8-year-old with a 5-year history of autoimmune neutropenia due to antibodies to FcγRIIIb who was resistant to treatment to IVIG and corticosteroids. While G-CSF was given, levels of soluble FcγRIIIb in the plasma increased and the antibody disappeared.[257] When the G-CSF was discontinued, the FcγRIIIb antibodies reappeared and the neutrophil count fell. It is likely that a G-CSF–induced increase in soluble FcγRIIIb levels contributes to the efficiency of G-CSF therapy in patients with antibodies specific to FcγRIIIb.

Antibodies to granulocytes can be detected in up to 98% of affected patients,[207] most commonly directed to NA1 antigen (10% to 46% of patients).[202, 207, 253] Anti-NA2 has been found in 2% to 3% of patients.[30, 202, 207] Disappearance of granulocyte antibodies has been associated with the recovery of neutrophil counts.[202, 207, 253] Finally, autoantibodies specific for anti-NA1 have been associated with the expression of HLA-DR2 antigen phenotype.[258]

Autoimmune Neutropenia in Adults

Neonatal autoimmune neutropenia is also called primary autoimmune neutropenia because it is not associated with other immunological or hematological abnormalities. Although primary autoimmune neutropenia of adults has been described, autoimmune neutropenia in adults has usually been associated with other autoimmune disorders or hematological malignancies[202, 268–263] (Table 12–9). Such secondary autoimmune neutropenia is most commonly seen in people between 40 and 80 years of age and commonly (78% of patients) causes no symptoms of infection.[202]

In many cases of secondary neutropenia, granulocyte antibodies cannot be detected: however, there have been several reports of secondary autoimmune neutropenia in which antibodies to granulocytes have been detected. One patient with primary biliary cirrhosis and neutropenia had an autoantibody specific for NA1 antigen.[262] Hartman and colleagues[264] found that sera from 7 of 50 neutropenic adults reacted with neutrophil actin. Klaassen and associates[263] studied 15 patients infected with human immunodeficiency virus (HIV) and found that sera from 3 patients immunoblotted granulocyte membrane proteins of approximately 50 to 70 kD. Rothko and colleagues[260] immunoblotted sera from 17 patients with secondary autoimmune neutropenia and found that the sera of 16 reacted with a variety of granulocyte membrane proteins between 30 and 120 kD. Immunoprecipitation studies with sera from seven adults from one county in Wisconsin who had secondary autoimmune neutropenia found that the sera of three reacted with an 80-kD protein, serum from one reacted with a 60-kD protein, and serum from one reacted with both 60-kD and 80-kD proteins.[261] Using a monoclonal antigen capture assay, Hartman and Wright[265] found that antibodies from 7 of 50 neutropenic patients reacted with CD11b/CD18 molecules.[265]

Table 12–9. Diseases Associated With Secondary Autoimmune Neutropenia

Disease	Reference(s)
Autoimmune Disorders	
Rheumatoid arthritis	202, 258, 259
Felty's syndrome	202, 258, 260
Systemic lupus erythematosus	202, 258–260
Sjögren's disease	258, 261
Mixed connective tissue syndrome	202
Polymyalgia rheumatica	202
Hashimoto's thyroiditis	258, 259
Immune-complex glomerulonephritis	258
Wegener's granulomatosis	202
Primary biliary cirrhosis	202, 262
Myasthenia gravis	258, 261
Autoimmune Hematologic Disorders	
Autoimmune thrombocytopenia	202, 258, 261
Autoimmune hemolytic anemia	202, 261
Evans' syndrome	202, 258, 261
Hematologic Malignancies	
Leukemia	202
Hodgkin's disease	202
Non-Hodgkin's lymphoma	202
Immune deficiencies	
HIV infection	202, 263
Common variable immune deficiency	202
Other	
Myelodysplastic syndrome	259
Crohn's disease	259
Acute rheumatic fever	258

HIV, human immunodeficiency virus.

Whereas antibodies to granulocyte antigens have been found in many patients, increased levels of circulating immune complexes may be inducing the neutropenia in some patients with secondary neutropenia. One study found that granulocyte antibodies could be detected in only 11% to 19% of the patients with secondary neutropenia, but circulating immune complexes could be detected in 58% of patients with secondary neutropenia.[258] Furthermore, the presence of circulating immune complexes correlated with low neutrophil counts, but the presence of neutrophil antibodies did not.

Severe or life-threatening infections are not common in patients with secondary autoimmune neutropenia, but an occasional patient has been treated with intravenous immunoglobulin, steroids, or granulocyte-macrophage colony-stimulating factor, with resultant transient increments in neutrophil counts.[261, 266–268] A single patient with pure white cell aplasia had a transient response to high-dose intravenous immunoglobulin treatment.[269] Five patients with Felty's syndrome were treated with high-dose intravenous immunoglobulin, but no improvement in neutropenia was seen.[270]

Plasma levels of soluble FcγRIIIb correlate with total body neutrophil mass. Plasma levels of FcγRIIIb are elevated in some patients with chronic neutropenia and may indicate which patients with chronic neutropenia are at risk for infection. In a study of 66 patients with chronic neutropenia but without neutrophil autoantibodies or an autoimmune disease, the 51 patients who did not have bacterial infections were found to have higher levels of soluble FcγRIIIb than were the 15 patients with bacterial infections.[271]

Drug-Induced Immune Granulocytopenias

Drug-induced granulocytopenias are common.[272–295] Although some cases of drug-induced granulocytopenias probably result from direct marrow toxicity, immune-mediated processes may also occur. Drugs implicated in immune-mediated granulocytopenia are listed in Table 12–10. Drug-dependent granulocyte antibodies have been

systemic lupus erythematosus and are often specific for elastase.[115] P-ANCA have also been detected in patients with giant cell arteritis and Felty's syndrome.[333] P-ANCA antibodies specific for lactoferrin have been found in fewer than 5% of patients with necrotizing glomerulonephritis and rarely in patients with systemic lupus erythematosus.[331] Finally, patients with rheumatoid arthritis and ulcerative colitis have been found to have ANCA.[133, 331]

Both clinical and laboratory data suggest that ANCA may play a role in the pathogenesis of these vasculitides. In Wegener's granulomatosis, the ANCA titer is associated with disease activity, and patients with active Wegener's granulomatosis have increased total blood granulocyte pools and turnover rates.[334] Although the antigenic targets of ANCA are not normally expressed on granulocyte plasma membranes, it has been shown that granulocytes primed with inflammatory agents such as TNF express small amounts of cytoplasmic antigens on their surfaces.[118, 335] When these TNF-primed granulocytes are incubated with ANCA, granulocyte stimulation results, and the granulocytes produce toxic oxygen species and release proteolytic enzymes.[334] Granulocytes primed with in vitro TNF and stimulated with ANCA specific for myeloperoxidase have been found to damage cultured human umbilical vein endothelial cells.[334] Because stimulated neutrophils are known to mediate numerous inflammatory reactions, it has been hypothesized that ANCA may not only be markers of disease activity but may also be involved in the pathogenesis of these diseases.[118, 335]

Leukocyte Adhesion Deficiency

Leukocyte adhesion deficiency (LAD) is an inherited syndrome characterized by recurrent infections, impaired wound healing, diminished pus formation, and granulocytosis.[336–339] Affected patients have delayed separation of the umbilical cord after birth and recurrent skin and soft tissue infections in childhood. Later in life, chronic gingivitis and periodontitis lead to tooth loss. Severe pneumonias and fungal infections can occur. Granulocytes from affected patients function abnormally in several respects: decreased ability to aggregate; decreased adhesion to C3bi-coated erythrocytes and to plastic and human endothelial cells; decreased chemotaxis[340]; decreased natural killer cell cytotoxicity; and decreased antibody-dependent cellular cytotoxicity.[341]

LAD syndrome is inherited in an autosomal recessive manner and has been linked to changes in chromosome 21.[338] Granulocytes from affected patients lack integrins CR3, LFA-1, and p150, 90.[342] Monocytes and lymphocytes are also affected. The defect in the expression of integrins results from either absence or abnormal synthesis of the β2 subunit. Although α subunits are synthesized in affected patients, they are not detected on mature leukocytes. A clinically less severe form of the disease that is associated with abnormally low levels of synthesis, but not a complete absence, of the β2 subunit has been reported.[326] Patients with this form have reduced levels, but not absence, of CR3 on their granulocytes. The severity of the patient's clinical symptoms correlates directly with the degree of glycoprotein deficiency.[340]

FcγRIIIb Deficiency

There have been several reports of deficiencies of granulocyte FcγRIIIb and the absence of granulocyte-specific antigens NA1 and NA2. Blood cells from patients with paroxysmal nocturnal hemoglobinuria (PNH) not only lack the GPI-linked complement regulatory protein decay accelerating factor (DAF) but also express decreased amounts of other GPI-linked membrane proteins. Granulocytes from patients with PNH express reduced amounts of the GPI-linked membrane protein FcγRIIIb[21] and the NA antigens.[18]

Genetic deficiencies of granulocyte FcγRIIIb and NA1 and NA2 antigens have also been reported. FcγRIIIb could not be detected on granulocytes from one person with systemic lupus erythematosus through the use of monoclonal and polyclonal antibodies specific for FcγRIIIb.[343] Granulocytes from three mothers of children with ANN[33, 34–36] and from one healthy blood donor[34] have been found to express neither NA1 or NA2 antigens. These granulocytes failed to react with monoclonal antibodies to FcγRIIIb. None of these people had clinical evidence of PNH, and granulocytes from all of them expressed other GPI-linked membrane proteins such as DAF and CD67. Granulocyte FcγRIIIb function was tested in several of these individuals, and their granulocytes bound dimeric IgG[34] or IgG-coated erythrocytes normally.[34, 36] Natural killer cells from two persons were tested for the expression of FcγRIIIa and natural killer cells from both persons expressed FcγRIIIa.[34, 36]

Initial studies found that despite the FcγRIIIb deficiency, all four people (except for the one person with systemic lupus erythematosus) were healthy, had no circulating immune complexes, and showed no increased susceptibility to infections.[33, 34, 36] All three alloimmunized women produced antibodies that reacted with granulocyte FcγRIIIb but did not show allospecificity for NA1 or NA2.[33, 34–36] Analysis of messenger RNA and DNA from patients with FcγRIIIb deficiency found that granulocytes lacked messenger RNA encoding the *FcγRIIIB* gene and that the granulocyte *FcγRIIIB* gene was abnormal or absent[34, 343]; the natural killer *FcγRIIIA* gene, however, is normal in these people.[34, 343] Both parents of one affected patient had one chromosome that expressed a normal granulocyte *FcγRIIIB* gene and one chromosome that expressed an abnormal granulocyte *FcγRIIIB* gene.[34]

The *FcγRIIIB* gene was analyzed in 21 people from 14 families with FcγRIIIb deficiency, and all affected persons were found to lack the *FcγRIIIB* gene.[344] In addition, an adjacent gene, *FcγRIIC,* was also deleted. Two of the 21 people were found to have autoimmune thyroiditis, and 4 had multiple episodes of bacterial infections.[344]

Other Examples of Abnormal Granulocyte Antigen Expression

Several diseases have been associated with decreased expression of granulocyte antigens. Patients with chronic myelogenous leukemia have been reported to have decreased expression of granulocyte-specific antigens NA1, NA2, NB1, and NC1[345, 346] and of 31D8 antigen.[154] The absence of these antigens has been associated with progression of the disease to blast phase. Granulocytes from patients with PNH have decreased expression of or totally lack DAF, FcγRIIIb, acetylcholinesterase, granulocyte alkaline phosphatase, and neutrophil-specific antigens NA1, NA2, and NB1.[18, 347]

Finally, granulocytes from normal full-term neonates have impaired chemotaxis owing to the inability of the granulocytes to upregulate CR3,[348] but the expression of CR3 on resting neonatal granulocytes is normal. Granulocyte phagocytosis and bacterial killing are abnormal in preterm neonates, and their granulocytes have been found to have reduced expression of FcγRIIIb.[349] Neonatal umbilical cord granulocytes have also been found to have a decreased percentage of cells that react with monoclonal antibody 31D8.[152]

CONCLUSION

Since the introduction of Metchnikoff's "theory of immunity" and his recognition of the importance of phagocytosis in this process, much has been learned about the pivotal role of granulocytes in host defense. Furthermore, significant advances have also been made in understanding the immune specificity of granulocyte antigens and their respective antibodies. In this regard, the scientific foundation of granulocyte immunology has been well defined; however, many of the essential features and processes of granulocyte immunobiology are still unknown. The clinical significance of granulocyte antigens and antibodies has been well documented, but little is known about the underlying pathophysiological disease mechanisms. The fields of granulocyte immunochemistry and molecular biology are in their infancy; as these fields mature, results of future studies will further enhance the understanding of granulocyte immunology.

REFERENCES

1. Metchnikoff E. Untersuchungen über die intracellulare verdauung bei wirbellosen thieren. Arb Zool Inst Univ Wien 1883; 5:141.
2. Lalezari P, Nussbaum M, Gelman S, Spaet TH. Neonatal neutropenia due to maternal isoimmunization. Blood 1960; 15:236.
3. Bodmer JG, Marsh SGE, Albert ED, et al. Nomenclature for factors of the HLA system, 1996. Tissue Antigens 1997; 297–321.
4. von dem Borne AEGKr, Decary F. Nomenclature of platelet-specific antigen. Hum Immunol 1990; 29:1.
5. Lalezari P. Alloantigens specific to blood polymorphonuclear neutrophils. *In* Cohen E, Singal D (eds): Non-HLA Antigens in Health, Aging and Malignancy. New York: AR Liss, 1984, pp 23–30.
6. Kline WE, Press C, Clay ME, et al. Three sera defining a new granulocyte–monocyte–T-lymphocyte antigen. Vox Sang 1986; 50:181.
7. Engelfriet CP, Tetteroo PAT, van der Veen JPW, et al. Granulocyte-specific antigens and methods for their detection. *In* McCullough J, Sandler SG (eds): Advances in Immunobiology: Blood Cell Antigens and Bone Marrow Transplantation. New York: AR Liss, 1984, pp 121–54.
8. van Leeuwen A, Ernise JG, van Rood JJ. A new leukocyte group with two alleles: leukocyte group five. Vox Sang 1964; 9:431.
9. Ohto H, Matsuo Y. Neutrophil-specific antigen and gene frequencies in Japanese [Letter]. Transfusion 1989; 29:654.
10. Fromont P, Bettaieb A, Skouri H, et al. Frequency of the polymorphonuclear neutrophil Fcγ receptor III deficiency in the French population and its involvement in the development of neonatal alloimmune neutropenia. Blood 1992; 79:2131.
11. Warkentin PI, Clay ME, Kersey JH, et al. Successful engraftment of NA1 positive bone marrow in a patient with a neutrophil antibody, anti-NA1. Hum Immunol 1981; 2:173.
12. Verheugt FWA, von dem Borne AEGKr, van Noord-Bokhorst JC, et al. Serological immunochemical and immunocytological properties of granulocyte antibodies. Vox Sang 1978; 35:294.
13. Boxer LA, Yokoyama M, Lalezari P. Isoimmune neonatal neutropenia. J Pediatr 1972; 80:782.
14. Madyastha PR, Glassman AB, Levine DH. Incidence of neutrophil antigens on human cord neutrophils. Am J Reprod Immunol 1984; 6:124.
15. Lalezari P, Radel E. Neutrophil-specific antigens: immunology and clinical significance. Semin Hematol 1974; 11:281.
16. Lalezari P, Bernard GE. An isologous antigen-antibody reaction with human neutrophils, related to neonatal neutropenia. J Clin Invest 1966; 45:1741.
17. Werner G, von dem Borne AEGKr, Bos MJE, et al. Localization of human NA1 alloantigen on neutrophil Fcγ-receptors. *In* Reinherz EL, Haynes BF, Nadler LM, Bernstein ID (eds): Leukocyte Typing II: Human Myeloid and Hematopoietic Cells. New York: Springer-Verlag, 1986, pp 109–121.
18. Huizinga TWJ, Kleijer M, Tetteroo PAT, et al. Biallelic neutrophil NA-antigen system is associated with a polymorphism on the phospho-inositol–linked Fcγ-receptor III (CD16). Blood 1990; 75:213.
19. Stroncek DF, Shankar R, Litz C, Clement L. The expression of the NB1 antigen on myeloid precursors and neutrophils from children and umbilical cords. Transfus Med 1998; 8:119–123.
20. Low MG. Biochemistry of glycosyl-phosphatidylinositol membrane protein anchors. Biochem J 1987; 244:1.
21. Huizinga TWJ, van der Schoot CE, Jost C, et al. The PI-linked receptor for FcRIII is released on stimulation of neutrophils. Nature 1988; 333:37.
22. Huizinga TWJ, de Haas M, Kleijer M, et al. Soluble Fcγ-receptor III in human plasma originates from release by neutrophils. J Clin Invest 1990; 86:416.
23. Trounstine ML, Peitz GA, Yssel H, et al. Reactivity of cloned, expressed human FcRIII isoforms with monoclonal antibodies which distinguish cell type specific and allelic forms of Fc-gamma-RIII. Int Immunol 1990; 2:303.
24. Ory PA, Clark MR, Kwoh EE, et al. Sequences of complementary DNAs that encode the NA1 and NA2 forms of Fc receptor III on human neutrophils. J Clin Invest 1989; 84:1688.
25. Scallon BJ, Scigliano E, Freedman VH, et al. A human immunoglobulin G receptor exists in both polypeptide-anchored and phosphatidylinositol-glycan–anchored forms. Proc Natl Acad Sci U S A 1989; 86:5079.
26. Bux J, Stein EL, Santoso S, Mueller-Eckardt C. NA gene frequencies in the German population, determined by polymerase chain reaction with sequence-specific primers. Transfusion 1995; 35:54–57.
27. Hessner MJ, Curtis BR, Endean DJ, Aster RH. Determination of neutrophil antigen frequencies in five ethnic groups by polymerase chain reaction with sequence-specific primers. Transfusion 1996; 36:895–899.
28. Ravetch JV, Perussia B. Alternative membrane forms of FcγRIII (CD16) on human natural killer cells and neutrophils. J Exp Med 1989; 170:481.
29. Salmon JE, Edberg JC, Kimberly RP, et al. FcγRIII on human neutrophils. Allelic variants have functionally distinct capacities. J Clin Invest 1990; 85:1287.
30. Lalezari P, Jiang AF, Yegen L, Santorineou M. Chronic autoimmune neutropenia due to anti-NA2 antibody. N Engl J Med 1975; 293:744.
31. McCullough J, Clay M, Press C, Kline W. Granulocyte Serology: A Clinical and Laboratory Guide. Chicago: American Society of Clinical Pathology, 1988, pp 52–53.
32. Schnell M, Halligan G, Herman J. A new granulocyte antibody directed at a high frequency antigen causing neonatal alloimmune neutropenia [Abstract]. Transfusion 1989; 29(suppl):46S.

33. Huizinga TWJ, Kuijpers RWAM, Kleijer M, et al. Maternal genomic neutrophil FcRIII deficiency leading to neonatal isoimmune neutropenia. Blood 1990; 76:1927.
34. Carfron J, Celton JL, Gane P, Cantron JP. Antibody against the FcγRIII of neutrophils in alloimmune neonatal neutropenia [Abstract]. Blood 1990; 76(suppl 1):177a.
35. Stroncek DF, Skubitz KM, Plachta LB, et al. Alloimmune neonatal neutropenia due to an antibody to the neutrophil Fcγ-receptor III with maternal deficiency of CD16 antigen. Blood 1991; 77:1572.
36. Bux J, Stein E-L, Bierling P, et al. Characterization of a new alloantigen (SH) on the human neutrophil Fcγ-receptor IIIb. Blood 1997; 89:1027–1034.
37. Koene HR, Marron M, Roos D, et al. *FcγRIIIB* gene duplication: evidence for presence and expression of three distinct *FcγRIIIB* genes NA(1+, 2+) SH(+) individuals. Blood 1998; 91:673–679.
38. Lalezari P, Murphy GB, Allen FH. NB1, a new neutrophil antigen involved in the pathogenesis of neonatal neutropenia. J Clin Invest 1971; 50:1108.
39. Huang ST, Lin J, McGowan EI, Lalezari P. NB2, a new allele of NB1 antigen involved in febrile transfusion reaction [Abstract]. Transfusion 1982; 22:426.
40. Lalezari P, Petrosova M, Jiang AF. NB2, an allele of NB1 neutrophil specific antigen: relationship to 9a [Abstract]. Transfusion 1982; 22:433.
41. McCullough J, Clay M, Press C, Kline W. Granulocyte Serology: A Clinical and Laboratory Guide. Chicago: American Society of Clinical Pathology, 1988, p 54.
42. Lalezari P, Khorshidi M. Detection of neutrophil and platelet antibodies: agglutination, immunofluorescence and flow cytometry. *In* Greenwalt TJ (ed): Blood Transfusion; Methods in Hematology. New York: Churchill Livingstone, 1988, pp 149–162.
43. Stroncek DF, Shankar RA, Noren PA, et al. Analysis of the expression of NB1 antigen using two monoclonal antibodies. Transfusion 1996; 36:168–174.
44. Stroncek DF, Plachta LB, Herr GP, Dalmasso AP. Analysis of the expression of neutrophil-specific antigen NB1: characterization of neutrophils that react with but are not agglutinated by anti-NB1. Transfusion 1993; 33:656–660.
45. Stroncek DF, Jaszcz W, Herr G, et al. Expression of neutrophil antigens after 10 days of granulocyte colony-stimulating factor. Transfusion 1998; 38:663–668.
46. Stroncek DF, Skubitz KM, McCullough JJ. Biochemical characterization of the neutrophil-specific antigen NB1. Blood 1990; 75:744.
47. Skubitz KM, Stroncek DF, Sun B. The neutrophil-specific antigen NB1 is anchored via a glycosyl-phosphatidylinositol linkage. J Leukoc Biol 1991; 49:163.
48. Goldschmeding R, van Dalen CM, Faber N, et al. Further characterization of the NB1 antigen as a variably expressed 56–62 kDa GPI-linked glycoprotein of plasma membranes and specific granules of neutrophils. Br J Haematol 1992; 81:336.
49. Stroncek DF, Shankar RA, Plachta LB, et al. Polycolonal antibodies against the NB1-bearing 58- to 64-kDa glycoprotein of human neutrophils do not identify an NB2-bearing molecule. Transfusion 1993; 33:399.
50. Lalezari P, Thalenfeld B, Weinstein WJ. The third neutrophil antigen. *In* Terasaki PI (ed): Histocompatibility Testing. Baltimore: Williams & Wilkins, 1970, pp 319–322.
51. Lalezari P. Neutrophil antigens: immunology and clinical implications. *In* Greenwalt TJ, Jamieson GA (eds): The Granulocyte: Function and Clinical Utilization [Progress in Clinical and Biological Research]. New York: AR Liss, 1977, pp 209–225.
52. Verheugt FWA. Neutrophil antigens and antibodies [Thesis]. Amsterdam, University of Amsterdam, 1977.
53. Schacter B, Preis P, Kadushin JM, et al. Family studies of neutrophil alloantigens in bone marrow transplantation. Tissue Antigens 1980; 16:267.
54. Schacter B, Kadushin J, Hsieh K. Neutrophil antigens: population and family studies Caucasians and blacks [Abstract]. Hum Immunol 1980; 1:280.
55. Kline WE, Press C, Uhlich A, et al. Association of neutrophil specific antigens NA2 and NC1 [Abstract]. Transfusion 1984; 24:431.
56. McCullough J, Clay M, Press C, Kline W. Granulocyte Serology: A Clinical and Laboratory Guide. Chicago: American Society of Clinical Pathology, 1988, pp 54–55.
57. Verheugt FWA, von dem Borne AEGKr, van Noord-Bokhorst JC, et al. ND1, a new neutrophil granulocyte antigen. Vox Sang 1978; 35:13.
58. Claas FHJ, Langerak J, Sabbe LJM, van Rood JJ. NE1, a new neutrophil specific antigen. Tissue Antigens 1979; 13:129.
59. Helmerhorst FM, Claas FHJ, van Dalen C, et al. Neutrophil specific antigen NE1 is not the antithetical allele of ND1. Tissue Antigens 1981; 18:139.
60. Clay ME, Kline WE, McCullough J. Granulocyte antigens and antibodies: current concepts of detection and histocompatibility testing. *In* Dutcher JP (ed): Modern Transfusion Therapy, vol 2. Boca Raton, FL: CRC Press, 1990, pp 171–225.
61. Bux J, Chapman J. Report of the Second International Granulocyte Serology Workshop. Transfusion 1997; 37:977–983.
62. van Rood JJ, van Leeuwen A, Schippers AMJ, et al. Immunogenetics of the group four, five and nine systems. *In* Curtoni ES, Mattiuz PL, Tosi RM (eds): Histocompatibility Testing 1967. Baltimore: Williams & Wilkins, 1967, pp 203–219.
63. Van Kessel AHMG, Stoker K, Claas FHJ, et al. Assignment of the leukocyte group five surface antigens to human chromosome 4. Tissue Antigens 1983; 21:213.
64. Warren RP, Storb R, Nguyen DD, Thomas ED. Association between leukocyte group-5a antigen and acute lymphoblastic leukemia. Lancet 1977; 1:509.
65. Warren RP, Lum LG, Storb R. Is the leukocyte group-5a antigen associated with reduced NK cell function? Tissue Antigens 1985; 25:107.
66. Lalezari P, Bernard GE. Identification of a specific leukocyte antigen: another presumed example of 5b. Transfusion 1965; 5:135.
67. Lawler SD, Shatwell HS. Some comments on the leukocyte antigen 5b. *In* Curtoni ES, Mattiuz PL, Tosi RM (eds): Histocompatibility Testing 1967. Baltimore: Williams & Wilkins, 1967, pp 247–250.
68. Nordhagen R, Conradi M, Dromtorp SM. Pulmonary reaction associated with transfusion of plasma containing anti-5b. Vox Sang 1986; 51:102.
69. Seeger W, Schneider U, Kreusler B, et al. Reproduction of transfusion related acute lung injury in an ex vivo lung model. Blood 1990; 76:1438.
70. van Rood JJ, van Leeuwen A, Schippers AMJ, et al. Leukocyte groups, the normal lymphocyte transfer test and homograft sensitivity. *In* Amos DB, van Rood JJ (eds.) Histocompatibility Testing 1965. Copenhagen: Munksgaard, 1965, pp 37–50.
71. Lalezari P. Granulocyte antigen systems. *In* Engelfreit CP, van Loghem JJ, von dem Borne AEGKr (eds): Immunohaematology. Amsterdam: Elsevier Scientific Publishers, 1984, pp 33–43.
72. van Rood JJ, van Leeuwen A, Rubinstein P. Isoantigens of leukocytes and platelets. *In* Miescher P, Muller-Eberhard H (eds): Textbook of Immunopathology II. New York: Grune & Stratton, 1969, pp 469–499.
73. Jager MJ, Claas FHJ, Witvliet M, van Rood JJ. Correspondence of the monocyte antigen HMA-1 to the non-HLA antigen 9a. Immunogenetics 1986; 23:71.
74. Kline WE, Press C, Clay ME, et al. Three sera defining a new granulocyte-monocyte–T-lymphocyte antigen. Vox Sang 1986; 50:181.
75. Simsek S, van der Schoot CE, Daams M, et al. Molecular characterization of antigenic polymorphisms (Ond^{a} and Mart^{a}) of the β2 family recognized by human leukocyte alloantisera. Blood 1996; 88:1350.
76. Thompson JS. Antileukocyte capillary agglutinating antibody in pre and post-transplantation sera. *In* Rose NR, Friedman H (eds): Manual of Clinical Immunology. Washington DC: American Society for Microbiology, 1976, pp 868–873.
77. Dausset J. Leuco-agglutinins IV: leuco-agglutinins and blood transfusion. Vox Sang 1954; 4:190.
78. Metzgar RS, Zmijewski CM, Siegler HF, et al. A comparison of the leukocyte agglutination and mixed agglutination techniques to detect human tissue antigens. Transplantation 1968; 6:84.
79. Engelfriet CP, Tetteroo PAT, van der Veen JPW, et al. Granulocyte-specific antigens and methods for their detection. *In* McCullough J, Sandler SG (eds): Advances in Immunobiology: Blood Cell Antigens and Bone Marrow Transplantation. [Progress in Clinical and Biological Research]. New York: AR Liss, 1984, pp 121–154.
80. Thompson JS, Severson CD. Granulocyte antigens. *In* Bell CA

(ed): A Seminar on Antigens on Blood Cells and Body Fluid. Washington DC: American Association of Blood Banks, 1980, pp 151–169.
81. Dunstan RA, Simpson MB, Sanfilippo FP. Absence of specific HLA-DR antigens on human platelets and neutrophils [Abstract]. Blood 1984; 64:85a.
82. Minchinton RM, Waters AH. Chloroquine stripping of HLA antigens from neutrophils without removal of neutrophil-specific antigens. Br J Haematol 1984; 57:703.
83. Kline WE, Jackson N, Boese C, et al. Comparison of granulocytes, neutroplasts and frozen-stored neutroplasts for granulocyte antibody identification [Abstract]. Transfusion 1986; 26:583.
84. McCullough J, Clay M, Press C, Kline W. Granulocyte Serology: A Clinical Laboratory Guide. Chicago: American Society of Clinical Pathology, 1988, p 60.
85. Dutcher JP, Schiffer CA, Johnson GS, et al. Alloimmunization prevents the migration of transfused indium-111–labeled granulocytes to sites of infection. Blood 1983; 62:354–360.
86. Dutcher JP, Riggs C, Fox JJ, et al. Effect of histocompatibility factors on pulmonary retention of ^{111}indium labeled granulocytes. Am J Hematol 1990; 33:238.
87. McCullough J, Clay M, Press C, Kline W. Granulocyte Serology: A Clinical Laboratory Guide. Chicago: American Society of Clinical Pathology, 1988, pp 58–59.
88. Berroche L, Maupin B, Hervier P, Dausset J. Mise en evidence des antigènes A et B dans les leucocytes humains par des épreuves d'absorption et d'élution. Vox Sang 1955; 5:82.
89. Gurner BW, Coombs RRA. Examination of human leukocytes for the ABO, MN, Rh, Tja, Lutheran and Lewis systems of antigens by means of mixed erythrocyte-leukocyte agglutination. Vox Sang 1958; 3:13.
90. Lalezari P, Bernard G. Studies on human leukocyte antigens. *In* Proceedings of the 9th Conference of the European Society of Haematologists. New York: S Karger, 1963, pp 1084–1087.
91. Kelton JG, Bebenek G. Granulocytes do not have surface ABO antigens. Transfusion 1985; 25:567.
92. Gaidulis L, Branch DR, Lazar GS, et al. The red cell antigens A, B, D, U, Ge, Jk3, and Yta are not detected on human granulocytes. Br J Haematol 1985; 60:659.
93. Dunstan RA, Simpson MB, Borowitz M. Absence of ABH antigens on neutrophils. Br J Haematol 1985; 60:651.
94. Karhi KK, Andersson LC, Vuopio P, Gahmberg CG. Expession of blood group A antigens in human bone marrow cells. Blood 1981; 57:147.
95. Lalezari P. Biological roles of tissue-specific and systemic alloantigens. *In* McCullough J, Sandler SG (eds): Advances in Immunobiology: Blood Cell Antigens and Bone Marrow Transplantation [Progress in Clinical and Biological Research]. New York: AR Liss, 1984, pp 55–75.
96. Dunstan RA. Status of major red cell blood group antigens on neutrophils, lymphocytes and monocytes. Br J Haematol 1986; 62:301.
97. Braman AM, Davis J, Schwartz KA. A radioimmune microfilter plate assay for the detection of anti-granulocyte antibodies. Am J Hematol 1992; 39:194.
98. McCullough J, Clay M, Hurd D, et al. Effect of leukocyte antibodies and HLA matching on the intravascular recovery, survival, and tissue localization of 111-indium granulocytes. Blood 1986; 67:522.
99. Lucas GF, Carrington PA. Results of the First International Granulocyte Serology Workshop. Vox Sang 1990; 59:251.
100. Bux J, Chapman J. Report on the Second International Granulocyte Serology Workshop. Transfusion 1997; 37:977.
101. Madyastha PR, Glassman A, Levine D, et al. Identification of a new neutrophil antigen (CN1) more prevalent among American blacks [Abstract]. Transfusion 1983; 23:426.
102. Madyastha PR, Glassman AB. Neutrophil antigens and antibodies in the diagnosis of immune neutropenias. Ann Clin Lab Sci 1989; 19(3):146.
103. Herman JH, Williams JK, Keashen-Schnell M, Stroncek D. Neutrophil NA-locus antigen typing of a large donor population: preliminary data [Abstract]. Blood 1991; 78(suppl 1):102a.
104. Rodwell RL, Tudehope DI, O'Regan P, et al. Alloimmune neonatal neutropenia in Australian aboriginals: an unrecognized disorder? Transfus Med 1991; 1:63.
105. Stroncek D, Ramsey G, Eiber G, et al. Identification of a new granulocyte-specific antigen [Abstract]. Transfusion 1991; 31:655.
106. Faber V, Elling P, Norup G, et al. An antinuclear factor specific for leukocytes. Lancet 1964; 2:344.
107. Wiik A, Munthe E. Restriction among heavy and light chain determinants of granulocyte-specific antinuclear factors. Immunology 1972; 23:53.
108. van der Woude FJ, Rasmussen N, Lobatto S, et al. Autoantibodies against neutrophils and monocytes: tool for diagnosis and marker of disease activity in Wegener's granulomatosis. Lancet 1985; 1:425.
109. Rasmussen N, Wiik A. Autoimmunity in Wegener's granulomatosis. Immunobiology autoimmunity and transplantation in otorhinolaryngology. *In* Veldman JE, McCabe BF, Houzing EH, Mygind N (eds): Proceedings, 1st International Conference, Utrecht, The Netherlands, 1984. Amsterdam: Kugler, 1985, pp 231–236.
110. Jennette JC, Falk RJ. Diagnostic classification of antineutrophil cytoplasmic autoantibody-associated vasculitides. Am J Kidney Dis 1991; 18(2):184.
111. Wieslander J: How are antineutrophil cytoplasmic autoantibodies detected? Am J Kid Diseases 1991; 18(2):154.
112. Proceedings of the First International Workshop on Anti-Neutrophil Cytoplasm Antibodies (ANCA), Copenhagen, 1988. APMIS Suppl 1989; 6:1.
113. Proceedings of the Second International Workshop on Antineutrophil Cytoplasmic Antibodies (ANCA), Noordwijkerhout, 1989. Neth J Med 1990; 36:87.
114. Falk RJ, Jennette JC. The Third International Workshop on Antineutrophil Cytoplasmic Autoantibodies. Am J Kidney Dis 1991; 18(2):145.
115. Goldschmeding R, van der Schoot CE, ten Bokkel Huinink D, et al. Wegener's granulomatosis autoantibodies identify a novel diisopropylfluorophosphate-binding protein in the lysosomes of normal human neutrophils. J Clin Invest 1989; 84:1577.
116. Niles JL, McCluskey RT, Ahmad MF. Wegener's granulomatosis autoantigen is a novel neutrophil serine proteinase. Blood 1989; 74:1888.
117. Wieslander J, Rasmussen N, Bygren P. An ELISA for ANCA and preliminary studies of the antigen involved. Acta Pathol Microbiol Immunol Scand 1989; 97:42.
118. Ludemann J, Utecht B, Gross WL. Anti-neutrophil cytoplasm antibodies in Wegener's granulomatosis recognize an elastinolytic enzyme. J Exp Med 1990; 171:357.
119. Kao RC, Wehner NG, Skubitz KM, et al. Proteinase 3. A distinct human polymorphonuclear leukocyte proteinase that produces emphysema in hamsters. J Clin Invest 1988; 82:1963.
120. Jenne DE, Tschopp J, Ludemann J, et al. Wegener's autoantigen decoded [Letter]. Nature 1990; 346:520.
121. Jennette JC, Hoidal JH, Falk RJ. Specificity of antineutrophil cytoplasmic autoantibodies for proteinase 3. Blood 1990; 75:2263.
122. Lesavre P. Antineutrophil cytoplasmic autoantibodies antigen specificity. Am J Kid Dis 1991; 18(2):159.
123. Falk RJ, Jennette JC. Anti-neutrophil cytoplasmic autoantibodies with specificity for myeloperoxidase in patients with systemic vasculitis and idiopathic necrotizing and crescentic glomerulonephritis. N Engl J Med 1988; 318:1651.
124. Locke IC, Cambridge G. Autoantibodies to neutrophil granule proteins: Pathogenic potential in vasculitis? Br J Biomed Sci 1996; 53:302–316.
125. Calafat J, Goldschmeding R, Ringeling PL, et al. In situ localization by double-labeling immunoelectron microscopy of anti-neutrophil cytoplasmic autoantibodies in neutrophils and monocytes. Blood 1990; 75:242.
126. Pereira HA, Spitznagel JK, Winton EF, et al. The ontogeny of a 57 kDa cationic antimicrobial protein of human polymorphonuclear leukocytes: Localization to a novel granule population. Blood 1990;76: 825–34.
127. Falk RJ, Becker M, Terrell R, Jennette JC. Antigen specificity of p-ANCA and of c-ANCA. Am J Kidney Dis 1991; 18(2):197.
128. Nassberger L, Jonsson H, Sjoholm AG, et al. Circulating anti-elastase in systemic lupus erythematosus. Lancet 1989; 1:509.
129. Thompson RA, Lee SS. Antineutrophil cytoplasmic antibodies [Letter]. Lancet 1989; 1:670.
130. Dolman KM, Goldschmeding R, Sonnenberg A, von dem Borne AEGKr. ANCA related antigens. APMIS Suppl 1990; 19:28.
131. Pozzi C, Radice A, Rota S, et al. Clinical significance of anti-lactoferrin antibodies in renal disease. Am J Kidney Dis 1991; 18(2):202.

132. Flesch BK, Lampe M, Rautman A. Anti-elastase cathepsin G and lactoferrin antibodies in sera with c-ANCA or with atypical fluorescence staining pattern. Am J Kidney Dis 1991; 18(2):201.
133. Jennette JC, Falk RJ. Antineutrophil cytoplasmic autoantibodies and associated diseases: a review. Am J Kidney Dis 1990; 15:517.
134. Knapp W, Dörken B, Rieber P, et al. CD antigens 1989. Blood 1989; 74:1448.
135. van der Schoot CE, Visser FJ, Bos MJE, et al. Serological and biochemical characterization of myeloid-specific antibodies of the myeloid panel. *In* McMichael AJ, Beverley PCL, Cobbold S, et al (eds): Leukocyte Tying III. White Cell Differentiation Antigens. Oxford, UK: Oxford University Press, 1987, pp 603–611.
136. Tetteroo PAT, van der Schoot CE, Visser FJ, et al. Three different types of Fcγ receptors on human leukocytes defined by workshop antibodies; $Fc\gamma R_{low}$ of neutrophils, $Fc\gamma R_{low}$ of K/NK lymphocytes, and FcγRII. *In* McMichael AJ, Beverley PCL, Cobbold S, et al (eds): Leukocyte Typing III. White Cell Differentiation Antigens. Oxford, UK: Oxford University Press, 1987, pp 702–706.
137. Huizinga TWJ, Kleijer M, Roos D, von dem Borne AEGKr. Differences between FcRIII of human neutrophils and human K/NK lymphocytes in relation to the NA antigen system. *In* Knapp W, Dorken B, Gilks WR, et al (eds): Leucocyte Typing IV. White Cell Differentiation Antigens. Oxford, UK: Oxford University Press, 1989, pp 582–585.
138. Selvaraj P, Hibbs ML, Carpen O, Springer TA. Reactivity of workshop CD16 mAb with distinct membrane-anchored forms of CD16. *In* Knapp W, Dorken B, Gilks WR, et al (eds): Leucocyte Typing IV. White Cell Differentiation Antigens. Oxford, UK: Oxford University Press, 1989, pp 595–597.
139. Clement LT, Lehmeyer JE, Gartland GL. Identification of neutrophil subpopulations with monoclonal antibodies. Blood 1983; 61:326.
140. Berkow RL, Baehner RL. Volume-dependent human polymorphonuclear leukocyte heterogeneity demonstrated with counterflow centrifugal elutriation. Blood 1985; 65:71.
141. Miyagawa H, Okada C, Sugiyama H, et al. Heterogeneity in chemotaxis of neutrophils with different densities. Biochem Biophys Res Commun 1990; 172:1094.
142. Fritzsche R, DeWeck AL. Chemiluminescence microscopy reveals functional heterogeneity in single neutrophils undergoing oxygen burst. Eur J Immunol 1988; 18:817.
143. Fletcher MP, Seligmann BE. PMN heterogeneity: long-term stability of fluorescent membrane potential responses to the chemoattractant *N*-formyl-methionyl-leucyl-phenylalanine in healthy adults and correlation with respiratory burst activity. Blood 1986; 68:611.
144. Seligmann B, Chused TM, Gallin JI. Human neutrophil heterogeneity identified using flow microfluorometry to monitor membrane potential. J Clin Invest 1981; 68:1125.
145. Klempner MS, Gallin JI. Separation and functional characterization of human neutrophil subpopulations. Blood 1978; 51:659.
146. Fanger MW, Shen L, Pugh J, Bernier GM. Subpopulations of human peripheral granulocytes and monocytes express receptors for IgA. Proc Natl Acad Sci U S A 1980; 77:3640.
147. Whited SC, Santaella M, Frank MM, et al. Binding of immunoglobulin- and complement-coated erythrocytes to human neutrophil subpopulations. Inflammation 1981; 5:103.
148. Broxmeyer HE, Ralph P, Bognacki J, et al. A subpopulation of human polymorphonuclear neutrophils contains an active form of lactoferrin capable of binding to human monocytes and inhibiting production of granulocyte-macrophage colony stimulating activities. J Immunol 1980; 125:903.
149. Harvath L, Leonard EJ. Two neutrophil populations in human blood with different chemotactic activities: separation and chemoattractant binding. Infect Immunol 1982; 36:443.
150. Seligmann B, Malech HL, Melnick DA, Gallin JI. An antibody binding to human neutrophils demonstrates antigenic heterogeneity early in myeloid maturation which correlates with functional heterogeneity of mature neutrophils. J Immunol 1985; 135:2647.
151. McCormack RT, Nelson RD, Chenoweth DE, LeBien TW. Identification and characterization of a unique subpopulation (CALLA/CD10-negative) of human neutrophils manifesting a heightened chemotactic response to activated complement. Blood 1987; 70:1624.
152. Seligmann B, Malech HL, Melnick DA, Gallin JI. An antibody to a subpopulation of neutrophils demonstrates antigenic heterogeneity which correlates with response heterogeneity. Trans Assoc Am Physicians 1984; 97:319.
153. Krause PJ, Malech HL, Kristie J, et al. Polymorphonuclear leukocyte heterogeneity in neonates and adults. Blood 1986; 68:200.
154. Gallin JI, Jacobson RJ, Seligmann BE, et al. A neutrophil membrane marker reveals two groups of chronic myelogenous leukemia and its absence may be a marker of disease progression. Blood 1986; 68:343.
155. Krause PJ, Maderazo EG, Bannon P, et al. Neutrophil heterogeneity in patients with blunt trauma. J Lab Clin Med 1988; 112:208.
156. Brown CC, Malech HL, Gallin JI. Intravenous endotoxin recruits a distinct subset of human neutrophils, defined by monoclonal antibody 31D8, from bone marrow to the peripheral circulation. Cell Immunol 1989; 123:294.
157. Krause PJ, Todd MB, Hancock WW, et al. The role of cellular maturation in neutrophil heterogeneity. Blood 1990; 76:1639.
158. Lalezari P, Bernard GE. Improved leukocyte antibody detection with prolonged incubation. Vox Sang 1964; 9:664.
159. Lalezari P, Jiange A, Lee S. A microagglutination technique for detection of leukocyte agglutinins. *In* Ray JG, Hare DB, Pederson PD, Mallally DI (eds): NIAID Manual of Tissue Typing Techniques [DHEW Publication (NIH) 77-545]. Bethesda, MD: U.S. Office of Health, Education and Welfare, 1976–1977, pp 4–6.
160. Lalezari P, Pryce SC. Detection of neutrophil and platelet antibodies in immunologically induced neutropenia and thrombocytopenia. *In* Rose NR, Friedmann H (eds): Manual of Clinical Immunology. Washington, DC: American Society for Microbiology, 1980, pp 744–749.
161. Thompson JS, Severson CD, Lavender AR, et al. Assay of human leukoagglutinins by capillary migration. Transplantation 1968; 6:728.
162. Severson CD, Greazel NA, Thompson JS: Micro-capillary agglutination. J Immunol Methods 1974; 4:369.
163. McCullough J, Burke ME, Wood N, et al. Microcapillary agglutination for the detection of leukocyte antibodies: evaluation of the method and clinical significance in transfusion reactions. Transfusion 1974; 14:425.
164. Hasegawa T, Graw RG, Terasaki PI. A microgranulocyte cytotoxicity test. Transplantation 1974; 15:492.
165. Caplan SN, Berkman EM, Babior BM. Cytotoxins against a granulocyte antigen system: detection by a new method employing cytochalasin-B–treated cells. Vox Sang 1977; 33:206.
166. Drew SI, Bergh O, McClelland J, et al. Antigenic specificities detected on papainized human granulocytes by microgranulocytotoxicity. Transplant Proc 1977; 9:639.
167. Drew SI, Carter BM, Guidera D, et al. Further aspects of microgranulocytotoxicity. Transfusion 1979; 19:434.
168. Hasegawa T, Bergh OJ, Mickey MR, Terasaki PI. Preliminary human granulocyte specificities. Transplant Proc 1975; 7:75.
169. Takasugi M. Improved fluorochromatic cytotoxic test. Transplantation 1971; 12:148.
170. Logue GL, Kurlander R, Pepe P, et al. Antibody-dependent lymphocyte-mediated granulocyte cytotoxicity in man. Blood 1978; 51:97.
171. Richards K, Sadrzadeh SMH, Clay M, McCullough J. Antibody-dependent lymphocyte-mediated granulocytotoxicity (ADLG) for the detection of granulocyte antibodies. J Immunol Methods 1983; 63:93.
172. Verheugt FWA, von dem Borne AEGKr, Decary S, et al. The detection of granulocyte alloantibodies with an indirect immunofluorescence test. Br J Haematol 1977; 36:533.
173. Verheugt FWA, von dem Borne AEGKr, van Noord-Bokhorst JC, et al. Autoimmune granulocytopenia: the detection of granulocyte autoantibodies with the immunofluorescence test. Br J Haematol 1978; 39:339.
174. von dem Borne AEGKr, van dem Plas-van Dalen C, Engelfriet CP. Immunofluorescence antiglobulin test. *In* McMillan R (ed): Immune Cytopenias. New York: Churchill Livingstone, 1983, pp 106–127.
175. Zaroulis CG, Jaramillo S. A microimmunofluorescent assay to detect human granulocyte antigens and antibodies. Am J Hematol 1981; 10:65.
176. Press C, Kline WE, Clay ME, McCullough J. A microtiter modification of granulocyte immunofluorescence. Vox Sang 1985; 49:110.

177. Henke M, Yonemoto LM, Lazar GS, et al. Visual detection of granulocyte surface antigens using the avidin-biotin complex. J Histochem Cytochem 1984; 32:712.
178. Mannoni P, Janowska-Wieczorek A, Turner AR, et al. Monoclonal antibodies against human granulocytes and myeloid differentiation antigens. Hum Immunol 1982; 5:309.
179. Rustagi PK, Currie MS, Logue GL. Complement-activating antineutrophil antibody in systemic lupus erythematosus. Am J Med 1985; 78:971.
180. Cines DB, Pessaro F, Guerry D, et al. Granulocyte-associated IgG in neutropenic disorders. Blood 1982; 59:124.
181. McCallister JA, Boxer LA, Baehner RL. The use and limitation of labeled staphylococcal protein A for study of antineutrophil antibodies. Blood 1979; 54:1330.
182. Lazar GS, Gaidulis L, Henke M, Blume KG. A sensitive screening method of detecting anti-granulocyte antibodies employing radiolabeled staphylococcal protein A. J Immunol Methods 1984; 68:1.
183. Bux J, Kober B, Kiefel V, Mueller-Eckhardt C. Analysis of granulocyte-reactive antibodies using an immunoassay based upon monoclonal antibody-specific immobilization of granulocyte antigens. Transfus Med 1993; 3:157.
184. Boxer LA, Stossel TP. Effects of anti-human neutrophil antibodies in vitro. Quantitative studies. J Clin Invest 1974; 53:1534.
185. Boxer LA, Greenberg SM, Boxer GJ, Stossel SP. Autoimmune neutropenia. N Engl J Med 1975; 293:748.
186. Drew S, Terasaki PI. Autoimmune cytotoxic granulocyte antibodies in normal persons and various diseases. Blood 1978; 52:941.
187. McCullough J, Clay ME, Priest JR, et al. A comparison of methods for detecting leukocyte antibodies in autoimmune neutropenia. Transfusion 1981; 21:483.
188. Thompson JS, Overlin VL, Herbick JM, et al. New granulocyte antigens demonstrated by microgranulocytotoxicity assay. J Clin Invest 1980; 65:1431.
189. McCullough J, Clay M, Press C, Kline W. Granulocyte Serology: A Clinical and Laboratory Guide. Chicago: American Society of Clinical Pathology, 1988, pp 155–195.
190. Hagen Ec, Andrassy K, Csernok E, et al. Development and standardization of solid phase assays of the detection of anti-neutrophil cytoplasmic antibodies (ANCP). A report of the second phase of an international cooperative study on the standardization of ANCA assays. J Immunol Methods 1996; 196:1–15.
191. Wiik A. Delineation of a standard procedure for indirect immunofluorescence detection of ANCA. APMIS 1989; 67:12.
192. Wiik A. Granulocyte specific antinuclear antibodies. Allergy 1980; 35:263.
193. Savige JA, Yeung SP, Gallicchio M, Davies DJ. Two ELISAs to detect antineutrophil cytoplasm antibodies (ANCA) in various vasculitides. Pathology 1989; 21:282.
194. Rasmussen N, Ludermann J, Utecht B. ELISA examination for IgG-ANCA in sera submitted for the First International Workshop on ANCA. APMIS 1989; 97:21.
195. Bygren P, Wieslander J, Rasmussen N, et al. An ELISA for the detection of anti-neutrophil cytoplasm antibodies (ANCA). J Immunol Methods 1990; 127:139.
196. Ludemann J, Utecht B, Gross WL. Detection and quantitation of anti-neutrophil cytoplasm antibodies in Wegener's granulomatosis by ELISA using affinity purified antigen. J Immunol Methods 1988; 114:167.
197. Savage CO, Winearls CG, Jones S, et al. Prospective study of radioimmunoassay for antibodies against neutrophil cytoplasm in diagnosis of systemic vasculitis. Lancet 1987; 1:1389.
198. Hammerberg G, Keren DF. Detection of antineutrophil cytoplasm antibodies in Wegener's granulomatosis. Lab Med 1991; 22:783.
199. Gunawen S, Clay M, Kline W, et al. Role of granulocyte Fc receptor in granulocyte agglutination [Abstract]. Transfusion 1987; 27:513.
200. Bux J, Jung KD, Kauth T, Mueller-Eckhardt C. Serological and clinical aspects of granulocyte antibodies leading to alloimmune neonatal neutropenia. Transfus Med 1992; 2:143.
201. Blaschke J, Goeken NE, Thompson JS, et al. Acquired agranulocytosis with granulocyte specific cytotoxic autoantibody. Am J Med 1979; 66:862.
202. Bux J, Kissel K, Nowak K, et al. Autoimmune neutropenia: clinical and laboratory studies in 143 patients. Ann Hematol 1991; 63:243.
203. Yomtovian R, Kline W, Press C, et al. Severe pulmonary hypersensitivity associated with passive transfusion of a neutrophil specific antibody. Lancet 1984; 1:244.
204. Popovsky MA, Moore SB. Diagnostic and pathogenetic considerations in transfusion-related acute lung injury. Transfusion 1985; 25:573.
205. Tam DA, Morton LD, Stroncek DF, Leshner RT. Neutropenia in a patient receiving intravenous immune globulin. J Neuroimmunol 1996; 64:175–178.
206. Van Buren NL, Stroncek DF, Clay ME, et al. Transfusion-related acute lung injury caused by an NB2 granulocyte-specific antibody in a patient with thrombotic thrombocytopenic purpura. Transfusion 1990; 30:42.
207. Lalezari P, Khorshidi M, Petrosova M. Autoimmune neutropenia of infancy. J Pediatr 1986; 109:764.
208. McCullough J, Clay M, Press C, Kline W. Granulocyte Serology: A Clinical and Laboratory Guide. Chicago: American Society of Clinical Pathology, 1988, pp 47–48.
209. McCullough J, Weiblen BJ, Clay ME, Forstrom L. Effect of leukocyte antibodies on the fate in vivo of indium-111–labeled granulocytes. Blood 1981; 58:164–170.
210. Chow HS, Alexander DL, Epstein RB. Detection and significance of granulocyte alloimmunization in leukocyte transfusion therapy on neutropenic dogs. Transfusion 1983; 23:15.
211. Dahlke MB, Keashen M, Alavi JB, et al. Granulocyte transfusions and outcome of alloimmunized patients with gram-negative sepsis. Transfusion 1982; 22:374.
212. Ruoslahti E. Integrins. J Clin Invest 1991; 87:1.
213. Albelda SM, Buck CA. Integrins and other cell adhesion molecules. FASEB J 1990; 4:2868.
214. Hemler ME. VLA proteins in the integrin family: structures, functions and their role on leukocytes. Annu Rev Immunol 1990; 8:365.
215. Wright SD, Detmers PA. Adhesion-promoting receptors on phagocytes. J Cell Sci Suppl 1988; 9:99.
216. Springer TA, Anderson DC. Antibodies specific for the Mac-1, LFA-1, p150, 95 glycoproteins or their family, or for other granulocyte proteins in the 2nd International Workshop on Human Leukocyte Differentiation Antigens. *In* Reinherz EL, Haynes BJ, Nadler LM, Bernstein ID (eds): Leukocyte Typing II: Human Myeloid and Hematopoietic Cells. Springer-Verlag, 1986, pp 55–68.
217. Springer TA. Adhesion receptors of the immune system. Nature 1990; 346:425.
218. Arnaout MA. Structure and function of the leukocyte adhesion molecules CD11/CD18. Blood 1990; 75:1037.
219. Nathan C, Srimal S, Farber C, et al. Cytokine-induced respiratory burst of human neutrophils: dependence on extracellular matrix proteins and CD11/CD18 integrins. J Cell Biol 1989; 109:1341.
220. Wallis WJ, Hickstein DD, Schwartz BR, et al. Monoclonal antibody defined functional epitopes on the adhesion-promoting glycoprotein complex (CD18) of human neutrophils. Blood 1986; 67:1007.
221. Schwartz BR, Ochs HD, Beatty PG, Harlan JM. A monoclonal antibody defined membrane antigen complex is required for neutrophil-neutrophil aggregation. Blood 1985; 65:1553.
222. Bohnsack JF, Akiyama SK, Damsky CH, et al. Human neutrophil adherence to laminin in vitro. Evidence for a district neutrophil receptor for laminin. J Exp Med 1990; 171:1221.
223. Bohnsack JF. CD11/CD18-independent neutrophil adherence to laminin is mediated by the integrin VLA-6. Blood 1992; 79:1545.
224. Gresham HD, Goodwin JL, Allen PM, et al. A novel member of the integrin receptor family mediates Arg-Gly-Asp stimulated neutrophil phagocytosis. J Cell Biol 1989; 108:1935.
225. Gallatin WM, Weisman IL, Butcher EC. A cell-surface molecule involved in organ-specific homing of lymphocytes. Nature 1983; 304:30.
226. Lewinsohn DM, Bargatze RF, Butcher EC. Leukocyte-endothelial cell recognition: evidence of a common molecular mechanism shared by neutrophils, lymphocytes, and other leukocytes. J Immunol 1987; 138:4313.
227. Tedder TF, Isaacs CM, Ernst TS, et al. Isolation and chromosomal localization of cDNAs encoding a novel human lymphocyte cell surface molecule, LAM-1: homology with the mouse lymphocyte homing receptor and other human adhesion proteins. J Exp Med 1989; 170:123.
228. Kishimoto TK, Jutila MA, Butcher EC. Identification of a human peripheral lymph node homing receptor: a rapidly down-regulated adhesion molecule. Proc Natl Acad Sci U S A 1990; 87:2244.

229. Griffin JD, Spertini O, Ernst TJ, et al. Granulocyte-macrophage colony-stimulating factor and other cytokines regulate surface expression of the leukocyte adhesion molecule-1 on human neutrophils, monocytes and their precursors. J Immunol 1990; 145:576.
230. Jutila MA, Kishimoto TK, Butcher EC. Regulation and lectin activity of the human neutrophil peripheral lymph node homing receptor. Blood 1990; 76:178.
231. Spertini O, Kansas GS, Munro M, et al. Regulation of leukocyte migration by activation of the leukocyte adhesion molecule-1 (LAM-1) selectin. Nature 1991; 349:691.
232. Johnston GI, Cook RG, McEver RP. Cloning of GMP-140, a granule membrane protein of platelets and endothelium: sequence similarity to proteins involved in cell adhesion and inflammation. Cell 1989; 56:1033.
233. Bevilacqua MP, Stengelin S, Gimbrone MA Jr, Seed B. Endothelial leukocyte adhesion molecule-1: an inducable receptor for neutrophils related to complement regulatory proteins and lectins. Science 1989; 243:1160.
234. Lawrence MB, Springer TA. Leukocytes roll on a selectin at physiologic flow rates: distinction from and prerequisite for adhesion through integrins. Cell 1991; 65:849.
235. Zhou Q, Moore KL, Smith DF, et al. The selectin GMP-140 binds to sialyated, fucosylated lactosaminoglycans on both myeloid and non-myeloid cells. J Cell Biol 1991; 115:557.
236. Springer TA, Lasky LA. Sticky sugars for selectins. Nature 1991; 349:196.
237. Smith CW, Kishimoto TK, Abbassf IO, et al. Chemotactic factors regulate lectin adhesion molecule-1 (LECAM-1)–dependent neutrophil adhesion to cytokine-stimulated endothelial cells in vitro. J Clin Invest 1991; 87:609.
238. Spertini O, Kansas GS, Reiman KA, et al. Function and evolutionary conservation of distinct epitopes on the leukocyte adhesion molecule-1 (TQ1, Leu-8) that regulate leukocyte migration. J Immunol 1991; 147:942.
239. Stamenkovic I, Amiot M, Pesando JM, Seed B. A lymphocyte molecule implicated in lymph node homing is a member of the cartilage link protein family. Cell 1989; 56:1057.
240. Goldstein LA, Zhou DFH, Picker LJ, et al. A human lymphocyte homing receptor, the Hermes antigen, is related to cartilage proteoglycan core and link proteins. Cell 1989; 56:1063.
241. Newman PJ, Berndt MC, Gorski J, et al. PECAM-1 (CD31) cloning and relation to adhesion molecules of the immunoglobulin gene superfamily. Science 1990; 247:1219.
242. Kishimoto TK. A dynamic model for neutrophil localization to inflammatory sites. J NIH Res 1991; 3:75.
243. Kishimoto TK, Warnock RA, Jutila MA, et al. Antibodies against human neutrophil LECAM-1 (LAM-1/LEU-8/DREG-56 antigen) and endothelial cell ELAM-1 inhibit a common CD18-independent adhesion pathway in vitro. Blood 1991; 78:805.
244. Furie B, Furie BC. Molecular and cellular biology of blood coagulation. N Engl J Med 1992; 326:800.
245. Larsen E, Celi A, Gilbert GE, et al. PADGEM protein: a receptor that mediates the interaction of activated platelets with neutrophils and monocytes. Cell 1989; 59:305.
246. Lalezari P. Alloimmune neonatal neutropenia. *In* Engelfriet CP, Van Logham JJ, von dem Borne AEGKr (eds): Immunohaematology. Amsterdam: Elsevier Science Publishers, 1984, pp 179–186.
247. Fasth A. Immunoglobulin for neonatal agranulocytosis. Arch Dis Child 1986; 61:86.
248. Verheugt FWA, van Noord-Bokhorst JC, von dem Borne AEGKr, Engelfriet CP. A family with alloimmune neonatal neutropenia: group-specific pathogenicity of maternal antibodies. Vox Sang 1979; 36:1.
249. van der Weerdt CM, Lalezari P. Another example of isoimmune neonatal neutropenia due to anti-NA1. Vox Sang 1972; 22:438.
250. Levine DH, Madyastha PR. Isoimmune neonatal neutropenia. J Perinatol 1986; 3:231.
251. Clay M, Kline W, McCullough J. The frequency of granulocyte-specific antibodies in postpartum sera and a family study of 6B antigen. Transfusion 1984; 24:232.
252. Skacel PO, Stacey TE, Tidmarsh CEF, Contreras M. Maternal alloimmunization to HLA, platelet and granulocyte-specific antigens during pregnancy: its influence on cord blood granulocyte and platelet counts. Br J Haematol 1989; 71:119.
253. Conway LT, Clay ME, Kline WE, et al. Natural history of primary autoimmune neutropenia in infancy. Pediatrics 1987; 79:728.
254. Ducos R, Madyastha PR, Warrier RP, et al. Neutrophil agglutinins in idiopathic chronic neutropenia of early childhood. Am J Dis Child 1986; 140:65.
255. Bux J, Behrens G, Welte K. Diagnosis and clinical course of autoimmune neutropenia in infancy: analysis of 240 cases. Blood 1998; 91:181.
256. Bussel J, Lalezari P, Fibrig S. Intravenous treatment with gamma-globulin of autoimmune neutropenia of infancy. J Pediatr 1988; 112:298.
257. Kuijpers TW, de Haas D, de Groot CJ, et al. The use of fh-G-CSF in chronic autoimmune neutropenia: reversal of autoimmune phenomena, a case history. Br J Haematol 1996; 94:464.
258. van der Veen JPW, Hack CE, Engelfriet CP, et al. Chronic idiopathic and secondary neutropenia: clinical and serological investigations. Br J Haematol 1986; 63:161.
259. Eastlund DT, Charbonneau TT, Steinmetz J. Granulocyte antibody detection to diagnose immune granulocytopenia and transfusion reactions due to leukocyte incompatibility. Hematol Rev 1992; 6:201.
260. Rothko K, Kickler TS, Clay ME, et al. Immunoblotting characterization of neutrophil antigenic targets in autoimmune neutropenia. Blood 1989; 74:1698.
261. Beatty PA, Stroncek DF. Autoimmune neutropenia in Sheboygan County, Wisconsin. J Lab Clin Med 1992; 119:718.
262. Bux J, Robertz-Vaupel GM, Glasmacher A, et al. Autoimmune neutropenia due to NA1 specific antibodies in primary biliary cirrhosis. Br J Haematol 1991; 77:121.
263. Klaassen RJH, Vlekke ABJ, von dem Borne AEGKr. Neutrophil-bound immunoglobulin in HIV infection is of autoantibody nature. Br J Haematol 1991; 77:403.
264. Hartman KR, Mallet MK, Nath J, Wright DG. Antibodies to actin in autoimmune neutropenia. Blood 1990; 75:736.
265. Hartman KR, Wright DG. Identification of autoantibodies specific for the neutrophil adhesion glycoproteins CD11b/CD18 in patients with autoimmune neutropenia. Blood 1991; 78:1096.
266. Gasner A, Ottmann OG, Erdmann H, et al. The effect of recombinant human granulocyte-macrophage colony-stimulating factor on neutropenia and related morbidity in chronic severe neutropenia. Ann Intern Med 1989; 111:887.
267. Pollack S, Cunningham-Rundles C, Smithwick EM, et al. High-dose intravenous gamma globulin for autoimmune neutropenia [Letter]. N Engl J Med 1982; 307:253.
268. Ricevuti G, Mazzone A, Rizzo SC. A study of neutrophil function in a case of associated autoimmune neutropenia and thrombocytopenia treated with high doses of intravenous gamma globulin (HDIGG). Clin Lab Haematol 1986; 8:325.
269. Barbui T, Bassan R, Viero P, et al. Pure white cell aplasia treated by high dose intravenous immunoglobulin. Br J Haematol 1984; 58:554.
270. Breedveld FC, Brand A, van Aken WG. High dose intravenous gamma globulin for Felty's syndrome. J Rheumatol 1985; 12:700.
271. Koene HR, de Haas M, Kleijier M, et al. Clinical value of soluble IgG Fc receptor type III in plasma from patients with chronic idiopathic neutropenia. Blood 1998; 91: 3962–3966.
272. Pisciotta AV, Cronkite C. Aprindine-induced agranulocytosis: evidence for immunologic mechanism. Arch Intern Med 1983; 143:241.
273. Samlowski WE, Frame RN, Logue GL. Flecanide-induced immune neutropenia. Documentation of a hapten-mediated mechanism of cell destruction. Arch Intern Med 1987; 147:383.
274. Weitzman SA, Stossel TP, Desmond M. Drug-induced immunological neutropenia. Lancet 1978; 1:1068.
275. Yomtovian R, Kline W, Press C, et al. Evidence for granulocyte antibody activity in two cases of procainamide-associated neutropenia [Abstract]. Blood 1984; 64:(suppl 1):92a.
276. Kelton JG, Huang AT, Mold N, et al. The use of in vitro techniques to study drug-induced pancytopenia. N Engl J Med 1979; 301:621.
277. Eisner EV, Carr RM, MacKinney AA. Quinidine-induced agranulocytosis. JAMA 1977; 238:884.
278. Ascensao JL, Flynn PJ, Slungaard A, et al. Quinidine-induced neutropenia: report of a case with drug-dependent inhibition of granulocyte colony generation. Acta Haematol 1984; 72:349.
279. Chong BH, Berndt ME, Koutts J, Castaldi PA. Quinidine-induced thrombocytopenia and leukopenia: demonstration and characterization of distinct antiplatelet and antileukocyte antibodies. Blood 1983; 62:1218.

280. Rouveix B, Lassoued K, Vittecoq D, Regnier B. Neutropenia due to β lactamine antibodies. BMJ 1983; 287:1832.
281. Lawson AA, McArdle T, Ghosh S. Cephadrine-associated immune neutropenia [Letter]. N Engl J Med 1985; 312:651.
282. Murphy MF, Metcalfe PC, Grint PCA, et al. Cephalosporin-induced immune neutropenia. Br J Haematol 1985; 59:9.
283. Salama A, Schutz B, Kiefel V, et al. Immune-mediated agranulocytosis related to drugs and their metabolites: mode of sensitization and heterogeneity of antibodies. Br J Haematol 1989; 72:127.
284. Murphy MF, Riordan T, Minchinton RM, et al. Demonstration of an immune-mediated mechanism of penicillin-induced neutropenia and thrombocytopenia. Br J Haematol 1983; 55:155.
285. Rouveix B, Coulombel L, Aymard JP, et al. Amodiaquine-induced immune agranulocytosis. Br J Haematol 1989; 75:7.
286. Stroncek DF, Vercellotti GM, Hammerschmidt DE, et al. Characterization of multiple quinine-dependent antibodies in a patient with episodic hemolytic uremic syndrome and immune agranulocytosis. Blood 1992; 80:241.
287. Mamus SW, Burton JD, Groat JD, et al. Ibuprofen-associated pure white-cell aplasia. N Engl J Med 1986; 314:624.
288. Berkman EM, Orlin JB, Wolfsdorf J. An anti-neutrophil antibody associated with a propylthiouracil-induced lupus-like syndrome. Transfusion 1983; 23:135.
289. Fibbe WE, Claas FHJ, van der Star-Dijkstra W, et al. Agranulocytosis induced by propylthiouracil: evidence of a drug dependent antibody reacting with granulocytes, monocytes and haematopoietic progenitor cells. Br J Haematol 1986; 64:363.
290. Sato K, Miyakawa M, Han DC, et al. Graves' disease with neutropenia and marked splenomegaly: autoimmune neutropenia due to propylthiouracil. J Endocrinol Invest 1985; 8:551.
291. Wall JR, Fang SL, Kuroki T, et al. In vitro immunoreactivity to propylthiouracil, methimazole, and carbimazole in patients with Graves' disease: a possible cause of antithyroid drug-induced agranulocytosis. J Clin Endocrinol Metab 1984; 58:868.
292. Levitt LJ. Chlorpropamide-induced pure white cell aplasia. Blood 1987; 69:394.
293. Thompson JS, Herbick JM, Klassen LW, et al. Studies on levamisole-induced agranulocytosis. Blood 1980; 56:388.
294. Drew SI, Carter BM, Nathanson DS, Tarasaki PI. Levamisole-associated neutropenia and autoimmune granulocytotoxins. Ann Rheum Dis 1980; 39:59.
295. Stroncek DF, Shankar RA, Herr GP. Quinine-dependent antibodies to neutrophils react with a 60-kD glycoprotein on which neutrophil-specific antigen NB1 is located and an 85-kD glycosyl-phoshatidylinositol–linked *N*-glycosylated plasma membrane glycoprotein. Blood 1993; 81:2758.
296. Menitove JE, McElligott MC, Aster RH. Febrile transfusion reactions: what blood component should be given next? Vox Sang 1989; 42:318.
297. Brittingham TE, Chaplin H. Febrile transfusion reactions caused by sensitivity to donor leukocytes and platelets. JAMA 1957; 165:819.
298. Payne R. The association of febrile transfusion reactions with leuko-agglutinins. Vox Sang 1957; 2:233.
299. Perkins HA, Payne R, Ferguson J, Wood M. Non-hemolytic febrile transfusion reactions. Quantitative effects of blood components with emphasis on isoantigenic incompatibility of leukocytes. Vox Sang 1966; 11:578.
300. Thulstrup H. The influence of leukocyte and thrombocyte incompatibility on non-haemolytic transfusion reactions. Vox Sang 1971; 21:233.
301. Decary F, Ferner P, Giavedoni L, et al. An investigation of nonhemolytic transfusion reactions. Vox Sang 1984; 46:277.
302. de Rie MA, van der Plas-van Dorlen CM, Engelfriet CP, von dem Borne AEGKr. The serology of febrile transfusion reactions. Vox Sang 1985; 49:126.
303. Goldfinger D, Lowe C. Prevention of adverse reactions to blood transfusions by the administration of saline-washed red blood cells. Transfusion 1981; 21:277.
304. Sirchia G, Wenz B, Rebulla P, et al. Removal of white cells from red cells by transfusion through a new filter. Transfusion 1990; 30:30.
305. Swank DW, Moore SB. Role of the neutrophil and other mediators in adult respiratory distress syndrome. Mayo Clin Proc 1989; 64:1118.
306. Lalezari P. Leukocyte antigens and antibodies. *In* Hoffman R, Benz EJ, Shattil SJ, et al (eds): Hematology: Basic Principals and Practices. New York: Churchill Livingstone, 1991, pp 1566–1572.
307. Popovsky MA, Abel MD, Moore SB. Transfusion-related acute lung injury associated with passive transfer of antileukocyte antibodies. Am Rev Respir Dis 1983; 128:185.
308. Ward HN. Pulmonary infiltrates associated with leukoagglutinin transfusion reactions. Ann Intern Med 1970; 73:689.
309. Thompson JS, Severson CD, Parmely MJ. "Pulmonary hypersensitivity" reactions induced by transfusion of non-HLA leukoagglutinins. N Engl J Med 1971; 284:1120.
310. Dubois M, Lotze MT, Diamond WJ, et al. Pulmonary shunting during leukoagglutinin-induced noncardiac pulmonary edema. JAMA 1980; 244:2186.
311. Campbell DA Jr, Swartz RD, Waskerwitz JA, et al. Leukoagglutination with interstitial pulmonary edema. A complication of donor-specific transfusion. Transplantation 1982; 34:300.
312. Gans ROB, Duurkens VAM, van Zundert AA, Hoorntje SJ. Transfusion-related acute lung injury. Intensive Care Med 1988; 14:654.
313. Wolf CFW, Canale VC. Fatal pulmonary hypersensitivity reaction to HL-A incompatible blood transfusion: report of a case and review of the literature. Transfusion 1976; 16:135.
314. Andrews AT, Zimijewski CM, Bowman HS, Reihart JK. Transfusion reaction with pulmonary infiltration associated with HL-A specific leukocyte antibodies. Am J Clin Pathol 1976; 66:483.
315. Carilli AD, Ramanamurty MV, Chang YS, et al. Noncardiac pulmonary edema following blood transfusion. Chest 1978; 74:310.
316. Goeken NE, Schulak JA, Nghiem DD, et al. Transfusion reactions in donor-specific blood transfusion patients resulting from transfused maternal antibody. Transplantation 1984; 38:306.
317. Eastlund R, McGrath PC, Britten A, Proopp R. Fatal pulmonary transfusion reaction to plasma containing donor HLA antibody. Vox Sang 1989; 57:63.
318. Brittingham TE. Immunologic studies of leukocytes. Vox Sang 1957; 2:242.
319. Reese EP Jr, McCullough JJ, Craddock PR. An adverse pulmonary reaction to cryoprecipitate in a hemophiliac. Transfusion 1975; 15:583.
320. Popovsky MA, Chaplin HC, Moore SB. Transfusion-related acute lung injury: a neglected, serious complication of hemotherapy. Transfusion 1992; 32:499.
321. Craddock PR, Hammerschmidt DE, Moldow CF, et al. Granulocyte aggregation as a manifestation of membrane interactions with complement: possible role in leukocyte margination, microvascular occlusion, and endothelial damage. Semin Hematol 1979; 16:140.
322. Jacob HS, Craddock PR, Hammerschmidt DE, Maldow CF. Complement induced granulocyte aggregation: an unsuspected mechanism of disease. N Engl J Med 1980; 302:789.
323. Goldblum SE, Reed WP. Distribution of pneumococcus-induced augmentation of tissue leukostasis in rabbits: specificity for the pulmonary vascular bed. J Lab Clin Med 1985; 105:374.
324. Tvedten TW, Till GO, Ward PA. Mediators of lung injury in mice following systemic activation of complement. Am J Pathol 1985; 119:92.
325. Hammerschmidt DE, Craddock PR, McCullough J, et al. Complement activation and pulmonary leukostasis during nylon fiber filtration leukapheresis. Blood 1978; 51:721.
326. Seeger W, Schneider U, Kreusler B, et al. Reproduction of transfusion-related acute lung injury in an ex vivo lung model. Blood 1990; 76:1438.
327. Jennette JC. Antineutrophil cytoplasmic autoantibody-associated diseases: a pathologist's perspective. Am J Kidney Dis 1991; 18:164.
328. Cohen-Tervaert JWC, Huitema MG, Hene RJ, et al. Prevention of relapses in Wegener's granulomatosis by treatment based on antineutrophil cytoplasmic antibody titre. Lancet 1990; 336:709.
329. Nolle B, Ulrich S, Ludemann J, et al. Anticytoplasmic autoantibodies: their immunodiagnostic value in Wegener granulomatosis. Ann Intern Med 1989; 111:28.
330. Specks U, Wheatley CL, McDonald TJ, et al. Anticytoplasmic autoantibodies in the diagnosis and follow-up of Wegener's granulomatosis. Mayo Clin Proc 1989; 64:28.
331. Lesavre P. Antineutrophil cytoplasmic autoantibodies antigen specificity. Am J Kidney Dis 1991; 18:159.
332. Hoffman GS, Kerr GS, Leavitt RY, et al. Wegener granulomatosis: an analysis of 158 patients. Ann Intern Med 1992; 116:488.

333. Gross WL, Schmitt WH, Csernok E. Anti-neutrophil cytoplasmic autoantibody-associated diseases: a rheumatologist's perspective. Am J Kidney Dis 1991; 18:175.
334. Ewert BH, Jennette JC, Falk RJ. The pathogenic role of anti-neutrophil cytoplasmic autoantibodies. Am J Kid Dis 1991; 18:188.
335. Falk RJ, Terrell RS, Charles LA, Jennette JC. Anti-neutrophil cytoplasmic autoantibodies induce neutrophils to degranulate and produce oxygen radicals in vitro. Proc Natl Acad Sci U S A 1990; 87:4115.
336. Arnaout MA, Pitt J, Cohen HJ, et al. Deficiency of a granulocyte membrane glycoprotein (gp 150) in a boy with recurrent bacterial infections. N Engl J Med 1982; 306:693.
337. Styrt B. History and implications of the neutrophil glycoprotein deficiencies. Am J Hematol 1989; 31:288.
338. Malech HL, Gallin JI. Current concepts: immunology. Neutrophils in human disease. N Engl J Med 1987; 317:687.
339. Anderson DC, Schmalsteig FC, Finegold MJ, et al. The severe and moderate phenotypes of heritable Mac-1, LFA-1 deficiency: their quantitative definition and relation to leukocyte dysfunction and clinical features. J Infect Dis 1985; 152:668.
340. Wright SD, Detmers DA. Adhesion promoting receptors on phagocytes. J Cell Sci 1988; Suppl 9:99.
341. Kohl S, Springer TA, Schmalstieg FC, et al. Detective natural killer cytotoxicity and polymorphonuclear leukocyte antibody-dependent cellular cytotoxicity in patients with LFA-1/OKM-1 deficiency. J Immunol 1984; 133:2972.
342. Dana N, Todd RF, Pitt J, et al. Deficiency of a surface membrane glycoprotein (Mo1) in man. J Clin Invest 1984; 73:153.
343. Clark MR, Liu L, Clarkson SB, et al. An abnormality of the gene that encodes neutrophil Fc receptor III in a patient with systemic lupus erythematosus. J Clin Invest 1990; 86:341.
344. De Haas, Kleijer M, Zwieten RV, et al. Neutrophil FcγRIIIb deficiency, nature, and clinical consequences: a study of 21 individuals from 14 families. Blood 1995; 86:2403.
345. Yokoyama MM, Nishiki M, Matsui Y, et al. Neutrophil surface markers in chronic myelocytic leukemia. Kurume Med J 1980; 27:43.
346. Reijden HJ, von dem Borne AEGKr, Verheught FW, et al. Granulocyte-specific alloantigen loss in chronic granulocytic leukemia. Br J Haematol 1979; 43:589.
347. Kawakami Z, Ninomiya H, Tomiyama J, Abe T. Deficiency of glycosyl-phosphatidylinositol anchored proteins on paroxysmal nocturnal haemaglobinuria (PNH) neutrophils and monocytes: heterogeneous deficiency of decay-accelerating factor (DAF) and CD16 on PNH neutrophils. Br J Haematol 1990; 74:508.
348. Anderson DC, Becker Freeman KL, et al. Abnormal stimulated adherence of neonatal granulocytes: impaired induction of surface MAC-1 by chemotactic factors or secretagogues. Blood 1987; 70:740.
349. Carr R, Davies JM. Abnormal FcRIII expression by neutrophils from very preterm neonates. Blood 1990; 76:607.

SECTION

V Platelets

CHAPTER 13

Platelet Storage and Metabolism

Edward L. Snyder
Patricia T. Pisciotto

PLATELET STRUCTURE AND FUNCTION

Platelets are anucleate, disc-shaped, membrane-encapsulated fragments of cytoplasm derived from bone marrow megakaryocytes. They play an essential role in preserving vascular integrity and in maintaining hemostasis. On Wright-stained smears, platelets appear as small particles consisting of pale blue cytoplasm with occasional azurophilic granules. Electron microscopy shows the presence of several distinguishable structures, including membranes, mitochondria, microtubules, and granules of various densities.

The platelet plasma membrane serves two important roles in hemostasis: it provides the means for cell-to-cell or cell-to-matrix interactions, and it furnishes a surface for enhancing the fluid phase of coagulation. The lipid bilayer consists of phospholipids asymmetrically arranged between the outer and inner leaflets. In the resting state, the outer leaflet is composed primarily of the neutral phospholipids, phosphatidylcholine and sphingomyelin, whereas the inner leaflet is composed of the negatively charged phosphatidylserine and phosphatidylethanolamine. On activation, an elevation of intracellular Ca^{2+} causes a "flip-flop," resulting in an increase in phosphatidylserine in the outer leaflet. This alteration in the membrane accounts for the increased procoagulant activity, formerly referred to as platelet factor 3 activity. The phospholipid surface promotes the activation of both factor X and prothrombin.[1] The platelet membrane also contains numerous glycoproteins (GPs), which function as adhesive proteins, including glycoprotein Ib-IX-V complex (GPIb-IX-V), which acts as a platelet receptor for von Willebrand factor (vWF) in platelet adhesion and facilitates the ability of thrombin, at low concentrations, to activate platelets[2,3]; the glycoprotein IIb-IIIa (GPIIb-IIIa) complex, which spans the platelet membrane and is the functional receptor for fibrinogen, vWF, fibronectin, and vitronectin[3,4]; glycoprotein Ia-IIa complex (GPIa-IIa), the receptor for collagen[3]; and glycoprotein Ic-IIa (GPIc-IIa), the receptor for fibronectin.[3] The last three glycoprotein receptors are integrins, which are a large family of related heterodimers grouped on the basis of the β subunit.[3] P-selectin (also known as CD62P, GMP-140, PADGEM) is an integral membrane protein of the alpha granule that becomes expressed on the surface of activated platelets on granule release.[3,5] CD62P is an adhesive protein that mediates interactions of neutrophils and monocytes to activated platelets.[6] P-selectin is also found on the Weibel-Palade body of the endothelial cell.[7] The external plasma membrane of the platelet invaginates to form a surface-connected canalicular or collecting system (SCCS). This creates a means for plasma components to enter the platelet as well as for internal granule contents to be externalized (released). It also greatly increases the surface area of the platelet.

The platelet is laced with submembranous microfilaments that serve as a constituent of the cytoskeletal network. Actin filaments, along with a peripheral microtubule coil, serve to maintain the platelet's discoid shape. The contractile proteins, consisting mainly of actin and myosin filaments, are also involved in motor activities, such as pseudopod formation and secretion, which are essential to platelet function. Actin and myosin have also been found to be structurally linked to transmembrane glycoproteins.[8] The dense tubular system is an enclosed system consisting of membrane-limited tubules. It serves as the storage site for ionized calcium and the site of prostaglandin synthesis.[9]

Mitochondria, peroxisomes, lysosomes, and two major secretory granules, alpha granules and electron-dense granules (dense bodies), are present within the cytoplasm of the platelet. The alpha granules contain a broad range of proteins and require the least stimulation to release their contents. These granules contain adhesive proteins (vWF, fibrinogen, fibronectin, thrombospondin, vitronectin, P-selectin), anticoagulants (antiheparins: platelet factor 4, and β-thromboglobulin, procoagulants [factors V, XI, XIII]), protein S, plasminogen activator inhibitor-1, and growth-promoting factors for angiogenesis and repair (platelet-derived growth factor, and transforming growth factor-β).[10,11] Stronger stimulation is required to release the content of the dense bodies that contain substances such as storage pool adenosine diphosphate (ADP), adenosine triphosphate (ATP), serotonin, and the major portion of the platelet's calcium.[11]

Platelets in the "resting" state circulate in the blood stream, without adhering to vessel walls, for approximately 10 days and are then removed, primarily in the spleen. In the resting state, granules are found dispersed throughout the platelet cytoplasm. Platelets rapidly respond to an appropriate stimulus, such as denuded endothelium with exposed collagen, by adhering to the subendothelial matrix, undergoing a change in shape from a disc to a sphere with multiple extended pseudopods, and spreading to increase surface contact. Interaction between agonists in the microenvironment and specific receptors on the platelet surface results in the transmission of signals from the outside of the cell to the interior, generating secondary messengers that induce protein phosphorylation and the opening of ion channels.[12] Platelet granules are brought together centrally by activated contractile proteins. Granule membranes then fuse with the SCCS of the platelet, and the granule contents exit the platelet and enter the extracellular environment. Secretion of the dense granules will induce vasoconstriction (serotonin), platelet aggregation (ADP), and increased localization of Ca^{2+}, which further augments activation, adhesion, and aggregation of platelets. Release of alpha granules contributes adhesive proteins and coagulation factors. The release reaction can be defined as the platelet's response to a stimulus resulting in the externalization of granule contents associated with the appearance of ligands on the platelet surface. This process culminates in the formation of a hemostatic platelet plug, which becomes interlaced with fibrin.

Adhesion, the binding of platelets to a nonplatelet surface, is the initial event in the formation of the platelet plug. Shear forces within the vessel influence the deposition of platelets on exposed endothelium.[13] At high shear stress, such as within the microcirculation, the primary adhesive event is mediated by the interaction of the subendothelial-bound vWF with the platelet GPIb receptor. The vWF bound to the subendothelial matrix is believed to undergo a conformational change revealing the binding site for the GPIb-IX-V complex.[14] The binding site for GPIb resides in the A1 domain of vWF. This bond is transient, and the interaction induces a transmembrane flux of Ca^{2+}, which results in a conformational change and activation of GPIIb-IIIa. Activated GPIIb-IIIa binds irreversibly to vWF, producing a firm adhesion of the platelet to the vessel wall, and mediates spreading. The activated GPIIb-IIIa integrin recognizes and binds to the RGD (Arg-Gly-Asp) peptide sequences of circulating vWF and fibrinogen, resulting in platelet aggregation.[15] At low shear stress, which occurs in larger vessels, the role of vWF is of less significance. Platelet glycoproteins will adhere to exposed subendothelial matrix proteins such as collagen, fibronectin, and fibrinogen by means of the receptors GPIa-IIa, GPIc-IIa, and GPIIb-IIIa, respectively. These bonds will initiate intracellular signaling to induce platelet activation.[12]

Platelet aggregation is defined as the binding of platelets to other platelets. The integrin GPIIb-IIIa ($\alpha_{IIb}\beta_3$) is essential for platelet aggregation. The structure of the integrins consists of a large extracellular domain, a transmembrane segment, and a short cytoplasmic segment that mediates signal transduction to intracellular proteins. The integrin is capable of bidirectional activation across the plasma membrane.[12] In the unstimulated or resting platelet, however, GPIIb-IIIa is relatively unavailable to its ligands. Interaction with an extracellular ligand such as fibrinogen bound to exposed subendothelium will induce a conformational change in the receptor. This, in turn, sends a signal into the interior of the platelet, resulting in cytoskeletal shape change and cytoplasmic phosphokinase activity with platelet activation and release of granule contents. Alternatively, platelet activation by an agonist such as thrombin will transmit a cytoplasmic signal that reaches the cytoplasmic tail of the integrin, producing a conformational change in the extracellular binding site, thus making it available to circulating ligands such as fibrinogen and vWF. Fibrinogen, which is an elongated protein, can thus crosslink platelets by means of their receptor sites. The activation of GPIIb-IIIa and binding of fibrinogen results in clustering of fibrinogen IIb-IIIa on the platelet surface, establishing a link between platelets, referred to as aggregates.[12, 16] Activated platelets participate in the generation of thrombin by providing a favorable external surface charge for the prothrombinase complex (X-Va), thereby localizing fibrin generation in the area of the platelet plug.[17]

Agonist-induced platelet activation initiates a series of events in the membrane and cytosol. Agonist (i.e., thrombin or ADP) and antagonist (i.e., prostaglandin I_2) receptor interactions are modulated by guanine nucleotide-binding regulatory proteins (G proteins).[18] The G proteins consist of three units: α, β, and γ. The α subunit is specific and when linked to guanosine triphosphate (GTP) can activate membrane-associated signal generating enzymes, phospholipase C (PLC) and phospholipase A_2 (PLA_2), which are both platelet activating, and adenyl cyclase, which is platelet inhibitory.[19, 20] In turn, these will trigger the generation of "second messengers": inositol triphosphate (IP_3), diacylglycerol (DAG), Ca^{2+}, thromboxane A_2 (TxA_2), and cyclic adenosine monophosphate (AMP), respectively. There are many different G proteins coupled to various receptors.[18]

The membrane phospholipid phosphoinositol (PIP_2), present in the inner leaflet, is hydrolyzed by the activation of PLC, forming IP_3 and DAG. The IP_3 is responsible for the release of intracellular Ca^{2+} from the dense tubular system and increased transmembrane Ca^{2+} flux. DAG activates the protein kinase C pathway, which induces granule secretion and upregulation of GPIIb-IIIa. PLA_2 can be activated directly by G protein–coupled receptors or by increasing cytosolic Ca^{2+}. Activated PLA_2 hydrolyzes platelet phospholipid with release of arachidonic acid. Arachidonic acid is rapidly metabolized to cycloendoperoxidases (prostaglandins G_2 and H_2) by the aspirin-sensitive enzyme cyclooxygenase, with the major portion of prostaglandin H_2 being further converted to TxA_2.[21] Both the cycloendoperoxidases and TxA_2 are potent stimulators of platelet activation.[22] In the endothelial cells, the endoperoxidase of arachidonic acid metabolism forms prostacyclin (PGI_2), an inhibitor of platelet aggregation and platelet release as well as a vasodilator.[23]

The enzyme adenyl cyclase converts ATP into cyclic AMP, which in turn activates cyclic AMP–dependent protein kinases.[24] Agents that induce platelet activation and release (agonists) inhibit platelet enzyme adenyl cyclase, resulting in a decrease in cyclic AMP and an increase in ionized calcium.[25] Conversely, agents that activate adenyl cyclase raise cyclic AMP levels, decrease ionized calcium levels, and inhibit platelet aggregation and release.[26] Intracellular calcium ions in conjunction with calmodulin, a calcium-binding protein, play an important role in the regulation of platelet function. Calmodulin becomes activated on the binding of Ca^{2+} to four available sites. In turn, calmodulin binds to an apoenzyme, transforming it to an active holoenzyme.[27] Ionized calcium-induced binding of calmodulin to platelet myosin light-chain kinase activates the latter to phosphorylate myosin and to facilitate the actin-myosin interaction that controls the initial change in platelet shape.[28] Protein kinase C, PLC, and PLA_2 are all Ca^{2+} dependent and, at least as they relate to PLA_2 activation, calmodulin independent.[29] Several other Ca^{2+}-dependent proteases participate in platelet function. One of these, calpain, can proteolyze many components of the platelet cytoskeleton (see later).

A critical level of ATP is required for each aspect of platelet function, including shape change, aggregation, and release. ATP is generated, in part, by glucose metabolism through the glycolytic and oxidative pathways. During platelet stimulation, an increase in glycolysis and Krebs cycle metabolism serves to replenish ATP levels. Platelet adhesion is not an energy-dependent function; even though the first phase of platelet aggregation requires a high basal level of ATP, very little ATP is consumed during adhesion.[30, 31] Although the basal level of ATP required to support shape change is less than is required for aggregation, ATP consumption occurs primarily at this step.[32] Adenine nucleotides present in platelets are found in two pools: ADP in the metabolic pool, which is constantly turning over, and storage pool ADP, which is found in the dense bodies and released during platelet activation. Plasma glucose metabolism generates approximately 15% of the ATP required during normal aerobic storage, largely through glycolytic catabolism to lactate.[33, 34] Oxidative phosphorylation, perhaps utilizing plasma free fatty acids by means of β oxidation, contributes the remaining 85%.[33, 34]

The importance of O_2 and CO_2 exchange across a plastic storage bag has been examined by Murphy and Gardner.[35] If deprived of oxygen, platelets increase lactate production through anaerobic glycolysis (Pasteur effect) in an attempt to compensate for the loss of energy normally derived from oxidative phosphorylation.[33–35] The ability to transport gases across the platelet storage bag is critical to normal platelet metabolism and thus to platelet survival after transfusion.

PREPARATION AND STORAGE OF PLATELET CONCENTRATES

Platelets are prepared from individual units of whole blood or from a single donor by automated blood cell processors using apheresis technology.[36] For whole blood collection, the donor blood is drawn into CPD, CPDA-1, or CP2D preservatives, each containing a specific combination of citrate, phosphate, dextrose, and/or adenine solutions. Citrate, the anticoagulant agent in the various preservative solutions, functions by chelating calcium and inhibiting the coagulation cascade. The other ingredients of the preservative solution have different functions. Phosphate is used as a buffer, and dextrose is used as a source of energy. Adenine actually serves no purpose in platelet storage; its primary role is to produce ATP for red cell survival during storage. After a holding period of up to 8 hours, the unit of blood is spun at a low speed (2200 × g) for 3 to 4 minutes to prepare platelet-rich plasma (PRP). The PRP thus prepared is then spun again at a higher speed (4000 × g) for 5 minutes to pellet the platelets. All but about 60 mL of PRP is removed, and the pellet is left undisturbed for about 1 hour.[37] It is then resuspended by gentle kneading of the bag or by placement of the unit on a platelet agitator.[38] Generally, the pellet smoothly resuspends within several hours and the unit is then stored for up to 5 days at 20°C to 24°C with continuous gentle agitation. Apheresis platelets are prepared in an ACD-A (citric acid, trisodium citrate, dextrose) preservative using automated apheresis technology. Citric acid is used to provide a lower pH. In some apheresis systems, the platelets are collected as PRP and do not require resuspension, whereas other apheresis systems yield a concentrated platelet pellet that requires resuspension. Apheresis platelets are stored in a manner similar to random donor platelets. Advances in apheresis technology have resulted in improved collection efficiencies for various apheresis machines.[39, 40]

Criteria have been established for a minimal acceptable unit of platelet concentrate (PC).[41] For a random donor unit of platelets (RDP), the minimum platelet count is 5.5×10^{10}/bag. The volume of platelet-poor plasma needed is not specified. However, it is usually 50 to 65 mL/bag and must be able to maintain a pH greater than 6.0 on the fifth (last) day of storage. Single-donor platelets (SDP) must have a minimum of 3.0×10^{11} platelets/bag. The volume of a unit of SDP varies from 200 to 300 mL. It, too, can be stored for only 5 days. A variety of factors that affect the ability to store platelets and maintain their viability during storage[36] include the storage plastic bag container, type of agitation, anticoagulant/preservative solution used, and temperature of storage (Table 13–1).[42]

PLATELET STORAGE LESION

The platelet storage lesion can be defined as the sum of the changes that occur in platelets after their collection, preparation, and storage as platelet concentrate for use in clinical transfusion practice. The storage lesion is not a single defect per se but rather a group of defects that affect a wide range of platelet structures and functions.[42] These include the platelet cytoskeleton, surface membrane antigen and ligand integrity, metabolic activity, release of granule contents, discharge of cytosolic contents, morphology, recovery from osmotic stress, and in vivo post-transfusion recovery and survival.[36, 43, 44]

Platelet Storage

Platelet storage technology has advanced to the point where we can reliably store 5 to 7 × 10^{11} apheresis

Table 13-1. Factors Affecting In Vitro Characteristics of Stored Platelet Concentrates

Factor	Characteristic(s) Affected
Phlebotomy conditions	Release reaction; platelet lysis
Anticoagulant/preservative solution	pH; metabolism of glucose, HCO_3, and lactate
Preparative centrifugation conditions	Release reaction; platelet lysis
Storage temperature	pH; metabolism; glucose consumption; lactate production
Plastic container composition or size	Oxygenation; metabolism; pH; glucose consumption; lactate metabolism
Type of agitation	Release reaction; platelet lysis
Number of platelets/volume of plasma	Metabolism; oxygenation; glucose consumption; pH; lactate generation
Storage time	pH; metabolism; release reaction; platelet lysis
Cryopreservation	Release reaction; platelet lysis; metabolism; freeze injury
Gamma irradiation	None at levels below 5000 cGy

platelets in a plastic container for 5 days and achieve a clinically acceptable post-transfusion increment in a nonrefractory recipient. Despite the advances made in transfusion medicine, however, key problems with platelet storage still remain. These include failure to maintain appropriate pH and thus platelet function during storage and the presence of bacterial contamination. Dealing with these issues poses challenges when developing innovative technology to enhance the safety and efficacy of platelet storage. That platelets can be stored beyond 5 days is known. Concerns regarding the risk of bacterial contamination, however, have limited U.S. Food and Drug Administration (FDA) approval of longer storage periods. In addition, in vitro evaluation of platelet function aimed at predicting post-transfusion in vivo viability has serious limitations. There are a myriad of in vitro platelet assays,[42, 45] and various researchers have their favorite tests. Some prefer measurement of pH or platelet swirl, whereas others prefer to assay the platelet hypotonic shock response (osmotic recovery), evaluate the extent of shape change, or use a morphology scoring system. None of these in vitro assays, however, is as reliable as radiolabeled in vivo platelet survival studies.[45, 46] Although some have suggested using other markers for in vivo survival studies (e.g., biotinylation[47]), the basic concept is unchanged. No one in vitro assay accurately predicts in vivo recovery and survival as does a paired labeled trial in human volunteers.

PRESERVATIVE

To prepare platelet concentrates, as described previously, whole blood is drawn into one of several anticoagulant-preservative solutions, the most common being CPD or CPDA-1. Ethylenediaminetetraacetic acid (EDTA) EDTA, although a better calcium chelator than citrate, cannot be used because it causes platelets to lose their normal discoid shape and become spherical. This shape change is associated with reduced in vivo platelet viability. Furthermore, EDTA has adverse effects on cardiac and skeletal muscle. Heparin is not acceptable because it activates platelets, causing clumping; and in conjunction with antithrombin III, heparin produces systemic anticoagulation. The citrate in the CPD or CPDA-1 preservative, however, is metabolized to bicarbonate and has no systemic in vivo anticoagulant effect.

Although platelets stored in citrated plasma are satisfactory for clinical use, several investigators have evaluated the possibility of replacing the plasma with a buffered salt solution containing various additives that would be capable of storing platelets for 5 days or longer.[36, 42, 48–51] The solutions being studied include commercial glucose-free crystalloid solution, synthetic media with glucose and bicarbonate, and synthetic phosphate-buffered solutions. Some investigators also have suggested placing various additives in the platelet storage bag, such as prostaglandin E_1, theophylline, aprotinin, and hirudin.[49–51] The potential for harmful side effects from use of such additives especially in infants and pregnant women has caused the FDA to take a very cautious approach to the addition of such compounds to blood components.

CENTRIFUGATION

Centrifugation conditions also affect platelet function. The shear stresses associated with the first "soft" spin (to prepare PRP) and the second "hard" spin (to pellet the platelet into the platelet concentrate) not only produce a discharge of cytosolic lactate dehydrogenase (LDH) but also stimulate the platelet release reaction.[52] Release of β-thromboglobulin into the plasma and the appearance of P-selectin (CD62P, GMP-140) on the platelet membrane surface are both evidence of the release of platelet granule contents after platelet preparation.[7, 42, 53, 54]

Various spin protocols have been developed in an attempt to decrease any adverse impact of the preparative technique on development of the platelet storage lesion. Research has shown that using a hard spin first to spin the platelets into a buffy coat on a cushion of red cells, and then using a slow spin to isolate the platelets from the separated buffy coat, yields a platelet product with less evidence of in vitro activation.[50] After 5 days of storage, however, this preparative technique does not appear to have any better in vivo survival or function characteristics than do platelets made by the soft spin followed by a hard spin method. The soft spin/hard spin method is favored in the United States, whereas the buffy coat technique is preferred in Europe.

TEMPERATURE

The optimal platelet storage temperature appears to be 20°C to 24°C with continuous gentle agitation. Cold storage at 1°C to 6°C, such as is used for red cells, is not acceptable for long-term storage of platelets.[36] Whereas cold storage would likely inhibit bacterial growth compared with the warmer temperatures currently used, cold storage markedly reduces post-transfusion platelet viability. In the cold, the platelet's microtubule apparatus disassembles, producing platelet dysfunction. Some researchers believe, however, that if changes in the platelet cytoskeleton, especially actin, can be prevented, long-term cold storage of platelets could become a reality.[55–58] Researchers[55–58] have shown that platelets treated with cytochalasin B, an agent that inhibits the assembly of new actin filaments, do not develop pseudopods, undergo spreading, or retract clots. They do, however, aggregate with ADP. Hartwig and Winokur[55, 56] have shown that when EGTA-AM is added to stored platelets, it prevents increases in calcium flux into the platelet, thus inhibiting platelet actin assembly. When EGTA-AM is combined with cytochalasin B and added to human platelets stored at 4°C for 21 days, the resulting platelets retained excellent activity. Again, however, concerns have arisen regarding the wisdom of including such additives in stored platelet concentrates. Although further research may fully allay this concern, it is unclear what role cold stored platelets will play in the future of clinical transfusion practice. Temperature cycling, a technique in which platelets are stored at 4°C and periodically warmed to 37°C for brief periods,[59, 60] is not clinically useful.[61] Furthermore, the equipment necessary to produce and monitor the changes in temperature required is too cumbersome and expensive.

PROTEOLYSIS OF PLATELET CYTOSKELETAL PROTEINS DURING STORAGE

The platelet cytoskeleton plays a major role in the maintenance of platelet shape and in ensuring the integrity of the external platelet membrane with its associated ligands and receptors.[62–66] The role of cytoskeletal proteolysis in the development of the platelet storage lesion is unknown. Deterioration of cytoskeletal proteins could have a substantial negative impact on platelet structure and function and could play a role in the development of microvesicle formation.[67–69] There are a large number of platelet cytoskeleton proteins, including actin, actin-binding protein (ABP), talin, vinculin, gelsolin, tubulin, myosin heavy chain, and profilin. Of these, actin is present in greatest abundance, constituting 15% to 20% of total platelet protein.

Actin present in platelet concentrates stored under blood bank conditions is cleaved into at least two fragments of approximately 28 kD, called storage proteins 1 and 2 (SP1 and SP2).[70, 71] Amino acid sequencing identified these proteins as fragments of actin formed by cleavage on the N-terminal side of residues Thr-106 (SP1) and Ala-114 (SP2).[71] Generation of these proteins was stimulated by the calcium ionophore A23187 and was inhibited by nonspecific protease inhibitors. These findings are consistent with proteolysis of actin by calpain, the calcium-dependent neutral protease.[72–78] Degradation of platelet cytoskeletal proteins ABP, talin, and vinculin during storage is also due to calpain activation. ABP degradation products have been seen on immunoblots of 1-day-old platelet concentrates, implying that activation of platelets actually begins with the preparative centrifugation and resuspension procedures, before storage of the concentrate. The shear stresses that are generated during these processes are known to produce the release reaction[52, 53] and to stimulate calpain generation.[79–81] Continued proteolysis during storage under blood bank conditions is reflected by the further generation of lower-molecular-weight breakdown products of ABP by day 6 of storage. The increased proteolysis over time may be the result of the initial generation of calpain due to the preparative protocol and/or the continued generation of calpain during storage by shear stress induced by the continued shaking of platelets on a blood bank agitator.

Calpain activation during storage may also promote microvesicle formation by altering the actin-membrane interface through cleavage of actin, ABP, talin, and vinculin. Microvesicles, pieces of platelet membrane, are known to form in platelet concentrate during storage.[68] Some researchers suggest that formation of microvesicles requires the fixation of complement.[82, 83] Other mechanisms have also been postulated.[84] Whether calpain is released as a result of shear stress or by the fixation of the C5-9 component of complement, however, it is activated during blood bank storage and digests a variety of major cytoskeletal proteins, including ABP, talin, vinculin,[85, 86] spectrin,[63] and band 4.1. Actin and actin fragments (SP1 and SP2) are also present in microvesicles. Activated calpain may thus degrade actin and other cytoskeleton elements, leading to a weakening of the actin–cytoplasmic membrane interface, with resultant formation of microvesicles. Caspases are proteins produced by cells undergoing apoptosis-programmed cell death.[87] Caspase 9 is known to degrade a variety of proteins.[88] The role played by caspases in the degradation of actin and other parts of the platelet cytoskeleton, if any, is unclear because platelets are anucleate cytoplasmic fragments. However, study of megakaryocyte apoptosis will likely prove to be very rewarding in this regard.

ACTIVATION OF PLATELET CONCENTRATE DURING PREPARATION AND STORAGE

A variety of markers have been employed to examine platelet activation during storage of platelet concentrates.[42, 45, 89] These include proteins associated with the alpha granule, such as β-thromboglobulin,[52] platelet factor 4, and P-selectin (CD62P)[53]; dense granule proteins such as serotonin[45]; cytosolic enzymes such as LDH[52]; and membrane ligands, including GPIb[90–92] and GPIIb-IIIa[93] (Table 13–2). Yet, despite evidence for significant platelet activation during storage, platelets stored for 5 days and subsequently transfused circulate, correct the bleeding time, produce acceptable corrected count increments, and arrest bleeding.[38, 94–97]

P-Selectin

P-selectin (CD62P, previously known as GMP-140 or PADGEM) is an important adhesive protein involved in platelet/leukocyte/endothelial interactions involving leukocyte attachment, rolling, extravasation, and regulation of cytokine synthesis in the leukocyte.[7] This alpha granule membrane protein is sequestered on the internal membrane of the alpha granule in resting platelets. With platelet activation and fusion of the alpha granule with the

Table 13–2. Markers of Platelet Activation in Stored Platelets

Release of alpha granule contents: β-thromboglobulin, platelet factor 4, thrombospondin, fibronectin, and platelet-derived growth factor
Release of dense granule contents: Ca^{2+}, serotonin, and ADP/ATP
Generation of P-selectin (GMP-140, PADGEM, CD62P) on external membrane
Discharge of cytosolic enzymes such as lactate dehydrogenase
Conformational change in GPIIb-IIIa
Binding of fibrinogen to platelet membrane receptor complex GPIIb-IIIa
Increases in generation and release of platelet microvesicles
Increased degradation of cytoskeletal proteins by calpain, including actin, actin-binding protein, talin, vinculin, and spectrin
Cleavage of GPIb-IX with generation of glycocalicin

ADP, adenosine diphosphate; ATP, adenosine triphosphate; GP, glycoprotein.

platelet membrane, P-selectin becomes an integral membrane glycoprotein on the platelet surface.[98] The presence of P-selectin allows quantitation of the percentage of platelets that have undergone alpha granule release; the total surface content of P-selectin may correlate with the released alpha granule contents.[7, 44]

Using monoclonal antibodies that recognize P-selectin, several investigators have examined this selectin in stored platelet concentrates.[53, 99, 100] Fijnheer and associates[100] found that pelleting of platelets from platelet-rich plasma resulted in expression of P-selectin by 20% of platelets, compared with only 8% when platelets were isolated from the buffy coat without pelleting. Interestingly, after 5 days of storage, the percentages of activated platelets in the two preparations approached 50%. These data suggest that whereas the pelleting step significantly contributes to alpha granule release, ongoing platelet activation occurs during storage and significantly increases the degree of platelet activation, regardless of the preparative methodology used.

Fijnheer and coworkers[101] also found that the higher the platelet count in the platelet concentrate, the greater the percentage of activated platelets at any given time. After 5 days of storage, platelet activation averaged 15% in stored platelets at the lower counts (1×10^9/mL) and 30% at counts of 1.4×10^9/mL; these percentages increased to 60% and 70%, respectively, by 10 days of storage. P-selectin on the surface of activated platelets (and endothelial cells) has been demonstrated to function as a ligand for neutrophils and monocytes.[102] It has been shown by some researchers that P-selectin–positive platelets might be preferentially removed from the circulation after transfusion, being cleared by the mononuclear-phagocyte system as bound conjugates with leukocytes.[7, 53] Platelets isolated from normal donors were stored for 2 to 4 days under standard blood bank conditions and were subsequently examined for P-selectin expression, labeled with indium-111, and reinfused into the autologous donors.[53] Platelet recoveries at 1 hour demonstrated an inverse correlation with the percentage of activated platelets expressing P-selectin; the r value was -0.55 ($r^2 = 0.30$; $p<.05$). With the r^2 being low, even though P-selectin expression may affect early platelet recovery, there are clearly other factors (pH, temperature, agitation) influencing platelet recovery.

Rinder and associates[53] also studied the recovery of activated platelets after transfusion into thrombocytopenic cancer patients. By quantitating the percentage of activated platelets in patients before and after transfusion and in the platelet concentrate, they compared the observed recovery of activated platelets with the predicted recovery, which was based on the increment in platelet count after transfusion. They found that the observed recovery of activated platelets was always lower than predicted (average: 38% of the predicted values), implying that activated platelets may be cleared preferentially after transfusion.

These data again suggest that P-selectin expression on the platelet surface may be only one factor influencing platelet recovery after transfusion of platelet concentrates. This hypothesis of preferential clearance of activated platelets is also supported by their differential ability to bind to monocytes and neutrophils in whole blood. Circulating activated platelets bind to fixed tissue macrophages, or circulating leukocyte-platelet conjugates, and may consequently be cleared from the blood stream. However, platelets may later dissociate from leukocyte conjugates and reenter the circulating platelet pool. Other possibilities for the continued circulation of activated platelets include loss of P-selectin from the platelet membrane, possibly by cleavage or endocytosis.[103] Platelet activation results in proteolysis of the platelet cytoskeleton.[70, 71, 104] Interactions between the platelet cytoskeleton and the platelet external membrane have been demonstrated, and activation could affect receptor expression or receptor/ligand interactions. Gamble and associates[105] have shown that soluble P-selectin affects neutrophil adhesion to endothelium; similar mechanisms function for platelet adhesion to the reticuloendothelial system after transfusion. Despite alterations in the quantity and function of platelet surface adhesion receptors, membrane glycoproteins, and platelet granule contents, stored platelet concentrates retain remarkably normal function after transfusion. However, there are data that post-transfusion platelet count increments decline during storage. Hogge and associates[106] showed that the 1-hour corrected count increment for fresh platelets transfused into thrombocytopenic patients averaged 20,000, compared with 12,000 and 10,000 for platelets transfused after being stored for 3 days and 7 days, respectively.

Glycoprotein Ib

Changes in platelet surface expression of glycoprotein Ib (GPIb) with storage have been studied by several laboratories. Michelson and colleagues[90–92] have demonstrated that the extracellular portion of GPIb was cleaved during platelet storage and that the level of cleaved segment, glycocalicin, increased in the cell-free supernatant over 5 days of storage. They reported that surface GPIb was degraded by proteases, such as plasmin, that are present in stored platelet concentrates. Despite this increase in plasma glycocalicin, surface GPIb content remained relatively constant, although a subpopulation of GPIb-negative platelets did appear over time. They postulated that replacement of surface GPIb must occur by relocation of GPIb to the surface from an intracellular pool or a sequestered surface population. They found that total platelet GPIb content was four times higher than surface amounts, suggesting the presence of an intraplatelet pool of GPIb. Using flow cytometry and ristocetin function studies, Michelson and Barnard[92] confirmed that plasmin was capable of degrading surface GPIb; incubation of plasmin-treated platelets with fresh autologous plasma caused surface GPIb to be replenished. This relocation of GPIb appeared functionally linked to the platelet cytoskeleton, because treatment with cytochalasin B inhibited the plasma effect on GPIb.

George and associates[99] showed that storage conditions may play a significant role in platelet surface receptor changes. They demonstrated that platelet concentrates stored on an elliptical rotator lost nearly 50% of their surface GPIb, whereas membrane GPIb on platelets stored on a circular tumbler rotator did not significantly decrease. Therefore, comparisons between studies of stored platelet concentrates must carefully examine not only detection methods but also the storage and preparation protocols. Manipulation of platelet concentrates may also result in decreased surface GPIb. In platelet concentrates exposed to high-dose (10,000 mJ/cm^3) ultraviolet B irradiation, surface GPIb declined on average by 60%, compared with a 20% decrease in untreated platelet concentrates.[107] By contrast, there was no significant difference in GPIIb-IIIa surface density between the two treatment groups. Bertolini and colleagues[108] examined the effect of different blood filters on GPIb and GPIIb-IIIa expression in platelet concentrates. They determined that blood filters did not significantly change the density of surface adhesion receptors.

The ability of fresh plasma to restore platelet GPIb and its adhesive properties may be one avenue by which stored platelets retain their function after transfusion. GPIb is critical to platelet function, serving as the primary receptor for von Willebrand factor and mediating platelet adhesion to the vasculature at high shear rates. Relocation of GPIb to the platelet surface from an intraplatelet pool or from a sequestered surface site may well occur after transfusion to preserve platelet function. In addition, the levels of GPIb after storage, although low, are not as low as those seen on platelets from patients with Bernard-Soulier syndrome. Thus, there may be a critical level of surface GPIb below which platelet adhesion is significantly impaired but above which normal function can be anticipated.

Glycoprotein IIb-IIIa

In a study by George and associates,[99] 7 days of storage on both the elliptical and tumbler rotators caused surface GPIIb-IIIa to increase slightly, as measured by iodine-125–labeled monoclonal antibodies. Fijnheer and coworkers[101] used flow cytometry and two monoclonal antibodies to GPIIb-IIIa to examine surface expression of the complex in stored platelet concentrates. After 5 days of storage, mean surface expression of GPIIb-IIIa increased 50% to 70% from baseline; expression increased by 300% or more when storage was continued for 5 days longer (10 days total).

In a separate study, Fijnheer and associates[100] found that preparation of platelets (especially the pelleting step) was largely responsible for the initial increase in surface GPIIb-IIIa. The increased surface GPIIb-IIIa in these studies paralleled increases in β-thromboglobulin release and surface expression of P-selectin, both indicative of alpha granule release. Because alpha granules contain a pool of GPIIb-IIIa, it seems likely that the increase in platelet surface expression of GPIIb-IIIa is due to relocation to the surface from alpha granule stores. Loss of surface GPIIb-IIIa may be occurring with storage, owing to protease degradation or to formation of microparticles from the platelet membrane, as demonstrated by Bode and colleagues,[109] but any potential loss appears to be well compensated by release of intracellular pools on platelet activation.

Platelet Cold Storage and Cryopreservation

Although platelets are traditionally stored at 20°C to 24°C with continuous gentle agitation, other forms of platelet storage include that in the frozen state and storage of lyophilized platelets.[110] The successful application of the principles of cryobiology to the freezing and preservation of red blood cells for transfusion was achieved in the 1960s. Techniques for cryopreservation of platelets, however, have been less successful. Cryoinjury to a cell is minimized by using the highest possible concentration of a cryoprotectant. However, that concentration is usually limited by the deleterious effects of the cryoprotectant. These effects can be the result either of direct chemical damage, usually dependent on both the concentration of cryoprotectant and the temperature, or of osmotic changes that occur secondary to the rate at which the cryoprotectant crosses the cell membrane.

Glycerol and dimethylsulfoxide (DMSO) are the two cryoprotective agents in clinical use. Glycerol, used extensively for red cell cryopreservation, is a physiological compound with relatively little direct chemical toxicity at the doses used. However, the relatively slow intracellular penetrance of this compound can result in severe osmotic effects. Use of a 5% glycerol/4% glucose solution results in minimal freeze/thaw platelet loss and, in initial studies, good preservation of platelet function.[111] However, subsequent reports of the effects of freezing on in vitro platelet function have varied, perhaps reflecting problems with the glucose/glycerol freezing methodology that may be detrimental to platelets. In particular, several in vitro studies have shown significant platelet damage after freezing. The damage consists of morphological and ultrastructural changes, decreased ATP levels, inability to undergo the release reaction or aggregation, and decreased recovery from hypotonic stress.[112–114] In vivo recovery of platelets cryopreserved in glucose/glycerol is significantly decreased compared with liquid-stored platelets and platelets frozen in DMSO.[112, 114] Modifications of the original procedure, including optimizing the platelet count before freezing and use of a nonplasma diluent, have improved in vitro function.[115] However, optimum conditions for platelet cryopreservation are not yet defined. Despite promising early results, platelet cryopreservation using glucose/glycerol solutions has not successfully been adapted for use in clinical transfusion practice.[116] DMSO, which rapidly penetrates the platelet membrane, produces less of an osmotic effect than does glucose/glycerol. Moreover, DMSO has been shown by both in vitro and in vivo studies to be a more effective cryoprotective agent than glycerol.[113, 117] Indeed, attempts at freezing platelets in 5% to 6% DMSO have been successful. Valeri[118] reported that DMSO preserved platelets remain functional after 3 years at −80°C; Schiffer has reported similar success with DMSO cryopreservation.[110, 119] However, cryopreservation with 5% to 6% DMSO still results in a substantial loss of platelet viability associated with changes in morphology, decreased aggregation, and decreased platelet recovery.[120, 121] Furthermore, there are safety concerns regarding the general usefulness of DMSO as a cryoprotectant that have yet to be addressed. The average post-transfusion recovery of cryopreserved platelets has been reported to be 50% to 70% of that for fresh platelets, with those platelets circulating showing a normal survival.[110, 118, 119] Studies have reported that approximately 50% of platelets show cryopreservation damage and become unresponsive to various agonists. Platelets affected by cryopreservation show a reduction in the content of secretory granules and an almost complete absence of the metabolic activity usually seen after platelet activation.

It has been postulated that these findings reflect a defect in the stimulus-response coupling mechanism as a result of plasma membrane damage. Although these effects generally appear to be equally distributed among subpopulations of platelets of different sizes, the largest platelets have been found to retain a better platelet aggregation response than have the smallest platelets.[122] Platelets stored frozen in liquid nitrogen with DMSO as a cryoprotectant have also been shown to have lower adhesive capacity in vitro, compared with fresh platelets from the same platelet unit.[123]

Another concern about the use of DMSO as a cryoprotective agent is the incidence of clinical side effects such as nausea, vomiting, and local vasospasm. However, there are relatively few data evaluating the use of other cryoprotective agents for freezing platelets. Propane-1,2-diol (propylene glycol), which has been shown to be an effective agent for other hematopoietic elements and has a higher permeability rate than glycerol, has been shown to be an ineffective cryoprotectant for platelets.[124, 125] Other cryoprotectants that have been investigated, including various combinations of glycerol, polyvinylpyrrolidone, mannitol, nitroprusside, amiloride, trehalose, and glucose, have not been fully successful in protecting platelets from freeze-induced injury.[110] Lyophilized platelets have been studied by Bode's group.[126] They reported that rehydrated lyophilized human platelets correct hemostatic abnormalities in an aspirin-treated dog cardiopulmonary bypass model.

PLASTIC CONTAINERS AND PLASTICIZER TOXICITY

First-generation platelet storage bags composed of polyvinyl chloride (PVC) containing a 2-diethylhexyl phthalate (DEHP) plasticizer did not permit storage of platelets beyond 3 days.[127] The walls of such plastic bags were too thick to permit adequate gas exchange; insufficient oxygen entered the bag to sustain aerobic metabolism. After 3 days of storage, anaerobic metabolism produces so much lactic acid that the pH of the concentrate routinely decreased to less than 6.0, and in vivo platelet recovery and survival were markedly decreased.[33–35] Platelet concentrate pH can be adequately maintained for 5 days by storing 50 to 65 mL of platelet concentrate in more gas-permeable, second-generation blood bags, made of either PVC with a trimellitate, non-DEHP plasticizer such as TOTM (Fenwal PL-1240 or Cutter CLX)[96] or blow-molded polyolefin (Fenwal PL-732).[38, 128] A third type of second-generation platelet storage bag uses a thin-film PVC with a 2-DEHP plasticizer (XT-612, Terumo). A fourth type of second-generation blood bag is made of PVC with a citrate-based non-DEHP plasticizer (butyryl-tri-hexyl citrate [BTHC], Fenwal PL-2209); a COBE Spectre Apheresis System licensed by the FDA also uses this plastic. PL-2209 also is able to store 5 to 7 × 10^{11} platelets/bag, in 400 mL of plasma for 5 days at 20°C to 24°C with acceptable in vitro and in vivo storage characteristics.[97]

The importance of an oxygen-permeable platelet storage bag cannot be overemphasized. The entrance of oxygen into the bag during storage permits platelets to maintain energy metabolism through mitochondrial oxidative phosphorylation. If oxygen in the storage bag is insufficient, platelet metabolism is channeled through the anaerobic, glycolytic pathway. This pathway produces large amounts of lactic acid, which reacts with the bicarbonate buffer in the plasma. When the bicarbonate is exhausted, at levels of 20 to 25 mmol/L of lactic acid, there is a rapid reduction in pH and a loss of platelet viability.[33–35] This effect can be ameliorated by using a gas-permeable storage bag that permits the influx of oxygen as well as the efflux of carbon dioxide. Although 6.0 is the minimum acceptable pH, a fall in pH below 6.2 is associated not only with an increase in the expression of CD62 but also with abnormal platelet morphology and a loss of reactivity to hypotonic stress (osmotic recovery).[36] Optimal pH for platelet concentrate approximates 7.0. An excessively alkaline pH, greater than 7.6, is also associated with platelet damage and release.

Some blood storage bags are still composed of PVC plastic with a DEHP plasticizer. Despite its use since the 1950s, concerns have been raised regarding the potential adverse effects of the administration of large amounts of DEHP plasticizer, which leaches into blood when DEHP-plasticized containers are used for blood storage.[127, 129–131] These concerns, which include the potential carcinogenicity of DEHP and also of its monoethylhexyl phthalate (MEHP) metabolite, have led to development of the various alternative plasticizers for use in blood storage containers.[132–134] A number of animal model studies have demonstrated various forms of DEHP toxicity, including reduced fertility, testicular atrophy, teratogenesis, and hepatic enlargement.[133, 135] DEHP, however, also confers a beneficial membrane-stabilizing antihemolytic effect on the red cell during storage.[136–138] Indeed, DEHP has been found to exert a significant red cell protective effect and to reduce hemolysis by approximately 50% during a given period of storage compared with other plasticizers and with storage in glass containers.[136–138] Although platelet concentrates prepared from units of whole blood or from plateletpheresis collections may be stored in blood bags composed of blow-molded polyolefin plastic without a plasticizer, or with a tri-2-ethylhexyl trimellitate plasticizer,[139–142] these alternative storage containers are unacceptable as red cell storage bags. The greater degree of hemolysis measured during storage of red cells in non-DEHP plasticized containers[143–147] is unacceptable.

Toxicological studies of BTHC have shown the plasticizer to be safe.[148, 149] BTHC leaches into plasma at a level 60% to 70% less than DEHP. Moreover, BTHC differs from the phthalate plasticizer in that BTHC is metabolized to the physiological compounds citric acid, butyric acid, and hexanol. Extensive toxicological testing has shown that BTHC has a very low level of toxicity, with an oral median lethal dose (LD_{50}) of more than 20 g/kg for rats and more than 48 g/kg for mice. Neither the BTHC plasticizer nor the PVC plastic polymer produces local toxic effects, as determined by dermal, ocular, and intramuscular implantation testing; extensive testing in a number of species demonstrates the lack of significant intravenous toxicity as well. The chemical compound is not mutagenic and, unlike with DEHP, repeated oral administration does not induce peroxisome proliferation in the liver. BTHC plasticizer and its degradation products are rapidly eliminated from the body by pulmonary, fecal, and urinary routes; 70% of a single dose is excreted in 44 hours. Although gas permeability of the material is slightly less than that of PL-732 plastic,[139, 140, 144] there is sufficient transmission of oxygen into, and carbon dioxide out of, the platelet container to ensure aerobic oxidative metabolism and maintenance of an acceptable pH.

PLATELET AGITATORS

Platelets must be stored with continuous gentle agitation. Rotators are available in a face-over-face (circular) angle of rotation[38] or flatbed agitators. Not all agitators have been compatible with all types of plastic bags, however. For example, the use of 6-rpm elliptical rotators for storage of the PL-732 blow-molded polyolefin bags was found to show a decreased post-transfusion recovery and survival,[128] perhaps related to platelet-plastic storage bag interactions at various shear stresses. All of the various storage bag-rotator combinations are associated with increasing levels of CD62P over the time of storage. It is clear that the shear stress associated with the required continuous gentle agitation results in progressive release of β-thromboglobulin from alpha granules and appearance of CD62P on the platelet plasma membrane.[44, 52–54] Agitation is also associated with discharge of cytosolic LDH, suggesting that some degree of platelet lysis occurs during agitation.[52]

PLATELET AGE

Fresh platelets have better in vivo recovery and survival rates than do stored platelets. The post-transfusion corrected count increments of fresh platelets are generally better than those of platelets stored for 3 to 7 days. However, in one study, the corrected count increments of platelets stored 3 days were no different from those of platelets stored for 7 days.[106] Thus, it would appear that whatever the cause of the platelet storage defect, it likely occurs early in storage. Furthermore, once it has occurred, its effects persist for the rest of the storage period. Although platelets stored for 5 days function in vivo and correct bleeding times, they generally have worse in vivo recovery and survival than fresh (less than 24 hours old) platelets. However, stored platelets still function sufficiently well for use in clinical practice.

LEUKOREDUCTION

Until the mid-1980s, filtration of blood occurred primarily at the bedside. In the 1980s, the development of the techniques of spin-cool-filter for microaggregate removal popularized the concept of depleting a unit of blood of leukocytes at the bedside.[150] In the 1990s, the concept of high-efficiency filtration became accepted, as filters designed to remove 3 to 4 $\log_{10}$ or more of white cells from a unit of red blood cells and platelets became available.[151–153]

There has been a growing interest in preventing the multiple adverse effects attributable to leukocytes in stored platelet concentrates as well as in preventing in vivo post-transfusion reactions ascribed to the inflammatory cytokines produced by leukocytes contained within the units of infused platelets. For example, lysosomal enzymes present in neutrophils are known to digest various platelet proteins; elastase, for example, digests GPIb. During storage, the NADPH oxidase system in platelets is activated by released platelet activating factor (PAF).[154] Cytokines released from lymphocytes are known to produce a variety of adverse effects in vivo. Heddle and colleagues[155] showed that the platelet-poor supernatant plasma from stored platelet concentrates is more likely to produce febrile reactions than are the platelets contained in the cellular fraction of the stored units of concentrates. Several groups have shown that lymphocytes present in units of stored platelets produce cytokines.[156, 157] These cytokines likely produce, in turn, febrile transfusion reactions. Generation of the lymphokine interleukin (IL)-8 during storage of platelet concentrates could produce symptoms of nonhemolytic transfusion reactions.[156] Removal of leukocytes early in storage (prestorage leukoreduction), however, eliminates this risk because it removes the lymphocytes before the cells have had a chance to deteriorate or synthesize and release various enzymes and cytokines. Degenerating basophils release histamine and other vasoactive substances and leukocytes, such as antigen-presenting cells (APCs) present in platelet concentrate, to promote human leukocyte antigen (HLA) alloimmunization and platelet refractoriness.[153, 158] The adverse effects from the discharge of neutrophilic enzymes, from release of cytokines from lymphocytes during storage, and from the initiation of HLA alloimmunization by donor APCs can all be reduced by prestorage leukocyte depletion, which would remove the offending leukocytes before they could produce the adverse effects described earlier.

Blajchman and coworkers[159] showed, in a rabbit model, that supernatant plasma obtained from blood stored before filtration induced a significantly higher degree of alloimmunization than did plasma filtered before whole blood storage. These results imply that prefiltration may further decrease the incidence of HLA alloimmunization by preventing generation of soluble biological response modifiers as well as by preventing the formation of platelet or red cell microparticles during storage. The applicability of these data to humans, however, is uncertain. It is generally believed that viable donor APCs are needed to present donor HLA antigen to the recipient's T cells.[158] Whether this mechanism would function with the infusion of plasma without donor APCs is not clear. In such cases the recipient's APCs can also present transfused donor antigens. If so, removal of leukocytes before they shed HLA antigens into the stored plasma may be beneficial. Blood bags with red cell and platelet leukoreduction filters integrally attached so as to provide a closed system for prestorage leukocyte depletion at the time of collection are available and being used more extensively.

Leukocyte Removal Filters and Biological Response Modifiers

There is a misconception among some clinicians that platelets should not be transfused through a filter because the filter will remove a significant percentage of platelets.[160] This is not only false, but it is actually a violation of FDA regulations, which require that all blood components be infused through an administration set containing a filter. Platelets transfused through a first-generation 170-μm standard filter pass through with less than 5% loss of platelets owing to the filter void volume. Similarly, platelet concentrates also pass through second-generation screen and depth microaggregate filters with a small degree of loss (less than 10%).[160] Moreover, any platelets retained in the second-generation filter's dead space can be recovered by flushing the filter with normal saline.[160] Second-generation filters, however, are designed primarily to remove microaggregate debris from units of red cells. Because there are few microaggregates in units of platelet concentrate, and because second-generation filters do not remove individual white cells, the use of such filters for platelet transfusions is not indicated.

Third-generation leukocyte depletion filters are designed to remove individual white cells. These filters are generally manufactured from a polyester fiber matrix to which various polymer chemicals are linked. The size of the polymer affects the degree of surface tension removal, and thus the degree of leukocyte removal. Filters that are specifically designed for red cells remove white cells as well as platelets from units of red blood cells.[161] On the other hand, filters that are specifically designed for leukocyte depletion of units of platelets will remove only white cells and not platelets. The use of the wrong filter can result in removal of a significant percentage of the desired cells.[161]

The transfusion of platelets through blood filters can produce other effects. Holme and associates[162] showed that infusion of platelets through cotton-wool filters as well as polyester filters stimulates the production of $C3a_{desarg}$ during filtration. A rise in $C3a_{desarg}$ production is also seen in older units of platelet concentrates during storage. After infusion into patients, no adverse effect attributable to the infusion of the pre-formed $C3a_{desarg}$ was noted, presumably because it was inactivated in vivo. The occurrence of frequent and substantial pulmonary compromise or other adverse effects related to infusion of activated complement components has not been widely reported.

Anaphylactic reactions after some platelet and red cell transfusions have been reported. Although the pathogenesis of this syndrome is unclear, it appears in some cases to involve generation of plasma kallikrein by some types of biomaterials that stimulate the generation of bradykinin. Bradykinin produces adverse effects in vivo, such as hypotension, abdominal pain, and facial flushing, without fever or chills.[163] A percentage of these cases involve patients receiving blood through bedside leukoreduction filters, especially if such patients are receiving an angiotensin-converting enzyme (ACE) inhibitor medication.[163, 164] ACE is identical to kininase II, an enzyme that degrades bradykinin. Blockage of kininase II thus prolongs the half-life of bradykinin in these patients and can profoundly worsen the clinical symptomatology. Because bradykinin has a half-life of 15 to 30 seconds, prestorage leukoreduction as opposed to bedside leukoreduction should eliminate reactions due to bradykinin generation from contact with the filter biomaterials. Although these anaphylactic reactions occur infrequently, blood bank physicians should inform house staff and nurses about this potential problem. Clinicians need to be aware when a patient on an ACE inhibitor is to receive a platelet or a red blood cell transfusion through a bedside leukoreduction filter, so that the patient can be monitored closely. Such patients could benefit from receiving blood that has been either prestorage or in-laboratory leukoreduced, as opposed to being infused through a bedside leukoreduction filter. This area is under active study.

Bacterial Contamination

Concern over the risk of bacterial contamination of stored platelet concentrates is becoming a serious public health issue. The number of case reports of sepsis and death from units of platelet concentrate contaminated with bacteria has increased over the past years, as the FDA has increased its surveillance activities.[165, 166] The organisms implicated include skin contaminants such as *Staphylococcus epidermidis* as well as enteric organisms such as *Enterobacter* and *Escherichia coli.*[167] Use of incorrect technique for donor arm preparation as well as use of inappropriate venipuncture technique can lead to disastrous consequences for the recipient of such an improperly collected unit of blood. Passage of the venipuncture needle through a dimple in donor skin could result in increased risk of bacterial seeding of the collected unit of blood by organisms buried in the skinfolds in the dimple. Morrow and coworkers[166] reviewed their experience with septic platelet transfusions and concluded that the risk of septic platelet transfusion was real and would likely increase. Commercial assays for bacteria, including polymerase chain reaction (PCR) techniques, chemical tests, and tests aimed at detection of radioactive CO_2, are under various stages of development. A major problem is the lack of a suitable and rapid point-of-care, or point-of-sign-out, method to determine whether platelets are contaminated. A Gram stain is insensitive unless more than 10^5 to 10^6 organisms/mL are found. Third-generation filters have been shown to have an inconsistent protective effect on units of platelets contaminated with bacteria.[168] These filters have been shown to remove some types of bacteria from units of platelets contaminated with bacteria in vitro. However, even leukoreduction filters capable of removing 4 to 5 logs of leukocytes cannot remove all types and strains of bacteria. Accordingly, filters cannot be labeled or recommended for this indication. The overall risk rate for bacterial contamination of a unit of blood is 1:1500 to 1:2000.

Concern over the transmission of viral and bacterial pathogens influences much of the research carried out in the field of platelet storage. The use of psoralen compounds and other pathogen inactivation systems may well do much to eliminate this concern.[169] Other agents are also being evaluated. For all of these technologies, however, it must be shown that post-transfusion platelet function and survival are not adversely affected. Despite advances in pathogen inactivation, once the unit of platelets is entered, as per current FDA guidelines, if it is not used within 4 hours, it must be discarded. The loss of a unit of SDP or a pool of RDP is becoming less tolerable, owing to the financial impact of this wastage on the transfusion service. Thus, despite pathogen inactivation technology designed for use at the point of manufacture, such as a blood center, there is still likely to be a future role for bacterial pathogen testing systems. When perfected, such a system will help ensure that units of blood components that are entered but not transfused within the current shelf life for open system products can still be used for transfusion. This system will facilitate component salvage and decrease wastage.

Single-Donor Platelets

Apheresis permits collection of 5 to 7 $\times$ 10^{11} platelets, well in excess of the minimum of 3 $\times$ 10^{11} platelets from a single donor. Storage of such a large number of platelets in a 300-mL container at 20°C to 24°C is inadequate, however, because the pH rapidly decreases. Thus, 1000-mL apheresis platelet storage bag containers are used to store 1.5 to over 3.0 $\times$ 10^{11} platelets in 100 to 200 mL of plasma. This larger bag permits improved gas transport of oxygen. Inability to provide adequate transport of oxygen into the storage bag and, to a lesser degree, adequate transport of carbon dioxide out limits the number of platelets that can be stored. Current citrate-based plasticizer bags can store up to 7 $\times$ 10^{11} platelets in a bag. Apheresis products must also be stored with continuous gentle agitation. Generally, apheresis platelets are collected in ACD-A solutions rather than the standard whole blood anticoagulants CPD, CPDA-1, or CP2D.

Apheresis platelets show in vitro characteristics comparable to those of random-donor platelets prepared from whole blood donation. A major benefit of single-donor plateletpheresis technology has been the ability to collect a large number of HLA-matched single-donor platelets needed for patients who had become HLA-alloimmunized. Refinements in apheresis technology permit a 3 to 4 log reduction in the number of white cells contained in single-donor platelets. Thus, a level of approximately 10^5 to 10^6 white cells is currently present in most apheresis platelets, as opposed to the 10^8 to 10^9 seen previously. Some physicians believe it is prudent to use third-generation filters to administer machine (process) leukocyte-reduced single-donor platelets to remove as many remaining white cells as possible in an attempt to lower the number of leukocytes by about 1 more $\log_{10}$; many others believe this is unnecessary and ineffective.

Controversy continues regarding the benefit of exclusive use of single-donor platelets. Benefits from use of single-donor versus random-donor platelets relate (1) to the decreased risk of transfusion-related infections achieved with the use of SDP and (2) to the lower degree of allogeneic donor antigenic stimulation with use of SDP. Future FDA licensure of pathogen inactivation technologies currently under development will help to reduce the concerns related to the first issue.[169] The transfusion community, however, is not currently able to provide all platelet products as SDPs, and random-donor platelets prepared from whole blood collection remain in major demand. Although it would appear that random-donor platelets will continue to be a major platelet product for the foreseeable future, the use of SDPs is increasing, either as HLA-matched, crossmatched, or random SDPs.

Platelet Substitutes

A variety of platelet substitutes are in various stages of development.[110, 126, 170–174] The term *platelet substitute* is really a misnomer. These products are not in truth substitutes for platelets. Although they may provide some type of platelet function, none of these products under development really replaces a platelet. Because we do not fully understand platelet function, any product developed can only be a partial substitute at best. As outlined by Lee and Blajchman,[172] a novel platelet product should be hemostatically effective, nonthrombogenic, nonimmunogenic, and sterile and not transmit infection; have a clinically significant duration of hemostatic action; have a long biologically active shelf life; have no or few specialized requirements for storage; and be easy to prepare and administer when needed. The military is especially interested in a platelet substitute that has most of these characteristics.

Several products are under development. One of these is a preparation known as "infusible platelet membrane."[170] This material is made from outdated platelets that are then lysed by freeze-thawing, then heat inactivated for 20 hours at 60°C and subsequently sonicated.

The fragments are then formulated with a preservative solution, lyophilized, and stored at 4°C. Much of the product is in the form of spherical vesicles with a mean modal diameter of 600 nm; the product is reported to be stable at 4°C for 2 years. It contains detectable GPIb but not GPIIb-IIIa. This preparation has a phospholipid content similar to that of natural platelets, retains PF3 activity, and has been reported to have reduced class I HLA expression.[172] Studies showed a shortening of the bleeding time in thrombocytopenic rabbits.[170, 172] There are several preliminary reports of its hemostatic effectiveness in humans as well.[172] One problem with this product relates to demonstration of efficacy for possible FDA licensure. Because measurement of a postinfusion platelet count increment is not possible with this material, because it consists of platelet fragments, the question of how to ascertain efficacy has been raised. This issue is germane to several types of platelet substitutes and is under active discussion. Lyophilized platelets have also been described.[126] Concerns regarding some of the issues raised earlier are being evaluated with reconstituted lyophilized platelets, including toxicity, in vivo survival, thrombogenicity, and reticuloendothelial system blockade.[126, 172]

Other substitutes include modified red cells named thromboerythrocytes.[171] These are red cells covalently coupled with RGD (Arg-Gly-Asp)-containing peptides, about 10^6/cell. These peptides are designed to bind to activated GPIIb-IIIa molecules, which limit thromboerythrocyte reactivity to platelets activated at the site of vascular injury. These RGD-peptide–coated red cells are not in active clinical trials. Other platelet substitutes being studied include inert polyacrylonitrile beads coated with fibrinogen, red cells with fibrinogen covalently bound to the membrane, fibrinogen-coated albumin microspheres, and liposome-based agents.[172] Although many of these products face long research and development times, problems with current platelet preparations and antigenicity of the current formulations of thrombopoietic cytokines (see later) may make a second look at these types of products prudent. Other types of nontraditional platelet preparations include frozen platelets, described earlier.

Thrombopoietic Growth Factors

There are three major hematopoietic cell lines for which physicians have traditionally treated deficiencies by transfusion, rather than by the stimulation of hematopoiesis.[175] These are the red cell, leukocyte (granulocyte), and platelet cell lines. Many molecules are now known to affect hematopoiesis; currently, several of them are licensed. Thrombopoietin (TPO) and a form known as megakaryocyte growth and development factor (MGDF) have been described.[175–180] Three growth factors are known to influence platelet production: IL-6, IL-11, and TPO. IL-6 is a 212-amino acid glycoprotein whose gene is located on chromosome 7p. It works with many other factors, including IL-1 or IL-3, to stimulate thrombopoiesis; a recombinant form is available. IL-11 is a 199-amino acid glycoprotein with its gene located on chromosome 19q. Recently licensed, IL-11 (oprelvekin) increases the platelet count by directly stimulating the proliferation of hematopoietic stem cells and megakaryocyte progenitor cells and by inducing increased megakaryocyte maturation.

IL-11 is indicated for preventing severe chemotherapy-induced thrombocytopenia and for reducing the need for platelet transfusions after myelosuppressive chemotherapy in patients with nonmyeloid malignancies. TPO is composed of approximately 350 amino acids, and its gene is located on chromosome 3q. Its receptor c-*mpl* was discovered during study of a viral oncogene v-*mpl* in the myeloproliferative (mpl) leukemia virus. Once this receptor was identified, the ligand (TPO) could then be isolated directly. The structure of TPO shows that there are two domains. The first is an erythropoietin-like domain of 163 amino acids. The second is a long carbohydrate chain. In the native form the carbohydrate chain remains intact. However, a truncated form in which the carbohydrate chain was cleaved and replaced with polyethylene glycol (PEG) was evaluated in clinical trials. Without the presence of the PEG moiety, or the carbohydrate chain, the half-life of the molecule in the circulation is too low. TPO also enhances the action of erythropoietin on red cells.

Thrombocytopenia is normally treated with platelet transfusions. The use of TPO to stimulate the production of platelets in thrombocytopenic oncology patients has been evaluated as part of animal trials.[181] Another aspect of the trial was use of TPO for treating normal volunteers.[182] TPO was evaluated in an attempt to increase the yield of platelets in donors who were enrolled in a volunteer plateletpheresis donation program.[183–186] This indication was evaluated carefully because it would be unacceptable to have any serious side effects resulting from injection of a thrombopoietic cytokine in a normal volunteer donor. A variety of treatment regimens were used, including one-cycle and three-cycle injections of TPO. Data showed that the platelet count in a normal individual receiving 1 dose of 3 μg/kg of TPO was approximately doubled. Apheresis platelets collected from such donors were stored and when transfused improved the platelet corrected count increment in the recipient. However, the development of an antibody to TPO that cross-reacted with endogenous TPO resulted in severe thrombocytopenia in several normal volunteer donors and has suspended the evaluation of this material for use in normal volunteer donors. The PEG-rHuMGDF clinical trials have been canceled, and this material is no longer under study in its present configuration. The full-length TPO (glycosylated) molecule is about to enter clinical trials. Because it is the natural molecule (i.e., not pegylated), there is hope that antibody formation will not be a problem with this thrombopoietic growth factor.

Interestingly, there has been a published report of a cytokine ligand mimic. Cwirla and colleagues[187] described a peptide agonist of the TPO receptor that was a 14-amino acid peptide with a high affinity for the TPO receptor. This molecule was shown to be equipotent to the 332-amino acid natural cytokines in cell-based assays. These small molecules, which can activate receptors, replacing the need for large peptide ligands, may open the way for production of new types of hematopoietic stem cell growth factors.

EFFECTS OF IRRADIATION ON PLATELETS

Gamma Irradiation

Cellular blood components are exposed to gamma irradiation to prevent the development of transfusion-associated graft-versus-host disease (TA-GVHD) in susceptible high-risk patients. Ionizing radiation affects cells adversely by damaging nuclear DNA or producing deleterious effects on cell membrane integrity.[188] Until recently, the dose of irradiation used varied from 1500 to 5000 cGy (1 rad = 1 cGy), with doses between 1500 and 3500 cGy most widely used in transfusion centers.[188–190] The FDA has recommended that a dose of 2500 cGy be delivered to the midplane of a free-standing irradiation canister with a minimum dose of 1500 cGy delivered to any other point in the canister.[191] Platelets stored for 1 to 5 days and subsequently irradiated with 5000 cGy have been shown to have normal platelet function in vitro, including morphology, platelet factor 3 activity, response to hypotonic stress and synergistic aggregation, β-thromboglobulin release, and thromboxane B_2 formation.[190] Irradiation with 5000 cGy caused a decrease in initial recovery of fresh and stored platelets transfused into normal volunteers but with normal platelet survival.[192] The circulating platelets also failed to neutralize the effects of aspirin on recipient's bleeding time; however, the hemostatic effectiveness of these platelets in thrombocytopenic patients did not appear to be compromised.[192] Subsequent studies have not confirmed any damaging effect of irradiation on platelets. Exposure of platelet concentrates to 3000 cGy followed by storage for 5 days has been shown to have no significant effect on either in vivo platelet recovery or platelet survival.[193] Similarly, no detrimental effects on in vitro function were demonstrated in platelet units irradiated with 2000 cGy and stored for up to 5 days.[194] Evaluation of paired apheresis platelets stored for 5 days after receiving 2500 cGy on days 1 or 3 showed no deleterious effects on in vivo recovery or survival or in vitro properties of platelets.[195] In contrast to the observed effects of irradiation on the storage of red cell products,[195, 196] the storage period of irradiated platelets is not affected and therefore does not need to be modified. These are important findings because many transfusion services are not equipped to irradiate blood components just before transfusion and therefore must maintain an inventory of irradiated platelets obtained from the collecting facility.

Ultraviolet Irradiation

Contaminating donor leukocytes in platelet concentrates have been found to play a significant role in primary alloimmunization of recipients to class I major histocompatibility complex (MHC) antigens, which in turn may result in refractoriness to platelet transfusions.[197] Lindahl-Keissling and Søfwenberg[198] showed in 1971 that lymphocytes exposed to ultraviolet (UV) irradiation at appropriate dosages are unable to stimulate allogeneic cells in mixed lymphocyte culture (MLC) or to respond to mitogenic stimulation. UVC, which has the shortest wavelength (200 to 280 nm) and the greatest biological activity, has been found to induce aggregation of human blood platelets and formation of pseudopods at the platelet surface.[199] Medium-wavelength UV light (UVB, 280 to 320 nm) has been shown to inactivate leukocytes in platelet concentrates at various doses, depending on the UV source, the type of plastic container used, and the cross-sectional depth of the platelet concentrate volume.[200–202] Platelet concentrates irradiated with 3000 J/m^2 of UVB and then stored for 5 days showed no difference in pH, hypotonic stress, or aggregation responses.[201] Irradiation of pooled platelet concentrates with high-dose UVB (100,000 J/m^2), however, resulted in a significant decrease in morphology score and osmotic recovery after 96 hours of storage. The expression of GPIb was also found to have declined by 60% at 96 hours after irradiation at the high dose, with no alteration observed in the level of surface GPIIb-IIIa.[107] Therefore, long-term storage of platelets after irradiation with high-dose UVB is not recommended. Autologous platelets stored for 1 to 5 days and then irradiated with 26,000 J/m^2 UVB showed normal recovery and survival compared with paired, nonirradiated controls. The hemostatic effectiveness of these platelets, measured by corrected platelet count increments in paired transfusions to thrombocytopenic patients, was not impaired.[203]

In vivo recovery and survival of autologous platelet concentrates irradiated with 15,000 J/m^2 of UVB showed a modest reduction in survival compared with controls (7 vs. 7.75 days), but all values for survival were acceptable.[204] In the Trial to Prevent Alloimmunization to Platelets (TRAP), UVB irradiation at 1480 mJ/cm^2 was shown to be equivalent to use of a leukoreduction filter for decreasing the incidence of refractoriness to platelet transfusions in patients with acute myelogenous leukemia.[205] Long-wavelength (320 to 400 nm) UV light (UVA) by itself is insufficient to inactivate leukocytes. However, at low doses, UVA activates 8-methoxypsoralen (8-MOP), transforming it into a potent DNA crosslinking agent capable of abolishing MLC activity.[206] The pretreatment of platelet concentrates with 8-MOP and UVA irradiation can reduce the allogenicity of class I MHC antigens in mice.[207] Platelet aggregation was unaffected in the system tested.

Platelet Photochemical Treatment

A platelet photochemical treatment (PCT) system for inactivation of infectious pathogens and leukocytes in platelet concentrates is under development.[169] This system uses a synthetic form of psoralens known as S-59, which is photoactivated by long-wavelength UVA light. In the absence of UVA light, S-59 reversibly intercalates into helical regions of DNA and RNA. With the addition of UVA light, S-59 binds to thymidine and forms nonreversible covalent monoadducts with DNA and RNA, resulting in the inactivation of viruses, bacteria, and leukocytes. The PCT system for platelets calls for the thrombocytes to be resuspended in approximately 35% plasma and 65% platelet additive solution (PAS III) in a total volume of 300 mL. After this, S-59 (150 μM) is added to the platelets through an integral closed container system.

After a 5-minute incubation, the platelets are illuminated with shaking for 3 minutes. All procedures are performed using a plastic storage bag transparent to UVA. After illumination, the platelets are transferred to another plastic platelet storage bag, containing an S-59 reduction device (SRD). The platelets are incubated with the SRD device for 6 hours with shaking to reduce the residual levels of S-59 and any free photoproducts. Although preclinical toxicology studies have been performed without S-59 reduction treatment, and have shown no clinically relevant toxicity, further reduction of S-59 levels enhances the safety margins associated with use of this pathogen inactivation system. After SRD incubation, the platelets are transferred to the final storage container for up to 5 days of storage. All transfers are made within an integral closed plastic bag system.

PCT with S-59 has demonstrated inactivation of high titers (10^5 to 10^6) of cell free human immunodeficiency virus (HIV), proviral HIV, duck hepatitis B virus (DHBV; a surrogate for HBV), bovine viral diarrhea virus (BVDV; a surrogate for hepatitis C virus), cytomegalovirus, gram-positive bacteria, and gram-negative bacteria. These studies were previously reported in detail.[169, 208, 209] In addition, recent studies were presented demonstrating inactivation of community-acquired inocula of hepatitis B and C viruses using a chimpanzee infectivity model.[210] Other studies have demonstrated inactivation of *Trypanosoma cruzi, Plasmodium malariae, Borrelia burgdorferi,* and *Rickettsia tsutsugamushi* in platelet concentrates.[169]

Leukocyte Inactivation

Leukocytes contaminating platelet concentrates have been associated with a spectrum of adverse immune reactions, including fever, alloimmunization, and graft-versus-host disease (TA-GVHD). Photochemical treatment of platelet concentrates has demonstrated inhibition of T cell proliferation and synthesis of cytokines.[169] Additional studies have demonstrated prevention of TA-GVHD using a mouse marrow transplantation model.[169] The TRAP trial[205] showed that UVB irradiation of platelet concentrates without leukoreduction filtration resulted in a reduced incidence of alloimmunization. Thus, the PCT process appears to have the potential for reduction of febrile transfusion reactions, reduction of alloimmunization, and inhibition or prevention of TA-GVHD.[169]

Clinical Trial Program

Preclinical studies demonstrated preservation of in vitro platelet properties and pH during 5 days of storage. PCT-treated platelets have been in clinical trials since June 1995. Four clinical trials (phases 1A, 1B, 2A, and 2B) were completed in healthy subjects without problems. These studies showed that PCT platelets appear to be well tolerated, are safe, and provide adequate platelet support of thrombocytopenic patients.[169] A fifth clinical trial to assess the hemostatic efficacy of PCT platelets in profoundly thrombocytopenic patients has been completed. A large phase 3 study using pooled random-donor PCT platelets was initiated in Europe in 1998, and a similar trial using SDP is planned for the United States in 1999–2000.

Merocyanine 540 (MC 540), which is a heterocyclic polymethine dye, has also been shown to photoinactivate viruses through an oxygen-dependent mechanism directed against the viral membrane.[169] In both the presence and absence of visible light, MC 540 has deleterious in vitro effects on platelets. Immediate effects on the ability of platelets to aggregate have been observed, as well as declining pH and morphology scores on storage of platelet concentrates.[211, 212] Platelets may be too sensitive to the membrane damage that is associated with this mechanism of photoinactivation.

STORAGE OF PLATELET CONCENTRATES FOR NEONATES

Platelet concentrates that are stored at room temperature (20°C to 24°C) in second-generation containers require a volume between 45 and 60 mL to maintain an appropriate pH. At a pH below 6.0, platelet viability is impaired.[213] The overall quality of platelet concentrates may also be affected, even at pH levels above 6.0.[36, 42]

The routine volume-reduction of platelet concentrates for neonates is not necessary because an adequate platelet increment should be achieved after transfusion of 10 mL/kg of a standard platelet concentrate.[214] There may be selected clinical situations, however, when the use of volume-reduced platelets may be considered.[215] Transfusion of incompatible plasma is of greater concern in infants, with their small blood volume, than in adults. If it is necessary to give an ABO incompatible platelet unit, plasma can be reduced or removed and replaced with saline or albumin. This would be applicable for any antibody present in the plasma directed against an antigen present on a neonatal blood cell (i.e., anti-HPA-1a). Situations in which circulatory overload is a major concern, necessitating volume restriction of all intravenous fluids, also would warrant the use of volume-reduced platelets, particularly if repeated transfusions were anticipated.

Recentrifugation of platelets stored for up to 5 days, at either 1500 × g for 7 minutes, 2000 × g for 10 minutes, or 5000 × g for 6 minutes, and then resuspension in 10 mL of plasma after a 1-hour rest period resulted in a platelet loss of between 5% and 20%.[132] At the latter two centrifuge speeds, in vivo survival was found to be normal in normal volunteers. A study by Moroff and colleagues,[216] using a softer spin for a longer time (580 × g for 20 minutes), found the platelet loss to be less than 15% after a 20-minute rest period. Platelets stored for either 1 or 5 days either on a flatbed or an end-over-end tumbler agitator and then volume reduced showed no adverse effects on in vitro function, as assessed by morphology and volume, response to hypotonic stress, aggregation, platelet factor 3 activity, pH, and discharge of LDH. Acceptable platelet increments were also obtained in critically ill, thrombocytopenic neonates transfused with volume-reduced platelet concentrates. The use of the softer spin technique to produce volume-reduced single platelet concentrates also allows the product to be available in a shorter time.

Neonates usually require small-volume transfusions; therefore, blood components are often dispensed or transfused using a syringe. For platelets to be maintained at an appropriate pH, it is imperative that the storage container allow for sufficient gas exchange. Platelet concentrates stored for up to 5 days and then maintained in gas-impermeable polypropylene syringes for 6 hours showed increases in consumption of glucose and production of lactic acid. The resultant decline in pH was associated with a switch from aerobic to anaerobic metabolism.[217] Similar results were observed when platelets were stored in syringes for 6 hours at 37°C, which was evaluated to simulate conditions if a syringe was placed in an isolette in the nursery. The pH in all these situations, however, never fell below 6.5, which is well within the accepted range for platelets stored in gas-permeable blood bags. Volume-reduced platelets produced by soft-spin technique[216] were stored in syringes at room temperature and at 37°C for 6 hours and evaluated.[217, 218] The latter condition produced the greatest and most rapid decline in pH. Other in vitro parameters of platelet function, such as morphology score, response to hypotonic stress, and LDH discharge, were not adversely affected under any of the conditions studied; in vivo studies were not performed. Therefore, on the basis of in vitro analysis, it appears that platelet concentrates, either standard or volume reduced, that are dispensed to neonatal nurseries in syringes for transfusion maintain acceptable in vitro platelet function.

CONCLUSION

The search for the platelet "holy grail"—a truly useful in vitro assay that will predict in vivo platelet recovery, survival, and function—must continue because this sought-after ideal still eludes our best efforts at discovery. Pathogen inactivation systems, both at the point of manufacture and at or near the point of care in the transfusion service, will continue to occupy much research time and attention into the next century. Such studies are difficult because the goal is to only inactivate the pathogens and not the platelets. Research into the ability to freeze or freeze-dry whole platelets or platelet membrane fragments will continue because there is a need for a stable platelet preparation for use in trauma venues, be they civilian or military. The role of TPOs in transfusion medicine is in question, owing to antigenicity concerns. However, a need to have a thrombopoietic growth factor in the physicians' armamentarium will remain. Clearly, much research into the structure and function of platelets remains to be done.

REFERENCES

1. Zwaal RFA, Schroit AJ. Pathophysiologic implications of membrane phospholipid asymmetry in blood cells. Blood 1997; 89:1121.
2. Lopez JA, Andrews RK, Afshar-Kharghan V, Berndt MC. Bernard-Soulier syndrome. Blood 1998; 91:4397.
3. Keiffer N, Phillips DR. Platelet membrane glycoproteins: functions in cellular interactions. Annu Rev Cell Biol 1990; 6:329.
4. Nachman RL, Leung LLK. Complex formation of platelet membrane glycoproteins IIb and IIIa with fibrinogen. J Clin Invest 1982; 69:263.
5. Berman CL, Yeo EL, Wencel-Drake JD, et al: A platelet alpha granule membrane protein that is associated with the plasma membrane after activation. J Clin Invest 1986; 78:130.
6. Hamburger SA, McEver RP. GMP-140 mediates adhesion of stimulated platelets to neutrophils. Blood 1990; 75:550.
7. Dumont LJ, VandenBroeke T, Aultl, KA, et al. Platelet surface P-selectin measurements in platelet preparations: an international collaborative study. Transfus Med Rev 1999; 13:31.
8. Fox JEB. The platelet cytoskeleton. Thromb Haemost 1993; 70:884.
9. Gerrard JM, White JG, Peterson DA. The platelet dense tubular system: its relationship to prostaglandin synthesis and calcium flux. Thromb Haemost 1978; 40:224.
10. Holt JC, Niewiarowski S. Biochemistry of α-granule proteins. Semin Hematol 1985; 22:151.
11. Fukami MH, Salganicoff L. Human platelet storage organelles. Thromb Haemost 1977; 38:963.
12. Clemetson KJ. Platelet activation: signal transduction via membrane receptors. Thromb Haemost 1995; 74:111.
13. Weiss HJ. Flow-related platelet deposition on subendothelium. Thromb Haemost 1995; 74:117.
14. Perutelli P, Biglino P, Mori PG. von Willebrand factor: biological function and moleular defects. Pediatr Hematol Oncol 1997; 14:499.
15. Ruggeri ZM. Mechanisms initiating platelet thrombus formation. Thromb Haemost 1997; 78:611.
16. Nurden P, Heilman E, Paponneau A, Nurden A. Two-way trafficking of membrane glycoproteins on thrombin-activated human platelets. Semin Hematol 1994; 3:240.
17. Rosing J, van Rijn JLML, Bevers EM, et al. The role of activated human platelets in prothrombin and factor X activation. Blood 1985; 65:319.
18. Brass LF, Hoxie JA, Manning DR. Signaling through G-proteins and G-protein–coupled receptors during platelet activation. Thromb Haemost 1993; 70:217.
19. Casey, PJ, Gilman AG. G protein involvement in receptor effector coupling. J Biol Chem 1988; 263:2577.
20. Kroll MH, Schafer AI. Biochemical mechanisms of platelet activation. Blood 1989; 74:1181.
21. Longenecker GL. Platelet arachidonic acid metabolism. *In* Longenecker GL (ed): The Platelets: Physiology and Pharmacology. New York: Academic Press, 1985, pp 159–185.
22. Smith JB, Ingerman CM. Effects of arachidonic acid and some of its metabolites on platelets. *In* Silver MJ, Smith JB, et al (eds): Prostaglandins in Hematology. New York: Spectrum Publications, 1977, pp 277–292.
23. Weksler BB, Marcus AJ. Synthesis of prostaglandin I_2 (prostacyclin) by cultured human and bovine endothelial cells. Proc Natl Acad Sci U S A 1977; 74:3922.
24. Nairn AC, Hemmings HC Jr, Greengard P. Protein kinases in the brain. Annu Rev Biochem 1985; 54:931.
25. Mills D, Macfarlane D. Stimulation of human platelet adenylate cyclase by prostaglandin D_2. Thromb Res 1974; 5:401.
26. Michel H, Caen JP, Born GVR, et al. Relation between the inhibition of aggregation and the concentration of cAMP in human rat platelets. Br J Haematol 1976; 33:27.
27. Cheung WY. Calmodulin plays a pivotal role in cellular regulation. Science 1980; 207:19.
28. Hathaway DR, Adelstein RS. Human platelet myosin light chain kinase requires the calcium-binding protein calmodulin for activity. Proc Natl Acad Sci U S A 1979; 76:1653.
29. Murer EH. The role of platelet calcium. Semin Hematol 1985; 22:313.
30. Lyman B, Rosenberg L, Karpatkin S. Biochemical and biophysical aspects of human platelet adhesion to collagen fibers. J Clin Invest 1971; 50:1854.
31. Mills DCB. Changes in the adenylate energy charge in human blood platelets induced by adenine diphosphate. Nature 1973; 243:220.
32. Holmsen H, Setkowsky CA, Day HJ. Effects of antimycin and 2-deoxyglucose on adenine nucleotides in human platelets: a role of metabolic adenine triphosphate in primary aggregation, secondary aggregation and shape change of platelets. Biochem J 1974; 144:385.
33. Kilkson H, Holme S, Murphy S. Platelet metabolism during storage of platelet concentrates at 22°C. Blood 1984; 64:406.
34. Moroff G, Friedman A, Robkin-Klin L. Factors influencing changes in pH during storage of platelet concentrates at 20–24°C. Vox Sang 1982; 42:33.
35. Murphy S, Gardner FH. Platelet storage at 22°C: role of gas

transport across platelet containers in maintenance of viability. Blood 1975; 46:209.
36. Moroff G, Holme S. Concepts about current conditions for the preparation and storage of platelets. Transfus Med Rev 1991; 5:48.
37. Mourad N. A simple method for obtaining platelet concentrates free of aggregates. Transfusion 1968; 8:48.
38. Snyder EL, Pope C, Ferri PM, et al. The effect of mode of agitation and type of plastic bag on storage characteristics and in vivo kinetics of platelet concentrates. Transfusion 1986; 26:125.
39. Burgstaler EA, Pineda AA, Potter BM, Brown R. Plateletapheresis with a next generation blood cell separator. J Clin Apheresis 1997; 12:55.
40. Yockey C, Murphy S, Eggers L, et al. Evaluation of the Amicus Separator in the collection of apheresis platelets. Transfusion 1998; 38:848.
41. Menitove JE (ed). Standards for Blood Banks and Transfusion Services, 18th ed. Bethesda, MD: American Association of Blood Banks, 1997.
42. Seghatchian J, Krailadsiri P. The platelet storage lesion. Transfus Med Rev 1997; 11:130.
43. Chernoff A, Snyder EL. The cellular and molecular basis of the platelet storage lesion: a symposium summary. Transfusion 1992; 32:386.
44. Rinder HM, Snyder EL. Activation of platelet concentrate during preparation and storage. Blood Cells 1992; 18:445.
45. Murphy S, Rebulla P, Bertolini F, et al. In vitro assessment of the quality of stored platelet concentrates. Transfus Med Rev 1994; 8:29.
46. Snyder EL, Moroff G, Simon T (eds). Symposium on radiolabeling of stored platelet concentrates. Transfusion 1986; 26:1.
47. Heilman E, Friese P, Anderson S, et al. Biotinylated platelets: a new approach to the measurement of platelet life span. Br J Haemtaol 1993; 85:729.
48. Gulliksson H, Sallander S, Pedajas I, et al. Storage of platelets in additive solutions: a new method for storage using sodium chloride solution. Transfusion 1992; 32:435.
49. Murphy S, Kagen L, Holme S, et al. Platelet storage in synthetic media lacking glucose and bicarbonate. Transfusion 1991; 31:16.
50. Fijnheer R, Veldman HA, van den Eertwegh AJM, et al. In vitro evaluation of buffy-coat–derived platelet concentrates stored in a synthetic medium. Vox Sang 1991; 60:16.
51. Bode AP, Holme S, Heaton WA, Swanson MS. Extended storage of platelets in an artificial medium with the platelet activation inhibitors prostaglandin E_1 and theophylline. Vox Sang 1991; 60:105.
52. Snyder EL, Hezzey A, Katz AJ, Bock J. Occurrence of the release reaction during preparation and storage of platelet concentrates. Vox Sang 1981; 41:172.
53. Rinder HM, Murphy M, Mitchell JG, et al. Progressive platelet activation with storage: evidence for shortened survival of activated platelets after transfusion. Transfusion 1991; 31:409.
54. Triulzi DJ, Kickler TS, Braine HG. Detection and significance of GMP 140 expression on platelets collected by apheresis. Transfusion 1992; 32:529.
55. Hartwig JH. Mechanisms of actin rearrangements mediating platelet activation. J Cell Biol 1992; 118:1421.
56. Winokur R, Hartwig JH. Mechanism of shape change in chilled human platelets. Blood 1995; 85:1796.
57. Vostal JG, Mondoro TH. Liquid cold storage of platelets: a revitalized possible alternative for limiting bacterial contamination of platelet products. Transfus Med Rev 1997; 11:286.
58. Janmey P, Stossel T. Gelsolin-polyphosphoinositide interaction. J Biol Chem 1989; 264:4825.
59. Hutchinson RE, Kunkel KD, Schell MJ, et al. Beneficial effect of brief pre-transfusion incubation of platelets at 37°C. Lancet 1989; 1:986.
60. McGill M. Temperature cycling preserves platelet shape and enhances in vitro test scores during storage at 4°C. J Lab Clin Med 1978; 92:970.
61. Husain MA, Schiffer CA, Lee EJ. Incubation of platelet concentrates prior to transfusion does not improve posttransfusion recovery [Abstract 673]. Blood 1989; 74(suppl 1):179A.
62. Fox JEB. Identification of actin-binding protein as the protein linking the membrane skeleton to glycoproteins on platelet plasma membranes. J Biol Chem 1985; 260:11970.
63. Fox JEB, Reynolds CC, Morrow JS, Phillips DR. Spectrin is associated with membrane-bound actin filaments in platelets and is hydrolysed by the Ca^{2+}-dependent protease during platelet activation. Blood 1987; 69:537.
64. Pollard TD, Cooper JA. Actin and actin-binding proteins: a critical evaluation of mechanisms and functions. Annu Rev Biochem 1986; 55:987.
65. Fox JEB. The platelet cytoskeleton. *In* Verstraet M, Verylen J, Lijnen HR, Arnout J (eds): Thrombosis and Hemostasis. Leuven: Leuven University Press, 1987, pp 175–225.
66. Hartwig JH, DeSisto M. The cytoskeleton of the resting human blood platelet: structure of the membrane skeleton and its attachment to actin filaments. J Cell Biol 1991; 112:407.
67. Abrams CS, Ellison N, Budzynski AZ, Shattil SJ. Direct detection of activated platelets and platelet-derived microparticles in humans. Blood 1990; 75:128.
68. Bode AP, Orton SM, Frye MJ, Udis BJ. Vesiculation of platelets during in vitro aging. Blood 1991; 77:887.
69. George JN, Pickett EB, Heinz R. Platelet membrane glycoprotein changes during the preparation and storage of platelet concentrates. Transfusion 1988; 28:123.
70. Snyder EL, Dunn BE, Biometti CS, et al. Protein changes occurring during storage of platelet concentrates: a two-dimensional gel electrophoretic analysis. Transfusion 1987; 27:335.
71. Snyder EL, Horne WC, Napychank P, et al. Calcium-dependent proteolysis of actin during storage of platelet concentrates. Blood 1989; 73:1380.
72. Mehdi S. Cell-penetrating inhibitors of calpain. Trends Biochem Sci 1991; 16:150.
73. McGowan EB, Becker E, Detwiler TC. Inhibition of calpain in intact platelets by the thiol protease inhibitor E-64d. Biochem Biophys Res Commun 1989; 158:432.
74. Tsujinaka T, Sakon M, Kambayashi J, Kosaki G. Cleavage of cytoskeletal proteins by two forms of Ca^{2+} activated neutral proteases in human platelets. Thromb Res 1982; 28:149.
75. Robey FA, Freitag CM, Jamieson GA. Disappearance of actin binding protein from human blood platelets during storage. FEBS Lett 1979; 102:257.
76. Phillips DR, Jakobova M. Ca^{2+}-dependent protease in human platelets: specific cleavage of platelet polypeptides in the presence of added Ca^{2+}. J Biol Chem 1977; 252:5602.
77. Fox JEB, Goll DE, Reynolds CC, Philips DE. Identification of two proteins (actin-binding protein and P235) that are hydrolysed by endogenous Ca^{2+}-dependent protease during platelet aggregation. J Biol Chem 1985; 260:1060.
78. Fox JEB, Reynolds CC, Phillips DR. Calcium-dependent proteolysis occurs during platelet aggregation. J Biol Chem 1983; 258:9973.
79. Hellums JD, Peterson DM, Stathopoulos NA, et al. Studies on the mechanisms of shear-induced platelet activation. *In* Hartmann A, Kuchinsky W (eds): Cerebral Ischemia and Hemorrheology. Berlin: Springer-Verlag, 1987, pp 80–89.
80. Hellums JD, Giorgio TD. A cone and plate viscometer for the continuous measurement of blood platelet activation. Biorheology 1988; 25:605.
81. Moake JL, Turner NA, Stathopoulos NA, et al. Shear-induced platelet aggregation can be mediated by vWF released from platelets, as well as by exogenous large or unusually large vWF multimers, requires adenosine diphosphate and is resistant to aspirin. Blood 1988; 71:1366.
82. Weidmer T, Shattil SJ, Cunningham M, Sims PJ. Role of calcium and calpain in complement-induced vesiculation of the platelet plasma membrane and in the exposure of the platelet Va receptor. Biochemistry 1990; 29:623.
83. Sims PJ, Weidmer T, Esmon CT, et al. Assembly of the platelet prothrombinase complex is linked to vesiculation of the platelet plasma membrane. Studies in Scott syndrome: an isolated defect in platelet procoagulant activity. J Biol Chem 1989; 264:17049.
84. Fox JEB, Reynolds CC, Austin CD. The role of calpain in stimulus-response coupling: evidence that calpain mediates agonist-induced expression of procoagulant activity in platelets. Blood 1990; 76:2510.
85. Kilic F, Ball EH. Partial cleavage mapping of the cytoskeletal protein vinculin: antibody and talin binding sites. J Biol Chem 1991; 266:8734.
86. Horvath AR, Asijee GM, Muszbek L. Cytoskeletal assembly and

vinculin-cytoskeleton interaction in different phases of the activation of bovine platelets. Cell Motil Cytoskel 1992; 21:123.
87. Green DR, Reed JC. Mitochondria and apoptosis. Science 1998; 281:1309.
88. Thornberry NA, Lazebnik Y. Caspases: enemies within. Science 1998; 281:1312.
89. Devine DV. Novel markers for the detection of platelet activation. Trans Med Rev 1990; 6:115.
90. Michelson AD, Adelman B, Barnard MR, et al. Platelet storage results in a redistribution of glycoprotein Ib molecules; evidence for a large intraplatelet pool of glycoprotein Ib. J Clin Invest 1988; 81:1734.
91. Adelman B, Michelson AD, Handin RI, Ault KA. Evaluation of glycoprotein Ib by fluoresence flow cytometry. Blood 1985; 66:423.
92. Michelson AD, Barnard MR. Plasmin-induced redistribution of platelet glycoprotein Ib. Blood 1990; 76:2005.
93. Wencel-Drake JD. Plasma membrane GPIIb/IIIa: evidence for a cycling receptor pool. Am J Pathol 1990; 136:61.
94. Snyder EL, Ezekowitz MD, Malech HL, et al. In vitro characteristics and in vivo viability of platelets contained in granulocyte-platelet apheresis concentrate. Transfusion 1987; 27:10.
95. Snyder EL, Stack G, Napychank PA, Roberts S. Storage of pooled platelet concentrates, in vitro and in vivo analysis. Transfusion 1989; 29:390.
96. Snyder EL, Ezekowitz MD, Aster R, et al. Extended storage of platelets in a new plastic container. Transfusion 1985; 25:209.
97. Snyder EL, Aster R, Heaton A, et al. Five-day storage of platelets in a non-DEHP plasticized container. Transfusion 1992; 32:736.
98. McEver RP. GMP-140: a receptor for neutrophils and monocytes on activated platelets and endothelium. J Cell Biochem 1991; 45:156.
99. George JN, Pickett EB, Heinz R. Platelet membrane glycoprotein changes during the preparation and storage of platelet concentrates. Transfusion 1988; 28:123.
100. Fijnheer R, Pietersz RNI, DeKorte D, et al. Platelet activation during preparation of platelet concentrates: a comparison of the platelet-rich plasma and the buffy coat methods. Transfusion 1990; 30:634.
101. Fijnheer R, Modderman PW, Veldman H, et al. Detection of platelet activation with monoclonal antibodies and flow cytometry: changes during platelet storage. Transfusion 1990; 30:20.
102. Rinder HM, Bonan JL, Rinder CS, et al. Dynamics of leukocyte-platelet adhesion in whole blood. Blood 1991; 78:1730.
103. Leistikow EA, Barnhart MI, Escolar G, White JG. Receptor-ligand complexes are cleared to the open canalicular system of surface-activated platelets. Br J Haematol 1990; 74:93.
104. Snyder EL, Prodouz K, McGowan E, Napychank PA. Presence of calpain-induced actin fragments in microvesicles formed during storage of platelet concentrate. Blood 1991; 78(suppl 1):388a.
105. Gamble JR, Skinneer MP, Bermdt MC, Vadas MA. Prevention of activated neutrophil adhesion to endothelium by soluble adhesion protein GMP140. Science 1990; 249:414.
106. Hogge DF, Thompson BW, Schiffer CA. Platelet storage for 7 days in second generation blood bags. Transfusion 1986; 26:131.
107. Snyder EL, Beardsley DS, Smith BR, et al. Storage of platelet concentrates after high-dose ultraviolet B irradiation. Transfusion 1991; 31:491.
108. Bertolini F, Rebulla P, Porretti L, Sirchia G. Comparison of platelet activation and membrane glycoprotein Ib and IIb-IIIa expression after filtration through three different leukocyte removal filters. Vox Sang 1990; 59:201.
109. Bode AP, Orton SM, Frye MJ, Udis BJ. Vesiculation of platelets during in vitro aging. Blood 1991; 77:887.
110. Alving BM, Reid TJ, Fratantoni JC. Frozen platelets and platelet substitutes in transfusion medicine. Transfusion 1997; 37:866.
111. Dayian G, Pert JH. A simplified method for freezing human blood platelets in glycerol-glucose using a statically controlled cooling rate device. Transfusion 1979; 19:255.
112. Ridgway RL, Usry RT. Cryopreservation of platelets simplified: a modified glycerol-glucose method. Transfusion 1980; 20:427.
113. Kotelba-Witkowska B, Schiffer CA. Cryopreservation of platelet concentrates using glycerol-glucose. Transfusion 1982; 22:121.
114. Redmond J III, Bolin RB, Cheney BA. Glycerol-glucose cryopreservation of platelets: in vivo and in vitro observations. Transfusion 1983; 23:213.
115. Dayian G, Harris HL, Vlahides GD, Pert JH. Improved procedure for platelet freezing. Vox Sang 1986; 51:292.
116. Arnaud FG, Pegg DE. Cryopreservation of human platelets with 1.4M glycerol at −75°C in PVC blood packs. Thromb Res 1990; 57:919.
117. Taylor MA. Cryopreservation of platelets: an in-vitro comparison of our methods. J Clin Pathol 1981; 34:71.
118. Handin RI, Valeri RR. Improved viability of previously frozen platelets. Blood 1972; 40:509.
119. Daly PA, Schiffer CA, Aisner J, Wiernik PH. Successful transfusion of platelets cryopreserved for more than 3 years. Blood 1979; 54:1023.
120. van Prooijen HC, van Heugten JG, Mommersteeg ME, Akkerman JWN. Acquired secretion defect in platelets after cryopreservation in dimethyl sulfoxide. Transfusion 1986; 26:358.
121. Towell BL, Levine SP, Knight WA III, Anderson JL. A comparison of frozen and fresh platelet concentrates in the support of thrombocytopenic patients. Transfusion 1986; 26:525.
122. van Prooijen HC, van Heugten MI, Riemens MI, Akkerman JWN. Differences in the susceptibility of platelets to freezing damage in relation to size. Transfusion 1989; 29:539.
123. Owens M, Cimino C, Donnelly J. Cryopreserved platelets have decreased adhesive capacity. Transfusion 1991; 31:160.
124. Arnaud FG, Hunt CJ, Pegg DE. Some effects of propane-1,2-diol on human platelets. Cryobiology 1990; 27:119.
125. Arnaud FG, Pegg DE. Cryopreservation of human platelets with propane-1,2-diol. Cryobiology 1990; 27:130.
126. Read MS, Reddick RL, Bode AP, et al. Preservation of hemostatic and structural properties of rehydrated lyophilized platelets: potential for long term storage of dried platelets for transfusion. Proc Natl Acad Sci U S A 1995; 92:397.
127. Rubin RJ, Ness PM. What price progress? An update on vinyl plastic blood bags. Transfusion 1989; 29:358.
128. Murphy S, Kahn RA, Holme S, Phillips GL. Improved storage of platelets for transfusion in a new container. Blood 1982; 60:194.
129. Jaeger RJ, Rubin RJ. Migration of a phthalate ester plasticizer from polyvinyl chloride blood bags into stored human blood and its localization in human tissues. N Engl J Med 1972; 287:1114.
130. Jaeger RJ, Rubin RJ. Di-2-ethylhexyl phthalate, a plasticizer contaminant of platelet concentrates. Transfusion 1973; 13:107.
131. Sasakawa S, Mitomi Y: Di-2-ethylhexylphthalate (DEHP) content of blood or blood components stored in plastic bags. Vox Sang 1978; 34:81.
132. Rock G, Secours VE, Franklin CA, et al. The accumulation of mono-2-ethylhexylphthalate (MEHP) during storage of whole blood and plasma. Transfusion 1978; 18:553.
133. Conway JG, Tomaszewski KE, Olson MJ, et al. Relationship of oxidative damage to the hepatocarcinogenicity of the peroxisome proliferators di-(2-ethylhexyl) phthalate and Wy-14,643. Carcinogenesis 1989; 10:513.
134. Peck CC, Odom DG, Friedman HI, et al. Di-2-ethylhexylphthalate (DEHP) and mono-2-ethylhexylphthalate (MEHP) accumulation in whole blood and red cell concentrates. Transfusion 1979; 19:137.
135. Albro PW, Chapin RE, Corbett JT, et al. Mono-2-ethylhexyl phthalate, a metabolite of di-(ethylhexyl) phthalate, causally linked to testicular atrophy in rats. Toxicol Appl Pharmacol 1989; 100:193.
136. AuBuchon JP, Estep TN, Davey RJ. The effect of the plasticizer di-2-ethylhexylphthalate on the survival of stored RBCs. Blood 1988; 71:448.
137. Horowitz B, Stryker MH, Waldman AA, et al. Stabilization of red blood cells by the plasticizer diethylhexylphthalate. Vox Sang 1985; 48:150.
138. Rock G, Tocchi M, Ganz PR, Tackaberry ES. Incorporation of plasticizer into red cells during storage. Transfusion 1984; 24:493.
139. Snyder EL, Ezekowitz M, Aster R, et al. Extended storage of platelets in a new plastic container: II. In vivo response to infusion of platelets stored for 5 days. Transfusion 1985; 25:209.
140. Murphy S, Kahn RA, Holme S, et al. Improved storage of platelets for transfusion in a new container. Blood 1982; 60:194.
141. Simon TL, Nelson EJ, Carmen R, Murphy S. Extension of platelet concentrate storage. Transfusion 1983; 23:207.
142. Snyder EL, Pope C, Ferri PM, et al. The effect of mode of agitation and type of plastic bag on storage characteristics and in vivo kinetics of platelet concentrates. Transfusion 1986; 26:125.
143. Simon TL, Sierra ER, Ferdinando B, Moore R. Collection of

platelets with a new cell separator and their storage in a citrate-plasticized container. Transfusion 1991; 31:335.
144. Gulliksson H, Shanwell A, Wikman A, et al. Storage of platelets in a new plastic container. Vox Sang 1991; 61:165.
145. Seidl S, Gosda W, Reppucci AJ. The in vitro and in vivo evaluation of whole blood and red cell concentrates drawn on CPDA-1 and stored in a non-DEHP plasticized container. Vox Sang 1991; 61:8.
146. Hogman CF, Eriksson L, Ericson A, Reppucci AJ. Storage of saline-adenine-glucose-mannitol suspended red cells in a new plastic container: polyvinyl chloride plasticized with butyryl-n-trihexyl-citrate. Transfusion 1991; 31:26.
147. Buchholz D, Aster R, Menitove J, et al. Red blood cell storage studies in a citrate-plasticized polyvinyl chloride container [Abstract]. Transfusion 1989; 29(suppl):8S.
148. Hull EH, Jacobson M, Kevy SV. Medical grade citrate ester plasticizers. *In* Proceedings of the Society of Plastic Engineers. Medical Plastic Conference, January 29–30, 1990, Anaheim, CA, pp 1–3.
149. Jacobson MS, Kevy SV, Ausprunk D, Kaplan M. Citroflex B-6, a safe PVC plasticizer for the storage of red blood cells, platelets and plasma [Abstract P-Th-7-54]. *In* Book of Abstracts of the XX Congress of the International Society of Blood Transfusion. London: Karger, 1988.
150. Parravicini A, Rebulla P, Apuzzo J, et al. The preparation of leukocyte-poor red cells for transfusion by a simple cost-effective technique. Transfusion 1984; 24:508.
151. Kickler TS, Bell W, Ness PM, et al. Depletion of white cells from platelet concentrates with a new adsorption filter. Transfusion 1989; 29:411.
152. Sirchia G, Wenz B, Rebulla P, et al. Removal of white cells from red cells by transfusion through a new filter. Transfusion 1990; 30:30.
153. Snyder EL. Clinical use of white cell-poor blood components. Transfusion 1989; 29:568.
154. Silliman CC, Dickey WO, Paterson AJ, et al. Analysis of the priming activity of lipids generated during routine storage of platelet concentrates. Transfusion 1996; 36:133.
155. Heddle NM, Klama L, Singer J, et al. The role of plasma from platelet concentrates in transfusion reactions. N Engl J Med 1994; 331:625.
156. Stack G, Snyder EL. Cytokine generation in stored platelet concentrates. Transfusion 1994; 34:20.
157. Aye MT, Palmer DS, Giulivi A, Hashemi S. Effect of filtration of platelet concentrates on the accumulation of cytokines and platelet release factors during storage. Transfusion 1995; 35:117.
158. Snyder EL. Prevention of HLA alloimmunization: role of leukocyte depletion and UVB irradiation. Yale J Biol Med 1990; 60:419.
159. Blajchman MA, Bardossy L, Carmen RA, et al. An animal model of allogeneic donor platelet refractoriness: the effect of the time of leukodepletion. Blood 1992; 79:1371.
160. Snyder EL, Hezzey A, Cooper-Smith M, James R. Effect of microaggregate blood filtration on platelet concentrates in vitro. Transfusion 1981; 21:427.
161. Snyder EL, DePalma L, Napychank P. Use of polyester filters for the preparation of leukocyte-poor platelet concentrates. Vox Sang 1988; 54:21.
162. Holme S, Snyder E, Heaton A, et al. In vitro and in vivo evaluation of cotton wool filtration of platelet concentrates obtained by automated and manual apheresis. Transfusion 1992; 32:328.
163. Hild M, Soderstrom T, Egberg N, Lundahl J. Kinetics of bradykinin levels during and after leucocyte filtration of platelet concentrates. Vox Sang 1998; 75:18.
164. Scott CF, Brandwein H, Whitbread J, Colman RW. Lack of clinically significant contact system activation during platelet concentrate filtration by leukocyte removal filters. Blood 1998; 92:616.
165. Centers for Disease Control. Bacterial contamination of platelet pools—Ohio. MMWR 1991; 41:36.
166. Morrow JF, Braine HG, Kickler TS, et al. Septic reactions to platelet transfusions: a persistent problem. JAMA 1991; 266:555.
167. Goldman M, Blajchman MA. Blood product–associated bacterial sepsis. Transfus Med Rev 1991; 5:73.
168. Buchholz DH, AuBuchon JP, Snyder E, et al. Effects of white cell reduction on the resistance of blood components to bacterial multiplication. Transfusion 1994; 34:852.
169. Corash L. Inactivation of viruses, bacteria, protozoa and leukocytes in platelet concentrates: current research perspectives. Transfus Med Rev 1999; 13:18.
170. Chao FC, Kim BK, Houranieh AM, et al. Infusible platelet membrane microvesicles: a potential transfusion substitute for platelets. Transfusion 1996; 36:536.
171. Coller BS, Springer KT, Beer JH, et al. Thromboerythrocytes. In vitro studies of a potential autologous, semi-artificial alternative to platelet transfusions. J Clin Invest 1992; 89:546.
172. Lee DH, Blajchman MA. Novel platelet products and substitutes. Transfus Med Rev 1998; 12:175.
173. Alving B. Potential for synthetic phospholipids as partial platelet substitutes. Transfusion 1998; 38:997.
174. Galan AM, Hernandez MR, Bozzo J, et al. Preparations of synthetic phospholipids promote procoagulant activity on damaged vessels: studies under flow conditions. Transfusion 1998; 38:1004.
175. Ramsey G. Hematopoietic growth factors and transfusion medicine. Transfus Med Rev 1998; 12:195.
176. Kaushansky K. Thrombopoietin and the hematopoietic stem cell. Blood 1998; 92:1.
177. Hoelzer D. Hematopoietic growth factors—not whether, but when and where. N Engl J Med 1997; 336:1822.
178. Farese A, Schiffer CA, MacVittie TJ. The impact of thrombopoietin and related mpl-ligands on transfusion medicine. Transfus Med Rev 1997; 11:243.
179. Fielder PJ, Gurney AL, Stefanich E, et al. Regulation of thrombopoietin levels by c-mpl–mediated binding to platelets. Blood 1996; 87:2154.
180. Kuter DJ. Thrombopoietin: biology, clinical applications, role in the donor setting. J Clin Apheres 1996; 11:149.
181. Harker LA, Marzec UM, Novembre F, et al. Treatment of thrombocytopenia in chimpanzees infected with human immunodeficiency virus by pegylated recombinant human megakaryocyte growth and development factor. Blood 1998; 91:4427.
182. Miller YM, Klein HG. Growth factors and their impact on transfusion medicine. Vox Sang 1996; 71:196.
183. Tomita D, Petrarca M, Paine T, et al. Effect of a single dose of pegylated human recombinant megakaryocyte growth and development factor (PEG-rHuMGDF) on platelet counts: implications for platelet apheresis [Abstract S8]. Transfusion 1997; 37(suppl 1):2S.
184. Goodnough LT, DiPersio J, McCullough J, et al. Pegylated recombinant human megakaryocyte growth and development factor (PEG-rHuMGDF) increases platelet (PLT) count (CT) and apheresis yields of normal PLT donors [Abstract S266]. Transfusion 1997; 37(suppl 1):67S.
185. Kuter D, McCullough J, Romo J, et al. Treatment of platelet (PLT) donors with pegylated recombinant human megakaryocyte growth and development factor (PEG-rHuMGDF) increases circulating platelet counts and platelet apheresis yields and increases platelet increments in recipients of platelet transfusions [Abstract 2579]. Blood 1997; 90(suppl 1):579a.
186. Snyder EL, Perrotta P, Rinder H, et al. Effect of recombinant human megakaryocyte growth and development factor coupled with polyethylene glycol on the platelet storage lesion. Transfusion 1999; 39:258.
187. Cwirla SE, Balasubramanian P, Duffin DJ, et al. Peptide agonist of the thrombopoietin receptor as potent as the natural cytokine. Science 1997; 276:1696.
188. Davey RJ. The effect of irradiation on blood components. *In* Baldwin ML, Jefferies LC (eds): Irradiation of Blood Components. Bethesda, MD: American Association of Blood Banks, 1992, pp 51–62.
189. Anderson KC, Goodnough LT, Sayers M, et al. Variation in blood component irradiation practice: implications for prevention of transfusion-associated graft-versus-host disease. Blood 1991; 77:2096.
190. Moroff G, George VM, Siegel AM, Luban NLC. The influence of irradiation on stored platelets. Transfusion 1986; 26:453.
191. Center for Biologics Evaluation and Research, Food and Drug Administration: Recommendations regarding license amendments and procedures for gamma irradiation of blood products. Washington, DC: U.S. Department of Health and Human Services, July 22, 1993.
192. Button LN, DeWolf WC, Newburger PE, et al. The effects of irradiation on blood components. Transfusion 1981; 21:419.
193. Read EJ, Kodis C, Carter CS, Leitman SF. Viability of platelets following storage in the irradiated state: a pair-controlled study. Transfusion 1988; 28:446.

194. Rock G, Adams GA, Labow RS. The effects of irradiation on platelet function. Transfusion 1988; 28:451.
195. Sweeney JD, Holme S, Moroff G. Storage of apheresis platelets after gamma irradiation. Transfusion 1994; 34:779.
196. Moroff G, Luban NLC. The irradiation of blood and blood components to prevent graft-versus-host disease: Technical issues and guidelines. Transfus Med Rev 1997; 11:15.
197. Sniecincki I, O'Donnell MR, Nowicki IB, Hill LR. Prevention of refractoriness and HLA alloimmunization using filtered blood products. Blood 1988; 71:1402.
198. Lindahl-Keissling K, Søfwenberg J. Inability of UV-irradiated lymphocytes to stimulate allogenic cells in mixed lymphocyte culture. Int Arch Allergy Appl Immunol 1971; 41:670.
199. Doery JCG, Dickson RD, Hirsh J. Induction of aggregation of human blood platelets by ultraviolet light: action spectrum and structural changes. Blood 1973; 42:551.
200. Kahn RA, Duffy BR, Rodey CG. Ultraviolet irradiation of platelet concentrates abrogates lymphocyte activation without affecting platelet function in vitro. Transfusion 1985; 25:547.
201. Pamphilon DH, Corbin SA, Saunders J, Tandy NP. Applications of ultraviolet light in the preparation of platelet concentrates. Transfusion 1989; 29:379.
202. Pamphilon DH. Platelet concentrates and ultraviolet light. Transfus Sci 1990; 11:149.
203. Buchholz DH, Miripol J, Aster RH, et al. Storage of platelet concentrates after high-dose ultraviolet B irradiation [Abstract]. Transfusion 1988; 28(suppl):26S.
204. Andreu G, Boccaccio C, Lecrubier C, et al. Ultraviolet irradiation of platelet concentrates: feasibility in transfusion practice. Transfusion 1990; 30:401.
205. TRAP Study Group. Leukocyte reduction and ultraviolet B irradiation of platelets to prevent alloimmunization and refractoriness to platelet transfusions. N Engl J Med 1997; 337:1861.
206. Kraemer KH, Levis WR, Cason JC, Tarone RE. Inhibition of mixed leukocyte reaction by 8-methoxypsoralen and long-wavelength ultraviolet radiation. J Invest Dermatol 1981; 77:235.
207. Grana NH, Kao KJ. Use of 8-methoxypsoralen and ultraviolet-A pretreated platelet concentrates to prevent alloimmunization against class I major histocompatibility antigens. Blood 1991; 77:2530.
208. Lin L, Cook DN, Wiesehahn GP, et al. Photochemical inactivation of viruses and bacteria in platelet concentrates by use of a novel psoralen and long-wavelength ultraviolet light. Transfusion 1997; 37:423.
209. Lin L, Londe H, Janda M, et al. Photochemical inactivation of pathogenic bacteria in human platelet concentrates. Blood 1994; 83:2698.
210. Lin L, Corten L, Murthy KK, et al. Photochemical inactivation of hepatitis B (HBV) and hepatitis C (HCV) virus in human platelet concentrates as assessed by a chimpanzee infectivity model [Abstract 2066]. Blood 1998; 92(suppl 1):502a.
211. Dodd RY, Moroff G, Wagner S, et al. Inactivation of viruses in platelet suspensions that retain their in vitro characteristics: comparison of psoralen-ultraviolet A and merocyanine 540-visible light methods. Transfusion 1991; 31:483.
212. Prodouz KN, Lytle CD, Keville EA, et al. Inhibition by albumin of merocyanine 540–mediated photosensitization of platelets and viruses. Transfusion 1991; 31:415.
213. Kunicki TJ, Tuccelli M, Becker GA, Aster RH. A study of variables affecting the quality of platelets stored at "room temperature." Transfusion 1975; 15:414.
214. Blanchette VS, Kuhne T, Hume H, Hellman J. Platelet transfusion therapy in newborn infants. Transfus Med Rev 1995; 9:215.
215. Simon TL, Sierra ER. Concentration of platelet units into small volumes. Transfusion 1984; 24:173.
216. Moroff G, Friedman A, Robkin-Kline L, et al. Reduction of the volume of stored platelet concentrates for use in neonatal patients. Transfusion 1984; 24:144.
217. Pisciotto PT, Snyder EL, Napychank PA, Hopfer SM. In vitro characteristics of volume-reduced platelet concentrate stored in syringes. Transfusion 1991; 31:404.
218. Pisciotto PT, Snyder EL, Snyder JA, et al. In vitro characteristics of white cell–reduced single-unit platelet concentrates stored in syringes. Transfusion 1994; 34:407.

CHAPTER 14
Platelet Immunology

Thomas Kickler

The immune-mediated platelet disorders include alloimmunization to platelet alloantigens, autoimmune thrombocytopenia, and drug-induced thrombocytopenia.[1] Platelets are destroyed by immune-mediated processes that are similar to those that destroy red cells but have distinctive clinical and immunological features. Like red cell transfusion recipients, patients who receive multiple platelet transfusions form alloantibodies against transfused cells that complicate transfusion management. Unlike red cell alloantibodies, platelet alloantibodies do not lead to acute reactions but do shorten the survival of the transfused platelets and diminish their therapeutic effectiveness. Just as mothers sensitized to paternal red cell antigens may have infants with hemolytic disease of the newborn, mothers immunized to paternal human platelet antigens (HPAs) can have thrombocytopenic newborns. Autoimmune thrombocytopenia is a relatively common disorder compared with autoimmune hemolytic anemia. Its molecular targets are relatively well characterized because of their presence on important glycoprotein receptors.[2] Drug-induced immune thrombocytopenia is caused by many of the same drugs associated with drug-related immune hemolysis, as well as many other drugs not producing hemolytic anemia. This chapter's purpose is to provide an overview of relevant platelet immunology to understand the unique clinical and immunological bases of these immune-mediated platelet disorders.

PLATELET ALLOANTIGEN DISORDERS

Human Platelet Antigens

HPAs arise as the result of polymorphisms of platelet membrane glycoproteins.[3] Alloimmunization to the HPAs cause neonatal alloimmune thrombocytopenia and post-transfusion purpura and accounts for approximately 8% of platelet transfusion refractoriness in multiply transfused platelet recipients.[4, 5] These antigenic differences arise as a result of single nucleotide substitution. Table 14–1 shows the well-characterized platelet-specific antigens, their associated platelet glycoproteins, and the nucleotide substitution associated with the epitope.[3] These glycoproteins, which belong to the integrin family, are characterized by two-chain membrane heterodimer complexes involved in cellular adhesive interaction and may be found on the cell surface of many different cell types. The HPAs were thought to be unique to platelets and megakaryocytes and were originally called platelet-specific antigens. Because these antigens are epitopes on integrins, some HPAs are expressed on endothelial cells, fibroblasts, and smooth muscle cells. For example, antigens associated with platelet glycoprotein IIIA have this diverse tissue distribution. In contrast, other antigens, such as those associated with glycoprotein IIB, seem restricted to platelets.

Table 14–2 summarizes the immunogenetic data for platelet-specific antigen systems.[6] Extensive studies in all ethnic groups have not been conducted; nonetheless, there appear to be important phenotypic differences in different populations.

Neonatal Alloimmune Thrombocytopenia

Neonatal alloimmune thrombocytopenia is the result of maternal alloimmunization to fetal platelet antigens. Its pathogenesis is analogous to that of hemolytic disease of the newborn caused by maternal alloimmunization to red cell antigens. With transplacental transfer of maternal platelet antibodies to the developing fetus, thrombocytopenia may result. The evaluation of a newborn baby with thrombocytopenia requires serological investigation to document whether the thrombocytopenia has an immunological basis. With improved serological and immunological methods, a growing number of platelet antigen systems have been etiologically linked to neonatal alloimmune thrombocytopenia.[7, 8]

Clinical Aspects

The true incidence of neonatal alloimmune thrombocytopenia in the United States is not known.[7, 8] Although much has been written about the disorder, most series

Table 14–1. Human Platelet Antigens

Antigen	Glycoprotein Location	Amino Acid Substitution
HPA-1a	IIIA	Leu33
HPA-1b		Pro33
HPA-2a	IB alpha	Thr145
HPA-2b		Met145
HPA-3a	IIB	Ile843
HPA-3b		Ser843
HPA-4a	IIIA	Arg143
HPA-4b		Gln143
HPA-5a	IA	Lys505
HPA-5b		Glu505

Table 14–2. Gene Frequencies of Human Platelet Antigens Calculated From Genotype Frequencies

Haplotype	Whites	African Americans	Koreans	Dutch*
HPA-1a	0.89	0.92	0.995	0.846
HPA-1b	0.11	0.08	0.005	0.154
HPA-2a	0.92	0.82	0.87	0.934
HPA-2b	0.09	0.18	0.13	0.066
HPA-3a	0.67	0.63	0.67	0.555
HPA-3b	0.33	0.37	0.33	0.445
HPA-4a	1.00	1.00	1.00	1.000
HPA-4b	0.00	0.00	0.00	0.000
HPA-5a	0.89	0.79	0.97	0.902
HPA-5b	0.11	0.21	0.03	0.098

*From Semsek S, Faber NM, Bleeker PM, et al. Determination of human platelet antigen frequencies in the Dutch population by immunophenotyping and DNA analyses. Blood 1993; 81:835.

are compiled by referral centers. Unless platelet counts are routinely performed, some cases may not be recognized, because thrombocytopenia is not always severe. With the development of improved serological techniques for platelet antibody identification and increased awareness of the condition, a better estimate of the true incidence of the syndrome may be possible.

In a carefully performed Canadian study, Blanchette and colleagues documented eight cases of neonatal alloimmune thrombocytopenia out of 8197 admissions to a single neonatal intensive care unit.[7] It is unknown whether there are racial differences in the incidence of neonatal alloimmune thrombocytopenia. More careful studies of the epidemiology of this disease in different populations are needed.

In contrast to Rh hemolytic disease of the newborn, neonatal alloimmune thrombocytopenia may affect first-born infants. Between 20% and 59% of cases of neonatal alloimmune thrombocytopenia occur in the first-born. Because the child of a primigravida may be affected, and because prenatal screening for platelet alloantibodies is not routine, serious bleeding complications may develop, either during gestation or during vaginal delivery. Subsequent children born to a couple with a previously affected child are also likely to be affected, although this generalization depends on the zygosity of the father for the immunizing platelet alloantigen. In second-born infants, obstetricians are aware of the possibility of thrombocytopenia and can manage the pregnancy expectantly. In general, women who are alloimmunized have cesarean sections to prevent severe bleeding and head trauma to the infant during vaginal delivery.

Although neonatal alloimmune thrombocytopenia is a self-limited disorder, mortality due to bleeding approaches 15%. Infants may be asymptomatic at birth and develop hemorrhagic symptoms within the first few postnatal hours. Platelet counts less than 10,000 cells/mm^3 are seen in children with severe hemorrhagic symptoms. By day 21, the platelet count is usually greater than 50,000 cells/mm^3. Some affected children may remain unrecognized because of only moderate thrombocytopenia, or they may develop bleeding when invasive procedures such as circumcision are performed.

Because severe thrombocytopenia may develop, life-threatening central nervous system (CNS) bleeding complications can occur. CNS hemorrhage is a well-recognized complication of neonatal alloimmune thrombocytopenia that may occur in utero, during delivery, or postnatally. Approximately 20% of cases of neonatal alloimmune thrombocytopenia are complicated by intracranial hemorrhage, with 50% of these in utero. Intracranial bleeding may occur as early as the first trimester. As a result of in utero bleeding, porencephalic cysts, hydrocephalus, and intracerebral or spinal cord hematomas may occur. These complications may be diagnosed antenatally by ultrasonography.[9]

Immunological Aspects

Neonatal alloimmune thrombocytopenia is caused by antibodies to HPAs, expressed on fetal platelets as early as 16 weeks of gestation. Systematic studies on the importance of antibody titer, the immunoglobulin G (IgG) subtype, and the role of antibody-dependent cytotoxicity have not been performed. Some small studies suggest that the titer of platelet-specific antibodies does not predict the severity of thrombocytopenia in a newborn.

In white patients, 80% to 90% of cases of neonatal alloimmune thrombocytopenia are due to anti-HPA-1a. Anti-HPA-5b is the second most common cause. Only rarely have antibodies to the HPA-3 antigens been implicated in the disorder. The role of human leukocyte antigen (HLA) antibodies is unclear. A compelling argument that HLA antibodies do not play a role in neonatal alloimmune thrombocytopenia is the large number of pregnant women with HLA antibodies who give birth to nonthrombocytopenic infants.[8]

All serological testing can be performed with serum from the mother and platelets from both parents. Testing against the father's platelets is recommended to avoid missing low-incidence antigens. Isoagglutinins may result in positive antiplatelet antibody tests when tested against ABO-incompatible platelets, especially in women who are group O with high isoagglutinin titers. As in red cell serology, identification of platelet antibodies is done with a panel of group O platelets. A platelet panel ideally should present the major platelet-specific antigens as well as negative platelets to aid in characterizing the specificity of the antibodies.

Phenotyping or genotyping mothers for platelet-specific antigens is crucial for confirming an antibody's specificity. Immunophenotyping with clinically obtained antisera has been widely used for decades. Unfortunately, these antisera are either not widely available or not well standardized. Because the HPA differences are due to single nucleotide substitutions, it has been relatively easy to develop DNA-based methods to genotype for the major antigen. The ability to determine the father's zygosity is especially important in counseling a couple. This may be accomplished most reliably by means of DNA-based testing. If the father is heterozygous, it may be necessary to harvest amniocytes from a fetus to determine whether the fetus is at risk for intrauterine bleeding due to thrombocytopenia.[6]

One puzzling question has been why more patients, based on the gene frequencies for HPA-1a and HPA-

1b, are not alloimmunized to these antigens. In several serological studies, certain HLA class II specificities were significantly overrepresented in the patients who became alloimmunized to HPA-1a. The most frequent association is with HLA-DR52a. There is no known association between response to the HPA-1b form of platelet glycoprotein IIIA and the DR52a phenotype, suggesting that the immune response is remarkably specific to a single amino acid residue in the context of the conformation of the glycoprotein IIIA molecule.

More recently, through restriction fragment length polymorphism analysis by Valentin's and Decary's groups, all HPA-1b homozygous responders were found to be HLA-DR52a positive. However, about one third of nonresponders were also HLA-DR52a positive, suggesting that other determinants may be important. Subsequently, L'Abbe and coworkers refined the description of the involved HLA alleles by using polymerase chain reaction and sequence-specific oligonucleotide probes. In these studies, they demonstrated that the DRB3*0101 allele is not an absolute determinant for responsiveness and that another allele, DQB1*0201, is also overrepresented in the responders. These studies suggest that the alloimmune response to glycoprotein IIIA depends on the differential binding of HPA-1a and HPA-1b antigens with HLA-DR52a class II molecules. Defining the precise interaction of these molecules may lead to therapeutic approaches by immune modulation of the alloimmune response to HPA-1a.[10–14]

Treatment

Most blood centers do not maintain a registry of donors typed for HPAs, so the mother is generally used as the platelet donor. Most mothers can safely donate platelets in the immediate postpartum period. If a woman has already had an affected baby, platelets can be collected before delivery and made available in the labor and delivery suite in case the baby is born with signs of serious bleeding. Transfusion of 1 unit of platelets may be sufficient to increase the platelet count above 200,000 cells/mm^3. Some babies have shortened platelet survival, particularly when bleeding is severe. In these cases, daily platelet transfusions may be required.[15]

Because intrauterine bleeding may occur, in utero platelet transfusions have been given. This approach was originally proposed as a method of allowing safe delivery and was used immediately before delivery. In the last decade, investigators have advocated giving weekly platelet transfusions until an early delivery is feasible, to prevent possible intrauterine bleeding.[8]

In anecdotal reports, intravenous γ globulin has been useful both antenatally and postnatally in cases of neonatal alloimmune thrombocytopenia.[16, 17] The usual postnatal dose of intravenous γ globulin is 0.4 g/kg/day for 5 days or 1 g/kg/day for 2 days. A response is usually seen within 48 hours, with the count rising to above 50,000/μL. Occasionally, subsequent doses of intravenous γ globulin are required. It is unclear whether intravenous immunoglobulin therapy alone is preferable to simply transfusing maternal platelets. Certainly, if maternal platelets are not available, intravenous γ globulin should be used. In more persistent or severe cases of neonatal alloimmune thrombocytopenia, intravenous γ globulin may be of benefit in reducing the duration of thrombocytopenia. If platelet transfusions are needed and platelets lacking the offending antigen are not available, intravenous γ globulin may prolong the survival of transfused platelets.

Antenatal intravenous γ globulin has been given to alloimmunized mothers to protect the fetus from maternal platelet alloantibodies. Lynch and coworkers treated mothers antenatally who were immunized to platelet-specific antigens.[18] Eighteen women who had previously delivered infants with severe alloimmune thrombocytopenia were treated with weekly infusions of intravenous γ globulin from the diagnosis of fetal thrombocytopenia until birth; nine were also treated with corticosteroids. The dose of immunoglobulin was 1 g/kg/week. There were no intracranial hemorrhages in the treated fetuses, compared with 10 cases among the 21 untreated siblings (48%). Only three treated fetuses, compared with 16 of 20 untreated siblings, had platelet counts of less than 30,000/μL, with no bleeding complications. These investigators concluded that weekly γ globulin treatment of fetuses with alloimmune thrombocytopenia effectively improves the fetal platelet count and prevents intracranial hemorrhage. One case report, however, documents that intravenous immunoglobulin treatment may not prevent intracranial hemorrhage in fetal alloimmune thrombocytopenia.

In a second large study, Murphy and coworkers investigated the use of antenatal immunoglobulin.[19] They studied 15 pregnancies in 11 women who had previously given birth to infants with alloimmune thrombocytopenia due to anti-HPA-1a. The antenatal management included fetal platelet transfusions and maternal steroids and/or high-dose intravenous immunoglobulin. In the first pregnancy, intracranial hemorrhage occurred between 32 and 35 weeks gestation, before any treatment had been given, emphasizing the need for earlier intervention. Five of the 14 subsequent pregnancies in this study were considered to be severely affected (severe hemorrhagic complications in previous infants and initial fetal platelet count <20,000/μL); four were managed successfully with weekly fetal platelet transfusions started between 18 and 29 weeks and continued until delivery at 33 to 35 weeks, and one case referred at 36 weeks was managed successfully with a single platelet transfusion before delivery. Five pregnancies were considered to be mildly affected (previous infants unaffected by severe bleeding and initial fetal platelet count >50,000/μL). The platelet counts were maintained in one case with steroids and in three cases with immunoglobulin without the need for repeated platelet transfusions; in the fifth case, however, the fetal platelet count fell despite steroids and immunoglobulin, and serial platelet transfusions were required. Four pregnancies were unsuccessful: two pregnancies were terminated after severe intracranial hemorrhage occurred at an early stage, before fetal blood sampling had been carried out; one fetus died after the mother had a severe fall, despite the successful initiation of fetal platelet transfusions; and one fetus died from a cord hematoma that occurred during the initial fetal blood sampling. The optimal management of neonatal alloimmune thrombocytopenia to reduce the risk of antenatal intracranial hemorrhage remains uncertain. Steroids and immunoglobulin may be effective in some mildly affected cases, but serial fetal platelet transfusions are the preferred therapy for those who are severely affected.

Post-transfusion Purpura

The syndrome of post-transfusion purpura was initially described by Shulman and associates.[1] This disorder was first described in patients who were HPA-1b homozygous, although other platelet-specific antigens have since been implicated.[5] Thrombocytopenia occurs after transfusion with HPA-1a blood in individuals previously sensitized by pregnancy or transfusion. With development of thrombocytopenia, anti-HPA-1a antibody is found in the patient's blood.[1]

Clinical Aspects

Typically, patients who have post-transfusion purpura are female. Thrombocytopenia usually develops 7 to 10 days after transfusion. Thrombocytopenia is usually severe, with platelet counts of less than 5000 cells/mm^3 not uncommon. Most types of blood products have been implicated, including whole blood, red cell concentrates, and fresh frozen plasma. As many as 50% of patients experience severe transfusion reactions when the blood products are administered. Symptoms include hypotension, hypertension, chills, bronchospasm, and fever. The thrombocytopenia may last from 4 to 40 days, although it is unclear whether those patients with longer durations have other clinical conditions leading to more prolonged thrombocytopenia.[20]

In patients known to be HPA-1b homozygous, the occurrence of post-transfusion purpura is not predictable. Some patients with documented episodes of post-transfusion purpura have received transfusions several months after recovery to normal platelet counts without recurrence of thrombocytopenia. In contrast, other patients have had second episodes of post-transfusion purpura after subsequent transfusions.

Immunological Aspects

The mystery of post-transfusion purpura is why patients should destroy their own as well as transfused HPA-1b homozygous platelets. Shulman and associates pointed out the similarity to drug purpura, in which there is an abrupt onset and resolution of thrombocytopenia despite the presence of an antibody.[1] They proposed that a foreign antigen-antibody complex binds to platelets, as in drug purpura, leading to thrombocytopenia. Morrison and Mollison proposed that a second antibody with autoimmune specificity reacts with HPA-1b homozygous platelets.[21]

In carefully performed studies by Gengozian and McLaughlin involving transfusion of platelets from one species of marmosets to another, the appearance of IgG-coated platelets coincided with the development of serum antibody, which preceded the onset of thrombocytopenia.[22] Eluates prepared from the recipient marmoset platelets reacted not only with the platelets of all tested marmosets of the same species as the immunized animals but also with the platelets of the immunizing species. These studies suggest that autoantibodies may develop as a result of the transfusion of homologous blood. Whether a similar situation occurs in humans is unknown. To date there have been no well-documented cases of post-transfusion purpura caused by autoantibodies.

Another proposed mechanism for destruction of both HPA-1a-positive and HPA-1a-negative platelets is that transfused antigenic material may bind to circulating platelets, thereby rendering them reactive with the alloantibody. It has been shown in vitro that centrifuged plasma from stored units of HPA-1a blood can promote the binding of anti-HPA-1a to HPA-1b homozygous platelets. This HPA-1a material binds to circulating platelets during transfusion, leading to their destruction by alloantibody. This hypothesis does not fully explain the long duration of thrombocytopenia and is in conflict with the observation that patients transfused more heavily do not have longer durations of thrombocytopenia.[23]

Treatment

Treatment of post-transfusion purpura should be individualized. If the patient is not bleeding and is not at risk for bleeding because of invasive procedures, observation may be all that is required. High-dose intravenous γ globulin may promptly correct the thrombocytopenia in bleeding patients. Platelet transfusions, even if platelets are negative for the immunizing platelet-specific antigen, usually are not effective. Although corticosteroids and plasma exchange are commonly used in post-transfusion purpura, their efficacy has not been established.[20]

Human Leukocyte Antigens

HLA antibody sensitization is the major cause of immune-mediated platelet transfusion refractoriness in patients receiving long-term platelet transfusion therapy. Platelets express only class I HLAs.[24–26] HLA class I gene products are composed of two different glycoprotein chains. The lower-molecular-weight β_2-microglobulin chain, of 12 kD, noncovalently binds to the larger heavy chain, of approximately 45 kD. Both of these proteins belong to the immunoglobulin superfamily of gene products. β_2-microglobulin is a single domain, whereas the class I heavy chain consists of three domains (α_1, α_2, and α_3). There are three well-characterized HLA class I gene products: HLA-A, HLA-B, and HLA-C. Only HLA-A and HLA-B have been shown to be important in causing immune-mediated refractoriness to transfusion. Table 14–3 lists currently described HLA-A and HLA-B class I antigens.[26–28]

Considering the relatively large size of the HLA heavy chain and the number of variable regions, one can predict that antibodies with multiple specificities may be induced by a single HLA molecule. HLA antibodies that are formed can be classified into two groups. The first group recognizes an epitope unique to a particular HLA

Table 14–3. Recognized HLA Class I Specificities

HLA-A Loci Antigens	HLA-B Loci Antigens		
A1	B5		Bw49
A2	B7		Bw50
A3	B8		Bw51
A9	B12		Bw52
A10	B13		Bw53
A11	B14		Bw54
Aw19	B15		Bw55
A23	B16		Bw56
A24	B17		Bw57
A25	B18		Bw58
A26	B21		Bw59
A28	Bw22	Bw60	
A30	B27		Bw61
A31	B35		Bw62
A32	B37		Bw63
Aw33	B38		Bw64
Aw34	B39		Bw65
Aw36	B40		Bw67
Aw43	Bw41	Bw71	
Aw66	Bw42	Bw73	
Aw68	B44		Bw75
Aw69	B45		Bw76
Aw74	Bw46	Bw77	
A29	Bw47	Bw4	
	Bw48	Bw6	

allele. Antibodies to A2 or B12 belong to this group. The second group of HLA antibodies recognizes structural similarities between gene products (cross-reactive) or identical epitopes present on different gene products (public epitopes). These distinctions have been defined serologically rather than molecularly. Several laboratories have demonstrated biochemically that most public specificities represent distinct antigenic epitopes controlled by the class I loci. With continued elucidation of the molecular structure of HLA proteins, these differences should be clarified.

Traditionally, HLA serology has placed the greatest emphasis on classifying the private antigens and defining serological variations of these private antigens, known as splits. These investigations have led to major advances in identifying the large number of polymorphisms controlled by the class I HLA loci and have formed the basis of donor-recipient matching for organ transplantation as well as platelet transfusion therapy.

More importance has been placed on the clinical importance of public HLA specificities. The best-known examples of public specificities are Bw4 and Bw6. These antigens are encoded by a diallelic system and are associated with two different groups of HLA-B class I antigens. Other public antigens carried by HLA-B class I antigens have been divided into four cross-reactive groups: B5, B7, B8, and B12 (Table 14–4). The importance of matching for these public epitopes in the selection of platelets for alloimmunized patients was first documented for the Bw4 and Bw6 antigens. The relevance of matching for other public antigens in platelet transfusion therapy is only beginning to be investigated.[27–29]

Matching for certain private HLA class I antigens does not ensure compatibility for all public antigens. The observations that 20% to 40% of platelet transfusions selected by the matching of private antigens are failures and that the specificities of HLA antibodies in multitransfused individuals are generally against public specificities suggest that matching for these public antigens will prove to be important. With improved serological approaches for the identification of antibody specificities to class I HLAs, selection of platelets may be simplified by using a process based on public specificities.[30]

Immune Platelet Transfusion Refractoriness

Clinical and Laboratory Aspects

Serial measurement of lymphocytotoxic antibodies is useful in documenting alloimmune transfusion refractoriness. Leukemic patients who are undergoing induction chemotherapy and become alloimmunized usually do so by the third week of transfusion support. When antibodies are detected, transfusion failures usually occur, although in a small number of patients transfusions may continue to succeed.

Lee and colleagues carefully studied the natural history of alloimmunization during platelet transfusion support.[31] Serial evaluations of lymphocytotoxic antibodies and responsiveness to random donor platelet transfusions were reviewed in 234 patients who had developed lymphocytotoxic antibodies at some time during treatment. Seventy (30%) of these patients had significant falls in antibody levels during the course of treatment. In 44 patients, these declines occurred after further antigenic exposure was reduced, either because no transfusions were administered or because only histocompatible platelets were transfused. Forty patients who were previously refractory to platelet transfusion underwent rechallenge with random donor platelets when they had declining levels of lymphocytotoxic antibodies. Thirty-four of 35 clinically evaluable patients had good responses to these unmatched transfusions for 2 weeks to 36 months, and antibodies did not return despite repeated transfusions to 21 patients. Thus, serial lymphocytotoxic antibody measurements are helpful in the management of alloimmunized patients. Many patients will have decreases or loss of lymphocytotoxic antibodies, either permanently or transiently, and can be successfully supported with more readily available unmatched random donor platelet transfusions. The pathophysiology of this antibody loss is unknown.

HLA antibodies that react with public epitopes require special techniques for their detection. These antibodies cannot be detected by standard, complement-dependent cytotoxicity testing. They can be detected with a ligand-binding assay employing a labeled antiglobulin

Table 14–4. Class I Cross-Reactive HLA Groups (Associated Private Epitopes)

A1C (1, 3, 11, 10, W19, 9, 28)
A2C (2, 28, 9, 17, 10, 33)
B5C (5, 53, 35, 18, 15, 17, 70, 49)
B7C (7, 27, 22, 42, 48, 40, 41, 13, 47)
B8C (8, 14, 16, 22, 42, 48, 40, 41, 13, 47)
B8C (8, 14, 16, 22, 52)
B12C (12, 21, 40, 41, 13)

reagent or by antiglobulin-enhanced complement-dependent cytotoxicity. Therefore, it is important that these newer techniques be used in both clinical management and investigations of platelet alloimmunization.

Despite close HLA matching of platelet transfusions for patients alloimmunized to HLAs, some transfusion failures occur that cannot be explained by nonimmune causes. The rate of failure in HLA-identical transfusions has been reported to be between 12% and 39%. The importance of platelet-specific antigens has not been widely investigated as a cause of HLA-identical platelet transfusion failure, because the serological identification of platelet-specific antibodies is difficult in patients who may also have HLA antibodies.

Newly developed solid-phase assays, which use immobilized glycoproteins carrying the platelet-specific antigens, permit specific identification of antibodies to platelet-specific antigens in the presence of HLA antibodies. Kickler and coworkers prospectively studied the rate of alloimmunization to platelet-specific antigens associated with platelet glycoproteins IIB-IIIA and IB-IX in 293 multitransfused thrombocytopenic patients.[32] Antibodies to platelet-specific antigens were measured with a solid-phase assay by using platelet glycoprotein IIB-IIIA or IB-IX as the antigenic target. Nine patients were found to have antibodies to platelet glycoprotein IIB-IIIA, but none had antibodies to platelet glycoprotein IB-IX. In six of the nine patients,[32] antibodies recognizing known polymorphisms of IIB-IIIA were found; in the remaining three, no specificity could be identified. The rate of alloimmunization to platelet-specific antigens associated with glycoprotein IIB-IIIA was 2%, compared with 23% for HLA alloimmunization. Of the patients alloimmunized to HLAs, 9% also had antibodies to platelet-specific antigens. These results suggest that the incidence of antibodies to platelet-specific antigens carried on glycoprotein IIB-IIIA is low. Platelet-specific antibodies may be found more commonly in patients who are alloimmunized to HLAs than in patients who are not.

Selecting Platelets for the Alloimmunized Patient

Once it is determined that a patient is alloimmunized to HLAs, compatible platelets are required for transfusion.[5, 25] The large number of polymorphisms in the HLA system complicate the provision of HLA-matched platelets. With approximately 70 antigens to consider, the probability of finding matched donors is low, unless a large number of HLA-typed plateletpheresis donors are available. Because of this, different degrees of HLA similarity are used. These are defined in Table 14–5.

Traditional selection guidelines are as follows:

1. If HLA-identical platelets are unavailable, platelets from donors whose HLA types are serologically cross-reactive with the recipient's may be substituted.
2. Matching for antigens of the HLA-C locus is not necessary.
3. Mismatching for some HLA-B locus antigens that are weakly expressed on platelets is acceptable for some donor-recipient pairs.
4. If cross-reactive platelets are ineffective for some patients, attention to linked HLA specificities (e.g., Bw4/Bw6) may be important.
5. Although ABO is expressed on platelets, ABO matching is usually not critical.

This approach has remained relatively unchallenged for several years and is still in widespread use. However, in evaluating this approach, several investigators have reported shortcomings. In studies by Kickler and coworkers, 20% of 50 HLA-identical platelet transfusions were unsuccessful. Of the transfusions selected on the basis of cross-reactivities without regard to matching of public specificities, 41% were failures (23 of 56 transfusions). Approximately one third of platelet transfusions in which one or two antigens were mismatched were failures. These observations indicate that matching platelets solely on the basis of HLA private antigens is frequently ineffective. Furthermore, even if a patient is alloimmunized, mismatched platelets may produce successful transfusion outcomes.[33]

For these reasons, refining the selection process for platelet transfusion in alloimmunized patients is the subject of much investigation. As previously discussed, one approach may be to characterize the public specificity of antibodies and then select platelets on the basis of this identification. A more direct strategy involves performing platelet crossmatching. Numerous investigators have evaluated the usefulness of crossmatching a recipient's serum with that of potential platelet donors. A variety of labeled antiglobulin techniques exist that are proving clinically useful in improving transfusion outcome.[34] A simple, standardized method entailing the use of anti–human IgG-coated red cells that can detect antibody bound to immobilized platelets has been developed. This method permits platelet crossmatching to be performed in most blood banks. Using platelet crossmatching in patients who are alloimmunized can significantly reduce the refractoriness to platelet transfusion. With the availability of standardized platelet crossmatching techniques, many blood centers now routinely perform platelet compatibility testing. Guidelines to the selection of compatible platelets are given in Table 14–6.

Table 14–5. Donor and Recipient HLA Match Grades

Grade	Definition
A	All four donor antigens are identical to those in the recipient
B1U	All donor antigens are identical to those in the recipient; only three antigens are detected in the donor
B2U	All donor antigens are identical to those in the recipient; only two antigens are detected in the donor
B1X	Three donor antigens are identical to those in the recipient, and the fourth is serologically cross-reactive with a recipient antigen
B2UX	Two donor antigens are identical to those in the recipient; a third is cross-reactive; only three antigens are detected in the donor
B2X	Two antigens are identical to those in the recipient; two are cross-reactive
C	One donor antigen is mismatched with a recipient antigen
D	Two or more donor antigens are mismatched with recipient antigens

Table 14–6. Approach to Selection of Platelets for Alloimmunized Patients

Determine HLA phenotype and ABO type of the recipient
Screen patient's serum for lymphocytotoxic antibody, or antibodies to human platelet antigens if there is a history of failed transfusion with HLA-identical platelets
Select from the donor pool those units with the most compatible HLAs and, if possible, ABO systems
or
Crossmatch available platelet units without regard to patient or donor HLA type (circumvents the need for HLA typing and is a means of finding compatible platelets when antibodies to human platelet antigens are present)
Obtain 1-hour and 18- to 24-hour post-transfusion platelet counts, not only to assess transfusion outcome but also to guide the selection of future transfusions

AUTOIMMUNE THROMBOCYTOPENIA

Chronic Autoimmune Thrombocytopenia

Early observations by Harrington and coworkers showed that thrombocytopenic pregnant women frequently delivered babies with thrombocytopenia.[35] This suggested that some plasma factor crossing the placenta mediated the newborn's thrombocytopenia. Plasma infusions from patients with thrombocytopenia were shown to produce thrombocytopenia in normal volunteers. Subsequently, Shulman showed that the degree of thrombocytopenia was dependent on the amount of plasma infused, with splenectomized or corticosteroid-treated subjects being more resistant to the effects of the infused autoimmune thrombocytopenic plasma.[1] The pathogenic factor present in the plasma reacted with normal and autologous platelets and could be isolated and removed from the γ globulin fraction of plasma by adsorption with platelets. These early studies provided us with a basic understanding of the pathogenic mechanisms of the factors involved in platelet destruction.

The first direct evidence that autoantibodies are present on platelets was the observation that eluates prepared from the platelets of patients with autoimmune thrombocytopenia bind to normal platelets.[36] These eluate studies also documented that the major antigenic target for these antibodies was platelet glycoprotein IIB-IIIA. This observation was based on the failure of the eluates to react with platelets from patients who are deficient for platelet glycoprotein IIB-IIIA (Glanzmann's thrombasthenia). Subsequent studies with western blotting or immunoprecipitation demonstrated that the autoantigens were principally found on platelet glycoprotein IIIA. Some patients may have autoantibodies that react with one or more platelet glycoproteins, including platelet glycoprotein IB-IX or IA-IIA.[37–39]

The distribution of the heavy-chain type of autoantibodies present on the platelets, frequently referred to as platelet-associated immunoglobulin, is as follows: 95% of patients have IgG either alone or in combination with IgA or IgM, and 5% have IgM alone. A variety of studies have shown a broad range for the IgG subclass distribution. However, subclass determination has not been shown to have prognostic importance. Although immune complexes may be measured in patients with chronic autoimmune thrombocytopenia, there is little evidence that they are of pathogenic importance.[40]

Clinical Aspects

Patients with chronic autoimmune thrombocytopenia typically present with petechiae and mucosal bleeding. Symptoms may be present for months, or some patients may experience more acute manifestations. If bleeding has been significant, anemia may be present. Alternatively, some patients may have concomitant autoimmune hemolytic anemia, which accounts for the associated anemia. Physical examination is unremarkable except for bleeding manifestations. The peripheral smear shows reduced to absent platelets with an increased mean platelet volume. The bone marrow is normal.[39]

Acute Immune Thrombocytopenia

Acute immune thrombocytopenia occurs primarily in children, with a peak age of 2 to 6 years. Typically there is a history of an antecedent viral infection followed by the acute onset of bruising, petechiae, and mucosal bleeding. If thrombocytopenia persists for longer than 6 months despite therapy, the child should be considered to have chronic autoimmune thrombocytopenia. The risk of chronicity increases with the age of the child. Otherwise, there are no prognostic features, either clinical or laboratory, that will predict whether a child with acute immune thrombocytopenia will recover spontaneously. Our understanding of the pathogenic mechanisms of acute immune thrombocytopenia is incomplete. It appears that viral illnesses are responsible for evoking an immune response and that antibodies to platelets or immune complexes are involved in shortened platelet survival. Increased levels of immunoglobulin found on the platelets of these patients may reflect the deposition of immune complexes that have bound to the platelet Fc receptor. It is also possible that transient production of autoantibodies may be induced by viral infections. There is little evidence to suggest that microbial agents produce some factor that alters the surface of platelets, making them immunogenic.[39]

Platelet Autoantibody Detection

For over a half a century, the measurement of either IgG or complement on the red cell membrane has been done reliably with the antiglobulin test (Coombs' test) for the diagnosis of autoimmune hemolytic anemia. It was once thought that this agglutination technique would prove equally useful in the diagnosis of autoimmune thrombocytopenia. This has not been the case because of the natural tendency of platelets to clump and the relatively high amount of immunoglobulins on the platelet surface, contributing to a high background. In many cases, it appears that the amount of pathological antibody may be relatively low. The normal high-background membrane-bound immunoglobulin makes the distinction between positive and negative test results difficult.[40–42]

Although the measurement of platelet autoantibodies has provided important insights into the immunopathology of autoimmune thrombocytopenia, this laboratory determination should not be considered either specific or sensitive for the diagnosis of autoimmune thrombocytopenia. The antibody titer, immunoglobulin class, or glycoprotein to which the antibody is directed is not predictive of severity, response to therapy, or any particular clinical manifestation. The limiting factor in measuring membrane-bound immunoglobulin is the degree of thrombocytopenia, because the harvest of sufficient platelets may be impossible. The platelets of patients with autoimmune thrombocytopenia typically are larger than normal; consequently, the increased platelet size contributes to elevated levels of immunoglobulin on the membrane surface. Thus, quantitative determination of surface immunoglobulin is a function of platelet size rather than the amount of antibody being produced.

The specificity of tests for membrane-bound immunoglobulin is low because the platelet membrane permits the adsorption of normal plasma protein constituents. Patients with increased platelet turnover for any reason may adsorb normal serum immunoglobulins from the plasma, leading to increased platelet-associated immunoglobulin. When platelet glycoproteins are used as antigenic targets for the measurement of circulating antiplatelet antibodies, this problem is circumvented.

A variety of methods are available to measure antiplatelet antibodies. The earlier assays employing complement fixation or platelet lysis lacked sensitivity and are no longer used. Quantitative measurements based on antiglobulin consumption give falsely high values for platelet-associated immunoglobulin because antiglobulin binds differently to membrane-bound IgG than to the IgG in solution used to calibrate the standard curve.[43]

Currently, several quantitative assays employing radiolabeled antiglobulin reagents are used in clinical laboratories.[44] These have the advantage of being relatively simple to perform. The wide variety of commercially available antiglobulin reagents, either monoclonal or polyclonal, makes such testing widely available. Radiolabeled monoclonal antibodies have been employed in these assays to estimate the number of molecules of immunoglobulin on the platelet surface. If the radioactivity of the monoclonal antibody is expressed as activity per microgram of protein, and if one assumes a binding ratio of 1:1, the average number of molecules of immunoglobulin per platelet can be estimated.

Currently, a great deal of work is being done to standardize the use of tests that incorporate platelet glycoproteins as antigenic targets. These assays are referred to as platelet glycoprotein capture assays. In these assays, the binding of patient serum to specific platelet glycoproteins is measured by isolation of the platelet glycoproteins with monoclonal antibodies. The test can be performed with the patient's platelets to determine whether there is increased immunoglobulin bound to them. Alternatively, serum antibody can be tested against normal platelets. The isolation of the platelet glycoproteins may occur before or after incubation of the platelets with the patient's serum. Platelet glycoproteins can be solubilized from normal group O platelet donors and captured by specific monoclonal antibodies bound to microtiter wells. For example, one can use monoclonal antibodies to platelet glycoprotein IIIA, IB-IX, or IIA-IIIA to individually capture these platelet glycoproteins to a plastic surface. Binding of the platelet autoantibody can be detected by using an enzyme-labeled secondary antibody, with anti-IgG, -IgM or -IgA. In most investigators' experience, this testing has increased the specificity of testing for platelet autoantibodies. When a patient's own platelets are used, approximately 80% will have detectable antibody identified by a panel of captive monoclonal antibodies. The relative sensitivity for serum antibodies is approximately 50%.[40, 45]

Antigen capture assays have advantages over the previously mentioned tests for detecting autoimmune antibodies, because interference by nonspecific immunoglobulin is reduced, native conformation of platelet antigens is maintained by using nondenaturing detergents, and determination of target platelet glycoprotein is possible.

DRUG-INDUCED IMMUNE THROMBOCYTOPENIA

A variety of drugs have been implicated in drug-induced immune thrombocytopenia, which can develop after the patient has been taking a drug for a sufficient period to develop an antibody. For unknown reasons, a patient may receive a drug for several years and then unpredictably develop drug-induced immune thrombocytopenia. After the patient has recovered and the drug has been restarted, purpura may occur after a single dose, presumably secondary to an anamnestic response.

The characterization of the platelet membrane receptor involved in the binding of drug-antibody complexes has been best studied in quinidine/quinine-induced immune thrombocytopenia. Kunicki and associates first showed that quinine/quinidine-dependent antibodies failed to react with Bernard-Soulier syndrome platelets. This observation suggests that the drug-dependent antibodies bind to membrane glycoproteins that are absent in platelets from persons with Bernard-Soulier syndrome. These include glycoprotein IB-IX and glycoprotein V. Subsequently, other investigators have shown that the antibodies bind to glycoprotein IB-IX. There have also been reports that glycoprotein IIB-IIIA may serve as a receptor for drug-dependent antibodies.[46–48]

Heparin is one of the most widely studied drugs implicated in immune thrombocytopenia. The development of heparin-induced thrombocytopenia in patients with heparin-dependent antibodies still is not entirely understood. The antibodies can trigger platelet activation and aggregation, leading to thrombosis. The mechanism underlying this activation phenomenon involves Fc gamma RII receptors. The target antigen identified is a complex of heparin and platelet factor 4. In 5% to 10% of cases of heparin-induced thrombocytopenia, measurable antibodies to platelet factor 4–heparin complex are absent. This implies involvement of other antigens. The presence of autoantibodies to two other chemokines has been reported. These include neutrophil activation peptide and interleukin-8.[49]

SUMMARY

Significant work in characterizing the alloantigens and autoantigens and antibodies involved in immune-mediated thrombocytopenic disorders has led to a better understanding of these conditions. As in other areas of medicine, scientific discoveries in immunology, membrane chemistry, and molecular biology have led to advances in diagnosis and treatment. Further characterization of the structural characteristics of platelet alloantigens may yield a better understanding of their relative immunogenicity. The predisposing factors for the formation of either alloantibodies or autoantibodies to platelets remain undefined. Further studies of the immune response to platelets will devise novel approaches for the prevention and therapy of immune-mediated autoimmune thrombocytopenic disorders.

REFERENCES

1. Shulman NR, Marder V, Hiller M, Collier EM. Platelet and leukocyte isoantigens and their antibodies: clinical, physiologic and clinical studies. Prog Hematol 1964; 4:222.
2. Kunicki TJ. Biochemistry of platelet associated isoantigens and alloantigens. *In* Kunicki TJ, George JN (eds): Platelet Immunobiology. Philadelphia: JB Lippincott, 1989, p 99.
3. Newman PJ. Nomenclature of human platelet alloantigens: a problem with the HPA system? Blood 1992; 83:1447.
4. Kickler TS, Kennedy SD, Braine HG. Alloimmunization to platelet specific antigens on glycoprotein IIB-IIIA and IB/IX in multitransfused thrombocytopenic patients. Transfusion 1990; 30:622.
5. McFarland J. Matched apheresis platelets. *In* McLeod BC, Price TJ, Drew MJ (eds): Apheresis: Principles and Practice. Bethesda, MD: AABB Press, 1997, p 171.
6. Bray PR, Jin Y, Kickler T. Rapid genotyping of the five major platelet alloantigens by reverse dot blot hybridization. Blood 1996; 84:4361.
7. Blanchette V, Peters MA, Pegg-Feige K. Alloimmune thrombocytopenia. Review from a neonatal intensive care unit. *In* Decary F, Rock GA (eds): First Canadian Workshop and Conference on Platelet Serology, Ottawa. Current Studies in Hematology and Blood Transfusion. Basel: Karger, 1986.
8. Bussel J, Kaplan C, McFarland J. Recommendations for the evaluation and treatment of neonatal autoimmune and alloimmune thrombocytopenia. Thromb Haemost 1991; 65:631.
9. Herman JH, Ancona RJ, Jumbelic MI, et al. In vitro cerebral hemorrhage in isoimmune thrombocytopenia. Am J Pediatr Hematol Oncol 1986; 8:312.
10. Decary F. Is HLA DR 3 a risk factor in Pl^{A1} negative pregnant women? *In* DeCary F, Rock GA (eds): First Canadian Workshop and Conference on Platelet Serology, Ottawa. Current Studies in Hematology and Blood Transfusion. Basel: Karger, 1986.
11. Rexnikoff-Etievant MF, Dangu C, Lobet R. HLA-B8 antigen and anti-Pl^{A1} alloimmunization. Tissue Antigens 1981; 18:66.
12. Decary FM, L'Abbe D, Tremblay L, Chartrand P. The immune response to the HPA-1a antigen: association with HLA-DRw52a. Br J Haematol 1991; 1:55.
13. Valentin N, Vergracht A, Bignon JD, et al. HLA-DRw52a is involved in alloimmunization against Pl^{A1} antigen. Hum Immunol 1990; 27:79.
14. L'Abbe D, Tremblay L, Filion M, et al. Alloimmunization to platelet antigen HPA-1a (PIA1) is strongly associated with both HLA-DRB3*0101 and HLA-DQB1*0201. Hum Immunol 1992; 34:107.
15. Kickler TS. Neonatal alloimmune thrombocytopenia. Reprod Med 1992; 12:577.
16. Bussel JB, McFarland JG, Berkowitz RL. Antenatal management of fetal alloimmune and autoimmune thrombocytopenia. Transfus Med Rev 1990; 4:149.
17. Bussel JB, Berkowitz RL, McFarland JG, et al. Antenatal treatment of neonatal alloimmune thrombocytopenia. N Engl J Med 1992; 319:1374.
18. Lynch L, Bussel JB, McFarland JG, et al. Antenatal treatment of alloimmune thrombocytopenia. Obstet Gynecol 1992; 80:67.
19. Murphy MF, Waters AH, Doughty HA, et al. Antenatal management of fetomaternal alloimmune thrombocytopenia—report of 15 affected pregnancies. Transfus Med 1994; 4:281.
20. Vogelsang G, Kickler TS, Bell WR. Post-transfusion purpura. Am J Hematol 1986; 21:259.
21. Morrison FS, Mollison PL. Post transfusion purpura. N Engl J Med 1966; 275:243.
22. Gengozian N, McLaughlin C. Actively induced platelet bound IgG associated with thrombocytopenia in the marmoset. Blood 1978; 51:1197.
23. Kickler TS, Ness PM, Herman JH, Bell WR. Studies on the pathophysiology of post transfusion purpura. Blood 1986; 68:347.
25. Heyman MR, Schiffer CA. Platelet transfusion to patients receiving chemotherapy. *In* Rossi EC, Simon TL, Moss GS, Gould SA (eds): Principles of Transfusion Medicine, 2nd ed. Baltimore: Williams & Wilkins, 1996, p 263.
26. Hogge DE, Dutcher JP, Aisner J, et al. Lymphocytotoxicity antibody is a predictor of response to random donor platelet transfusion. Am J Hematol 1993; 14:363.
27. Rodey GE. Class I antigens: HLA-A, -B, -C and cross reactive groups. *In* Moulds J, Fawcett KJ, Garner RJ (eds): Scientific and Technical Aspects of the Major Histocompatibility Complex. Arlington, VA: American Association of Blood Banks, 1989, p 23.
28. Rodey GE, Park M, Fuller T, et al. Analysis of sera that define public or crossreactive HLA class I epitopes. *In* Dupont B (ed): Immunobiology of HLA, vol 1. Basel: Springer Verlag, 1989, p 288.
29. Duquesnoy RJ. HLA humoral allosensitization. Clinical significance of humoral allosensitization of HLA antigens. *In* Lee J (ed): The First HLA Symposium. Proceedings of the First Red Cross International Workshop. New York: Springer Verlag, 1990, p 27.
30. Schiffer CA, O'Connell B, Lee EJ. Platelet transfusion therapy for alloimmunized patients: selective mismatching for HLA B12, an antigen with variable expression on platelets. Blood 1989; 74:1172.
31. Lee EJ, Schiffer CA. Serial measurement of lymphocytotoxic antibody and response to non-matched platelet transfusions in alloimmunized patients. Blood 1992; 70:1727.
32. Kickler TS, Kennedy SD, Braine HG. Alloimmunization to platelet specific antigens on glycoprotein IIB-IIIA and IB/IX in multitransfused thrombocytopenic patients. Transfusion 1990; 30:622.
33. Kickler TS, Braine HG, Ness PM. The predictive value of crossmatching platelet transfusion for alloimmunized patients. Transfusion 1985; 25:385.
34. Moroff G, Garraty G, Heal JM, et al. Selection of platelets for refractory patients by HLA matching and prospective crossmatching. Transfusion 1992; 32:633.
35. Harrington WJ, Minnich V, Hollingsworth JW, et al. Demonstration of a thrombocytopenic factor in the blood of patients with thrombocytopenic purpura. J Lab Clin Med 1951; 38:1.
36. Leeuwen EF van, Ven JTM, van der Engelfriet CP, Borne AEGK von dem. Specificity of autoantibodies in autoimmune thrombocytopenia. Blood 1982; 59:23.
37. McMillan R. Antigen-specific assays in immune thrombocytopenia. Trans Med Rev 1990; 4:136.
38. McMillan R, Tani P, Millard F. Platelet associated and plasma antiglycoprotein autoantibodies in chronic ITP. Blood 1987; 70:1040.
39. George JN, El-harangue MA, Rasion GE. Chronic idiopathic thrombocytopenic purpura. N Engl J Med 1995; 331:1207.
40. He R, Reid DM, Jones CE, Shulman NR. Spectrum of Ig classes, specificities and titers of serum antiglycoproteins in chronic idiopathic thrombocytopenic purpura. Blood 1994; 83:1024.
41. Tsubakio T, Tani P, Woods VL, McMillan R. Autoantibodies against platelet GPIIb/IIIa in chronic ITP react with different epitopes. Br J Haematol 1987; 67:345.
42. Woods VL, Oh EH, Mason D, McMillan R. Autoantibodies against the platelet glycoprotein IIb/IIIa complex in patients with chronic ITP. Blood 1984; 64:368.
43. Rosse WF, Devine DV, Ware R. Reactions of immunoglobulin G binding ligands with platelets and platelet associated immunoglobulin G. J Clin Invest 1984; 73:489.
44. LoBuglio AF, Court WS, Vinocur L, et al. Immune thrombocytopenic purpura: Use of a 125-I–labeled antihuman IgG monoclonal antibody to quantify platelet-bound IgG. N Engl J Med 1983; 309:459.

45. Kiefel V, Santoso S, Weisheit M, Mueller-Ecklhardt C. Monoclonal antibody-specific immobilization of platelet antigens (MAIPA): a new tool for the identification of platelet reactive antibodies. Blood 1987; 70:1722.
46. Kunicki TJ, Johnson MM, Aster RH. Absence of the platelet receptor for drug dependent antibodies in the Bernard-Soulier syndrome. J Clin Invest 1978; 62:716.
47. Chong BH, Du X, Berndt MC, et al. Characterization of the binding domains on platelet glycoproteins IB/IX and IIB/IIIA complexes for the quinine/quinidine dependent antibodies. Blood 1991; 77:2190.
48. Visentin GP, Newman PJ, Aster RH. Characteristics of quinine and quinidine induced antibodies specific for platelet glycoproteins IIB and IIIA. Blood 1991; 77:2668.
49. Visentin GP, Ford SE, Scott JP, Aster RH. Antibodies from patients with heparin induced thrombocytopenia are specific for platelet factor four complexed with heparin bound to endothelial cells. J Clin Invest 1994; 93:81.
50. Semsek S, Faber NM, Bleeker PM, et al. Determination of human platelet antigen frequencies in the Dutch population by immunophenotyping and DNA analysis. Blood 1993; 81:835.

SECTION

VI Plasma Proteins

CHAPTER 15

Biochemistry of Plasma Proteins

David H. Bing
Chester A. Alper

Plasma is a highly complex mixture of more than 100 proteins, many of which have been purified and their primary structures determined either by amino acid or DNA sequencing. Approximately 25 proteins have been crystallized. Three-dimensional models have been constructed on the basis of x-ray diffraction data for transthyretin, α_1-antitrypsin, retinol-binding protein, the C3a fragment of C3, the F 1.2 fragment of prothrombin, immunoglobulin G (IgG), and the complex of hirudin with thrombin. The list of purified plasma proteins includes at least 25 for which the physiological function has never been determined.[1–4]

The definition of a plasma protein has become more difficult with the advent of new methods demonstrating that trace components in plasma are often proteins shed from the cell membranes in a variety of tissues. Moreover, some proteins are found in two or more distinct forms, one associated with cells and the other present in blood or urine. To date, no systematic attempt has been made to classify all of the plasma proteins according to an international convention. There has been progress, however, in naming certain groups of proteins that are related either structurally or functionally. These include the immunoglobulins, the complement proteins, the coagulation proteins, and the lipoproteins. Standard nomenclature is based on historical as well as international conventions.[3, 5]

Almost all plasma proteins, with the major exception of the immunoglobulins, are produced by hepatocytes. Plasma cells and B lymphocytes synthesize immunoglobulins. Plasma proteins are, in general, synthesized on polyribosomes and discharged into the rough endoplasmic reticulum. If carbohydrate is part of the circulating protein, it is added during passage through the cisternae of the endoplasmic reticulum and the Golgi apparatus. As it is synthesized, each polypeptide chain may have extra peptides at the amino-terminus, called pre and pro fragments. Release from the ribosomes of newly synthesized polypeptide chains involves cleavage during processing, which removes the pro fragment. The latter may serve as a signal for passage through the endoplasmic reticulum. Some proteins are synthesized as single-polypeptide chains but then are cleaved intracellularly by a protease to produce multichain structures that circulate as the major "natural" protein.

NOMENCLATURE

The genetic nomenclature used in this chapter is that endorsed by the International Society for Human Genetics.[2] By eliminating subscripts and superscripts and by using only capital letters and arabic numerals, it is meant to be easily used for computer storage and analysis. Gene loci are designated by two or more italicized letters and/or numbers (preferably four characters or fewer). Alleles are designated by the locus name, an asterisk, and one or more italicized letters and/or numbers (preferably four characters or fewer). All characters are on the same line. Gene products, genetic variants, and phenotypes are noted as alleles, except that the asterisk is replaced by a space and characters are not italicized. Null alleles or variants are designated "Q0" for "quantity zero" and hypomorphic variants are designated "QL" for "quantity lowered." Table 15–1 lists this nomenclature for the genetic loci and alleles and shows equivalents appearing in the literature.

CHROMOSOMAL LOCALIZATION OF PLASMA PROTEIN GENES

The genes for many of the plasma proteins have been assigned to specific chromosomes and chromosomal regions by somatic cell hybridization techniques, by family linkage studies, and most recently by recombinant DNA methods. Table 15–2 summarizes this information: PI (α_1-antitrypsin), GM (Ig heavy chain), C2 (complement component C2), BF (complement factor B), C4A (complement component C4, isotype A), C4B (complement component C4, isotype B), CR1 (complement receptor 1), FH (complement factor H), CR2 (complement receptor 2), C4BP (C4 binding protein), MCP (membrane cofactor protein), DAF (decay accelerating factor), ALB (albumin), and GC (Gc-globulin, vitamin D–binding protein).

Table 15–1. Gene Locus and Allele Designation Equivalents

Designation in this Chapter		Alternative and Prior Designations	
Locus	**Common or Selected Alleles**	**Locus**	**Common or Selected Alleles**
PI	M1, M2, M3, M4, Z, S, Q0, M MALTON	*Pi*	M_1, M_2, M_3, M_4, Z, S, null or –, M^{Malton}
OR	F, S	*Or*	F, S
HP	1F, 1S, 2	*Hp*	1αF, 1αS, 2α
GC	1F, 1S, 2, 1A1, 2A3	*Gc*	1F, 1S, 2, Ab, Japan
CP	A, B, C, NH	*Cp*	A, B, C, B^{NH}
E1	U, A, J, F, S, K	*E1*	u, a, j, f, s, k
TF	C1, C2, C3, C4, C5, B2, D1	*Tf*	C_1, C_2, C_3, C_4, C_5, B_2, D_1
AG	X, Y, A2, D, C, G, T, Z, H, I	*Ag*	x, y, a1, d, c, g, t, z, h, I
LP	A	*Lp*	a
G1M	A, Z, X, F, NONA	*G1m*	a or 1, z or 17, x or 2, f or 3, non-a n or 23
G2M	N	*G2m*	
G3M	B0, B1, B3, B4, B5, C3, C5, S, T, G	*G3m*	b^0 or 11, b^1 or 5, b^3 or 12, b^4 or 14, b^5 or 10, c^3 or 6, c^5 or 24, s or 15, t or 16, g or 21
A2M	1, 2	*A2m*	1, 2
KM	1, 2, 3	*Km, InV*	1, a, b
PLG	A, B	*Plg, PLGN*	1, 2
F13A	1, 2	*FXIIIA*	1, 2
F13B	1, 2, 3	*FXIIIB*	1, 2, 3, (S, F)
BG	N, Q0	*Bg*	N, D
C3	F, S, Q0	*C3*	F, S, null or –
BF	F, S, F1, S1	*Bf, Gb*	F, S, F1, S 0.7, F_1, S_1
C2	C, B, A1, A2	*C2*	1, 2, (3), (4)

Data from Shows TB, Alper CA, Bootsma D, et al. International system for human gene nomenclature. Cytogenet Cell Genet 1979; 28:96; and Putnam FW. Trace components of plasma: an overview. *In* Jamieson GA, Greenwall TA (eds): Trace Components of Plasma. New York: Alan R. Liss, 1976.

The normal abundance of plasma proteins of clinical interest encompasses a 50,000-fold concentration range. A tabulation of the normal concentration ranges of many plasma proteins can be found in several reviews.[2, 3] One method that is often used to depict the plasma proteins is illustrated in the scatter diagram in Figure 15–1, which shows the approximate mean concentration of approximately 50 human plasma proteins. Albumin (3500 to 4500 mg/dL) is the most abundant protein, accounting for 50% to 65% of the total protein content of plasma,[6] with IgG present at 600 to 1500 mg/dL. Other categories of plasma proteins, based on concentration in blood, are major (100 to 1000 mg/dL), minor (10 to 100 mg/dL), trace (1 to 10 mg/dL), and ultratrace (0.01 to 1 mg/dL). Many of the proteins have been used to assist clinicians in making diagnostic decisions about metabolic and genetic disorders.[7, 8]

ALBUMIN: PROPERTIES AND STRUCTURE

Albumin is a single-polypeptide chain with a molecular mass of 66 to 68 kD. It is one of the few plasma proteins that is not a glycoprotein. The gene for albumin is on

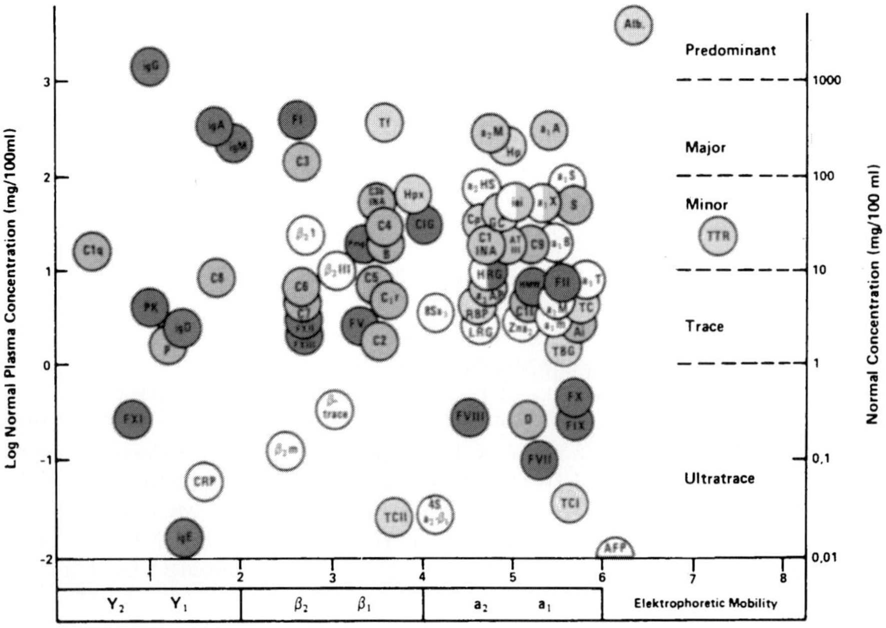

Figure 15–1. Scatter diagram of human plasma proteins. The *y*-axis is the log of normal concentration; the *x*-axis is the electrophoretic mobility. Coagulation proteins are indicated by the *dotted box*, proteinase inhibitors are *black*, transport proteins are *dark gray*, complement proteins are *medium gray*, immunoglobulins are *light gray*, and acute phase proteins are *white*. (From Schwick HG, Haupt H. Properties of acute phase proteins of human plasma. Behring Inst Mitt 1986; 80:1.)

Table 15–2. Chromosomal Localization of Genes for Some Plasma Proteins*

Locus	Protein	Location
A2M	α_2-Macroglobulin	12
AACT	α_1-Antichymotrypsin	14q31-qter
AHSG	α_2-HS globulin	3cen-q13
ALB	Albumin	4q11-q13
SAP	Serum amyloid P component	1q12-q23
APOLP1	Apolipoprotein cluster I	11q13
APOLP2	Apolipoprotein cluster II	19cen-q13.2
APOA2	Apolipoprotein AII	1p21-q23
APOB	Apolipoprotein B	2p24
APOD	Apolipoprotein D	3p14.2-qter
AT3	Antithrombin III	1q23.1-q23.9
B2M	β_2-Microglobulin	15q21-22
BF	Properdin factor B	6p21.3
C1I	C1 inhibitor	11p11.2-q13
C1QB	Clq β chain	1p
C1R	C1r	12
C1S	C1s	12
C2	C2	6p21.3
C3	C3	19p13.3-13.2
C4A, C4B	C4A, C4B	6p21.3
C81, C82	C8 α-γ, β	1p22
CP	Ceruloplasmin	3q21-q24
CRP	C-reactive protein	1q12-q23
FNZ	Fibronectin	4q12
GC	Gc-globulin	4q12
HP	Haptoglobin	16q-22.1
HPX	Hemopexin	11
F13A	Factor XIIIA	6pter-p23
F13B	Factor XIIIB	1
IGH	Heavy chains for IgG, A, M, D, and E	14q32-33
IGK	κ light chains	2p12
IGL	λ light chains	22q11-12
OR	α_1-Acid glycoprotein	9q34.3-qter
PI	α_1-Antitrypsin	14q32.1
RCAC	Regulator of complement activation cluster (DAF, H, C4BP, CR1, CR2)	1q32
SAA	Serum amyloid A component	11pter-p12
TBG	Thyroxine-binding globulin	Xq28
TBPA	Transthyretin	18q11.2-12.1
TC2	Transcobalamin II	22q11.2-2-qter
TF	Transferrin	3q21

Data from New Haven Gene Mapping Library Chromosome Plots, No. 4, HGM9.5, November 1988, Howard Hughes Medical Institute.
*Exclusive of the genes for most of the proteins of the coagulation system.

chromosome 4 (see Table 15–2). A variety of amino acids and hormones can affect the synthesis of albumin, but if the nutritional state and hormonal environment are normal, the principal regulator of albumin appears to be the osmotic pressure at or near the site of synthesis. Thus, depression of albumin synthesis can follow administration of synthetic blood expanders or human plasma or the stimulation of immunoglobulin biosynthesis. In addition, if there is an increase in colloid osmotic pressure, there will also be an increase in the catabolic rate of albumin, thus demonstrating the linkage between albumin synthesis and degradation.[9, 10] The degradation and distribution of albumin in comparison with IgG, IgM, fibrinogen, and transferrin are shown in Table 15–3. Compared with that of other major plasma proteins, the fractional catabolic rate of albumin is low (like that of IgG), and its distribution in the intravascular and extravascular space is similar to that of transferrin, which has almost the same molecular weight.[11, 12]

Structural studies of albumin are consistent with the protein's folding into three domains and nine subdomains. The regions in albumin that bind small molecules have been identified (Fig. 15–2*A*). This domain structure has been confirmed by x-ray diffraction analysis (see Fig. 15–2*B*).[13] The molecular dimensions of albumin are 3.8 × 15 nm. This symmetry (in contrast to the dimensions of IgG or fibrinogen) results in a relatively low viscosity for solutions of albumin. Thus, a 25% solution of albumin has a viscosity approximately equal to that of blood, a 15% solution of IgG, or a 2% solution of fibrinogen. Because the work performed by the heart depends in large part on the viscosity of whole blood, this becomes an important factor when albumin is used as a volume expander.[10–12]

The major function of albumin is its role in osmotic regulation. It is responsible for 75% to 80% of the osmotic effect of plasma, because it constitutes over half of the total protein in plasma by weight and has the lowest molecular weight of the major plasma proteins. Albumin has an isoelectric point of 4.7, and at pH 7.4 it has 18 net-negative charges per molecule. This net-negative charge at neutral pH results in albumin's exhibiting a

Table 15–3. Degradation and Distribution of Some Plasma Proteins*

Plasma Protein	Serum Concentration (mg/dL)	Fractional Catabolic Rate (% IVM/day)	Synthetic Rate (g/175 cm²/day)	Molecular Weight (kD)	Distribution Ratio (IVM as % of Total Mass)
Albumin	4200 (10%)	9 (9%)	11 (16%)	68	45 (8%)
Transferrin	220 (8%)	17 (7%)	1.1 (21%)	70	49 (5%)
IgG	1100 (17%)	7 (21%)	2.1 (28%)	160	58 (12%)
IgM	103 (35%)	11 (14%)	0.3 (41%)	900	74 (15%)
Fibrinogen	336 (35%)	25 (21%)	2.2 (41%)	360	84

From Jarnum S, Jensen KB. Distribution and degradation of albumin. *In* Yap SH, Majoor CLH, Van Tongeren JHM (eds): Clinical Aspects of Albumin. Boston: Martinus Nijhoff Medical Division, 1978.

*Percentages in parentheses in columns 2 to 4 and 6 represent the coefficients of variation.

IVM, Intravascular mass.

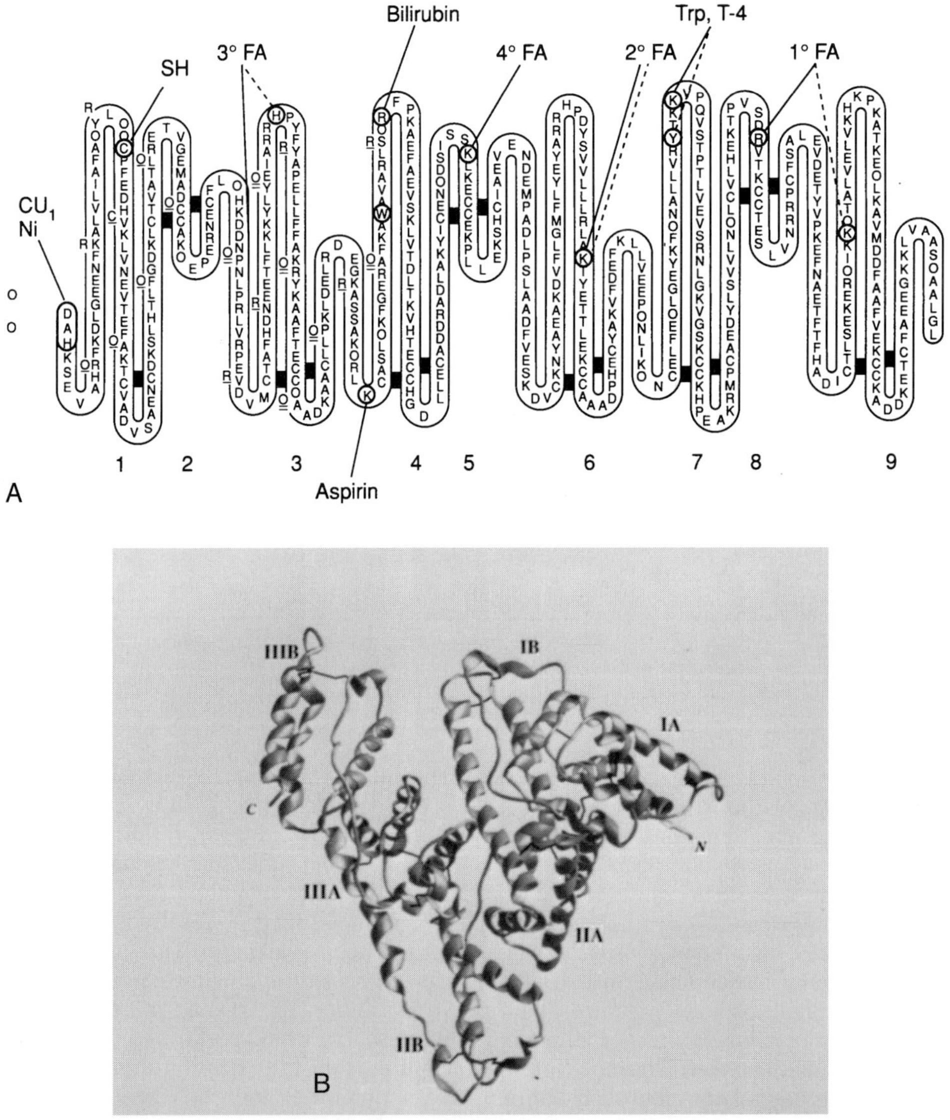

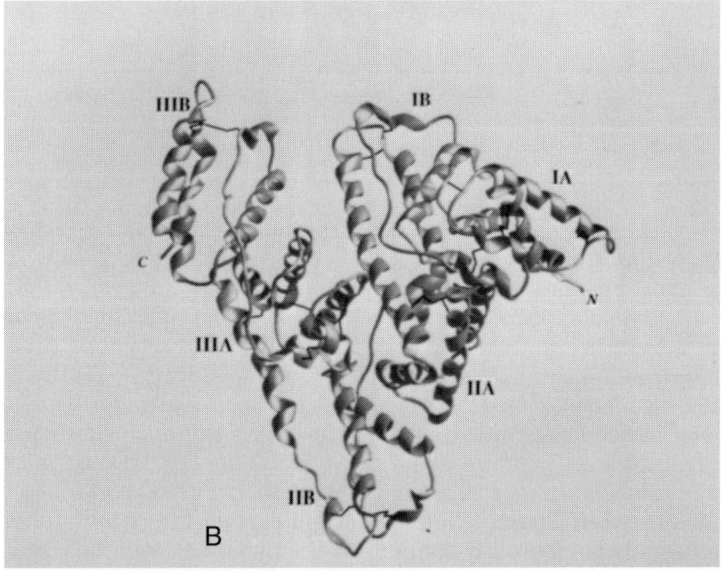

Figure 15–2. *A*, Diagrammatic representation of the proposed domains and subdomains of human albumin aligned on the basis of amino acid sequence. The three domains are enclosed, and all subdomains are indicated by the numbers *1* to *9*. The four binding sites for fatty acid (FA) are indicated by *1°*, *2°*, *3°*, and *4°*. The cysteine in domain 1 is a free sulfhydryl. The sites for binding Ca^{2+}, Ni^{2+}, tryptophan (TRP), aspirin, bilirubin, and the hormone T4 are indicated. The single-letter code is used to indicate amino acid sequence. *B*, Illustration of the molecular configuration of human serum albumin based on the interpretation of the 6.0-Å electron density. The high degree of primary and tertiary structural homology among domains I, II, and III provides a useful cross-check of the topology. The binding sites within subdomains IA and IIIA are represented by red spheres. (*A* from Bing DH. Plasma proteins: immunoglobulins. *In* Benz EJ Jr, Shattil SJ, Furie B, Cohen HJ [eds]: Hematology: Basic Principles and Practice. New York: Churchill Livingstone, 1991, p 1576. *B* from He XM, Carter DC. Atomic structure and chemistry of human serum albumin. Nature 1992; 358:6383.)

much greater osmotic effect in blood as a result of Gibbs-Donnan equilibrium effects. By this mechanism, albumin can markedly influence concentration of cations in plasma and have a greater effect on the overall osmotic pressure of plasma by directly modulating the movement of water between plasma and extravascular fluid.[12]

About 40% of the body's albumin is contained in the circulation, and the remainder is principally in the extravascular space associated with muscle, skin, and intestinal tissues. In addition to its osmotic functions, albumin serves an important role in transporting diverse substances, many of which are only sparingly soluble in water. Normal lipid metabolism requires albumin for the transport of fatty acids, cholesterol, phosphoglycerides, and lipoproteins. Albumin also binds bilirubin and transports it to the liver, where it is excreted in the bile. Other ligands in plasma bound by albumin include Ca^{2+}, steroid hormones, and amino acids such as tryptophan. Finally, albumin tightly binds to a broad spectrum of drugs.[4, 14] The principal therapeutic use of albumin is as a volume expander in the treatment of shock. Albumin has also been used in disorders associated with chronic protein loss and in cirrhosis associated with ascites and extreme hypoalbuminemia.[15, 16]

α_1-ANTITRYPSIN

α_1-Antitrypsin inhibits a number of serine proteases, including pancreatic and leukocyte elastase, trypsin, chymotrypsin, plasmin, and granulocyte proteases. It does so by forming stable equimolar complexes. The molecular weight of α_1-antitrypsin is 52 kD, and it contains 12.5% carbohydrate.[17] There are 30 or more genetic variants of α_1-antitrypsin, of which six occur in European populations with allele frequencies in excess of 1%.[18] Ten common variants are known and are designated PI (protease inhibitor) M1, M2, M3, S, Z, I, F, I, V, and W. Of clinical interest are the alleles *PI*Z*, *PI*Q0*, and *PI*S*, which are associated with markedly and moderately reduced serum concentrations of α_1-antitrypsin. Individuals doubly heterozygous or homozygous for these alleles have an increased risk of severe, early-onset chronic obstructive pulmonary disease (panlobular emphysema). Those homozygous for *PI*Z* or heterozygous for this allele and another moderately or severely deficient PI allele are susceptible to neonatal hepatitis, juvenile cirrhosis, and primary cancer of the liver. All subjects who have the *PI*Z* allele have characteristic inclusion bodies in their hepatocytes. These represent α_1-antitrypsin accumulated in the endoplasmic reticulum. There is normal synthesis of PI Z protein; there appears to be a problem in postsynthetic processing, and only about 10% of synthesized protein is released from the cell.[19] The structural differences between a number of PI variants involve single amino acid substitutions for Glu in PI M1. In PI M2 it is Asp,[20] in PI S it is Val,[21] and in PI Z it is Lys[22]; the substitutions are not all at the same Glu residue. PI Z has a second substitution at position 213 (Val, Ala).[23] The C-terminal 8- to 10-amino acid sequence of human α_1-antitrypsin is virtually identical to that of human and porcine antithrombin III, suggesting a common evolutionary origin for the genes of both protease inhibitors. The gene for α_1-antitrypsin is on chromosome 14 (see Table 15–2).

α_1-ACID GLYCOPROTEIN

α_1-Acid glycoprotein (orosomucoid) contains 37% carbohydrate and binds a number of basic drugs, including local anesthetics and propranolol. The gene for α_1-acid glycoprotein is on chromosome 9 (see Table 15–2). On electrophoresis near its isoelectric point or on isoelectric focusing, the protein exhibits marked microheterogeneity, largely ascribable to differences in sialic acid content. Treatment of whole serum with neuraminidase (to remove sialic acid from all serum proteins) followed by analysis with agarose gel electrophoresis at pH 8.6 and immunofixation with antiserum to α_1-acid glycoprotein[24] reveals a simple genetic polymorphism. Two alleles of nearly equal frequency are found in almost all populations studied.

HAPTOGLOBIN

Haptoglobin is an axially symmetrical molecule consisting of two β chains and two α chains.[25] The protein binds hemoglobin and thereby conserves iron released from red cell destruction. Each β chain of one molecule of haptoglobin binds one half-molecule of hemoglobin. The β chain has 245 amino acids and a molecular weight of 33,820 daltons, including about 6560 daltons for carbohydrate.[26] The α chain contains either 83 amino acids (molecular weight = 9189 daltons) or nearly twice this number, depending on genetic type. The β chain shows about 30% homology with serine proteases, suggesting its evolutionary origin from a primordial protease gene. The gene for haptoglobin is on chromosome 16 (see Table 15–2).

CERULOPLASMIN

The copper-containing blue protein ceruloplasmin has a molecular weight of approximately 160 kD. It is not a copper transport protein (that function is carried out by albumin), but it has amine oxidase activity and probably detoxifies superoxide and other reactive oxygen-containing species released during phagocytosis.

Ceruloplasmin concentration is markedly decreased in the serum of patients with Wilson's disease or with an inherited disorder called kinky hair disease. The latter is a rare autosomal disorder characterized by copper malabsorption and resulting copper deficiency, mental retardation, and microscopically kinky hair. The ceruloplasmin gene appears to have arisen by intragenic triplication. There is 50% identity between the complementary DNAs (cDNAs) for ceruloplasmin and coagulation factor VIII. Even more remarkably, the third homology unit of ceruloplasmin shows striking identity with the carboxy-terminal portion of the copper-containing protein lactase of *Neurospora crassa*.[27] The gene for ceruloplasmin is on chromosome 3 (see Table 15–2).

TRANSFERRIN

The protein responsible for iron transport in the blood is the β-globulin transferrin.[5] The molecule is a single chain with a molecular weight of 75 kD and two similar domains, each with an iron-binding site, suggesting evolution by gene duplication. Inherited deficiency of transferrin is rare but well documented. Affected patients are homozygous for null *TF* alleles and have severe, fatal iron-deficiency anemia. The gene for transferrin is on chromosome 3 (see Table 15–2).

IMMUNOGLOBULINS

The mammalian immune system responds to an almost unlimited array of antigens by producing antibodies, each of which reacts specifically with the molecule that induced its production. During the immune response, the structure of the inducing antigen is imprinted on the immune system through B cell clonal expansion; subsequent challenges with the same or structurally related molecule(s) cause a rapid rise in antibody levels to much greater concentrations than were achieved after the primary antigenic challenge. Thus, the hallmarks of the immune system include induction, specific protein interaction, and memory.[28]

Antibodies belong to the family of proteins called the immunoglobulins. The basic structure of every immunoglobulin (Ig) consists of a monomer that contains four polypeptide chains: two identical heavy (H) chains and two identical light (L) chains covalently linked by disulfide bonds (Fig. 15–3). A model of the monomeric form of Ig has been based on x-ray crystallographic data obtained on the IgG myeloma protein Dob.[29] The Ig monomer consists of a Y- or T-like structure. The size of the arms, called *fragment antigen binding* (Fab) of the Y or T, is 80 × 50 × 40 nm; the size of the base, called the *crystallizable fragment* (Fc), is approximately 70 × 45 × 40 nm.[30] The Ig molecule exhibits considerable flexibility; the angle between the Fabs has been observed by electron microscopy, low-angle x-ray scattering, transient electric birefringence, and resonance energy transfer studies to vary from

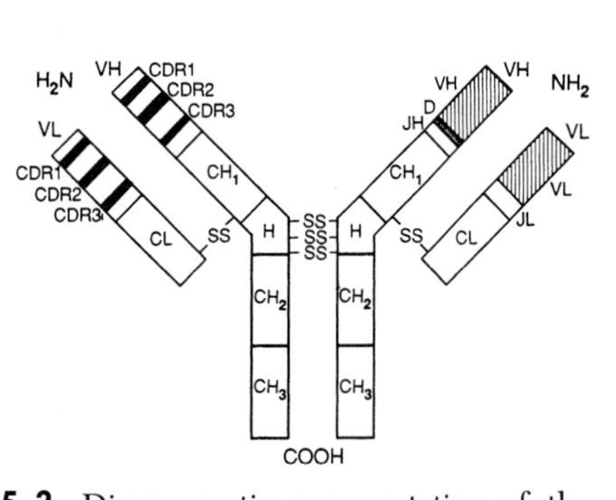

Figure 15–3. Diagrammatic representation of the structural features of an IgG molecule. H_2N indicates the amino-terminus and COOH indicates the C-terminus. The V_H, C_H, V_L, and C_L homology domains are shown as boxes, and the hinge region is denoted H. Only the disulfide linkages that join H and L chains are shown. *Left,* Approximate boundaries of the CDR regions in the V_L and V_H regions. *Right,* Sequences encoded by V_H, D, J_H, V_L, and J_L segments in the V_H and V_L regions.[30] (From Alt FW, Blackwell TK, Yancopoulos GD. Development of the primary antibody repertoire. Science 1987; 238:1079. Copyright by the American Association for the Advancement of Science.)

0 to 180 degrees. All antibodies have two identical combining sites for each antigen located at the ends of the Fab fragments.

The Fab and Fc represent functional domains in Ig. These were discovered by performing limited proteolytic digestion of the molecule. Both the H and L chains contribute amino acids that constitute the antigen-binding site in Fab. The Fab combines with but does not precipitate multivalent antigens. In contrast to native Ig, it is univalent and cannot form a lattice. A fragment called $F(ab')_2$ can be prepared; it is devoid of Fc but still precipitates antigen. This form of Ig consists of two Fab fragments disulfide bonded at the hinge region, the part of the Ig molecule that is responsible for the molecular flexibility exhibited by all immunoglobulins. Every immunoglobulin is a glycoprotein, with carbohydrate primarily attached to the H chain in the Fc region. Other major functions of Ig, such as binding to specific receptors on cells and the effector proteins, protein A of staphylococci and Clq, are associated with binding site(s) also found in Fc.

The chain structure of Ig does not explain antibody structural diversity or antibody binding to antigen. The discovery that there were variable and constant regions of amino acid sequence formed the basis for understanding both phenomena. Thus, in the L chain, the 100 or so amino acids in the amino-terminal half of the protein (V_L) vary among antibody molecules. In the second half (C_L) of all antibodies of a given isotype or isotype subclass, however, there is virtually complete correspondence in amino acid sequences (see Fig. 15–3). H chains exhibit the same pattern and can be divided likewise into V_H and C_H. Comparison of the amino acid sequence of many V_Ls has revealed that certain parts of the variable region exhibit excess variability and others have less variability. The former are called hypervariable or complementarity-determining regions (CDRs) and the latter framework regions (FRs). H chains exhibit the same pattern in their V_H regions. Amino acid sequence analysis of the C_H region has shown there are three homologous regions where the amino acid sequences show more similarity than could have occurred by chance. These are called C_H1, C_H2, and C_H3. The Fab region consists of the intact L chain and the Fd region of the H chain, which consists of V_H through C_H1 (see Fig. 15–3). The combining site for antigen is a trough or a cavity composed of parts of the hypervariable regions of both the H chain and the L chain. Thus, the variation in a relatively few amino acids in the hypervariable regions accounts for the specificity and contributes to the diversity of antibodies.[28, 30]

In addition to the amino acid sequence variations at the binding site responsible for antigen-binding activity, immunoglobulins can exhibit additional physical heterogeneity and thus impart to each Ig a unique biological effector function. Heterologous and autologous antisera raised against immunoglobulins have been used to classify three types of physical heterogeneity. The first kind is based on the antigenic heterogeneity exhibited by Ig when it is used as an immunogen in other species. This is called class or isotypic variation. In humans, five isotypes can be distinguished on the basis of unique antigenic (isotypic) determinants found on the H chain. These are designated by capital Roman letters: IgG, IgM, IgA, IgD, and IgE. The H chain of each class is designated by the small Greek letter corresponding to the Roman letter of the class and is encoded by a distinct gene or set of genes on chromosome 14 (see Table 15–2). Thus the H chain for IgG is γ, for IgM it is μ, for IgA it is α, for IgD it is δ, and for IgE it is ϵ. Some of the Ig classes are composed of polymers of the basic monomer and have an additional polypeptide, the 15-kD J chain. In humans, there are two antigenic varieties of the L chain, called kappa, κ, and lambda, λ, encoded on chromosomes 2 and 22, respectively (see Table 15–2). Each Ig has two identical L chains, κ or λ, which are shared by all classes of Ig. The monomeric form of any Ig is described by the structure of its H and L chains.

IgG is the most prevalent Ig isotype, constituting 75% of the total Ig in blood. It is present in normal adults at concentrations of 600 to 1500 mg/dL. IgG is designated $\gamma_2\kappa_2$ or $\gamma_2\lambda_2$. It is the only class of Ig that crosses the placenta. The isotype IgM is a pentamer consisting of five monomeric units disulfide linked at the C-terminus of the H chain; each monomer of IgM is 180 kD because of the presence of an additional, fourth C_H domain. The complete protein has a sedimentation coefficient of 19S, which corresponds to a molecular mass of 850 to 1000 kD. IgM is designated $(\mu_2\kappa_2)_5$ or $(\mu_2\lambda_2)_5$. IgM also contains a 15-kD protein called the J chain. In the current structural model of IgM, the J chain forms a disulfide-bonded clasp at the C-terminus of two H chains. The function of the J chain is not known.

The structures of the other isotypes of Ig are summarized as follows: The isotype IgA has a variable number of monomeric units and is designated $(\alpha_2\kappa_2)_n$ or $(\alpha_2\lambda_2)_n$, where n is 1 to 5. Serum IgA constitutes 20% of the total serum Ig, and 80% of this is monomeric. The other form of IgA is found in external secretions such as saliva, tracheobronchial secretions, colostrum, milk, and genitourinary secretions. Secretory IgA (IgA_{sec}) consists of four components: a dimer of two monomeric molecules, a 70-kD secretory component (derived from the poly-Ig receptor of secretory epithelium) that binds noncovalently to the IgA dimer, and a 15-kD J chain that is believed to form a disulfide-bonded clasp at the C-terminus of the H chains. The isotype IgD has a molecular weight of 180 kD. Its serum concentration is very low, approximately 3 mg/dL. IgD apparently functions as a membrane molecule, associated on mature but unstimulated B cells with IgM. IgE is the homocytotropic or reaginic Ig and mediates immediate hypersensitivity. It has a molecular weight of 180 kD and, like IgM, has four C_H domains. The Fc portion of IgE binds strongly to a receptor on mast cells, inducing cell degranulation. The overall properties of the immunoglobulins are summarized in Table 15–4.

Additionally, subclasses of the isotypes IgG, IgA, and IgM have been identified. The structural basis for this heterogeneity is antigenic variation (e.g., amino acid sequence differences) in the Fc portion of the H chain of a given class. The subclasses of IgG are the best characterized. These are called IgG1, IgG2, IgG3, and IgG4. Each has a slightly different structure, the most notable difference being the interchain disulfide bonding

Table 15–4. Human Immunoglobulin Properties and Functions

Property/Function	IgG1	IgG2	IgG3	IgG4	IgM	IgA1	IgA2	IgA_{SEC}	IgD	IgE
H chain	$\gamma1$	$\gamma2$	$\gamma3$	$\gamma4$	μ	$\alpha1$	$\alpha2$	$\alpha1, \alpha2$	δ	ϵ
Molecular weight (kD)	146	146	170	146	970	160	160	385	184	189
Molecular weight of H chain (kD)	51	51	60	51	65	56	52	52–56	70	73
Number of H chain domains	4	4	4	4	5	4	4	4	5	5
Carbohydrate (%)	2–3	2–3	2–3	2–3	12	7–11	7–11	7–11	9–14	12
Serum concentration (mg/dL)	90	30	10	0.5	1.5	30	0.5	0.5	0.3	0.0005
Classical complement fixation	+ +	+	+ + +	–	+ + +	–	–	–	–	–
Alternative pathway complement activity	–	–	–	–	–	±	±	–	–	–
Placental transfer	+	+	+	+	±	–	–	–	–	–
Binding to mononuclear cells	+	–	+	–	–	–	–	–	–	–
Binding to mast cells and to basophils	–	–	–	–	–	–	–	–	–	+ + +
Reaction with protein A from *Staphylococcus aureus*	+	+	–	+	–	–	–	–	–	–
Half-life (days)	21	20	7	21	10	6	6	ND	3	2
Distribution (% intravascular)	45	45	45	45	80	42	42	ND	75	50
Fractional catabolic rate (% intravascular pool catabolized/day)	7	7	17	7	9	25	25	ND	37	71
Synthetic rate (mg/kg/day)	33	33	33	33	3.3	24	24	ND	0.4	0.002

Data from several sources, particularly reference 28.
ND, Not determined.

pattern. IgG1 constitutes 70% of the total IgG, with that of IgG2 20%, IgG3 8%, and IgG4 2%. The subclasses of IgG exhibit different catabolic rates, and IgG2 crosses the placenta slightly more slowly than the other three. The other known subclasses of Ig isotypes are associated with IgM (IgM1 and IgM2) and IgA (IgA1 and IgA2). The properties and functions of these subclasses are less well known.

COMPLEMENT COMPONENTS C3 AND C4

C3 is a molecule of 190 kD. It is synthesized as a single polypeptide chain that is processed intracellularly by proteolysis to a disulfide-linked α chain (115 kD) and a smaller β chain (75 kD). The gene for C3 is encoded on chromosome 19 (see Table 15–2). Component C4, a molecule of 200 kD, is synthesized as a single polypeptide chain and is split post-translationally by a plasmin-like enzyme into three disulfide-linked chains (α, β, and γ) of 93, 75, and 32 kD, respectively.[31, 32] The gene for C4 is encoded on chromosome 6 (see Table 15–2). The evidence that C3 and C4 arose by gene duplication is summarized as follows: (1) the amino termini of each show considerable amino acid sequence homology; (2) there is sequence homology around a thioester bond involved in binding each protein to cell substrates; (3) both are synthesized as single polypeptide chains that are post-translationally processed into two or three disulfide-linked chains; (4) they are functional analogues—both C3 and C4 bind to the target surface and assemble the complement enzymes C3 and C5 convertase of the two complement pathways by combination with the analogous complement serine proteases, factor B (C3) and C2 (C4).

Electron microscopy has revealed that the native and activated C3 molecules are similar in shape and size. Both have an irregular and multidomain structure, the most conspicuous features being a large head-like region and a smaller tail-like structure. Electron microscopy of the C4 molecule shows it to be an irregular globular protein indistinguishable from C3.[33]

C-REACTIVE PROTEIN

C-reactive protein (CRP) is so named because it binds to phosphoryl choline in the C carbohydrate of *Streptococcus pneumoniae* in the presence of Ca^{2+}. CRP also binds to C1q, thereby activating the classical complement pathway. CRP is a pentraxin, or protein with a discoid organization of five noncovalently bound monomeric subunits. Native CRP is a single disc.[34] Nucleotide and derived amino acid sequences obtained from human CRP cDNA clones indicate that their mature product comprises 206 amino acids.[35] The analysis of the cDNA and genomic clones for a large number of mammalian pentraxins has established that they are highly conserved with respect to protein sequence and gene structure. The gene encoding CRP has been mapped to chromosome 1 (see Table 15–2).

Table 15–5. Normal Values for Serum Concentration of 14 Human Serum Proteins*

Serum Protein	Mean (mg/dL)	Range (mg/dL)
Albumin	4000	3200–5500
α_1-Antitrypsin	240	160–360
α_1-Acid glycoprotein (orosomucoid)	100	40–150
C1 inhibitor	18	11–26
Ceruloplasmin	32	18–45
α_1-Macroglobulin		
Pediatric	550	200–700†
Adult, female	300	120–540†
Adult, male	240	90–400†
Haptoglobin	108	25–180‡
Transferrin	280	200–350
Low-density lipoprotein	105	40–140§
C3	165	90–220‖
C4	30	10–40
IgA	240	60–360¶
IgM	105	25–170¶
IgG	1100	700–1500**

From Ritchie RF. Automated immunoprecipitation analysis of serum proteins. *In* Putnam FW (ed): The Plasma Proteins, 2nd ed, vol 2. New York: Academic Press, 1975.

*Values derived from a large northern New England white population.

†Varies markedly during and about the time of puberty.

‡Varies from 0 to normal adult levels during first 2 weeks of life.

§Varies from 10% of normal to normal adult levels during first year of life.

‖Varies from 50% of normal to normal adult levels during the first month of life.

¶Varies from 0 to normal adult levels during first year of life.

**Varies from adult normal levels at birth to 25% of normal at about 3 months, returning to adult normal during next several years.

α_2-MACROGLOBULIN

α_2-Macroglobulin is a large glycoprotein of 725 kD containing 8% to 10% carbohydrate that includes sialic acid and 4 to 8 atoms of zinc per molecule. There are four identical polypeptide chains covalently linked in pairs by S-S bonds, and these associate noncovalently to form an "H-shaped" tetramer. α_2-Macroglobulin inhibits metalloproteases, including both leukocyte and nonleukocyte collagenases, proteoglycanase, and gelatinase. Latent forms of enzymes do not bind to this inhibitor, because the formation of the α_2-macroglobulin/protease complex is initiated by specific limited proteolysis of α_2-macroglobulin in a region located near the middle of each of the four subunits. Following the cleavage in one of these regions, the irreversible entrapment of the protease ensues, and one molecule of α_2-macroglobulin is able to bind one to two molecules of protease. A fraction of the protease becomes covalently linked to the α_2-macroglobulin, and a protease once bound to the inhibitor cannot be displaced by another protease. The conformation of the tetramer changes on interaction with proteases. Additionally, the proteases become trapped within the molecule and can no longer digest large substrates, although low-molecular-weight substrates can still be hydrolyzed by the entrapped enzyme.[36] α_2-Macroglobulin is encoded on chromosome 12 (see Table 15–2).

Table 15–6. Effects of Selected Hormones and Clinical Conditions on Levels of Selected Plasma Proteins*

Hormone or Condition	Prealbumin (Transthyretin)	Albumin	α_1-Acid Glycoprotein	α_1-Antitrypsin	Ceruloplasmin	Haptoglobin	Transferrin	C3	C4	Complement Component Factor B	C-Reactive Protein
Inflammation or trauma	↓	↓	↑	↑	↑	↑	↓	↑	↑	↑	↑
Androgens	N	N	↑	↑	↑	↑	↑	↑	↑		N
Estrogens (pregnancy, contraceptive pills)	(↓)	(↓)	(↓)	↑	↑	↓	↑	N	N	N	N
Adrenal glucocorticoids (prednisone, etc.)	↑	N	↑	N	↑	↑	N	(↑)	(↑)		
Chronic hepatocellular disease	↓	↓	(↓)	↑	N	↓	↓	N	(↓)		N
Biliary obstruction						↑		↑			
Complement consumption†									↓		
Classical pathway								↓	↓	N	N
Alternative pathway								↓	(↓)	↓	(↓)
Malnutrition	↓	↓	(↓)	(↓)	(↓)	(↓)	↓	(↓)	(↓)		N
Iron deficiency	N	N	N	N	N	N	↑	N	N	N	N
In vivo hemolysis	N	N	N	N	N	↓	N	N‡	N‡	N‡	N
Nephrotic syndrome	↓	↓	↓	↓	(↓)	↑ ↓	↓	N	↓	↓	N
Increased immunoglobulins (polyclonal or monoclonal)	N‡	↓	N‡	N‡	N‡	N‡	↓	N‡	N‡	N‡	N‡
Hypomorphic genetic variants	Rare	Rare	?	Yes	No	Yes§	Rare	Rare	Yes	Yes	No

From Johnson AM. Plasma protein assays in clinical diagnosis and management. *In* Ritzmann SE, Daniels JC (eds): Beckman Bulletin 6215. Boston: Little, Brown, 1975, p 173.

*Symbols: ↑, usually increased; ↑ ↓, variable; ↓, usually decreased; (↑), may be increased; N, usually normal; (↓), may be decreased; ?, unknown. All proteins except immunoglobulins may be low in end-stage liver disease or in severe malnutrition.

†Complement may be consumed in autoimmune hemolytic anemia, transfusion reactions, and paroxysmal nocturnal hemoglobinuria.

‡Normal unless accompanied by acute phase response, liver disease, hemolysis, glomerulopathy, or complement consumption.

§Secondarily low in Wilson's disease and kinky-hair syndrome.

DIAGNOSTIC USE OF PLASMA PROTEINS

The clinician is interested in the deviations of plasma proteins from their normal concentration ranges, because such changes can be used to assist differential diagnosis, detect genetic deficiencies, track disease activity, and monitor therapy. Changes in the concentration of plasma proteins are generally due to four factors: rate of synthesis, rate of catabolism, dilutional effects, and distribution. Plasma proteins for which changes are associated with clinical diagnosis include albumin, α_1-acid glycoprotein (orosomucoid), α_1-antitrypsin (α_1 proteinase inhibitor), α_2-macroglobulin, ceruloplasmin, haptoglobin, transferrin, complement C3, complement C4, CRP, and the immunoglobulins IgG, IgM, and IgA.[37] The normal concentrations and ranges of these proteins are presented in Table 15–5.[7] The effects of hormones and clinical disorders on levels of these plasma proteins are summarized in Table 15–6.[8] In most clinical situations, with the exception of multiple myeloma and specific genetic deficiencies, variations occur in more than one plasma protein component, and the temporal aspects of the change can be different for each protein. Thus, in an inflammatory response, the increase in CRP occurs within 6 to 12 hours; haptoglobin, α_1-antitrypsin, α_1-acid glycoprotein, C4, and fibrinogen peak at about 4 days; but the increase in C3 and ceruloplasmin does not appear until 3 to 5 days after the initial insult. Estrogens and adrenal glucocorticoids lead to different patterns of plasma protein changes, as do liver disease, kidney disease, malnutrition, and transfusion reactions (see Table 15–6).

REFERENCES

1. Schwick HG, Haupt H. Human plasma proteins of unknown function. *In* Putnam FW (ed): The Plasma Proteins, 2nd ed, vol 4. New York: Academic Press, 1984.
2. Shows TB, Alper CA, Bootsma D, et al. International system for human gene nomenclature. Cytogenet Cell Genet 1979; 25:96.
3. Putnam FW. Trace components of plasma: an overview. *In* Jamieson GA, Greenwall TA (eds): Trace Components of Plasma. New York: Alan R. Liss, 1976.
4. Haupt H, Baudwen S. Kristallisierte human Plasma Proteine. *In* Seilar FR, Schwick HG (eds): Advances in Diagnosis and Therapy. Marburg: Medizinische Yerlagsgesellschaft, 1988; 82:104.
5. Putnam FW. Progress in plasma proteins. *In* Putnam FW (ed): The Plasma Proteins, 2nd ed, vol 4. New York: Academic Press, 1984.
6. Schwick HV, Haupt H. Purified plasma proteins of unknown function. *In* Bing DH, Rosenbaum RA (eds): Plasma and Cellular Modulatory Proteins. Boston: Center for Blood Research, 1981.
7. Ritchie RF. Automated immunoprecipitation analysis of serum proteins. *In* Putnam FW (ed): The Plasma Proteins, 2nd ed, vol 2. New York: Academic Press, 1975.
8. Johnson AM. Plasma protein assays in clinical diagnosis and management. *In* Ritzmann SE, Daniels JC (eds): Beckman Bulletin 6215. Boston: Little, Brown, 1975.
9. Brown JR, Scheckley P, Behrans PQ. Albumin: sequence evolution and structural models. *In* Bing DH (ed): The Chemistry and Physiology of the Human Plasma Proteins. New York: Pergamon Press, 1979.
10. Tullis JM. Albumin 2: guidelines for clinical use. JAMA 1977; 237:460.
11. Jarnum S, Jensen KB. Distribution and degradation of albumin. *In* Yap SH, Majoor CLH, Van Tongeren JHM (eds): Clinical Aspects of Albumin. Boston: Martinus Nijhoff Medical Division, 1978.
12. Peters T Jr. Serum albumin. Adv Protein Chem 1988; 37:161.
13. Carter DC, He X-M, Munson SH, et al. Three dimensional structure of human albumin. Science 1989; 244:1195.
14. Ariens EJ, Simonis AM. Changes in plasma albumin in concentration and drug action. *In* Yap SW, Majoor CLH, Van Tongeren JWM (eds): Clinical Aspects of Albumin. Boston: Martinus N. Hoff Medical Division, 1978.
15. Goris RJA. Use and abuse of albumin and plasma protein infusion in acute clinical situations. *In* Yap SW, Majoor CLH, Van Tongeren JWM (eds): Clinical Aspects of Albumin. Boston: Martinus N. Hoff Medical Division, 1978.
16. Alexander MR, Alexander B, Mustion AL, et al. Therapeutic use of albumin. JAMA 1981; 247:831.
17. Laurell C-B. Aspects of biochemistry and pathophysiology of α_1-antitrypsin. *In* Bing DH (ed): The Chemistry and Physiology of the Human Plasma Proteins. New York: Pergamon, 1979.
18. Cox DW, Johnson AM, Fagerhol MK. Report of nomenclature meeting for α_1-antitrypsin: INSERM, Rouen/Bois Guillaume—1978. Hum Genet 1980; 52:429.
19. Carlson JA, Rogers BB, Sifers RN, et al. Accumulation of PiZ α_1-antitrypsin causes liver damage in transgenic mice. J Clin Invest 1989; 83:1183.
20. Yoshida A, Taylor JC, Van den Brock WGM. Structural difference between the normal PiM_1 and the common PiM_2 variant of human α_1-antitrypsin. Am J Hum Genet 1979; 31:564.
21. Owen MC, Carrell RW. Alpha$_1$-antitrypsin: molecular abnormality of S variant. BMJ 1976; 1:130.
22. Jeppsson J-O. Amino acid substitution-Glu Lys in α1-antitrypsin PiZ. FEBS Lett 1976; 65:195.
23. Nukiwa T, Satoh K, Brantly ML, et al. Identification of a second mutation in the protein-coding sequence of the Z type α1-antitrypsin gene. J Biol Chem 1986; 261:15989.
24. Johnson AM, Schmid K, Alper CA. Inheritance of human α_1-acid glycoprotein (orosomucoid) variants. J Clin Invest 1969; 48:2293.
25. Smithies O, Connell GE, Dixon GH. Gene action in the human haptoglobins: I: dissociation into constituent polypeptide chains. J Mol Biol 1966; 21:213.
26. Kurosky A, Barnett DR, Lee T-H, et al. Covalent structure of human haptoglobin: a serine protease homolog. Proc Natl Acad Sci U S A 1980; 77:3388.
27. Germann UA, Lerch K. Isolation and partial nucleotide sequence of the lactase gene from *Neurospora crassa*: amino acid sequence homology of the protein to human ceruloplasmin. Proc Natl Acad Sci U S A 1986; 83:8854.
28. Golub ES. Immunology: A Synthesis. Sunderland: Sinauer Associates, 1987.
29. Getzoff ED, Tamer JA, Lerner RA, et al. The chemistry and mechanism of antibody binding to protein antigens. Adv Immunol 1988; 43:1.
30. Alt FW, Blackwell TK, Yancopoulos GD. Development of the primary antibody repertoire. Science 1987; 238:1079.
31. Hughes-Jones NC. The classical pathway. *In* Ross GD (ed): Immunobiology of Complement System. New York: Academic Press, 1986.
32. Law SKA, Reid KBM. Complement. Oxford: IRL Press, 1988.
33. Smith CA, Vogel C-W, Müller-Eberhard HJ. MHC class III products: an electron microscopic study of the C3 convertases of human complement. J Exp Med 1984; 159:324.
34. Osmand AP, Friedenson B, Gewurz H, et al. Characterization of C-reactive protein and the complement subcomponent C1t as homologous proteins displaying cyclic pentameric symmetry (pentraxins). Proc Natl Acad Sci U S A 1977; 74:739.
35. Woo P, Kornberg JR, Whitehead AS. Characterization of genomic and complementary DNA sequence of human C-reactive protein, and comparison with the complementary DNA sequence of serum amyloid P component. J Biol Chem 1985; 260:13384.
36. Camston TF. *In* Barrett AJ (ed): Proteinase in Mammalian Cells and Tissues, 2nd ed. Amsterdam: North Holland Publishing Company, 1985.
37. Bing DH. Plasma proteins: immunoglobulins. *In* Benz EJ Jr, Shattil SJ, Furie B, Cohen HJ (eds): Hematology: Basic Principles and Practice. New York: Churchill Livingstone, 1991.

CHAPTER 16

Hemostasis

Barbara M. Alving

Clot formation at the site of vessel injury is a dynamic event that involves localized adherence and activation of platelets and simultaneous activation of the coagulation cascade, resulting in thrombin generation, followed by fibrin deposition. The complex interaction between platelets and coagulation factors rapidly produces a localized clot that undergoes retraction to ensure stability. For the sake of simplicity in this chapter, the role of platelets in the hemostatic process is described first, and then the pathways by which newly exposed tissue factor generates thrombin are discussed. The final section is a discussion of the newer and very potent agents that are used clinically to block platelet function and thrombin activity.

ROLE OF PLATELETS IN HEMOSTASIS

Platelet function in hemostasis can be arbitrarily divided into three phases: adherence, activation, and aggregation (Fig. 16–1). *Adherence* of platelets to exposed collagen is modulated by the shear stress of the vessel. Under conditions of low shear, which occur in arteries, platelets adhere to collagen through their GPIa/IIa receptors and to collagen-associated von Willebrand factor (vWF)[1] through their GPIb/IX/V receptors.[2] In smaller arterial vessels with higher shear stresses, the binding of vWF to GPIb/IX/V activates signaling pathways within the platelet which results in conformational changes in the GPIIb/IIIa that provide binding sites for vWF.[3–6] Additional matrix proteins also bind to other specific platelet receptors, thus ensuring redundancy in adherence.[7]

During *activation* by agonists such as thrombin, platelets undergo secretion of granular contents, changes in shape, and activation of the GPIIb/IIIa receptors. In addition, the platelet membrane is altered by rearrangement of the phosphatidylserine from the inner surface of the membrane to the outer surface; phosphatidyl serine binds specific coagulation factors, thereby accelerating the rate of thrombin formation.[8] The interaction of agonists with specific membrane receptors induces the generation of second messengers, which are involved in altering cytoskeletal proteins, thereby transforming platelets from disks to spheres with extended pseudopods. The second messenger system is also involved in the release of the contents of the dense and alpha granules.[9] Release is an energy-dependent process and is mediated

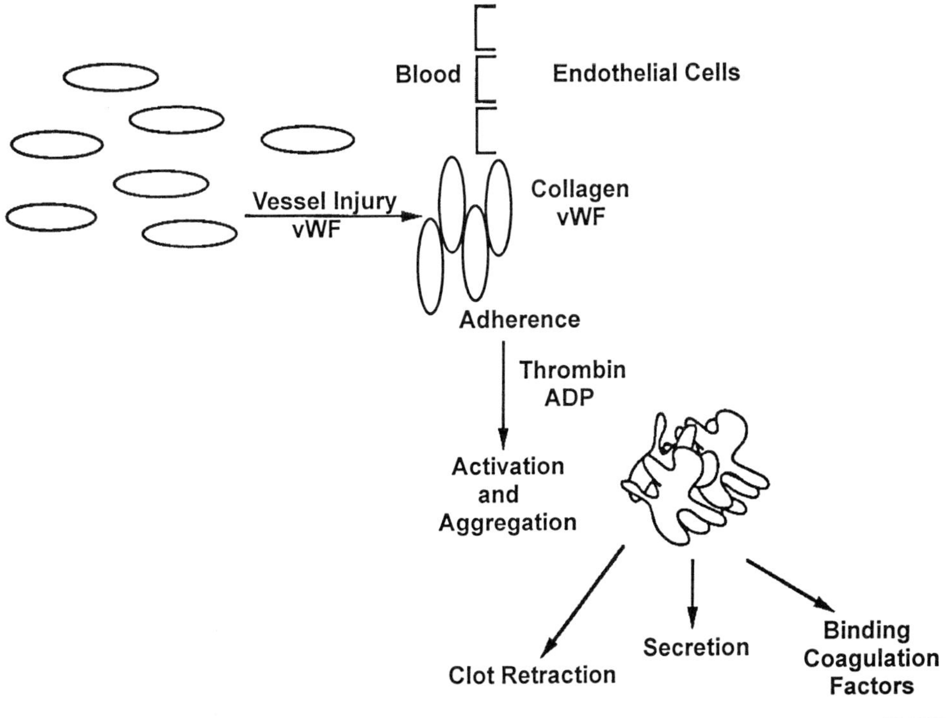

Figure 16–1. The major phases of platelet activation. When vascular injury occurs under conditions of high shear, circulating von Willebrand factor (vWF) binds to the exposed subendothelial collagen. Platelets adhere to the site of injury by binding to the extravascular vWF through their GPIb/IX/V receptors. Activation and aggregation are initiated by agonists such as adenosine diphosphate (ADP), collagen, and thrombin. Activated platelets secrete granular contents, express negatively charged phospholipids on their outer membrane for binding of procoagulant complexes, and promote clot retraction through the interaction of fibrinogen with the GPIIb/IIIa receptor.

by several mechanisms of signal transduction, including calcium and kinases such as protein kinase C and phosphatidylinositol kinase. The dense granules contain calcium, serotonin, and adenosine diphosphate (ADP), which promote continued aggregation. The secreted alpha granule contents include platelet factor 4, β-thromboglobulin, platelet-derived growth factor, thrombospondin, factor V, and plasma proteins such as fibrinogen and immunoglobulin G (IgG).[10]

Strong agonists, which are thrombin, prostaglandin endoperoxides, thromboxane A_2, collagen, platelet-activating factor, and vasopressin, do not require secretion of additional platelet contents to induce aggregation. Weak agonists such as ADP, serotonin, and epinephrine require release of granular contents in order to induce a full response. ADP-induced activation and aggregation involves the synthesis of thromboxane A_2 from arachidonic acid by cyclooxygenase; this process can be blocked by aspirin, which is a cyclooxygenase inhibitor.[11]

Aggregation occurs when fibrinogen, a dimeric molecule, forms a bond between adjacent platelets through interaction with the activated form of GPIIb/IIIa, which is composed of two glycoproteins with molecular weights of 136 kDa and 95 kDa. Fibrinogen binding occurs only after the complex has undergone a conformational change induced by platelet activation.[10] GPIIb/IIIa is a transmembrane complex associated on the inner surface of the platelet with actin, the major component of the platelet cytoskeleton; the actin–GPIIb/IIIa association is essential for clot retraction.[11]

INITIATION AND PROPAGATION OF THE CLOTTING CASCADE

The clotting cascade is activated when small amounts of circulating factor VIIa bind to tissue factor that is exposed on the subendothelium[12] or on monocytes and endothelial cells that have been exposed to thrombin or endotoxin.[13] The tissue factor/factor VIIa (TF/factor VIIa) complex converts small amounts of factor X to factor Xa, which in turn activates additional factor VII (Fig. 16–2).[14] TF/factor VIIa then activates additional factor X directly or through activation of factor IX.[15] TF/factor VIIa is regulated by tissue factor pathway inhibitor (TFPI).[16,17] Before TFPI can inhibit the TF/factor VIIa, it first binds to factor Xa (Fig. 16–3), thereby inhibiting factor Xa activity.[18] The TFPI/factor Xa complex then binds to TF/factor VIIa and blocks its procoagulant activity.

After the TF/factor VIIa pathway is inhibited, the ongoing activation of coagulation factors in the "intrinsic" system becomes dominant. Thrombin that has been initially generated activates factor XI; thrombin and factor Xa can each activate factor VIII and factor V by limited proteolysis, thereby greatly enhancing their binding to phospholipid membranes.[19] Factor VIIIa then combines

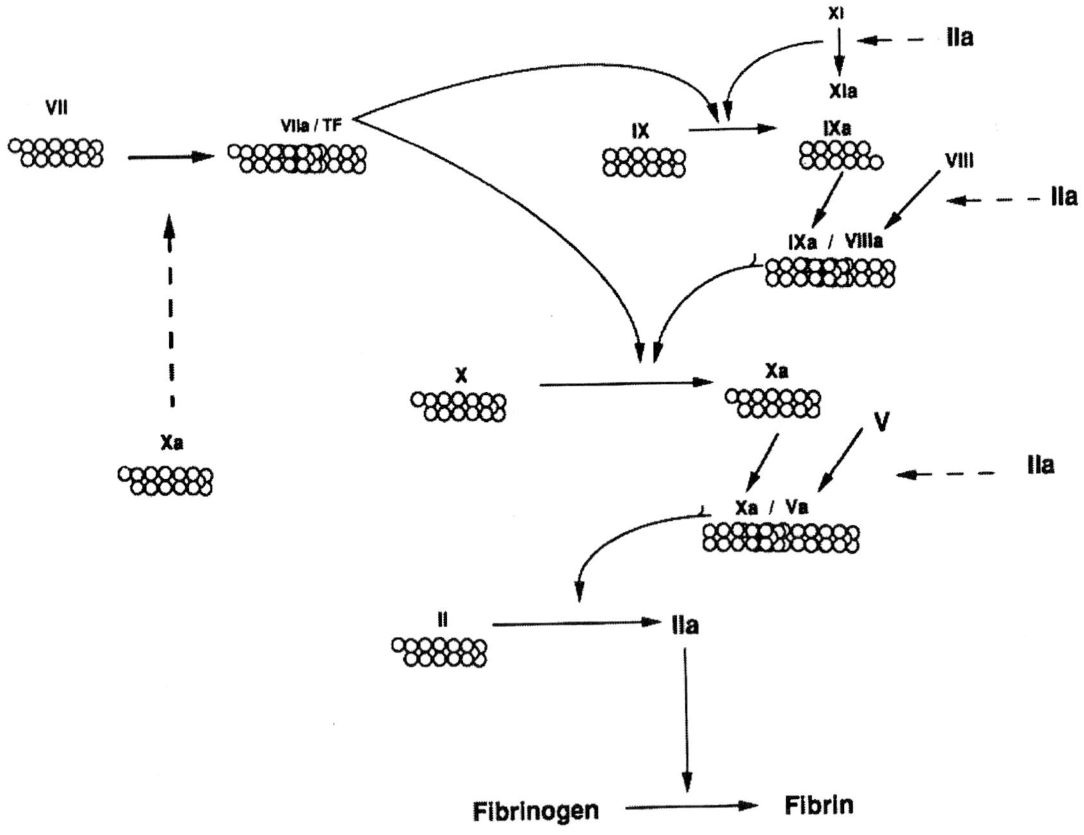

Figure 16–2. Proposed scheme of coagulation pathway under in vivo conditions. Coagulation is initiated by the tissue factor/factor VIIa complex (TF/factor VIIa), which can activate factor X directly or through activation of factor IX. Thrombin can reciprocally activate factors XI, V, and VIII. Factor Xa can promote activation of factor VII.

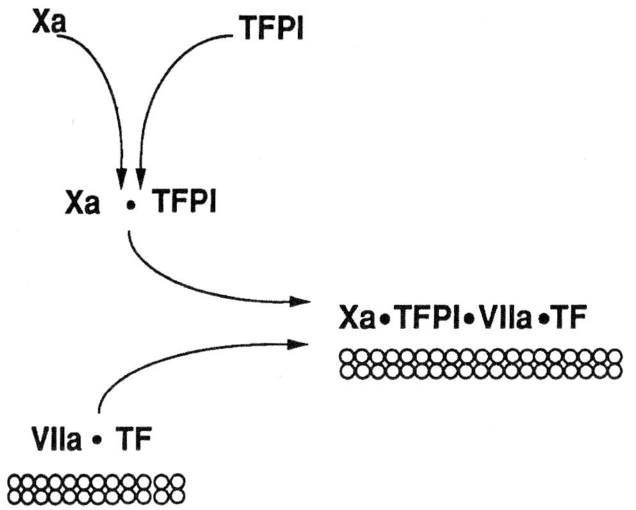

Figure 16–3. Inhibition of the tissue factor (TF) complex by factor Xa. Tissue factor pathway inhibitor (TFPI) first combines with factor Xa. The TFPI/factor Xa complex then binds on a phospholipid surface to inhibit TF/factor VIIa.

with factor IXa to activate factor X, and factor Va combines with factor Xa to activate prothrombin (see Fig. 16–2). Once bound to the platelet, factor Va acts as a specific receptor for factor Xa.[20]

The localization of factor IXa/factor VIIIa and factor Xa/factor Va complexes on platelet membranes increases their concentration at the injury site and allows substrates and intermediates to shuttle easily between neighboring complexes, thereby further amplifying reaction rates. In addition, binding to the lipid membrane increases the affinity of the proteinase-cofactor interaction (see Fig. 16–2).[21] The factor Xa/factor Va complex binds to prothrombin, which associates with the platelet membrane because of a calcium-dependent conformational change.[22]

The presence of these cofactors in their respective complexes is essential for maximal enzyme activity. In the presence of calcium alone, membrane-bound factor IXa can slowly activate factor X, but the factor IXa/factor VIIIa complex increases the reaction rate by more than 100,000-fold.[23] Similarly, prothrombin is converted to thrombin slowly by factor Xa; the conversion is accelerated 300,000-fold in the presence of factor Xa/factor Va and phospholipids.[24] Thrombin converts fibrinogen to fibrin and activates factor XIII, which catalyzes crosslinking of the fibrin clot. Included in the crosslinking is α_2-antiplasmin, which is the specific inactivator of plasmin.[25] The relative resistance of the clot to degradation by plasmin is a function of the α_2-antiplasmin in the crosslinked clot.[26]

VITAMIN K–DEPENDENT SERINE PROTEINASES, COFACTOR PROTEINS, AND FIBRINOGEN

The cofactors V and VIII are synthesized as high-molecular-weight precursors that exhibit significant sequence homology.[27] They are primarily produced by the liver and circulate in the plasma either uncomplexed (factor V) or in a noncovalent complex with vWF, which stabilizes the molecule (factor VIII). Factor V is also synthesized by megakaryocytes and stored in the alpha granules of platelets.[28, 29]

The vitamin K–dependent factors II, VII, IX, and X, which are synthesized by the liver, share sequence homology and structural features (Fig. 16–4).[30] These factors circulate as zymogens that undergo activation on a phospholipid surface by limited proteolysis. The carboxy-terminal portion of the factors contains the active serine site. Each factor has 9 to 12 gammacarboxyglutamic acid residues, known as Gla domains, at the amino terminus. The Gla domains are essential for the calcium-dependent binding of the factors to acidic phospholipids. Vitamin K is an essential cofactor in the post-translational gamma-carboxylation of these proteins.[30] The inhibition of this carboxylation reaction by warfarin or dietary vitamin K deficiency results in factors that are unable to bind to phospholipids and therefore lack procoagulant activity.[31] Prothrombin is unique among the vitamin K–dependent factors in that the active enzyme thrombin does not contain the Gla domain and therefore does not remain bound to the surface.

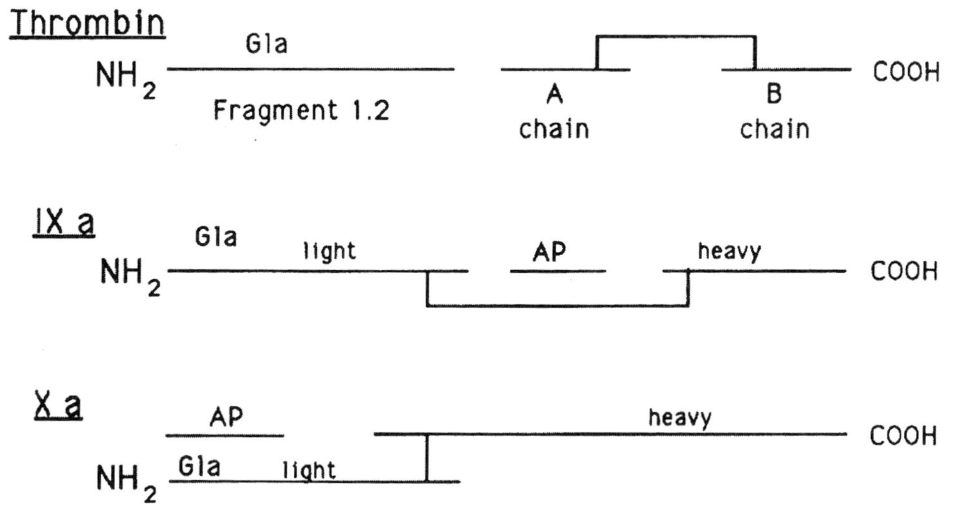

Figure 16–4. Examples of vitamin K–dependent enzymes. Because the activation peptide (AP) of prothrombin (which is fragment 1.2) and the AP of factors IXa and Xa can be measured in the circulation, they serve as sensitive markers of ongoing coagulation. Prothrombin is the only vitamin K–dependent factor that does not remain bound to the surface through its Gla domain after conversion to the active enzyme. (Gla domain is released as part of fragment 1.2.)

The conversion of prothrombin to thrombin requires cleavage of two peptide bonds, resulting in the formation of thrombin and fragment 1.2 (see Fig. 16–4). The fragment 1.2, which has a half-life of minutes, has been used as a marker of hemostatic activation.[32] Thrombin is one of the primary enzymes linking the coagulation system with the inflammatory response and tissue repair mechanisms. Thrombin stimulates secretion of prostacyclin,[33] which is an inhibitor of platelet activation and increases the synthesis and release of endothelial plasminogen activator inhibitor–1, the primary inhibitor of tissue-type plasminogen activator (t-PA).[34] It also promotes the release of platelet-derived growth factor from the endothelium.[35] Thrombin can stimulate smooth muscle contraction and act as a potent chemotaxin for monocytes and macrophages.[36]

Fibrinogen is a glycoprotein (340 kDa) composed of three pairs of polypeptide chains (Aα, Bβ, and γ) that are linked by disulfide bonds.[25, 37] It is generally depicted as a trinodular structure (Fig. 16–5) with the N-terminal portions of the polypeptide chains in the central or E domain. Fibrin monomer is formed when thrombin cleaves fibrinopeptides A and B from the N-terminal portions of the A and B chains in the E domain. Polymerization is initiated by the overlap of two fibrin monomers that are in a half-staggered formation due to the charge distribution of the E and D domains. This can be lengthened and then stabilized by the factor XIIIa, which crosslinks the protofibrils through catalyzing the formation of γ-glutamyl-ε-lysine bridges between adjacent fibrin molecules.

THE REGULATION OF HEMOSTASIS

Hemostasis is regulated by TFPI, thrombomodulin, antithrombin III (AT-III), as well as protein C and protein S. TFPI, a 40 kDa protein which has been described above as the inhibitor of the TF/factor VIIa complex, is associated with plasma lipoproteins. An even larger quantity of TFPI appears to be bound to the endothelial surface and can be released in the presence of heparin.[38] Thrombomodulin is an integral membrane protein (molecular weight 75 kDa) located on the luminal surface of endothelial cells and lymphatics in all organs except the brain.[39, 40] The amount of thrombomodulin expressed on the endothelial surface is decreased in the presence of agents such as tumor necrosis factor,[41] endotoxin, and interleukin-1.[42, 43] Thrombin that is bound to thrombomodulin does not clot fibrinogen, activate platelets, or activate factors V, VIII, and XIII.[44–46] Instead, thrombin becomes a highly efficient activator of protein C, which can then inhibit factors Va and VIIIa in the presence of the cofactor protein S.[47]

Protein C has significant homology to the vitamin K–dependent procoagulant factors and circulates as a two-chain zymogen. Activation by thrombin results in the cleavage of a 12–amino acid peptide from the amino-terminus of its heavy chain.[48] Activated protein C combines with its cofactor, protein S, to form an anticoagulant enzyme complex on phospholipid membranes (Fig. 16–6). Protein S is also a vitamin K–dependent protein, but it has no enzymatic activity and does not require proteolytic processing. Approximately 60% of protein S in the circulation is in an inactive form complexed to C4b-binding protein. The remaining 40%, which circulates as free protein S, is responsible for the cofactor activity.[49] Both activated protein C and protein S bind to anionic phospholipids through their respective Gla domains. Once assembled on the membrane surface, the protein C/protein S complex can inactivate factors Va and VIIIa by limited proteolysis.[50]

AT-III, a 58-kDa glycoprotein, is the primary inhibitor of thrombin and factor Xa.[51] It also inhibits factors XIIa, XIa, and IXa, but the physiological importance of its effect on these proteinases appears to be minor. A critical arginyl residue near the C-terminal end of AT-III interacts with the active site serine of thrombin or factor Xa to form a covalent bond. These reactions proceed slowly in the absence of heparin or related sulfate polysaccharides known as glycosaminoglycans. With heparin acting as a cofactor, the reaction rate increases by more than 1000-fold.[52] When AT-III interacts with heparin, it undergoes a conformational change that increases its affinity for factor Xa or thrombin. Once AT-III has formed a covalent complex with the serine proteinase, heparin

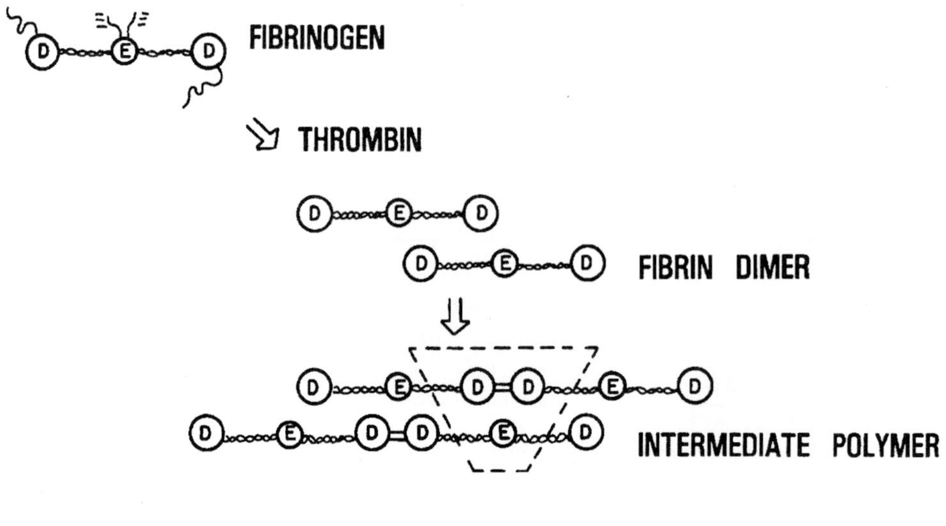

Figure 16–5. Fibrinogen is a trinodular structure with a central E domain that contains the N-terminal ends and two D domains. Thrombin initially cleaves fibrinopeptides A and B from the E domain, after which polymerization occurs, followed by crosslinking between the D domains catalyzed by factor XIIIa.

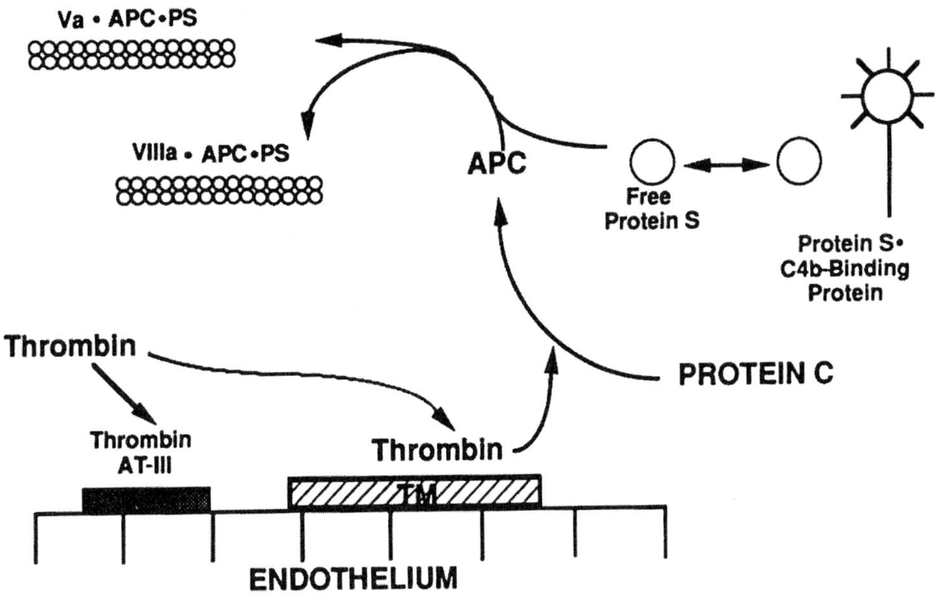

Figure 16–6. Inhibition of thrombin by antithrombin III (AT-III) bound to glycosaminoglycans on the endothelial surface and by the receptor thrombomodulin (TM). When bound to TM, thrombin converts protein C to activated protein C (APC). Together, APC and its cofactor, protein S inactivate factors Va and VIIIa. Free protein S (PS) is in equilibrium with protein S complexed with C4b-binding protein.

can disassociate and catalyze another AT-III inhibitory interaction. Heparin can also function as a catalytic surface or template to increase the probability of interaction of the two proteins.[53] Although heparin is not normally present in circulating blood, the endothelium is coated with a related glycosaminoglycan known as heparan sulfate. This heparin-like molecule accelerates AT-III activity and is presumably responsible for the "heparin" effect in vivo.[54]

THE CONTACT SYSTEM

The contact system is composed of factor XII, high-molecular-weight kininogen (HMWK), prekallikrein, and factor XI.[55] A deficiency of any one of the contact factors causes a prolonged activated partial thromboplastin time, which relies on a negatively charged surface such as silica to bind the factors and therefore accelerate their activation. The role of factor XII, prekallikrein, or HMWK in hemostasis in vivo appears to be negligible, inasmuch as a deficiency of these factors is not associated with a bleeding diathesis. As previously discussed, the major activator of factor XI in vivo is probably thrombin and not factor XIIa. Prekallikrein and factor XI circulate as a complex with HMWK, which can bind to a negatively charged surface. Contact activation is initiated when factor XII and the complexes of HMWK-prekallikrein and HMWK/factor XI bind to negatively charged surfaces, which may include collagen as well as many other biological and synthetic materials (Fig. 16–7). The surface-bound factor XII expresses a low level of enzymic activity, thereby converting small amounts of prekallikrein to kallikrein, which reciprocally activates additional factor XII to an active form. The factor XIIa then activates additional prekallikrein and converts factor XI to factor XIa.

The contact system is closely linked to the kinin system. Kallikrein can cleave surface-bound factor XIIa to a fragment (Hageman factor fragment, βXIIa) that is then released from the surface. The fragment cannot activate factor XI; however, it retains the ability to activate prekallikrein to kallikrein, which releases bradykinin from HMWK. The nonapeptide bradykinin has a circulation time in minutes, and is a highly potent vasodilator that can induce pain, flushing, bronchospasm, and hypotension when infused into humans.[56] Bradykinin can be generated in patients who receive rapid infusions of plasma fractionation products that contain high levels of activated factor XII. Reactions in the recipients can range from facial flushing to severe, transient hypotension.[57] The contact system is regulated by C1 esterase inhibitor, which is the

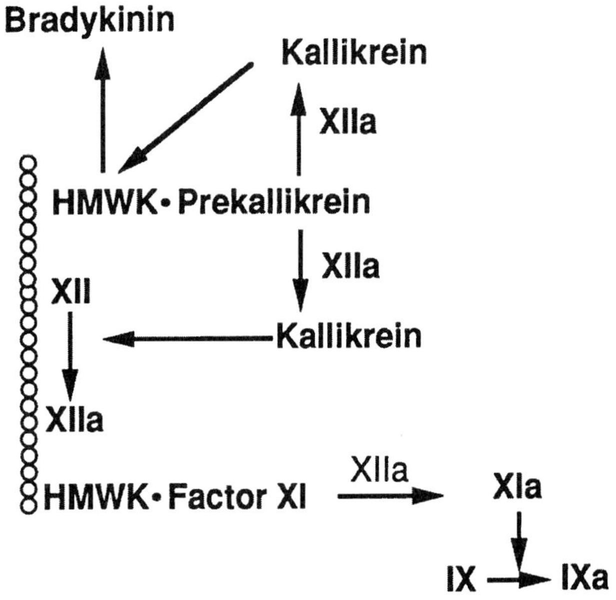

Figure 16–7. Contact system. The contact factors, which are factor XII, high-molecular-weight kininogen (HMWK), prekallikrein, and factor XI, can all bind to a negatively charged surface either directly (factor XII, HMWK) or through their association with HMWK (prekallikrein, factor XI). Once activated, factor XII converts prekallikrein to kallikrein, and factor XI to XIa. Kallikrein cleaves bradykinin from HMWK.

major inactivator of factor XIIa and kallikrein; factor XIa is primarily inhibited by α_1-antitrypsin.

PRODUCTS FOR CLINICAL USE IN HEMOSTASIS

Concentrates for Inhibitor Deficiencies

Persons with deficiencies in functional AT-III, protein S, or protein C are at increased risk for venous thrombosis. Concentrates of purified AT-III, which has been purified from pooled human plasma and heat-treated for viral inactivation, are used primarily for AT-III–deficient patients who are undergoing surgery and during parturition.[58, 59] The goal of therapy is to increase the AT-III activity above 90% until adequate anticoagulation can be resumed in the postoperative state. The half-life of the AT-III is biphasic; the initial phase is as short as 7 to 14 hours, and the terminal phase is 43 to 90 hours.[60]

Population studies suggest that a significant percentage of protein C–deficient persons may be asymptomatic.[61] The disorder is clinically manifested by recurrent venous thromboembolic phenomena, primarily deep venous thrombosis and pulmonary emboli, generally beginning in the third decade. In symptomatic persons, the condition is usually managed with long-term oral anticoagulation. Warfarin-induced skin necrosis is a rare complication that can occur in protein C–deficient patients who begin oral anticoagulation without receiving heparin concomitantly.[62] The skin necrosis can be explained by the fact that protein C has a short half-life (6 hours) in comparison with factors II, IX, and X. In the first few days of therapy with warfarin, there is a more rapid decrease in protein C than in these other factors, resulting in exacerbation of a hypercoagulable state. The histopathological process of the skin lesion is characterized by diffuse microvascular thrombosis of venules and capillaries and is similar to that seen in infants with neonatal purpura fulminans who are homozygous for protein C deficiency.[63] Protein C concentrates have been used for the treatment of infants who are homozygous for protein C deficiency and for patients with warfarin-induced skin necrosis.[64] The concentrates are not commercially available in the United States.

Protein S deficiency is also inherited in an autosomal dominant manner but is more predictably associated with thromboembolic complications.[65] The clinical manifestations are similar to those of protein C deficiency, and most patients become symptomatic in their late 20s. No purified concentrates of protein S are yet available as adjuvant treatment for these patients.

An additional common inherited cause for recurrent venous thrombosis is a mutation in the factor V gene (factor V Leiden, arginine to glutamine at amino acid position 506) which causes a relative resistance of the abnormal factor V to inhibition by activated protein C.[66] Another abnormality is a mutation in the prothrombin gene (a guanine to adenine change in base 20,210 of the 3′-untranslated region) that results in elevated levels of prothrombin and an increased risk for thrombosis.[67] Factor V Leiden and the prothrombin gene mutation can be diagnosed by commercially available DNA analysis. Both are relatively common in white patients presenting with deep venous thrombosis; factor V Leiden may be present in 14% of these patients and the prothrombin gene mutation in 5%.[68] Treatment decisions for these patients are similar to those for patients with other types of inherited hypercoagulability.

Agents That Are Direct Thrombin Inhibitors

Unlike heparin and low-molecular-weight heparins which require AT-III for anticoagulant activity, anticoagulants derived from leeches[69] directly inhibit specific proteins in the coagulation cascade. Hirudin, a specific inhibitor of thrombin, is a 7-kDa protein from the salivary glands of the leech *Hirudo medicinalis.* Hirudin binds to the active site of thrombin as well as to the exosite where thrombin interacts with fibrinogen.[70] In contrast to heparin, hirudin can inhibit thrombin that is bound to fibrin.[71] Hirudin, which is now available in recombinant form, and its analogs appear to provide effective anticoagulation without inducing bleeding in animal models in which venous or arterial thrombi are formed.[72, 73] Lepirudin (Refludan), which is a recombinant form of hirudin with a half-life of 2 hours in patients with normal renal function, is now available as an alternative drug for patients who have or who are at risk for heparin-induced thrombocytopenia.[74, 75] In Japan, the thrombin inhibitor argatroban (known in the United States as Novastan) is commercially available. The drug has undergone extensive testing in the United States in patients with heparin-induced thrombocytopenia but has not yet been approved by the U.S. Food and Drug Administration (FDA). Both drugs are monitored with the activated partial thromboplastin time (APTT) and have no antidotes.

Newer Antiplatelet Agents

Agents that block the interaction between fibrinogen and platelet GPIIb/IIIa have demonstrated efficacy in patients with coronary syndromes and are now in general use. Abciximab (ReoPro) is an antigen-binding fragment (Fab) of chimeric human-murine monoclonal antibody 7E3.[76] It is used in patients undergoing percutaneous transluminal angioplasty (PTCA) and unstable angina with PTCA planned in 24 hours. Abciximab treatment of patients undergoing angioplasty or stent procedures significantly reduces the combined end points of death, repeat myocardial infarction, and need for urgent revascularization during 30 days in comparison to those undergoing stent procedures in the absence of abciximab.[76] Two newer GPIIb/IIIa inhibitors have also been licensed; one is tirofiban (Aggrastat), a nonpeptide tyrosine derivative that is indicated for patients with unstable angina/non–Q wave myocardial infarction (with or without PTCA).[77, 78] The other drug is eptifibatide (Integrelin), a cyclic heptapeptide that is indicated for patients with unstable angina/non–Q wave myocardial infarction (with or without PTCA) and for patients undergoing PTCA.[79] Multiple other anti–GIIB/IIIa inhibitors are in clinical trials as oral agents; their safety and efficacy profiles have yet to be determined.

Agents that block the ADP receptor are ticlopidine and an analog known as clopidogrel.[80, 81] These agents have a prolonged half-life and must undergo metabolism before showing activity. They appear to be more potent than aspirin. Ticlopidine is indicated for the secondary prevention of stroke and to prevent abrupt closure of stents.[80] Clopidogrel appears to have a better safety profile than does ticlopidine,[81] which has been associated with neutropenia, agranulocytosis, aplastic anemia, and thrombotic thrombocytopenic purpura.[82]

SUMMARY

Advances in the understanding of the hemostatic process as it occurs in vivo have prompted the development of antithrombotic agents as well as biological agents for hemostasis. The potent antiplatelet agents described have gained immediate widespread use in cardiology. In the future, strategies will be developed to improve certain characteristics of the biological agents already available. For example, detailed knowledge of platelet function will facilitate the development of platelet products that can be frozen or stored in the cold and yet retain function when infused into patients.[83] Thus the discoveries of the intricate aspects of hemostasis, which include platelets, coagulation factors, and the environment in which they interact (conditions of high or low shear stress) will provide clues for modulation of the system by biological agents or drugs to preserve the delicate balance between hemorrhage and thrombosis.

REFERENCES

1. Rand JH, Patel ND, Schwartz E, et al. 150-kD von Willebrand factor binding protein extracted from human vascular subendothelium is type VI collagen. J Clin Invest 1991; 88:253.
2. Coller BS, Beer JH, Scudder LE, Steinberg MH. Collagen-platelet interactions: evidence for a direct interaction of collagen with platelet GPIa/IIa and an indirect interaction with platelet GPIIb/IIIa mediated by adhesive proteins. Blood 1989; 74:182.
3. Roth GJ. Developing relationships: arterial platelet adhesion, glycoprotein Ib, and leucine-rich glycoproteins. Blood 1991; 77:5.
4. Greco NJ, Tandon NN, Jones GD, et al. Contributions of glycoprotein Ib and the seven transmembrane domain receptor to increases in platelet cytoplasmic [Ca^{2+}] induced by alpha-thrombin. Biochemistry 1996; 35:906.
5. Schulte am Esch II J, Cruz MA, Siegel JB, et al. Activation of human platelets by the membrane-expressed AI domain of von Willebrand factor. Blood 1997; 90:4425.
6. Kroll MH, Hellums JD, McIntire LV, et al. Platelets and shear stress. Blood 1996; 88:1525.
7. Peershke EIB, Lopez JA. Platelet membranes and receptors. *In* Loscalzo J, Schafer AI (eds): Thrombosis and Hemorrhage, 2nd ed. Philadelphia: Williams & Wilkins, 1998, pp 229–260.
8. Gilbert GE, Arena AA. Activation of the factor VIIIa–factor IXa enzyme complex of blood coagulation by membranes containing phosphatidyl-*l*-serine. J Biol Chem 1996; 271:11120.
9. Kroll MH, Sullivan R. Mechanisms of platelet activation. *In* Loscalzo J, Schafer AI (eds): Thrombosis and Hemorrhage, 2nd ed. Philadelphia: Williams & Wilkins, 1998, pp 261–291.
10. Bennett JS, Shattil SJ. Platelet function. *In* Williams WJ, Beutler E, Erslev AJ, Lichtman MA (eds): Hematology, 4th ed. New York: McGraw-Hill, 1990, pp 1233–1250.
11. Majerus PW. Platelets. *In* Stamatoyannopoulos G, Nienhuis AW, Leder P, Majerus PW (eds): The Molecular Basis of Blood Diseases. Philadelphia: WB Saunders, 1987, pp 689–718.
12. Lawson JH, Kalafatis M, Stram S, Mann KG. A model for the tissue factor pathway to thrombin. J Biol Chem 1994; 269:23357.
13. Colucci M, Balconi G, Lorenzet R, et al. Cultured human endothelial cells generate tissue factor in response to endotoxin. J Clin Invest 1983; 71:1893.
14. Rapaport SI. The extrinsic pathway inhibitor: a regulator of tissue factor–dependent blood coagulation. Thromb Haemost 1991; 66:6.
15. Nemerson Y. Tissue factor and hemostasis. Blood 1988; 71:1.
16. Broze GJ, Jr, Warren LA, Novotny WF, et al. The lipoprotein-associated coagulation inhibitor that inhibits the factor VII–tissue factor complex also inhibits factor Xa: insight into its possible mechanism of action. Blood 1988; 71:335.
17. Rao LVM, Rapaport SI. Studies of a mechanism inhibiting the initiation of the extrinsic pathway of coagulation. Blood 1987; 69:645.
18. Rapaport SI. Inhibition of factor VIIa/tissue factor–induced blood coagulation: with particular emphasis upon a factor Xa–dependent inhibitory mechanism. Blood 1989; 73:359.
19. Nesheim ME. Factor VIII binds to platelets. J Biol Chem 1988; 263:16467.
20. Kane WH, Lindhout MJ, Jackson CM, Majerus PW. Factor Va–dependent binding of factor Xa to human platelets. J Biol Chem 1980; 255:1170.
21. Mann KG, Nesheim ME, Church WR, et al. Surface-dependent reactions of the vitamin K–dependent enzyme complexes. Blood 1990; 76:1.
22. Church WR, Boulanger LL, Messier TL, Mann KG. Evidence for a common metal ion-dependent transition in the 4-carboxyglutamic acid domains of several vitamin K–dependent proteins. J Biol Chem 1989; 264:17882.
23. van Dieijen G, Tans G, Rising J, Hemker HC. The role of phospholipid and factor VIIIa in the activation of bovine factor X. J Biol Chem 1981; 256:3433.
24. Mann KG, Jenny RJ, Krishnaswamy S. Cofactor proteins in the assembly and expression of blood clotting enzyme complexes. Annu Rev Biochem 1988; 57:915.
25. Francis CW, Marder VJ. Mechanisms of fibrinolysis. *In* Williams JW, Beutler E, Erslev AJ, Lichtman MA (eds): Hematology, 4th ed. New York: McGraw-Hill, 1990, pp 1313–1321.
26. Jansen JWCM, Haverkate F, Koopman J, et al. Influence of factor XIIIa activity on human whole blood clot lysis in vitro. Thromb Haemost 1987; 57:171.
27. Church WR, Jernigan RL, Toole J, et al. Coagulation factors V and VIII and ceruloplasmin constitute a family of structurally related proteins. Proc Natl Acad Sci U S A 1984; 81:6934.
28. Schick BP, Schick PK. Megakaryocyte biochemistry. Semin Hematol 1986; 23:68–87.
29. Tracy PB, Eide LL, Bowie EJW, Mann KG. Radioimmunoassay of factor V in human plasma and platelets. Blood 1982; 60:59.
30. Furie B, Furie BC. Molecular basis of vitamin K–dependent carboxylation. Blood 1990; 75:1753.
31. Esmon CT, Suttie JW, Jackson CM. The functional significance of vitamin K action. J Biol Chem 1978; 200:4095.
32. Bauer KA, Rosenberg RD. The pathophysiology of the prethrombotic state in humans: insights gained from studies using markers of hemostatic system activation. Blood 1987; 70:343.
33. Weksler BB, Ley CW, Jaffe EA. Stimulation of endothelial cell prostacyclin production by thrombin, trypsin, and the ionophore A 23187. J Clin Invest 1978; 62:923.
34. Gelehrter TD, Sznycer-Laszuk R. Thrombin induction of plasminogen activator-inhibitor in cultured human endothelial cells. J Clin Invest 1986; 77:165.
35. Daniell TO, Gibbs VC, Milfay DF, et al. Thrombin stimulates c-*sis* gene expression in microvascular endothelial cells. J Biol Chem 1986; 261:9579.
36. Bar-Shavit R, Kahn A, Fenton JW II, Wilner GD. Chemotactic response of monocytes to thrombin. J Biol Chem 1988; 96:282.
37. Hantgan RR, Francis CW, Scheraga HA, Marder VJ. Fibrinogen structure and physiology. *In* Colman RW, Hirsh J, Marder VJ, Salzman EW (eds): Hemostasis and Thrombosis: Basic Principles and Clinical Practice. Philadelphia: JB Lippincott, 1987, pp 269–288.

38. Sandset PM, Abilegaard U, Larsen ML. Heparin induces release of extrinsic coagulation pathway inhibitor (EPI). Thromb Res 1988; 50:803.
39. Dittman WA, Majerus PW. Structure and function of thrombomodulin: a natural anticoagulant. Blood 1990; 75:329.
40. Ishii H, Salem HH, Bell CE, et al. Thrombomodulin, an endothelial anticoagulant protein, is absent from the human brain. Blood 1986; 67:362.
41. Moore KL, Esmon CT, Esmon NL. Tumor necrosis factor leads to the internalization and degradation of thrombomodulin from the surface of bovine aortic endothelial cells in culture. Blood 1989; 73:159.
42. Moore KL, Andreoli SP, Esmon NL, et al. Endotoxin enhances tissue factor and suppresses thrombomodulin expression of human vascular endothelium in vitro. J Clin Invest 1987; 79:124.
43. Nawroth PP, Handley DA, Esmon CT, Stern DM. Interleukin 1 induces endothelial cell procoagulant while suppressing cell-surface anticoagulant activity. Proc Natl Acad Sci U S A 1986; 83:3460.
44. Esmon CT, Esmon NL, Harris KW. Complex formation between thrombin and thrombomodulin inhibits both thrombin-catalyzed fibrin formation and factor V activation. J Biol Chem 1982; 257:7944.
45. Esmon NL, Carroll RC, Esmon CT. Thrombomodulin blocks the ability of thrombin to activate platelets. J Biol Chem 1983; 258:12238.
46. Polgar J, Lerant I, Muszbek L, Machovich R. Thrombomodulin inhibits the activation of factor XIII by thrombin. Thromb Res 1986; 43:585.
47. Esmon CT, Owen WG. Identification of an endothelial cell cofactor for thrombin-catalyzed activation of protein C. Proc Natl Acad Sci U S A 1981; 78:2249.
48. Kisiel W. Human plasma protein C: isolation, characterization, and mechanism of activation by α-thrombin. J Clin Invest 1979; 64:761.
49. Dahlback B. Inhibition of protein Ca cofactor function of human and bovine protein S by C4b-binding protein. J Biol Chem 1986; 261:12022.
50. Solymoss S, Tucker MM, Tracy P. Kinetics of inactivation of membrane-bound factor Va by activated protein C. J Biol Chem 1988; 263:14884.
51. Bauer KA, Rosenberg RD. Role of antithrombin III as a regulator of in vivo coagulation. Semin Hematol 1991; 28:10.
52. Jordan RE, Oosta M, Gardner WT, Rosenberg RD. The kinetics of hemostatic enzyme–antithrombin interactions in the presence of low molecular weight heparin. J Biol Chem 1980; 255:10081.
53. Shore JD, Olson ST, Craig PA, et al. Kinetics of heparin action. Ann N Y Acad Sci 1989; 556:75.
54. Marcum JA, McKenney JB, Rosenberg RD. Acceleration of the thrombin-antithrombin complex formation in rat hindquarters via heparinlike molecules bound to the endothelium. J Clin Invest 1984; 74:341.
55. Schmaier AH, Silverberg M, Kaplan AP, Colman RW. Contact activation and its abnormalities. *In* Colman RW, Hirsh J, Marder VJ, Salzman EW (eds): Hemostasis and Thrombosis: Basic Principles and Clinical Practice. Philadelphia: JB Lippincott, 1987, pp 18–38.
56. Elliott DF, Horton EW, Lewis GP. Action of pure bradykinin. J Physiol 1960; 153:473.
57. Alving BM, Hojima Y, Pisano JJ, et al. Hypotension associated with prekallikrein activator (Hageman-factor fragments) in plasma protein fraction. N Engl J Med 1978; 299:66.
58. Menache D, O'Malley JP, Schorr JB, et al. Evaluation of the safety, recovery, half-life, and clinical efficacy of antithrombin III (human) in patients with hereditary antithrombin III deficiency. Blood 1990; 75:33.
59. Schwartz RS, Bauer KA, Rosenberg RD, et al. Clinical experience with antithrombin III concentrate in treatment of congenital and acquired deficiency of antithrombin. Am J Med 1989; 87:53S.
60. Jackson M, Olsen S, Gomez E, Alving B. Use of antithrombin III concentrates to correct antithrombin III deficiency during vascular surgery. J Vasc Surg 1995; 22:804.
61. Miletich J, Sherman L, Broze G Jr. Absence of thrombosis in subjects with heterozygous protein C deficiency. N Engl J Med 1987; 317:991.
62. McGehee WG, Klotz TA, Epstein DJ, Rapaport SI. Coumarin necrosis associated with hereditary protein C deficiency. Ann Intern Med 1984; 101:59.
63. Marciniak E, Wilson HD, Marlar RA. Neonatal purpura fulminans: a genetic disorder related to the absence of protein C in blood. Blood 1985; 65:15.
64. Dreyfus M, Magny JF, Bridey F, et al. Treatment of homozygous protein C deficiency and neonatal purpura fulminans with a purified protein C concentrate. N Engl J Med 1991; 325:1565.
65. Engesser L, Broekmans AW, Briet E, et al. Hereditary protein S deficiency: clinical manifestations. Ann Intern Med 1987; 106:677.
66. Middeldorp S, Henkens CMA, Koopman M, et al. The incidence of venous thromboembolism in family members of patients with factor V Leiden mutation and venous thrombosis. Ann Intern Med 1998; 128:15.
67. Poort SR, Rosendaal FR, Reitsma PH, Bertina RM. A common genetic variation in the 3′-untranslated region of the prothrombin gene is associated with elevated plasma prothrombin levels and an increase in venous thrombosis. Blood 1996; 88:3698.
68. Cumming AM, Keeney S, Salden A, et al. The prothrombin gene G20,210A variant: prevalence in a U.K. anticoagulant clinic population. Br J Haematol 1997; 98:353.
69. Sawyer RT. Thrombolytics and anticoagulants from leeches. Biotechnology 1991; 9:513.
70. Fenton JW II. Thrombin interactions with hirudin. Semin Thromb Hemost 1989; 15:265.
71. Weitz JI, Hudoba M, Massel D, et al. Clot-bound thrombin is protected from inhibition by heparin–antithrombin III but is susceptible to inactivation by antithrombin III–independent inhibitors. J Clin Invest 1990; 86:385.
72. Cadroy Y, Maraganore JM, Hanson SR, Harker LA. Selective inhibition by a synthetic hirudin peptide of fibrin-dependent thrombosis in baboons. Proc Natl Acad Sci U S A 1991; 88:1177.
73. Kaiser B, Simon A, Markwardt F. Antithrombotic effects of recombinant hirudin in experimental angioplasty and intravascular thrombolysis. Thromb Haemost 1990; 63:44.
74. Greinacher A, Volpel H, Potzsch B. Recombinant hirudin in the treatment of patients with heparin-induced thrombocytopenia (HIT). Blood 1996; 88:281.
75. Schlele F, Vuillemenot A, Kramarz P, et al. Use of recombinant hirudin as anti-thrombotic treatment in patients with heparin-induced thrombocytopenia. Am J Hematol 1995; 50:20.
76. The EPISTENT Investigators. Randomised placebo-controlled and balloon-angioplasty–controlled trial to assess safety of coronary stenting with use of platelet glycoprotein-IIb/IIIa blockade. Lancet 1998; 352:87.
77. PRISM-Plus Study Investigators. Inhibition of the platelet glycoprotein IIb/IIIa receptor with tirofiban in unstable angina and non–Q-wave myocardial infarction. N Engl J Med 1998; 338:1488.
78. The RESTORE Investigators. Effects of platelet glycoprotein IIb/IIIa blockade with tirofiban on adverse cardiac events in patients with unstable angina or acute myocardial infarction undergoing coronary angioplasty. Circulation 1997; 96:1445.
79. The PURSUIT Trial Investigators. Inhibition of platelet glycoprotein IIb/IIIa with eptifibatide in patients with acute coronary syndromes. N Engl J Med 1998; 339:436.
80. McTavish D, Faulds D, Goa KL. Ticlopidine. An updated review of its pharmacology and therapeutic use in platelet-dependent disorders. Drugs 1990; 40:238.
81. Gent M, Beaumont D, Blanchard J, et al. A randomised, blinded, trial of clopidogrel versus aspirin in patients at risk of ischaemic events (CAPRIE). Lancet 1996; 348:1329.
82. Bennett CL, Weinberg PD, Rozenberg–Ben-Dror K, et al. Thrombotic thrombocytopenic purpura associated with ticlopidine. A review of 60 cases. Ann Intern Med 1998; 128:541.
83. Alving BM, Reid TJ, Fratantoni JC, Finlayson JS. Frozen platelets and platelet substitutes in transfusion medicine. Transfusion 1997; 37:866.

CHAPTER 17

Fibrinolysis

Jeffrey J. Rade
William R. Bell

Recognition of the existence of an endogenous fibrinolytic system was first appreciated in the 4th century BC.[1] It was observed that postmortem coagulated blood underwent liquefaction after several hours. These observations were confirmed nearly 2000 years later by both the anatomist Malpighi in 1687 and the pathologist Morgagni in 1761. In 1794, the English physician John Hunter described the fibrinolytic effects of exercise when he noted that the blood of animals exercised before sacrifice failed to clot.[2] More than a century ago, Scherer and Green observed the spontaneous dissolution of fibrin clots under a variety of in vitro conditions.[3, 4] Dastre, in 1893, concluded that this phenomenon resulted from enzymatic digestion of fibrin and designated this transformation "fibrinolysis."[5]

Identification of the principal components of the fibrinolytic system occurred during the 1930s and 1940s. The first therapeutic utilization of the fibrinolytic system was made possible by Tillet and Garner in 1933, who discovered that an extract of α-hemolytic streptococci was capable of inducing lysis of human blood and plasma clots.[6] Milstone, in 1941, demonstrated that this streptococcal extract alone was insufficient to induce fibrinolysis and that a plasma "lytic factor" was also required.[7] Kaplan detailed the nature of this factor, but it was Christensen and MacLeod, in 1945, who named the extract from α-hemolytic streptococci "streptokinase" and renamed Milstone's lytic factor "plasmin."[8, 9]

The search for other activators of the fibrinolytic system led to the discovery of a number of naturally occurring substances that are able to activate plasminogen. The fibrinolytic activity of human urine was first noted in 1885 by Sahli, although it was not until 1951 that Williams identified a plasminogen activator in urine that was subsequently named "urokinase" by Sobel and colleagues in 1952.[10, 11] Astrup and Permin recognized a second naturally occurring plasminogen activator in 1947 and named it "tissue plasminogen activator."[12] Since that time several plasminogen activators have been adapted for clinical use as thrombolytic agents. Thrombolytic therapy is now an accepted treatment for a variety of thromboembolic disorders, including acute myocardial infarction, acute ischemic stroke, pulmonary embolism, deep vein thrombosis, and intra-arterial and intracardiac thromboembolic diseases.

The human fibrinolytic system is known to mediate two important, but very different, physiological processes. Intravascular fibrinolysis is the process by which plasmin degrades fibrin at the site of vascular injury, thus maintaining hemostatic homeostasis. Extravascular fibrinolysis is the process by which plasmin mediates extracellular matrix degradation, both directly and indirectly through the activation of matrix metalloproteinases.[13, 14] Matrix degradation is of critical importance to several physiological and pathological conditions, including angiogenesis, wound healing, tissue remodeling, ovulation, and neoplastic growth and metastasis. This review will focus almost exclusively on the components and regulation of intravascular fibrinolysis, with an emphasis on its therapeutic manipulation.

PLASMINOGEN AND PLASMIN

Biochemistry

Activation of the circulating glycoprotein plasminogen yields the fibrinolytic enzyme plasmin. Plasminogen is synthesized by the liver and has a serum concentration in humans of approximately 20 mg/dL. The major pathway for its elimination is by catabolic degradation rather than conversion to plasmin.[15] The molecule has a carbohydrate content of approximately 2% and exhibits a remarkable degree of microheterogeneity.[16] The tertiary structure of plasminogen is determined in large part by a total of 24 disulfide bonds. Sixteen of these bonds participate in folding the molecule into five homologous triple loops, called kringles domains, because of their resemblance to a type of Danish pastry. These kringles, numbered K1 through K5, each contain approximately 80 amino acids (Fig. 17–1). The gene for human plasminogen is located on chromosome 6.[17]

Two major forms of plasminogen exist based on molecular weight and affinity for both plasminogen activators and fibrin.[18] A native form, termed Glu-plasminogen because of its amino terminal glutamine residue, is a single chain 92-kD glycoprotein composed of 790 amino acids. A modified form, termed *Lys-plasminogen,* is an 84-kD protein formed by cleavage at Lys77 of an 8-kD amino acid preactivation peptide. Lys-plasminogen is activated 3- to 10-fold more efficiently by plasminogen activators and has a 2-fold higher affinity for fibrin than Glu-plasminogen.[19] The circulating half-life of Lys-plasminogen is 16 hours compared with 2.2 days for Glu-plasminogen.[20]

The conversion of plasminogen into plasmin by plasminogen activators involves the cleavage of a single bond between Arg560 and Val561, forming two polypeptide chains that remain connected by two disulfide bridges. A 63-kD A (heavy) chain, composed of 549 amino acids, is

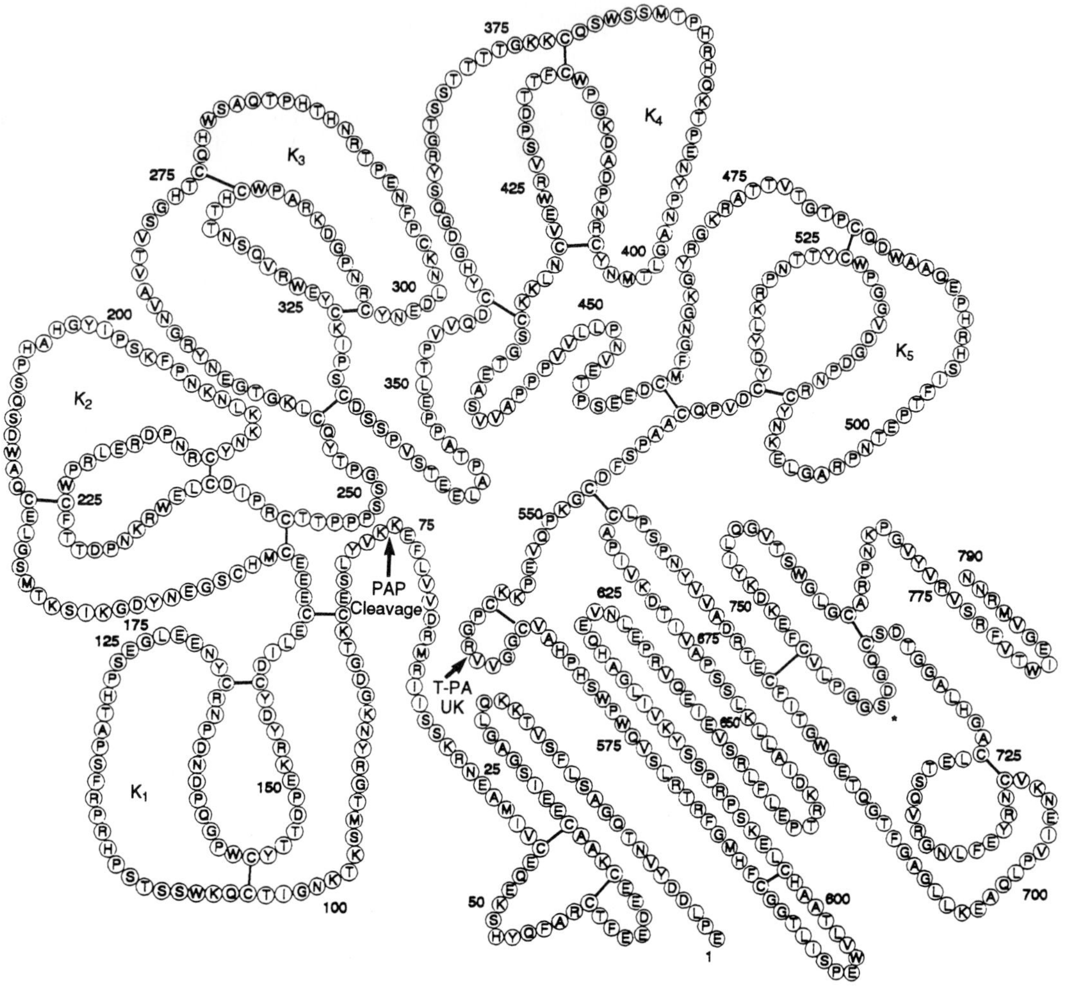

Figure 17–1. Schematic model of the structure of Glu-plasminogen. K_1 through K_5 are the kringles into which the molecule is folded with the aid of disulfide bridges. PAP, pre-activation peptide. (Adapted from Henkin T, Mancotte P, Yang H. The plasminogen-plasmin system. Prog Cardiovasc Dis 1991; 34:135.)

formed from the amino terminus of the plasminogen molecule and a 25-kD B (light) chain, composed of 241 amino acids, is formed from the carboxyl terminus. A possible second step involves the proteolytic cleavage of the preactivation peptide from the amino terminus of the Glu-plasmin(ogen) molecule to form Lys-plasmin(ogen).[21] The schematic of plasminogen activation is shown in Figure 17–2. Glu-plasmin is an inherently unstable molecule that quickly undergoes autocatalysis to Lys-plasmin, the predominant physiologic form of plasmin. Both Glu-plasmin and Lys-plasmin can cleave the preactivation peptide from Glu-plasminogen, thus forming Lys-plasminogen. The latter may then be converted to Lys-plasmin by any one of several plasminogen activators.

Within the five kringle domains located on the plasmin A chain are a number of allostearic effector sites that interact with several components and modulators of the fibrinolytic system. These sites are known as lysine-binding sites (LBS). An LBS with a very high affinity for lysine residues is located on K1 and mediates the interaction of

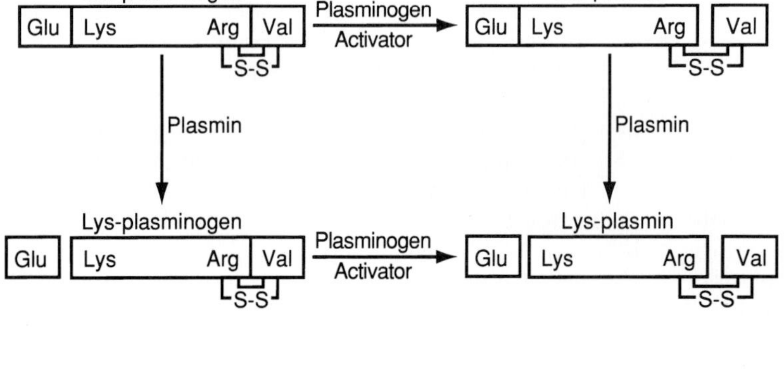

Figure 17–2. Mechanism of plasminogen activation. (Adapted from Bachmann F. Fibrinolysis. *In* Verstraete M, Vermylen J, Lienen HR, Arnout J [eds]: Thrombosis and Hemostasis. Leuven: Leuven University Press, 1978, pp 233–235.)

plasmin with fibrin and the plasma inhibitor α2-antiplasmin.[22] Five other LBS with lower affinity for lysine residues are found on K2 through K5 and mediate the binding of plasminogen activators.

The B chain contains the active site of the plasmin molecule, which is formed by the amino acid residues His602, Asp645, and Ser740. The active site is a serine protease, homologous in both structure and function to other serine proteases, including thrombin, factor Xa, and chymotrypsin. Fibrin is the principal physiologic substrate of plasmin, although any peptide containing an Arg-Lys sequence can be nonspecifically cleaved. Other elements of the coagulation cascade, including fibrinogen and factors VIII and V, are inactivated by plasmin whereas prekallikrein, HMW-kininogen, and elements of the complement cascade are activated by the enzyme.[23]

Action on Fibrin and Fibrinogen

Human fibrinogen is a glycoprotein with a molecular weight of 340 kD. The molecule is synthesized by the liver and has a plasma concentration of 200 to 400 mg/dL. Fibrinogen is also stored in hepatic parenchymal cells and can behave as an acute phase reactant, being released in response to various physiologic and pathologic stimuli.[24] Its half-life is approximately 4 days in humans.

The fibrinogen molecule (Fig. 17–3) is a dimer consisting of three nonidentical pairs of peptide chains represented by the formula AαBβ/2. The formation of fibrin involves a three-step process. In the first step, thrombin cleaves two pairs of peptides, known as fibrinopeptides A and B, from the amino termini of the Aα and Bβ chains, respectively, yielding the fibrin monomer αB/(2). The second step is the spontaneous polymerization of the fibrin monomers. The final step involves the cross-linking of the fibrin polymers by activated factor XIII, forming the insoluble fibrin clot.

Plasmin cleaves both fibrinogen and fibrin into a family of fragments known as fibrinogen-fibrin degradation products (FDP-fdp) (Fig. 17–4).[25] These FDP-fdp are known as fragments X, Y, D, and E, and are found in the circulation in various stages of digestion. Fragments D and E are the so-called terminal core fragments that are resistant to further proteolysis by plasmin. In contrast, fragments X and Y are intermediate fragments capable of further degradation by plasmin, eventually to fragments 2D and E. Degradation of fibrin and fibrinogen are similar but differ in several important respects. Fragment E derived from fibrinogen degradation contains fibrinopeptides A and B, whereas fragment E from fibrin degradation does not. Second, because the majority of fibrin within a clot exists as polymers cross-linked at the γ-chain carboxy terminus, degradation by plasmin results in liberation of D-D and D-Y dimerized fragments.

Several of the FDP-fdp possess biologic activity.[26, 27] Fragments D and Y both inhibit coagulation in the thrombin clotting time test. Fragment X retains the ability of

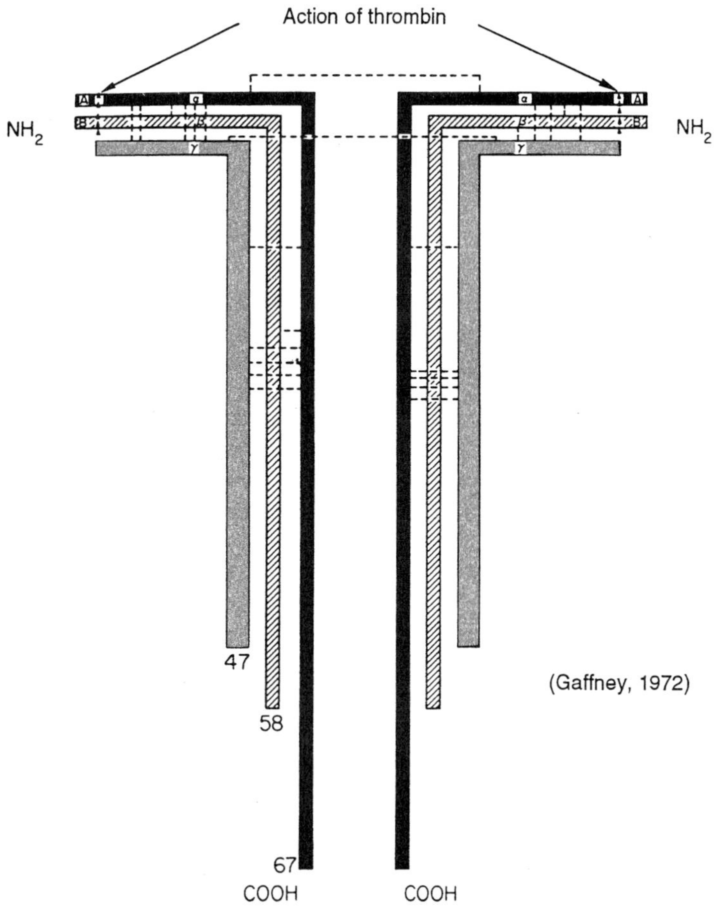

Figure 17–3. Schematic model of fibrinogen. *Solid bars,* Aα chain; *striped bars,* Bβ chain; *stippled bars,* γ chain; *dotted lines,* S-S bonds. (Adapted from Gaffney P. The biochemistry of fibrinogen and fibrin degradation products. *In* Hemostasis: Biochemistry, Physiology and Pathology. Chichester, UK: John Wiley & Sons, 1977, p 110.)

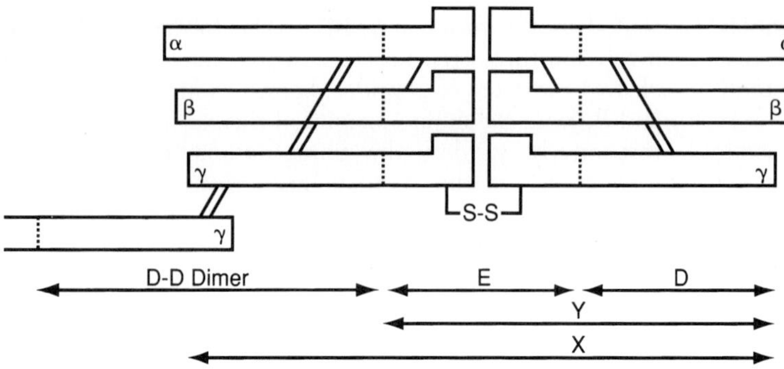

Figure 17–4. Fibrin degradation by plasmin with generation of fibrin degradation products. (Adapted from Henschen A. On the structure of functional sites in fibrinogen. Thromb Res 1983; Suppl V:27.)

the intact fibrinogen molecule to promote ADP-induced platelet aggregation and erythrocyte sedimentation and is thrombin coagulable. The terminal core fragments D and E have been shown to stimulate synthesis and release of fibrinogen by the liver, increase capillary permeability, and potentiate the vasoactive effects of bradykinin and angiotensin II.[28]

ENDOGENOUS ACTIVATORS OF FIBRINOLYSIS

A number of substances possess the ability to convert plasminogen to plasmin and are known generically as plasminogen activators. Endogenous plasminogen activators are physiologic constituents of the body's hemostatic mechanism and are classified as either intrinsic or extrinsic activators. Exogenous plasminogen activators are nonphysiological molecules, such as streptokinase and staphylokinase, which are used clinically as thrombolytic agents.

Intrinsic Activators

The intrinsic activators of plasmin are proteins that comprise the contact system of coagulation. Although their precise relationship is not clearly understood, factor XII (Hageman factor), prekallikrein, factor XI, and high-molecular-weight kininogen, when activated in response to contact with negatively charged surfaces, are able to initiate fibrinolysis.[29] Activated factor XII can activate plasminogen either directly or indirectly by activation of prekallikrein of factor XI, which then in turn are able to convert plasminogen to plasmin. The contribution of the contact system proteins to fibrinolysis is relatively minimal, accounting for only 15% of total plasma plasminogen activator activity.[30]

Extrinsic Activators

Extrinsic plasminogen activating factors have been identified in a number of tissues including neoplastic tissue. They are significantly more potent at activating plasminogen than are the intrinsic activators. The extrinsic plasminogen activators can be divided into two categories: tissue-type plasminogen activator (t-PA) and urokinase-type plasminogen activators (u-PA). Both types activate plasminogen directly through cleavage of the Arg560—Val561 bond. t-PA is the predominant plasminogen activator in the circulation responsible for mediating intravascular fibrinolysis whereas u-PA plays a greater role in cell-mediated or extravascular fibrinolysis. This distinction is by no means mutually exclusive. Mice genetically deficient for either t-PA or u-PA develop normally and manifest little or no spontaneous thrombosis, although both develop thrombosis in response to local inflammation.[31] This suggests that there is a relative degree of redundancy to the fibrinolytic system.

Tissue-Type Plasminogen Activators

The tissue-type plasminogen activators are ubiquitous molecules produced by nearly every tissue in the body but predominantly by the vascular endothelium. Increased expression may also be found in uterine smooth muscle and some malignant neoplasms.[32] The resting plasma concentration of t-PA is 5 to 7 ng/mL with a plasma half-life of 2.5 to 5 minutes.[33–35] Enhanced t-PA secretion by the vascular endothelium can occur in response to a number of vasoactive substances, including thrombin, catecholamines, histamine, bradykinin, and vasopressin, as well as in response to exercise and venous occlusion.[36, 37] Approximately one third of circulating t-PA at baseline is in the active state with the remainder complexed with various inhibitors, the most important being plasminogen activator inhibitor-1 (PAI-1).[38] Clearance of both free and complexed circulating t-PA is mainly by hepatic uptake and degradation.[39] The human t-PA gene is more than 20 kB in length, encompasses some 14 exons, and is located on chromosome 8.[40]

The t-PA molecule is translated as a 562-amino acid single-chain protein (Fig. 17–5). Post-translational modification consists of cleavage of the 32-amino acid "prepro" leader peptide and glycosylation at four potential N-glycosylation sites.[41] Mature t-PA has a molecular weight of 68 kD and exists in one of two variants, types I and II, based on their respective carbohydrate contents of 7% and 13%.[42] In vivo, the single-chain form of t-PA is converted to a double-chain form by several endogenous proteases, including factor Xa, tissue kallikrein, or on the surface of a thrombus by plasmin.[36] Single-chain t-PA is cleaved at Arg27-I/e 276, yielding two polypeptide chains that remain connected by a single disulfide bridge; an A chain with a molecular weight of 36 kD and a B chain with a molecular weight of 32 kD.

The A chain of t-PA chain is composed of a finger domain, an epidermal growth factor–like domain, and two

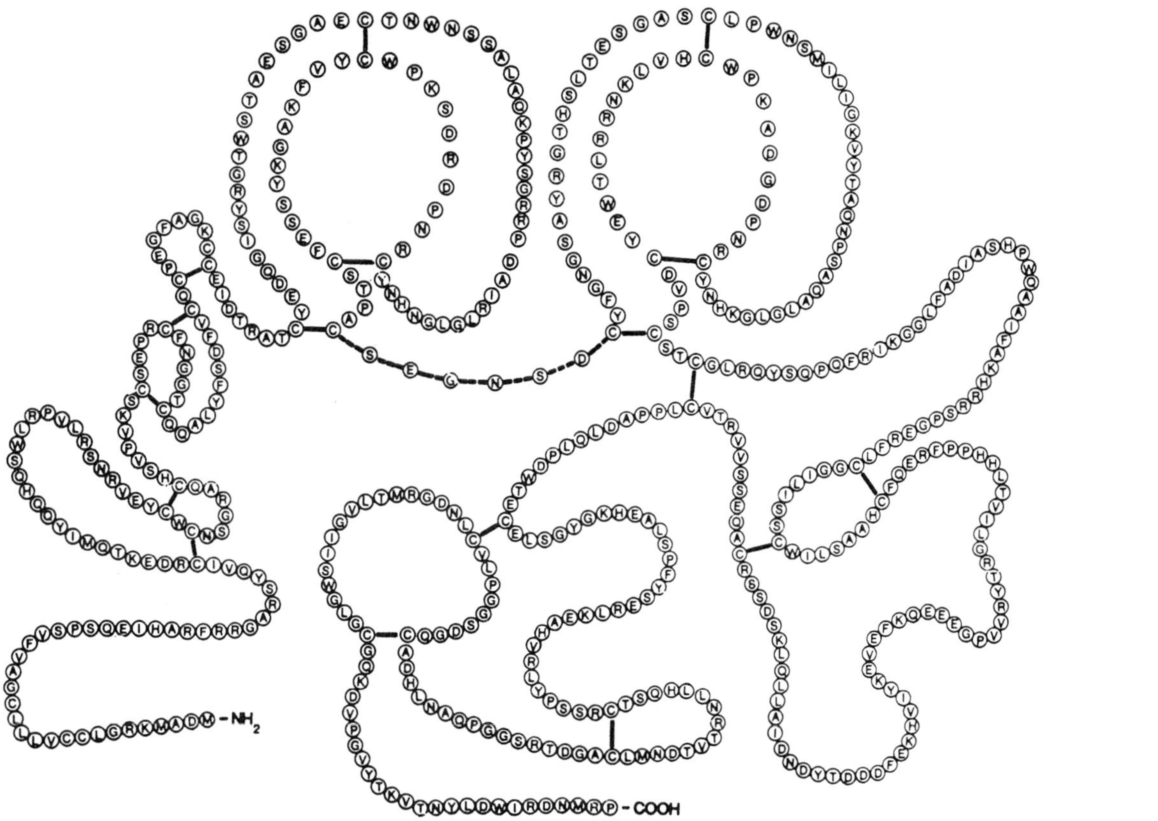

Figure 17–5. Schematic model of tissue plasminogen activator (t-PA). (Adapted from Ny T, Eigh F, Lund B. The structure of the human tissue-type plasminogen activator gene: correlation of intron and exon structure to functional and structural domains. Proc Natl Acad Sci U S A 1984; 81:5355.)

kringle loops that share homology with the fourth (K4) and fifth kringle (K5) loops of plasminogen. The second kringle domain contains a high-affinity lysine-binding site (LBS) that, along with the finger domain, mediates fibrin binding. The epidermal growth factor and first kringle domain mediate the binding of t-PA to high-affinity receptors on liver cells, thus facilitating its clearance from the circulation. The B chain contains the active site of the molecule, which is similar to other serine proteases.

An important physiological property of t-PA is its enhanced enzymatic activity in the presence of fibrin. In the absence of fibrin, both single- and double-chain t-PA are poor activators of Glu-plasminogen. The addition of physiological concentrations of fibrin to t-PA preparations in vitro markedly increases the rate of Glu-plasminogen activation nearly 400-fold.[43] Activation appears to occur through the formation of a ternary complex, formed first by binding of t-PA to fibrin followed by binding of plasminogen. The higher affinity of t-PA for plasminogen in the presence of fibrin enhances plasminogen activation at the site of a thrombus while minimizing free plasminogen activation in the circulation. The single- and double-chain forms of t-PA are nearly equal activators of plasminogen, although the double-chain form is more active against low-molecular-weight substrates.[44]

Urokinase-Type Plasminogen Activators

A second group of extrinsic plasminogen activators are the urokinase-type plasminogen activators. Urokinase is a glycoprotein produced by a variety of cell types but predominantly by renal parenchymal cells that mediate secretion into the urine. The concentration of urokinase in plasma during rest ranges from 2 to 5 ng/mL with a serum half-life of 10 to 15 minutes.[45–47] The concentration in human urine is about 2 μg/mL.[48] The human u-PA gene is 6.4 kB in length, contains 11 exons, and is located on chromosome 10.[40]

Urokinase is initially synthesized as a single-chain precursor (scu-PA), also called pro-urokinase (pro-UK), composed of 411 amino acids and having a molecular weight of 54 kD (Fig. 17–6). scu-PA is converted to its active form, u-PA, through cleavage of the Lys158—IIe 159 bond by plasmin, kallikrein, or factor XII. Activation of scu-PA can occur in the plasma phase but is accelerated nearly 20-fold on binding to a specific cellular u-PA receptor (uPAR).[49] uPAR is present on peripheral leukocytes, tumors, and other cells. Its function is to help control the spatial orientation of fibrinolysis, thus facilitating directional matrix degradation and cellular migration.

u-PA is similar in structure to t-PA but lacks the ability to bind fibrin. It is composed of an A and B chain linked by a disulfide bridge and having molecular weights of 20 kD and 34 kD, respectively. The A chain of u-PA consists of 158 amino acids and contains a single kringle as well as an epidermal growth factor–like domain similar to the t-PA A chain. The B chain consists of 252 amino acids and contains the serine protease active site.

The predominant form of u-PA is also called high-molecular-weight urokinase (HMW-UK), to differentiate

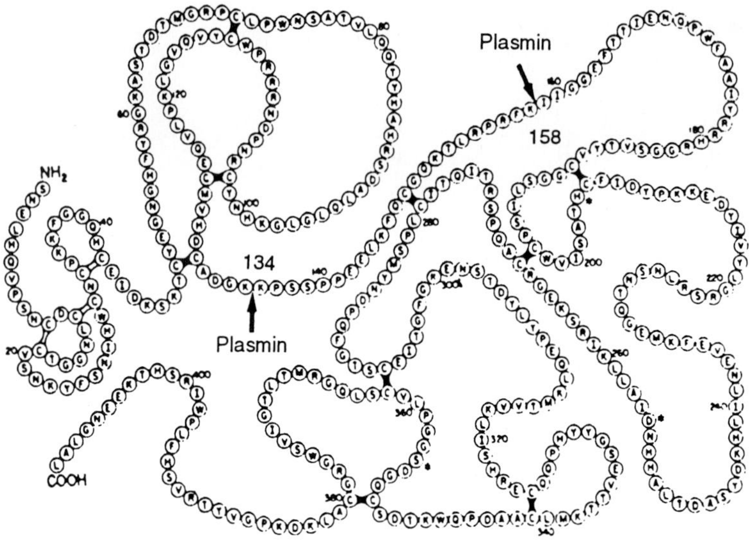

Figure 17–6. Schematic model of intact single-chain urokinase (scu-PA). (Adapted from Bachmann F. Fibrinolysis. *In* Verstraete M, Vermylen J, Lienen HR, Arnout J [eds]: Thrombosis and Hemostasis. Leuven: Leuven University Press, 1978, pp 233–235.)

it from a 32-kD low-molecular-weight form (LMW-UK) formed by partial degradation by plasmin and other proteolytic enzymes. LMW-UK is generated by cleavage of HMW-UK at Lys135—Lys136, leaving the 23 carboxy-terminal amino acids of the A chain connected by a disulfide bridge to an intact B chain.[50] LMW-UK is as active as HMW-UK as a plasminogen activator but lacks the epidermal growth factor–like domain, which mediates binding to the uPAR.

Although scu-PA is not a true zymogen, it does exhibit a small amount of intrinsic plasminogen-activating activity that is approximately 1% that of u-PA.[51] Unlike u-PA, scu-PA is not inhibited by PAI-1 or PAI-2 and thus is the predominant form found in the circulation. Although none of the u-PA species bind fibrin, scu-PA has been found to have a modest degree of thrombus specificity. Several hypotheses have been proposed to explain this, including (1) the presence of a competitive inhibitor in plasma that prevents binding of scu-PA to plasminogen, which is neutralized in the presence of fibrin,[51] (2) the enhanced ability of scu-PA to activate Lys-plasminogen, bound to partially digested fibrin on the surface of a thrombus compared with its ability to activate Glu-plasminogen in the circulation,[52] and (3) the negligible plasminogen-activating activity of scu-PA. Most conversion to active u-PA naturally occurs on the surface of a thrombus, where plasmin and fibrin concentrations are the highest.[53] Currently, a combination of the latter two hypotheses is the most favored explanation for the fibrin-specificity of scu-PA.

INHIBITION OF FIBRINOLYSIS

A number of substances, both endogenous and synthetic, have been identified as inhibitors of fibrinolysis in humans. Control of fibrinolysis occurs through inhibition of plasmin directly or by inhibition of plasminogen activation. The natural inhibitors of plasmin are members of a group of serine protease inhibitors, called serpins, that irreversibly bind to and inactivate a wide variety of plasma enzymes, including many components of the coagulation pathway.

Plasmin Inhibitors

α_2-Antiplasmin

The principal physiologic inhibitor of plasmin is α_2-antiplasmin. This serine protease inhibitor is synthesized in the liver as a 67-kD single-chain glycoprotein composed of 450 amino acids and having a carbohydrate content of 13%. α_2-Antiplasmin has a plasma concentration of approximately 7 mg/dL, although the molecule can behave as an acute-phase reactant.[54] The plasma half-life is approximately 2.5 days but may decrease to 12 hours during thrombolytic therapy.[55] Decreased levels, either congenital or acquired, are associated with bleeding.[56]

α_2-Antiplasmin inhibits plasmin by means of a two-step process.[54] In the first step, it forms a reversible 1:1 complex with plasmin through noncovalent binding to the high-affinity fibrin binding site located on K1 and a complementary binding site located in the carboxyl terminus of α_2-antiplasmin. This interaction is prevented by ϵ-aminocaproic acid (EACA). In the second step, serine residues in the plasmin active site covalently bind to and cleave the α_2-antiplasmin active site residues Arg354-Met355, with subsequent liberation of an 8-kD polypeptide fragment.

α_2-Antiplasmin inhibits fibrinolysis at the level of the fibrin clot via two mechanisms.[57] First, α_2-antiplasmin interferes with the binding of plasminogen to fibrin by competitive occupation of the plasmin high-affinity LBS. Second, α_2-antiplasmin is cross-linked to fibrin by factor XIII, thereby inhibiting fibrinolysis within the clot. α_2-Antiplasmin also inactivates several components of the coagulation cascade, including factors XII, XI, and X and thrombin.

The interaction between the high-affinity LBS of plasminogen and α_2-antiplasmin is a key regulatory point in the fibrinolytic cascade. When a thrombus is formed, plasminogen binds to fibrin via the LBS. t-PA released from the nearby vascular endothelium binds to and converts plasminogen into plasmin. Because the generated plasmin has both its LBS and active site occupied, inactivation by α_2-antiplasmin occurs relatively slowly. In the absence of fibrin, α_2-antiplasmin has access to both the LBS and active site, leading to quick inactivation of plasmin. In this way, fibrinolysis is enhanced at the site of clot formation and inhibited in the general circulation.

α_2-Macroglobulin

The second most important physiologic inhibitor of plasmin is α_2-macroglobulin. This serine protease is synthesized by hepatocytes, endothelial cells, and monocytes. α_2-Macroglobulin is a 725-kD glycoprotein that exists as a tetramer, composed of two pairs of identical 160-kD peptide chains linked by a disulfide bridge. The plasma concentration is approximately 2.5 mg/dL but exhibits age-dependent variation.[58] Concentrations are highest in infancy, reach a nadir in early adulthood, then rise thereafter. Increased levels are found in pregnancy, the nephrotic syndrome and with oral contraceptive use.[59] Decreased levels are found during thrombolytic therapy and in disseminated intravascular coagulation (DIC). The molecule is not an acute-phase reactant.

α_2-Macroglobulin has the unique ability to inhibit four different classes of endopeptidases, including serine, thiol, and metallo- and carboxy-proteases.[60] The molecule contains two reactive sites: a "bait" site that is briefly bound, then cleaved by the active site of plasmin, and a second thiol ester site that covalently binds to the plasmin molecule.[61] Each molecule of α_2-macroglobulin can bind two molecules of plasmin. Stearic hindrance of the active site of plasmin by α_2-macroglobulin selectively inhibits plasmin's ability to degrade fibrin, although not fibrinogen or factor VIII. α_2-Macroglobulin weakly inhibits many other components of the fibrinolytic and coagulation systems, including t-PA, streptokinase-plasminogen complexes, and kallikrein.[54]

α_2-Antiplasmin functions as the primary inhibitor of plasmin with α_2-macroglobulin functioning as a physiologic "back-up." Although α_2-antiplasmin is a 10-fold more powerful inhibitor of fibrinolysis than is α_2-macroglobulin, its serum concentration is only half as much.[62] During thrombolytic therapy or DIC the large amount of plasmin that is generated quickly saturates the binding capacity of α_2-antiplasmin, α_2-macroglobulin then becomes important in neutralizing the remaining free plasmin. Plasmin α_2-macroglobulin complexes are removed from the circulation by the reticuloendothelial system.[54]

Other Inhibitors

Several other inhibitors of fibrinolysis have been described, but their physiologic roles are less important. α_2-Antiprotease is a 45-kD single-chain glycoprotein, which is an important inhibitor of neutrophil elastase as well as a broad class of proteases. It is secreted by the liver with a serum concentration of approximately 2.5 mg/dL and a half-life of about 1 week.[57] α_1-Antiprotease levels rise during inflammation, neoplasia, pregnancy, and estrogen therapy, indicating that the inhibitor behaves as an acute-phase reactant. The well-described hereditary α_1-antiprotease deficiency is associated with emphysema and liver disease but not with any disorder of hemostasis.[63]

C-1 inhibitor is a protease that inhibits the activity of the first component of the complement cascade (C1) as well as plasmin, kallikrein, and activated factors XI and XIII. C1-inhibitor is a glycoprotein monomer, which exists in two forms having molecular weights of 96 and 105 kD. Normal plasma levels are between 18 and 22 mg/dL.[64] Deficiencies are associated with hereditary angioedema but not with bleeding tendencies.

Antithrombin III (ATIII) is principally an inhibitor of thrombin and other clotting factors, but it also exhibits plasmin inhibition that is enhanced by heparin. ATIII is a single-chain glycoprotein with a molecular weight of 60 kD. It is synthesized by hepatocytes and endothelial cells and is found in megakaryocytes. The plasma concentration is between 18 and 30 mg/dL, and the normal plasma half-life is approximately 24 hours.[57] ATIII inhibits plasmin by slow, irreversible binding. The binding of heparin to ATIII accelerates plasmin inhibition 50 to 100 times, inducing a conformational change that allows greater access of the ATIII active site to the serine active site of plasmin.[65] The contribution of ATIII to the inhibition of plasmin in vivo is small. Only about 1% of plasmin is bound to ATIII in the circulation, although this increases to 5% in the presence of heparin.[66]

Inhibitors of Plasminogen Activation

PAI-1

PAI-1 is a 52-kD, single-chain glycoprotein consisting of 379 amino acids with a carbohydrate content of 13%. It is synthesized by a variety of cell types, but endothelial cells are the major physiologic source. The molecule is also stored in the alpha granules of platelets, although mostly in the latent form.[67] The PAI-1 gene is 12.2 kB in length, contains 9 exons, and is located on chromosome 7, near the cystic fibrosis gene.[68] Analysis of the promoter region has demonstrated the presence of several enhancer elements that help to confer a high degree of tissue specificity to PAI-1 expression. In endothelial cells, in contrast to other cell types, PAI-1 expression is induced on exposure to a variety of growth factors and cytokines, including glucocorticoids, transforming growth factor-β, tumor necrosis factor-α, interleukin-1, fibroblast growth factor-2, thrombin, angiotensin II, lipoproteins, and bacterial endotoxin.[69]

PAI-1 is initially secreted by endothelial cells as an active molecule that slowly decays over 2 to 4 hours to a latent, or inactive, form.[70, 71] The basis for this latency is a spontaneous conformational change that renders the active site inaccessible to ligands.[72] Latent PAI-1 can be reactivated in vitro after treatment with a number of denaturing agents, and there is some evidence that this can also occur in vivo.[73, 74] Free PAI-1 in the plasma can be stabilized in the active conformation through noncovalent interaction with fibrin and vitronectin, the latter of which also mediates PAI-1 binding to extracellular matrix.[75] Active PAI-1, either free or bound to vitronectin and fibrin, is an effective inhibitor of t-PA and u-PA, although neither scu-PA nor streptokinase. Inhibition occurs, as with other serpins, through a two-step process in which PAI-1 forms a reversible complex with the plasminogen, followed by covalent attachment with subsequent cleavage of a 33-amino acid peptide from the carboxyl terminus of the PAI-1 molecule. t-PA/PAI-1 complexes are cleared from the circulation by the liver.[76]

PAI-1 has been shown to be the most important physiologic inhibitor of plasmin activation and, in concert with α_2-antiplasmin, accounts for the majority of physiologic inhibition of fibrinolysis. The free circulating plasma concentration of PAI-1 in the resting state ranges from 5 to 20 ng/mL, although the molecule exhibits diurnal variation with a morning peak and an afternoon nadir.[77] PAI-1 also behaves as an acute-phase reactant with serum levels increasing 10- to 20-fold during sepsis, DIC, and after surgery. Increased PAI-1 levels are also associated with pregnancy, deep venous thrombosis (DVT), and myocardial infarction.[78–80] Deficiency of PAI-1 is associated with a bleeding diathesis.[81]

PAI-2

PAI-2 is a serpin inhibitor of t-PA and u-PA that was discovered in extracts of placental tissue.[82] The molecule is a single-chain glycoprotein composed of 415 amino acids that exists in two forms: a 47-kD nonglycosylated intracellular form and a 60-kD glycosylated secreted form.[83] The PAI-2 gene is 1.9 kB in length, contains 8 exons, and is located on chromosome 18. PAI-2 inhibits the double-chain forms of both t-PA and u-PA in a manner similar to PAI-1 but does not appreciably inhibit single-chain t-PA and scu-PA at physiological concentrations.

PAI-2 is synthesized by trophoblastic epithelium of fetal origin as well as human monocytes and several monocytic cell lines.[83] In the normal resting state, plasma levels of PAI-2 are undetectable but rise during pregnancy to a mean of 250 ng/mL during the third trimester.[84] The physiological role of PAI-2 is not well understood. Rather than being a major inhibitor of intravascular fibrinolysis, PAI-2 mainly functions to inhibit u-PA that is secreted into the extracellular space.

Others

Several other molecules are known to inhibit plasminogen activators. Protease nexin I is a 43-kD glycoprotein that is produced by fibroblasts, cardiac muscle cells, and kidney epithelial cells.[77] It is an inhibitor of t-PA and u-PA as well as a number of serine proteases, including thrombin, plasmin, and trypsin. Protease nexin I is undetectable in human serum, and its physiological significance is unknown.

An inhibitor of u-PA that was isolated from human urine and termed *PAI-3* has been shown to be identical to protein C inhibitor.[85] PAI-3 is a single-chain glycoprotein with a molecular weight of 57 kD whose main function is to inhibit activated protein C, thus preventing inactivation of activated factors V and VIII. C1-inhibitor, by virtue of its inhibitory effect on plasmin activation, prevents the plasmin-mediated conversion of scu-PA to HMW-UK.

PHYSIOLOGY OF FIBRINOLYSIS

Normal Physiology

The activity of the intravascular fibrinolytic system in the human body exhibits normal physiological variation. A diurnal rhythm exists, with plasma fibrinolytic activity being lowest in the early morning hours and peaking in late afternoon.[86] The major determinant of plasma fibrinolytic activity is the relative plasma level of PAI-1 to t-PA. The levels of several other fibrinolytic inhibitors also exhibit diurnal variation but do not correspond to fluctuations in systemic fibrinolytic activity. Secretion of both t-PA and PAI-1 follow a circadian rhythm, although PAI-1 secretion exhibits a more marked variation (Fig. 17–7). In addition, both behave as acute-phase reactants. Because PAI-1 secretion in response to a physiological stress tends to be more pronounced than that of t-PA, the result is often a net decrease in plasma fibrinolytic activity.

Exercise has long been associated with an increase in fibrinolysis. John Hunter first demonstrated this in 1794 when he showed rapid dissolution of in vivo blood clots with subsequent lack of coagulability in blood from animals that had been exercised before death.[2] In 1947,

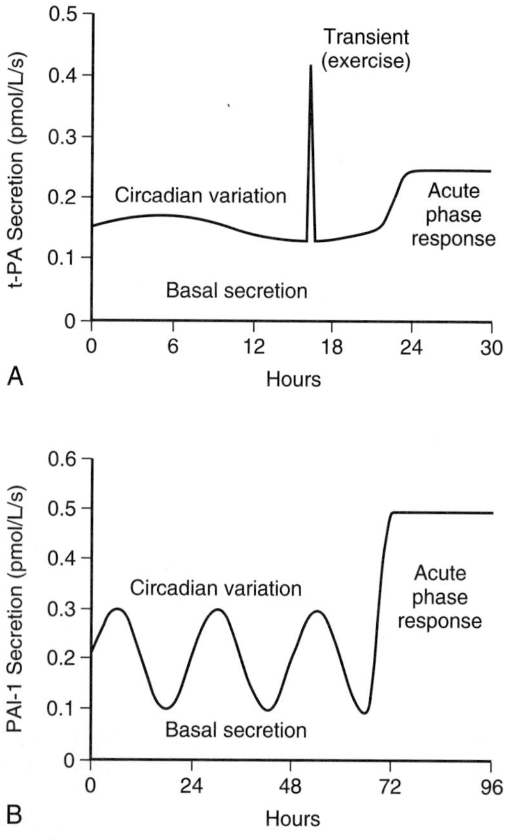

Figure 17–7. Diagram of the temporal secretion patterns for t-PA *(A)* and PAI-1 *(B)*. (Adapted from Chandler WL. The human fibrinolytic system. Crit Rev Oncol Hematol 1996; 24:27.)

Biggs demonstrated an increase in fibrinolytic activity in subjects who vigorously climbed steps of the Radcliffe Observatory at Oxford.[87] This enhancement of fibrinolysis during acute exercise is in part due to epinephrine-mediated release of t-PA from intravascular stores within vascular endothelial cells.[88] PAI-1 levels decrease during exercise, largely due to accelerated clearance of t-PA/PAI-1 complexes. Plasma plasminogen, fibrinogen, and α_2-antiplasmin levels remain unaltered during exercise, although plasminogen and fibrinogen turnover are increased.[89] This increase in fibrinolysis is proportional to the intensity and duration of the exercise. After moderate exercise, tissue plasminogen activator levels decrease rapidly to resting values. After prolonged strenuous exercise, however, fibrinolytic activity may fall below the pre-exercise baseline secondary to depletion of activator stores.[90] Long-term physical conditioning has been shown to enhance t-PA release in response to thrombotic stimuli (e.g., vascular occlusion) and may contribute to the beneficial effect of exercise in reducing the risk of coronary artery disease.[91]

There is no significant difference in fibrinolytic activity between the sexes, although exogenous estrogens and testosterone are known to stimulate fibrinolysis, whereas progestins and anabolic steroids inhibit it.[92] A decrease in fibrinolytic activity is observed during pregnancy and is thought to result from the release of PAI-2 from the placenta.[84] There is a steady decline in fibrinolytic activity with age. A study involving a large cohort of men demonstrated a steady decline in fibrinolytic activity between the ages of 20 and 50, followed by a modest rise until age 65.[33] Racial differences in fibrinolytic activity do exist and seem to be related to levels of tissue plasminogen activator.[93]

Diet, smoking, and alcohol consumption have also been shown to influence fibrinolytic activity. A low-fat diet and caffeine consumption are associated with an increase in fibrinolysis.[94, 95] Long-term consumption of moderate amounts of alcohol increases fibrinolytic activity. Consumption of beer or wine, but not other alcoholic beverages, lowers fibrinolytic activity, suggesting a component other than the alcohol is responsible.[96] Beer also abolishes the diurnal variation of fibrinolytic activity. Cigarette smoking is associated with a decrease in fibrinolytic activity.[97]

Pathologic Variation

Disseminated Intravascular Coagulation

Disseminated intravascular coagulation is not a primary disease entity but occurs secondary to various pathologic conditions. DIC is most often associated with severe infection, malignancy, severe burns or trauma, liver disease, and obstetrical complications including pre-eclampsia, placental abruption, amniotic fluid embolism, and abortion. The hallmark of DIC is the widespread deposition of fibrin clots in small blood vessels, often in association with clotting factor consumption, thrombosis, or a generalized bleeding diathesis. The pathophysiological trigger of DIC is the exposure of circulating blood to tissue factor from injured, necrotic, or neoplastic tissue. Exogenous substances such as bacterial endotoxin or some snake venoms can also activate the coagulation cascade directly or by induction of tissue factor expression on endothelial cells and circulating monocytes. The end result is widespread generation of thrombin, which converts fluid-phase fibrinogen into fibrin. As fibrin monomers are generated, they form circulating soluble complexes, which polymerize, forming fibrin microthrombi that become deposited in the microcirculation of the lungs, kidneys, liver, and skin.

Once the coagulation system is activated, concomitant fibrinolytic activation occurs through thrombin-mediated release of tissue plasminogen activators.[98] Fibrinolysis may also be initiated intrinsically through factor XIII–mediated pathways. The use of fibrinolytic inhibitors in models of DIC enhances deposition of microthrombi and increases the severity of end-organ damage.[99, 100] PAI-1 is also released during DIC and may modulate the overall degree of fibrinolysis.[101] As a result of diffuse activation of both the coagulation and fibrinolytic systems, many of their constitutive components are degraded or depleted. Plasminogen and fibrinogen levels are usually low, but the latter may be in the normal range because of its behavior as an acute-phase reactant.

The severity of DIC can range between a low-grade chronic form, often associated with malignancy, to an acute fulminant form as seen in sepsis, burns, and obstetrical complications. The two major clinical manifestations are bleeding and thrombosis. Which of these predominates depends on the degree of active fibrinolysis. Bleeding by far is the more common and can occur at any site of the body. It occurs secondary to depletion and inhibition of clotting factors, platelets, and lysis of existing hemostatic plugs. The generation of fibrinopeptides A and B further impairs coagulation by inhibiting thrombin-induced fibrin formation and platelet aggregation.[102] Thrombosis usually occurs in association with neoplasms or in states of diminished blood flow as seen during shock.

The diagnosis of DIC is made clinically and confirmed with laboratory studies. The thrombin time (TT), prothrombin time (PT), and activated partial thromboplastin times (aPTT) are usually prolonged but may be normal. Fibrinogen levels are often below 300 mg/dL but rarely may be within the normal range. Generally, a bleeding diathesis does not become manifest until the fibrinogen level falls below 100 mg/dL. Fibrin(ogen) degradation products and fibrinopeptides A and B are usually elevated. Measurement of the FDP D-D dimer is a reliable method for confirming the diagnosis when the fibrinogen levels are within the normal range.[103] The platelet count is often reduced secondary to direct platelet destruction and formation of platelet-fibrin thrombi, which lodge in peripheral small vessels. The peripheral blood smear may reveal red cell fragments consistent with microangiopathic hemolysis, but this finding is much less frequent than in thrombotic thrombocytopenic purpura. Anemia, when present, is not primarily usually due to hemolysis.

Treatment of DIC is aimed at reversal of the underlying condition. Supportive measures include maintenance of volume, correction of electrolytes and acid-base disturbances, and prevention of venous stasis. Transfusion of packed red blood cells and fresh frozen plasma or cryoprecipitate may be given with caution in severely ill patients, but platelet transfusions or replacement of individual clotting factors is of little help and may induce organ damage. The use of heparin remains controversial and is only of marginal benefit in patients experiencing DIC during treatment for promyelocytic leukemia or in patients with a low-grade chronic DIC secondary to malignancy.[104] The use of antifibrinolytic agents such as EACA or tranexamic acid are contraindicated because of the risk of inducing thrombosis.

Malignancy

A variety of hematologic abnormalities are associated with neoplasia. Fifty percent of all cancer patients and 95% of patients with metastatic disease manifest some laboratory abnormality of hemostasis.[105] Although impairment of coagulation, platelet abnormalities, and vascular disorders have been associated with malignancy, most hematologic abnormalities involve a chronic form of DIC.

Malignant tumors have been shown to express tissue factor as well as plasminogen activators. Most human solid and leukemic tumors studied produce urokinase-type plasminogen activators; however, some brain tumors and melanoma cells have been found to produce tissue-type plasminogen activators.[106–109] Over 90% of patients with metastatic disease have elevated fibrinopeptide A levels suggestive of DIC, and as many as 15% of patients with cancer will develop clinically significant DIC.[104]

The clinical manifestations of DIC depend on the balance between coagulation and fibrinolysis. In general, thromboembolic events are more common in patients with solid tumors while hemorrhagic events are more common with the leukemias. Venous thrombosis, either superficial, deep, or migratory (Trousseau's syndrome) is a well-recognized clinical entity and occurs in approximately 5% of cancer patients, especially those with metastatic disease and mucinous adenocarcinoma of the pancreas, lung, prostate, and stomach.[104] Arterial thrombosis is less common than venous thrombosis and usually secondary to embolism of ventricular thrombi (murantic endocarditis). Hemorrhage is a frequent complication of leukemia and accounts for approximately 10% of deaths.[110] DIC occurs in most patients with promyelocytic leukemia, especially during chemotherapy, owing to release of procoagulants and plasminogen activators from cytoplasmic granules. Some 14 to 26% of these patients die of cerebral hemorrhage.[104] Primary fibrinogenolysis without DIC has been described in association with prostate carcinoma but is very rare.[111]

Treatment of DIC in the cancer patient depends on whether thromboembolism or hemorrhage dominates the clinical picture. In patients with a chronic low-grade DIC manifested as recurrent venous thromboses, heparin is the treatment of choice. Unfractionated heparin has been shown to be far superior to warfarin in the treatment of thrombosis associated with malignancy.[112–114] More recently, low-molecular-weight heparin (LMWH) has been shown to be as efficacious as unfractionated heparin in the treatment of venous thromboses with a more favorable side-effect profile.[115] In addition, LMWH may have tumor growth inhibitory properties not associated with unfractionated heparin.[116] The use of antifibrinolytic agents such as EACA and tranexamic acid should not be used except in the rare instance where primary systemic fibrinolysis without intravascular coagulation occurs.

Liver Disease

Liver disease is frequently accompanied by a hemorrhagic diathesis. This bleeding tendency not only results from the coagulopathy secondary to decreased synthesis of coagulation factors by the liver but also from increased fibrinolysis. Several factors increase the plasma fibrinolytic activity in hepatocellular disease, including increased production of plasminogen activators, decreased hepatic clearance of plasminogen activators and activated coagulation factors, and decreased production of fibrinolytic inhibitors.[117, 118]

In contrast to hepatocellular disease, fibrinolytic activity in cholestatic liver disease is decreased proportional to the degree of cholestasis. This is thought to occur secondary to the increased serum β-lipoproteins and triglycerides, which are known to exert an antifibrinolytic effect.[119]

Renal Disease

Renal disease is associated with decreased fibrinolytic activity and elevated fibrinogen levels. This decrease is not related to the degree of renal failure and cannot be significantly improved by dialysis. Several factors are thought to contribute to the decrease in fibrinolytic activity. Renal disease is associated with increased levels of fibrinolytic inhibitors.[120] Second, glomerular injury may cause loss of plasma fibrinolytic proteins including plasminogen, plasminogen activator, fibrinogen, and fibrin degradation products.[121, 122]

Fibrin deposition in the glomeruli is known to occur in patients with acute glomerulonephritis. This deposition has been proposed to stimulate endothelial cell proliferation. The presence of fibrin degradation products in the urine appears to be an indicator of local fibrinolysis and correlates with disease severity.[123] Fibrinolytic therapy has been shown to decrease the amount of proteinuria and to retard the progression of some forms of glomerulonephritis.[124]

Atherosclerotic Vascular Disease

Several disturbances of the fibrinolytic system are associated both with the development of atherosclerotic plaques and with the pathological sequelae of their rupture. Low plasma fibrinolytic activity has been shown to be predictive of future cardiovascular events in young healthy men followed prospectively for up to 16 years.[125] Elevated PAI-1 levels are associated with several traditional risk factors for atherosclerosis, including obesity, hypertriglyceridemia, below-normal high-density-lipoprotein cholesterol, hypertension, and diabetes mellitus.[126] Interestingly, elevated t-PA antigen levels are also associated with many of these same risk factors.[127] This apparent paradox is because free t-PA is cleared from the circulation faster than inactive t-PA complexed with PAI-1.[128] A rise in plasma PAI-1 activity results in a rise of plasma t-PA antigen but a decrease in total plasma t-PA activity.

Diminished systemic fibrinolytic activity predisposes to a relative hypercoaguable state, promoting occlusive thrombus formation at the site of atherosclerotic plaque rupture that may lead to cerebral or myocardial infarction. Several studies have correlated elevated levels of PAI-1 with unstable angina and myocardial infarction.[129] Survivors of myocardial infarction with elevated levels of PAI-1 have been shown to be at increased risk for subsequent reinfarction.[130] Local perturbations in fibrinolytic activity may also play a role in the pathophysiology of plaque rupture. Endothelial cells that are overlying atherosclerotic plaques or adjacent to thrombi have been shown to produce more PAI-1 locally than healthy endothelium.[131]

Venous Occlusion

Venous occlusion is a potent stimulator of t-PA release from the vascular endothelium. The immediate mechanism appears to be increased hydrostatic pressure within the vessel lumen with release of t-PA being proportional to resting fibrinolytic activity[132] DVT, however, is associated with decreased fibrinolysis. Not only are patients with decreased fibrinolytic activity at risk for developing DVT, but many who develop idiopathic DVT have systemic fibrinolytic abnormalities related to defective release of t-PA.[46]

Postoperative DVT is related to fibrinolytic defects that develop in response to surgery.[133] The stress of surgery increases the fibrinolytic activity of circulating blood due to increased release of t-PA. However, fibrinolytic activity declines significantly during the first postoperative week due to depletion of intracellular stores of t-PA as well as a rise in PAI-1 activity.

Inflammation

Inflammation and response to injury invariably involves activation of the clotting and fibrinolytic cascades. Several connections between inflammation and fibrinolysis exist. During tissue injury, exposure of subendothelial collagen and basement membrane to the circulation activates factor XII. As previously described, activated factor XII not only triggers the extrinsic clotting cascade but also is capable of converting plasminogen to plasmin either directly or by activation of factor XI and prekallikrein. Conversely, plasmin is able to directly convert prekallikrein to kallikrein as well as cleave bradykinin from HMW-kininogen.

Plasmin has been shown to activate the complement cascade by two different mechanisms: by direct activation of C1 and by functioning as a C3 convertase, producing C3b and the anaphylatoxin C3a.[134] Non–plasmin-mediated fibrinolysis occurs at the site of injury by release of the proteolytic enzymes elastase and cathepsin G (chymotrypsin-like protease) from the primary granules of polymorphonuclear leukocytes.[135] Digestion of fibrin by these enzymes produces fibrin fragments similar to fdp D and E. Finally, many of the plasmin inhibitors including α_2-antiplasmin, α_2-macroglobulin, α_1-antiprotease, C1-inhibitor, and antithrombin III also function as inhibitors of thrombin, kallikrein, and other enzymes of the coagulation, kinin, and complement systems.

THROMBOLYTIC THERAPY

Thrombolytic Agents

A number of endogenous and exogenous activators of fibrinolysis have been developed for clinical use and have found applications in the treatment of a variety of thromboembolic disorders.

Streptokinase

One of the most extensively studied and clinically employed plasminogen activators is streptokinase. First isolated from group C β-hemolytic streptococci in 1933 by Tillett and Garner, streptokinase is a single-chain glycoprotein with a molecular weight of 47 kD, minimal carbohydrate content, and no intrachain disulfide bridges.[6] The secondary structure is mainly random coil with about 10% alpha helix.[136]

Streptokinase itself has no intrinsic enzymatic activity; therefore, it must form a 1:1 noncovalent complex with one of the various forms of plasminogen before it can become an active catalyst. Forms of plasminogen that can complex with streptokinase include Glu- and Lys-plasminogen or the plasmin B chain.[137] During formation of the streptokinase-plasminogen activator (SK-Plg) complex, an active site on the plasminogen molecule is exposed, without any peptide bond cleavage, that enables the activator complex to convert both complexed and free plasminogen to plasmin. The plasminogen molecule within the activator complex is also susceptible to gradual conversion to plasmin. During this conversion, the streptokinase molecule is cleaved into at least six identifiable fragments ranging in size from 10 to 44 kD.[138] These fragments remain complexed with the plasmin(ogen) moiety, with the resulting complex retaining some degree of activator activity.

In vitro studies have shown that the potency of the SK-Plg activator complex varies directly with the size of the streptokinase fragment and indirectly with the size and the form of plasmin(ogen) with which it is complexed. The intact SK-plasmin B-chain complex has the highest potency, followed by Lys- and then Glu-plasminogen.[139] In vivo, the potency of the activator complex is modulated by several components of the fibrinolytic and coagulation pathways. Fibrin degradation products Y and E bind to plasminogen, enhancing the potency of the activator complex, whereas the binding of α_2-antiplasmin has been found to act as an inhibitor.[140]

Streptokinase activity is quantitated by either clot-lysis or chromogenic substrate methods. The Christensen unit is defined as that quantity of streptokinase required to lyse a clot of defined weight in 10 minutes. This unit is equivalent to 1 IU. One milligram of streptokinase extract contains approximately 3100 IU.[141]

Streptokinase is not appreciably absorbed after repeated oral or rectal dosing.[142] It has a plasma half-life of 18 to 25 minutes after intravenous dosing, with elimination mainly by the reticuloendothelial system. The elimination half-life of the SK-Plg activator complex is much shorter, 1.5 to 2.5 minutes, with clearance also by the reticuloendothelial system.[143, 144]

The SK-Plg activator complex binds fibrin very weakly and slowly by means of the high-affinity LBS on the A chain of plasminogen. Because of its short elimination half-life, little or no clot adsorption occurs. Furthermore, the SK-Plg complex is not inhibited by α_2-antiplasmin. The net result is that degradation of fibrin, fibrinogen, and some clotting factors occurs nonselectively in the fluid phase, producing systemic fibrinogenolysis.

Streptokinase is of bacterial origin; it is antigenic and can induce the production of antistreptokinase antibodies. Most individuals possess low titers of antistreptokinase antibodies on the basis of previous streptococcal infections. Antibody titers can rise 100-fold 2 to 3 weeks after treatment with streptokinase.[145] Titers gradually return to baseline over a period of 4 to 6 months. Because of this preexisting immunity, most treatment protocols require a loading dose of streptokinase to neutralize any antistreptokinase antibodies that might be present. The average dose of streptokinase required to overcome circulating antibodies is about 200,000 IU but may range as high as 1 million IU.

Hypersensivity reactions, mild in degree, occur after streptokinase administration and may be either immediate (IgE-mediated) or delayed (IgG-mediated) type reactions. Fever occurs in 15% to 25% of patients, but body temperature is usually less than 40°C. Nausea, urticaria, pruritus, headache, and flushing occur in less than 15% of patients, with hypotension occurring in less than 5%.[146, 147]

Streptokinase is available in the United States as a lyophilized powder in 250,000-, 750,000- and 1.5 million-IU aliquots.

APSAC

p-Anisoylated plasminogen-streptokinase activator complex (APSAC) is a 131-kD thrombolytic agent derived from modifications of the streptokinase/plasminogen activator complex. The agent is an equimolar noncovalent complex of human plasminogen and streptokinase modified by acylation of the Ser740 residue of the plasminogen catalytic site.[148] Acylation of this catalytic site prevents both fibrinolytic activity and inactivation of the molecule by α_2-antiplasmin. Because the A chain of the plasminogen moiety remains unmodified, APSAC retains the ability to bind to fibrin through the high-affinity LBS on K1.

The fibrinolytic activity of APSAC requires hydrolysis of the acyl group. Deacylation occurs spontaneously in an aqueous environment, exhibits first-order kinetics, and is dependent on the structure of the acyl group. p-Anisoyl derivatives have serum deacylation half-lives of approximately 105 minutes in vitro.[149] The plasma elimination half-life of APSAC mostly depends on the deacylation rate, but administered dose, uptake by the reticuloendothelial system, and dissociation of streptokinase from plasminogen also influence clearance. Half-lives of 88 to 112 minutes have been reported in patients receiving 30 U for treatment of myocardial infarction.[144, 150]

APSAC has a thrombolytic potency 10 times that of streptokinase when measured by in vitro assays.[151] Direct measurement of the fibrinolytic activity half-life of APSAC in vitro using the fibrin plate method with pooled human plasma has been reported to be approximately 120 minutes.[152] This compares with 15 to 20 minutes for streptokinase or preformed streptokinase-plasmin complex. In vitro studies have also shown that, like streptokinase-plasminogen complex, APSAC does have increased fibrinolytic activity in the presence of fibrin (8-fold increase), although not as dramatic as t-PA (590-fold increase).[153]

Unlike streptokinase, the delay in deacylation of APSAC allows for binding of the agent to fibrin before production of an active complex, thus theoretically increasing fibrinolysis at the site of thrombus formation and decreasing systemic fibrinolysis. Unfortunately, the degree of fibrin specificity in vivo has proved to be considerably less than expected. Systemic activation of the fibrinolytic system in humans appears to be dose related with significant reductions in fibrinogen (up to 90% after a 30-U intravenous dose), plasminogen, α_2-antiplasmin, and elevation of fibrinogen-fibrin degradation products (greater than 100 mg/L).[149] These changes begin quickly after drug administration, peak at about 1 hour, and persist for 24 to 48 hours. Although many coagulation factors, including factors V and VIII, are potential substrates for plasmin, significant reductions do not occur, and therefore prolongation of clotting times are not usually seen after APSAC administration.

Like streptokinase, APSAC is immunogenic. Healthy volunteers given low doses of APSAC develop antistreptokinase antibody titers as high as 60-fold within 2 to 3 weeks, with persistence of significant titers at 3 months after administration.[154, 155] The thrombolytic potency of this agent is also dependent on the presence and titer of antistreptokinase antibodies. One study involved administration of APSAC to patients with myocardial infarction. Patients with low to moderate antistreptokinase titers (less than 1:50) had a dose-related response to low-dose APSAC (less than 10 U), whereas patients with high antistreptokinase titers (greater than 1:100) had little response.[156] In general, higher doses now routinely used in the treatment of patients with myocardial infarction easily overcome resistance and achieve a sufficient fibrinolytic effect.

APSAC (generic name: anistreplase) is supplied as a lyophilized powder in vials containing 30 U aliquots. One unit of APSAC is approximately 1 mg of material and contains approximately 36,000 IU of streptokinase.

Staphylokinase

Staphylokinase is a plasminogen activator produced by certain lysogenic strains of *Staphylococcus aureus*. The gene for staphylokinase (sakSTAR) is found in the genomic DNA of *S. aureus* as well as in the bacteriophages sak(C) and sak42D.[157–159] Staphylokinase is translated as a 163-amino acid nonglycosylated protein that contains a 27-amino acid signal peptide and no disulfide bonds. The mature molecule is composed of 136 amino acids and has a molecular weight of 18 kD.[157, 160] Several truncated forms of staphylokinase have been purified that differ in molecular weight and isoelectric points. Sak-(6) and Sak-(10) lack the respective 6 and 10 amino-terminal residues of sakSTAR and appear to be produced on interaction with plasmin(ogen).[161]

Like streptokinase, staphylokinase is an indirect activator of plasminogen, although the two molecules share no significant homology and have several distinct differences in their mechanisms of action. Staphylokinase binds to plasminogen to form a 1:1 noncovalent complex. Unlike the binding of streptokinase to plasminogen, which exposes the plasminogen active site, resulting in an active SK-Plg complex, binding of staphylokinase to plasminogen does not result in an active Sak-Plg complex. Plasminogen within the Sak-Plg complex must first be converted to plasmin to expose the active site.[161] The conversion of Sak-Plg to Sak-Pln occurs in a rate-limiting fashion that is accelerated by Sak-Pln itself. The staphylokinase molecule within the Sak-Plg/Pln complexes is also cleaved by plasmin to Sak-(10). Sak-(10) has been shown to have nearly identical plasminogen-activating as mature staphylokinase.[160]

A second major difference is that the Sak-Pln complex is rapidly inhibited by α_2-antiplasmin whereas the SK-Plg complex is not.[162] α_2-Antiplasmin dissociates staphylokinase, or Sak-(10), from the activator complex and forms an inactive covalent α_2-antiplasmin-plasmin complex. Binding of α_2-antiplasmin to plasmin occurs through the high affinity LBS, which also mediates the binding of plasmin to fibrin. The displaced staphylokinase, or Sak-(10) molecule, is available to bind other free plasminogen molecules.

A third major difference is the significant fibrin specificity of staphylokinase. This fibrin specificity is due mainly to the rapid inhibition of Sak-Pln in the free circulation of α_2-antiplasmin and prevention of plasmin-mediated conversion of Sak-Plg to Sak-Pln. In the presence of fibrin, α_2-antiplasmin cannot appreciably bind to plasmin and its ability to inhibit Sak-Pln or prevent conversion of Sak-Plg is inhibited nearly 100-fold.[163] The fibrin specificity of staphylokinase has been demonstrated in animal models of thrombosis, in which, on a molar basis, it was demonstrated to be equivalent to streptokinase in thrombolytic potency but without significant systemic fibrinogenolysis.[164] In addition, staphylokinase may be more active than streptokinase against platelet-rich clots.[165]

Recombinant staphylokinase produced in bacteria has a half-life of approximately 6 minutes after a 10-mg intravenous infusion in patients treated for myocardial infarction.[166] In these same patients, neutralizing antistaphylokinase antibodies were low at baseline but rose significantly 14 to 35 days after treatment. Significantly, no cross reactivity with streptokinase was observed. As with streptokinase and APSAC, the immunogenicity of staphylokinase precludes readministration of the drug. Several staphylokinase mutants have been produced that appear to have preserved thrombolytic potency in animal models but with reduced immunogenicity.[167, 168] Staphylokinase has not yet been approved for clinical use.

Urokinase

Urokinase for clinical use was initially obtained by purification of human urine. Because normal human urine contains only a small amount of urokinase, approximately 1500 L of urine was required to purify enough of the drug for a single thrombolytic treatment.[48] Urokinase is now produced in large quantities from tissue culture of human fetal kidney cells. Commercially available preparations are a mixture of high- and low-molecular-weight urokinase.

Several different activity units for urokinase have been used. In the United States, the activity of urokinase is standardized according to its ability to lyse a fibrin clot by plasmin activation.[169] A single milligram of urokinase contains approximately 2667 IU of activity.[170] Other expressions of activity include the Ploug unit (approximately 1.33 IU) and the Committee on Thrombolytic Agents (CTA) unit, which is approximately equal to the IU.

Although urokinase is not available for oral administration in humans, experiments in dogs have shown that significant oral absorption of enteric-coated urokinase does occur.[171] Various animal studies indicate that degradation and elimination of urokinase occur via hepatic pathways.[172] Determination of elimination half-lives has varied with the methodologies employed. Radiolabelling of urokinase molecules reveals elimination after a biexponential curve, with a first phase half-life of 13 to 20 minutes and a second phase half-life of 3 to 10 hours.[47] This extended phase possibly represents elimination of radiolabeled metabolites. When activity assays are employed, a half-life of 9 to 16 minutes is reported.[173] Like streptokinase, the in vivo effect of the drug is more consistent with rapid elimination.

Urokinase does have a weak affinity for fibrin, although the predominant in vivo effect is the production of a systemic fibrinolysis.[174] When measured by depletion of fibrinogen, plasminogen, and α_2-antiplasmin, or elevation of fibrinogen degradation products, urokinase appears to have about half the systemic fibrinolytic effects of streptokinase.[175] Unlike streptokinase, urokinase is not immunogenic. It can therefore be readministered at any time it is indicated. Approximately 15% of patients receiving urokinase may develop low-grade fevers.[176, 177]

Urokinase is supplied as a lyophilized powder in 250,000-IU aliquots. Urokinase for use to restore patency to clotted central intravenous catheters is supplied as a lyophilized powder of 500 IU/vial.

Recombinant scu-PA

Single-chain urokinase-type plasminogen activator is the physiologic precursor to urokinase. Unlike urokinase, scu-PA exhibits a modest degree of fibrin specificity that is not related to fibrin binding. Initially purified from human urine or cell culture, recombinant scu-PA (rscu-PA) is now obtained as a full-length unglycosylated protein from *Escherichia coli.*[178] The activity of scu-PA is assessed after conversion to the two-chain form by plasmin and expressed at latent urokinase activity. One milligram of recombinant scu-PA has a specific latent urokinase activity of approximately 160,000 IU.[179] Like urokinase, scu-PA is nonimmunogenic.

Recombinant scu-PA is rapidly cleared from the plasma by hepatic uptake with a half-life of 6 to 8 minutes.[180, 181] First-pass extraction by the liver is so efficient that hepatic blood flow becomes the rate-limiting step in scu-PA clearance. Patients with decreased hepatic blood flow, such as those with heart failure, have increased u-PA levels and systemic fibrinogenolysis after administration of scu-PA for the treatment of myocardial infarction.[182] Despite its theoretical clot specificity, rscu-PA exhibits substantial systemic fibrinolytic effects that appear to be dose-dependent. In a large trial comparing rscu-PA to streptokinase for the treatment of myocardial infarction, administration of 80 mg of rscu-PA resulted in a fall in the fibrinogen concentration from 250 mg/dL to 35 mg/dL, compared with a fall from 240 mg/dL to 15 mg/dL with 1.5 million IU of streptokinase. Fibrin(ogen) degradation products following rscu-PA rose from a median of 1.5 mg/dL to 144 mg/dL, whereas streptokinase resulted in a median increase from 1.5 mg/dL to more than 200 mg/dL.[183] In comparison with urokinase, rscu-PA has virtually identical effects on hemostatic components in patients treated for acute myocardial infarction.[184]

scu-PA is not yet approved for clinical use in the United States. In Europe, rscu-PA (generic name: saruplase) is available as a lyophilized powder in 10-mg aliquots.

Recombinant t-PA

Although identification of t-PA was first made by Astrup and Permin in 1947, it was not until the early 1980s that sufficient quantities for clinical studies could be isolated from the supernatant of a melanoma cell line.[185] In 1983, recombinant t-PA (rt-PA) became available and was shown to be nearly identical to that derived from cell culture except in the degree of glycosylation.[186] Several preparations of rt-PA exist that differ in the ratio of single- to double-chain species. Initial trials of rt-PA in humans employed preparations consisting of mainly double-chain species, although most trials in this country now employ preparations consisting of 70% to 80% single-chain rt-PA.[187]

rt-PA is standardized by the International Committee for Thrombosis and Hemostasis according to a clot lysis assay. t-PA derived from a melanoma cell line has an activity of about 500,000 IU/mg, whereas single- and double-chain rt-PA have activities of approximately 580,000 and 300,000 IU, respectively.[187]

rt-PA is not absorbed orally, and absorption after intramuscular administration is poor.[188] The onset of action of intravenously administered drug is rapid, and elimination is dose dependent and best described by a two-compartment model.[187] The initial half-life of single-chain rt-PA is 3 to 5 minutes with a terminal half-life of 40 to 55 minutes. The initial half-life of the double-chain form is 4 to 6 minutes with a comparable terminal half-life. The half-life of fibrinolytic activity of both forms ranges from 3 to 9 minutes. Clearance is predominantly by hepatic uptake and degradation.[128, 189] Renal failure does not affect steady-state concentrations of rt-PA.[190]

Because the enzymatic activity of the tissue-type plasminogen activators is greatly enhanced in the presence of fibrin, rt-PA manifests a degree of in vitro clot specificity modestly greater than seen with streptokinase or urokinase. The same degree of fibrin specificity has not been demonstrated in vivo. Studies in patients with myocardial infarction indicate that a modest degree of systemic activation of the fibrinolytic system does occur, resulting in moderate decreases of plasma fibrinogen (up to 50%) and plasminogen, with elevation of fibrinogen-fibrin degradation products.[191] Prolongation of clotting times is usually minimal, and bleeding times remain normal in over 60% of patients.[192] This systemic fibrinogenolytic effect is likely due to the high plasma concentrations of rt-PA achieved during thrombolytic therapy and is not as pronounced as that seen with streptokinase or urokinase administration. Fibrinogenolysis is slightly less with the single-chain than with the double-chain rt-PA species.

rt-PA is produced by several manufacturers. In the United States the single-chain species is the only product currently licensed. It is supplied as a lyophilized powder in 20-mg (11.6 million IU) and 50-mg (29 million IU) aliquots. Double-chain rt-PA is available only in Europe.

Novel Tissue-Type Plasminogen Activators

Although t-PA is modestly fibrin specific and nonantigenic, its short half-life and inactivation by PAI-1 are distinct disadvantages to its use as a thrombolytic agent. Several novel t-PA mutants have been developed that attempt to improve the efficacy and safety of thrombolytic therapy as well as the ease of administration.

r-PA (Fig. 17–8*A*) is a deletion mutant of t-PA that lacks the finger, epidermal growth factor, and first kringle (K1) domain of the wild-type molecule. Because r-PA is a recombinant protein produced in *E. coli,* it is nonglycosylated and is initially translated as an inert inclusion body that requires in vitro folding before being rendered enzymatically active.[193] Both the epidermal growth factor and K1 domains mediate the binding of t-PA to hepatic receptors, facilitating its clearance from the circulation. Their elimination greatly prolongs the plasma half-life of r-PA. After intravenous bolus administration in both healthy individuals and patients suffering from myocardial infarction, the plasma half-life of the r-PA antigen was found to be 14 to 19 minutes, some 4 to 5 times longer than the half-life of rt-PA.[194] The finger domain of t-PA contributes to fibrin binding. In vitro studies demonstrate that the binding of r-PA to fibrin is fivefold lower than rt-PA and that fibrin-mediated enhancement of plasminogenolytic activity is fourfold lower, despite the fact that both molecules have equivalent activities in the absence of fibrin.[193] In animal models of both arterial and venous thrombosis, r-PA was found to be 5 to 12 times more potent than rt-PA.[195, 196] Significantly, however, at equivalent doses (based on 50% thrombolytic efficacy) both molecules produced an approximate 25% fall in plasma fibrinogen concentration.[196]

r-PA (generic name: reteplase) is supplied as a lyophilized powder in 10.8-U (10.8 mg) aliquots. The drug has been approved in the United States for the treatment of acute myocardial infarction.

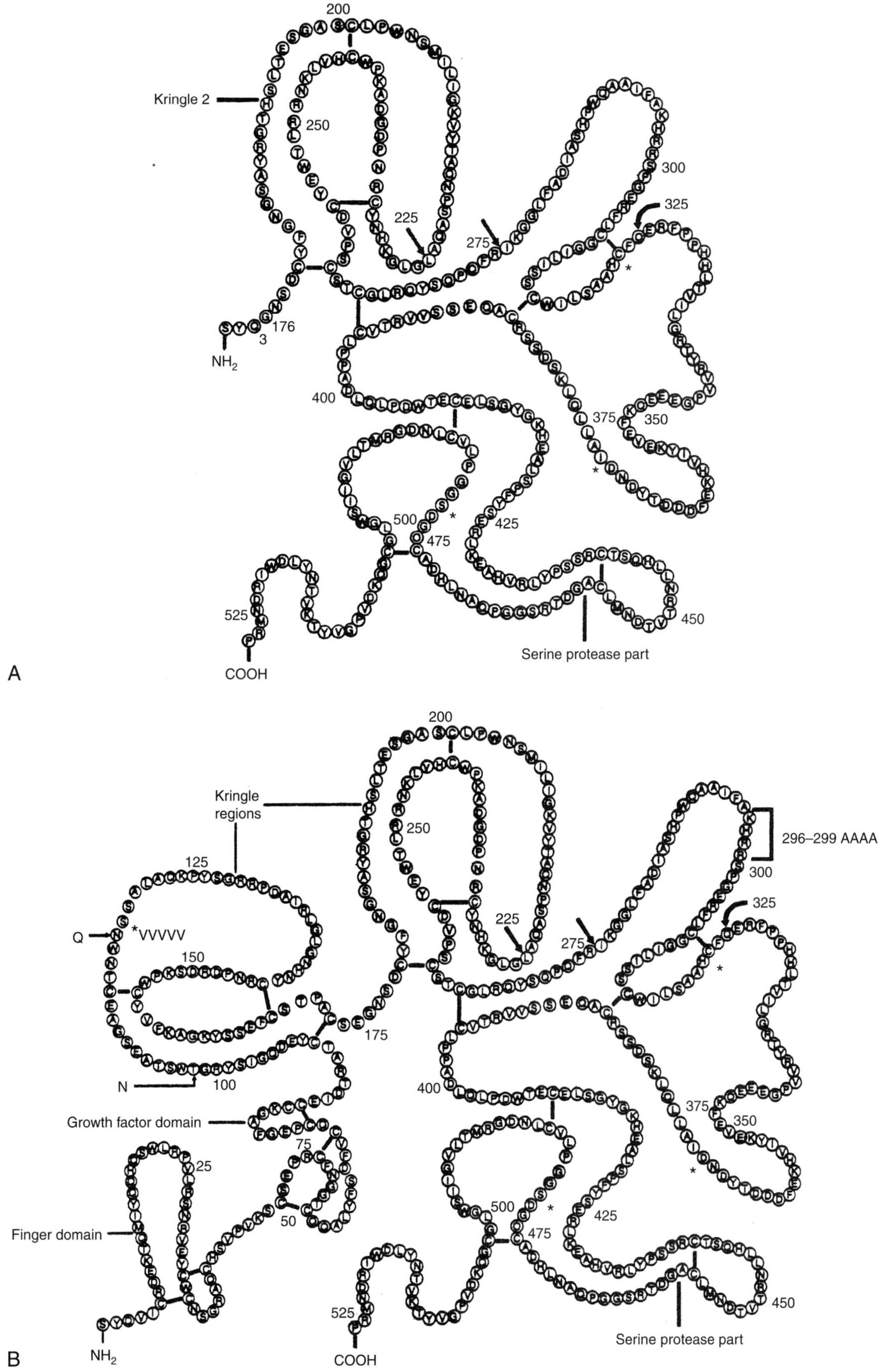

Figure 17–8. Schematic model of reteplase *(A)* and TNK-tPA *(B)*. The *arrows* indicate the plasmin cleavage sites. (Adapted from Verstraete M, Lijnen HR, Collen D. Thrombolytic agents in development. Drugs 1995; 50:29.)

Table 17–1. Comparative Features of Thrombolytic Agents Used in the Treatment of Myocardial Infarction

	Intracoronary Streptokinase	Streptokinase	Urokinase	APSAC	Alteplase	Reteplase	scu-PA	TNK-tPA	Lanoteplase	Staphylokinase
Dose	2000 IU/min	1.5 million IU	3 million IU	30 U	100 mg	20 mg	30 U	50 mg	120 IU/kg	30 mg
Duration of Infusion	90–120 min	60 min	60 min	Bolus	90 min	Double bolus	Bolus	Bolus	Bolus	Double bolus
Half-Life	18–25 min	18–25 min	9–16 min	90–110 min	3–5 min	14–19 min	90–110 min	18 min	30–45 min	6 min
Plasminogen Activation	Indirect	Indirect	Direct	Direct	Direct	Direct	Direct	Direct	Direct	Indirect
Fibrin Specificity	1+	1+	1+	1+	3+	2+	3+	4+	2+	4+
Fibrinogenolysis	1+	4+	3+	4+	1+	1+	2+	1+	1+	1+
90-Minute Patency	70%	50–60%	55–65%	65–75%	75–85%	80–85%	70–85%	80–85%	80–85%	80–85%
Allergic Reactions	Yes	Yes	No	Yes	No	No	No	No	No	Yes
Intracranial Hemorrhage	<0.3%	0.3–0.5%	<0.6%	0.6%	<1.0%	<1.0%	<1.0%	<1.0%	<1.0%	<1.0%
Cost ($) per Dose	1+	1+	4+	3+	3+	3+	3+	NA	NA	NA

Adapted from Marder VJ, Sherry S. Thrombolytic therapy: current status (second of two parts). N Engl J Med 1988; 318:1585; and White HD, Van de Werf FJJ. Thrombolysis for acute myocardial infarction. Circulation 1998; 97:1632.

TNK-tPA (see Fig. 17–8*B*) is a mutant of rt-PA containing three separate amino acid substitutions: Asp for Thr103, Gln for Asn117, and four Ala repeats for Lys296 through Arg299.[197] These first two-point mutations result in prolongation of the serum half-life by adding an additional glycosylation site at Asp113 and by eliminating the N-linked high mannose-type glycosylation site at Asn117, which mediates clearance of wild-type t-PA by high-affinity hepatic mannose receptors. After intravenous bolus administration in rabbits, TNK-tPA manifests biexponential clearance with α and β half-life values of 9 and 31 minutes, respectively. In humans, the plasma half-life is approximately 17 minutes, compared with a half-life of 3 minutes for rt-PA.[198] Substitution of Lys296-Arg299 for four alanine residues provides the molecule with greater fibrin specificity as well as an 80-fold greater resistance to PAI-1 inhibition compared with wild-type t-PA. In a rabbit model of arteriovenous shunt thrombosis, TNK-tPA was found to be 8- and 13-fold more potent than rt-PA in lysing whole blood and platelet-rich clots, respectively.[197] Administration of up to 50 mg of TNK-tPA in humans during myocardial infarction resulted in only 3% and 13% reductions in fibrinogen and plasminogen, respectively, confirming the molecule's relative fibrin specificity in humans.[198]

n-PA (generic name: lanoteplase) is a mutant of rt-PA where the finger and epidermal growth factor domains have been deleted and glutamine is substituted for Asn117.[199] Like TNK-tPA, substitution of Asn117 on the first kringle domain removes the high mannose-type N-linked glycosylation site, thus diminishing hepatic clearance of the molecule. In rabbits, the clearance of n-PA was found to be monoexponential with a half-life of 49 minutes after a single intravenous bolus injection. Like r-PA, n-PA has reduced fibrin binding, owing to deletion of the finger domain. In a rabbit venous thrombosis model, n-PA was found to be nearly ninefold more potent than rt-PA on a per weight basis. At equipotent doses, there were no significant differences in fibrinogen or α_2-antiplasmin depletion between the two compounds.[199]

Clinical Applications of Thrombolytic Therapy

Myocardial Infarction

Acute myocardial infarction (MI) is a major cause of morbidity and mortality in most western countries and accounts for over half a million deaths annually in the United States. The rationale for using a thrombolytic agent in the setting of acute MI is based on several principles. First, rupture of an atherosclerotic plaque with formation of an overlying occlusive thrombus is the proximate cause of the vast majority of myocardial infarctions. In the first hours of an acute MI, over 80% of patients have identifiable thrombi by coronary angiography.[200] Second, myocardial necrosis is proportional to the duration and the degree of myocardial hypoperfusion. Third, mortality is directly related to the extent of myocardial necrosis and severity of left ventricular dysfunction. Timely restoration of blood flow to ischemic myocardium with the use of thrombolytic therapy limits the extent of myocardial necrosis and preserves left ventricular function, thereby improving survival. To date, the U.S. Food and Drug Administration (FDA) has approved five agents for the treatment of acute MI. Streptokinase, urokinase, alteplase (single-chain rt-PA), anistreplase (APSAC), and reteplase (r-PA) are approved for systemic administration, while streptokinase and urokinase are also approved for intracoronary administration. Approval is expected shortly expected for intravenous administration of rscu-PA (saruplase) (Table 17–1).

The immediate goal of thrombolytic therapy is rapid and complete reperfusion of ischemic myocardium. Early attempts at thrombolytic therapy employed intracoronary infusions of streptokinase, which resulted in reperfusion of approximately 70% of occluded vessels.[200] This compares to spontaneous reperfusion rates of approximately 20%. Because of the obligate delays inherent in cardiac catheterization and the observation that thrombi become more resistant to lysis with age, focus quickly shifted away from intracoronary to systemic intravenous administration.

Conclusions about the comparative efficacies of the different thrombolytic agents come from a large number of clinical trials, many of which differ in study design, primary end-points, and use of adjunctive therapy. rt-PA, given in an accelerated "front-labeled" dosing regimen[201] manifests the fastest reperfusion velocity, with 90-minute patency rates of approximately 85% (Fig. 17–9).[202] Standard-dosed rt-PA and APSAC achieve patency in approximately 70%, similar to intracoronary streptokinase.[203] Intravenous streptokinase and urokinase are associated with significantly lower 90-minute patency rates (50–65%)

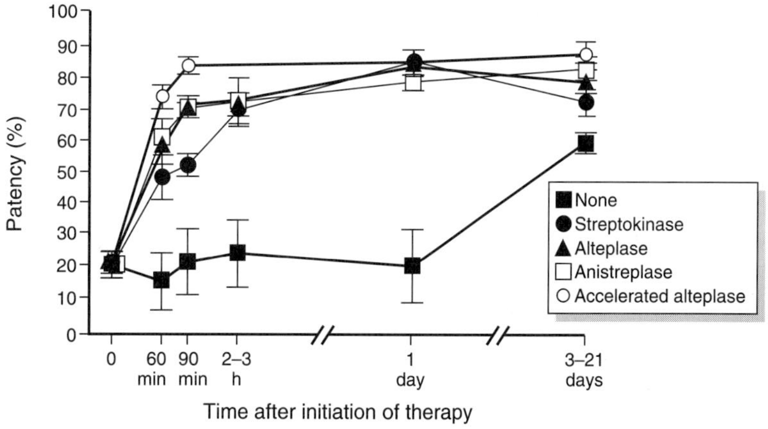

Figure 17–9. Pooled analysis of angiographic patency rates over time after administration of various thrombolytic agents. (Adapted from Granger CB, Califf RM, Topol EJ. Thrombolytic therapy for acute myocardial infarction. Drugs 1992; 44:293.)

compared with the other agents, especially when administered later than 4 hours in the course of an evolving MI.[203–205] Despite a slower reperfusion velocity, streptokinase administration results in late vessel patency rates comparable to other agents.[183, 203]

An important related issue is that of reocclusion after initial successful thrombolysis. Early reocclusion of an otherwise successfully reperfused infarct-related artery impairs recovery of left ventricular function and is associated with a doubling of the mortality rate.[206] Re-thrombosis occurs because of the persistence of thrombogenic stimuli associated with atherosclerotic plaque rupture as well as from thrombin released from the dissolving clot. Reocclusion occurs in 5% to 30%, depending on the thrombolytic agent and the adjunctive therapy.[207] Non–fibrin-selective agents (e.g., streptokinase) are less prone to reocclusion than are the fibrin-selective agents (e.g., rt-PA), in large part due to fibrinogen depletion and maintenance of a "systemic lytic state." In early studies, rt-PA was associated with up to a 30% risk of reocclusion, although with the concurrent use of intravenous heparin this rate has fallen to an average of 13%.[203] This compares to an average reocclusion rate of only 8% for intravenous streptokinase. The concurrent use of aspirin not only improves initial patency but has also been shown to decrease the incidence of re-thrombosis and reinfarction.[208, 209]

Survival after an acute MI is in large part dependent on preservation of left ventricular function. Numerous studies involving several different agents have demonstrated consistent improvement in global and regional ventricular function after successful thrombolytic therapy.[210–215] Improvement is most notable in patients with reperfusion within 1 to 3 hours after the onset of symptoms. The angiographic substudy of the GUSTO trial has conclusively demonstrated that both left ventricular function and survival vary proportionally with the speed and degree of reperfusion achieved, regardless of the thrombolytic agent employed.[216] In addition to limitation of actual infarct size, successful reperfusion may have a role in limiting infarct expansion and aneurysm formation through beneficial effects on ventricular remodeling.[217]

Over the past decade, nine large placebo-controlled trials have addressed the impact of thrombolytic therapy on survival in acute MI. Pooled results of these studies indicate that thrombolytic therapy results in the avoidance of 18 deaths per 1000 patients treated.[218] Patients who benefit the most from thrombolytic therapy are those treated within 1 to 3 hours of symptom onset, those with electrocardiographic evidence of transmural ischemia or new left bundle-branch block, and those with anterior infarcts. There is no benefit in patients treated 12 to 24 hours after symptom onset. Patients treated later than 24 hours after the onset of symptoms have an increased mortality risk, in part due to an increased risk of ventricular rupture.[219] Although the elderly (age older than 75 years) have an overall higher mortality, thrombolytic therapy significantly decreases mortality with the avoidance of 10 deaths per 1000 patients treated.[218]

There have also been three international "mega" trials directly comparing different thrombolytic agents and dosing regimens in terms of overall infarct survival. The GISSI-2 trial randomized 12,490 patients with ECG evidence of acute MI within 6 hours of symptom onset to receive either 1.5 million IU of streptokinase or 100 mg of rt-PA (altephase) with and without heparin as adjunctive therapy.[220] In-hospital mortality rates of approximately 9% were similar for both groups, irrespective of adjunctive heparin therapy, infarct site, time from symptom onset, age, or Killip class. The ISIS-3 trial randomized 46,092 patients with clinical suspicion of myocardial infarction within the previous 24 hours to receive either streptokinase, APSAC, or double-chain rt-PA (duteplase) with and without heparin.[221] There were no significant mortality differences at 35 days between the three agents, even among subgroups receiving heparin, having ST-segment elevations, or presenting within 6 hours of symptom onset.

One common criticism of these studies was that the rt-PA was not optimally administered. The GUSTO trial took this into account when randomizing 41,021 patients within 6 hours of onset of MI to "front-loaded" rt-PA (alteplase) plus intravenous heparin, streptokinase plus subcutaneous heparin, streptokinase plus intravenous heparin, or a combination of the thrombolytic agents plus intravenous heparin.[222] Mortality at 30 days was significantly lower in the "front-loaded" rt-PA group (Fig. 17–10) than in the other groups (6.3% vs. 7.0%–7.4%), resulting in the avoidance of 10 deaths per 1000 patients treated.

As a result of the GUSTO trial, front-loaded alteplase with concurrent intravenous heparin is now the "gold standard" against which newer thrombolytic agents and dosing regimens are compared. Studies suggest that several of the newer thrombolytic agents, including reteplase (r-PA), saruplase (scu-PA), and staphylokinase may achieve similar or slightly higher 90-minute patency rates than front-loaded altephase.[223–226] Despite a faster reperfusion velocity, reteplase has been shown to be equivalent, but not superior, to front-loaded alteplase in terms of 30-day mortality.[227] Saruplase, staphylokinase, n-PA, and TNK-PA have yet to be compared to front-loaded alteplase in trials of sufficient size to generate conclusions about effects on mortality.

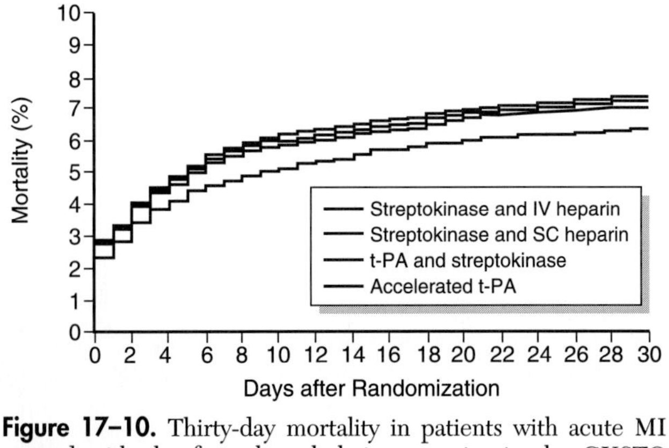

Figure 17–10. Thirty-day mortality in patients with acute MI treated with the four thrombolytic strategies in the GUSTO trial. (Adapted from the GUSTO investigations, an international randomized trial comparing four thrombolytic strategies for acute myocardial infection. N Engl J Med 1993; 329:673.)

Minor bleeding associated with thrombolytic therapy appears independent of the agent employed and is estimated at 15% to 25%.[146, 147] Serious bleeding occurs in 1% to 5% of patients.[218, 221, 222] Although streptokinase produces greater systemic fibrinogenolysis than the other more fibrin-selective agents, depletion of fibrinogen and production of fibrinogen degradation products correlates only weakly with overall bleeding complications. Bleeding is due more to disruption of hemostatic plugs at sites of vascular injury than to defects in blood coagulation.[228]

The most serious complication of thrombolytic therapy is intracranial hemorrhage. Most studies employing streptokinase report incidences of less than 0.5%. The use of rt-PA in doses up to 150 mg is associated with a higher risk of intracranial hemorrhage of approximately 1.6%.[229] rt-PA doses of 100 mg given in a front-loaded regimen are associated with rates slightly higher than with streptokinase. The GUSTO trial found the incidence of intracranial hemorrhage in the rt-PA group (0.72%) to be higher than those of the streptokinase groups (0.49% to 0.54%) but lower than the group receiving the combination of rt-PA and streptokinase (0.94%).[222]

Deep Venous Thrombosis

Deep venous thrombosis is a commonly encountered clinical entity that is frequently asymptomatic, although it can present as a life-threatening pulmonary embolus. The most common long-term sequela of proximal lower-extremity DVT remains the postphlebitic syndrome, which can occur in up to 94% of patients.[230] Caused mainly by disruption of the deep venous valvular system leading to venous hypertension, appearance of the postphlebitic syndrome is usually delayed for many years. Clinically, this syndrome is characterized by persistent swelling, pain, and pigmentation changes of the lower extremity that eventually lead to stasis ulceration. The risk of recurrent DVT is also increased in affected extremities.

Traditional therapy for DVT consists of symptomatic treatment combined with anticoagulation, mainly with unfractionated or low-molecular-weight heparin for the first 3 to 5 days followed by warfarin for a period of 3 to 6 months.[231] Although effective at preventing thrombus extension, these agents do not appreciably promote clot lysis. The rationale behind the use of thrombolytic therapy is to effect clot lysis rapidly, thus minimizing damage to venous valves and avoiding complications of the postphlebitic syndrome. Unfortunately, only 7% to 22% patients with proximal lower extremity DVT lack significant contraindications to thrombolytic therapy.[232, 233] There is no evidence to suggest that thrombolytic therapy is more efficacious in preventing pulmonary embolism than routine anticoagulation.[234]

The thrombolytic agents most widely studied for the treatment of proximal DVT are streptokinase and urokinase. Dosing schedules for streptokinase were adopted in the late 1960s and designed to overcome antistreptococcal antibody resistance that is present in over 90% of the population.[235] A standard regimen consists of a bolus infusion of 250,000 IU over 1 hour followed by an hourly infusion of 100,000 IU for up to 7 days. Based on a comprehensive review of multiple clinical trials using similar regimens, thrombolytic therapy results in complete or substantial lysis of lower extremity DVT in 50% to 90% of patients.[236] This compares to partial or complete clot lysis rates of 0% to 28% with heparin alone. Venogram-documented resolution of thrombosis occurs nearly four times more often with streptokinase and urokinase than with heparin but may be slightly more often associated with bleeding.[237] Factors associated with successful therapy include shorter duration of symptoms, lesser degree and length of occlusion, more proximal location of thrombus, and achievement of a systemic fibrinogenolytic state. Of these, age of thrombus appears to be the most critical, with the highest response rates seen in patients treated within the first 3 days.[238] There is a gradual decline in response rates from 3 to 14 days.

Pooled results of comparison trials demonstrate normal follow-up venograms in nearly 50% of patients treated with streptokinase and urokinase but in less than 5% of patients treated with heparin.[236] Valve function studies are normal in 40% to 75% of patients treated with urokinase. Patients with normal venograms are more likely to have normal valvular function and remain asymptomatic, whereas patients with thrombotic remnants and incompetent valves tend to develop symptoms of the postphlebitic syndrome. Although difficult to quantitate, successful thrombolysis with streptokinase and urokinase with preservation of valvular architecture appears to prevent the postphlebitic syndrome.

Urokinase is often used for the treatment of DVT when streptokinase is contraindicated or not tolerated. Several small prospective trials comparing the two agents have been conducted.[238, 239] van de Loo and colleagues randomized 40 patients with venogram-documented DVT to either streptokinase, 250,000 IU bolus followed by 100,000 IU/hour, or urokinase, 4000 U/kg IV loading dose over 30 minutes followed by 4000 U/kg IV per hour.[238] After an average of 5 days of therapy, 79% of the streptokinase group and 83% of the urokinase group had substantial clot lysis. Of note, 42% of patients in the streptokinase group and none in the urokinase group failed to complete therapy due to adverse effects. Fever and bleeding accounted for the majority of events in the streptokinase recipients.

There is less experience with rt-PA in the treatment of proximal DVT. Several small trials have been conducted using various dosing regimens of rt-PA. Goldhaber and associates employed 24-hour infusions of 0.05 mg/kg/hour of rt-PA (up to 150 mg) and found more than 50% thrombolysis in 10 of 36 (28%) of patients compared with none of 17 (0%) patients treated with heparin.[240] Turpie and colleagues randomized 83 patients to either heparin or 0.5 mg/kg rt-PA infused over 4 or 8 hours.[241] Fifty percent thrombolysis occurred in 58% of patients in the 4-hour rt-PA infusion group, in 21% of subjects in the 8-hour rt-PA infusion group, but in only 7% of patients in the heparin group. There have been no trials directly comparing the efficacy of rt-PA to streptokinase or urokinase. To date, streptokinase and urokinase are the only two agents with FDA approval for the treatment of DVT.

Pulmonary Embolism

Pulmonary embolism (PE) is reported in over 500,000 people in the United States each year, although the true incidence is likely much higher. In over 90% of patients the source of PE is proximal lower-extremity DVT. Approximately 10% of deaths occur within the first hour of a PE, before definitive diagnosis and institution of treatment.[242] Similar to DVT, traditional treatment of PE consists of supportive care and anticoagulation with heparin and warfarin (Coumadin). In those surviving to initiation of such treatment the survival rate is estimated to be 92%. In contrast, survival in similar patients in whom the diagnosis is not made and remain untreated is estimated to be only 70%.[243]

Studies on the natural history of PE indicate that resolution occurs by two mechanisms.[244] In the minutes to hours after massive embolization, fragmentation and remodeling of the thrombus occurs and probably accounts for the spontaneous recovery of consciousness and hemodynamic stability often seen clinically. Over the ensuing days to weeks the endogenous fibrinolytic system gradually completes clot lysis. Anticoagulation serves to prevent thrombus propagation and formation while endogenous thrombolysis is commencing. Pulmonary hypertension and cor pulmonale develop in less than 2% of adequately treated patients.[245] In most cases the cause is recurrent PE, although there have been rare cases due to persistence of unresolved emboli in the proximal pulmonary circulation.[246]

Initial enthusiasm for the use of thrombolytic agents in the treatment of PE grew out of several uncontrolled studies in the late 1960s demonstrating the effectiveness of streptokinase at achieving in vivo thrombolysis.[247–249] These studies resulted in the commission by the National Institutes of Health of two multicenter randomized prospective trials comparing urokinase and streptokinase with heparin. The first, completed in 1970, was the Urokinase Pulmonary Embolism Trial (UPET), which compared standard heparin therapy to intravenous urokinase therapy in 160 patients with massive and submassive PE.[250] Urokinase was administered in a loading dose of 2000 IU/lb with a 2000 IU/lb/hour infusion for 12 hours followed by standard heparin therapy. "Moderate or greater" qualitative angiographic improvement at 24 hours occurred in 53% of the urokinase group but in only 5% of the heparin group. No significant differences, however, were noted in recurrence rates (15% vs. 19%) or in 2-week mortality (7% vs. 9%) or 6-month mortality (10% vs. 12%). Normalization of lung scans at 1 year was also similar in both groups and approached 75%.

The follow-up Urokinase-Streptokinase Embolism Trial (USPET) compared 12- and 24-hour regimens of urokinase (same dosing as UPET) to 24 hours of streptokinase (250,000 IU bolus followed by 100,000 IU/hour) in 157 patients with angiographic evidence of PE.[251] Angiograms at 24 hours revealed nearly equal improvement in all three groups, although 24-hour infusions of urokinase were associated with a slightly higher resolution rate than in patients treated with streptokinase when assessed by serial lung perfusion scans. The amount of resolution at 3 and 6 months was not statistically different among the three treatment groups nor were 2-week (7% vs. 9%) or 6-month (10% vs. 15%) mortality rates. In a follow-up study of 40 patients from both UPET and USPET, pulmonary-capillary blood volumes and diffusion capacities at 2 weeks and 1 year were found to be significantly higher in patients receiving thrombolytics compared with those receiving heparin.[252]

As would be expected, thrombolytic therapy was associated with a higher frequency of bleeding complications. Forty five percent of patients receiving urokinase and 27% receiving heparin experienced moderate to severe bleeding in the UPET.[250] Bleeding complications in the USPET trial were similar in the three groups.[251] Transfusion of more than 1 unit of blood was needed in 13% to 18% of patients. The majority of bleeding complications occurred late and were attributable to conventional anticoagulation, rather than to thrombolytic therapy. No hemorrhagic strokes occurred in any group. As a result of these trials, both urokinase and streptokinase were approved by the FDA in 1977 for treatment of acute PE.

In 1990, the FDA approved the use of rt-PA (alteplase) for the treatment of acute PE. This was based largely on several nonrandomized studies demonstrating safety and efficacy, as well as a trial by Goldhaber and associates comparing intravenous rt-PA to urokinase in 46 patients with angiographically documented PE.[253–255] This latter study found that 100 mg of intravenous rt-PA given over 2 hours resulted in demonstrable clot lysis in 82% of patients at 2 hours, compared with 48% of patients receiving urokinase at 2000 U/lb/hour for 24 hours. Improvement in perfusion lung scans at 24 hours was identical in the two treatment groups.

More recently there have been several randomized prospective trials comparing intravenous rt-PA with heparin for the treatment of PE.[256–259] The PAIMS-2 trial randomized 36 patients to either a 2-hour infusion of alteplase (10-mg bolus followed by a 90-mg infusion over 2 hours) or a bolus of 10,000 U of heparin followed by a continuous infusion at 1750 U/hour. Pulmonary angiographic scores of PE severity at 2 hours compared with baseline demonstrated a mean improvement by 12% in the rt-PA group versus 0.4% in the heparin group.[258] Mean pulmonary artery pressure decreased by 29% in the rt-PA by 2 hours while it increased in the heparin group by 11%. Serial perfusion scans, however, performed at baseline, 7, and 30 days after treatment, failed to show any differences between the groups. Goldhaber and associates[254] randomized 101 hemodynamically stable patients to alteplase (100 mg over 2 hours) followed by heparin or to heparin alone. In patients with baseline right-ventricular hypokinesis on echocardiography, treatment with rt-PA was associated with wall-motion improvement at 24 hours in 89% compared with 44% of patients given heparin alone. Perfusion lung scans also performed at baseline and at 24 hours revealed mean absolute improvements in blood flow of 14.6% and 1.5% in patients receiving rt-PA and heparin, respectively. No patient in the rt-PA group suffered recurrent PE compared with 5 patients in the heparin group (with two fatalities).

From the previous studies, it is clear that thrombolytic therapy enhances clot resolution, which can result in significantly faster hemodynamic improvement, especially within the first 24 hours. Because of the inherent bleeding risks and the lack of a clear mortality advantage, thrombolytic therapy has traditionally been reserved for the most critically ill patients, that is, those presenting with hypotension, right ventricular failure, or severe refractory hypoxemia. Recent results of a multicenter registry have challenged this practice.[260] The registry included 719 patients presenting with major PE without evidence of cardiogenic shock. Primary thrombolytic therapy, within 24 hours of presentation, was performed in 169 patients whereas 550 patients were treated with heparin alone. Mortality at 30 days was significantly lower in patients treated with thrombolytic therapy (5% vs. 11%), as was the incidence of recurrent PE (8% vs. 19%). Although syncope, hypotension, and heart failure were associated with a higher death rate, by multivariate analysis only primary thrombolytic therapy was found to be an independent predictor of survival (odds ratio for death 0.46; 95% confidence level 0.21 to 1.00). There was an increased frequency of serious bleeding with thrombolytic therapy (22% vs. 8%), but the rate of intracranial hemorrhage was low and identical between the two groups (two patients each). These results suggest that hemodynamically stable patients presenting with PE might benefit from thrombolytic therapy. Further studies are needed to clarify this issue.

Arterial Thrombosis

Acute occlusion of native atherosclerotic arteries or arterial bypass grafts results mainly from thromboembolism or in situ thrombosis. When collateral blood flow is inadequate, the patient experiences pain, pallor, and numbness in the affected limb. Eventually gangrene may develop if measures are not taken to restore the blood supply. Such interventions have mainly included thrombectomy and surgical bypass grafting. In the past decade thrombolytic therapy has been increasingly employed in the treatment of native arterial and peripheral arterial graft occlusion.

Early uses of thrombolytic therapy in the 1960s employed intravenous administration of streptokinase at rates of approximately 100,000 U/hr to patients with arterial thrombosis.[261, 262] Successful thrombolysis occurred in fewer than half of treated patients, and bleeding complications were extremely common and often severe. In the mid-1970s, techniques were developed that allowed intra-arterial administration of relatively low doses of streptokinase at rates of 5000 to 10,000 IU/hour for up to 48 hours through an infusion catheter positioned adjacent to a thrombus.[263] This method achieved excellent results with acceptable bleeding complication rates and is now the preferred method of treatment when traditional surgical approaches are not feasible or as an adjunct to percutaneous transluminal angioplasty.

Success of thrombolytic therapy depends in large part on the age, location, and nature of the occlusion. Acute embolic occlusions are much more likely to respond than are chronic thrombotic occlusions. If intra-arterial thrombolytic therapy is administered within 3 days of the onset of symptoms, effective lysis of embolic occlusion approaches 80%.[264] Conversely, lysis of chronic thrombotic occlusions occurs in 50% to 60% of cases treated with intra-arterial administration and in only 20% to 30% of patients treated with intravenous infusions.[265, 266]

Because of the high rate of allergic side effects associated with prolonged infusions of streptokinase, urokinase has been used more recently at rates of 1000 to 2000 IU/min. As with streptokinase, adjunctive heparin therapy is usually begun at the termination of the urokinase infusion. Belkin and associates[267] compared intra-arterial streptokinase and urokinase for the treatment of occlusive arterial disease. Urokinase was found in this nonrandomized comparative study to be more efficacious than streptokinase (recanalization rate of 100% vs. 50%) and produced less bleeding complications (25% vs. 48%). Pooled data from multiple trials revealed that of 474 patients who received streptokinase for both embolic and thrombotic arterial occlusions, successful thrombolysis occurred in 316 (67%).[268] Of 162 patients receiving urokinase, successful thrombolysis occurred in 130 (81%). Major complication rates were 19% and 12% for streptokinase and urokinase, respectively. Based on these data, urokinase has largely supplanted streptokinase for the intra-arterial treatment of thrombosis. Recently, intra-arterial urokinase has been shown to be equivalent to vascular surgery for the initial treatment of acute arterial occlusion of the lower extremities.[269]

Several small trials have been published comparing intra-arterial rt-PA to streptokinase for the treatment of native and arterial bypass graft occlusions. In a small randomized trial of 60 patients with acute occlusion of native peripheral arteries, intra-arterial rt-PA (0.5 mg/hour) was found to be superior to both intravenous rt-PA (same dose) or intra-arterial streptokinase (5000 U/hour) in producing recanalization (100% vs. 45% vs. 80%, respectively), clinical improvement and in 30-day limb salvage (80% vs. 45% vs. 60%).[270] A follow-up series from this trial included additional patients receiving intra-arterial rt-PA or streptokinase for both native arterial and peripheral bypass-graft occlusion.[271] Intra-arterial rt-PA was superior to streptokinase in terms of successful thrombolysis (58% vs. 41%) and shorter median time to lysis (22 hr vs. 40 hr). Hemorrhagic complications were comparable. No randomized trial comparing intra-arterial rt-PA to urokinase has been published.

Ischemic Stroke

Ischemic stroke is the third leading cause of death in the United States, with an incidence of approximately 400,000 new cases annually. The majority of strokes are caused by in-situ thrombosis within atherosclerotic intracerebral arteries or from thromboembolism from extracranial arteries or from the cardiac chambers. Cerebral angiography performed shortly after the onset of symptoms has demonstrated thrombotic occlusion in nearly 80% of patients with ischemic stroke.[272, 273]

The use of thrombolytic therapy for the treatment of acute ischemic stroke was first reported in 1958.[274] Several studies performed in the 1980s on patients with completed stroke failed to demonstrate significant improvements in clinical outcome with the use of thrombolytic agents.[275–279] Based on animal studies, it is now known that neurons within the "ischemic core" suffer irreversible damage within several minutes of ischemia.[280, 281] The surrounding "penumbral zone" receives some collateral blood flow from adjacent vascular territories and remains viable for up to 4 to 6 hours. It is salvage of the neurons in this penumbral zone that is the goal of timely reperfusion of the infarct-related artery using thrombolytic therapy.

Several small studies have established the efficacy of intra-arterial administration of streptokinase, urokinase, and rt-PA in restoring patency to occluded cerebral blood vessels.[282–286] Recanalization occurred in 45% to 75% of patients and was associated with an improved clinical outcome. In a recent pilot study, intra-arterial scu-PA (6 mg) has been shown to result in significantly better recanalization compared with placebo (57.7% vs. 14.3%, respectively) in patients with acute middle cerebral artery stroke.[287] As with all thrombolytic agents, the incidence of hemorrhagic transformation was also significantly increased (15.4% vs. 7.1%).

Because of the inherent delays and resource requirements associated with intra-arterial thrombolytic therapy, recent attention has moved toward intravenous administration. There have been five large randomized, placebo-controlled trials of intravenous thrombolysis. Three of these trials used streptokinase (1.5 million U) in patients treated within 6 hours of the onset of symptoms and in whom there was no evidence of cerebral hemorrhage on computed tomography.[288–290] All three trials were stopped prematurely because of excess mortality in the streptokinase group, primarily due to hemorrhagic transformation of the infarct. Reasons for this possibly include the use of adjunctive heparin, the relatively late presentation of patients (beyond 3 hours after symptom onset), and the lack of appropriate dosing studies.[286, 291]

Two trials have been published examining the efficacy of intravenous rt-PA. The first of these was the European Cooperative Acute Stroke Study (ECASS), which randomized 620 patients presenting within 6 hours of symptom onset to either 1.1 mg/kg of alteplase (10% given as a bolus followed by a 60-minute intravenous infusion to a maximum of 100 mg) or placebo.[292] Neurologic recovery at 90 days was significantly better and hospital stays were shorter in the alteplase group compared with placebo. There was a significant difference in 30-day mortality (17.9% in the alteplase group vs. 12.7% in the placebo group, $p = .08$) but not in the incidence of intracranial hemorrhage (39.8% in the alteplase group vs. 40.1% in the placebo group). A major criticism of the study was that 109 patients (17.4%) were enrolled in the study despite signs of early infarct extension on computed tomography. When these patients were excluded, there was no longer a significant difference in 30-day mortality (14.6% in the alteplase group vs. 11.7% in the placebo group, $p = .36$) and treatment with alteplase was associated with a better functional outcome.

The second trial was the National Institute of Neurologic Disorder and Stroke (NINDS) rt-PA Stroke Study, which randomized 624 patients presenting within 3 hours of symptoms to either 0.9 mg/kg alteplase (10% given as a bolus followed by a 60-minute intravenous infusion to a maximum of 90 mg) or placebo.[293] Mortality rates of the two groups were similar (17% for the alteplase group vs. 21% for the placebo group; $p = .3$) although the alteplase group had greater neurologic recovery both at 24 hours (as assessed by the National Institutes of Health Stroke Scale) and at 90 days (50% in the alteplase group had no or minimal disability compared with 38% of the placebo group, as assessed by the Barthel Index). Treatment with alteplase was associated with a higher incidence of symptomatic intracerebral hemorrhage (6.4% vs. 0.6%, $p < .001$). The odds ratio for a favorable outcome with alteplase was 1.7 (95% confidence intervals, 1.2 to 2.6). Based on this study, the FDA, in June 1996, approved alteplase for use in patients presenting with ischemic stroke within 3 hours of symptom onset and meeting the other NINDS entry criteria.

The differences in the incidences of intracranial hemorrhage in the ECASS and NINDS trials raise concerns about selection of patients for thrombolytic therapy. In the ECASS trial, patients with early evidence of extensive infarction on initial computed tomography had a high mortality rate regardless of therapy (33.3% in the alteplase group vs. 22.1% in the placebo group, $p = .17$).[292] As a result, the American Heart Association recommends that if computed tomography reveals early changes of a recent major infarction such as sulcal effacement, mass effect, edema, or possible hemorrhage, thrombolytic therapy should be avoided.[294] The time to treatment may also predispose to an increased incidence of intracranial hemorrhage and mortality. Pooled results from both the streptokinase and rt-PA randomized trials suggests that patients treated within 3 hours of symptom onset had a lower risk of mortality than those treated between 3 and 6 hours (odds ratio 0.78 vs. 1.56, $p = .01$), regardless of the thrombolytic agent used.[295] Results from the on-going ECASS 2 and the Alteplase Thrombolysis for Acute Noninterventional Therapy in Ischemic Stroke (ATLANTIS) Study will help clarify some of these issues and further define the role of thrombolytic therapy.[296]

Other Uses

Thrombolytic therapy has been shown to be effective treatment for a number of arterial and venous occlusions.[297] Both renal and hepatic vascular occlusions have been successfully treated. Superior vena cava syndrome responds well to both regional and systemic thrombolytic therapy. Use of streptokinase for prosthetic valve thromboses has been shown to be a viable alternative to surgery, although the risk of embolism is increased.[298] Indwelling vascular catheters that become clotted frequently can be opened with the use of low-dose (5000 IU) urokinase.[299]

Guidelines for the Use of Thrombolytic Agents

Contraindications to Thrombolytic Therapy

By their very nature, thrombolytic agents produce a number of hemostatic defects that predispose to local and systemic bleeding complications. To minimize the incidence of these events, an NIH Consensus Conference in 1980 developed a list of absolute and relative contraindications to the use of thrombolytic therapy.[300] Since that time considerable clinical experience has been accumulated that supports these guidelines. The generally accepted contraindications to thrombolytic therapy are shown in Table 17–2.

Table 17–2. Contraindications to Thrombolytic Therapy

Absolute
Major trauma, surgery, or organ biopsy within 6 weeks
Active gastrointestinal or genitourinary bleeding within 6 months
Any history of hemorrhagic stroke
Nonhemorrhagic stroke within 1 year or other active intracranial process
Head trauma or brain surgery within 6 months
Active bleeding or known bleeding disorder
Traumatic cardiopulmonary resuscitation within 3 weeks
Known or suspected aortic dissection
Known or suspected pericarditis
Relative
Severe uncontrolled arterial hypertension (greater than 180 mm Hg systolic or greater than 110 mm Hg diastolic)
Recent puncture of noncompressible vessels within 2 weeks
Recent minor trauma, including cardiopulmonary resuscitation for more than 10 minutes
Bacterial endocarditis or intracardiac thrombi
Hemostatic defects, including those associated with severe hepatic or renal disease
Pregnancy or within 1 week post partum
Diabetic hemorrhagic retinopathy
Transient ischemic attack within 6 months
Acute pancreatitis

Adapted from White HD, Van der Werf FJJ. Thrombolysis for acute myocardial infarction. Circulation 1998; 97:1632.

Several specific conditions deserve comment. The current use of oral anticoagulants is considered a contraindication for the use of thrombolytic agents for the treatment of MI because the risk of intracranial hemorrhage is increased by twofold to fourfold.[301] If thrombolytic agents absolutely need to be given to a patient receiving warfarin, some authors advocate simultaneously administering fresh frozen plasma to replenish the vitamin K–dependent clotting factors.[302] Active menstruation is not a contraindication to thrombolytic therapy. Endometrial sloughing and bleeding is mediated by prostaglandin-induced arteriolar vasoconstriction in association with high local levels of plasminogen activators, not to a systemic hematologic abnormality. The GUSTO-I investigators found no increase in major bleeding in a small subset of women who were actively menstruating at the time they received thrombolytic therapy.[302] Finally, thrombolytic therapy can safely be given to diabetics, even those with proliferative retinopathy. The GISSI-2 investigators found no increase in complications in diabetics compared with nondiabetics.[303] None of the more than 6000 diabetics in the GUSTO-I trial developed intraocular hemorrhage, even though 300 of them were estimated to have proliferative retinopathy.[304]

Laboratory Monitoring

Thrombolytic agents activate the fibrinolytic system that results in the generation of plasmin. Plasmin that is generated on the surface of a thrombus enzymatically degrades the constitutive fibrin molecules leading to thrombolysis. Unfortunately, no agents exist that can differentiate between pathologic thrombi and protective hemostatic plugs that maintain vascular integrity. Concomitant lysis of hemostatic plugs along with pathologic thrombi results in bleeding at sites of vascular injury, especially associated with vascular access catheters. Plasmin that is generated in the circulation degrades circulating fibrinogen, leading to both its depletion and production of fibrinogen degradation products. Although both low fibrinogen and elevated fibrinogen degradation products predispose to bleeding, it is the primary dissolution of protective hemostatic plugs that is primarily responsible for the bleeding complications associated with thrombolytic therapy (Fig. 17–11).

A variety of laboratory tests have been used to assess the hemostatic defects produced by thrombolytic agents. Useful tests include the TT, PT, aPTT, fibrinogen level, and assays for fibrin(ogen) degradation products. In general, these tests are used to confirm the attainment of a lytic state, to monitor adjunctive anticoagulant therapy, and, in the event of a serious hemorrhage, to quantitate the hemostatic defect and help guide specific factor replacement.

Because derangements of laboratory tests do not predict either thrombolytic efficacy nor untoward bleeding complications, they are not generally employed with high-dose bolus or short-term infusion regimens where the attainment of a lytic state is assured.[305, 306] When prolonged infusions of low-dose streptokinase and urokinase

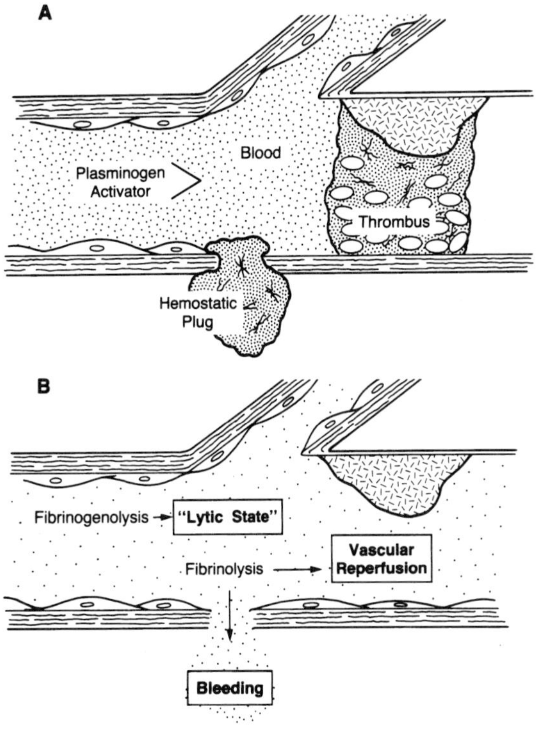

Figure 17–11. The three principal sites of action of thrombolytic agents. *A,* A pathologic thrombus composed of fibrin, platelets, and erythrocytes overlying a stenosed artery. A hemostatic plug composed of fibrin and platelets seals a site of previous vascular injury. *B,* The effects of thrombolytic therapy, which result in not only the dissolution of the pathologic thrombus but also of the protective hemostatic plug and generation of a generalized "lytic state." (From Marder VJ, Sherry S. Thrombolytic therapy [first of two parts]. N Engl J Med 1988; 138:1512.)

are employed in the treatment of PE or DVT, serial measurements of the thrombin time aid in attaining and maintaining a lytic state.

When employing streptokinase, a TT is obtained at baseline and at 4 hours after the 250,000 IU bolus and institution of the 100,000 IU/hour infusion. If an adequate lytic state has been achieved the TT will be within one and one-half to five times the control value. Because this regimen almost always overcomes any neutralizing antistreptokinase antibodies, the most common cause for a subtherapeutic TT is overuse of circulating plasminogen, resulting in inadequate amounts of free plasminogen available for conversion to plasmin. Reduction of the streptokinase infusion to 25,000 to 50,000 IU/hour will increase the amount of free plasminogen, thereby achieving a lytic state. A repeat TT is obtained in 4 hours, and if the TT is again less than 1.5, it is likely that high titers of neutralizing antibodies are present and one should change to urokinase. If the TT is within therapeutic range, it should be repeated at 12-hour intervals until the infusion is complete. Any TT over five times control or any further drop below one and one-half times control should prompt a reduction in the infusion rate by one half. After discontinuation of the infusion, the TT is assessed at 2-hour intervals. When the TT is less than two times control a heparin infusion is begun without a loading dose.

When urokinase is used, a TT is obtained at baseline and at 4 hours after a 4000-IU/kg loading dose and institution of a 4000-IU/kg/hour infusion. Unlike streptokinase, the infusion rate is increased if the TT is below one and one-half times control and decreased if greater than five times control. Serial TTs are obtained at 12-hour intervals. After discontinuation of UK, at approximately 2–5 hours and when the TT is less than two times control, heparin is begun without a loading dose at 1000 U/hour intravenously, and the final dose of heparin is identified by monitoring with the APTT.

Management of Bleeding Complications

Most bleeding associated with thrombolytic therapy occurs as a result of disruption of hemostatic plugs, as opposed to derangement of the plasma coagulation system.[228] This usually occurs at sites of vascular access and can be controlled with direct pressure or discontinuation of adjunctive therapy such as heparin. Spontaneous bleeding at a noninvaded site requires prompt discontinuation of the thrombolytic infusion and determination of the TT. Spontaneous hemorrhage in the presence of a therapeutic TT indicates a vascular structural abnormality, and the thrombolytic agent should not be restarted.

If after discontinuation of the thrombolytic agent severe bleeding persists, a fibrinogen level should be obtained; and if it is below 100 mg/dL, fresh frozen plasma or cryoprecipitate should be administered. Cryoprecipitate contains higher concentrations of fibrinogen and factor VIII than does fresh frozen plasma and is more efficacious in correcting the lytic state induced by thrombolytic agents.[307] Each bag of cryoprecipitate contains approximately 250 mg of fibrinogen and 80 units of factor VIII in a small volume. Adequate hemostasis is usually achieved with transfusion of 10 bags of cryoprecipitate, which will increase the fibrinogen level approximately by 70 mg/dL and the factor VIII level by 30% in an average adult.[308] Hemostasis is generally achieved by raising the fibrinogen level above 100 mg/dL and the factor VIII level above 30%.

ANTIFIBRINOLYTIC THERAPY

Antifibrinolytic Agents

During the 1950s the search for antifibrinolytic agents led to the discovery that several mono-substituted analogues of lysine could inhibit plasminogen activation.[309] Later, a protease inhibitor purified from bovine pancreas was also found to have antifibrinolytic activity.[310] Several of these agents have been developed for clinical use and have found wide application in the treatment of a variety of bleeding disorders (Fig. 17–12).

ϵ-Aminocaproic Acid

The most widely employed synthetic antifibrinolytic agent is ϵ-aminocaproic acid (EACA). EACA is monosubstituted carboxylic acid with a molecular weight of 146 kD. The substance is freely soluble in water and therefore has virtually complete absorption from the gastrointestinal tract.[311] Peak levels after oral dosing are reached within 2 hours and are comparable to those reached after intravenous administration. EACA is widely distributed, including passage into synovial fluid and accross the blood-brain barrier.[312, 313] About 75% of the drug is excreted unchanged in the urine, with only a small percentage of the drug being actively metabolized. The elimination half-life of EACA is approximately 2 hours, with a biological half-life of 77 minutes.[311, 314]

Like its analogue lysine, EACA at low concentrations (1–4 mol) binds competitively to the LBS on K1 of the plasminogen A chain.[315, 316] The main antifibrinolytic effect of EACA is to inhibit plasminogen binding to fibrin. Binding of EACA to plasminogen also induces a conformational change that actually renders the plasminogen molecule nonsusceptible to activation. However, at higher concentrations (1–2 mol), EACA noncompetitively inhibits the enzymatic activity of plasmin. Although plasmin may be formed in the presence of EACA, it has less access to and activity against its fibrin substrate. EACA has also been found to competitively inhibit the action of urokinase and to prevent binding of t-PA to fibrin.[317, 318] Plasma levels of about 64 μg/mL (range, 37 to 84 μg/mL) were required to inhibit 50% clot lysis in one study.[319] Serum levels of 130 μg/mL are generally taken to be adequate to control systemic fibrinolysis in humans.[314]

EACA is available as 20-mL or 96-mL vials containing 5 g and 24 g, respectively of an aqueous injectable solution; a 250-mg/mL syrup; or 500-mg tablets. The usual adult dose is 4 to 5 g orally or by slow intravenous infusion (in 250 mL of normal saline, D_5W or lactated Ringer's solution) followed by 1 g/hour or 4 to 5 g every 4 hours to a maximum of 30 g/day. Dosages should be reduced by 25% in patients with severe renal impairment.

The most common side effects of EACA are nausea,

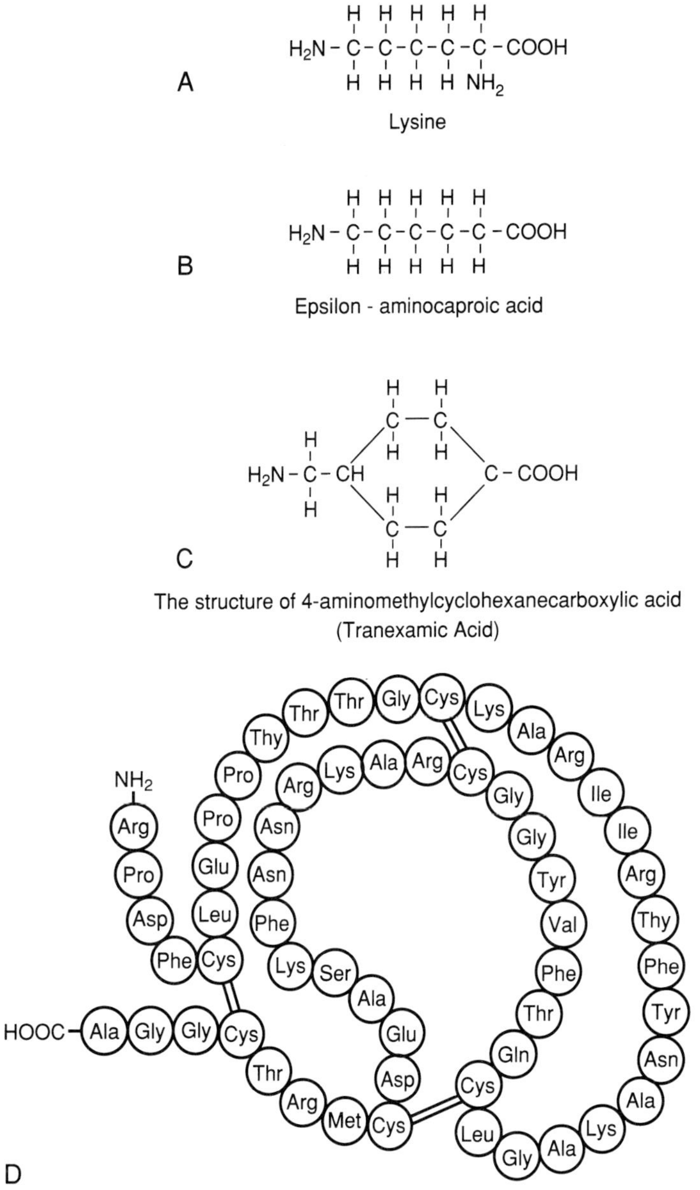

Figure 17–12. Schematic structures of the antifibrinolytic agents. *A,* Lysine. *B,* ε-aminocaproic acid (EACA). *C,* Tranexamic acid (AMCA). *D,* Aprotinin. (Adapted from Ogston D. Antifibrinolytic Drugs: Chemistry, Pharmacology and Clinical Usage. Chichester, UK: John Wiley & Sons, 1984, pp 47–51.)

vomiting, and diarrhea, which occur in approximately 20%.[320] They appear to be related to direct gastrointestinal irritation rather than toxic serum levels of the agent. Less common side effects are dizziness, pruritus, rash, and headache. Inflammatory myopathy has been reported rarely in a few patients taking large doses for prolonged periods of time.[321] By far the most serious complication is thrombosis, usually in patients with predisposing hypercoagulable states, especially DIC.

Tranexamic Acid

Tranexamic acid (trans-4-aminomethylcyclohexanoic acid; AMCA) is another lysine analogue that was found to be 10 times more potent on a molar basis than EACA. The mechanism of action is identical to EACA. AMCA is freely soluble, but oral bioavailability is only about 40% of the corresponding intravenous dose.[322] Tissue distribution and mechanism of elimination are the same as EACA. The plasma elimination half-life has been found to be about 2 hours with an apparent biologic half-life of 1.9 to 2.7 hours.[323, 324] AMCA levels of 10 μg/mL have been found to inhibit 80% of clot lysis.[322] Serum levels of 10 to 15 μg/mL have been found to control systemic fibrinolysis in humans.

AMCA is available as 500-mg tablets or 10-mL ampules containing 100 mg/mL of AMCA. The recommended intravenous dose of AMCA is 10 mg/kg every 3 to 4 hours. Because of poor absorption, an oral dose of 30 to 50 mg/kg is required. Intravenous dosages should be adjusted to the degree of renal failure. Patients with a serum creatinine level between 120 and 250 μmol/L should receive 10 mg/kg twice daily. With a creatinine level between 250 and 500 μmol/L this dose should be administered every 24 hours and for a creatinine level over 500 μmol/L the dose should be administered every 48 hours.[324] The side effect profile of AMCA is similar to that of EACA.

Aprotinin

Aprotinin is a plasmin inhibitor with substantial antifibrinolytic activity first isolated from bovine lung in 1936.[310] It was not until the 1960s that the compound was developed for clinical use. The molecule consists of a single polypeptide chain containing 58 amino acid residues and having a molecular weight of 65 kD. Aprotinin inhibits a wide array of proteases in addition to plasmin, including trypsin, chymotrypsin, and kallikrein. It exerts its antifibrinolytic effect by reversible binding to plasmin through a lysine residue in the molecule's active site.[325] Because kallikrein participates in the activation of factor XII, aprotinin also inhibits the contact-phase coagulation system. The drug does not affect platelet function.[326] Aprotinin activity is expressed in kallikrein inactivator units (KIU). One milligram of aprotinin contains approximately 7160 KIU.[327]

Aprotinin is not absorbed orally and has an elimination half-life of 150 minutes.[328] Elimination is through renal metabolism and excretion. The drug does not distribute across cell membranes and does not cross the blood-brain barrier. Because of its relatively short half-life compared with other antifibrinolytic agents and poor tissue distribution, use of aprotinin is mainly to reduce blood loss during cardiopulmonary bypass surgery. Aprotinin is available in 100-mL and 200-mL vials containing 1 and 2 million KIU, respectively. Side effects are rare and include a 1% incidence of allergic reactions, including anaphylaxis.[329]

Clinical Applications of Antifibrinolytic Agents

Antifibrinolytic agents have been found to be useful in the treatment of a wide variety of bleeding disorders that occur secondary to systemic hyperfibrinolysis, primary coagulopathies, localized bleeding conditions, surgery, and thrombocytopenia. They are generally contraindicated in disorders such as DIC, which manifest a hypercoagulable state as part of their pathophysiology. In these instances, inhibition of the fibrinolytic component may unmask the hypercoagulable state and lead to clinically significant thrombosis. Because disorders of pure hyperfibrinolysis are rare, antifibrinolytic agents must not be employed indiscriminately.

Bleeding After Thrombolytic Therapy

Antifibrinolytic agents have occasionally been useful in the treatment of bleeding complications associated with thrombolytic therapy. Thrombolytic agents not only cause bleeding by the induction of an active fibrinolytic state but also by impairment of the coagulation system by depletion of fibrinogen and the use of adjunctive agents such as heparin. Most bleeding will therefore respond to discontinuation of the thrombolytic agent and/or the adjunctive agent. Continued bleeding can be managed by repletion of fibrinogen if found to be low. The use of antifibrinolytic agents is generally reserved for severe refractory bleeding because of the risk of re-thrombosis. Although early studies demonstrated the efficacy of antifibrinolytic agents in controlling bleeding in patients receiving urokinase or streptokinase, no recent controlled studies have been done to evaluate their overall clinical benefit.[330, 331]

Congenital and Acquired Coagulopathies

Patients with bleeding secondary to both congenital and acquired coagulopathies may also benefit from antifibrinolytic therapy. Their use includes adjunct therapy to factor replacement in patients undergoing surgical procedures, prophylaxis against the frequency and severity of bleeding episodes, and treatment of hematuria. Saliva and the oral mucosa are rich sources of plasminogen activators.[332] Both EACA (50 mg/kg every 4 hours) and AMCA (25 mg/kg every 8 hours) have been shown to be efficacious in controlling bleeding after dental extraction in patients with hemophilia and Christmas disease.[333, 334] Most studies indicate that fibrinolytic activity is not generally increased by hemophilia and the beneficial effects of antifibrinolytic agents are a consequence of localized inhibition of fibrinolysis in injured areas.[335, 336] EACA has also been shown to help control bleeding in patients with both immune and nonimmune thrombocytopenia.[337, 338]

Gastrointestinal Bleeding

Gastrointestinal tract bleeding also responds to antifibrinolytic therapy. This observation is consistent with studies showing that gastric tissue contains plasmin activators that are released during pathologic states, such as surgical manipulation or active peptic ulcer disease.[339] Several well-designed studies have revealed that AMCA (1 g every 6 hours) reduces both blood loss and mortality in patients treated for acute upper-gastrointestinal bleeding.[340–343] A meta-analysis of 1267 patients with upper gastrointestinal bleeding found that treatment with AMCA was associated with 40% reduction in mortality, a 30% to 40% reduction in the need for surgery, and a 20% to 30% reduction in recurrent bleeding.[344] Lower gastrointestinal bleeding secondary to ulcerative colitis also has been shown to respond to EACA.[345]

Dysmenorrhea

Endometrial tissue contains large amounts of plasminogen activators, especially during the secretory phase of the menstrual cycle and with alterations of normal menses.[346] AMCA, in a small randomized trial, has been shown to reduce blood loss by 54% in women with menorrhagia.[347] Antifibrinolytic therapy has also been proven to reduce bleeding in patients with menorrhagia associated with intrauterine devices and postoperative bleeding after cervical conization.[348, 349] In general, antifibrinolytic agents are reserved for women with menorrhagia who fail or do not tolerate treatment with the more traditional estrogen and progesterone combinations.

Intracranial Hemorrhage

The indications for antifibrinolytic therapy in the treatment of intracranial hemorrhage are less clear. It is well established that plasminogen activator activity, which is normally absent from the cerebrospinal fluid, is increased after subarachnoid hemorrhage. This increased activity is thought to disrupt initial hemostasis after rupture of an aneurysm and be responsible for the 18% to 30% incidence of rebleeding that complicates a subarachnoid hemorrhage.[350] Because both EACA and AMCA cross the blood-brain barrier these agents should theoretically be of benefit in preventing rebleeding. Uncontrolled trials with EACA have demonstrated a slight reduction in the incidence of rebleeding over historical controls, although several small, controlled trials failed to demonstrate a consistent benefit.[351] One of the potential complications of antifibrinolytic therapy is increasing the incidence of hydrocephalus due to fibrin deposition and eventual fibrosis of the subarachnoid space. For these reasons, antifibrinolytic therapy is not routinely used in the treatment of subarachnoid hemorrhage.

Postoperative Bleeding

Antifibrinolytic agents are useful in controlling blood loss after several specific types of surgery. The urinary tract is rich in urokinase-type plasminogen activators.[352] Prostatic u-PA can dissolve clots and enhance bleeding after prostatectomy. EACA has been shown to reduce blood loss by up to 50% compared with placebo after prostatectomy.[353–355] Use of these agents in treatment of upper urinary tract bleeding can result in ureteral obstruction from enhanced clot formation and therefore should be accompanied with caution.[356]

Bleeding during orthotopic liver transplantation is often extensive, owing to preexisting coagulopathy, as well as to intraoperative fibrinolysis. In a small randomized study, AMCA was associated with a 50% reduction in blood loss compared with placebo.[357] Aprotinin has also had mixed results in controlling bleeding. In two small nonrandomized studies, a single bolus dose of 2 million KIU at the start of the procedure reduced blood loss by 35% whereas the same dose followed by an infusion of 0.5 million KIU/hour during the entire procedure reduced blood loss by over 60%.[358, 359] In a small randomized study, however, aprotinin was not more efficacious than placebo in controlling bleeding.[360]

Joint replacement surgery is often associated with significant blood loss. In a randomized placebo-control trial, a single dose of AMCA administered before tourniquet release in patients undergoing knee replacement resulted in a nearly 50% reduction in postoperative bleeding.[361] At present, the use of antifibrinolytic agents is reserved for patients at high risk of significant hemorrhage during joint replacement.

Cardiopulmonary Bypass

The use of cardiopulmonary bypass during cardiac surgery is associated with a myriad of hemostatic defects. The two major abnormalities are platelet dysfunction and hyperfibrinolysis. Plasma fibrinolytic activity increases dramatically during and after bypass and is likely due to several factors.[362] Fibrinogen is preferentially adsorbed onto the synthetic surfaces of the bypass circuit and, in conjunction with hemodilution, results in a nearly 50% reduction in circulating levels.[363] Heparinization before the initiation of bypass has been shown to result in a significant rise in plasmin activity.[364] Although the mechanism is not entirely clear, in vitro studies have demonstrated that high doses of unfractionated heparin are able to bind and activate prekallikrein, which may, in turn, directly activate plasminogen.[365] Cardiopulmonary bypass is also a major stimulus for the release of t-PA from the vascular endothelium.[366] Plasma t-PA levels increase during bypass but return to baseline shortly after the procedure. The major stimuli for t-PA release are thought to be thrombin and kallikrein, which are formed on contact of blood with the extracorporeal circuit.[362] Hypoxia, circulating epinephrine, angiotensin II, and leukotrienes may also stimulate t-PA release. Finally, the pericardial cavity is a rich source of tissue factor and plasminogen activators. Blood that accumulates in the pericardial cavity has high levels of t-PA, thrombin, and fibrin(ogen) degradation products.[367] When this blood is returned to the systemic circulation, it can stimulate systemic hyperfibrinolysis.

Because hyperfibrinolysis is a major cause of postoperative blood loss, there have been a number of trials examining the effects of antifibrinolytic agents. EACA, administered immediately before and during cardiopulmonary bypass (10 to 30 g bolus, with or without a 1-g/hour infusion), has consistently been shown in randomized trials to decrease 24-hour blood loss by 20% to 35%.[368–370] In several randomized trials, AMCA (10-g bolus with or without a 2-g/hour infusion) also reduced 24-hour blood loss by 35% to 48%.[371, 372] Although these agents reduce postoperative blood loss, they have inconsistently been shown to substantially reduce the need for blood transfusions, the primary indicator of efficacy.

Aprotinin is the only fibrinolytic agent that has been demonstrated to substantially reduce postoperative blood loss as well as the need for blood transfusions. Several small placebo-control studies have demonstrated that aprotinin administered in high doses (4 to 6 million KIU) during the entire procedure reduced postoperative bleeding by 30% to 80% and blood transfusion requirements by 40% to 90%.[373–378] In a prospective study of 1784 patients, high-dose aprotinin reduced blood loss by 35% and transfusion requirements by 53% compared with placebo.[379]

Because of the theoretical concern that aprotinin may increase the risk of thrombosis leading to graft occlusion and myocardial infarction, several low-dose aprotinin regimens have been evaluated.[380–382] In a recent multicenter trial, 287 patients undergoing coronary artery bypass surgery were randomized to either high-dose aprotinin (2 million KIU loading dose and 2 million KIU added to the pump prime followed an infusion of 0.5 million KIU/hour during surgery), low-dose aprotinin (1 million KIU loading dose and 1 million KIU added to the pump prime followed by a 0.25 million KIU/hour infusion), pump-prime only aprotinin (2 million KIU) or placebo.[383] The need for red cell transfusion was reduced by 26% in the pump-prime group and by 53% in the high- and low-dose groups compared with placebo. There were no differences between the four groups in the incidence of perioperative myocardial infarction. Furthermore, several studies using ultrafast computed tomography, magnetic resonance imaging, and coronary angiography have failed to demonstrate any detrimental effect of aprotinin on graft patency.[384–386]

REFERENCES

1. Smith JA, Ross WD. Translation of Aristotle's De Partibus Animalium. Oxford, Clarendon Press, 1912, p 4.
2. Hunter J. A Treatise on Blood, Inflammation, and Gunshot Wounds. London, 1794.
3. Scherer J. Chemish-physiologiscke untersuchungen. Ann Chem Pharm 184:1; 40:1.
4. Green JR. Note on the action of sodium chloride in dissolving fibrin. J Physiol 1887; 8:372.
5. Dastre A. Fibrinolyse dans le sang. Arch Physiol Norm Pathol 1893; 5:661.
6. Tillet WS, Garner RL. The fibrinolytic activity of hemolytic streptococci. J Exp Med 1933; 58:485.
7. Milstone H. A factor in normal human blood which participates in streptococcal fibrinolysis. J Immunol 1941; 42:109.
8. Kaplan MH. Nature and role of the lytic factor in hemolytic streptococcal fibrinolysis. Proc Soc Exp Biol Med 1944; 57:40.
9. Christensen LR, MacLeod CM. A proteolytic enzyme of serum: characterization, activation and reaction with inhibitors. J Gen Physiol 1945; 28:559.
10. Sahl W. Uber das Yorkommen von Pepsin und Trypsin in normalen menschlichen Harn. Pflugers Arch 1885; 36:209.
11. Sobel GW, Mohler SR, Jones NW, et al. Urokinase: an activator of plasma profibrinolysin extracted from urine. Am J Physiol 1952; 171:768.
12. Astrup T, Permin PM. Fibrinolysis in the animal organism. Nature 1947; 159:681.
13. Kwaan HC. The biologic role of components of the plasminogen-plasmin systems. Prog Cardiovasc Dis 1992; 34:309.
14. Mignatti P, Rifkin DB. Plasminogen activators and matrix metalloproteinases in angiogenesis. Enzyme Protein 1996; 49:117.
15. Tagnon HJ, Palade GE. Activation of proplasmin by a factor from mammalian tissue. J Clin Invest 1950; 29:317.
16. Wiman B, Wallen P. On the primary structure of human plasminogen and plasmin: purification and characterization of cyanogen-bromide fragments. Eur J Biochem 1975; 57:387.
17. Swisshelm K, Dyer K, Sadler E, Disteche C. Localization of the plasminogen gene (PLG) to the distal portion of the long arm of chromosome 6 by in situ hybridisation. Cytogen Cell Genet 1985; 40:756.
18. Robbins KC, Summaria L, Elwyn D, Barlow GH. Further studies on the purification and characterization of human plasminogen and plasmin. J Biol Chem 1965; 240:541.
19. Robbins KC, Summaria L, Hsieh B, Shah RJ. The peptide chains of human plasmin: mechanism of activation of human plasminogen to plasmin. J Biol Chem 1967; 242:2333.
20. Collen D, Verstraete M. Molecular biology of human plasminogen: II. Metabolism in physiological and some pathological conditions in man. Thromb Diath Haemorrh 1975; 34:403.
21. Castellino FJ. Biochemistry of human plasminogen. Semin Thromb Hemost 1984; 10:18.
22. Wiman B, Wallen P. The specific interaction between plasminogen and fibrin: a physiological role of the lysine binding site in plasminogen. Thromb Res 1977; 10:213.
23. Henkin J, Marcotte P, Yang H. The plasminogen-plasmin system. Prog Cardiovasc Dis 1991; 24:135.
24. Marsh N. Fibrinolysis. New York: John Wiley & Sons, 1982, pp 46–47.
25. Marder V, Budzynski AZ. The structure of fibrinogen degradation products. Prog Hemost Thromb 1974; 2:141–174.
26. Niewarowski S, Budzynski AZ, Lipinski B. Significance of the intact polypeptide chains of human fibrinogen in ADP-induced platelet aggregation. Blood 1977; 49:636.
27. Holt JC, Mahmoud M, Gaffney PJ. The ability of fibrinogen fragments to support ADP-induced platelet aggregation. Thromb Res 1979; 16:427.
28. LaDuca FM, Tinsley LA, Dang CV, Bell WR. Stimulation of fibrinogen synthesis in cultured rat hepatocytes by fibrinogen degradation product fragment D. Proc Natl Acad Sci U S A 1989; 86:8788.
29. Niewarowski S, Prou-Wartelle O. Role du facteur contact (facteur Hageman) dans la fibrinolyse. Thromb Diath Haemorrh 1959; 3:593.
30. Kluft C, Dooijewaard G, Emeis JJ. The role of the contact system in fibrinolysis. Semin Thromb Hemost 1987; 13:50.
31. Carmeliet P, Collen D. Gene manipulation and transfer of the plasminogen and coagulation system in mice. Semin Thromb Hemost 1996; 22:525.
32. Albrechtsen OK. The fibrinolytic agents in saline extracts of human tissues. J Clin Invest 1958; 10:91.
33. Rijken DC, Juhan-Vague I, deCock F, Collen D. Measurement of human tissue-type plasminogen activator by two-site immunoradiometric assay. J Lab Clin Med 1983; 101:274.
34. Matsuo O. Turnover of tissue plasminogen activator in man. Thromb Haemost 1983; 48:242.
35. Baughman RA. Pharmacokinetics of tissue plasminogen activator. *In* Sobel BE, Collen D, Grossbard EB (eds): Tissue Plasminogen Activator in Thrombolytic Therapy. New York, Marcel Dekker, 1987, pp 41–53.
36. Bachmann F, Kruitkoff EKO. Tissue plasminogen activator: chemical and physiological aspects. Semin Thromb Hemost 1984; 10:6.
37. Collen D, Lijnen HR, Todd PA, Goa KL. Tissue-plasminogen activator: a review of its pharmacology and therapeutic use as a thrombolytic agent. Drugs 1989; 38:346.
38. Chandler WL, Trimble SL, Loo SC, Mornin D. Effect of PAI-1 levels on the molar concentrations of active tissue plasminogen activator (t-PA) and t-PA/PAI-1 complex in plasma. Blood 1990; 76:930.
39. Otter M, Kuiper J, van Berkel TJC, Rijken DC. Mechanisms of tissue-type plasminogen activator (t-PA) clearance by the liver. Ann NY Acad Sci 1992; 667:431.
40. Rajput B, Degen SF, Reich E, et al. Chromosomal locations of human tissue plasminogen activator and urokinase genes. Science 1984; 230:672.
41. Berg DT, Grinnell BW. Signal and propeptide processing of human tissue plasminogen activator: activity of a pro-tPA derivative. Biochem Biophys Res Commun 1991; 179:1289.
42. Wallen P. Structural characterization of tissue plasminogen activator purified by immunosorbent chromatography. *In* Davidson F, Bachmann F, Bouvier CA, Kruitkoff EKO (eds): Progress in Fibrinolysis. New York: Churchill Livingstone, 1983, pp 338–343.
43. Bachmann F. Fibrinolysis. *In* Verstraete M, Vermylen J, Lijnen HR, Arnout J (eds): Thrombosis and Hemostasis. Leuven: Leuven University Press, 1987, pp 233–235.
44. Rijken DC, Hoylaerts M, Collen D. Fibrinolytic properties of one-chain and two-chain human extrinsic (tissue-type) plasminogen activator. J Biol Chem 1982; 257:2920.
45. Dooijewaard G, de Boer A, Turion PN, et al. Physical exercise induces enhancement of urokinase-type plasminogen activator (u-PA) levels in plasma. Thromb Haemost 1991; 65:82.
46. Binnema DJ, van Iersel JJ, Dooijewaard G. Quantitation of urokinase antigen in plasma and culture media by use of an ELISA. Thromb Res 1986; 43:569.
47. Ueno T, Kobayashi N, Maekawa T. Studies on metabolism of urokinase and mechanism of thrombolysis by urokinase. Thromb Haemost 1979; 42:885.
48. Verstraete M. Biochemical and clinical aspects of thrombolysis. Semin Hematol 1978; 15:35.
49. Ellis V, Scully MF, Kakkar VV. Plasminogen activation by single chain urokinase-type plasminogen activator: potentiation by U937 cells. J Biol Chem 1989; 264:2185.
50. Steffens G, Gunzler W, Otling F, et al. The complete amino acid sequence of low molecular mass urokinase from human urine. Hoppe-Seylers Z Physiol Chem 1982; 363:1043.
51. Lijnen HR, Van Hoef B, De Cock F, Collen D. The mechanism of plasminogen activation and fibrin dissolution by single chain urokinase-type plasminogen activator in a plasma milieu in vitro. Blood 1989; 73:1864.
52. Pannell R, Gurewich V. Pro-urokinase: a study of its stability in plasma and of a mechanism for its selective fibrinolytic effect. Blood 1986; 67:1864.

53. Husain SS. Single-chain urokinase-type plasminogen activator does not possess measurable intrinsic amidolytic or plasminogen activator activities. Biochemistry 1991; 30:5797.
54. Aoki N, Harpel PC. Inhibitors of the fibrinolytic system. Semin Thromb Hemost 1984; 10:24.
55. Collen D, Wiman B. Turnover of antiplasm, the fast acting plasmin inhibitor of plasma. Blood 1979; 53:313.
56. Aoki N. Genetic abnormalities of the fibrinolytic system. Semin Thromb Hemost 1984; 10:42.
57. Messmore HL. Natural inhibitors of the fibrinolytic system. Semin Thromb Hemost 1982; 8:267.
58. Tunstall AM, Merriman JM, Milne J, James K. Normal and pathological serum levels of α_2-macroglobulin in men and mice. J Clin Pathol 1975; 28:133.
59. Harpel PC, Rosenberg RD. α_2-macroglobulin and anti-thrombin-heparin cofactors: modulators of hemostatic and inflammatory reactions. *In* Spat TH (ed): Progress in Hemostasis. New York: Grune & Stratton, 1976, pp 145–189.
60. Barret A, Starkey PM. The interaction of alpha$_2$-macroglobulin with proteinases: characteristics and specificity of the reaction and a hypothesis concerning its molecular mechanism. Biochem J 1973; 133:709.
61. Travis J, Salvesen GS. Human plasma proteinase inhibitors. Ann Rev Biochem 1983; 52:655.
62. Harpel PC. Plasmin inhibitor reactions. J Exp Med 1977; 146:1033.
63. Morse JO. Alpha$_1$-antitrypsin deficiency. N Engl J Med 1978; 299:1045.
64. Harpel PC, Cooper NR. Studies on human plasma C1 inactivator-enzyme interactions: I. Mechanisms of interaction with C1s, plasmin and trypsin. J Clin Invest 1975; 55:593.
65. Highsmith RF, Rosenberg RD. The inhibition of human plasmin by human antithrombin heparin cofactor. J Biol Chem 1974; 249:4335.
66. Telesforo P, Semeraro N, Verstraete M, Collen D. The inhibition of plasmin by antithrombin III–heparin complex in vitro, in human plasma and during streptokinase therapy in man. Thromb Res 1975; 7:669.
67. Sprengers ED, Akkerman JWN, Jansen BG. Blood platelet plasminogen activator inhibitor: two different pools of endothelial cell type plasminogen activator inhibitor in human blood. Thromb Haemost 1986; 55:325.
68. Ginsburg D, Zeheb R, Yang H, et al. cDNA cloning of human plasminogen activator-inhibitor from endothelial cells. J Clin Invest 1986; 78:167.
69. Declerck PJ, Vaughan DE. Fibrinolysis regulation. *In* Thrombosis and Hemorrhage. Cambridge: Blackwell Scientific Publications, 1994, pp 145–160.
70. Kooistra T, Sprengers ED, van Hinsburgh VWM. Rapid inactivation of the plasminogen-activator inhibitors upon secretion from cultured human endothelial cells. Biochem J 1986; 239:497.
71. Hekman CM, Loskutoff DJ. Bovine plasminogen activator inhibitor: I. Specificity determinations and comparison of the active, latent and guanidine-activated forms. Biochemistry 1988; 27:2911.
72. Mottonen J, Strand A, Symersky J, et al. Structural basis of latency in plasminogen activator inhibitor-1. Nature 1992; 355:270.
73. Heckman CM, Loskutoff DJ. Endothelial cells produce a latent inhibitor of plasminogen activators that can be activated by denaturants. J Biol Chem 1985; 260:11581.
74. Vaughan DE, Decl, van Houtte E, de Mol M, Collen D. Studies of recombinant plasminogen activator inhibitor-1 in rabbits: pharmacokinetics and evidence for reactivation of latent plasminogen activator inhibitor-1 in vivo. Circ Res 1990; 67:1281.
75. Wiman B, Lindahl TL, Sigurdardottir O. Plasminogen activator inhibitor (PAI-1): interaction with vitronectin and plasminogen activators. *In* Takada A, Samama MM, Collen D (eds): Protease Inhibitors. Amsterdam: Elsevier Scientific, 1990, pp 37–44.
76. Emeis JJ. Fast hepatic clearance of plasminogen activator inhibitor. Thromb Haemost 1985; 54:230.
77. Sprengers ED, Kluft C. Plasminogen activator inhibitors. Blood 1987; 69:381.
78. Juhan-Vague I, Moerman B, De Cock F, et al. Plasma levels of a specific inhibitor of tissue-type plasminogen activator (and urokinase) in normal and pathologic conditions. Thromb Res 1984; 33:523.
79. Wiman B, Ljungberg B, Chmielewska J, et al. The role of the fibrinolytic system in deep venous thrombosis. J Lab Clin Med 1985; 105:265.
80. Nilsson IM, Ljungner H, Tengborn L. Two different mechanisms in patients with deep venous thrombosis and defective fibrinolysis: low concentrations of plasminogen activator or increased concentrations of plasminogen activator inhibitor. Br J Med 1985; 290:1453.
81. Schleef RR, Higgins DL, Pillemer E, Levitt LJ. Bleeding diathesis due to decreased functional activity of type 1 plasminogen activator inhibitor. J Clin Invest 1989; 83:1747.
82. Kawano T, Morimoto K, Uemura Y. Urokinase inhibitor in human placenta. Nature 1968; 217:253.
83. Kruitkoff EKO. Plasminogen activator inhibitor type 2: biochemical and biologic aspects. *In* Takada A, Samama MM, Collen D (eds): Protease Inhibitors. Amsterdam: Elsevier Science, 1990, pp 15–22.
84. Kruitkoff EKO, Tran-Thang C, Gudinchet A, et al. Fibrinolysis in pregnancy: a study of plasminogen activator inhibitors. Blood 1987; 69:460.
85. Suzuki K. Protein C inhibitor: structure and complex formation with activated protein C. *In* Takada A, Samama MM, Collen D (eds): Protease Inhibitors. Amsterdam: Elsevier Science, 1990, pp 91–104.
86. Fornasari PM, Gamba G, Dolci D, et al. Circadian rhythms in fibrinolysis. *In* Neri-Serneri GC, Prentice CRM (eds): Haemostasis and Thrombosis. London: Academic Press, 1979, pp 773–777.
87. Biggs R, MacFarlane RG, Pilling J. Observations on fibrinolysis: experimental activity produced by exercise or adrenaline. Lancet 1947; 1:402.
88. Streiff M, Bell WR. Exercise and hemostasis in humans. Semin Hematol 1994; 31:155.
89. Marsh N, Gaffney PJ. Some observations on the release of extrinsic and intrinsic plasminogen activators during exercise in man. Haemostasis 1980; 9:238.
90. Keber D, Stegnar M, Keber J, Accetto B. Influence of moderate and strenuous daily physical activity on fibrinolytic activity of blood: possibility of plasminogen activator store depletion. Thromb Haemost 1979; 41:745.
91. Williams RS, Logue EE, Lewis JL, et al. Physical conditioning augments the fibrinolytic response to venous occlusion in healthy adults. N Engl J Med 1986; 302:987.
92. Brakman P, Sobrero AJ, Astrup T. Effects of different systemic contraceptives on blood fibrinolysis. Am J Obstet Gynecol 1970; 106:187.
93. Walker WR. Fibrinolytic activity of whole blood from South African Banta and white subjects. Am J Nutr 1961; 9:461.
94. Meade TW, Chakrabarti R, Haines AP, et al. Characteristics affecting fibrinolytic activity and plasma fibrinogen concentrations. BMJ 1979; 1:153.
95. Al Samarrae W, Tuswell AS. Short term effect of coffee on blood fibrinolytic activity in healthy adults. Atherosclerosis 1977; 26:255.
96. Walter E, Birkholz L-B, Herenberg J, Weber E. Circadian rhythms of platelet function, fibrinolytic activity of plasma, and the influence of reduced food intake, fat loading and beer drinking on fibrinolytic activity. *In* Neri-Serneri GC, Prentice CRM (eds): Haemostasis and Thrombosis. London, Academic Press, 1977, pp 525–530.
97. Janzon L, Nilsson IM. Smoking and fibrinolysis. Circulation 1975; 51:1120.
98. Francis RB, Seyfert U. Tissue plasminogen activator antigen and activity in disseminated intravascular coagulation: clinicopathologic correlations. J Lab Clin Med 1987; 110:541.
99. Kwaan HC. The role of fibrinolysis in disease processes. Semin Thromb Hemost 1984; 19:71.
100. Suffredini AF, Harpel PC, Parillo JE. Promotion and subsequent inhibition of plasminogen activation after administration of intravenous endotoxin to normal subjects. N Engl J Med 1989; 320:1165.
101. Colucci M, Paramo JA, Collen D. Generation of a fast-acting inhibitor of plasminogen activator in response to endotoxin stimulation. J Clin Invest 1985; 75:818.
102. Bick BL. The clinical significance of fibrinogen degradation products. Thromb Haemost 1982; 8:302.
103. Elms MJ. Rapid detection of cross-linked fibrin degradation products in plasma using monoclonal antibody-coated latex particles. Am J Clin Pathol 1986; 85:360.

104. Nand S, Messmore HL. Hemostasis in malignancy. Am J Hematol 1990; 35:45.
105. Nand S, Fisher SG, Salgia R, Fisher RI. Hemostatic abnormalities in untreated cancer: incidence and correlation with thrombotic and hemorrhagic complications. J Clin Oncol 1987; 5:1998.
106. Wilson EL, Becker ML, Hoal EG. Molecular species of plasminogen activators secreted by normal and neoplastic cells. Cancer Res 1980; 40:933.
107. Wilson EL, Jacobs P, Dowdle EB. The secretion of plasminogen activators by myeloid cells in vitro. Blood 1983; 61:568.
108. Wu M, Arimura GK, Yunis AA. Purification and characterization of a plasminogen activator secreted by cultured human pancreatic cell carcinoma. Biochemistry 1977; 16:1908.
109. Markus G, Kohga S, Camiolo SM, et al. Plasminogen activators in human melanoma. J Natl Cancer Inst 1984; 2:1213.
110. Henderson ES. Acute leukemias—general considerations. *In* Williams WJ, Beutler E, Erslau AJ, Lichteman MA (eds): Hematology. New York: McGraw Hill, 1983, p 231.
111. Soong BC-F, Miller SP. Coagulation disorders in cancer: Fibrinolysis and inhibitors. Cancer 197; 25:867.
112. Zacharski LR. Basis for selection of anticoagulant drugs for therapeutic trials in malignancy. Haemostasis 1986; 16:300.
113. Mosesson MW, Coleman RW, Sherry S. Chronic intravascular coagulation syndromes. N Engl J Med 1968; 278:815.
114. Hull R, Delmore T, Carter C, et al. Adjusted subcutaneous heparin versus warfarin sodium in the long term treatment of venous thrombosis. N Engl J Med 1982; 306:189.
115. Walsh-McGonagle D, Green D. Low-molecular weight heparin in the management of Trousseau's syndrome. Cancer 1997; 80:649.
116. Green D, Hull RD, Brant R, Pineo GF. Lower mortality in cancer patients treated with low-molecular weight heparin versus standard heparin. Lancet 1992; 339:1476.
117. Astrup T, Rasmussen J, Amery A. Fibrinolytic activity of cirrhotic liver. Nature 1960; 185:619.
118. Tytgat GN, Collen D, de Vreker R. Investigations into the fibrinolytic system in cirrhosis. Acta Haematol 1968; 40:265.
119. Jedrychowski A, Hildebrand P, Ajdukiewicz AB, et al. Fibrinolysis in cholestatic jaundice. BMJ 1973; 1:640.
120. Larsson SO, Hedner U, Nilsson IM. On coagulation and fibrinolysis in acute renal insufficiency. Acta Med Scand 1971; 189:443.
121. Chen HF, Nakabayashi M, Satoh K, Sakamoto S. Studies on the purification and characterization of human urinary plasminogen and plasmin. Thromb Haemost 1980; 42:1536.
122. Hall CL, Blainey JD, Gaffney PJ. Origin of urinary fibrin-fibrinogen degradation products in renal glomerular disease. Nephron 1979; 23:6.
123. Nilsson IM. Fibrinogen degradation products and renal disease. Scand J Haematol 1971; 13(suppl 13):357.
124. Humair L, Potter EV, Kwaan HC. The role of fibrinogen in renal disease: II. Effects of anticoagulants and urokinase on experimental lesions in mice. J Clin Invest 1969; 74:72.
125. Meade TW, Ruddock V, Stirling Y, et al. Fibrinolytic activity, clotting factors and long-term incidence of ischaemic heart disease in the Northwick Park Heart Study. Lancet 1993; 342:1076.
126. Juhan-Vague I, Alessi MC. PAI-1, obesity, insulin resistance and risk of cardiovascular events. Thromb Haemost 1997; 78:656.
127. Juhan-Vague I, Alessi MC, Vague P. Thrombogenic and fibrinolytic factors and cardiovascular risk in non–insulin-dependent diabetes mellitus. Ann Med 1996; 28:371.
128. Brommer EJP, Derkx FHM, Schalekamp MADH, et al. Renal and hepatic handling of endogenous tissue-type plasminogen activator and its inhibitor in man. Thromb Haemost 1988; 59:404.
129. Juhan-Vague I, Alessi MC. Plasminogen activator inhibitor 1 and atherothrombosis. Thromb Haemost 1993; 70:138.
130. Hamsten A, de Faire U, Walldius G, et al. Plasminogen activator inhibitor in plasma: risk factor for recurrent myocardial infarction. Lancet 1987; 2:3.
131. Lijnen HR, Collen D. Endothelium in hemostasis and thrombosis. Prog Cardiovasc Dis 1997; 39:343.
132. Shaper AG, Marsh NA, Patel I, Kater F. Response of fibrinolytic activity to venous occlusion. BMJ 1975; 3:571.
133. Griffiths NJ, Woodford M, Irving MH. Alteration in fibrinolytic capacity after operation. Lancet 1977; 2:635.
134. Pottmeyer E, Vassar MJ, Holcroft JW. Coagulation, inflammation and response to injury. Crit Care Clin 1986; 2:683.
135. Moroz LA. Non–plasmin-mediated fibrinolysis. Semin Thromb Hemost 1984; 10:80.
136. Castellino FJ. Streptokinase. Methods Enzymol 1976; 45:244.
137. Summaria L, Robbins KC. Isolation of a human plasmin–derived functionally active, light (B) chain–streptokinase complex with plasminogen activator activity. J Biol Chem 1976; 251:5810.
138. Chesterman CN, Cederholm-Williams SA, Allington MJ. The degradation of streptokinase during the production of plasminogen activator. Thromb Res 1974; 5:413.
139. Markus G, Evers JL, Hobika GH. Activator activities of the human plasminogen-streptokinase complex during its proteolytic conversion to the stable activator complexes. J Biol Chem 1976; 251:6495.
140. Takada A, Takada Y. Potentiation of the activation of Glu-plasminogen by streptokinase and urokinase in the presence of fibrinogen degradation products. Thromb Res 1982; 25:229.
141. Bell WR, Sasahara A. Chemistry of thrombolytic agents. *In* Review of Thrombolytic Therapy and Thromboembolic Disease. Glenview, IL: Physicians and Scientists, 1990, pp 3–17.
142. Oliven A, Gidron E. Orally and rectally administered streptokinase: investigation of its absorption and activity. Pharmacology 1981; 22:135.
143. Mentzer RL, Budzynski AZ, Sherry S. High-dose, brief-duration intravenous infusion of streptokinase in acute myocardial infarction: Description of effects in circulation. Am J Cardiol 1986; 57:1220.
144. Nunn B, Esmail A, Fears R, et al. Pharmacokinetic properties of anisoylated plasminogen streptokinase activator complex and other thrombolytic agents in animals and humans. Drugs 1987; 33(suppl 3):88.
145. Brogden RN, Speight TM, Avery GS. Streptokinase: a review of its clinical pharmacology, mechanism of action and therapeutic uses. Drugs 1973; 5:357.
146. Nazari J, Davidson R, Kaplan K, Fintel D. Adverse reactions to thrombolytic agents: Implications for coronary reperfusion following myocardial infarction. Med Toxicol 1987; 2:274.
147. Thayer CF. Results of post-marketing surveillance program on streptokinase. Curr Ther Res 1981; 30:129.
148. Smith RAG, Dupe RJ, English PD. Fibrinolysis with acyl enzymes: a new approach to thrombolytic therapy. Nature 1981; 290:505.
149. Monk JP, Heel RC: Anisoylated plasminogen streptokinase activator complex (APSAC): A review of its mechanism of action, clinical pharmacology and therapeutic uses in acute myocardial infarction. Drugs 1987; 34:25–49.
150. Been M, deBoro DP, Muir AL, et al. Coronary thrombolysis with intravenous anisoylated plasminogen-streptokinase complex BRL 26921. Br Heart J 1985; 53:253.
151. Matsuo O, Collen D, Verstraete M. On the fibrinolytic and thrombolytic properties of active-site p-anisoylated streptokinase-plasminogen complex (BRL 26921). Thromb Res 1981; 24:347.
152. Fears R, Ferres H, Standring R. The protective effect of acylation on the stability of anisoylated plasminogen streptokinase activator complex in human plasma. Drugs 1987; 33:57.
153. Fears R. The effect of heparin and fibrin on the enzymatic efficiencies of thrombolytics in vitro. Drugs 1998; 33:69.
154. Staniforth DH, Smith RAG, Hibbs M. Streptokinase and anisoylated streptokinase plasminogen complex: their action on haemostasis in human volunteers. Eur J Clin Pharmacol 1983; 24:751.
155. Prowse CV, Honsey V, Ruckley CV, Boulton FE. A comparison of acylated streptokinase–plasminogen complex and streptokinase in healthy volunteers. Thromb Haemost 1984; 51:204.
156. Walker ID, Davidson JF, Rae AP, et al. Acylated streptokinase-plasminogen complex in patients with acute myocardial infarction. Thromb Haemost 1984; 51:204.
157. Collen D, Silence K, Demarsin E, et al. Isolation and characterization of natural and recombinant staphylokinase. Fibrinolysis 1992; 6:203.
158. Sako T, Sawaki S, Sakurai T, et al. Cloning and expression of the staphylokinase gene of *Staphylococcus aureus* in *E. coli.* Mol Gen Genet 1983; 190:271.
159. Behnke D, Gerlach D. Cloning and expression in *Escherichia coli, Bacillus subtillis,* and *Streptococcus sanguis* of a gene for staphylokinase-A bacterial plasminogen activator. Mol Gen Genet 1987; 210:528.
160. Lijnen HR, Van Hoef B, Vandenbossche L, Collen D. Biochemical properties of natural and recombinant staphylokinase. Fibrinolysis 1992; 6:214.

161. Collen D, Lijnen HR. Staphylokinase, a fibrin-specific plasminogen activator with therapeutic potential? Blood 195; 84:680.
162. Silence K, Collen D, Lijnen HR. Interaction between staphylokinase, plasmin(ogen) and α_2-antiplasmin: recycling of staphylokinase after neutralization of the plasmin-staphylokinase complex by α_2-antiplasmin. J Biol Chem 1993; 268:9811.
163. Lijnen HR, Van Hoef B, Matsuo O, Collen D. On the molecular interactions between plasminogen-staphylokinase, α_2-antiplasmin and fibrin. Biochem Biophys Acta 1992; 11118:144.
164. Lijnen HR, Stassen JM, Vanlinthout I, et al. Comparative fibrinolytic properties of staphylokinase and streptokinase in animal models of venous thrombosis. Thromb Haemost 1991; 66:468.
165. Collen D, De Cock F, Stassen JM. Comparative immunogenicity and thrombolytic properties toward arterial and venous thrombi of staphylokinase and streptokinase in baboons. Circulation 1993; 87:996.
166. Collen D, Van de Werf F. Coronary thrombolysis with recombinant staphylokinase in patients with evolving myocardial infarction. Circulation 1993; 87:1850.
167. Collen D, Bernaerts R, Declerck P, et al. Recombinant staphylokinase variants with altered immunoreactivity: I. Construction and characterization. Circulation 1996; 94:197.
168. Collen D, Moreau H, Stockx L, Vanderschuren S. Recombinant staphylokinase variants with altered immunoreactivity: II. Thrombolytic properties and antibody induction. Circulation 1996; 94:207.
169. McEvoy GK, McQuarrie GM, DiPietro-Heydron J. Thrombolytic agents. *In* McEvoy GK (ed): Drug Information '87. Bethesda, MD: American Society of Hospital Pharmacists, 1987, pp 700–705.
170. Wade A, Reynolds JEF, Prasad AB. Enzymes, choleretics and other digestive agents. *In* Reynolds JEF (ed): Martindale: The Extra Pharmacopoeia. London, Pharmaceutical Press, 1982, pp 644–661.
171. Sumi H, Sasaki K, Toki N, Robbins KC. Oral administration of urokinase. Thromb Res 1980; 20:711.
172. Collen D, De Cock F, Lijnen HR. Biological and thrombolytic properties of proenzyme and active forms of human urokinase: II. Turnover of natural and recombinant urokinase in rabbits and squirrel monkeys. Thromb Haemost 1984; 52:24.
173. Fletcher AP, Alkjaersig N, Sherry S, et al. The development of urokinase as a thrombolytic agent: maintenance of a sustained thrombolytic state in man by intravenous infusion. J Lab Clin Med 1965; 65:713.
174. Thorsen S, Glas-Greenwalt P, Astrup T. Differences in the binding to fibrin of urokinase and tissue plasminogen activator. Thromb Diath Haemorrh 1972; 28:65.
175. Bell WR, Sasahara A. Adverse events. *In* Review of Thrombolytic Therapy and Thromboembolic Disease. Glenview, IL: Physician and Scientists Publishing, 1990, pp 113–117.
176. Bell WR, Simon TL. A comparative analysis of pulmonary perfusion scans with pulmonary angiograms. Am Heart J 1976; 92:700.
177. Bell WR. Pulmonary embolism: progress and problems. Am J Med 1982; 72:181.
178. Holmes WE, Pennica D, Blaber M, et al. Cloning and expression of the gene for prourokinase in *Escherichia coli.* Biotechnology 1985; 3:923.
179. Stump DC. Pharmacokinetics of single chain forms of urokinase-type plasminogen activator. J Pharmacol Exp Ther 1987; 242:245.
180. de Boer A, Kluft C, Gerloff J, et al. Pharmacokinetics of saruplase, a recombinant unglycosylated human single-chain urokinase-type plasminogen activator and its effects on fibrinolytic and haemostatic parameters in healthy male subjects. Thromb Haemost 1993; 70:320.
181. Kuiper J, Rijken DC, de Munk GAW, van Berkel TJC. In vivo and in vitro interaction of high and low molecular weight single chain urokinase-type plasminogen activator with rat liver cells. J Biol Chem 1992; 267:1589.
182. van Griensven JMT, Koster R, Hopkins G, et al. Effect of changes in liver blood flow on the pharmacokinetics of saruplase in patients with acute myocardial infarction. Thromb Haemost 1997; 78:1015.
183. PRIMI Trial Study Group. Randomised double-blind trial of recombinant pro-urokinase against streptokinase in acute myocardial infarction. Lancet 1989; 1:863.
184. Michels HR, Hoffmann JML, Windeler J, Hopkins GR. Hemostatic changes after thrombolytic therapy with saruplase (unglycosylated single-chain urokinase-type plasminogen activator) and urokinase (two-chain urokinase-type plasminogen activator). Blood Coagul Fibrinolysis 1996; 7:766.
185. Rijken DC, Collen D. Purification and characterization of the plasminogen activator secreted by human melanoma cell lines in culture. J Biol Chem 1981; 156:7041.
186. Pennica D, Holmes WE, Kohr WJ, et al. Cloning and expression of human tissue-type plasminogen activator cDNA in *E. coli.* Nature 1983; 301:214.
187. Loscalzo J, Braunwald E. Tissue plasminogen activator. N Engl J Med 1988; 319:925.
188. Sobel BE, Saffitz JE, Fields LE, et al. Intramuscular administration of human tissue-type plasminogen activator in rabbits and dogs and its implications for coronary thrombolysis. Circulation 1987; 75:1261.
189. Bounameaux H, Stassen JM, Seghers C, Collen D. Influence of fibrin and liver flow on the turnover and the systemic fibrinogenolytic effects of recombinant human tissue-type plasminogen activator in rabbits. Blood 1986; 67:1493.
190. Brommer EJP, Schicht I, Wijngaards G, et al. Fibrinolytic activity and inhibitors in terminal renal insufficiency and in anephric patients. Thromb Haemost 1984; 52:311.
191. Topol EJ, Bell WR, Weisfeldt ML. Coronary thrombolysis with recombinant tissue plasminogen activator: a hematologic and pharmacologic study. Ann Intern Med 1985; 103:837.
192. Gimple LW, Gold HK, Leinbach RC, et al. Correlation between template bleeding times and spontaneous bleeding during treatment of acute myocardial infarction with recombinant tissue-type plasminogen activator. Circulation 1989; 80:581.
193. Kohnert U, Rudolph R, Verheijen JH, et al. Biochemical properties of the kringle 2 and protease domains are maintained in the refolded t-PA deletion variant BM 06.022. Protein Eng 1992; 5:93.
194. Noble S, McTavish D. Reteplase: a review of its pharmacologic properties and clinical efficacy in the management of acute myocardial infarction. Drugs 1996; 52:589.
195. Martin U, Fischer S, Kohnert U, et al. Coronary thrombolytic properties of a novel recombinant plasminogen activator (BM 06.022) in a canine model. J Cardiovasc Pharmacol 1991; 18:111.
196. Martin U, Fischer S, Kohnert U, et al. Pharmacokinetic properties of *Escherichia coli*–produced recombinant plasminogen activator (BM 06.022) in rabbits. Thromb Res 1991; 62:137.
197. Keyt BA, Paoni NF, Refino CJ, et al. A fast-acting and more potent form of tissue plasminogen activator. Proc Natl Acad Sci U S A 1993; 91:3670.
198. Cannon CP, McCabe CH, Gibson MS, et al. TNK-tissue plasminogen activator in acute myocardial infarction: results of the thrombolysis in myocardial infarction (TIMI) 10A dose-ranging trial. Circulation 1997; 95:351.
199. Larsen G, Timony GA, Horgan PG, et al. Protein engineering of novel plasminogen activators with increased thrombolytic potency in rabbits relative to Activase. J Biol Chem 1991; 266:8156.
200. O'Neill WW, Topol EJ, Pitt B. Reperfusion therapy of acute myocardial infarction. Prog Cardiovasc Dis 1988; 30:235.
201. Levine MN. Bolus, front-loaded, and accelerated thrombolytic therapy for myocardial infarction and pulmonary embolism. Chest 1991; 99:128S.
202. Lincoff AM, Topol EJ. Illusion of reperfusion: does anyone achieve optimal reperfusion during acute myocardial infarction? Circulation 1993; 87:1792.
203. Granger CB, Califf RM, Topol EJ. Thrombolytic therapy for acute myocardial infarction. Drugs 1992; 44:293.
204. Topol EJ. Thrombolytic intervention. *In* Topol EJ (ed): Textbook of Interventional Cardiology. Philadelphia: WB Saunders, 1998, pp 68–111.
205. Chesebro JH, Knatterud G, Roberts R, et al. Thrombolysis in myocardial infarction (TIMI) trial, phase 1: a comparison between intravenous tissue plasminogen activator and intravenous streptokinase. Circulation 1987; 76:142.
206. Califf RM, Topol EJ, Candele RJ, et al. Consequences of reocclusion after successful reperfusion therapy in acute myocardial infarction. Circulation 1990; 82:781.
207. Lavie CJ, Gersh BJ, Chesbro JH. Reperfusion in acute myocardial infarction. Mayo Clin Proc 1990; 65:549.
208. Popma JJ, Topol EJ. Adjuncts to thrombolysis for myocardial reperfusion. Ann Intern Med 1991; 115:34.

209. ISIS-2 (Second International Study of Infarct Survival) Collaborative Group. Randomised trial of intravenous streptokinase, oral aspirin, both, or neither among 17,187 cases of suspected myocardial infarction: ISIS-2. Lancet 1988; 2:349.
210. ISAM study group. A prospective trial of intravenous streptokinase in acute myocardial infarction (ISAM). N Engl J Med 1986; 314:1465.
211. White HD, Norris RM, Brown MA, et al. Effect of intravenous streptokinase on left ventricular function and early survival after acute myocardial infarction. N Engl J Med 1987; 317:850.
212. National Heart Foundation of Australia Coronary Thrombolysis Group. Coronary thrombolysis and myocardial salvage by tissue plasminogen activator given up to 4 hours after onset of myocardial infarction. Lancet 1988; 1:203.
213. Van de Werf F, Arnold AER. Intravenous tissue plasminogen activator and size of infarct, left ventricular function, and survival in acute myocardial infarction. BMJ 1988; 297:1374.
214. Bassand J-P, Machecourt J, Cassagnes J, et al. Multicenter trial of intravenous anisoylated plasminogen streptokinase activator complex (APSAC) in acute myocardial infarction: effects on infarct size and left ventricular function. J Am Coll Cardiol 1989; 13:988.
215. Armstrong PW, Baigrie RS, Daly PA, et al. Tissue plasminogen activator: Toronto (TPAT) placebo-controlled randomized trial in acute myocardial infarction. J Am Coll Cardiol 1989; 13:1469.
216. The GUSTO Angiographic Investigators. The effects of tissue plasminogen activator, streptokinase, or both on coronary-artery patency, ventricular function, and survival after acute myocardial infarction. N Engl J Med 1998; 329:1615.
217. Lamas GA, Flaker GC, Mitchell G, et al. Effect of infarct artery patency on prognosis after acute myocardial infarction. Circulation 1995; 92:1101.
218. Fibrinolytic Therapy Trialists' (FTT) Collaborative Group. Indications for fibrinolytic therapy in suspected acute myocardial infarction: collaborative overview of early mortality and major morbidity results from all randomised trials of more than 1000 patients. Lancet 1994; 343:311.
219. Honan MB, Harrell FE, Reimer KA, et al. Cardiac rupture, mortality and the timing of thrombolytic therapy: a meta-analysis. J Am Coll Cardiol 1990; 16:359.
220. Gruppo Italiano per lo Studio Della Sopravvivenza Nell'Infarto Microcardio. GISSI-2: a factorial randomised trial of alteplase versus streptokinase and heparin versus no heparin among 12,490 patients with acute myocardial infarction. Lancet 1990; 336:65.
221. ISIS-3 (Third International Study of Infarct Survival Collaborative Group). ISIS-3: a randomised comparison of streptokinase vs tissue plasminogen activator vs anistreplase and of aspirin plus heparin vs aspirin alone among 41,299 cases of suspected myocardial infarction. Lancet 1992; 339:753.
222. The GUSTO Investigators. An international randomized trial comparing four thrombolytic strategies for acute myocardial infarction. N Engl J Med 1993; 329:673.
223. Tebbe U, Michels R, Adgey J, et al. Randomized, double-blind study comparing saruplase with streptokinase therapy in acute myocardial infarction: the COMPASS equivalence trial. J Am Coll Cardiol 1998; 31:487.
224. Bode C, Smalling RW, Berg G, et al. Randomized comparison of coronary thrombolysis achieved with double-bolus reteplase (recombinant plasminogen activator) and front-loaded, accelerated alteplase (recombinant tissue plasminogen activator) in patients with acute myocardial infarction. Circulation 1996; 94:891.
225. Smalling RW, Bode C, Kalbfleisch JM, et al. More rapid, complete, and stable coronary thrombolysis with bolus administration of reteplase compared with alteplase infusion in acute myocardial infarction. Circulation 1995; 91:2725.
226. Bar F, Meyer J, Vermeer F, Michels R, et al. Comparison of saruplase and alteplase in acute myocardial infarction. Am J Cardiol 1997; 79:727.
227. GUSTO Investigators: A comparison of reteplase with alteplase for acute myocardial infarction. N Engl J Med 1997; 337:1118.
228. Sane DC, Califf RM, Topol EJ, et al. Bleeding during thrombolytic therapy for acute myocardial infarction: mechanisms and management. Ann Intern Med 1989; 111:1010.
229. Bovill EG, Terrin ML, Stump DC, et al. Hemorrhagic events during therapy with recombinant tissue-type plasminogen activator, heparin, and aspirin for acute myocardial infarction. Ann Intern Med 1991; 115:256.
230. Albrechtsson U, Anderson J, Einarsson E, et al. Streptokinase treatment of deep venous thrombosis and the postphlebitic syndrome. Arch Surg 1981; 116:33.
231. Weinmann EE, Salzman EW. Deep-vein thrombosis. N Engl J Med 1994; 331:1630.
232. Brown WD, Goldhaber SZ. How to select patients with deep vein thrombosis for t-PA therapy. Chest 1989; 95:276S.
233. Markel A, Manzo RA, Strandness E. The potential role of thrombolytic therapy in venous thrombosis. Arch Intern Med 1992; 152:1265.
234. Ott P, Eldrup E, Oxholm P, et al. Streptokinase therapy in routine management of deep venous thrombosis in the lower extremities: a retrospective study of phlebographic results and therapeutic complications. Acta Med Scand 1986; 219:295.
235. Verstraete M, Vermylen J, Amery A, Vermylen C. Thrombolytic therapy with streptokinase using a standard dosing scheme. BMJ 1966; 1:454.
236. Rogers LQ, Lutcher CL. Streptokinase therapy for deep vein thrombosis: a comprehensive review of the English literature. Am J Med 1990; 88:389.
237. Goldhaber SZ, Buring JE, Lipnick RL, Hennekens CH. Pooled analysis of randomized trials of streptokinase and heparin in phlebographically documented acute deep venous thrombosis. Am J Med 1984; 76:393.
238. Theiss W, Wirtzfeld A, Fink U, Maubach P. The success rate of fibrinolytic therapy in fresh and old thrombosis of the iliac and femoral veins. Angiology 1983; 34:61.
239. van de Loo JCW, Kriessmann A, Trubestein G, et al. Controlled multicenter pilot study of urokinase-heparin and streptokinase in deep venous thrombosis. Thromb Haemost 1983; 50:660.
240. Goldhaber SZ, Meyerovitz MF, Green D, et al. Randomised controlled trial of tissue plasminogen activator in proximal deep venous thrombosis. Am J Med 1990; 88:235.
241. Turpie AGG, Levine MN, Hirsh J, et al. Tissue plasminogen activator (rt-PA) vs. heparin in deep vein thrombosis. Chest 1990; 97:172S.
242. Dalen JE, Alpert JS. Natural history of pulmonary embolism. Prog Cardiovasc Dis 1975; 17:259.
243. Hermann RE, Davis JH, Holden WD. Pulmonary embolism: a clinical and pathologic study with emphasis on the effect of prophylactic therapy with anticoagulants. Am J Surg 1961; 102:19.
244. Benotti JR, Dalen JE. The natural history of pulmonary embolism. Clin Chest Med 1984; 5:403.
245. Paraskos JA, Adelstein SJ, Smith RE, et al. Late prognosis of acute pulmonary embolism. N Engl J Med 1973; 289:55.
246. Benotti JR, Ockene IS, Alpert JS, Dalen JE. The clinical profile of unresolved pulmonary embolism. Chest 1983; 84:669.
247. Sasahara A, Cannilla JE, Belko JS, et al. Urokinase therapy in clinical pulmonary embolism. N Engl J Med 1967; 277:1168.
248. Sautter RD, Emanuel DA, Fletcher FW, et al. Urokinase for the treatment of acute pulmonary thromboembolism. JAMA 1967; 202:215.
249. Tow DE, Wagner HN, Holmes REA. Urokinase in pulmonary embolism. N Engl J Med 1967; 277:1161.
250. Urokinase Pulmonary Embolism Trial Study Group. Urokinase pulmonary embolism trial: phase 1 results. JAMA 1970; 214:2163.
251. Urokinase Pulmonary Embolism Trial Study Group. Urokinase:streptokinase embolism trial: phase 2 results. JAMA 1974; 229:1606.
252. Sharma GVRK, Burleson VA, Sasahara AA. Effect of thrombolytic therapy on pulmonary-capillary blood volume in patients with pulmonary embolism. N Engl J Med 1980; 303:842.
253. Goldhaber SZ, Markis JE, Meyerovitz MF, et al. Acute pulmonary embolism treated with tissue plasminogen activator. Lancet 1986; 2:886.
254. Goldhaber SZ, Heit J, Sharma GVRK, et al. A randomized trial of recombinant tissue plasminogen activator versus urokinase in the treatment of acute pulmonary embolism. Lancet 1988; 2:293.
255. Verstraete M, Miller GAH, Bounameaux H, et al. Intravenous and intrapulmonary recombinant tissue-type plasminogen activator in the treatment of acute massive pulmonary embolism. Circulation 1988; 77:353.
256. Levine M, Hirsh J, Weitz J, et al. A randomized trial of a single bolus dosage regimen of recombinant tissue plasminogen activator in patients with acute pulmonary embolism. Chest 1990; 98:1473.

257. Goldhaber SZ, Haire WD, Feldstein ML, et al. Alteplase versus heparin in acute pulmonary embolism: randomised trial assessing right-ventricular function and pulmonary perfusion. Lancet 1993; 341:507.
258. Dalla-Volta S, Palla A, Santolicandro A, et al. Alteplase combined with heparin versus heparin in the treatment of acute pulmonary embolism: plasminogen activator Italian multicenter study 2. J Am Coll Cardiol 1992; 20:520.
259. PIOPED Investigators. Tissue plasminogen activator for the treatment of acute pulmonary embolism. Chest 1989; 97:528.
260. Konstantinides S, Geibel A, Olschewski M, et al. Association between thrombolytic treatment and the prognosis of hemodynamically stable patients with major pulmonary embolism: results of a multicenter registry. Circulation 1997; 96:882.
261. McNichol GP, Douglas AS. Treatment of peripheral vascular occlusion by streptokinase perfusion. Scand J Clin Lab Invest 1964; 16:23.
262. Earnshaw JJ. Thrombolytic therapy in the management of acute limb ischaemia. Br J Surg 1991; 78:261.
263. Dotter CT, Rosch J, Seaman AJ. Selective clot lysis with low dose streptokinase. Radiology 1974; 111:31.
264. Amery A, Deloof W, Vermylen J, Verstraete M. Outcome of recent thromboembolic occlusions of limb arteries treated with streptokinase. BMJ 1970; 4:639.
265. Towne JBBDF. Application of thrombolytic therapy in vascular occlusive disease: a surgical view. Am J Surg 1987; 154:548.
266. Poliwoda H, Alexander K, Buhl V, et al. Treatment of chronic arterial occlusions with streptokinase. N Engl J Med 1969; 280:689.
267. Belkin M, Belkin B, Bucknam CA, et al. Intra-arterial fibrinolytic therapy. Arch Surg 1986; 121:769.
268. Olin JW, Graor RA. Thrombolytic therapy in the treatment of peripheral arterial occlusions. Ann Emerg Med 1988; 17:1210.
269. Ouriel K, Veith FJ, Sasahara AA. A comparison of recombinant urokinase with vascular surgery as initial treatment for acute arterial occlusion of the legs. N Engl J Med 1998; 338:1105.
270. Berridge DC, Gregson RHS, Hopkinson BR, Makin GS. Randomized trial of intra-arterial recombinant tissue plasminogen activator, intravenous recombinant tissue plasminogen activator and intra-arterial streptokinase in peripheral arterial thrombolysis. Br J Surg 1991; 78:988.
271. Lonsdale RJ, Berridge DC, Earnshaw JJ, et al. Recombinant tissue-type plasminogen activator is superior to streptokinase for local intra-arterial thrombolysis. Br J Surg 1992; 79:272.
272. Fieschi C, Argentino C, Lenzi GL, et al. Clinical and instrumental evaluation of patients with ischemic stroke within the first six hours. J Neurol Sci 1989; 91:311.
273. del Zoppo GJ, Poeck K, Pessin MS, et al. Recombinant tissue plasminogen activator in acute thrombotic and embolic stroke. Ann Neurol 1992; 32:78.
274. Sussman BJ, Fitch TSP. Thrombolysis with fibrinolysin in cerebral arterial occlusion. JAMA 1959; 167:1705.
275. Abe T, Kazama M, Naito I. Clinical effect of urokinase (60,000 units/day) on cerebral infarction: comparative study by means of multiple center double blind test. Blood Vessel 1981; 12:342.
276. Atarashi J, Otomo E, Araki G. Clinical utility of urokinase in the treatment of acute stage of cerebral thrombosis: multi-center double-blind study in comparison to placebo. Clin Eval 1985; 13:659.
277. Otomo E, Araki G, Itoh E. Clinical efficacy of urokinase in the treatment of cerebral thrombosis. Clin Eval 1985; 13:711.
278. Abe T, Terashi A, Tohgi H. Clinical efficacy of intravenous administration of SM-9527 (t-PA) in cerebral thrombosis. Clin Eval 1990; 18:39.
279. Otomo E, Tohgi H, Hirai S. Clinical efficacy of AK-124 (tissue plasminogen activator) in the treatment of cerebral thrombosis: study by means of multi-center double blind comparison with urokinase. Yakuri To Chiryo 1988; 16:3775.
280. Pulsinelli WA, Jacewicz M, Levy DE, et al. Ischemic brain injury and the therapeutic window. Ann NY Acad Sci 1997; 835:187.
281. Zivin JA. Factors determining the therapeutic window for stroke. Neurology 1998; 50:599.
282. del Zoppo GJ, Ferbert A, Otis SM, et al. Local intra-arterial fibrinolytic therapy in acute carotid territory stroke: a pilot study. Stroke 1988; 19:307.
283. Mori E, Tabuchi M, Yoshida T, Yamadori A: Intracarotid urokinase with thromboembolic occlusion of the middle cerebral artery. Stroke 1988; 19:802.
284. Theron J, Courtheoux P, Casasco A, et al. Local intraarterial fibrinolysis in the carotid territory. AJNR 1989; 10:753.
285. Hacke W, Zeumer H, Ferbert A, et al. Intra-arterial thrombolytic therapy improves outcome in patients with acute vertebrobasilar occlusive disease. Stroke 1988; 19:1216.
286. del Zoppo GJ. Thrombolytic therapy in the treatment of stroke. Drugs 1997; 54:90.
287. del Zoppo GJ, Higashida RT, Furlan AJ, et al. PROACT: a phase II randomized trial of recombinant pro-urokinase by direct arterial delivery in acute middle cerebral artery stroke. Stroke 1998; 29:4.
288. Multicentre Acute Stroke Trial-Italy (MAST-I) Group. Randomised controlled trial of streptokinase, aspirin, and a combination of both in treatment of acute ischemic stroke. Lancet 1995; 346:1509.
289. Multicentre Acute Stroke Trial-Europe (MAST-E) Study Group. Thrombolytic therapy with streptokinase in acute ischemic stroke. N Engl J Med 1996; 335:145.
290. Geoffrey D, Davis SM, Chambers BR, et al. Streptokinase for acute ischemic stroke with relationship to time of administration. JAMA 1996; 276:961.
291. Fisher M, Bogousslavsky J. Further evolution toward effective therapy for acute ischemic stroke. JAMA 1998; 279:1298.
292. Hacke W, Kaste M, Fieschi C, et al. Intravenous thrombolysis with recombinant tissue plasminogen activator for acute hemispheric stroke: the European Cooperative Acute Stroke Study (ECASS). JAMA 1995; 274:1017.
293. The National Institutes of Neurological Disorders and Stroke rt-PA Study Group. Tissue plasminogen activator for acute ischemic strokc. N Engl J Med 1995; 333:1581.
294. Adams HP, Brott TG, Furlan AJ, et al. Guidelines for thrombolytic therapy for acute stroke: a supplement to the guidelines for the management of patients with acute ischemic stroke. Circulation 1996; 94:1167.
295. Wardlaw JM, Warlow CP, Counsell C. Systematic review of evidence on thrombolytic therapy for acute ischaemic stroke. Lancet 1997; 350:607.
296. Alberts MJ. Hyperacute stroke therapy with tissue plasminogen activator. Am J Cardiol 1997; 80:29D.
297. Marder VJ, Sherry S. Thrombolytic therapy: current status (second of two parts). N Engl J Med 1988; 318:1585.
298. Kurzrok S, Singh AK, Most AS, Williams DO. Thrombolytic therapy for prosthetic cardiac valve thrombosis. J Am Coll Cardiol 1987; 9:592.
299. Hurtubise MR, Bottino JC, Lawson M, McCredie KB. Restoring patency of occluded central venous catheters. Arch Surg 1980; 115:212.
300. Sherry S, Bell WR, Duckert FH. Thrombolytic therapy in thrombosis: a National Institutes of Health consensus development conference. Ann Intern Med 1980; 93:141.
301. De Jaegere PP, Arnold AA, Balk AH, Simoons ML. Intracranial hemorrhage in association with thrombolytic therapy: incidence and clinical predictive factors. J Am Coll Cardiol 1992; 19:289.
302. Karnash SL, Granger CB, White HD, et al. Treating menstruating women with thrombolytic therapy: insights from the global utilization of streptokinase and tissue plasminogen activator for occluded coronary arteries (GUSTO-I) trial. J Am Coll Cardiol 1995; 26:1651.
303. Barbash GI, White HD, Modan M, Van de Werf F. Significance of diabetes mellitus in patients with acute myocardial infarction receiving thrombolytic therapy. J Am Coll Cardiol 1997; 22:707.
304. Mahaffey KW, Granger CB, Toth CA, et al. Diabetic retinopathy should not be a contraindication to thrombolytic therapy for acute myocardial infarction: review of ocular hemorrhage incidence and location in the GUSTO-I trial. J Am Coll Cardiol 1997; 30:1606.
305. Rao AK, Pratt C, Berke A, et al. Thrombolysis in Myocardial Infarction (TIMI) Trial-Phase I: hemorrhagic manifestations and changes in plasma fibrinogen and the fibrinolytic system in patients treated with recombinant tissue plasminogen activator and streptokinase. J Am Coll Cardiol 1988; 11:1.
306. Califf RM, Topol EJ, George BS, et al. Hemorrhagic complications associated with the use of intravenous tissue-plasminogen activator in the treatment of acute myocardial infarction. Am J Med 1988; 85:353.
307. Ness PM, Perkins HA. Cryoprecipitate as a reliable source of fibrinogen replacement. JAMA 1979; 241:1690.

308. Salzmann EW. Hemostatic problems in the surgical patient. *In* Hirsh RW, Marder VJ, Salzmann EW (eds): Hemostasis and Thrombosis: Basic Principles. Philadelphia: JB Lippincott, 1987, p 922.
309. Okamoto S, Nakajima T, Okamoto U. A suppressing effect of ε-amino-n-caproic acid on the bleeding of dogs produced with the activation of plasmin in the circulating blood. Keio J Med 1959; 8:247.
310. Kunitz M, Northrup JH. Isolation from beef pancreas of crystalline trypsinogen, trypsin, a trypsin inhibitor, and an inhibitor-trypsin compound. J Gen Physiol 1936; 19:991.
311. McNicol GP, Fletcher AP, Alkjaersig N, Sherry S. The absorption, distribution, and excretion of ε-aminocaproic acid following oral or intravenous administration in man. J Lab Clin Med 1962; 59:15.
312. Ahlberg A. Diffusion of epsilon aminocaproic acid to the joints. Proc Soc Exp Biol Med 1970; 134:988.
313. Levy BJ, Silver D. Treatment of subarachnoid haemorrhage: the ability of epsilon aminocaproic acid to cross the blood–brain barrier and reduce spinal fluid fibrinolytic activity. Surg Forum 1968; 19:413.
314. Nilsson IM. Clinical pharmacology of aminocaproic acid and tranexamic acid. J Clin Pathol 1980; 33:41.
315. Alkjaersig N, Fletcher AP, Sherry S. ε-Aminocaproic acid: an inhibitor of plasminogen activation. J Biol Chem 1959; 234:832.
316. Ablondi FB, Hagan JJ, Philips M, De Renzo EC. Inhibition of plasmin, trypsin and the streptokinase-activated fibrinolytic system by ε-aminocaproic acid. Arch Biochem Biophys 1959; 82:153.
317. Lorand L, Condit EV. Ester hydrolysis by urokinase. Biochemistry 1965; 4:265.
318. Rakoczi I, Wiman B, Collen D. On the biological significance of the specific interaction between fibrin, plasminogen and antiplasmin. Biochem Biophys Acta 1978; 540:295.
319. Frederickson MC, Bowsher DJ, Ruo TI, et al. Kinetics of epsilon-aminocaproic acid distribution, elimination and antifibrinolytic effect in normal subjects. Clin Pharmacol Ther 1984; 35:387.
320. Nilsson IM, Anderson L, Bjorkman SE. Epsilon-aminocaproic acid as a therapeutic agent: based on 5 years' clinical experience. Acta Med Scand 1966; Suppl 448:1.
321. Ogston D. Antifibrinolytic Drugs. New York: John Wiley & Sons, 1966, pp 84–86.
322. Andersson L, Nilsson IM. Experimental and clinical studies on AMCA, the antifibrinolytically active isomer of a *p*-aminomethyl cyclohexane carboxylic acid. Scand J Haematol 1965; 2:230.
323. Eriksson O, Kjellman H, Pilbrant A, Schannong M. Pharmacokinetics of tranexamic acid after intravenous administration to normal volunteers. Eur J Clin Pharmacol 1974; 7:375.
324. Andersson L. Special considerations with regard to the dosage of tranexamic acid in patients with chronic renal disease. Urol Res 1978; 6:83.
325. Dubber AHC. In vitro and in vivo studies with Trasylol, an anticoagulant and a fibrinolytic inhibitor. Br J Haematol 1968; 14:31.
326. van Oeveren W, Eijman L, Roozendaal KJ, Wildevuur CR. Platelet preservation by aprotinin during cardiopulmonary bypass. Lancet 1988; 1:644.
327. Ogston D. Antifibrinolytic Drugs. New York: John Wiley & Sons, 1984, p 52.
328. Bellar FK, Epstein MD, Kaller H. Distribution, halflife time and placental transfer of the protease inhibitor Trasylol. Thromb Diath Haemorrh 1966; 16:302.
329. Freeman JG, Turner GA, Venables CW, Latner AL. Serial use of aprotinin and incidence of allergic reactions. Curr Med Res Opin 1983; 8:559.
330. Meyer JS. Lysis of cerebrovascular blood clots. NY State J Med 1962; 62:3750.
331. Kakkar VV, Flanc C, O'Shea MJ, et al. Treatment of deep-vein thrombosis with streptokinase. Br J Surg 1969; 56:178.
332. Sindet-Pedersen S. Distribution of tranexamic acid to plasma and saliva after oral administration and mouth rinsing: a pharmacokinetic study. J Clin Pharmacol 1987; 27:1005.
333. Walsh PN, Rizza CR, Mathews JM, et al. Epsilon-aminocaproic acid therapy for dental extractions in haemophilia and Christmas disease: a double blind controlled trial. Br J Haematol 1971; 20:463.
334. Forbes CD, Barr RD, Reid G, et al. Tranexamic acid in control of haemorrhage after dental extraction in haemophilia and Christmas disease. BMJ 1972; 2:311.
335. Kamel K, Cumming RA, Davies SH. Fibrinolytic system in certain congenital and hereditary haemorrhagic disorders, a critical evaluation of the theory of dynamic haemostasis. Nature 1963; 200:478.
336. Ogston D. Antifibrinolytic Drugs. New York: John Wiley & Sons, 1984, pp 103–109.
337. Gardner FH, Helmer REI. Aminocaproic acid: use in control of hemorrhage in patients with amegakaryocytic thrombocytopenia. JAMA 1980; 243:35.
338. Bartholomew JR, Salgia R, Bell WR. Control of bleeding in patients with immune and nonimmune thrombocytopenia with aminocaproic acid. Arch Intern Med 1989; 149:1959.
339. Cox HT, Poller L, Thompson JM. Gastric fibrinolysis: a possible aetiologic link to peptic ulcer. Lancet 1967; 1:1300.
340. Cormack F, Jouhar AJ, Chakrabarti RR, Fearney GR. Tranexamic acid in upper gastrointestinal haemorrhage. Lancet 1973; 1:1207.
341. Biggs JC, Hugh TB, Dodds AJ. Tranexamic acid and upper gastrointestinal bleeding—a double blind trial. Gut 1976; 17:729.
342. Engvist A, Brestrom O, Feilitzen FV, et al. Tranexamic acid in massive haemorrhage from the upper gastrointestinal tract: a double blind study. Scand J Gastroenterol 1979; 14:839.
343. Barer D, Ogilvie A, Henry D, et al. Cimetidine and tranexamic acid in the treatment of acute upper-gastrointestinal-tract bleeding. N Engl J Med 1983; 308:1571.
344. Henry DA, O'Connell DL. Effects of fibrinolytic inhibitors on mortality from upper gastrointestinal haemorrhage. BMJ 1989; 298:1142.
345. Mowat NAG. Epsilon-aminocaproic acid therapy in ulcerative colitis. Am J Dig Dis 1973; 18:959.
346. Albrechtsen OK. The fibrinolytic activity of the human endometrium. Acta Endocrinol 1956; 3:207.
347. Bonnar J, Sheppard BL. Treatment of menorrhagia during menstruation: randomised controlled trial of ethamsylate, mefenamic acid, and tranexamic acid. BMJ 1996; 313:579.
348. Bonnar J, Kasonde K, Haddon M, et al. Fibrinolytic activity in utero after bleeding complications with intrauterine devices. Br J Obstet Gynecol 1976; 83:160.
349. Rybo G, Westerberg H. The effect of tranexamic acid on postoperative bleeding after conization. Acta Obstet Gynecol Scand 1972; 51:347.
350. Ogston D. Antifibrinolytic Drugs. New York: John Wiley & Sons, 1984, pp 128–137.
351. Fodstad H, Ljunggren B. Antifibrinolytic drugs in subarachnoid hemorrhage. *In* Sawaya R (ed): Fibrinolysis and the Central Nervous System. Philadelphia: Hanley & Belfus, 1990, pp 257–273.
352. McNichol GP, Fletcher AP, Alkjaersig N, Sherry S. Impairment of hemostasis in the urinary tract: the role of urokinase. J Lab Clin Med 1961; 58:34.
353. Miller RA, May MW, Hendry WF, et al. The prevention of secondary haemorrhage after prostatectomy: the value of antifibrinolytic therapy. Br J Urol 1980; 52:26.
354. Gamba G, Fornasari PM, Grignani G, et al. Haemostasis during transvesical prostatic adenomectomy: a controlled trial on the effects of drugs with antifibrinolytic and thrombin-like activities. Blut 1979; 39:89.
355. Stefanini M, English HA, Taylor AE. Safe and effective, prolonged administration of epsilon aminocaproic acid in bleeding from the urinary tract. J Urol 1990; 143:559.
356. Ogston D. Antifibrinolytic Drugs. New York: John Wiley & Sons, 1984, pp 114–122.
357. Boylan JF, Klinck JR, Sandler AN, et al. Tranexamic acid reduces blood loss, transfusion requirements, and coagulation factor use in primary orthotopic liver transplantation. Anesthesiology 1996; 85:1043.
358. Neuhaus P, Bechstein WO, Lefebre B, et al. Effect of aprotinin on intraoperative bleeding and fibrinolysis in liver transplantation. Lancet 1989; 2:924.
359. Mallet SV, Cox D, Burroughs AK, Rolles K. Aprotinin and reduction of blood loss and transfusion requirements in orthotopic liver transplantation. Lancet 1990; 336:886.
360. Groh J, Welte M, Azad SC, et al. Does aprotinin affect blood loss in liver transplantation? Lancet 1992; 340:173.
361. Benoni G, Fredin H. Fibrinolytic inhibition with tranexamic acid reduces blood loss and blood transfusion after knee arthroplasty: a prospective, randomised, double blind study of 86 patients. J Bone Joint Surg Br 1996; 78:434.

362. Khuri SF, Michelson AD, Valeri CR. Effects of cardiopulmonary bypass on hemostasis. *In* Loscalzo J, Schafer Al (eds): Thrombosis and Hemorrhage. Baltimore: Williams & Wilkins, 1998, pp 1091–1117.
363. Khuri SF, Wolfe JA, Josa M, et al. Hematologic changes during and after cardiopulmonary bypass and their relationship to the bleeding time and non-surgical blood loss. J Thorac Cardiovasc Surg 1992; 104:94.
364. Khuri SF, Valeri CR, Loscalzo J, et al. Heparin causes platelet dysfunction and induces fibrinolysis before cardiopulmonary bypass. Ann Thorac Surg 1995; 60:1008.
365. Kongsgaard UE, Smith-Erichsen N, Geiran O, Bjornskau L. Changes in the coagulation and fibrinolytic systems during and after cardiopulmonary bypass surgery. Thorac Cardiovasc Surg 1989; 37:158.
366. Stibbe J, Kluft C, Brommer EJP, et al. Enhanced fibrolytic activity during cardiopulmonary bypass in open-heart surgery in man is caused by extrinsic (tissue-type) plasminogen activator. Eur J Clin Invest 1984; 14:375.
367. Tabuchi N, de Haan J, Boonstra PW, van Oeveren W. Activation of fibrinolysis in the pericardial cavity during cardiopulmonary bypass. J Thorac Cardiovasc Surg 1993; 106:828.
368. DelRossi AJ, Cernaianu AC, Botros S, et al. Prophylactic treatment of postperfusion bleeding using EACA. Chest 1989; 96:27.
369. Daily PO, Lamphere JA, Dembitsky WP, et al. Effect of prophylactic epsilon-aminocaproic acid on blood loss and transfusion requirements in patients undergoing first-time coronary artery bypass grafting: a randomized, prospective, double-blind study. J Thorac Cardiovasc Surg 1994; 108:99.
370. Vander Salm TJ, Kaur S, Lancey RA, et al. Reduction of bleeding after heart operations through the prophylactic use of epsilon-aminocaproic acid. J Thorac Cardiovasc Surg 1996; 112:1098.
371. Karski JM, Teasdale SJ, Norma P, et al. Prevention of bleeding after cardiopulmonary bypass with high-dose tranexamic acid: double-blind, randomized trial. J Thorac Cardiovasc Surg 1995; 110:835.
372. Katsaros D, Petricevic M, Snow NJ, et al. Tranexamic acid reduces postbypass blood use: a double-blinded, prospective, randomized study of 210 patients. Ann Thorac Surg 1996; 61:1131.
373. Dietrich W, Barankay A, Dilthey G, et al. Reduction of homologous blood requirement in cardiac surgery by intraoperative aprotinin application: clinical experience in 152 cardiac surgery patients. Thorac Cardiovasc Surg 1989; 37:92.
374. Harder MP, Eijsman L, Roozendaal KJ, et al. Aprotinin reduces intraoperative and postoperative blood loss in membrane oxygenator cardiopulmonary bypass. Ann Thorac Surg 1991; 51:936.
375. Fraedrich G, Weber C, Bernard C, et al. Reduction of blood transfusion requirement in open heart surgery by administration of high doses of aprotinin: preliminary results. Thorac Cardiovasc Surg 1989; 37:89.
376. Royston D, Bidstrup BP, Taylor KM, Sapsford RN. Effect of aprotinin on need for blood transfusion after repeat open-heart surgery. Lancet 1987; 2:1289.
377. Bidstrup BP, Royston D, Sapsford RN, Taylor KM. Reduction in blood loss and blood use after cardiopulmonary bypass with high dose aprotinin (Trasylol). J Thorac Cardiovasc Surg 1989; 97:364.
378. Blauhut B, Gross C, Necek S, et al. Effects of high-dose aprotinin on blood loss, platelet function, fibrinolysis, complement, and renal function after cardiopulmonary bypass. J Thorac Cardiovasc Surg 1991; 101:958.
379. Dietrich W, Barankay A, Hahnel C, Richter JA. High-dose aprotinin in cardiac surgery: Three years' experience in 1,784 patients. J Cardiothorac Vasc Anesth 1992; 6:324.
380. Cosgrove DM, Heric B, Lytle BW, et al. Aprotinin therapy for reoperative myocardial revascularization: a placebo-controlled study. Ann Thorac Surg 1993; 54:1031.
381. Speekenbrink RG, Wildevuur CR, Sturk A, Eijman L. Low-dose and high-dose aprotinin improve hemostasis in coronary operations. J Thorac Cardiovasc Surg 1996; 112:523.
382. Lemmer JH, Dilling EW, Morton JR, et al. Aprotinin for primary coronary artery bypass grafting: a multicenter trial of three dose regimens. Ann Thorac Surg 1996; 62:1659.
383. Levy JH, Pifarre R, Schaff HV, et al. A multi-center, double-blind, placebo-controlled trial of aprotinin for reducing blood loss and the requirement for donor-blood transfusion in patients undergoing repeat coronary artery bypass grafting. Circulation 1995; 92:2236.
384. Bidstrup BP, Underwood SR, Sapsford RN: Effect of aprotinin (Trasylol) on aorta-coronary bypass graft patency. J Thorac Cardiovasc Surg 1993; 105:147.
385. Lemmer JH, Stanford W, Bonney SL, et al. Aprotinin for coronary bypass surgery: efficacy, safety, and influence on early saphenous vein graft patency: a multicenter, randomized, double-blind, placebo-controlled study. J Thorac Cardiovasc Surg 1994; 107:543.
386. Havel M, Grabenwoger F, Schneider J, et al. Aprotinin does not decrease early graft patency after coronary artery bypass grafting despite reducing postoperative bleeding and use of donated blood. J Thorac Cardiovasc Surg 1994; 107:807.

CHAPTER 18

Plasma Protein Products

William N. Drohan
David B. Clark

PLASMA PROTEINS FOR CLINICAL USE

The preparation of plasma proteins has evolved from an ad hoc effort to provide specific products for individual patients into a global industry, with a large number of organizations throughout the world involved in the fractionation of plasma into a variety of derivatives for clinical use. Among the products licensed for use in the United States are albumin products, immunoglobulins, factor VIII and factor IX concentrates, α_1-proteinase inhibitor, and antithrombin III (AT-III). Other products available in Europe include fibrin sealant, von Willebrand factor (vWF), C_1-esterase inhibitor, and several other coagulation factors. This chapter focuses primarily on human plasma-derived products available in the United States. However, it also includes information on new or improved plasma protein products that are still in development or clinical evaluation, products available in other countries that have not yet been approved in the United States, and products produced by genetic engineering technologies.

There have been major improvements in plasma fractionation since World War II. Two major areas of advance should be emphasized as fundamental to modern plasma product therapy, process technology, and product safety. Advances in process technology have led to an ability to provide more products in more highly purified form at reasonable cost. Traditional precipitation-based processes have been supplemented and sometimes replaced by chromatographic and other techniques. Major advances in process technology have included improved methods for the concentration and diafiltration of proteins, better resins for chromatography, and the development of large-scale affinity chromatography including immunoaffinity methods, a technique made possible by large-scale preparation of monoclonal antibodies.[1] Today, each unit of plasma can be used to produce a large number of products at high yield and purity.

The second major area of advance, and probably the area of greatest focus in the plasma industry today, has been the development of effective techniques for the inactivation or removal of viruses that may be present in the starting plasma. Current techniques include heat treatment or pasteurization, chemical inactivation, and physical removal. Together they have significantly reduced the probability of transmitting viral infection with most plasma derivatives.

Progress has also come in the raw material; several plasma protein products are no longer derived from plasma. Extraordinary advances in genetic technology have led to the molecular cloning and expression of many important human plasma proteins. Recombinant versions of both factor VIII and factor IX are currently available, and experience shows them to be safe and efficacious. Additional recombinant plasma proteins are being developed. Another active area of development is the production of recombinant proteins in the milk of large transgenic farm animals.[2] This technology, if successful, will offer an additional means of providing large quantities of safe, economically produced therapeutic products.

HISTORY OF PLASMA FRACTIONATION

The development of methods for the large-scale preparation of plasma proteins began over 50 years ago.[3, 4] In the spring of 1940, after the outbreak of war in Europe, a meeting was held in Washington, D.C., to discuss the United States armed forces' request for 300,000 units of whole blood or plasma for transfusion. At that time, such a request seemed impossibly large. Alternatively, the armed forces needed a safe and effective blood substitute that would be stable under a wide variety of climatic conditions, compact for convenient transport, and easy to administer under field conditions. It was recognized that albumin, responsible for 80% of plasma's colloid osmotic pressure, would be the most effective plasma volume expander, and there was evidence in the literature that albumin might be less antigenic than some of the other plasma proteins.[3]

Dr. Edwin J. Cohn of the Harvard Medical School was approached to determine whether animal plasma could be made safe for human use. Cohn's Laboratory of Physical Chemistry had been devoted to studies of factors governing the solubility of amino acids, peptides, and proteins. He created a task force of investigators who continued to work together throughout the war to study the physical properties of plasma protein fractions. A method was developed for the fractionation of bovine plasma based on the differential precipitation of the various plasma proteins by appropriate combinations of ethanol concentration, pH, low temperature, ionic strength, and protein concentration. The use of ethanol as the protein precipitant permitted operations at temperatures below 0°C, which diminished the chance of bacterial growth. Moreover, the ethanol could be removed from the precipitated proteins by drying under vacuum in the frozen state. This was a much better system than those previously used for large-scale purification of plasma proteins.[3]

Within a short time, highly purified preparations of bovine serum albumin were available for clinical trials. Although there were no immediate reactions after the injection of these preparations, severe and prolonged serum sickness developed in some recipients, making it obvious that this preparation was unsuitable for therapeutic use. Meanwhile, Cohn had arranged with the American Red Cross, which was setting up blood collection centers in various cities, to provide his laboratory with a supply of human plasma. The ethanol method was quickly adapted to human plasma fractionation, and concentrated solutions of highly purified human serum albumin were prepared. Before all the intended clinical studies could be performed, battle casualties necessitated that the total supply of human serum albumin available from the Harvard Pilot Plant be flown to Pearl Harbor. Although albumin was the only plasma product distributed during the war, the remaining plasma fractions were preserved, and other preparations, including immunoglobulins and fibrinogen, were later developed.

FRESH FROZEN PLASMA

Plasma that is separated from the red blood cells of a donated whole blood unit, frozen within 6 hours of collection, and stored at −18°C or colder meets the criteria for therapeutic use as fresh frozen plasma (FFP).[5] The indications for the use of FFP are generally limited to the treatment of deficiencies of coagulation proteins for which appropriate concentrates are unavailable. These include the treatment of certain isolated deficiencies (e.g., factors V and XI), the reversal of anticoagulation due to warfarin therapy, and situations in which multiple factor deficiencies occur.[6] However, FFP, as well as other blood components, is often used for unlabeled indications, such as as a volume expander or a nutritional source.[6, 7] A consensus panel at the National Institutes of Health observed a large increase in the use of FFP and determined that its use for many unlabeled indications was inappropriate. A major educational effort is under way in many hospitals to make physicians aware of the risks involved in the inappropriate use of FFP.[8]

The major risk in the administration of FFP is the transmission of viral infection. At present, the viral safety of FFP depends entirely on donor selection and donor blood screening methods. However, a method has recently been developed for the solvent-detergent treatment of plasma to inactivate any lipid-enveloped viruses that might be present.[9, 10] The plasma is treated with 1% tri-*n*-butyl phosphate (TNBP) and 1% Triton X-100 for 4 hours at 30°C. The solvent and detergent are then removed by extraction with soybean oil, with any residual amounts removed in a subsequent chromatographic step. The coagulation factor content of solvent-detergent–treated plasma (SD-plasma) has been found to be comparable to that of untreated FFP.[11] Clinical trials have shown that SD-plasma is efficacious when treating acquired or inherited coagulation factor deficiencies and thrombotic thrombocytopenic purpura.[12, 13] SD-plasma was recently licensed in the United States, and is currently available in Europe.

ALBUMIN AND PLASMA PROTEIN FRACTION

Albumin, which is used as a plasma volume expander, is one of the major products of plasma fractionation. Since the initial use of human serum albumin in treating the casualties at Pearl Harbor, massive quantities of albumin have been isolated, and millions of units of albumin solutions have been infused.[14] Most manufacturers prepare albumin by some modification of the Cohn ethanol fractionation method (known as method 6),[15] but chromatographic methods[16] are also being used.

A fractionation scheme designed around Cohn's method 6 is shown in Figure 18–1. Most manufacturers start by thawing the plasma at a low temperature to collect a cryoprecipitate that is rich in factor VIII, vWF, fibrinogen, and other proteins. The cryosupernatant or cryo-poor plasma can then be treated to remove the vitamin K–dependent clotting factors, AT-III, or C_1-esterase inhibitor before it is processed by the Cohn method to obtain albumin, immunoglobulins, and other products. Albumin, having the highest solubility and the lowest isoelectric point of all the major plasma proteins, remains in solution as the ethanol concentration is raised in stages from zero to 40%, with an overall decrease in pH from neutral to 5.8 and a temperature adjustment to −5°C. Other proteins, such as fibrinogen (fraction I), immunoglobulins (fraction II + III), and α and β globulins (fractions IV_1 and IV_4) are precipitated during this process and are separated from those remaining in solution by conventional liquid-solid separation techniques such as centrifugation and filtration. It is only when the pH is adjusted to a value near its isoelectric point (pH 4.8) in the presence of 40% ethanol at −5°C that the majority of albumin is precipitated in fraction V.[14, 17] After the removal of ethanol and salts by lyophilization or diafiltration, sodium acetyltryptophanate and sodium caprylate are added to stabilize the product during heat treatment. The albumin preparation is sterile filtered, bottled, and then heated for 10 hours at 60°C to inactivate blood-borne viruses. Recently manufacturers have also been working on methods to decrease the aluminum content of albumin products because of aluminum's implication in several diseases.[18]

The original version of Cohn's method 6 requires five precipitation and separation steps to reach fraction V. Over the years, automation has been increased, and numerous improvements have resulted in better yields, shorter processing times, and enhanced process consistency. Many of the modifications have been aimed at reducing the volume of liquid that is processed and at combining steps. These include precipitating fraction I and II + III together and fractions IV_1 and IV_4 together. Such improvements have the potential to reduce both capital requirements and operating expenses.[19]

Three albumin products are currently manufactured

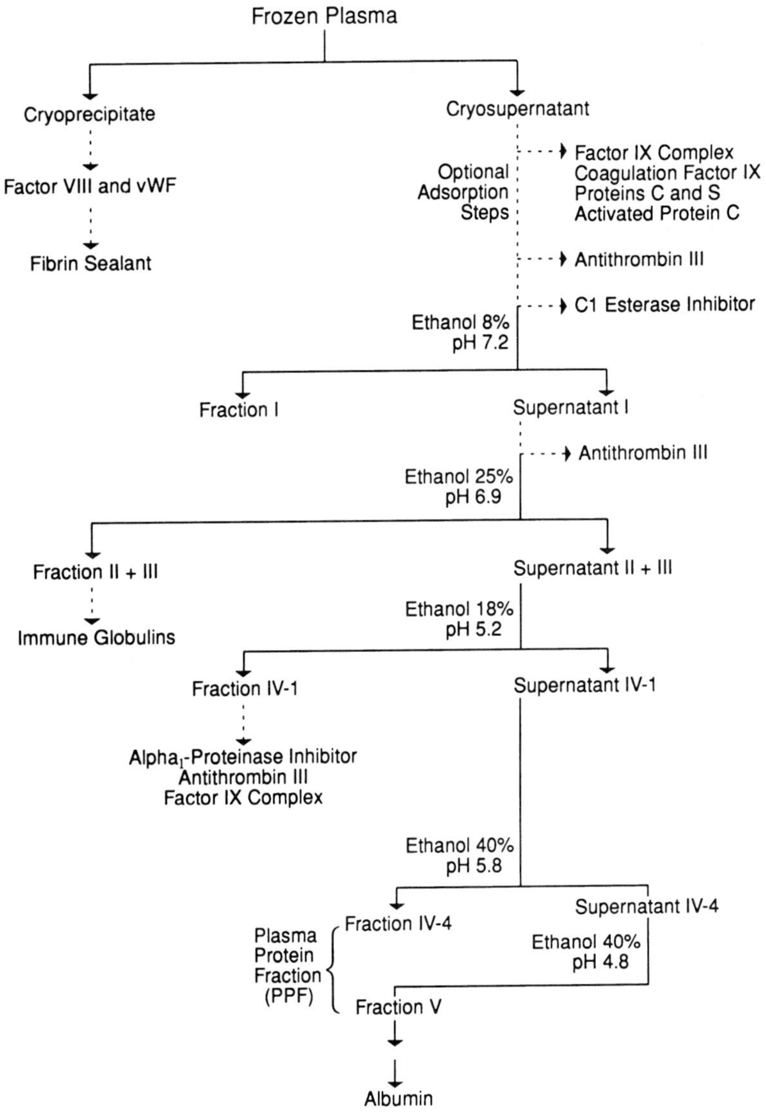

Figure 18–1. Plasma fractionation scheme. (From Drohan WN, Clark DB. Preparation of plasma-derived and recombinant human plasma proteins. *In* Hoffman R, Benz EJ Jr, Shattil SJ, et al [eds]: Hematology: Basic Principles and Practice, 3rd ed. Philadelphia: WB Saunders, in press.)

in the United States: albumin (human) 25%, albumin (human) 5%, and plasma protein fraction (PPF). To be designated albumin (human), at least 96% of the protein content must be albumin.[20] PPF, introduced in 1962, is an albumin product of lower purity that can still be heat-treated for 10 hours at 60°C. PPF is obtained in a simpler fractionation scheme by coprecipitating fractions IV_4 and V.[21] The additional proteins present in PPF are largely α and β globulins. The total protein in PPF must be at least 83% albumin, with no more than 17% globulins and no more than 1% γ globulin. PPF is more economical to produce than albumin and can be recovered in higher yields.[22] However, the rapid infusion of PPF has been associated with hypotensive episodes,[23, 24] and the use of PPF is therefore more limited than the use of albumin.[14] Albumin (human) 25% is also often used as a stabilizer in the formulation of other highly purified plasma products.

Chromatographic methods are being used to prepare albumin for clinical use, primarily outside the United States. After a pretreatment to remove lipids, cryo-poor plasma is processed by anion exchange chromatography on diethylaminoethyl (DEAE)-Sepharose, cation exchange chromatography on carboxymethyl (CM)-Sepharose, and gel filtration on Sephacryl S-200. The entire process takes about 5 days and yields a product of approximately 99% purity.[16, 25, 26] It is unknown whether the higher purity is clinically relevant, but recoveries are similar to those of Cohn fractionation.[19] This method has not been adopted in the United States, because of previous capital investments in Cohn fractionation.

IMMUNE GLOBULINS

Therapeutic use of immune globulins began in the 1950s when immune globulin concentrates were prepared from the fraction II + III precipitate obtained with Cohn's method.[15] In this process, known as Cohn-Oncley fractionation, the fraction II + III precipitate is first extracted with 20% ethanol, at pH 7.2, to solubilize lipoproteins.[27] The immune globulin-rich precipitate is then dissolved and brought to 17% ethanol at pH 5.2 to precipitate fraction III, which contains immune globulin M (IgM), IgA, and β globulins. The ethanol content of the supernatant is further increased to 25% at pH 7.4 to precipitate IgG as fraction II. The pH, ethanol concentration, and salt content at the fraction III precipitation step have a significant impact on purity, recovery, and viral safety of the product.[28] Variations of this purification scheme continue to be used by fractionators worldwide to prepare immune globulin concentrates.[29]

Two types of immune globulin preparations are produced: normal immune globulins from unselected donors, and hyperimmune products from donors selected because they have higher levels of specific antibodies. Hyperimmune globulin products are prepared from the plasma of donors with high antibody titers against antigens such as tetanus, hepatitis B, and Rh_o-D blood group antigen. These donors either have been identified in the convalescent period after infection or have been specifically immunized to produce the antibody.

The original immune globulin concentrates were known as immune serum globulin (ISG)—now immune globulin (human)—and were administered by the intramuscular route with the associated problems of limited injectable volume, poor bioavailability, and discomfort at the injection site.[30] Intravenous injection of ISG caused serious clinical reactions, attributed to complement-activating aggregates in these products.[31] To overcome these limitations, immune globulin intravenous (human) (IGIV) products have been developed with a variety of methods to remove or inactivate anticomplementary aggregates. Today, most intramuscular ISG usage is limited to hyperimmune products.

The first IGIV was prepared in 1962 by the digestion of ISG with pepsin to remove the complement-binding Fc portion of the molecule, leaving primarily $F(ab')_2$ fragments.[32] Although the product could be given intravenously, the IgG did not bind complement or initiate phagocytic clearance after combining with antigen, and the half-life in vivo was shortened from 21 days to less than 1 day.[33, 34] These deficiencies prevented acceptance of IGIV in the United States, although it was used widely in Europe.

In the ensuing years, several types of IGIV products were developed with less severe methods to remove or inactivate anticomplementary aggregates, such as mild proteolysis with plasmin[35] or pepsin,[33] precipitation of aggregates with polyethylene glycol (PEG),[36] chemical modification of lysine and histidine side chains with β-propiolactone,[37] and cleavage of interchain disulfide bonds by sulfonation or by reduction and alkylation.[38, 39] These IGIV products retain complement-binding and opsonic capabilities and have clearance rates similar to those of native IgG.[28, 29]

Although aggregate removal results in a product that can be used intravenously, additional aggregates were found to form during storage. Therefore, subsequent efforts focused not only on changes to improve processing but also on improved formulations to inhibit aggregate formation.[28, 40] For example, gentler processing methods have been introduced, such as concentration by ultrafiltration rather than precipitation and the removal of ethanol by diafiltration rather than lyophilization. Ion-exchange chromatography is also used to remove aggregates and contaminants. Suspension of the purified IgG in buffers that contain glycine, albumin, PEG, or carbohydrates inhibits aggregate formation and improves stability.[27, 28] Conditions have also been identified that permit IGIV products to be stored in the liquid state, such as formulation at pH 4.25 or with 5% albumin and glucose, and treatment with β-propiolactone.[28] A number of IGIV products are available in the United States (Table 18–1).

The introduction of IGIV permitted administration of much higher doses, with a subsequent expansion in immune globulin therapy. In addition to providing passive immune protection as replacement therapy, IGIV was found to modulate the immune response in autoimmune blood cell diseases such as idiopathic thrombocytopenic purpura (ITP).[41–43] Established indications for IGIV include primary antibody deficiencies (congenital agammaglobulinemia, common variable immunodeficiency, X-linked agammaglobulinemia, severe combined immunodeficiency, Wiskott-Aldrich syndrome), ITP, and B cell

Table 18–1. Intravenous Immune Globulin Products Available in the United States*

Manufacturer or Distributor	Product Name	Removal of Anticomplementary Activity	Viral Inactivation/Removal Process	Storage Form
Alpha Therapeutic Corporation	Venoglobulin-S	PEG precipitation of aggregates	S/D (TNBP/polysorbate 80), purification steps	Liquid
American Red Cross	Polygam S/D†	Ion exchange, PEG	S/D, purification steps	Lyophilized
Centeon	Gammar-P IV	Ultrafiltration	Pasteurization at 60°C for 10 hours, purification steps	Lyophilized
Baxter Healthcare Corporation	Gammagard S/D	Ion exchange, PEG	S/D, purification steps	Lyophilized
Immuno-U.S.	Iveegam	Hydrobase treatment, PEG precipitation	Not available	Lyophilized
Bayer Corporation	Gamimune N S/D Treated	Diafiltration at pH 4	S/D, low pH, purification steps	Liquid
Novartis Pharmaceuticals Corporation	Sandoglobulin	Pepsin at pH 4	Pepsin at pH 4, 37°C, purification steps	Lyophilized

From Drohan WN, Clark DB. Preparation of plasma-derived and recombinant human plasma proteins. *In* Hoffman R, Benz EJ Jr, Shattil SJ, et al (eds): Hematology: Basic Principles and Practice, 3rd ed. Philadelphia: WB Saunders, in press.

*Data obtained from manufacturers, distributors, and available literature regarding products marketed in the United States in 1997.

†Manufactured by Baxter Healthcare Corporation from plasma obtained from volunteer donors.

PEG, polyethylene glycol; S/D, solvent detergent; TNBP, tri-*n*-butyl phosphate.

chronic lymphocytic leukemia. Other conditions in which clinical benefit has been reported are secondary immunodeficiencies (multiple myeloma, protein-losing enteropathy, nephrotic syndrome), Kawasaki syndrome, and viral diseases (human immunodeficiency virus [HIV] and cytomegalovirus infections), as well as in burn therapy.[42] One recent survey identified 53 off-label indications for which IGIV therapy appears to have some efficacy.[44]

Immune globulin products tend to be self-protecting from viral transmission owing to the large pools of antibodies they contain.[45] However, postinfusion viral infections have occurred in a few instances. As a result, most manufacturers have incorporated viral inactivation or removal steps in the production of IGIV.[46]

The use of high-dose IGIV to manipulate the immune response is likely to grow and is expected to further increase immune globulin utilization. Moreover, it is likely that manufacturers will develop more hyperimmune IGIV products that are tailored for specific indications.

COAGULATION FACTOR CONCENTRATES

The distinction between hemophilia A and B was unknown when it was first shown that the transfusion of whole blood could be used to curtail bleeding in patients with hemophilia.[47, 48] By 1940, bleeding episodes were treated routinely, though relatively unsuccessfully, with plasma. Large amounts of plasma were needed to control hemorrhages, but this therapy could not provide adequate factor VIII levels without producing hypervolemia.[49] Since then, the development of coagulation factor concentrates has resulted in a dramatic increase in the life expectancy and quality of life of patients with hemophilia.

Factor VIII and factor IX concentrates are available for the treatment of hemophilia A and B, respectively. In addition, some factor VIII concentrates contain appreciable amounts of vWF and may be used for the treatment of von Willebrand's disease. Factor IX complex concentrates can also be used for the treatment of other congenital or acquired deficiencies of vitamin K–dependent clotting factors. Coagulation factor concentrates have been developed for the treatment of patients with inhibitors to factor VIII and for patients with other congenital deficiencies.

The major issues regarding the preparation and use of the various coagulation factor concentrates are viral safety and purity. With the exception of cryoprecipitate, all concentrates are now subjected to some form of treatment for the inactivation or removal of viruses that might be present in the starting materials. The purity may be important for both immediate and long-term safety. As discussed later, the purity of factor IX concentrates has definitely been shown to affect product safety, but the situation for factor VIII products is less clear. Whereas in vitro testing has shown deleterious effects on immunocompetence with less pure products, the few in vivo studies performed have shown no signs of immunomodulation.[50] The development of new or improved coagulation factor concentrates continues to be a major focus of research and development.[51]

ANTIHEMOPHILIC FACTOR CONCENTRATES

Factor VIII concentrates, termed antihemophilic factor (human) (AHF), for the treatment of hemophilia A have evolved from cryoprecipitate to high-purity immunoaffinity-purified products. Several recombinant products have also been licensed for clinical use.[52] The various AHF concentrates available in the United States are shown in Table 18–2.

Cryoprecipitate

In 1959, Pool and Robinson[53] reported that when frozen plasma is slowly thawed, a residual cryoprecipitate, or "cryo," results that contains much of the factor VIII activity from the input plasma. Pool and Shannon[54] used this finding to develop a process that blood centers could use to produce a concentrate with factor VIII concentrations 5 to 20 times that of plasma. Single-donor cryoprecipitate as a source of factor VIII for therapeutic use became widely available by 1965.

Single-donor cryoprecipitate is made by thawing FFP at 2°C to 4°C in the blood bag. The bag is then centrifuged to separate the cryoprecipitate, which is stored frozen at −20°C and thawed immediately before use. Depending on the way the plasma is collected, frozen, stored, and thawed, as much as half of the factor VIII activity and one third of the fibrinogen and factor XIII in whole plasma can be recovered in cryoprecipitate.[55] However, because of the variation among donors, individual cryoprecipitate units are not uniform in their factor VIII content.

Single-donor cryo is not currently treated for viral inactivation and must be considered potentially infectious. Interestingly, during the early days of the acquired immunodeficiency syndrome (AIDS) epidemic, before the development of good viral inactivation methods for pooled AHF, cryo was a recommended treatment for hemophilia A. The patient would be exposed to viruses from only a single donor rather than those from the thousands of donors represented in a pool. However, with the development of good viral inactivation methods, pooled products, with their additional advantages of higher purity, consistency, and convenience, have become the treatment of choice. Although single-donor cryoprecipitate now has only limited clinical use, large-scale cryoprecipitation is still the first step in most procedures for the preparation of plasma derivatives containing high concentrations of the factor VIII–vWF complex, fibrinogen, fibronectin, and factor XIII.[56]

Intermediate-Purity AHF Concentrates

The next significant advance in treatment of hemophilia A came with the development of intermediate-purity AHF concentrates purified from pooled cryoprecipitate obtained from a large number of plasma units. A variety of purification methods were developed to remove fibrinogen, immunoglobulins, and other proteins from the cryoprecipitate. For example, fibrinogen and fibronectin can

Table 18–2. Antihemophilic Factor Concentrates Available in the United States*

Manufacturer or Distributor	Product Name	Specific Activity (Factor VIII IU/mg)	Manufacturing Process	Viral Inactivation/Removal Process
Alpha Therapeutic Corporation	Alphanate	~140†	Cryoprecipitation, IEC, heparin-affinity chromatography	S/D (TNBP/polysorbate 80), dry heat at 80°C for 72 hours, purification steps
American Red Cross	MONARC-M‡	≥2000†	Cryoprecipitation, cold precipitation, IAC, IEC	S/D (TNBP/Triton X-100), purification steps
Baxter Healthcare Corporation	Hemofil M	≥2000†	Cryoprecipitation, cold precipitation, IAC, IEC	S/D (TNBP/Triton X-100), purification steps
	Recombinate	≥3000†	Cell culture, IAC, IEC	Purification steps§
Bayer Corporation	Koāte-HP	>50†	Cryoprecipitation, SEC	S/D (TNBP/polysorbate 80)
	KoGENate	>3000†	Cell culture, IAC, SEC, IEC	Purification steps§
Centeon	Bioclate‖	>3000†	Cell culture, IAC, IEC	Purification steps§
	Helixate¶	>3000†	Cell culture, IAC, SEC, IEC	Purification steps§
	Humate-P	2–5	Cryoprecipitation, $Al(OH)_3$ adsorption, glycine precipitation	Pasteurization at 60°C for 10 hours
	Monoclate P	>3000†	Cryoprecipitation, cold purification, $Al(OH)_3$ adsorption, IAC, AH-Sepharose chromatography	Pasteurization at 60°C for 10 hours, purification steps
Speywood Pharmaceuticals, Inc.	Hyate:C	>50**	Polyelectrolyte fractionation	Porcine source, in-process and final product viral testing

From Drohan WN, Clark DB. Preparation of plasma-derived and recombinant human plasma proteins. *In* Hoffman R, Benz EJ Jr, Shattil SJ, et al (eds): Hematology: Basic Principles and Practice, 3rd ed. Philadelphia: WB Saunders, in press.

*Data obtained from manufacturers, distributors, and available literature regarding products marketed in the United States in 1997.

†Before addition of human albumin in product formulation.

‡Manufactured by Baxter Healthcare Corporation from plasma obtained from volunteer donors.

§Recombinant source.

‖Manufactured by Baxter Healthcare Corporation.

¶Manufactured by Bayer Corporation.

**Porcine factor VIII μg/mg protein.

IAC, immunoaffinity chromatography; IEC, ion exchange chromatography; S/D, solvent detergent; SEC, size exclusion chromatography; TNBP, tri-*n*-butyl phosphate.

be precipitated at specific conditions of temperature and pH,[57] or by precipitation with ethanol or PEG.[58] Aluminum hydroxide can be used to adsorb and remove the vitamin K–dependent proteins,[58] and glycine has been used to precipitate factor VIII in order to separate it from residual PEG.[19]

Unlike cryo, intermediate-purity concentrates are freeze-dried in vials and can be stored in a refrigerator, making home treatment possible. However, even though these concentrates are enriched approximately 400-fold over plasma, factor VIII is still less than 1% of the total protein present.[59] Thus, hemophilic patients receiving these concentrates are exposed to very large quantities of other plasma proteins. In addition, each lot of AHF concentrate is prepared from cryoprecipitate obtained from the plasma of several thousand donors. Until effective methods were developed for viral inactivation, patients receiving these concentrates were exposed to all the blood-borne viruses in this donor population. It is not surprising that frequently treated patients uniformly became infected with hepatitis[60, 61] and often with HIV later.[62]

High-Purity AHF Concentrates

Intermediate-purity AHF concentrates were the mainstay of hemophilia A treatment until the development of high-purity concentrates in the late 1980s. Various ion exchange and gel filtration techniques have been added to the precipitation methods to produce concentrates with specific activities of 50 to 200 IU/mg of protein, in contrast to 1 to 50 IU/mg for intermediate-purity AHF and less than 1 IU/mg for cryoprecipitate.[50] However, even though these concentrates are highly purified in comparison with the intermediate-purity concentrates, high-molecular-weight proteins such as fibrinogen, fibronectin, and vWF tend to copurify with factor VIII and remain in these preparations.[63]

Very High Purity AHF Concentrates

Immunoaffinity-Purified AHF Concentrates. The next major advance in the preparation of AHF concentrates was the use of murine monoclonal antibodies (MAbs) that bind factor VIII for purification by immunoaffinity chromatography. Two different methods have been developed, both starting with low-purity factor VIII concentrates partially purified by conventional means.[64–66] One procedure uses a MAb that binds to the vWF portion of the factor VIII–vWF complex; the other uses a MAb that binds directly to factor VIII. In both processes, the columns are loaded with the low-purity intermediate, washed extensively to remove unwanted proteins, and then eluted, respectively, by separation of factor VIII from the vWF-MAb complex or directly from the MAb itself. Both processes use a final chromatography step to remove the strong elution solutions as well as any MAb that might have leached off the column. These processes produce factor VIII that is essentially pure before the addition of albumin as a stabilizer. Both processes also include several steps that inactivate or remove viruses.

Recombinant AHF Concentrates. One of the remarkable accomplishments of molecular biology has been the elucidation of the structure of factor VIII, its molecular cloning, and the successful production of recombinant human factor VIII (rFVIII). Almost simultaneously, two groups cloned the entire factor VIII gene, the largest gene cloned at that time, and isolated a cDNA encoding the structural regions of the factor VIII molecule.[67–70]

Because post-translational processing is essential to factor VIII functionality, both groups expressed the rFVIII molecule in mammalian cells. One process uses baby hamster kidney cells to express rFVIII that is purified by immunoaffinity, size exclusion, and ion exchange chromatography.[71] The other uses Chinese hamster ovary cells that coexpress rFVIII and recombinant vWF (rvWF). The rvWF substantially increases the recovery of rFVIII from the culture medium but is completely removed during downstream processing by immunoaffinity and ion exchange chromatography.[72] Both products contain only trace quantities of mouse immunoglobulin, hamster protein, and cellular DNA. The products are essentially pure before the addition of human albumin to stabilize the rFVIII. These AHFs have been shown to be similar to plasma-derived factor VIII in in vitro[72–75] as well as clinical[76–78] studies. Recombinant AHF products are termed antihemophilic factor (recombinant).

A recombinant AHF lacking the factor VIII B domain is also under development.[52] The B domain is a large portion of the factor VIII molecule with no known function. Clinical studies to date have demonstrated efficacy similar to that of plasma-derived AHF. A fully functional rFVIII has also recently been expressed in the milk of transgenic pigs.[79] The large amounts of protein that can be produced relatively inexpensively in transgenic animals may someday permit the widespread prophylactic treatment of hemophilic patients so that joint and soft tissue bleeds can be prevented rather than treated.

FACTOR IX CONCENTRATES

Two types of factor IX concentrates are available today: factor IX complex, which contains significant amounts of the other vitamin K–dependent proteins, including factors II, VII, and X; and coagulation factor IX (human), a preparation substantially free of these other proteins. The factor IX concentrates available in the United States are shown in Table 18–3.

Factor IX Complex Concentrates

The vitamin K–dependent clotting factors, because of their similar structures, tend to copurify by most of the methods used to isolate them from plasma. Thus the initial preparations containing factor IX for treatment of hemophilia B were complex mixtures of all the vitamin K–dependent proteins. Because the protein in highest concentration in these materials is prothrombin, they have also been identified as prothrombin complex concentrates. However, factor IX complex is the generic name in the United States.

Table 18–3. Factor IX and Anti-Inhibitor Coagulant Complex Concentrates Available in the United States*

Manufacturer or Distributor	Product Name (Product Type)	Specific Activity (Factor IX IU/mg)	Manufacturing Process	Viral Inactivation/Removal Process
Alpha Therapeutic Corporation	AlphaNine SD (CFIX)	≥150	DEAE adsorption, barium citrate adsorption, AC	S/D (TNBP/polysorbate 80), purification steps
	Profilnine SD (FIXC)	4–5	DEAE cellulose adsorption	S/D (TNBP/polysorbate 80), purification steps
Baxter Healthcare Corporation	Proplex T (FIXC)	Not available	Tricalcium phosphate adsorption	Dry heat at 60°C for 144 hours
Bayer Corporation	Konȳne 80 (FIXC)	~1	IEC	Dry heat at 80°C for 72 hours
Centeon	Mononine (CFIX)	≥190	IEC, IAC, AH-Sepharose chromatography	Sodium thiocyanate, ultrafiltration, purification steps
Genetics Institute	BeneFix (rCFIX)	≥200	Q Sepharose, cellufine sulfate, ceramic hydroxyapatite chromatography, IMAC	Nanofiltration, purification steps†
Immuno	Bebulin VH (FIXC)	Not available	IEC	Vapor heating at 60°C, 10 hours, 190 mbar; then 80°C, 1 hour, 375 mbar‡
	Feiba VH (AIC)	NA	IEC, activation	Vapor heating at 60°C, 10 hours, 190 mbar, then 80°C, 1 hour, 375 mbar
Nabi	Autoplex T§	NA	Not available	Dry heat at 60°C for 144 hours

From Drohan WN, Clark DB. Preparation of plasma-derived and recombinant human plasma proteins. *In* Hoffman R, Benz EJ Jr, Shattil SJ, et al (eds): Hematology: Basic Principles and Practice, 3rd ed. Philadelphia: WB Saunders, in press.

*Data obtained from manufacturers, distributors, and available literature regarding products marketed in the United States in 1997.

†Recombinant source.

‡Excess pressure above atmospheric.

§Manufactured by Baxter Healthcare Corporation.

AC, affinity chromatography; AIC, anti-inhibitor coagulant complex; CFIX, coagulation factor IX; DEAE, diethylaminoethyl; FIXC, factor IX complex; IAC, immunoaffinity chromatography; IEC, ion exchange chromatography; IMAC, immobilized metal affinity chromatography; NA, not applicable; rCFIX, recombinant CFIX; S/D, solvent detergent; TNBP, tri-*n*-butyl phosphate.

The first factor IX complex concentrate used for the treatment of hemophilia B was developed in France over 35 years ago[80] and termed PPSB, an acronym for *p*rothrombin (factor II), *p*roconvertin (factor VII), *S*tuart factor (factor X), and antihemophilic factor *B* (factor IX). It was produced by adsorption of the plasma vitamin K–dependent clotting factors with tricalcium phosphate (TCP) and was successfully used to treat hemophilia B for a number of years. However, the original production process had a number of disadvantages, including the need to collect the plasma in ethylenediaminetetraacetic acid (EDTA), which prevents preparation of AHF from the plasma. Because of these issues, the process was eventually discontinued.[81] This demonstrates a general goal in the development of new products and processes: because of the need to maximize use of the limited plasma resource, processes should not interfere with the production of other products from the same plasma pool.[51]

The PPSB method was adapted, however, to the development of several other processes based on adsorption of cryosupernatant plasma fractions with TCP in ways that do not interfere with the purification of other products.[82] Factor IX complex produced by this method contains approximately equal amounts of factors II, VII, IX, and X by activity units.

The next major development in the production of factor IX complex concentrates was the introduction of ion exchange chromatography with DEAE-cellulose or DEAE-Sephadex,[83] representing one of the first major uses of chromatography in plasma fractionation. As shown in Figure 18–1, the vitamin K–dependent clotting factors can be removed from cryosupernatant plasma by adsorption onto DEAE-cellulose or DEAE-Sephadex, and the plasma can then be further fractionated by the Cohn method for the production of immunoglobulins and albumin. The eluate from the DEAE resin may be further purified by additional precipitation or adsorption steps.[84, 85] Such processes give 100-fold or more purification of factors II, IX, and X. Factor VII does not bind to the DEAE ligand under the conditions used, however, and is present only at very low concentrations in concentrates prepared this way.

Coagulation Factor IX

With the widespread use of factor IX complex, it soon became apparent that serious thromboembolic episodes and acute myocardial infarctions were major complications of its use, especially when it was infused in large quantities over extended periods, such as for surgical procedures, or used in patients with liver disease.[86, 87] The cause of the thrombogenicity has not been determined. Potential causes include the presence of activated clotting factors,[88, 89] contaminating phospholipids,[90] or zymogen overload.[91] Zymogen overload refers to the coadministration of large, incidental quantities of factors II and X in the factor IX complex preparations.[91, 92] These factors persist in the circulation (half-lives of about 4 days and 30 to 50 hours, respectively, compared with about 20 hours for factor IX[93]) and accumulate after repeated infusions of the complex. Supranormal levels may upset the normal hemostatic balance and lead to a hypercoagulable state.[87]

On the basis of these hypotheses, methods have been developed for the preparation of factor IX concentrates that are more highly purified and essentially free of the other vitamin K–dependent clotting factors. These have been designated coagulation factor IX (human). Coagulation factor IX (CFIX) concentrates are manufactured from factor IX complex by one or more additional steps, such as chromatography on sulfated dextran,[92] a second DEAE column and a heparin-Sepharose column,[94] or barium citrate adsorption followed by an affinity column.[95] CFIX concentrates are also prepared by immunoaffinity chromatography with monoclonal antibodies to factor IX.[96, 97] All these methods also include viral inactivation steps. These preparations have been shown to be nonthrombogenic when compared with factor IX complex in animal models[98] and in clinical studies.[99, 100]

A recombinant CFIX has also been developed and licensed in the United States. Recombinant factor IX is produced by cell culture in Chinese hamster ovary cells, which coexpress a protease needed for proper post-translational modification of the factor IX molecule.[101] It is purified with several chromatography steps plus a viral removal step.[102] The final product has been shown to be structurally and functionally similar to plasma-derived factor IX.[103, 104] For reasons not yet determined, however, it has a lower recovery when infused into patients.[105]

OTHER COAGULATION FACTOR CONCENTRATES

Anti-Inhibitor Coagulant Complex. One of the major complications of hemophilia treatment is the development of inhibitors, antibodies directed against factor VIII or factor IX. Although low-titer inhibitors can be saturated by the administration of larger amounts of AHF or factor IX, this is not usually feasible when the inhibitor level is greater than 5 to 10 Bethesda units per milliliter of plasma.[106, 107] In that case, one method of treatment for hemophilia A patients who have developed inhibitors is "bypass therapy," the administration of either factor IX complex or a specially activated factor IX complex, termed anti-inhibitor coagulant complex, to bypass the factor VIII step in the coagulation cascade.[108, 109] These concentrates are effective in 50% to 60% of cases, but thromboembolic complications have occurred in some patients treated in this way. The two products available in the United States are listed in Table 18–3.

Recombinant Factor VIIa. The bypass rationale has also led to the use of activated factor VII (FVIIa) for the treatment of both hemophilia A and B patients with inhibitors.[110] Factor VII or FVIIa may be the active substance in the anti-inhibitor coagulant complexes.[111] Early work with plasma-derived FVIIa produced good results.[112] However, because it is impossible to purify enough FVIIa from plasma for widespread patient use, recombinant FVIIa was developed.[113] Recombinant Factor VII is produced in tissue culture in baby hamster kidney cells and spontaneously activates during purification by immunoaffinity chromatography.[113, 114] Recombinant FVIIa has been used successfully in a number of clinical trials[110, 112, 115, 116] but is not yet licensed in the United States. However, the manufacturer has made the product available on a compassionate-use basis for several years.[107]

Porcine Factor VIII. As an alternative to bypass therapy, porcine factor VIII is generally effective in restoring hemostasis in hemophilia A patients. Because some inhibitor antibodies inactivate porcine factor VIII less readily than the human protein,[117] a porcine factor VIII concentrate was developed that has been quite effective in the treatment of some patients.[117–120] The product is free of porcine vWF to prevent thrombocytopenia, and adverse reactions are minimal. Although most reactions require no treatment, the rest are easily controlled with antihistamine or hydrocortisone treatment. The critical reaction to repeated use of porcine factor VIII, anamnesis with development of high titers of inhibitors of porcine factor VIII, is seen in approximately one third of patients.[119]

von Willebrand Factor. Patients with von Willebrand disease have been treated with plasma, with cryoprecipitate, and with some AHF concentrates that contain vWF. Cryoprecipitate has a population of vWF multimers similar to that of normal plasma, whereas AHF concentrates are often deficient in the multimeric forms. However, during the past 10 years, the ratios of ristocetin cofactor activity (vWF:Rco) to vWF antigen (vWF:ag) in many plasma-derived AHFs have increased to the point that they are now preferred over cryoprecipitate because of their viral safety.[121] The vWF:Rco-vWF:ag ratio appears to be a good indicator of treatment efficacy. Current AHF products vary considerably, with vWF:Rco-vWF:ag ratios ranging from 0.25 to 1.4 and with 0.5 to 5.3 units of vWF:Rco per unit of factor VIII.[121] A vWF concentrate depleted of factor VIII has also been developed in Europe with plans to seek licensure in the United States.

Other Coagulation Factors. Patients deficient in vitamin K–dependent clotting factors other than factor IX are also currently treated with factor IX complex. However, such treatment carries the risk of thrombosis, as described previously. Several more purified coagulation factor concentrates are currently available outside the United States. Factor VII[122, 123] concentrates are available in Europe. Factor X concentrates have been investigated by two U.S. companies but are not currently available.[124, 125] A factor XI concentrate is available in Europe, but there is increasing concern about potential thrombogenic risks associated with its use.[126] Factor XIII concentrates are also available or in development in Europe,[127, 128] as are fibrinogen concentrates in some countries.[129]

FIBRIN SEALANTS

Fibrin sealants, or fibrin glues, are topical hemostatic agents that have been used in a variety of surgical situations for their hemostatic and adhesive properties.[130] The preparations consist of two components that are mixed together immediately before use. The first component is derived from human plasma and contains fibrinogen, along with factor XIII, fibronectin, and other plasma proteins. Depending on the manufacturer, the fibrinogen component may be isolated from Cohn fraction I or from cryoprecipitate as a by-product of AHF manufacture.[130] These fibrinogen concentrates also typically either contain an added plasmin inhibitor to delay clot lysis[130, 131] or are purified to remove endogenous plasminogen.[131, 132] The second component contains either bovine or human plasma-derived thrombin and possibly other proteins. Although bovine thrombin has been in widespread use for many years, recent research suggests that it may be responsible for many postsurgical hemostatic problems.[131, 133]

The use of fibrinogen as a hemostatic agent began in the early 1900s, with the direct application of fibrin preparations to bleeding tissue surfaces. A combination of fibrinogen and thrombin was used for anchoring skin grafts in the 1940s, but the adhesive effect was poor, probably because of inadequate fibrinogen concentration.[134] The current concept of using a two-component fibrin sealant system in which the fibrinogen and thrombin components are well defined was developed in the early 1970s, when techniques for the isolation and concentration of clotting factors were being improved.[135] Although preparations of fibrin sealant have been available in Europe since the mid-1970s, the U.S. Food and Drug Administration revoked all licenses for the manufacture of fibrinogen concentrates in 1978 owing to frequent viral contamination.[136] However, several manufacturers have developed improved, virally inactivated products, one of which was recently licensed in the United States. Additional products containing fibrin sealant, such as a fibrin sealant–coated bandage, are also being developed.[131, 137]

Fibrin sealant has been advocated by many surgeons as the material that best approaches the ideal operative sealant.[135] It appears to have no tissue toxicity, forms a firm seal within seconds, is completely readsorbed within days or weeks after application, and may promote local tissue growth and repair.[134, 135, 138] In the absence of licensed products, a variety of methods have been used by surgeons to prepare fibrin sealant from single-donor cryoprecipitate plus bovine thrombin.[139, 140] However, the methods are somewhat cumbersome, the concentration of fibrinogen is highly variable, and, most importantly, the products are not treated to prevent viral transmission.[130] The use of a standardized manufactured product should increase the likelihood of safe, uniform performance in the surgical field.

PLASMA PROTEINASE INHIBITORS

The proteinase inhibitors present in human plasma play a critical role in the regulation of the proteolytic cascades of the coagulation, fibrinolytic, complement, and kinin systems. Most of these inhibitors have similar amino acid and structural properties and are members of a superfamily of proteins designated serine proteinase inhibitors, or serpins.[141] Hereditary deficiencies of α_1-antitrypsin, AT-III, and C_1-esterase inhibitor can cause specific disease states, and inhibitor concentrates have been developed.

Alpha$_1$-Proteinase Inhibitor

The first of the serpins to be isolated and characterized was α_1-antitrypsin.[142] Although the protein was originally named for its antitrypsin activity, it inhibits several serine proteinases, and the generic name for concentrates in the United States is alpha$_1$-proteinase inhibitor (human) (API). Its primary physiological function appears to be the inhibition of neutrophil elastase. Patients with hereditary deficiencies of this inhibitor develop pulmonary emphysema and liver disease.[143, 144]

API therapy is indicated for the long-term treatment of individuals with hereditary deficiency who have clinical evidence of panacinar emphysema. Weekly intravenous infusions are recommended to maintain an adequate level of functional API in the epithelial lining of the lower respiratory tract.[145] Although an effect can be demonstrated, intravenous administration is an inefficient therapy. It has been estimated that only 2% of the infused API is present in the lung. Clinical studies suggest that aerosol delivery of API directly into the lungs by inhalation would require much less API, would be efficacious, and could replace intravenous administration because of its lower cost and greater convenience.[146] API is also currently in clinical trials for the treatment of cystic fibrosis.

An API concentrate prepared from human plasma is licensed for use in the United States. The product is prepared from Cohn fraction IV$_1$ by fractional precipitation with PEG, followed by ion exchange chromatography on DEAE-Sepharose. It is pasteurized by heating in solution for 10 hours at 60°C to ensure viral inactivation.[147, 148] Several new plasma-derived API concentrates are being developed, as are recombinant concentrates from both cell culture[149, 150] and transgenic animals. The large amounts of API that can be produced in the milk of transgenic animals may be important in the future. Owing to the relatively large doses of API that are needed even with aerosol delivery, the amount available from plasma will be insufficient, especially with additional indications being studied. With the use of recombinant DNA techniques, it may also be possible to modify the API molecule to give it advantageous new properties, such as resistance to oxidation and a broader antiprotease inhibitory spectrum.[146]

ANTITHROMBIN III

AT-III is a coagulation inhibitor that plays a crucial role in the regulation of hemostasis as the major physiological inhibitor of thrombin and factor Xa.[151] It also inhibits other serine proteinases, including factors IXa, XIa, and XIIa and plasmin. Heparin binds to AT-III to increase the rates of inactivation and is required for a physiologically significant effect.

Heterozygous hereditary deficiency of AT-III has been linked with an increased tendency for thrombosis. Unlike hemophilias, in which symptoms occur only at factor levels less than 5% to 20% of normal, a moderate decrease in the AT-III blood concentration to 50% to 70% of normal significantly increases the risk of thrombosis.[152] Acquired deficiencies of AT-III have also been reported in women taking oral contraceptives and as a consequence of pregnancy, surgery, cirrhosis, and hepatic malignancies.

Binding of heparin to AT-III, essential for the pharmacological effect of the drug, is also used to purify AT-III. Immobilized heparin as an affinity adsorbent for AT-III[153] is the key to the large-scale preparation of AT-III concentrates for clinical use.[154] As shown in Figure 18–1, AT-III can be isolated from cryo-poor plasma,[155] Cohn fraction I supernatant,[156, 157] or Cohn fraction IV$_1$.[158] Although heparin-based adsorbents are not specific for AT-III, other plasma proteins are bound less tightly and may be washed off with medium-ionic-strength buffers before the elution of AT-III with a high-ionic-strength buffer. Although these eluates may contain small amounts of other proteins, an additional purification step produces concentrates that contain greater than 95% AT-III.[154]

All AT-III concentrates currently being manufactured are pasteurized by heating in solution for 10 hours at 60°C to inactivate blood-borne viruses. With respect to viral safety, the pasteurized AT-III concentrates have an impeccable record: no patient has been reported as being infected with HIV or hepatitis viruses.

Clinical studies by a number of investigators have shown that AT-III concentrates are effective in the prophylaxis or treatment of thromboembolic disorders in patients with hereditary AT-III deficiency.[151, 159] The benefit of AT-III therapy in acquired deficiencies is as yet unproved in clinical trials.

C$_1$-Esterase Inhibitor

C$_1$-esterase inhibitor plays an important role in the regulation of the complement system cascade. It is believed to be the only inhibitor of the activated form of the first component of complement. In 1963, deficiency of C$_1$-esterase inhibitor was established as the underlying biochemical defect in hereditary angioedema,[160] an autosomal dominant disease characterized by episodic swelling of the subcutaneous tissues and the mucosa of the gastrointestinal and respiratory tracts. The swelling can lead to acute airway obstruction, a major cause of mortality among patients with this disease.[161] FFP has been used in replacement therapy for the treatment of acute attacks of hereditary angioedema, as well as for short-term prophylaxis before surgery.[162] However, the volume of plasma needed and the time required for thawing and infusion are drawbacks to this approach.

C$_1$-esterase inhibitor concentrates are not available in the United States. Preparations have been available in Europe for several years, where they have been used for short-term and long-term prophylaxis, as well as for the treatment of acute episodes of hereditary angioedema.[156, 163–165]

PROTEIN C

Protein C is a vitamin K–dependent protein that is an important anticoagulant. Activated protein C with its cofactor protein S inhibits the generation of factor Xa and thrombin by inactivating factors VIIIa and Va.[166, 167] Hereditary heterozygous deficiencies of protein C or protein S are associated with recurrent venous thrombosis in some individuals.[168–171] In a more severe disorder, infants with homozygous protein C deficiency have a characteristic hemorrhagic skin necrosis termed neonatal purpura fulminans and usually succumb to disseminated intravascular coagulation. Some factor IX complex products contain appreciable amounts of protein C and protein S and have been used to treat patients successfully. However, as described earlier, their use is often associated with severe thromboembolic complications, an even greater problem in these patients, who already have an increased risk of thrombosis.[172, 173]

Because of their similar structures, proteins C and S usually copurify into the factor IX complex with the other vitamin K–dependent proteins.[174] Protein C concentrates are usually prepared from factor IX complex by affinity or immunoaffinity chromatography.[175, 176] Recombinant protein C has also been produced in cell culture[177, 178] and in the milk of transgenic animals.[179] Plasma-derived protein C concentrates are currently available in Europe[180, 181] but not in the United States.

Activated protein C (APC) also has a number of potential indications, including treatment of acute thrombosis, warfarin-induced skin necrosis, heparin-induced thrombocytopenia, myocardial ischemia and infarction, and possibly septic shock.[182] In myocardial infarction, APC may increase the effectiveness of tissue plasminogen activator by its role in inactivating plasminogen activator inhibitors. Processes for making APC concentrates from immunoaffinity-purified protein C have been developed,[183, 184] but none is currently available.

FUTURE DIRECTIONS IN THE PREPARATION OF THERAPEUTIC PROTEINS

Almost all plasma proteins licensed for human use have been cloned and expressed in biologically active form in animal cells, and several of these have been developed into licensed products.[52] The main advantages of recombinantly produced plasma proteins are freedom from human viruses and a supply not limited by the availability of donated plasma. Recombinant proteins can also be produced in modified forms that may give them advantageous new properties, such as increased potency, longer half-life, or varied specificity. Challenges include reducing production costs and obtaining correct post-translational modification of the recombinant protein.[185, 186] However, these problems may be solved by the use of transgenic animals as bioreactors for protein production.

Transgenic Animal Production of Human Plasma Proteins

Advances in molecular biology and embryology have led to the production of plasma proteins in the milk of genetically engineered farm animals.[187–189] This technology has overcome at least one of the apparent shortcomings of tissue culture production systems. Transgenic cows, goats, pigs, and sheep can produce large quantities of human proteins, typically 1 to 10 g/L in milk, whereas animal tissue culture systems routinely produce substantially less protein, typically 10 to 100 mg/L.[190] In addition, transgenic animals appear to be able to perform most of the post-translational modifications required for protein activity, even when the protein is being made at relatively high levels of production.[190] Most recently, even the highly modified factor VIII protein has been made in the milk of pigs in a biologically active form.[79] Proteins produced in transgenic animals should be free of human viruses, less expensive to produce, and available in unlimited quantities. Thus, the production of human plasma proteins in transgenic animals is an attractive alternative to their isolation from human plasma or their production in tissue culture systems.

Gene Therapy

The most satisfying solution to human genetic deficiencies would be the replacement of the dysfunctional gene in the affected individual so that the consequence of the gene abnormality goes unnoticed. This approach, termed gene therapy, is the subject of intense research, especially for treatment of hemophilia A and B.[191–194] Although the number of hemophilia B patients is relatively small, the characteristics of both the disease and the factor IX molecule are such that it has become an excellent model system for the development of generic gene therapies.[191] There are two general approaches. Fully functional new genes may be inserted into various body cells by means of a modified virus or other carrier. Alternatively, cells containing functional genes may be implanted into various body tissues. The main issues with either approach are the production of sufficient protein and the persistence of the production. In addition, hemophiliacs could still develop inhibitors to these proteins. Although these problems are far from being solved, the pace of the research has been rapid, and an actual cure for diseases such as hemophilia may be in sight.

REFERENCES

1. Köhler G, Milstein C. Continuous cultures of fused cells secreting antibody of predefined specificity. Nature 1975; 256:495.
2. Lubon H, Paleyanda RK, Velander WH, et al. Blood proteins from transgenic animal bioreactors. Transfus Med Rev 1996; 10:131.
3. Janeway CA. Human serum albumin: historical review. *In* Sgouris JT, René A (eds): Proceedings of the Workshop on Albumin (DHEW Publication No. [NIH] 76-925). Washington, DC: U.S. Government Printing Office, 1976, pp 3–21.
4. Palmer JW. The evolution of large-scale human plasma fractionation in the United States. *In* Sgouris JT, René A (eds): Proceedings of the Workshop on Albumin (DHEW Publication No. [NIH] 76-925). Washington, DC: U.S. Government Printing Office, 1976, pp 255–269.
5. Code of Federal Regulations, 21CFR640.34(b), 1997.
6. Consensus Conference. Fresh-frozen plasma: indications and risks. JAMA 1985; 253:551.
7. The Sanguis Study Group. Use of blood products for elective surgery in 43 European hospitals. Transfus Med 1994; 4:251.
8. Tuckfield A, Haeusler MN, Grigg AP, et al. Reduction of inappropriate use of blood products by prospective monitoring of transfusion request forms. Med J Aust 1997; 167:473.
9. Horowitz B, Bonomo R, Prince AM, et al. Solvent/detergent-treated plasma: a virus-inactivated substitute for fresh frozen plasma. Blood 1992; 79:826.
10. Piquet Y, Janvier G, Selose P, et al. Virus inactivation of fresh

frozen plasma by a solvent detergent procedure: biological results. Vox Sang 1992; 63:251.
11. Josic D, Schulz P, Biesert L, et al. Issues in the development of medical products based on human plasma. J Chromatogr B Biomed Appl 1997; 694:253.
12. Kohler M, Wieding JU. Virusinaktiviertes Plasma. Infusionsther Transfusionsmed 1994; 21(suppl 1):73.
13. Harrison CN, Lawrie AS, Iqbal A, et al. Plasma exchange with solvent/detergent-treated plasma of resistant thrombotic thrombocytopenic purpura. Br J Haematol 1996; 94:756.
14. Finlayson JS. Albumin products. Semin Thromb Hemost 1980; 6:85.
15. Cohn EJ, Strong LE, Hughes WL Jr, et al. Preparation and properties of serum and plasma proteins: IV. A system for the separation into fractions of the proteins and lipoprotein components of biological tissues and fluids. J Am Chem Soc 1946; 68:459.
16. Curling JM. Albumin purification by ion exchange chromatography. *In* Curling JM (ed): Methods of Plasma Protein Fractionation. New York: Academic Press, 1980, pp 77–91.
17. More JE, Harvey MJ. Purification technologies for human plasma albumin. *In* Harris JR (ed): Blood Separation and Plasma Fractionation. New York: Wiley-Liss, 1991, pp 261–306.
18. Inoue M, Yoshihiko G, Hirokazu I, et al. Reduction of aluminum concentration in albumin products. Vox Sang 1994; 66:249.
19. Vandersande J. Current approaches to the preparation of plasma fractions. *In* Goldstein J (ed): Biotechnology of Blood. Boston: Butterworth-Heinemann, 1991, pp 165–176.
20. Code of Federal Regulations, 21CFR640.82(b), 1997.
21. Hink JH Jr, Hidalgo J, Seeberg VP, et al. Preparation and properties of a heat-treated human plasma protein fraction. Vox Sang 1957; 2:174.
22. Ng PK, Fournel MA, Lundblad JL. Plasma protein fraction: product improvement studies. Transfusion 1981; 21:682.
23. Bland JHL, Laver MB, Lowenstein E. Vasodilator effect of commercial 5% plasma protein fraction solutions. JAMA 1973; 224:1721.
24. Alving BM, Hojima Y, Pisano JJ, et al. Hypotension associated with prekallikrein activator (Hageman-factor fragments) in plasma protein fraction. N Engl J Med 1978; 299:66.
25. Berglöf JH, Eriksson S, Suomela H, Curling JM. Albumin from human plasma: preparation and in vitro properties. *In* Curling JM (ed): Separation of Plasma Proteins. Uppsala: Pharmacia Fine Chemicals AB, 1983, pp 51–58.
26. Jeans ERA, Marshall PJ, Lowe CR. Plasma protein fractionation. Trends Biotechnol 1985; 3:267.
27. Oncley JL, Melin M, Richert A, et al. The separation of the antibodies, isoagglutinins, prothrombin, plasminogen and $\exists_1$-lipoprotein into subfractions of human plasma. J Am Chem Soc 1949; 71:541.
28. Rousell RH, McCue JP. Antibody purification from plasma. *In* Harris J (ed): Blood Separation and Plasma Fractionation. New York: Wiley-Liss, 1991, pp 307–340.
29. Stryker MH, Bertolini MJ, Hao Y. Blood fractionation: proteins. *In* Mizrahi A, Van Wezel AL (eds): Advances in Biotechnological Processes 4. New York: Wiley-Liss, 1985, pp 275–336.
30. Nydegger UE. Immunoglobulins in clinical medicine. *In* Rossi EC, Simon TL, Moss GL (eds): Principles of Transfusion Medicine. Baltimore: Williams & Wilkins, 1991, pp 383–393.
31. Barandun S, Kistler P, Jeunet F, et al. Intravenous administration of human γ-globulin. Vox Sang 1962; 7:157.
32. Schultze HE, Schwick G. Über neue Möglichkeiten intravenöser Gammaglobulin-Applikation. Deutsch Med Wschr 1962; 87:1643.
33. Barandun S, Kistler P, Jeunet F, et al. Intravenous administration of human γ-globulin. Vox Sang 1962; 7:157.
34. Janeway CA, Merler E, Rosen FS, et al. Intravenous gamma globulin: metabolism of gamma globulin fragments in normal and agammaglobulinemic persons. N Engl J Med 1968; 278:919.
35. Sgouris JT. The preparation of plasmin-treated immune serum globulin for intravenous use. Vox Sang 1967; 13:71.
36. Polson A. Removal of anti-complementary material and Australia antigen from immunoglobulin. Prep Biochem 1973; 3:327.
37. Stephan W. Beseitigung der Komplementfixierung von γ-Globulin durch chemische Modifizierung mit β-Propiolacton. Z Klin Chem Klin Biochem 1969; 7:282.
38. Masuho Y, Tomibe K, Matsuzawa K, et al. Development of an intravenous γ-globulin with Fc activities. I. Preparation and characterization of S-sulfonated human γ-globulin. Vox Sang 1977; 32:175.
39. Fernandes PM, Lundblad JL. Preparation of a stable intravenous gamma-globulin: process design and scale-up. Vox Sang 1980; 39:101.
40. Tankersley DL. Intravenous Immunoglobulins: Past, Present, and Future. NIH Consensus Conference on Intravenous Immunoglobulin: Prevention and Treatment of Disease, Bethesda, MD, May 21–23, 1990.
41. Nydegger UE. Immunoglobulins in clinical medicine. *In* Rossi EC, Simon TL, Moss GL (eds): Principles of Transfusion Medicine. Baltimore: Williams & Wilkins, 1991, pp 383–393.
42. Dwyer JM. Manipulating the immune system with immune globulin. N Engl J Med 1992; 326:107.
43. Nydegger UE. Intravenous immunoglobulin in combination with other prophylactic and therapeutic measures. Transfusion 1992; 32:72.
44. Ratko TA, Burnett DA, Foulke GE, et al. Recommendations for off-label use of intravenously administered immunoglobulin preparations. University Hospital Consortium Expert Panel for Off-Label Use of Polyvalent Intravenously Administered Immunoglobulin Preparations. JAMA 1995; 273:1865.
45. NIH Consensus Conference. Intravenous immunoglobulin: prevention and treatment of disease. JAMA 1990; 264:3189.
46. Hamalainen E, Suomela H, Ukkonen P. Virus inactivation during intravenous immunoglobulin purification. Vox Sang 1992; 63:6.
47. Lane S. Haemorrhagic diathesis. Successful transfusion of blood. Lancet 1840; 1:185.
48. Menache D. Coagulation factor IX concentrate: historical perspective. Haemophilia 1995; 1(suppl 3):7.
49. Roberts HR. Highly purified factor VIII concentrates. *In* Kasper CK (ed): Recent Advances in Hemophilia Care. New York: AR Liss, 1990, pp 167–176.
50. Berntorp E. Why prescribe highly purified factor VIII and IX concentrates? Vox Sang 1996; 70:61.
51. Clark DB, Drohan WN, Miekka SI, et al. Strategy for purification of coagulation factor concentrates. Ann Clin Lab Sci 1989; 19:196.
52. Roddie PH, Ludlam CA. Recombinant coagulation factors. Blood Rev 1997; 11:169.
53. Pool JG, Robinson J. Observations on plasma banking and transfusion procedures for haemophilic patients using a quantitative assay for antihaemophilic globulin (AHG). Br J Haematol 1959; 5:24.
54. Pool JG, Shannon AE. Production of high-potency concentrates of antihaemophilic globulin in a closed bag system. N Engl J Med 1965; 273:1443.
55. Feldman P, Winkelman L. Preparation of special plasma products. *In* Harris JR (ed): Blood Separation and Plasma Fractionation. New York: Wiley-Liss, 1991, pp 301–383.
56. Farrugia A, Grasso S, Douglas S, et al. Modulation of fibrinogen content in cryoprecipitate by temperature manipulation during plasma processing. Transfusion 1992; 32:755.
57. Smith JK, Evans DR, Stone V, et al. A factor VIII concentrate of intermediate purity and higher potency. Transfusion 1979; 19:299.
58. Newman J, Johnson AJ, Karpatkin MH, et al. Methods for the production of clinically effective intermediate- and high-purity factor-VIII concentrates. Br J Haematol 1971; 21:1.
59. Weinstein RE. Immunoaffinity purification of factor VIII. Ann Clin Lab Sci 1989; 19:84.
60. Gerety RJ, Eyster ME, Tabor E, et al. Hepatitis B virus, hepatitis A virus, and persistently elevated aminotransferases in hemophiliacs. J Med Virol 1980; 6:111.
61. Kim HC, Saidi P, Ackley AM, et al. Prevalence of type B and non-A, non-B hepatitis in hemophilia: relationship to chronic liver disease. Gastroenterology 1980; 79:1159.
62. Bloom AL. AIDS and haemophilia. Biomed Pharmacother 1985; 39:355.
63. Gomperts ED, de Biasi R, De Vreker R. The impact of clotting factor concentrates on the immune system in individuals with hemophilia. Tranfus Med Rev 1992; 6:44.
64. Tuddenham EGD, Trabold NC, Collins JA, et al. The properties of factor VIII coagulant activity prepared by immunoadsorbent chromatography. J Lab Clin Med 1979; 93:40.
65. Zimmerman TS. Purification of factor VIII by monoclonal antibody affinity chromatography. Semin Hematol 1988; 25(suppl 1):25.

66. Griffith MJ. Biochemical characterization of method M AHF process developed to reduce the risk of hepatitis transmission. *In* Roberts HH (ed): Proceedings of the Symposium on Biotechnology and the Promise of Pure Factor VIII. Brussels: Baxter Healthcare Publications, 1988, pp 69–85.
67. Gitschier J, Wood WI, Goralka TM, et al. Characterization of the human factor VIII gene. Nature 1984; 312:326.
68. Wood WI, Capon DJ, Simonsen CC, et al. Expression of active human factor VIII from recombinant DNA clones. Nature 1984; 312:330.
69. Vehar GA, Keyt B, Eaton D, et al. Structure of human factor VIII. Nature 1984; 312:337.
70. Toole JJ, Knopf JL, Wozney JM, et al. Molecular cloning of a cDNA encoding human antihaemophilic factor. Nature 1984; 312:342.
71. Boedeker BGD. The manufacturing of the recombinant factor VIII, KoGENate. Trans Med Rev 1992; 6:256.
72. Gomperts E, Lundblad R, Adamson R. The manufacturing process of recombinant factor VIII, Recombinate. Trans Med Rev 1992; 6:247.
73. Eaton DL, Hass PE, Riddle L, et al. Characterization of recombinant human factor VIII. J Biol Chem 1987; 262:3285.
74. Giles AR, Tinlin S, Hoogendoorn H, et al. In vivo characterization of recombinant factor VIII on a canine model of hemophilia A (factor VIII deficiency). Blood 1988; 72:335.
75. Fournel MA. Preclinical and in vitro studies of recombinant factor VIII. Semin Hematol 1991; 28:22.
76. Schwartz RS. Clinical trials of factor VIII produced by recombinant technology. *In* Hoyer LW, Drohan WN (eds): Recombinant Technology in Hemostasis and Thrombosis. New York: Plenum Press, 1991, pp 229–233.
77. White GC II, McMillan CW, Gomperts ED, et al. Clinical trials of recombinant factor VIII. *In* Hoyer LW, Drohan WN (eds): Recombinant Technology in Hemostasis and Thrombosis. New York: Plenum Press, 1991, pp 235–241.
78. Mannucci PM, Gringeri A, Cattaneo M. Use of recombinant factor VIII in the management of hemophilia. *In* Albertini A, Lenfant CL, Mannucci PM, Sixma JJ (eds): Biotechnology of Plasma Proteins. Basel: Karger, 1991, pp 46–51.
79. Paleyanda RK, Velander WH, Lee TK, et al. Transgenic pigs produce functional human factor VIII in milk. Nature Biotechnol 1997; 15:971.
80. Didisheim P, Loeb J, Blatrix C, Soulier JP. Preparation of a human plasma fraction rich in pro-thrombin, proconvertin, Stuart factor, and PTC and a study of its activity and toxicity in rabbits and man. J Lab Clin Med 1959; 53:322.
81. Soulier JP. The history of PPSB. Vox Sang 1984; 46:58.
82. White GC, Lundblad RL, Kingdon HS. Prothrombin complex concentrates: preparation, properties, and clinical uses. Curr Top Hematol 1979; 2:203.
83. Heysteck J, Brummelhuis HGJ, Krijnen HW. Contributions to the optimal use of human blood. II. The large-scale preparation of prothrombin complex. A comparison between two methods using the anion exchangers DEAE-Cellulose DE 52 and DEAE-Sephadex A-50. Vox Sang 1973; 25:113.
84. Bidwell E, Dike GW, Snape TJ. Therapeutic materials. *In* Biggs R (ed): Human Blood Coagulation, Haemostasis and Thrombosis, 2nd ed. Oxford: Blackwell Scientific, 1976, pp 275–309.
85. Aronson DL. Factor IX concentrates. *In* Sandberg HE (ed): Proceedings of the International Workshop on Technology for Protein Separation and Improvement of Blood Plasma Fractionation (DHEW Publication No. [NIH] 78-1422). Washington, DC: U.S. Government Printing Office, 1977, pp 345–357.
86. Kasper CK. Thromboembolic complications. Thromb Diathes Haemorrh 1975; 33:640.
87. Lusher JM. Thrombogenicity associated with factor IX complex concentrates. Semin Hematol 1991; 28(suppl 6):3.
88. Hultin MB. Activated clotting factors in factor IX concentrates. Blood 1979; 54:1028.
89. Seligsohn U, Kasper CK, Osterud B, et al. Activated factor VII: presence in factor IX concentrates and persistence in the circulation after infusion. Blood 1979; 53:828.
90. Giles AR, Nesheim ME, Hoogendoorn H, et al. The coagulant-active phospholipid content is a major determinant of in vivo thrombogenicity of prothrombin complex (factor IX) concentrates in rabbits. Blood 1982; 59:401.
91. Magner A, Aronson DL. Toxicity of factor IX concentrates in mice. Dev Biol Stand 1979; 44:185.
92. Menache D, Behre HE, Orthner CL, et al. Coagulation factor IX concentrate: method of preparation and assessment of potential in vivo thrombogenicity in animal models. Blood 1984; 64:1220.
93. Murano G. Commercial preparations of vitamin K–dependent factors and their use in therapy. *In* Seegers WH, Walz DA (eds): Prothrombin and Other Vitamin K Proteins, vol 2. Boca Raton, FL: CRC Press, 1986, pp 131–142.
94. Burnouf T, Michalski C, Goudemand M, et al. Properties of a highly purified human plasma factor IX:c therapeutic concentrate prepared by conventional chromatography. Vox Sang 1989; 57:225.
95. Herring S, Abramson S, Kasper C, et al. A highly purified factor IX concentrate. Presented at the XVIIIth International Congress of the World Federation of Hemophilia, Madrid, 1988.
96. Tharakan J, Strickland D, Burgess W, et al. Development of an immunoaffinity process for factor IX purification. Vox Sang 1990; 58:21.
97. Hrinda ME, Huang C, Tarr GC, et al. Preclinical studies of a monoclonal antibody-purified factor IX, Mononine. Semin Hematol 1991; 28(suppl 6):6.
98. Macgregor IR, Ferguson JM, McLaughlin LF, et al. Comparison of high purity factor IX concentrates and a prothrombin complex concentrate in a canine model of thrombogenicity. Thromb Haemost 1991; 66:609.
99. Menache D, Clark DB, Miekka SI, et al. Coagulation factor IX (human). *In* Lusher JM, Kessler CM (eds): Hemophilia and von Willebrand's Disease in the 1990's. Amsterdam: Elsevier, 1991, pp 301–305.
100. Kasper CK, Lusher JM. Recent evolution of clotting factor concentrates for hemophilia A and B. Transfusion 1993; 33:422.
101. Harrison S, Clancy B, Brodeur S, et al. Development of a serum-free process for recombinant factor IX expression in Chinese hamster ovary cells [Abstract]. Presented at the XVth Congress of the International Society of Thrombosis and Haemostasis, Jerusalem, Israel, June 11–16, 1995.
102. Foster WB, Anagnostopoulos A, Bonam D, et al. Development of a process for purification of recombinant human factor IX [Abstract]. Presented at the 37th Annual Meeting of the American Society of Hematology, Seattle, WA, December 1–5, 1995.
103. Bond MD, Jankowski MA, Huberty MC, et al. Structural analysis of recombinant human factor IX [Abstract]. Presented at the 36th Annual Meeting of the American Society of Hematology, Nashville, TN, December 2–6, 1994.
104. Steckert J, Amphlett G. Comparative biophysical characterization of recombinant human factor IX [Abstract]. Presented at the XXIIth International Congress of the World Federation of Hemophilia, Dublin, Ireland, June 23–28, 1996.
105. White G, Shapiro A, Ragni M, et al. Phase I/II pharmacokinetics, safety and efficacy data of recombinant human factor IX in previously treated patients with hemophilia B [Abstract]. Presented at the 37th Annual Meeting of the American Society of Hematology, Seattle, WA, December 1–5, 1995.
106. Aledort L. Inhibitors in hemophilia patients: current status and management. Am J Hematol 1994; 47:208.
107. Lusher JM. Transfusion therapy in congenital coagulopathies. Hematol Oncol Clin North Am 1994; 8:1167.
108. Bloom AL. Management of factor VIII inhibitors: evolution and current status. Hemostasis 1992; 22:268.
109. Lusher JM, Blatt PM, Penner JA, et al. Autoplex versus Proplex: a controlled double-blind study of effectiveness in acute hemarthroses in hemophiliacs with inhibitors to factor VIII. Blood 1983; 62:1135.
110. Hedner U. Experiences with recombinant factor VIIa in hemophiliacs. *In* Hoyer LH, Drohan WN (eds): Recombinant Technology in Hemostasis and Thrombosis. New York: Plenum Press, 1991, pp 223–228.
111. Hellstern P, Beeck H, Fellhauer A, et al. Factor VII and activated-factor-VII content of prothrombin complex concentrates. Vox Sang 1997; 73:155.
112. Hedner U, Kisiel W. Use of human FVIIa in the treatment of two haemophilia A patients with high titre inhibitors. J Clin Invest 1983; 71:1836.
113. Hagen FS, Gray CL, O'Hara P, et al. Characterization of a cDNA coding for human factor VII. Proc Natl Acad Sci U S A 1986; 83:2412.

114. Pedersen AH, Lund-Hansen T, Bisgaard-Frantzen H, et al. Autoactivation of human recombinant coagulation factor VII. Biochemistry 1989; 28:9331.
115. Macik BG, Hohneker J, Roberts HR, et al. Use of recombinant activated factor VII for treatment of a retropharyngeal hemorrhage in a hemophilic patient with a high titer inhibitor. Am J Hematol 1989; 32:232.
116. Shapiro AD. American experience with home use of NovoSeven recombinant factor VIIa in hemophiliacs with inhibitors. Haemostasis 1996; 26(suppl 1):143.
117. Kernoff PBA, Thomas ND, Lilley PA, et al. Clinical experience with polyelectrolyte-fractionated porcine factor VIII concentrate in the treatment of hemophiliacs with antibodies to factor VIII. Blood 1984; 63:31.
118. Hultin MB, Hennessey J. The use of polyelectrolyte-fractionated porcine factor VIII in the treatment of a spontaneously acquired inhibitor to factor VIII. Thromb Res 1989; 55:51.
119. Brettler DB, Forsberg AD, Levine PH, et al. The use of porcine factor VIII concentrate (Hyate:C) in the treatment of patients with inhibitor antibodies to factor VIII: a multicenter US experience. Arch Intern Med 1989; 149:1381.
120. Kernoff PBA. The clinical use of porcine factor VIII. *In* Kasper CK (ed): Recent Advances in Hemophilia Care. New York: AR Liss, 1990, pp 47–56.
121. Menache D, Aronson DL. New treatments of von Willebrand disease: plasma derived von Willebrand factor concentrates. Thromb Haemost 1997; 78:566.
122. Menache D. New concentrates of factors VII, IX and X. *In* Kasper CK (ed): Recent Advances in Hemophilia Care. New York: AR Liss, 1990, pp 177–187.
123. Cohen LJ, McWilliams NB, Neuberg R, et al. Prophylaxis and therapy with factor VII concentrate (human) Immuno, vapor heated in patients with congenital factor VII deficiency: a summary of case reports. Am J Hematol 1995; 50:269.
124. Miekka SI, Clark DB, Menache D. Development of a coagulation factor X concentrate as a by-product of coagulation factor IX production [Abstract]. Thromb Haemost 1987; 58:306.
125. Herring SW, Castruita JJ, Shitanishi KT, et al. A highly purified factor X concentrate. Presented at the XVIIIth International Congress of the World Federation of Hemophilia, Madrid, 1988.
126. Evans G, Pasi KJ, Mehta A, et al. Recurrent venous thromboembolic disease and factor XI concentrate in a patient with severe factor XI deficiency, chronic myelomonocytic leukaemia, factor V Leiden and heterozygous plasminogen deficiency. Blood Coagul Fibrinolysis 1997; 8:437.
127. Karges HE, Metzner HJ. Therapeutic factor XIII preparations and perspectives for recombinant factor XIII. Semin Thromb Hemost 1996; 22:427.
128. Rodeghiero F, Tosetto A, Di Bona E, et al. Clinical pharmacokinetics of a placenta-derived factor XIII concentrate in type I and type II factor XIII deficiency. Am J Hematol 1991; 36:30.
129. Smith JK, Snape TJ. Therapeutic materials in the management of haemorrhagic disorders. *In* Biggs R, Rizza CR (eds): Human Blood Coagulation, Haemostasis and Thrombosis, 3rd ed. Oxford: Blackwell Scientific, 1984, pp 242–272.
130. Radosevich M, Goubran HI, Burnouf T. Fibrin sealant: scientific rationale, production methods, properties, and current clinical use. Vox Sang 1997; 72:133.
131. Alving BM, Weinstein MJ, Finlayson JS, et al. Fibrin sealant: summary of a conference on characteristics and clinical uses. Transfusion 1995; 35:783.
132. Hoots K, McLeod J, Eggers E, et al. Pilot study to evaluate efficacy of fibrin sealant (human) on hemostasis in hemophiliacs undergoing tooth extractions [Abstract]. Blood 1993; 82a(suppl):598.
133. Ortel TL, Charles LA, Keller FG, et al. Topical thrombin and acquired coagulation factor inhibitors: clinical spectrum and laboratory diagnosis. Am J Hematol 1994; 45:128.
134. Matras H. Fibrin seal: the state of the art. J Oral Maxillofac Surg 1985; 43:605.
135. Gibble JW, Ness PM. Fibrin glue: the perfect operative sealant? Transfusion 1990; 30:741.
136. Bove JR. Fibrinogen: is the benefit worth the risk? Transfusion 1978; 18:129.
137. Jackson MR, MacPhee MJ, Drohan WN, et al. Fibrin sealant: current and potential clinical applications. Blood Coagul Fibrinolysis 1996; 7:737.
138. Toti F, Follea G, Delannee C, et al. Biological glues: present status and further prospects. *In* Stoltz JF, Rivat C (eds): Biotechnology of Plasma Proteins: Fractionation and Applications. Paris: INSERM, 1989, pp 81–87.
139. Reiss RF, Oz MC. Autologous fibrin glue: production and clinical use. Transfus Med Rev 1996; 10:85.
140. Silver FH, Wang MC, Pins GD. Preparation and use of fibrin glue in surgery. Biomaterials 1995; 16:891.
141. Carrell R, Travis J. α_1-antitrypsin and the serpins: variation and countervariation. Trends Biochem Sci 1985; 10:20.
142. Schultze HE, Heide K, Haupt H. Alpha$_1$-antitrypsin aus Humanserum. Klin Wochenschr 1962; 40:427.
143. MacDonald JL, Johnson CE. Pathophysiology and treatment of α_1-antitrypsin deficiency. Am J Health Syst Pharm 1995; 52:481.
144. van Steenbergen W. α_1-antitrypsin deficiency: an overview. Acta Clin Belg 1993; 48:171.
145. Hubbard RC, Crystal RG. Alpha-1-antitrypsin augmentation therapy for alpha-1-antitrypsin deficiency. Am J Med 1988; 84:52.
146. Hubbard RC, Crystal RG. Strategies for aerosol therapy of α_1-antitrypsin deficiency by the aerosol route. Lung 1990; 168(suppl):565.
147. Hein RH, Van Beveren SM, Shearer MA, et al. Production of alpha$_1$-proteinase inhibitor (human). Eur Respir J 1990; 3(suppl 9):16s.
148. Coan MH, Dobkin MB, Brockway WJ, et al. Characterisation and virus safety of alpha$_1$-proteinase inhibitor. Eur Respir J 1990; 3(suppl 9):35s.
149. Hubbard RC, McElvaney NG, Sellers SE, et al. Recombinant DNA–produced α_1-antitrypsin administered by aerosol augments lower respiratory tract antineutrophil elastase defenses in individuals with α_1-antitrypsin deficiency. J Clin Invest 1989; 84:1349.
150. Courtney M, Jallat A, Tessier L-H, et al. Synthesis in *E. coli* of alpha 1-antitrypsin variants with potential in the therapy of emphysema and thrombosis. Nature 1985; 313:149.
151. Menache D, Grossman BJ, Jackson CM. Antithrombin III: physiology, deficiency, and replacement therapy. Transfusion 1992; 32:580.
152. Bock SC. Antithrombin III, genetics, structure and function. *In* Hoyer LW, Drohan WN (eds): Recombinant Technology in Hemostasis and Thrombosis. New York: Plenum Press, 1991, pp 25–47.
153. Miller-Andersson M, Borg H, Andersson L-O. Purification of antithrombin III by affinity chromatography. Thromb Res 1974; 5:439.
154. Nunez H, Drohan WN. Purification of antithrombin III (human). Semin Hematol 1991; 28:24.
155. Wickerhauser M, Williams C, Mercer J. Development of large scale fractionation methods. VII. Preparation of antithrombin III concentrate. Vox Sang 1979; 36:281.
156. Fuhge P, Gratz P, Geiger H. Modern methods for the manufacture of coagulation factor concentrates. Transfus Sci 1990; 11:23S.
157. Eketorp R, Engman L, Johansson L, Marschall R. A large-scale purification method for antithrombin III (applied to the Cohn fractionation procedure). *In* Sandberg HE (ed): Proceedings of the International Workshop on Technology for Protein Separation and Improvement of Blood Plasma Fractionation (DHEW Publication No. [NIH] 78-1422). Washington, DC: U.S. Government Printing Office, 1977, pp 321–325.
158. Hoffman DL. Purification and large-scale preparation of antithrombin III. Am J Med 1989; 87(suppl 3B):23S.
159. Hathaway WE. Clinical aspects of antithrombin III deficiency. Semin Hematol 1991; 28:19.
160. Donaldson VH, Evans RR. A biochemical abnormality in hereditary angioneurotic edema: absence of serum inhibitor of C_1-esterase. Am J Med 1963; 35:37.
161. Atkinson JP. Diagnosis and management of hereditary angioedema (HAE). Ann Allergy 1979; 42:348.
162. van Aken WG. Preparation of plasma derivatives. *In* Rossi EC, Simon TL, Moss GL (eds): Principles of Transfusion Medicine. Baltimore: Williams & Wilkins, 1991, pp 323–334.
163. Bork K, Witzke G. Long-term prophylaxis with C_1-inhibitor (C_1 INH) concentrate in patients with recurrent angioedema caused by hereditary and acquired C_1-inhibitor deficiency. J Allergy Clin Immunol 1989; 83:677.
164. Laxenaire M-C, Audibert G, Janot C. Use of purified C_1 esterase

inhibitor in patients with hereditary angioedema. Anesthesiology 1990; 72:956.
165. Waytes AT, Rosen FS, Frank MM. Treatment of hereditary angioedema with a vapor-heated C_1 inhibitor concentrate. N Engl J Med 1996; 334:1630.
166. Esmon CT. Regulation of coagulation: the nature of the problem. *In* Bruley DF, Drohan WN (eds): Protein C and Related Anticoagulants. Houston: Gulf Publishing, 1990, pp 3–27.
167. Marlar RA, Adcock DM. Protein C replacement therapy as a treatment modality for homozygous protein C deficiency. *In* Bruley DF, Drohan WN (eds): Protein C and Related Anticoagulants. Houston: Gulf Publishing, 1990, pp 165–178.
168. Miletich J, Sherman L, Broze G Jr. Absence of thrombosis in subjects with heterozygous protein C deficiency. N Engl J Med 1987; 317:991.
169. Gladson CL, Scharrer I, Hach V, et al. The frequency of type I heterozygous protein S and protein C deficiency in 141 unrelated young patients with venous thrombosis. Thromb Haemost 1988; 59:18.
170. Bovill EG, Bauer KA, Dickerman JD, et al. The clinical spectrum of heterozygous protein C deficiency in a large New England kindred. Blood 1989; 73:712.
171. Marlar RA, Mastovich S. Hereditary protein C deficiency: a review of the genetics, clinical presentation, diagnosis and treatment. Blood Coagul Fibrinolysis 1990; 1:319.
172. Mannucci PM, Vigano S. Protein C concentrates for therapeutic use. Lancet 1983; 1:875.
173. Marlar RA, Montgomery RR, Broekmans AW. Report on the diagnosis and treatment of homozygous protein C deficiency. Report of the Working Party on Homozygous Protein C Deficiency of the ICTH-Subcommittee on Protein C and Protein S. Thromb Haemost 1989; 61:529.
174. Vukovich T, Auberger K, Weil J, et al. Replacement therapy for a homozygous protein C deficiency-state using a concentrate of human protein C and S. Br J Haematol 1988; 70:435.
175. Schwarz HP, Schramm W, Dreyfus M. Monoclonal antibody purified protein C concentrate: initial clinical experience. *In* Bruley DF, Drohan WN (eds): Protein C and Related Anticoagulants. Houston: Gulf Publishing, 1990, pp 83–89.
176. Velander WH, Morcol T, Clark DB, et al. Technological challenges for large-scale purification of protein C. *In* Bruley DF, Drohan WN (eds): Protein C and Related Anticoagulants. Houston: Gulf Publishing, 1990, pp 11–27.
177. Grinnell BW, Walls JD, Gerlitz B, et al. Native and modified recombinant human protein C: function, secretion, and posttranslational modifications. *In* Bruley DF, Drohan WN (eds): Protein C and Related Anticoagulants. Houston: Gulf Publishing, 1990, pp 29–63.
178. Sugiura T, Maruyama HB. Production of recombinant protein C in serum-containing and serum-free perfusion culture. Cytotechnology 1991; 7:159.
179. Van Cott KE, Lubon H, Russell CG, et al. Phenotypic and genotypic stability of multiple lines of transgenic pigs expressing recombinant human protein C. Transgenic Res 1997; 6:203.
180. Smith OP, White B, Vaughan D, et al. Use of protein-C concentrate, heparin, and haemodiafiltration in meningococcus-induced purpura fulminans. Lancet 1997; 350:1590.
181. Dreyfus M, Masterson M, David M, et al. Replacement therapy with a monoclonal antibody purified protein C concentrate in newborns with severe congenital protein C deficiency. Semin Thromb Hemost 1995; 21:371.
182. Comp PC. The clinical potential of protein C and activated protein C. *In* Bruley DF, Drohan WN (eds): Protein C and Related Anticoagulants. Houston: Gulf Publishing, 1990, pp 181–186.
183. Orthner CL, Ralston AH, McGriff JD, et al. Large scale purification and preclinical studies of activated protein C (APC) as an antithrombotic agent. Blood 1990; 76(suppl 1):517a.
184. Heeb MJ, Schwarz HP, White T, et al. Immunoblotting studies of the molecular forms of protein C in plasma. Thromb Res 1988; 52:33.
185. Saunders CW, Schmidt BJ, Mallonee RL, et al. Secretion of human serum albumin from *Bacillus subtilis*. J Bacteriol 1987; 169:2917.
186. Latta M, Kanpp M, Sarmientos P, et al. Synthesis and purification of mature human serum albumin from *E. coli*. Bio/Technology 1987; 5:1309.
187. Echelard Y. Recombinant protein production in transgenic animals. Curr Opin Biotechnol 1996; 7:536.
188. Hoyer LW, Drohan WN, Lubon H. Production of human therapeutic proteins in transgenic animals. Vox Sang 1994; 67(suppl 3):217.
189. Paleyanda R, Young J, Velander W, Drohan W. The expression of therapeutic proteins in transgenic animals. *In* Hoyer LW, Drohan WN (eds): Recombinant Technology in Thrombosis and Hemostasis. New York: Plenum Press, 1991, pp 197–212.
190. Wright G, Carver A, Cottom D, et al. High level expression of active human alpha-1-antitrypsin in the milk of transgenic sheep. Bio/Technology 1991; 9:830.
191. Eisensmith RC, Woo SLC. Viral vector-mediated gene therapy for hemophilia B. Thromb Haemost 1997; 78:24.
192. Walter J, High KA. Gene therapy for the hemophilias. Adv Vet Med 1997; 40:119.
193. Connelly S, Kaleko M. Gene therapy for hemophilia A. Thromb Haemost 1997; 78:31.
194. Kay MA, Liu D, Hoogerbrugge PM. Gene therapy. Proc Natl Acad Sci U S A 1997; 94:12744.

SECTION

VII Intrauterine and Neonatal Transfusion

CHAPTER 19

Intrauterine Transfusion

J. M. Bowman

Hemolytic disease of the fetus and newborn is the principal disorder for which intrauterine transfusion is used. Hydrops fetalis (generalized fetal anasarca) and severe jaundice (icterus gravis) causing neonatal death (kernicterus) were first reported in 1609 in a set of twins, but the relationship between the two conditions was not defined until 1932. In that year, Diamond and colleagues[1] stated that icterus gravis (kernicterus) and hydrops fetalis were simply different spectra of the same disease characterized by hemolysis of the fetal red cells, with compensating medullary and extramedullary erythropoiesis. The outpouring of primitive nucleated red cells (Fig. 19–1) led to the original descriptive term for this disorder, *erythroblastosis fetalis.*

The cause of the fetal red cell hemolysis was elucidated in 1940, when Landsteiner and Wiener discovered the Rh blood group system.[2] Levine and colleagues[3] in 1941 determined that a woman who had had several hydropic fetal deaths was Rh(D)-negative and her husband was Rh(D)-positive. She had in her serum a powerful antibody that agglutinated her husband's red cells, as well as the red cells of Landsteiner and Wiener's Rh(D)-positive experimental subjects.[3] The etiology and pathogenesis of hemolytic disease of the newborn (HDN) were

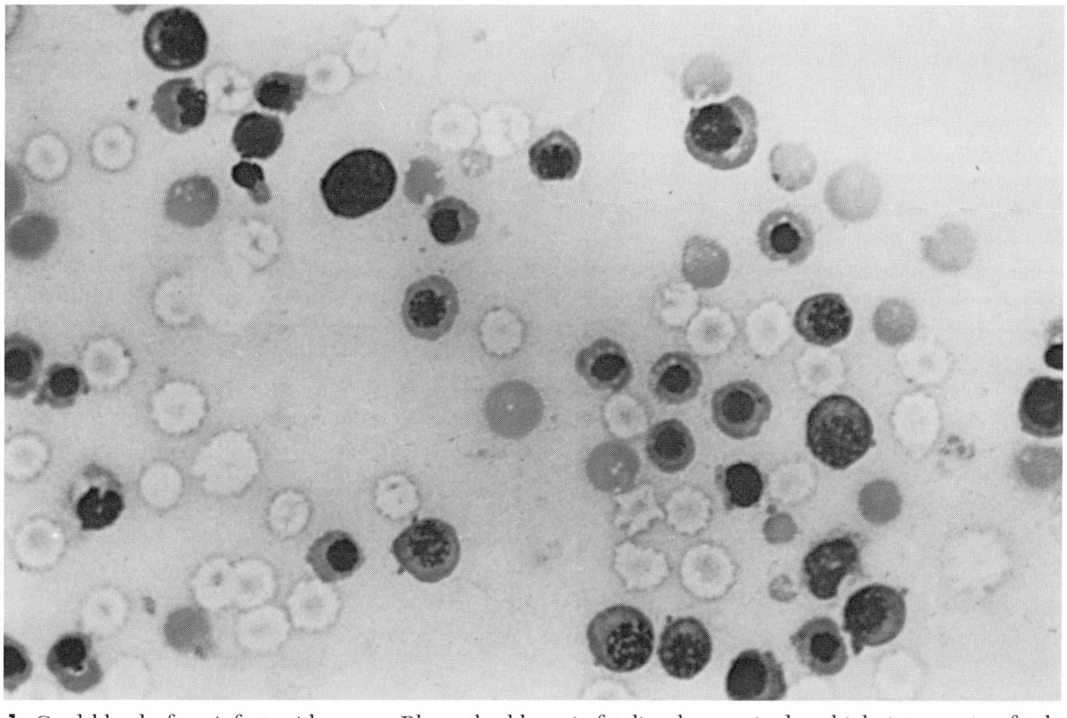

Figure 19–1. Cord blood of an infant with severe Rh erythroblastosis fetalis who required multiple intrauterine fetal transfusions and exchange transfusions. Smear treated by Kleihauer's technique and Wright's stain. Note adult unstained donor "ghost" red cells, dark-stained fetal red cells, and fetal erythroid series from erythroblasts through normoblasts. (From Bowman JM. Blood-group incompatibilities. *In* Iffy L, Kaminetzky HA [eds]: Principles and Practice of Obstetrics and Perinatology. New York: John Wiley & Sons, 1981, p 1201.)

then clear. An Rh(D)-negative mother, when exposed to Rh(D)-positive red cells (usually owing to a transplacental fetal hemorrhage), develops an Rh(D) antibody. If the antibody is an immunoglobulin G (IgG), it crosses the placenta, coats the fetus's Rh(D)-positive red cells, and causes extravascular hemolysis primarily in the fetal spleen.

In the most serious form of the disorder (20% to 25% of cases), hemolysis is severe. Compensatory extramedullary erythropoiesis becomes extreme. Portal hypertension causes ascites. With increasing anemia and obstruction to the intrahepatic circulation, hepatocellular damage occurs. Hypoalbuminemia develops, along with generalized edema, ascites, and pleural and pericardial effusions, the full-blown picture of hydrops fetalis (Fig. 19–2). In the past, most hydropic fetuses died in utero, and the few born alive died promptly. Rarely, affected newborns were salvaged with exemplary neonatal care. About half of fetuses destined to become hydropic do so between 18 and 34 weeks of gestation; the remainder become hydropic between 34 and 40 weeks.[4]

Between 25% and 30% of affected fetuses have less severe hemolysis. Anemia is not severe, and compensatory extramedullary erythropoiesis is not so extreme that portal hypertension and hepatocellular damage result. The babies are born at or near term and are in good condition, with only moderate anemia. However, hemolysis is such that the newborn infant's immature hepatic bilirubin conjugation system cannot cope with the increased amounts of indirect bilirubin produced. Albumin bilirubin binding sites become saturated. Free bilirubin penetrates the neuron lipid membrane, interfering with vital metabolic processes, and the neuron dies. As jaundice deepens, the infant becomes listless and lethargic and stops feeding. Ultimately the infant becomes spastic, lying in a position of opisthotonos (Fig. 19–3). Ninety percent of such infants then become apneic and die. At postmortem examination, yellow staining (bilirubin) can be seen in certain areas of the brain (substantia nigra, hypocampal gyrus, eighth nerve nucleus). The descriptive term *kernicterus* was derived from this yellow staining of the brain. The 10% of such infants who survive have devastating neurological sequelae, profound sensory neural deafness, spastic choreoathetosis, and varying degrees of developmental retardation.[4]

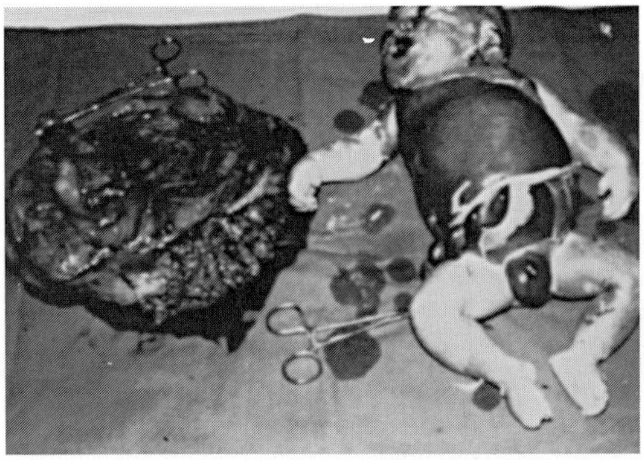

Figure 19–2. Stillborn fetus with hydrops fetalis. Note the edema and markedly enlarged placenta. (From Bowman JM. Rh-isoimmunization 1977. Mod Med Can 1977; 32:17–25.)

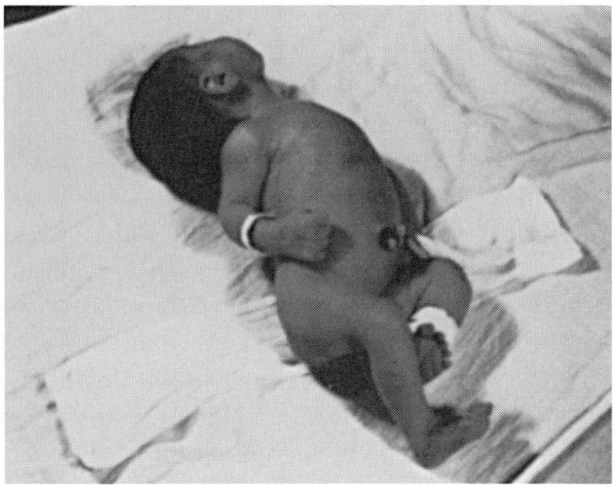

Figure 19–3. Infant with kernicterus. Note spasticity and opisthotonos. (From Bowman JM. Rh-isoimmunization 1977. Mod Med Can 1977; 32:17–25.)

The remaining 45% to 55% of infants with Rh(D) hemolytic disease are only mildly affected. They are born in good condition at term. They may become moderately hyperbilirubinemic and anemic but recover without requiring treatment. Their prognosis for intact survival was as good in the early 1940s, when no treatment was available, as it is today.[4]

PARAMETERS OF NEONATAL TREATMENT

The outlook for infants born in good condition but with hemolytic disease severe enough for kernicterus to develop was completely altered after the introduction of exchange transfusion in 1945 by Wallerstein.[5] Ancillary methods of management include phototherapy to convert neurotoxic bilirubin to water-soluble, nontoxic photoisomers; phenobarbital administration to hasten glucuronyl transferase induction and thus increase bilirubin conjugation and excretion; and albumin administration to increase albumin indirect bilirubin binding. However, exchange transfusion is the keystone of treatment after birth. Exchange transfusion, which in the late 1940s and early 1950s reduced the perinatal mortality due to HDN from 50% to 25%, requires no further discussion. Our remaining concern is to reduce or, if possible, eliminate mortality (and morbidity) in fetuses affected so severely that they will become hydropic, either by preventing hydrops fetalis or by reversing it after it has developed.

ANTIGEN-ANTIBODY SYSTEMS CAUSING ALLOIMMUNE HYDROPS

The development of prevention programs, through administration of Rh immune globulin (RhIG), has decreased the prevalence of Rh(D) immunization.[6] The Rh antigen D is still the most important cause of hemolytic disease, but non-D blood group immunization is assuming greater importance. Some non-Rh(D) alloantibodies have the same hemolytic potential in the pregnant woman and her fetus as anti-D, and they should be managed in a similar fashion.

In Manitoba, the mean annual prevalence of Rh(D) immunization in pregnant women dropped from 194 cases in the 5-year period ending October 1967 to 27 cases in the 8-year period ending October 31, 1990. In these two periods, the mean annual prevalence of non-Rh(D) immunization rose from 14 cases to 88 cases. Although many non-Rh(D) alloantibodies are of little or no clinical significance (for example, anti-Lu^a, Lu^b, P, Le^a, Le^b, and Fy^b), Mollison and associates[7] state that the following antibodies have been implicated in producing moderate to severe hemolytic disease: anti-C, anti-E, anti-c, and anti-e in the Rh system; and anti-K1, Jk^a, Js^a, Js^b, Ku, Fy^a, M, N, s, U, PP_1P^k, Di^b, Lan, LW, Far, Good, Wr^a, and Zd. There are also reports of severe hemolytic disease caused by anti-Kp^b and anti-M,[8, 9] and we and others have observed severe disease due to anti-K2 (k, Cellano).[10] Although this list is intimidating, it must be considered in conjunction with the frequency with which these antibodies occur and the frequency with which they cause significant HDN.

In our experience with Manitoban patients and those referred to our unit for management (Table 19–1), anti-c and anti-K1 (Kell) are by far the most common non-Rh(D) antibodies that can cause severe disease.[11] One patient each with severe disease caused by anti-Fy^a, Jk^a, C, and E was referred to us for fetal transfusions. In our own population, over a 26-year period, we have had 13 infants with hemolytic disease due to anti-E, 45 due to anti-c, 7 due to anti-C or C^w, 1 due to anti-Kp^a, 1 due to anti-K2(k), 1 due to anti-Fy^a, and 2 due to anti-S who required treatment. Twelve cases due to anti-c either demonstrated hydrops or required fetal transfusions. Of 396 babies delivered from Kell-alloimmunized women over a 43-year period in Manitoba (1948 to 1990), 20 were Kell-positive and affected. One died of kernicterus (1951), three were hydropic and died (1948, 1953, and 1954), four required transfusions or phototherapy, and 12 did not require treatment.

Table 19–1 lists the non-Rh(D) alloantibodies encountered by the Rh laboratory as of October 31, 1990, in both Manitoban pregnant women and women referred to our unit because of HDN. Pregnant women with alloantibodies listed in the first two columns of the table should be managed in the same way as pregnant Rh(D)-alloimmunized women, as should the women with the rare antibodies listed in the second footnote. Women with the alloantibodies listed in the fourth column do not require investigation, because their fetuses will be unaffected. Those with the antibodies listed in the third column, in our experience, have not produced fetuses or babies affected severely enough to require treatment. Nevertheless, on rare occasions, these antibodies (e.g., anti-M) have caused severe disease. Therefore, investigation is indicated if the titer is very high (indirect antiglobulin [IAT] ≥128) or if the mother has a high-titer antibody (IAT ≥32 to 64) of unknown hemolytic potential.

Table 19–1. Non-Rh(D) Alloantibodies and Severity of Hemolytic Disease of the Newborn (HDN)

Severe HDN (Hydrops or Requiring IUT)		Alloantibodies Causing HDN Requiring Neonatal Treatment	Alloantibodies Causing HDN Not Requiring Treatment	Alloantibodies Found Without HDN
Alloantibody*	**No. of Patients†**			
c	19	s	F_Y^b	Le^a
Kell	18	c^W	Jk^b	Le^b
k	1	Kp^a	s	Lu^a
C	1		M	Lu^b
E	1		LW	P
F_Y^a	1			
Jk^a	1			

*Alloantibodies reported by others as causing severe HDN: Js^a, Js^b, Ku, M, N, s, U, PP_1P^k, Di^a, Lan, LW, Far, Good, Wr^a, Zd, and Kp^b.[6–8] Most are extremely rare.

†Manitoban patients and other pregnant women referred to our Rh laboratory because of non-Rh(D) immunization during the following periods: November 1, 1962, through October 31, 1988, for immunizations other than anti-Kell; 1948 through 1990 for anti-Kell immunization.

IUT, intrauterine transfusion.

DETERMINATION OF SEVERITY OF HEMOLYTIC DISEASE

Invasive investigative and treatment measures carry some risk to the fetus. It is therefore important that they be reserved for pregnancies in which the fetuses are at risk.

Past Pregnancy History

There are two common patterns of severity in hemolytic disease: it may remain the same in subsequent pregnancies, or, just as often, it may become progressively more severe (from not requiring treatment to hydropic fetal death). Occasionally (5% to 10% of cases), disease may be less severe in a succeeding pregnancy. Nevertheless, in a woman with a history of hydrops, there is a 90% chance that hydrops will develop in the next affected fetus. In a first Rh(D)-sensitized pregnancy, there is an 8% to 10% risk that hydrops will develop.

Alloantibody Titers

Antibody titrations, carried out in the same laboratory by experienced personnel using the same methods and test cells, are of some help in identifying fetuses at risk. Unfortunately, such tests are not accurate enough by themselves to justify invasive treatment measures, but they do suggest the need for further investigative measures. History and titer alone, in one series, were only 62% accurate in predicting impending hydrops fetalis.[12]

In the author's experience, further investigation is required if there is a prior history of hydrops or of a fetus or infant requiring treatment (intrauterine or exchange transfusions), no matter what the alloantibody titer. Without such a history, investigative procedures are required if a critical antibody titer is reached (in the Rh laboratory, ≥16 by an albumin method, ≥32 to 64 by IAT). Repeated antibody titrations are required, because a sharp rise in titer may herald increasing severity of disease.

Invasive investigative tests are not required before 16 to 18 weeks of gestation. After the initial titration in the first trimester, a second titration should be carried out at

16 weeks; titrations should be repeated thereafter at 4-week intervals until 26 weeks, and then every 2 weeks. If the critical history is present, further investigation is undertaken at 16 to 18 weeks of gestation. If the critical titer is reached after 16 to 18 weeks, further investigation is undertaken within 7 days.

Cellular Bioassays

Certain cellular bioassays have been developed to try to improve the accuracy of predicting the severity of HDN and thereby further restricting the need for invasive investigative measures.[13] These include antibody-dependent, cell-mediated cytotoxicity with monocytes (ADCCM) or with killer lymphocytes (ADCCL), monocyte-mediated chemiluminescence, and adherence to and phagocytosis of antibody-coated red cells by peripheral monocytes or cultured macrophages. Although such tests, particularly ADCCM and ADCCL, may be slightly more accurate in predicting the severity of hemolytic disease than antibody titers, they are not readily available and are quite inaccurate in the presence of an antigen-negative, unaffected fetus. If available, they may modestly reduce the number of fetuses requiring more invasive investigative procedures.[13] However, such tests in no way supplant the three investigative measures that follow: amniotic fluid spectrophotometry,[14] real-time fetal ultrasonography,[15] and percutaneous umbilical blood sampling (PUBS).[16]

Amniotic Fluid Spectrophotometry

In 1961, Liley[14] introduced amniotic fluid spectrophotometry as a means of accurately determining the severity of HDN. Although Bevis[17] was the first to use amniotic fluid spectrophotometry, Liley developed a method of measuring the deviation from linearity at 450 nm (the ΔOD 450), the absorption spectrum of bilirubin, which allowed communication among centers of an easily interpreted reading. Readings are made in a good-quality spectrophotometer and plotted on semilogarithmic graph paper (Fig. 19–4). Readings falling into zone 3 indicate severe disease, with hydrops present within 7 to 10 days; readings falling into zone 1 suggest either no disease or no anemia but a 10% chance that the baby will require treatment after birth; readings in zone 2 indicate moderate disease, becoming more severe as the zone 3 boundary is approached.

Serially performed ΔOD 450 readings are more accurate (Fig. 19–5). The slope of subsequent readings falling or rising in zone 2 is measured. The accuracy of ΔOD 450 readings in mid-trimester has been questioned.[18] In the author's experience, the predictive accuracy of ΔOD 450 measurements is 98% when the last reading falls into zone 1 or zone 3, but only 90% if the last reading falls into zone 2. The readings are even less accurate before 24 weeks of gestation. These inaccuracies are undoubtedly due to the fact that the Liley zone boundaries (determined by Liley from 29 weeks of gestation to term) cannot be extended backward in gestation without loss of

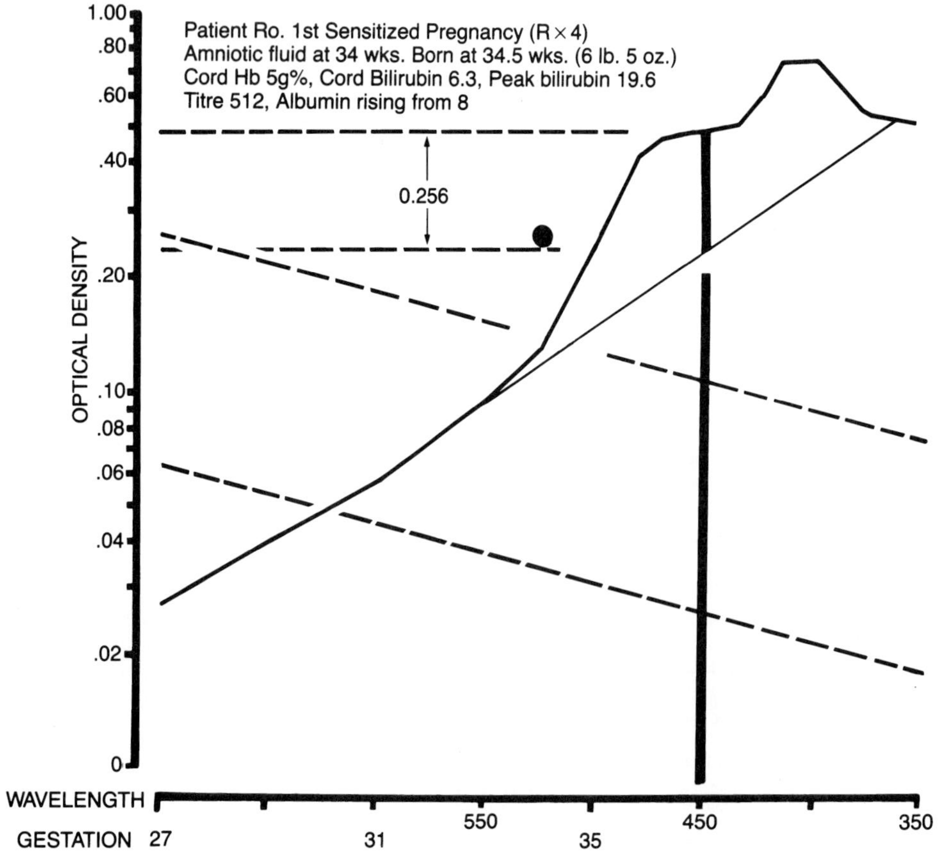

Figure 19–4. Amniotic fluid spectrophotometric reading. Liley method ΔOD 450 (0.256 in this example) falls into zone 3, indicating impending fetal death. A second pigment peak at 405 nm denotes the presence of heme pigment, further evidence of severe erythroblastosis. (From Bowman JM, Pollock JM. Amniotic fluid spectrophotometry and early delivery in the management of erythroblastosis fetalis. Pediatrics 1965; 35:822.)

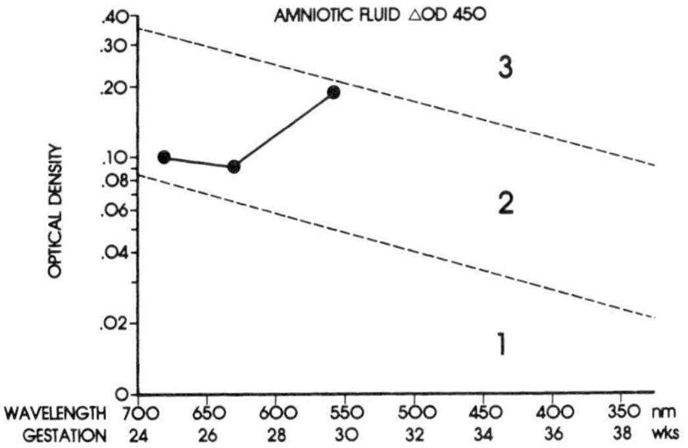

Figure 19–5. Serial ΔOD 450 readings. The first intrauterine transfusion was indicated when the third ΔOD 450 reading was at the 90% level in zone 2 at 29 weeks of gestation. (From Bowman JM. Rh immune disease: diagnosis, management and prevention. *In* Depp R [ed]: Chapter 66: Maternal and fetal medicine. *In* Sciarra JJ [ed]: Gynecology and Obstetrics, vol 3. Philadelphia: Harper & Row, 1998, pp 1–35.)

accuracy. Amniotic fluids in unaffected pregnancies have bilirubin levels that peak at 23 to 24 weeks of gestation.[18] The author has modified the Liley zone boundaries before 24 weeks of gestation, declining them downward at the same angle as the angle of inclination after 24 weeks (Fig. 19–6).

Amniocentesis is not without some hazard to the fetus. In the pre-ultrasonography era, there was a 10% risk of placental trauma producing amniotic fluid oxyhemoglobin peaks, which obscure the 450-nm bilirubin peak and render the fluid inaccurate for predicting the severity of hemolytic disease. Even more serious, such placental trauma produces a high risk of fetomaternal transplacental hemorrhage (TPH), raising alloantibody titers and increasing the severity of HDN. Ultrasonography-guided placental localization reduces the risk of placental trauma to 2%. At present, ultrasonographic evidence of an anterior placenta, which cannot be avoided by the amniocentesis needle, is an absolute contraindication to amniocentesis.

Maternal urine or fetal ascitic fluid is occasionally aspirated instead of amniotic fluid. Urine produces no 450-nm peak. Ascitic fluid is clear, bright yellow, and more viscous than amniotic fluid. The absorption peak of ascitic fluid is much higher, often requiring dilution before it can be measured. The absorption peak is deviated toward 460 nm.

Congenital abnormalities of the fetus such as anencephaly, open spina bifida, and obstructive lesions of the gastrointestinal tract such as tracheoesophageal fistula and duodenal atresia produce hydramnios and marked rises in the ΔOD 450, which may be misleading if the mother is Rh-immunized.

Perinatal Ultrasonography

The introduction of real-time fetal ultrasonography in the late 1970s was a major advance in management of maternal alloimmunization.[15] Ultrasonography allows an estimation of placental and hepatic size and indicates the presence or absence of hydrops (ascites, edema) (Fig. 19–7). It is of value in assessing fetal well-being (biophysical profile). By allowing accurate delineation of the placental implantation site, it has reduced the incidence of placental trauma during amniocentesis.

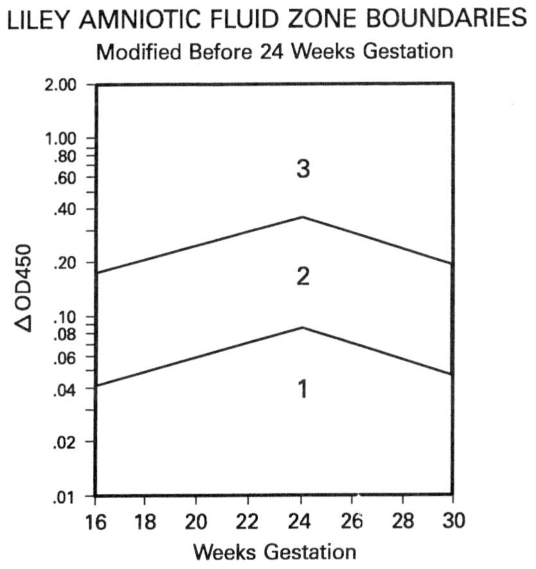

Figure 19–6. Modification of zone boundaries of Liley ΔOD 450 readings before 24 weeks of gestation. The zone boundary angle of inclination before 24 weeks of gestation is the same as the zone boundary angle of declination after 24 weeks of gestation. (From Bowman JM, Pollock JM, Manning FA, et al. Maternal Kell blood group alloimmunization. Obstet Gynecol 1992; 79:239).

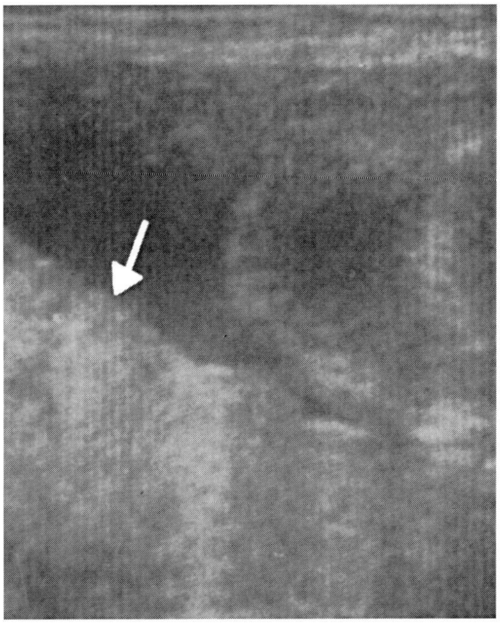

Figure 19–7. Sonogram of fetus with hydrops fetalis. The placenta is enormously thickened and edematous *(arrow)*. The fetal abdomen, which is grossly distended with ascitic fluid, can be seen to the right of the arrow. (From Bowman JM. Maternal blood group immunization. *In* Creasy RK, Resnik R [eds]: Maternal-Fetal Medicine: Principles and Practice. Philadelphia: WB Saunders, 1984, pp 561–602.)

phatic lacunae, up the right lymphatic duct and into the venous circulation. Diaphragmatic movements are necessary for absorption to occur.[27] In the absence of hydrops, 10% to 12% of infused red cells will be absorbed daily. The presence of ascites per se does not prevent absorption,[28] although the rate of absorption becomes more variable. If the hydropic fetus is moribund and not breathing, no donor red cells will be absorbed.[27]

Peritoneal capacity limits the volume of red cells infused. If the volume is such that intraperitoneal pressure exceeds umbilical venous pressure, placental blood flow to the fetus stops and the fetus dies.[29] Infusion red cell volumes can, in nearly every instance, be given safely if calculated by the following formula: (number of weeks of gestation − 20) × 10 mL (e.g., 50 mL at 25 weeks, 100 mL at 30 weeks).

Accurate calculation of donor hemoglobin concentration in the fetus at any time after transfusion allows appropriate spacing of IPTs and selection of the proper point in gestation (after 33 to 34 weeks) for delivery. After IPT, 85% of the transfused red cells will be in the fetoplacental circulation. Residual donor hemoglobin levels in the fetus may be estimated within 1.5 g/dL in 90% of cases using the following parameters: 0.85 as the fraction of donor red cells in the fetoplacental circulation; fetal weight at the point at which donor hemoglobin levels are to be estimated; 125 mL/kg body weight as fetoplacental blood volume; and 1/120th as the daily attrition rate of donor red cells. For example, the donor red cell hemoglobin concentration at 30 weeks of gestation (fetal weight estimated to be 1500 g) 10 days after intrauterine transfusion (IUT) of 85 mL of donor red cells with a hemoglobin concentration of 28 g/dL can be determined as follows:

$$\frac{85 \times 28}{125 \times 1.5} \times \frac{120 - 10}{120} \times 0.85 \text{ g/dL} = 9.9 \text{ g/dL}$$

After subsequent IPTs, estimations of residual circulating donor hemoglobin concentrations for each fetal transfusion at any time after the last transfusion can be made and added together to give the estimated donor hemoglobin level at that point in gestation.

These calculations can be used to determine the time for the next fetal transfusion (or for delivery), with the requirement that the donor hemoglobin level be kept above 10 to 11 g/dL at all times. Because one transfusion rarely raises donor hemoglobin levels above 10 g/dL, a second transfusion is carried out 9 to 12 days after the first. Subsequent transfusion intervals are 3.5 to 4 weeks, with the last transfusion rarely being given after 32 weeks. Delivery is carried out 3.5 to 4 weeks after the last transfusion, usually between 34 and 36 weeks of gestation.

Technique

The mother is premedicated with an analgesic and muscle relaxant but is not anesthetized. After aseptic and local anesthetic preparation, the operator directs an 18-cm, 16-gauge Tuohy needle through a 5-mm skin incision into the fetal peritoneal cavity under direct ultrasonographic guidance, having selected the site and depth of needle insertion on the basis of real-time ultrasonographic assessment. Often, but not invariably, the real-time image shows the needle tip in the fetal abdomen. As the needle enters the fetal abdominal wall, the operator may note a feeling of resistance that disappears as the tip enters the peritoneal cavity. The stylet is removed, and an epidural catheter, with its tip and side holes removed, is passed down the needle. If the catheter passes through the end of the needle, it is lying free in the fetal peritoneal cavity (Fig. 19–9). Between 25 and 30 cm of catheter is passed down the needle. The needle is pulled back over the catheter to lie on the maternal abdomen, and 1 to 1.5 mL of radiopaque contrast medium is injected through the catheter. An anteroposterior radiograph is taken. If the catheter lies free in the fetal peritoneal cavity, the contrast-filled catheter is seen to be within the peritoneal cavity, and contrast appears within the cavity, outlining the negative shadow of liver and semilunes of small bowel (Fig. 19–10).

Diagnosis of hydrops fetalis should be made by ultrasonography before the IPT. Ascitic fluid obtained at IPT is characteristic. It is bright yellow, clear, and slightly viscous because of its protein content. It looks quite different from the dull yellow, slightly turbid, less viscous amniotic fluid. If ascites is present at the second and subsequent fetal transfusions, the fluid is mixed with residual donor blood to various degrees. When ascites is present, a radiograph, after injection of contrast medium, reveals characteristic diffusion of dye into the ascitic fluid with no visible small bowel semilunes or other landmarks (Fig. 19–11).

Since the development of highly sophisticated ultra-

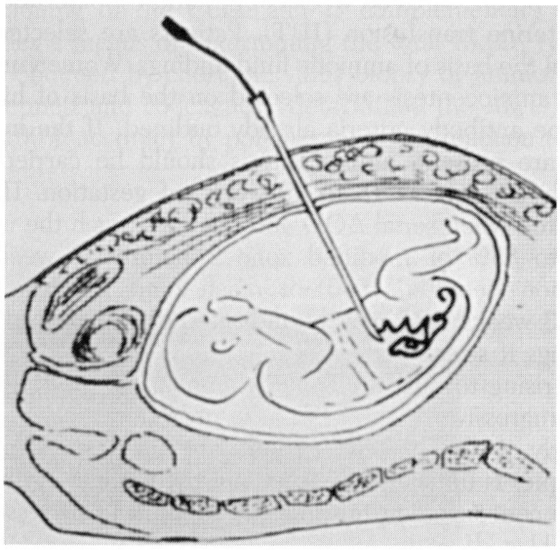

Figure 19–9. Intrauterine transfusion. The Tuohy needle has been inserted across the maternal abdominal wall and uterine wall into the fetal peritoneal cavity, and the epidural catheter has been threaded into the peritoneal cavity of the fetus. The safest position for the fetus during intraperitoneal transfusion is not with the abdomen anterior (as shown in this diagram), because the fetal umbilical vessels would then lie in the center of the target area. (From Bowman JM. Blood-group incompatibilities. *In* Iffy L, Kaminetzky HA [eds]: Principles and Practice of Obstetrics and Perinatology. New York: John Wiley & Sons, 1981, pp 1193–1239.)

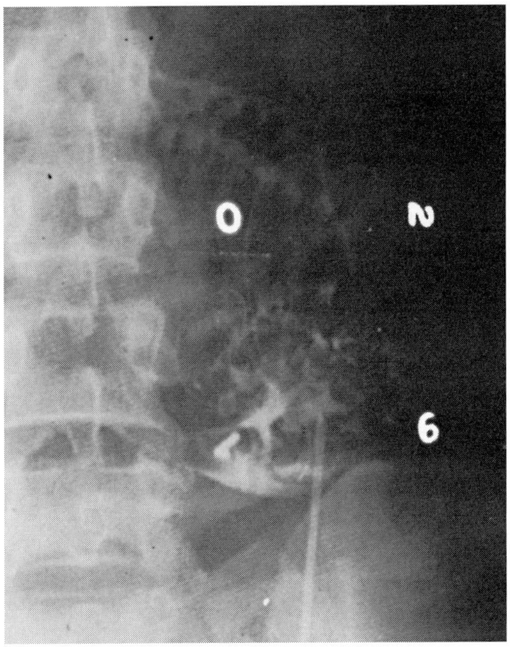

Figure 19–10. Successful catheterization of fetal peritoneal cavity as shown by radiopaque contrast medium outlining negative shadows of small bowel. (From Bowman JM. Maternal blood group immunization. *In* Creasy RK, Resnik R [eds]: Maternal-Fetal Medicine: Principles and Practice. Philadelphia: WB Saunders, 1984, pp 561–602.)

sonography equipment, we have confirmed the proper placement of the catheter tip free in the fetal peritoneal cavity by the injection of 1 mL of aerated sterile saline and the observation by ultrasonography of the bubble rising to the top of the fetal abdomen. However, on one occasion this method led to a mistaken confirmation of proper placement when the catheter tip was actually in the fetal colon. For this reason, although x-ray amniograms and preliminary radiographs are no longer necessary, we believe that it is essential that proper placement of the catheter tip be confirmed radiographically after the injection of 1 to 1.5 mL of radiopaque contrast medium (see Fig. 19–10).

Because of the additional risk of trauma and needle dislodgment, the intrauterine team of the University of Manitoba and Rh Laboratory does not inject blood into the peritoneal cavity directly down the needle, despite reports of success with this method.[30] We advise against this method of IPT, because we believe that the epidural catheter transfusion technique pioneered by Liley is safer and more reliable than the direct needle transfusion technique.

When the contrast injection radiograph demonstrates the catheter to be lying in the fetal peritoneal cavity (see Fig. 19–10), the transfusion is started. Infusion of compatible red cells is carried out in 10-mL aliquots, each 10-mL injection taking 3 to 6 minutes. The fetal heart rate is monitored by Doppler ultrasonography at the end of each 10-mL injection and continuously for the last 10 to 15 mL of the infusion. The volume infused is calculated according to the formula given earlier. If the fetus is in good condition, fetal heart rate increases to 160 to 190 beats per minute during the procedure. Fetal bradycardia early in the transfusion is ominous, indicating the probability of transfusion trauma and fetal death. Fetal bradycardia toward the end of the transfusion is an indication for prompt termination of the procedure, because intraperitoneal pressure may be approaching umbilical venous pressure.

If gross ascites is noted (see Fig. 19–11), every effort should be made to aspirate a significant quantity of fluid (35 to 120 mL) through the needle before the catheter is passed. If the postinjection radiograph reveals a considerable amount of residual ascitic fluid after passage of the catheter and injection of contrast, more fluid (as much as possible) should be aspirated through the catheter before the IPT is begun.

If a greater volume of ascitic fluid is aspirated than the planned red cell volume to be injected, the total volume to be transfused may be increased, but it should always be 15 to 20 mL less than the volume of ascitic fluid removed. IPT is no longer recommended for treatment of the hydropic fetus; IVT is the preferred method of transfusion.

Problems With IPT

Although IPT was a major advance in the management of severe erythroblastosis fetalis, it has serious problems.

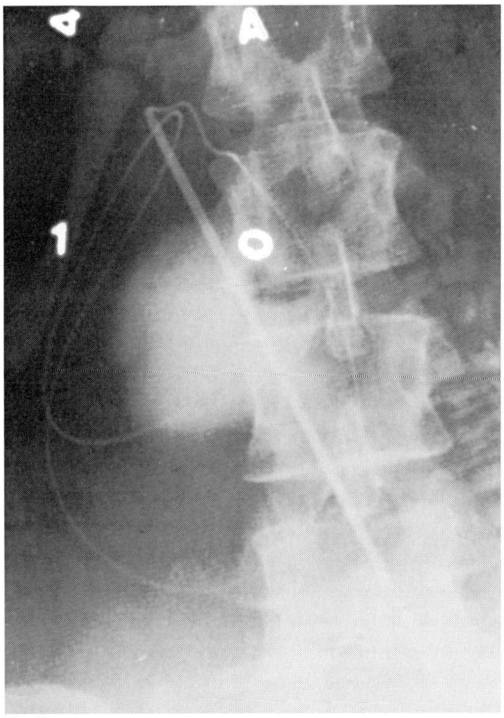

Figure 19–11. Hydrops fetalis found at intrauterine transfusion. Note gross ascites at this first transfusion (31.5 weeks of gestation), which was more severe at the second transfusion 4 days later (not shown). Severe residual hydrops was seen at emergency cesarean section (33.5 weeks of gestation). Cord hemoglobin, 6.2 g/100 mL (99% donor in origin); cord bilirubin, 5.4 mg/100 mL. Five exchange transfusions, respirator care for 4 days, and 3 weeks of intensive nursery care were required. (From Bowman JM. Maternal blood group immunization. *In* Creasy RK, Resnik R [eds]: Maternal-Fetal Medicine: Principles and Practice. Philadelphia: WB Saunders, 1984, pp 561–602.)

IPT is of no value for the nonbreathing, moribund hydropic fetus. In this situation, red cells are not absorbed and the fetus dies. Also, if the placenta is implanted on the anterior uterine wall and must be transfixed by the Tuohy needle in order to enter the fetal peritoneal cavity, the traumatic death rate, in our hands, is 7%. Moreover, after IPT, there is a 30% spontaneous labor rate, with delivery earlier than otherwise planned. Fortunately, most such deliveries occur after 30 weeks of gestation, and 70% of fetuses born after spontaneous labor survive.

IPT of the Hydropic Fetus

Although the aim in immunized mothers is to predict impending hydrops and prevent it by beginning fetal transfusions before hydrops develops, hydrops is present at IUT in 28% to 33% of cases either because of late referral or because it develops between the first and second IPT. The latter occurs when one IPT does not raise donor hemoglobin levels high enough to "shut off" hepatic erythropoiesis and interrupt the hepatic events that lead to the development of ascites and hydrops fetalis.

Although direct IVT is the procedure of choice when hydrops is encountered, IPT has achieved significant salvage rates in hydropic fetuses in the past. In the ultrasound era at our center, 60% (18 of 30) of hydropic fetuses were salvaged with IPT. However, none of eight moribund, nonbreathing hydropic fetuses subjected to IPT survived.

Hydrops fetalis may be reversed by fetal transfusions. Reversal is more common when hydrops is first found at the second IPT. Reversal is quite common when hydrops is encountered at the first direct IVT. As hemoglobin levels rise after transfusion, erythropoietin levels drop. If the fetus remains alive, hepatic erythropoiesis decreases, intrahepatic circulation improves, portal and umbilical venous pressures fall, hepatocellular function improves, serum albumin levels rise, and both ascites and anasarca disappear.

DIRECT INTRAVASCULAR FETAL TRANSFUSION

Pioneering attempts at direct IVT into either a fetal or a placental vessel approached through a hysterotomy incision were made in the mid-1960s.[31–33] The results were poor because the mothers almost invariably went into labor. Rodeck and colleagues,[34] in 1981, introduced direct transfusion through a fetoscope. Few others have achieved their skill with the fetoscope. Blood, meconium, or turbidity in the amniotic fluid makes fetoscopic visualization of the fetal blood vessels difficult. With the advent of fetal blood sampling,[16] it became possible by the early to mid-1980s to follow the sampling procedure with direct IVT.[35–38] Under ultrasonographic guidance, the tip of a 22- or 20-gauge spinal needle is introduced into an umbilical blood vessel, preferably the vein but occasionally the artery, at its insertion into the placenta or, rarely, at its insertion into the fetal abdomen.

Advantages of Fetal Blood Sampling and IVT

As stated earlier, in the absence of hydrops, direct measurement of fetal blood parameters is the most accurate method of determining the severity of hemolytic disease—more accurate than ΔOD 450 measurements and ultrasonographic assessments. Those two methods, however, combined with past history and maternal antibody titers, identify a fetus at risk that requires a fetal blood sampling procedure. Direct IVT does not rely on diaphragmatic movement to increase hemoglobin levels. It is capable of salvaging a moribund, nonbreathing fetus, provided the fetus still has umbilical blood flow. Also, direct IVT raises circulating hemoglobin levels in the fetus immediately, rather than the 8 to 10 days required for IPT.

Technique of PUBS and IVT

Because of the previously reported problems with IPT, direct IVT has become the fetal transfusion procedure of choice. When it has been decided that PUBS and direct IVT are required, the mother is premedicated. A highly skilled, experienced, perinatal ultrasonographer is an essential component of the IVT group. Great care and considerable time are spent in identifying the target blood vessel (see Fig. 19–8). Concentrated red cells used for IVT are of the same hemoglobin and maternal crossmatch compatibility as those used for IPT. Immediately before the planned procedure, 5 to 10 mL of sterile saline are added to the red cell unit. The red cells can be readily infused through a 22- or 20-gauge spinal needle without hemolysis.

After careful aseptic preparation of the maternal abdomen, the obstetrician drapes the maternal abdomen, infiltrates the skin with local anesthetic, and inserts a 20- or 22-gauge spinal needle tip through the maternal skin, immediately over the target site selected by the ultrasonographer. The ultrasound transducer, enclosed in sterile plastic, is applied to the maternal abdomen immediately adjacent to the needle insertion site. The ultrasonographer and the venipuncturist select a plane and position the transducer to allow simultaneous ultrasonographic identification of both the blood vessel target site and the needle tip. The needle is guided toward the blood vessel with appropriate ultrasonography-guided corrections in needle direction to keep the tip on target.

In most instances, the needle tip can be identified as it penetrates the blood vessel. Because the needle tip is being advanced in a three-dimensional plane using ultrasonography, which is in two dimensions, one cannot always be certain that the needle tip has been correctly inserted into the lumen of the vessel. When the tip is at the proper depth, the needle stylet is withdrawn and aspiration is attempted using a lightly heparinized 1-mL tuberculin syringe. If nothing is obtained, or if amniotic fluid is aspirated, withdrawal but not removal of the needle tip and its reinsertion under ultrasonographic guidance are carried out. If a free-flowing blood sample is aspirated, the tip of the needle is probably properly positioned in the fetal blood vessel. At initial fetal blood sampling, placement can be confirmed by determining that the blood is fetal using the alkaline denaturation method.

After the first IVT, the amount of donor blood present in the fetal circulation obscures the alkaline denaturation test result, so it cannot be used to confirm fetal origin of sampled blood. Proper needle tip placement is readily confirmed, however, by injecting 0.5 mL of sterile saline. If the needle tip is in the vein, streaming ultrasound turbulence is seen as the saline passes down the vein. Conversely, if the needle tip is in the artery, the turbulence of the saline may be seen moving in the opposite direction, onto the surface of the placenta. If turbulence can be seen in the amniotic fluid, the needle tip is in the amniotic cavity. If no turbulence can be seen, the needle tip may be dislodged and embedded in the umbilical cord. In this situation, injection of blood should not be carried out because life-threatening umbilical vein compression may occur. Only if streaming of saline in the vessel can be seen should blood infusion be begun.

Hemoglobin is measured immediately in the fetal blood sample. Subsequently, complete investigation of the fetal blood sample is carried out in the laboratory. If the immediate hemoglobin reading is below 10 to 11 g/dL, the IVT proceeds. If fetal movements are likely to disturb the needle insertion (posterior cord insertion), the fetus is paralyzed by the intravenous injection of pancuronium. The venipuncturist holds the filled blood transfusion tubing connector in the needle hub firmly. The ultrasonographer continually watches the blood flow turbulence in the fetal blood vessel. The transfusionist (the third member of the transfusion team) transfuses the red cells in 10-mL aliquots. Because there are only 2 to 3 mm of needle tip within the fetal blood vessel, which may be as small as 2 to 3 mm in diameter, the tip is in danger of dislodgment. For this reason, transfusion of red cells is carried out as rapidly as possible. Each 10 mL is transfused in 1 to 2 minutes, until the desired volume is attained. The usual transfusion volume is 50 mL/kg of estimated nonhydropic fetal weight. The expansile placental vascular bed can tolerate these large red cell volumes transfused at a rapid rate.

The ultrasonographer monitors fetal heart rate and cardiac ventricular size. If there is evidence of significant bradycardia or marked ventricular dilatation (a rare event), the transfusion is discontinued before the full volume is administered. Because the aim is to shut off erythropoiesis so that hepatosplenomegaly will diminish and hydrops will be prevented or reversed, a second procedure is carried out as soon as it is estimated that the total circulating hemoglobin concentration has dropped into the range of 9 to 10 g/dL. The average donor hemoglobin attrition rate is 0.4 g/dL/day. Subsequent IVTs are usually required every 3 to 4 weeks, again when the estimated residual circulating hemoglobin concentration has dropped into the range of 9 to 10 g/dL. Because of the relative safety of IVT, the last procedure is carried out at 33.5 to 34.5 weeks of gestation to allow delivery at 37 to 38 weeks.

IVT in the presence of hydrops fetalis is much preferred over IPT. IVT has the potential to salvage all hydropic fetuses, even those that are moribund and not breathing, with the exception of those that are dying and have no umbilical blood flow. The procedure is no different from IVT of a nonhydropic fetus, other than that the volume administered in the first transfusion is frequently confined to 30 to 40 mL/kg estimated nonhydropic fetal body weight.

When the transfusion has been completed, the needle is cleared with 0.5 mL of normal saline. A 1-mL post-transfusion blood sample is withdrawn, again into a heparinized tuberculin syringe. All blood samples, both before and after transfusion, are tested for hemoglobin, hematocrit, bilirubin, Kleihauer fetal-adult red cell ratios, platelet counts, and plasma protein and blood gas estimations. The initial pretransfusion sample is tested for blood group and direct antiglobulin reactivity.

Simple IVT Versus Exchange IVT

In some centers, exchange IVTs have been carried out rather than simple IVTs.[39] In the author's opinion, because of the expansile fetoplacental vascular bed, exchange IVT, which prolongs the IVT procedure and increases the risk of needle tip dislodgment, is not necessary. Even with severe hydrops and extreme anemia (circulating hemoglobin level as low as 1 g/dL on one occasion), fetal rescue and ultimate nonhydropic delivery are possible with repeated, relatively small, simple IVTs (30 to 40 mL/kg estimated nonhydropic fetal weight).

INTRACARDIAC FETAL TRANSFUSION

IVT into an umbilical blood vessel is the method of choice. However, when the umbilical blood vessels are inaccessible or too small for a successful venipuncture, or when hemolytic disease is so severe that fetal circulatory flow is compromised, intracardiac blood sampling and intracardiac transfusion may be feasible and life-saving. On two occasions, using intracardiac transfusion, our transfusion team was able to rescue severely affected fetuses with circulatory compromise after failed IVT. Both fetuses subsequently underwent successful IVT and survived. On three other occasions, intracardiac transfusion was unsuccessful. Westgren and coworkers[40] reported salvage of four of six severely affected fetuses with intracardiac transfusions when venous access was impossible.

Because of the real hazards of cardiac puncture (tamponade), the author believes that cardiac puncture and intracardiac transfusion should be used only as a last resort, when venous access is not possible and the fetus is so severely compromised that immediate transfusion is imperative.

IUT SURVIVAL RATES

Our center's overall salvage rate with IPT from January 1964 to October 1986 (the last date that a fetus was given IPT alone) was 63% (222 of 353 fetuses transfused 862 times). Survival rates with IPT and IVT in the modern ultrasonography era are shown in Table 19–2. As can be

Table 19–2. Salvage Rates With Intrauterine Transfusion

	204 IPTs July 1980–October 1986	707 IVTs May 1986–January 1998
All fetuses	57 of 75 (76%)	142 of 164* (87%)
Nonhydrops	39 of 45 (87%)	106 of 113* (94%)
Hydrops	18 of 30 (60%)	36 of 51 (71%)
Nonmoribund	18 of 22 (82%)	24 of 31 (77%)
Moribund	0 of 8 (0%)	12 of 20 (60%)
Traumatic deaths	7 (10.3%)	5 (3%)
Risk per IUT	3.5%	0.7%
Risk when placenta anterior	7.0%	0.0%

*One in utero expected to survive.

IPT, intraperitoneal transfusion; IUT, intrauterine transfusion; IVT, intravascular transfusion.

seen, IVT survival rates are superior to IPT survival rates in every category. Three of the IVT hydropic deaths were in fetuses of intravenous drug abusers who were Rh-immunized by sharing needles with Rh-positive boyfriends. They presented with hydropic, moribund fetuses at 17 weeks 5 days to 22 weeks of gestation. If these three hydropic deaths and two other deaths unrelated to IVT (death after placental abruption at 35 weeks of gestation, 6 days after an uneventful IVT; and neonatal death after elective cesarean section delivery at 36 weeks 1 day of gestation) are excluded, the corrected overall survival rate after IVT in our center is 90%.

IVT VERSUS IPT

There is little doubt that IVT, if feasible, is the procedure of choice. Only through IVT can the moribund, nonbreathing, hydropic fetus be salvaged—12 of 20 (60%) in our series. What is gratifying is the lower overall risk with IVT versus IPT (0.7% versus 3.5% per procedure). This is illustrated even more dramatically when the placenta is anterior (0 risk to date for IVT, versus 7% for IPT).

Although the risk of IVT is much less, this low risk can be achieved only when the ultrasonographer and the venipuncturist have great skill and experience with the procedure. Otherwise, the following hazards will increase the risks of IVT: overtransfusion, with cardiac failure (not observed in our series); exsanguination (a problem particularly if the fetus is hydropic or thrombocytopenic and if the cord insertion is posterior)[41]; and inadvertent injection of blood into the cord around the vein, producing a cord hematoma that compresses and interferes with umbilical blood flow. This third hazard has caused fetal deaths. It can be prevented only by an alert, experienced ultrasonographer.

Despite the advantages of IVT, there are two situations in which IPT is still required. One is the rare situation early in pregnancy, before 20 to 21 weeks of gestation, when the cord vessels may be too small for a successful venipuncture. The second is the more common situation late in pregnancy when, after 30 weeks of gestation and after several successful IVTs, increasing fetal size totally obscures a posterior cord vessel insertion, making venipuncture impossible.

DEVELOPMENT IN IUT SURVIVORS

Physical and intellectual development in most fetal transfusion survivors is normal. Because prematurity may be marked (as early as 27 weeks of gestation) and residual severity of disease may be great, some problems may be anticipated. Of 101 children tested at 18 months or later in the Winnipeg Rh Laboratory, 87 appeared completely normal, 10 had minor developmental delay (probably transient and due to prematurity), and 4 were definitely abnormal—1 with a normal IQ but spastic hemiparesis; 2 with IQs of 75 and 85; and 1, in whom fetal hydrops had been reversed, with cerebral agenesis that was probably unrelated to the hydrops.

ATTEMPTS TO AMELIORATE ALLOIMMUNE HEMOLYTIC DISEASE

Although IUTs are capable of salvaging the majority of severely affected fetuses that would otherwise become hydropic and die, it appears that even with our best efforts, they will salvage only 90% to 95% of infants. The major residual problem is the fetus that is so severely affected that hydrops develops before 20 to 21 weeks of gestation (in one instance, at 17 weeks 5 days). We have been successful in carrying out IVT as early as 18 weeks 5 days of gestation. However, successful PUBS and IVT may be impossible as late as 21 to 22 weeks of gestation, leading to attempts at cardiac puncture and intracardiac transfusion that were successful in only two of five instances.

Attempts have been made to reduce maternal alloantibody levels and to interfere with macrophage-coated red cell binding to ameliorate fetal hemolytic disease and to delay PUBS and IVT until later in gestation. The two suppressive modalities of some benefit are intensive plasma exchange[42, 43] and administration of intravenous immune globulin (IGIV).[44, 45] With intensive plasma exchange (10 to 20 L weekly), maternal alloantibody levels can be reduced as much as 75%. However, after 6 to 8 weeks, even with continual plasma exchange, antibody levels tend to rebound. Venous access often becomes a problem, with the need for placement of arterial venous shunts. The plasma removed must be replaced, at least partially, with blood fractions (albumin and IGIV), to reduce antibody feedback rebound and to keep maternal serum albumin and IgG at adequate levels (≥3 g/dL and 300 mg/dL, respectively). Plasma exchange is tedious, costly, and uncomfortable. It is not without some risk to the mother, including bacterial sepsis, particularly if arterial venous shunts have been implanted. The only expectation with the use of intensive plasma exchange is that fetal treatment measures may be delayed until after 22 to 24 weeks of gestation.

The institution of plasma exchange must never preclude or delay the use of definitive investigative procedures such as amniocentesis and PUBS. Plasma exchange should be reserved for the mother whose partner is homozygous for the antigen to which she is immunized and who has a prior history of fetal hydrops occurring at or before 24 to 26 weeks of gestation. In this situation, intensive plasma exchange is begun at 10 to 12 weeks of gestation, when transfer of maternal IgG is beginning, with initial amniocentesis at 18 weeks or PUBS at 19 to 20 weeks. At present, plasma exchange is seldom carried out for fetal hemolytic disease.

There have been reports of the benefits of high-dose IGIV administration in severely alloimmunized pregnant women.[44, 45] With doses of 2 g/kg maternal body weight, circulating maternal alloantibody levels can be reduced by as much as 50%, primarily as a result of the negative feedback produced by total circulating maternal IgG levels of 2.5 to 3 g/dL. Further benefits of IGIV therapy may be due to interference with transfer of maternal antibody across the placenta by trophoblastic Fc receptor saturation and, similarly, reduction of IgG-coated fetal red cell hemolysis by fetal reticuloendothelial Fc saturation with the injected IGIV.

If IGIV therapy is considered, it should be used only for the same indications as intensive plasma exchange, again beginning at 9 to 10 weeks of gestation. The recommended dose is 1 g/kg maternal body weight weekly. This form of therapy appears to benefit the fetuses of severely alloimmunized women and is preferable to plasma exchange. In one instance, a mother who had had one hydropic fetal loss and an infant who survived only after multiple fetal transfusions begun at 22.5 weeks of gestation delivered an antigen-positive, direct Coombs' test–positive, but otherwise unaffected infant at 36 weeks gestation after administration of 1 g/kg of IGIV per week, beginning at 9 weeks of gestation (unpublished case, 1997).

CONCLUSION

Rh prophylaxis has reduced the prevalence of Rh alloimmunization by 85% to 90% but will never eradicate it. There are no prophylactic measures available to reduce the incidence of non-D alloimmunization. Therefore, the need to maintain skilled IUT teams and facilities will persist into the foreseeable future.

Over the past 45 years, great strides have been made in the treatment of alloimmune hemolytic disease. Intrauterine fetal transfusions have reduced the perinatal mortality from this disease to 3%. With increased experience with IVT and earlier referral before hydrops develops, perinatal mortality may be reduced even further.

REFERENCES

1. Diamond LK, Blackfan KD, Baty JM. Erythroblastosis fetalis and its association with universal edema of the fetus, icterus gravis neonatorum and anemia of the newborn. J Pediatr 1932; 1:269.
2. Landsteiner K, Wiener A. An agglutinable factor in human blood recognized by immune sera for rhesus blood. Proc Soc Exp Biol Med 1940; 43:223.
3. Levine P, Katzin E, Burnham L. Isoimmunization in pregnancy: its possible bearing on the etiology of erythroblastosis fetalis. JAMA 1941; 116:825.
4. Bowman JM. Rh immune disease: diagnosis, management and prevention. *In* Sciarra JJ (ed): Gynecology and Obstetrics, vol 3. Philadelphia: Harper & Row, 1998, pp 1–35.
5. Wallerstein H. Treatment of severe erythroblastosis by simultaneous removal and replacement of blood of the newborn. Science 1946; 103:583.
6. Bowman JM. The prevention of Rh immunization. Transfus Med Rev 1988; 2:129.
7. Mollison PL, Engelfriet CP, Contreras M. Blood Transfusion in Clinical Medicine, 8th ed. Oxford: Blackwell Scientific, 1987, p 639.
8. Dacus JV, Spinnato JA. Severe erythroblastosis fetalis secondary to anti-Kp[b] sensitization. Am J Obstet Gynecol 1984; 150:888.
9. MacPherson CR, Christiansen MJ, Newton WA, et al. Anti-M antibody as a cause of intrauterine death. Am J Clin Pathol 1961; 35:31.
10. Bowman JM, Harman C, Manning F, Pollock JM. Erythroblastosis fetalis produced by anti-k. Vox Sang 1989; 56:187.
11. Bowman JM. Treatment options for the fetus with alloimmune hemolytic disease. Transfus Med Rev 1990; 4:191.
12. Bowman JM, Pollock J. Amniotic fluid spectrophotometry and early delivery in the management of erythroblastosis fetalis. Pediatrics 1965; 35:815.
13. Mollison P (collaborative study). Results of tests with different cellular bioassays in relation to severity of RhD haemolytic disease. Report from nine collaborating laboratories. Vox Sang 1991; 60:225.
14. Liley A. Liquor amnii analysis in management of the pregnancy complicated by rhesus sensitization. Am J Obstet Gynecol 1961; 82:1359.
15. Chitkara U, Wilkins I, Lynch L, et al. The role of sonography in assessing severity of fetal anemia in Rh- and Kell-isoimmunized pregnancies. Obstet Gynecol 1988; 71:393.
16. Daffos F, Capella-Pavlovsky M, Forestier F. Fetal blood sampling during pregnancy with use of a needle guided by ultrasound: a study of 606 consecutive cases. Am J Obstet Gynecol 1985; 153:655.
17. Bevis D. Blood pigments in haemolytic disease of the newborn. J Obstet Gynaecol Br Emp 1956; 63:68.
18. Nicolaides KH, Rodeck CH, Mibashan MD, Kemp JR. Have Liley charts outlived their usefulness? Am J Obstet Gynecol 1986; 155:90.
19. Nicolaides KH, Fontanarosa M, Gabbe SG, Rodeck CH. Failure of ultrasonographic parameters to predict the severity of fetal anemia in rhesus isoimmunization. Am J Obstet Gynecol 1988; 158:920.
20. Le Van Kim C, Mouro I, Cherif-Zahar B, et al. Molecular cloning and primary structure of the human blood group RhD polypeptide. Proc Natl Acad Sci U S A 1992; 89:10925.
21. Bennett PR, Le Van Kim C, Colin Y, et al. Prenatal determination of fetal RhD type by DNA amplification. N Engl J Med 1993; 329:607.
22. Hyland CA, Wolter LC, Saul A. Identification and analysis of Rh genes: application of PCR and RFLP typing tests. Transfus Med Rev 1995; 9:289.
23. Avent ND, Martin PG. Kell typing by allele-specific PCR (ASP). Br J Haematol 1996; 93:728.
24. Lo Y-MD, Bowel PJ, Selinger M, et al. Prenatal determination of fetal RhD status by analysis of peripheral blood of rhesus negative mothers [Letter]. Lancet 1993; 341:1147.
25. Chown B, Bowman WD. The place of early delivery in the prevention of foetal death from erythroblastosis. Pediatr Clin North Am 1958; May:279.
26. Liley AW. Intrauterine transfusion of fetus in haemolytic disease. BMJ 1963; 2:1107.
27. Menticoglou SM, Harman CR, Manning FA, Bowman, JM. Intraperitoneal fetal transfusion: paralysis inhibits red cell absorption. Fetal Ther 1987; 2:154.
28. Lewis M, Bowman JM, Pollock JM, et al. Absorption of red cells from the peritoneal cavity of a hydropic twin. Transfusion 1973; 13:37.
29. Crosby WM, Brobmann GF, Chang ACK. Intrauterine transfusion and fetal death: relationship of intraperitoneal pressure to umbilical vein blood flow. Am J Obstet Gynecol 1970; 108:135.
30. Watts DH, Luthy DA, Benedetti TJ, et al. Intraperitoneal fetal transfusion under direct ultrasound guidance. Obstet Gynecol 1988; 71:84.
31. Adamsons K Jr, Freda VJ, James LS, et al. Prenatal treatment of erythroblastosis fetalis following hysterotomy. Pediatrics 1965; 35:848.
32. Asensio SH, Figueroa-Longo JG, Pelegrina A. Intrauterine exchange transfusion. Am J Obstet Gynecol 1966; 95:1129.
33. Seelen J, Van Kessel H, Eskes T, et al. A new method of exchange transfusion in utero: cannulation of vessels on the fetal side of the human placenta. Am J Obstet Gynecol 1966; 95:872.
34. Rodeck CH, Holman CA, Karnicki J, et al. Direct intravascular

fetal blood transfusion by fetoscopy in severe rhesus isoimmunization. Lancet 1981; 1:625.
35. De Crespigny LC, Robinson HP, Quinn M, et al. Ultrasound-guided blood transfusion for severe rhesus isoimmunization. Obstet Gynecol 1985; 66:529.
36. Berkowitz RL, Chikara U, Goldberg JD, et al. Intrauterine intravascular transfusions for severe red blood cell isoimmunization: ultrasound guided percutaneous approach. Am J Obstet Gynecol 1986; 155:574.
37. Nicholaides KH, Soothill PW, Clewell W, et al. Rh disease: intravascular fetal blood transfusion by cordocentesis. Fetal Ther 1986; 1:185.
38. Seeds JW, Bowes WA. Ultrasound-guided intravascular transfusion in severe rhesus immunization. Am J Obstet Gynecol 1986; 154:1105.
39. Grannum PAT, Copel JA, Moya FR, et al. The reversal of hydrops fetalis by intravascular intrauterine transfusion in severe isoimmune fetal anemia. Am J Obstet Gynecol 1988; 158:914.
40. Westgren M, Selbing A, Stangenberg M. Fetal intracardiac transfusions in patients with severe rhesus isoimmunisation. BMJ 1988; 296:885.
41. Harman CR, Bowman JM, Menticoglou SM, et al. Profound fetal thrombocytopenia in rhesus disease: serious hazard at intravascular transfusion. Lancet 1988; 2:741.
42. Graham-Pole J, Barr W, Willoughby MLN. Continuous flow plasmapheresis in management of severe rhesus disease. BMJ 1977; 1:1185.
43. Robinson EAE, Tovey LAD. Intensive plasma exchange in the management of severe Rh disease. Br J Haematol 1980; 45:621.
44. Berlin G, Selbing A, Ryden G. Rhesus haemolytic disease treated with high-dose intravenous immunoglobulin [Letter]. Lancet 1985; 1:1153.
45. de la Camara C, Arrieta R, Gonzalez A, et al. High-dose intravenous immunoglobulin as the sole prenatal treatment for severe Rh immunization. N Engl J Med 1988; 318:519.

CHAPTER 20

Neonatal Transfusion

Ronald G. Strauss

NEONATES AS BLOOD TRANSFUSION RECIPIENTS

Extremely preterm neonates (birth weight, <1.0 kg) require multiple blood transfusions, and the adverse effects of allogeneic transfusion, although uncommon in frequency, may have grave consequences. Depending on local blood banking practices (e.g., use of fresh versus stored red blood cells), many infants requiring transfusions may be exposed to multiple blood donors. Although each donor exposure poses only a small risk, the potential for compounding adverse effects via multiple transfusions obtained from multiple donors is of concern. Transfusion practices for neonates are controversial, variable, and often based on logical assumptions rather than on sound scientific information generated by controlled studies. Thus, firm indications for neonatal blood component transfusions do not exist, and efforts to expand knowledge of neonatal transfusion medicine are crucial for developing optimal practices.

Need for Neonatal Transfusions

Neonates, particularly when extremely preterm, have one of the highest transfusion rates of all patient groups. In 1989, approximately 80% of the 38,000 premature neonates with birth weight less than 1.5 kg born annually in the United States[1, 2] required multiple red blood cell (RBC) transfusions; many infants were given cumulative transfusion volumes in excess of their total blood volumes at birth.[3] A smaller percentage received other blood components such as fresh frozen plasma, cryoprecipitate, platelet and neutrophil (granulocyte) concentrates.

As is true for patients of all ages, efforts have been made to reduce the number of transfusions given to neonates and to limit donor exposures. Two studies of blood use for neonates, conducted at the University of Iowa, illustrate these changing practices. The first study, performed retrospectively during 1983–1984,[4] reported substantial use of blood components from multiple donors. During the first 4 months of life, 53 infants received 683 RBC transfusions (mean transfusions per infant = 12.9) from 503 donors (mean number of donors per infant, 9.5). In addition, 53 fresh frozen plasma, 62 platelet, and four neutrophil transfusions were given.[4] To more completely assess long-term patterns in neonatal transfusions, a second study reviewed transfusions in 1982, 1989, and 1993.[5] The mean number of transfusions per infant (birth weight, <1.5 kg) declined from 7.0 in 1982 to 5.0 in 1989 and to 2.7 in 1993 ($p < .001$). Of interest, the percentage of relatively large infants (birth weight, 1.0 to 1.5 kg) who were managed without need for transfusions increased from 17% in 1982 to 32% in 1989 and to 64% in 1993. In contrast, with rare exceptions, all extremely preterm infants (birth weight, <1.0 kg) required RBC transfusions.[5] Seventy percent of transfusions were given during the first month of life. Of importance is that as the survival of extremely preterm infants continues to increase, a great number of these tiny survivors will require blood component transfusions. Thus blood component transfusions provide a genuine benefit to many preterm infants, and their availability is indispensable to the neonatologist.

Risks of Neonatal Transfusions

It seems inescapable that the need for multiple transfusions, especially when obtained from multiple blood donors, increases the risk of transfusion-transmitted infections in infants. Moreover, the severity of these acquired infections may be greater because of immaturity of neonatal immunity. Accordingly, in addition to measures employed to improve the safety of blood component collection and manufacturing, efforts to diminish the frequency of transfusions and donor exposures must continue.

In early studies, the percentage of infants and children with human immunodeficiency virus (HIV) infection acquired via transfusion rather than by other routes was disproportionately high, in comparison with the percentage of adults who acquired HIV infection through transfusions. In one survey, even when children with hemophilia were excluded, 15% of childhood cases of HIV infection were found to have resulted from blood transfusion, in comparison with 2% of adult cases.[6] These rates were determined before current methods of donor screening and testing and thus certainly overestimate the current rate of HIV transmission through transfusion, which is stated to be about 1 in 680,000 donor exposures.[7] Expression of HIV has been reported to be both of greater[8] and of lesser[9] severity in infants than in adults. Regardless of the controversy, efforts must continue to eliminate this rare complication of blood transfusions in infants.

The current rate of transfusion-transmitted hepatitis has not been determined accurately in infants. Although the incidence of non-A, non-B hepatitis (the majority of which cases are now known to be hepatitis C) was believed to be low,[10] the current rate caused by transfusions is difficult to establish accurately. There is no reason to think that the rate of transmission to infants differs from that in general (i.e., about 1 in 100,000 donor exposures).[7] Disorders related to hepatitis C that lead to long-term morbidity (e.g., posthepatitic cirrhosis and hepatic cancer) are particularly alarming when hepatitis C is acquired during infancy, because of the possibility of a costly period of extended treatment and/or disability.[11]

The importance of transfusion-transmitted cytomegalovirus (CMV) in neonates is controversial. Studies conducted during the 1970s and early 1980s reported a disturbingly high incidence (25% to 50%) of CMV in infants who received transfusions of cellular blood components.[12] The incidence was particularly high in those who received the most transfusions, some of whom died of severe CMV disease. Several studies performed more recently suggested a diminishing, almost negligible risk of CMV.[12–14] However, these studies were criticized,[15] and the importance of transfusion-transmitted CMV in infancy is somewhat controversial. Regardless of the controversy, once the decision has been made to transfuse blood components with low risk of transmitting CMV, cellular products transfused should be either obtained from donors who are seronegative for antibody to CMV[12–18] or effectively leukocyte-reduced.[19, 20] Frozen deglycerolized RBCs are used by some centers and appear to pose little, if any, risk of CMV.[16, 21] However, frozen RBCs are expensive, and RBC loss is unavoidable during deglycerolization; this situation could lead to exposure to even greater numbers of donors. Similarly, frozen platelets would not transmit CMV, but this product is not available at most centers. Thus, as a more practical alternative, cellular blood components, consistently depleted of leukocytes to a level of less than 5×10^6 leukocytes per unit, offer safety comparable with that of blood products supplied by seronegative donors.[19, 20, 22] Inability to consistently achieve marked leukocyte reduction is the probable reason for the occasional failure by some leukocyte-reduction techniques (e.g., washed blood products) to prevent CMV.[12, 16] Obviously, leukocyte reduction is not an option when neutrophil (granulocyte) concentrates are to be transfused, and concentrates from CMV antibody–negative donors must be used. Finally, plasma products that have been frozen (e.g., fresh frozen plasma and cryoprecipitate) or pasteurized (e.g., albumin solutions) do not transmit CMV and do not have to be leukocyte-reduced or obtained from donors who are seronegative for antibody to CMV.[23]

Other transfusion-associated risks of a noninfectious nature that may occur in infants include fluid overload, graft-versus-host disease,[24, 25] electrolyte and acid-base imbalances, iron overload,[26] increased susceptibility to oxidant damage,[27] exposure to plasticizers,[28] hemolysis after plasma transfusions when T activation of RBCs has occurred,[29] immunosuppression,[30] and alloimmunization (although alloimmunization to RBC and leukocyte antigens seems to be rare in infants[4, 19]). Some adverse effects are seen only in the setting of massive transfusions—such as exchange transfusions, in which relatively large quantities of blood are needed—and would rarely occur with the small-volume transfusions commonly given.

The potential risks of transfusion are not trivial, and blood components should be transfused only when indicated and with use of optimal blood banking techniques. Unfortunately, these principles are not easily achieved because neonatal transfusion practices are controversial, variable,[31] and based on limited knowledge of the cellular and molecular biology of hematopoiesis during the perinatal period and of the neonate's response to severe cytopenia. Data from clinical studies of infants are sparse and difficult to interpret because of the precarious and heterogeneous medical conditions of these tiny patients. Even the deceptively simple task of obtaining sufficient blood to conduct definitive studies is a major impediment because of small total blood volumes and difficulty in obtaining vascular access. Although in some instances the value of transfusions is clear (e.g., transfusing RBCs to treat anemia that has caused congestive heart failure, or PLTs to treat severe thrombocytopenia that has led to bleeding), in others it is not. With these limitations in mind, the following discussion offers transfusion guidelines that would be accepted by most experts as being reasonable for the transfusion of neonates.

NEONATAL ANEMIA

Clearly established indications for neonatal RBC transfusions, based on controlled scientific studies, do not exist. In many clinical situations, the need for RBCs seems logical enough, but efficacy has not been established, and a complete understanding of the benefit:risk ratio is lacking. In general, RBC transfusions are given to maintain a level of hematocrit believed to be most desirable for each neonate's clinical status.[32, 33] It is widely recognized that this clinical approach is imprecise, and more physiological indications such as RBC mass, available oxygen, and measurements of oxygen delivery and tissue extraction have been suggested. However, the means by which these more demanding techniques can best be applied to everyday practice remain to be defined. Because definitive data to guide RBC transfusion practice are limited, it is important that pediatricians critically evaluate their use of RBCs in light of the pathophysiological processes involved and the standards of neonatal practice at their respective institutions.

Pathophysiology of Neonatal Anemia

All infants experience a decline in hemoglobin concentration, hematocrit, and circulating RBC volume (mass) in the first weeks of life. This decline results from physiological factors and, in sick preterm infants, from phlebotomy blood losses for monitoring. In healthy full-term infants, the nadir hemoglobin value is rarely below 9 g/dL at the age of 10 to 12 weeks. This decline is more rapid (i.e., nadir at 4 to 6 weeks of age) and falls to lower levels in infants born prematurely. Without transfusion, the mean hemoglobin concentration falls from approximately 16 g/dL at birth to approximately 8 g/dL in infants with birth weights of 1.0 to 1.5 kg and to approximately 7 g/dL in infants with birth weights of less than 1 kg.[32–34] Because this postnatal drop in hemoglobin level is universal and is well tolerated in full-term infants, it is commonly referred to as the "physiological anemia of infancy." However, the pronounced decline in hemoglobin concentration that occurs in many extremely preterm infants is associated with abnormal clinical signs and the need for RBC transfusions, and the acceptance of this "anemia of prematurity" as a normal, benign event has been questioned.[35, 36]

Physiological Factors

Many interacting physiological factors are at play in neonatal anemia. Of major importance is that marrow erythropoiesis decreases shortly after birth; this phenomenon cannot be prevented by hematinic nutrients such as iron, folic acid, vitamin B_{12}, and vitamin E. A key reason that the hemoglobin nadir is lower in preterm than in full-term infants is the former group's diminished plasma erythropoietin (EPO) level in response to anemia.[34, 37–40] Although anemia provokes EPO production in premature infants, the plasma levels achieved in anemic infants, at any given blood hemoglobin concentration, are lower than those observed in comparably anemic older persons.[39] When related quantitatively, rising EPO levels and falling blood hemoglobin concentrations correlate weakly in preterm infants.[40] Low plasma EPO levels, although accepted as part of physiological anemia, may limit compensation for anemia in the newborn that is due to "nonphysiological" mechanisms (e.g., blood loss, hemolysis). Erythroid progenitor cells in blood[41] and bone marrow[42] of preterm infants are quite responsive to EPO in vitro; this finding suggests that inadequate EPO production, not marrow unresponsiveness, is the major cause of physiological anemia.

The mechanisms responsible for the diminished erythropoietin output by preterm neonates are only partially defined. One mechanism is that the primary site of EPO production in preterm infants is in the liver, rather than the kidneys.[43] In normal fetuses, EPO is produced first by the liver and then by the kidneys. Studies in lambs show that EPO production by the fetal liver begins to decrease after 120 to 130 days of gestation (normal ovine term is 145 to 150 days), at which time renal EPO production increases.[43] At term, however, 70% to 75% of EPO produced in response to anemia continues to be contributed by the liver. This dependency on hepatic EPO is important, because the liver is less sensitive to anemia and tissue hypoxia—hence, a relatively sluggish EPO response to the falling RBC mass. In sheep, the switch to renal EPO production is complete by about 40 days after birth, an age after which the liver contributes less than 10% of EPO output. The timing of the switch is set at conception and is not accelerated by preterm birth. From a teleological perspective, decreased hepatic production of EPO under in utero conditions of tissue hypoxia may be an advantage for the fetus. If this were not the case, normal levels of fetal hypoxia could trigger high levels of EPO and produce erythrocytosis and consequent hyperviscosity in utero. After birth, however, diminished EPO responsiveness to tissue hypoxia would be disadvantageous and would lead to anemia—not unlike that routinely observed as the "physiological anemia of infancy."

Diminished EPO production cannot entirely explain low plasma EPO levels in preterm infants. Extraordinarily high plasma levels of EPO have been reported in some fetuses of postconceptional age that are comparable with those of neonates treated in intensive care settings,[44, 45] and macrophages from human cord blood were found to produce normal quantities of EPO messenger RNA and protein.[46] These studies document intact synthetic capability under some circumstances. Thus, additional mechanisms probably contribute to diminished EPO plasma levels. For example, plasma levels of EPO undoubtedly are influenced by metabolism (clearance) as well as by production. Thus, pharmacokinetic studies of EPO during the perinatal period are likely to be important both for understanding the physiological processes involved and for designing successful therapeutic trials for use of recombinant human erythropoietin (rHuEPO). Data from studies of human infants[47, 48] and neonatal monkeys[49] have demonstrated that low plasma EPO levels may result from increased plasma clearance and volume of distribution and from shorter fractional elimination and mean residence times for EPO in neonates in comparison with those of adults.

Physiological factors contribute to neonatal anemia because neonatal and adult RBCs differ with respect to a number of biochemical (enzymatic) and physical (membrane) properties, which shorten RBC survival during infancy.[50, 51] In addition, neonates and adults differ in the delivery of tissue oxygen. The position of the neonatal hemoglobin-oxygen dissociation curve (ODC) is shifted to the left in comparison with that of the adult (oxygen half-saturation pressure, 16 to 18 versus 24 to 26 mm Hg). This left shift is caused by several factors, including the neonate's higher levels of fetal hemoglobin. Fetal hemoglobin does not react well with 2,3-diphosphoglycerate (2,3-DPG) and fails to move the ODC rightward. In addition, neonatal RBCs contain lower levels of 2,3-DPG to react with the relatively few molecules of adult hemoglobin that are present.[33, 34] Thus a number of physiological factors contribute to the pathogenesis of neonatal anemia and alter the means by which infants adapt to this condition.

Phlebotomy Blood Losses

The complex practice of neonatology requires critically ill neonates to be monitored closely with serial laboratory studies such as blood gases, electrolytes, blood counts, and cultures. Small preterm infants are the most critically ill and therefore require the most frequent blood sampling. Obviously, the smallest infants suffer the greatest proportional loss of RBCs because their circulating RBC volumes are smallest. In the past, the mean volume of blood removed for sampling has been reported to range from 0.8 to 3.1 mL/kg/day during the first few weeks of life for preterm infants requiring intensive care.[52, 53] Expressed in terms of total RBCs lost in volumes removed for analysis, the quantities during an entire hospitalization ranged from 30% to more than 300% of the entire neonatal red cell volume present at birth. The hope that noninvasive monitoring might greatly diminish the need for blood sampling has yet to be realized. Although transcutaneous oxygen tension and saturation measurements have been in widespread use in neonatal intensive care, they have had limited impact because of the continuing need to monitor pH and other studies. "In-line" devices that withdraw blood, measure multiple analytes, and then reinfuse the sampled blood hold great promise. However, until they are proved effective and safe for infants, the need to replace blood losses due to phlebotomy will remain a critical factor responsible for multiple RBC transfusions in critically ill neonates.

Treatment of the Anemia of Prematurity

The major approach to treating the anemia of prematurity is to transfuse allogeneic RBCs. Indications for transfusing RBCs to neonates are controversial, and practices vary.[31, 32] The lack of a consistent approach stems from limited knowledge of the cellular and molecular biology of erythropoiesis during the perinatal period as well as an incomplete understanding of infants' responses to anemia. The usual indications for RBC transfusion are based on clinical criteria (i.e., hematocrit or hemoglobin values and the clinical condition of the infant). These are discussed first, after which RBC transfusions given on the basis of so-called physiological criteria are considered. Finally, therapeutic alternatives to allogeneic RBC transfusions are discussed.

Clinical Criteria for RBC Transfusions

A set of clearly established indications for neonatal RBC transfusions, based on results of randomized clinical trials, does not exist. In general, red blood cell transfusions are given to maintain a level of hemoglobin or hematocrit believed to be most desirable for each neonate's clinical condition. Broad guidelines for RBC transfusions during early infancy are listed in Table 20–1.[54] These guidelines are very general, and it is important that terms such as *severe* and *symptomatic* be defined to fit local practices.

Most RBC transfusions given to neonatal patients are small in volume (10 to 20 mL/kg) and often are repeated frequently to replace blood drawn for laboratory studies. There is no proven benefit to routine replacement of phlebotomy blood losses milliliter for milliliter. Instead, RBCs should be transfused to maintain a hematocrit level deemed appropriate for the clinical condition of each infant. In neonates with severe respiratory disease, such as those requiring high volumes of oxygen with ventilator support, it is customary to maintain the hematocrit above 40% (hemoglobin concentration, >13 g/dL), particularly when blood is being drawn frequently for testing. This practice is based on the belief that transfused donor RBCs containing adult hemoglobin will provide optimal oxygen delivery throughout the period of diminished pulmonary function. Although this seemingly logical practice is widely recommended, little evidence is available to establish its efficacy.[32] In one study, 10 infants with severe (oxygen-dependent) bronchopulmonary dysplasia demonstrated improvement of physiological end points (increased systemic oxygen transport and decreased oxygen use) after small-volume RBC transfusions.[55]

In accordance with this rationale for ensuring optimal oxygen delivery in neonates with pulmonary failure, it seems logical to maintain the hematocrit above 40% in infants with congenital heart disease that is severe enough to cause either cyanosis or congestive heart failure. With regard to the latter, Lister and colleagues reported on the use of isovolemic exchange transfusions to treat nine anemic infants with ventricular septal defects and large left-to-right shunts.[56] Exchange transfusion increased the mean hemoglobin level from 9.9 to 14.6 g/dL; this change increased pulmonary vascular resistance, decreased left-to-right shunting and pulmonary blood flow, and lowered heart rate and left ventricular stroke volume. Applying these observations to neonatal patients with patent ductus arteriosus, Rosenthal[57] suggested that RBC transfusions might increase pulmonary vascular resistance, enhance ductal closure, and alleviate high-output cardiac failure. This suggestion seems tenuous and requires more study.

Definitive studies are not available to establish the optimal hemoglobin level for neonates facing major surgery. However, it seems reasonable to maintain the hemoglobin above 10 g/dL (hematocrit, >30%) because of limited ability of the neonate's heart, lungs, and vasculature to compensate for anemia. Additional factors include the inferior offloading of oxygen as a result of the diminished interaction between fetal hemoglobin and 2,3-DPG and the developmental impairment of neonatal renal, hepatic and neurologic function. This transfusion guideline is simply a recommendation—not a firm indication—and it should be applied with flexibility to individual infants facing surgical procedures of varying complexity.

The clinical indications for RBC transfusions in preterm infants who are not critically ill but nonetheless develop moderate anemia (hematocrit, <24%, or blood hemoglobin level, <8 g/dL) are extremely variable. In general, infants who are clinically stable with moderate anemia do not require RBC transfusions unless they exhibit significant problems either ascribed to the presence of anemia or predicted to be corrected by RBC transfusions. As an example of such a clinical problem, proponents of RBC transfusions to treat disturbances of cardiopulmonary rhythms believe that a low blood level of

Table 20–1. Guidelines for Neonatal Blood Component Transfusions*

Red Blood Cells
Hemoglobin < 130 g/L (HCT < 40%) with *severe* cardiopulmonary disease
Hemoglobin < 100 g/L (HCT < 30%) with *moderate* cardiopulmonary disease
Hemoglobin < 100 g/L (HCT < 30%) with *major* surgery
Hemoglobin < 80 g/L (HCT < 24%) with *symptomatic* anemia
Bleeding with >25% loss of circulating blood volume
Platelets
Platelets < 100 × 10^9/L and bleeding
Platelets < 50 × 10^9/L and invasive procedure
Platelets < 20 × 10^9/L and no bleeding, but clinically *stable*
Platelets < 100 × 10^9/L and no bleeding, but clinically *unstable*
Neutrophils
Neutrophils < 3 × 10^9/L and *fulminant* sepsis during first week of life
Neutrophils < 1 × 10^9/L and *fulminant* sepsis after first week

*Words in italics must be defined per local practices.

RBCs contributes to tachypnea, dyspnea, apnea, and tachycardia or bradycardia, because of decreased oxygen delivery to the respiratory center of the brain.[58] Transfusions of RBCs might decrease the number of apneic spells by improving oxygen delivery to the central nervous system. To support this practice, RBC transfusions were shown in one study to diminish irregular breathing patterns and episodes of bradycardia in infants when the mean hematocrit was increased from 27% to 36%.[59] However, other researchers have reported no beneficial effects of RBC transfusions on breathing patterns.[60]

Another controversial clinical indication for RBC transfusions is to maintain a reasonable hematocrit level as treatment for unexplained growth failure. Some neonatologists consider poor weight gain to be an indication for RBC transfusion, particularly if the hematocrit is below 24% (hemoglobin, <8 g/dL) and if other signs of distress are evident (e.g., tachycardia, respiratory difficulty, weak sucking and crying, diminished activity). In this setting, growth failure is ascribed to the increase in metabolic expenditure required to support the work of labored breathing. In the past, a hematocrit below 30% was of concern, and Stockman and Clark investigated the effects of RBC transfusion on weight gain in stable but moderately anemic low-birth-weight infants.[61] Thirteen infants with birth weights less than 1.5 kg were studied for 1 week before and 1 week after RBC transfusions. Mean hemoglobin concentration was raised from 8.5 to 11.4 g/dL, mean daily weight increased from 20.8 to 28.0 g after the transfusions, and weight gain was associated with decreased metabolic rates. The authors regarded anemia as only one of several possible causes for growth failure, and they recommended RBC transfusions for growth failure in symptomatic anemic infants provided that nothing else could explain the poor weight gain. In support of this recommendation, Blank and associates[62] found no clinical advantages for prophylactic small-volume RBC transfusions in stable premature infants. Fifty-six premature infants were randomly assigned to either a mandatory "prophylactic" transfusion group (hemoglobin level kept above 10 g/dL) or a control "elective" transfusion group in which RBCs were given only for marked clinical manifestations of anemia. At discharge, infants in the elective group exhibited significantly ($p < .01$) lower hemoglobin levels (9.10 ± 1.67 versus 11.75 ± 1.72 g/dL) and higher reticulocyte counts (6% ± 3% versus 3% ± 2%) than those receiving prophylactic transfusions. Despite these hematological differences, the two groups were comparable in the number of days required to regain birth weight, in weight at discharge, in the length and cost of hospitalization, and in the frequency and severity of clinical problems. Thus no apparent rationale exists to justify maintaining a given hematocrit level by prophylactic, small-volume RBC transfusions in stable, growing infants who seem to be otherwise healthy.

Physiological Criteria for RBC Transfusions

In practice, the decision to transfuse RBCs is based on the desire to maintain the hematocrit or hemoglobin concentration at a level judged to be most beneficial for the infant's clinical condition. Investigators who believe this clinical approach is too imprecise have suggested the use of physiological criteria such as RBC mass,[63] available oxygen,[64] mixed venous oxygen saturation, and measurements of oxygen delivery and use[55] to develop guidelines for transfusion decisions. Physiological indications for RBC transfusion have shown promise in experimental studies.[65–69] However, these promising but technically demanding methods are, at present, difficult to apply in the day-to-day practice of neonatology. The application of data obtained from studies of animals and adult humans that attempt to correlate tissue oxygenation with the clinical effects of anemia and the need for RBC transfusions is confounded by the differences between infants and adults in hemoglobin oxygen affinity, ability to increase cardiac output, and regional patterns of blood flow.

The most critical physiological consequence of anemia is inadequate delivery of oxygen to the tissues. This adverse effect is difficult to assess accurately during infancy. Manifestations of anemia exhibited by animals and adult humans include increases in cardiac output and whole-body fractional oxygen extraction, enhanced blood flow to the brain and heart,[70–74] and higher oxygen extraction in the liver, kidneys, and gut.[71, 75] These manifestations represent normal physiological responses to anemia and are not necessarily harmful, unless the limits of these compensatory measures are insufficient to meet the needs of the anemic subject. However, these normal compensatory changes, when pushed to the limit, may be harmful in critically ill infants. As suggested by animal studies,[76] increasing cardiac output in response to anemia may not be possible in neonates because heart rate and stroke volume are already near maximum. When cardiopulmonary work does increase, it is accompanied by increased energy expenditure, and calories are diverted for this purpose rather than being used for growth.

Another physiological factor to be considered in the transfusion decision is use of the circulating RBC volume (mass) rather than the blood hematocrit or hemoglobin level.[36, 63, 77] Although circulating RBC volume is a potentially useful index of the blood's oxygen-carrying capacity, it cannot be predicted accurately from blood hemoglobin concentration or hematocrit in infants.[55] Low circulating RBC volume identifies, better than hemoglobin or hematocrit, infants who will respond to transfusion with a decrease in cardiac output.[78] At present, circulating RBC volume measurements are not widely available. However, the use of a nonradioactive biotin label to tag RBCs, which has already shown promise in other subjects, may be adapted for infant studies.[77, 79]

It is clear that extremely preterm infants currently receive many RBC transfusions. Existing clinical information is inadequate for making sound scientific decisions regarding firm indications for RBC transfusions in these infants. An understanding of the physiological effects of anemia is crucial for defining the best criteria for neonatal RBC transfusions and in identifying infants most likely to benefit from alternative therapies such as rHuEPO.

Transfusion Therapy of Neonatal Anemia

The RBC product of choice for small-volume (10 to 20 mL/kg) neonatal transfusions is RBCs collected from allogeneic donors, suspended in anticoagulant/preservative solution, and, often, concentrated before transfusion. Some physicians use relatively fresh RBCs for transfusion in preterm infants because of concerns regarding the increase in extracellular concentrations of potassium, the decrease in pH, and decrease in RBC levels of 2,3-DPG during storage. The need to use fresh RBCs for small-volume transfusions has been questioned,[33] and four reports documented that RBCs stored for extended periods could be safely transfused to neonates.[80–83] The findings of these reports indicated that the occurrence of donor exposure was decreased, without incidences of hyperkalemia or acidosis. However, in three of the reports, relatively few transfusions with RBCs stored longer than 20 days were included.[80–82] Furthermore, these three reports did not address use of AS-1 extended storage (42-day) RBC preservative medium, which contains mannitol. Liu and associates[80] stored RBCs in CPDA1, a standard 35-day storage medium. Although the other two studies did not indicate which RBC storage solutions were used, AS-1 was probably not used, inasmuch as mannitol was not listed as an ingredient.[81, 82] Because nearly all RBCs are routinely stored in a 42-day preservative medium, additional information is needed for neonates with regard to the potential for toxicity associated with adenine (hepatic) and mannitol (renal) as constituents of extended-storage RBC preservative media and with regard to the possibility of a deficiency in RBC levels of 2,3-DPG caused by repeated transfusion of stored RBCs. Accordingly, the transfusion of stored AS-1 RBCs was studied.[83]

In a two-arm, randomized, single-blinded study, the feasibility and safety of two techniques used to provide small-volume RBC transfusions to infants of very low birth weight (VLBW) (0.6 to 1.3 kg) were compared. In one arm of the study, infants received AS-1 RBCs stored up to 42 days (stored AS-1 RBCs); in the other, infants received CPDA1 RBCs stored up to 7 days (fresh CPDA1 RBCs). The results have been reported in detail elsewhere,[83] and only the safety aspects are summarized here. None of the CPDA1 RBCs were stored longer than 7 days, whereas 47% of AS-1 RBCs were stored 15 days or longer before transfusion. No clinical reactions occurred during 66 AS-1 RBC transfusions given to 15 infants or during 58 CPDA1 RBC transfusions given to 14 infants. Clinically significant changes in vital signs were infrequent and occurred at similar rates in infants in both groups. No significant differences occurred in the comparative changes between pretransfusion and posttransfusion blood chemistry levels, whether fresh CPDA1 or stored AS-1 RBCs were given. The hematocrit increased as expected. Changes in levels of glucose, lactate, pH, calcium, sodium, and potassium were very slight and not of clinical importance. No statistically significant differences in results of renal and hepatic chemistry levels were detected between infants who received fresh CPDA1 and those who received stored AS-1 RBCs. Levels of 2,3-DPG were similar, whether fresh CPDA1 or stored AS-1 RBCs were transfused. Thus AS-1 RBCs, collected from one donor and stored for up to 42 days, can safely provide all RBC transfusions needed by an individual infant.

In conclusion, several studies have documented the feasibility and safety of transfusing stored RBCs to preterm infants.[80–83] At the DeGowin Blood Center at the University of Iowa College of Medicine, therefore, newborn infants are assigned to long-term support with a fresh unit (stored <7 days) of RBCs in extended storage (42-day) media as follows: (1) Infants with birth weight of less than 1.0 kg are assigned to a half unit; (2) infants with a birth weight of 1.0 to 1.3 kg are assigned to a quarter to half unit; and (3) infants with a birth weight of more than 1.3 kg are assigned to varying volumes of RBC units, depending on transfusion needs estimated by neonatal intensive care unit (NICU) staff. When RBC transfusions are ordered, aliquots are issued.[83] Once a unit has been stored 14 days, it has become relatively aged, and no new neonates are assigned to it. When all infants originally assigned to a unit no longer require RBC transfusions, the remainder of the unit is placed into the general inventory for transfusion to older children. Although several clinical studies have documented the safety of selecting stored RBCs for small-volume transfusions, this approach does not apply to large-volume (>25 mL/kg) transfusions, in which greater doses of extracellular constituents (e.g., potassium) may be harmful, especially if infused rapidly. Fresh or washed RBCs are preferred for large-volume transfusions given to infants.

Alternatives to Allogeneic RBC Transfusions

Recognition of the low plasma EPO levels in preterm infants provides a rational basis for the use of rHuEPO as treatment for the anemia of prematurity. More than 20 controlled trials have tested several doses and treatment schedules in preterm infants, and results are mixed; hence consensus on the optimal treatment with rHuEPO is impossible.[32, 84] Unquestionably, proper doses of rHuEPO and iron are biologically effective in stimulating erythropoiesis, as evidenced by increased marrow erythroid activity and blood reticulocyte counts. However, the efficacy of rHuEPO in substantially diminishing RBC transfusions, the major goal for which it is prescribed, has not been convincingly demonstrated.[85] In many trials, relatively large preterm infants or those in stable clinical condition—infants who currently receive few RBC transfusions when given standard care (i.e., not given rHuEPO)—were studied.[5] Currently, even without use of rHuEPO, fewer than 50% of infants with birth weight of more than 1.0 kg receive RBC transfusions. Nearly all infants weighing less than 1.0 kg at birth are given RBCs, and most transfusions are given during the first 3 to 4 weeks of life. To illustrate this problem, the multicenter, randomized American trial, in which infants received either rHuEPO or placebo during a 6-week study period, reported statistically significant but only modest success.[86] Although significantly fewer RBC transfusions were given to rHuEPO-treated infants during the study phase (1.1 transfusions versus 1.6 for placebo), all infants required multiple transfusions during the 3-week prestudy phase. Therefore, rHuEPO exerted only a modest effect on total RBC transfusions given throughout the entire study (4.4 for rHuEPO versus 5.3 for placebo) and did not resolve the problem of severe neonatal anemia.[86]

Thus physicians wishing to prescribe rHuEPO are in a dilemma. The relatively large or stable preterm infants who respond best to rHuEPO plus iron are given relatively few RBC transfusions and, accordingly, have little need for rHuEPO to avoid transfusions.[5, 32] Extremely preterm infants who are sick and have the greatest need for RBC transfusions shortly after birth have not consistently responded to rHuEPO plus iron; this too raises questions about the efficacy of rHuEPO.[85] However, extremely preterm infants are beginning to be evaluated in therapeutic trials of rHuEPO and iron, both given intravenously.[87, 88] Although preliminary review of these promising studies suggests success in avoiding transfusions, data are insufficient to clearly establish efficacy or to detect potential toxicity. Thus, firm guidelines for the use of rHuEPO in the treatment of the anemia of prematurity cannot be made at this time.

Another alternative to allogeneic RBC transfusions is use of placental blood as a source of autologous RBCs.[89, 90] Although collection, storage, and transfusion of placental blood after delivery deserves careful consideration, at least three obstacles must be overcome before autologous transfusions of stored placental RBCs can be adopted for clinical use. One concern is that a sufficient number of RBCs will not be obtained consistently from placental blood to avoid later allogeneic transfusions. The second issue is the sterility of placental blood: because bacterial contamination of placental blood is a distinct possibility,[89] extensive testing is needed to ensure absolute safety. Third, acceptable quality of stored placental blood must be maintained. Neonatal RBCs differ from those of adults in many respects,[50, 51] and collection and storage of placental blood must be performed carefully.[90] Because of these concerns, collection and storage of placental blood has not been encouraged.[91] Instead, interest has been renewed in delayed clamping of the umbilical cord immediately after delivery.[92] In a small pilot study, delayed cord clamping increased blood volume and circulating red cell mass and improved cardiovascular hemodynamics.[92] However, many questions regarding feasibility, efficacy, and possible risks remain to be answered.

NEONATAL BLEEDING

Hemostasis in the neonate is quantitatively and qualitatively different from that in the older child or adult, and the potential exists for either serious hemorrhage or thrombosis. A comprehensive discussion of neonatal hemostasis is beyond the scope of this chapter; the following sections focus on neonatal thrombocytopenia and its treatment with platelet transfusions. However, because primary hemostasis (platelet plug formation) and fibrin clot formation are intimately intertwined, it is important to summarize a few important facts about neonatal clotting proteins before addressing issues of neonatal thrombocytopenia.

Maternal clotting factors do not cross the placenta, and fetal levels depend on endogenous production. Clotting proteins are synthesized by the fetus beginning in the first trimester, with concentrations gradually increasing throughout gestation.[93] At birth, the mean levels of the contact factors (factors XII and XI, prekallikrein, and high-molecular-weight kininogen) are about 40% to 50% of adult values in full-term infants and about 30% to 40% of adult values in preterm infants. The vitamin K–dependent factors (II, VII, IX, and X) are about 40% to 50% of adult values in full-term infants and about 30% to 50% of adults in preterm infants; levels are strikingly low in very immature neonates. Neonatal levels of factors VIII and XIII and fibrinogen are comparable with adult levels, although factor XIII are quite low in occasional infants at birth. The levels of natural anticoagulant proteins (antithrombin III and proteins C and S) are at 30% to 50% of adult values. Fibrinolysis is not as well studied but probably is diminished to a significant degree because of moderately low plasminogen levels.

Pathophysiology of Neonatal Thrombocytopenia

Blood platelet counts greater than 150 $\times$ 10^9/L are present in normal fetuses ($\geq$17 weeks of gestation) and neonates.[94–98] Lower platelet counts indicate potential problems, and high-risk infants—usually low-birth-weight premature infants—commonly exhibit thrombocytopenia.[97–101] In one neonatal intensive care unit, 22% of infants had blood platelet counts lower than 150 $\times$ 10^9/L at some time during hospitalization.[100] Although multiple pathogenic mechanisms are involved in these sick neonates, the predominant one is accelerated platelet destruction, as shown by shortened platelet survival, increased mean platelet volume, normal number of megakarocytes, and an inadequate increment in blood platelets after platelet transfusion.[100, 102] In individual infants, the mechanism underlying accelerated platelet destruction cannot always be identified, but increased levels of platelet-associated immunoglobulin G (IgG) and disseminated intravascular coagulation are commonly evident. Also contributing to neonatal thrombocytopenia is diminished platelet production, as evidenced by decreased numbers of clonogenic megakaryocyte progenitors[103] and relatively low levels of thrombopoietin[104] in comparison with the levels in children and adults.

Blood platelet counts lower than 100 $\times$ 10^9/L pose significant clinical risks for premature neonates. In one study, infants with birth weights of less than 1.5 kg and blood platelet counts lower than 100 $\times$ 10^9/L were compared with nonthrombocytopenic control infants of similar size.[101] The bleeding time was prolonged when platelet counts were below 100 $\times$ 10^9/L, and in many infants, platelet dysfunction was suggested by bleeding times that were disproportionately long for the degree of thrombocytopenia present. Hemorrhage was greater in thrombocytopenic infants than in controls. Of particular importance, the incidence of intracranial hemorrhage in thrombocytopenic infants with birth weights of less than 1.5 kg was 78% for thrombocytopenic infants, in contrast to 48% for nonthrombocytopenic infants of similar size. Moreover, the extent of hemorrhage and neurological morbidity was greater in the group of thrombocytopenic infants.[101]

Thrombocytopenia is not the only hemorrhagic risk factor related to neonatal platelets. Extensive controversy exists regarding the function of fetal and neonatal platelets. As reviewed by Whaun,[105] fetal and neonatal platelets have diminished aggregation to collagen, adenosine diphosphate, thrombin, and epinephrine, the last of which is associated with diminished α-adrenergic binding sites on the platelet membrane. Not all investigators found diminished aggregation, and some have reported enhanced responses, particularly to ristocetin, a finding ascribed to increased plasma von Willebrand factor.[106] Other reported abnormalities of neonatal platelets include decreased adhesion to glass, low platelet factor 3, defective clot retraction, low serotonin levels, deficient cytoplasmic granulation, decreased release of adenine nucleotides, and abnormalities of arachidonic acid metabolism (i.e., small quantities of cyclooxygenase metabolites in comparison with large amounts of lipoxygenase products).[105]

The pathogenic mechanisms proposed to mediate neonatal platelet dysfunction are not precisely defined, but they include developmental abnormalities intrinsic to the platelet membrane plus the extrinsic effects of gestation or parturition.[107] Platelet dysfunction is even more pronounced when infants or their mothers receive medications that affect platelet function.[108, 109] Despite the abnormal results of in vitro platelet function tests, the bleeding time of normal neonates has been found to be comparable with that of adults.[110, 111] When obtained by a modified template technique, the bleeding time provides useful clinical information because it is inversely related to the blood platelet count, is prolonged by drugs that produce platelet dysfunction, and may identify particular groups of neonates at increased risk of hemorrhage. Regarding the last, the accuracy of the bleeding time in predicting individual neonates at risk of bleeding requires more extensive study to define its true value, particularly if prolonged bleeding time results are used as criteria for platelet transfusions.[110]

Thrombocytopenia occurs most commonly in sick preterm infants. When severe thrombocytopenia is noted in neonates who appear otherwise well, immune thrombocytopenia caused by placental transport of maternal antiplatelet antibodies must always be suspected. The platelet antibodies involved are either autoimmune, with broad reactivity against platelets from all individuals, including the mother, or alloantibodies, with reactivity against an antigen inherited by the fetus from the father to which the mother has been immunized because her platelets lack the antigen. In general, the diagnosis of passively acquired autoimmune thrombocytopenia in a neonate is readily apparent because of a history of thrombocytopenia or the presence of elevated platelet-associated immunoglobulin levels in the mother.[112] The diagnosis of neonatal alloimmune thrombocytopenia is less obvious, but it should be suspected whenever unexplained thrombocytopenia is noted in an infant whose mother has a normal platelet count without increased amounts of platelet-associated immunoglobulin.[113–115] The reported frequency of neonatal alloimmune thrombocytopenia is variable, ranging from approximately 1 per 1000 to 1 per 10,000 births. The rarity of this disorder is surprising in view of the relatively common frequency of maternal-fetal platelet incompatibility (i.e., up to 14% of pregnant women lack platelet antigens expressed by their infants[114]) and the finding that approximately 2% of pregnant women have platelet-specific alloantibodies in their plasma.[114] Although antibodies to many platelet antigens have been implicated, the most common in the United States is anti-HPA-1a (anti-PL^{A1} or anti-Zw^{a}). About 50% of affected infants are firstborns, and more than 90% of subsequent siblings are affected.[114]

A complete discussion of the approach to immune thrombocytopenia is beyond the scope of this chapter. It is important to remember that alloimmune thrombocytopenia can be extremely serious for the fetus and newborn, necessitating careful management during both gestation and the perinatal period. In contrast, autoimmune thrombocytopenia is almost never severe for the fetus and is only occasionally severe for the neonate. Thus it is important to detect autoimmune thrombocytopenia during gestation so that it can be distinguished from the more severe alloimmune thrombocytopenia. However, neonates born of women with autoimmune thrombocytopenia only occasionally require therapy during the postpartum period. Finally, mild to moderate thrombocytopenia detected in women only during gestation does not pose a risk either to the pregnant woman or to her fetus and newborn and necessitates no intervention.[114–116]

Treatment of Neonatal Thrombocytopenia

Although the use of prophylactic platelet transfusions in an attempt to prevent bleeding in preterm neonates has been studied systematically,[98] no randomized clinical trials have been reported to establish the efficacy of therapeutic platelet transfusions as treatment for bleeding thrombocytopenic neonates. Thus even basic questions regarding the relative risks of different degrees of thrombocytopenia in various clinical settings during infancy remain unanswered. However, it seems logical to perform transfusions of platelets in thrombocytopenic infants, and guidelines acceptable to many neonatologists are listed in Table 20–1. Two firm indications for neonatal platelet transfusions are to treat hemorrhage that is ongoing and to prevent it from complicating an invasive procedure. Little disagreement exists over using a blood platelet count of less than 50 × 10^9/L as a "transfusion trigger" in these instances. However, platelet transfusions are given to infants by some physicians to treat bleeding that occurs at higher platelet counts (between 50 and 100 × 10^9/L) or to diminish the threat of intracranial hemorrhage in high-risk preterm infants whenever the platelet count is less than 100 × 10^9/L.

Prophylactic platelet transfusions can be given under one of two circumstances: to prevent bleeding when thrombocytopenia is severe or to maintain a normal platelet count. Most neonatologists agree that it is reasonable to give platelets to any neonate whose blood platelet count is less than 20 × 10^9/L. First, at this level of thrombocytopenia, an established risk of spontaneous hemorrhage is widely accepted.[117] Second, this risk is even more threatening because of developmental abnormalities of both platelets and clotting proteins that compound the risk of bleeding. Almost any stress can accentuate these abnormalities to increase the potential for hemorrhage beyond that expected for the degree of thrombocytopenia alone. Third, severe thrombocytopenia occurs most commonly in sick infants who, because of their illnesses, receive medications that may further compromise platelet function. Because all of these factors are pronounced in extremely preterm infants, some neonatologists favor prophylactic platelet transfusion whenever the platelet count falls below 50 × 10^9/L, or even below 100 × 10^9/L, in critically ill infants.[101] However, the need to maintain a truly normal platelet count in preterm infants without bleeding is unproven. Intracranial hemorrhage occurs commonly in sick preterm infants and, although the etiological role of thrombocytopenia and the therapeutic benefit of platelet transfusions have not been conclusively established in this disorder,[98, 101] it seems logical to consider thrombocytopenia as a risk factor.[118, 119] However, in a randomized trial designed to address this issue—transfusing platelets whenever the platelet count fell to less than 150 × 10^9/L and maintaining the average platelet count above 200 × 10^9/L versus transfusing platelets only when the platelet count fell to less than 50 × 10^9/L—did not diminish the incidence of intracranial hemorrhage (28% versus 26%).[98] Thus there is no documented benefit from transfusing prophylactic platelets to maintain a normal platelet count.

The goal of most platelet transfusions is to raise the platelet count to above 100 × 10^9/L. This goal can be achieved consistently by the infusion of 5 to 10 mL/kg of standard platelet suspensions prepared either from fresh units of whole blood or by automated plateletpheresis. Platelet suspensions should be transfused as rapidly as the baby's overall condition permits, certainly within 2 hours. Routinely reducing the volume of platelet concentrates by additional centrifugation steps is neither necessary nor wise.[98] In general, 5 to 10 mL/kg is not an excessive transfusion volume, provided that intake of other intravenous fluids, medications, and nutrients is monitored and adjusted as needed. Although methods have been reported to reduce the volume of platelet concentrates,[120, 121] additional processing must be subject to very careful quality control because of probable platelet loss, clumping, and dysfunction caused by the additional handling. Platelet concentrates contain viable lymphocytes—even when prepared as leukocyte-reduced components—and, like all cellular blood products, they should be considered for gamma irradiation to prevent graft-versus-host disease, especially when the donor and infant recipient are first-degree relatives.[24, 25]

NEONATAL NEUTROPENIA AND SEPSIS

Neonates are unusually susceptible to severe bacterial infections, and several defects of neonatal body defenses have been reported as possible contributing factors. Neutrophils (polymorphonuclear leukocytes [PMNs]) isolated from the blood of neonates exhibit both quantitative and qualitative abnormalities that may be related to the increased incidence of and morbidity and mortality from bacterial infections. The remainder of this discussion focuses on the physiology of neonatal PMNs and the possible role of PMN (granulocyte) transfusions to treat neonatal sepsis and alternatives to PMN transfusions, such as intravenous immunoglobulin (IVIG) and cytokine therapy. Abnormalities of neonatal PMNs include absolute and relative neutropenia, diminished chemotaxis, abnormal adhesion and aggregation, defective cellular orientation and receptor capping, decreased deformability, inability to alter membrane potential during stimulation, imbalances of oxidative metabolism, and a diminished ability to withstand oxidant stress.[122, 123] These abnormalities are accentuated in sick premature neonates, and it is logical to consider transfusing normal PMNs to augment neonatal body defenses. However, success of PMN transfusion therapy has not been uniform, this therapy is not user-friendly, and alternatives (IVIG and cytokines) seem promising. Thus PMN transfusions are prescribed infrequently.

Physiology of Neonatal Neutrophils

Neutropenia can occur during neonatal bacterial infections, particularly with fulminant sepsis. Because physiological neutrophilia occurs in normal neonates, it is considered quite abnormal for the absolute blood PMN count to fall below 3.0 × 10^9/L in the first week of life. Although an abnormally low PMN count can occur in neonates with disorders as diverse as sepsis, asphyxia, and maternal hypertension, suspicion of severe bacterial infection must be high whenever relative neutropenia (PMN count, <3.0 × 10^9/L) occurs. The mechanisms responsible are only partially defined, but abnormalities of neonatal granulopoiesis are frequently involved. As one factor, the postmitotic marrow PMN storage pool (metamyelocytes and mature, segmented PMNs) is small. The PMN storage pool accounts for 26% to 60% of all nucleated cells in the bone marrow of normal neonates. Neonates with sepsis may exhibit a storage pool numbering less than 10% of nucleated marrow cells and are considered to have severely diminished marrow PMN reserves.[123, 124] Second, storage pool PMNs are released at an excessively rapid and, apparently, poorly regulated rate from the marrow during stress. Third, PMN production in response to infection is decreased. Numbers of committed (clonogenic) FMN precursors in neonatal marrow are lower in neonates than in older patients, and a high percentage of these cells are proliferating even when studied at an apparently basal state.[125, 126] Thus, neonatal marrow is functioning at capacity and is unable to rapidly expand production to meet the increased demands of infection.[127]

Although abnormalities of nearly every aspect of function have been reported in studies of neonatal PMNs, diminished chemotaxis is one of the most consistently demonstrated defects.[123, 124] The initiating cellular event in chemotaxis is the binding of chemotactic factor molecules to specific receptors located on the neutrophil plasma membrane. Although not all investigators agree, the number and affinity of receptors for the chemotaxin F-Met-Leu-Phe (FMLP) is probably normal on neonatal PMNs, when they are studied as intact cells under steady-state conditions.[128–130] An aspect of chemotactic factor binding that requires additional study in neonatal PMNs is the ability to increase binding during stimulation through mobilization of intracellular receptors to the cell surface: a state of upregulation. Some evidence suggests that neonatal PMNs exist in a partially degranulated state (upregulated), even when they have received no recognized stimulation and are supposedly at rest.[131] The ability of neonatal PMN to increase binding, beyond that present in the apparent resting stage, with chemotactic factor stimulation needs more study. Of note, diminished expression of the C3bi receptor, important for PMN adherence and chemotaxis, has been reported in neonatal neutrophils.[132]

Adhesion and aggregation of neonatal PMNs have been studied, and defective chemotaxis may be caused in part by abnormalities of these functions. Neonatal PMNs stimulated with chemotactic factors exhibit abnormal adherence.[130] Stimulated neonatal PMNs also aggregate abnormally.[133, 134] Some studies have found aggregation to be abnormal because of its irreversible nature. When PMNs from adults are stimulated by chemotactic factors, a biphasic response occurs with an initial aggregation followed by disaggregation. Reports of irreversible aggregation of neonatal PMNs have been questioned by a study that ascribes the earlier findings to a technical artifact.[135] Finally, abnormalities of the cytoskeleton may contribute to the chemotactic defect. Neonatal PMNs fail either to undergo polarization when exposed to a gradient of chemotactic factor or to reorient themselves (change their direction of polarization and movement) when chemotactic factor concentration gradients are reversed.[136] These abnormalities of movement may be caused by defective interaction of the neutrophil plasma membrane and cytoskeleton, as evidenced by decreases of concanavalin A and latex bead capping,[130, 137, 138] decreased assembly of tubulin units,[136] and diminished ability to increase actin polymerization during stimulation.[139]

Although an occasional investigator may disagree, neonatal PMNs have been found to ingest bacteria and form phagolysosomes satisfactorily, provided that adequate quantities of opsonins are present. Ingested microorganisms that lie within phagolysosomes are killed by one of several mechanisms, both oxygen dependent and oxygen independent. Oxidative metabolism of neonatal PMNs exhibits inconsistencies in comparison with adult PMNs.[122] In neonatal PMNs, the relatively early aspects of oxidative metabolism are enhanced by greater oxygen consumption, superoxide anion, and H_2O_2 production and by increased activity of the hexose monophosphate shunt. In contrast, aspects that depend on later reactions, such as chemiluminescence and hydroxyl radical formation, are decreased.

Both the rate of activation and the activity of the superoxide-generating system were evaluated in one study during the stimulation of neonatal PMNs through the use of a continuous or kinetic assay.[140] Neonatal PMNs, isolated in an apparently basal state from healthy neonates, exhibited a more rapid activation when stimulated than did cells from adults. This finding suggests that neonatal PMNs (presumably unstimulated at rest) either exist in a state of partial activation or are prone to rapid activation. In another study, H_2O_2 production was increased in unstimulated neonatal PMNs,[141] but chemiluminescence was diminished.[142, 143] Chemiluminescence depends on the formation of highly reactive molecules, and the diminished ability of neonatal PMNs to produce these moieties may be related to lactoferrin deficiency.[131] The exact age at which neonatal PMN oxidative metabolism becomes normal is unknown. Abnormal chemiluminescence, however, has been documented throughout the first month of life.[142]

Neonatal PMNs may be prone to auto-oxidation with dysfunction caused, at least in part, by oxidant damage. Production of certain oxidizing molecules is increased in neonatal neutrophils. As a second factor, the ability to withstand oxidant stress seems diminished, as a result of deficiencies of oxygen-detoxifying enzymes and glutathione reserves.[144, 145] Thus the combination of the increased production of superoxide anion and H_2O_2, the imbalance of oxygen-detoxifying enzymes, and the seemingly limited glutathione reserves suggest that neonatal PMN dysfunction can, in part, be a consequence of oxidant damage to vital cellular structures.

Treatment of Neonatal Sepsis

Neutrophil (PMN) Transfusions

PMN transfusions have been used to treat neonatal sepsis regardless of whether neutropenia is present. Neonates exhibiting fulminant sepsis, relative neutropenia (PMN count, $<3.0 \times 10^9$/L during the first week of life or $<1.0 \times 10^9$/L thereafter), and a severely diminished PMN marrow storage pool (less than 10% of nucleated marrow cells are postmitotic PMNs) are at increased risk of dying if treated only with antibiotics. Results of 11 studies on the use of PMN transfusions to treat infected neonates,[124, 146–155] 6 of which were designed as controlled studies,[124, 145–148, 153, 154] have been reported. The fact that four of the six controlled studies noted significant benefit from PMN transfusion is encouraging.[124, 146–148] However, the controlled studies contain several experimental flaws. Although five professed to be randomized trials, two included nontransfused subjects who were deemed ineligible for randomization.[124, 154] In addition, two of the six reports dealt with the same study, reported first as a somewhat preliminary trial[147] and again later after it was expanded and slightly modified.[148] Also, the patients evaluated in all six studies were quite heterogeneous; relatively few neonates exhibited the complete clinical picture considered to be most indicative of poor prognosis (culture-proven sepsis, neutropenia severe for age, and a markedly depleted marrow PMN storage pool). Finally, the dosages and quality of the PMN concentrates transfused were quite variable, and in some instances, they were almost certainly inadequate.[153–155]

Because of these scientific imperfections, PMN transfusions in treating neonatal sepsis cannot be firmly recommended at this time. Although antibiotics are the key to successful treatment of neonatal sepsis, antibiotic therapy is not 100% successful, and attempts to bolster body defenses are warranted. Unfortunately, PMN transfusions have not provided a complete answer. Although efficacious for infants with neutropenia and fulminant sepsis,[156] only PMN transfusions obtained by automated leukapheresis have demonstrated effectiveness.[155, 156] Moreover, in many instances, standard supportive care with antibiotics seems adequate. Each institution must assess its own experience with neonatal sepsis. If nearly all infants survive without apparent long-term morbidity when treated only with antibiotics, PMN transfusions are unnecessary, and attention should be focused on prompt diagnosis and optimal antibiotic therapy. If the outcome of standard therapy is not optimal, alternative therapies such as PMN transfusions must be considered.

The characteristics of an ideal PMN concentrate for neonatal transfusions are as follows: dose of PMNs per infusion, 1 to 2 × 10^9/kg; volume for infusion, 10 to 15 mL/kg; seronegativity of donor for cytomegalovirus and for all required infectious disease tests; and erythrocyte compatibility between donor and neonate. Local practices should be followed with regard to gamma irradiation of cellular blood products for neonates. PMN concentrates must be infused promptly, certainly within a few hours of donation. Until more information becomes available, the only PMN product of proven efficacy is a PMN concentrate prepared by automated leukapheresis.[155, 156]

Alternatives to Neutrophil Transfusions

Not all neonatologists prescribe PMN transfusions. Their proper role has not been irrefutably established by controlled clinical trials. Moreover, the preparation of PMN concentrates by leukapheresis can be cumbersome and expensive, and the process of collecting and transfusing PMNs can pose risks for both neonates and donors. Accordingly, alternative therapies have been suggested. However, their efficacy has not been clearly established, their risks are only partially defined, and they require extensive study before being widely accepted. Two modalities that have been suggested are IVIG and myeloid cytokines.

Use of IVIG either to prevent or to treat neonatal sepsis has appeal because it may correct abnormalities both of humoral immunity and of PMN function. IVIG was found to be of benefit, particularly when given in combination with antibiotics, in experimental infections caused by a variety of microorganisms.[157–161] The expected increases in opsonic activity were observed with IVIG infusion, and PMN kinetics were also improved.[160, 161] Specifically, neither neutropenia nor depletion of the PMN storage pool occurred, and PMNs were released from marrow reserves to accumulate quickly at inflammatory sites. Although clinical trials in human infants have yielded conflicting results, IVIG has been given with promising effects both to prevent and to treat infections.

Most studies evaluating IVIG to prevent infections have found little or only modest benefit.[162–173] However, results are inconsistent, and a few studies have suggested some prophylactic benefit.[162, 163, 165] In contrast, of the therapeutic studies reviewed,[174–180] several demonstrated a benefit from adding IVIG to antibiotics in the treatment of neonatal infections.[174–177, 180] Overall, data are insufficient to justify the use of IVIG routinely in premature neonates to prevent or treat sepsis. However, modest "physiological" doses (0.3 to 0.4 mg/kg) may lessen the severity of bacterial sepsis in VLBL newborns, who are likely to be hypogammaglobulinemic as a result of extreme premature birth (i.e., born before the major placental transport of IgG has taken place).

However, caution must be used in prescribing IVIG therapy to prevent or treat neonatal sepsis. IVIG therapy, particularly at high doses, may impair body defense mechanisms.[181–183] In leukopenic mice, IVIG at 0.8 g/kg impaired clearance of bacteria from the blood stream and lowered the median lethal dose.[181] In neonatal rats, IVIG at a dose of 2.7 g/kg delayed bacterial clearance, whereas lower doses (0.15 g/kg) enhanced bacterial clearance and survival.[183] It has been suggested that infections in humans may be exacerbated by intravenous IgG.[181, 183] Finally, in a comparative study of infected human infants,[184] survival in the group receiving 1.0 g/kg/day of IVIG on 3 consecutive days plus antibiotics was 52%, in contrast to 97% in the group receiving PMN transfusions plus antibiotics ($p < .004$ favoring PMN transfusions over IVIG). Because of the ease with which IVIG can be prescribed for neonates, its apparent benefits to many body defense systems, and its safety in terms of only rarely transmitting infectious diseases, it is easy to become enthusiastic about its potential uses. However, it is crucial that the genuine benefits and risks of IVIG be examined carefully before it is used with impunity. For example, in a randomized study of 235 preterm infants, no significant reduction in either certain or probable infections was observed in those given 500 mg of IVIG on days 0, 1, 2, 3, 17, and 31 of life, in comparison with controls given albumin. There was actually a suggestion of more frequent infections in the IVIG group, possibly because of the large quantity of IgG given.[185]

Cytokine therapy may be very useful for preventing and/or treating neonatal sepsis in the future. A large number of cytokines—soluble molecules, including growth factors and interleukins, produced by a variety of cells—regulate the production of blood cells (hematopoiesis) and modulate their activities. The cytokine primarily responsible for PMN production and activation is granulocyte colony-stimulating factor (G-CSF). Studies of cytokine production in human neonates have yielded conflicting results; investigators have found values that are higher than, equal to, and lower than adult values.[186–193] Although results are quite variable, G-CSF levels are generally lower in premature than in full-term neonates, and the ability of neonatal leukocytes to increase production when stimulated, under many experimental conditions, is diminished in preterm infants. Plasma levels of G-CSF are reported by some investigators to be markedly elevated in neonates with infection,[187, 188] but many investigators have found G-CSF messenger RNA expression and protein production to be decreased in neonatal leukocytes, particularly when attempts are made to increase production by activating the cells.[189–191] Similar findings have been reported for production of granulocyte-macrophage colony-stimulating factor (GM-CSF) by neonatal leukocytes.[192, 193]

The mechanisms responsible for diminished G-CSF and GM-CSF production have not been defined. In one study, the decrease in messenger RNA expression was not caused by defective transcription, and abnormalities in posttranscriptional events, such as instability of messenger RNA, were suggested as possible mechanisms.[191] Although data are limited to date, studies of growth factor receptors and the growth of clonogenic myeloid progenitors in cultures stimulated with recombinant growth factors have not detected an impaired ability of neonatal myeloid progenitors to respond to exogenous myeloid growth factors.[189, 192, 193] Thus it seems likely that human neonates will respond to the administration of recombinant G-CSF or GM-CSF.

In preclinical studies, the administration of recombinant G-CSF and GM-CSF to neonatal animals with infections induced experimentally was beneficial.[192–198] Combination therapy with G-CSF plus either stem cell factor or interleukin-6 was reported to be superior to therapy with G-CSF alone.[197, 198] Improvements both in the resolution of infections and in survival rates were accompanied by correction both of neutropenia and of abnormal PMN kinetics. It is interesting that G-CSF, given to pregnant rats, crossed the placenta and improved neonatal survival of experimentally induced infection.[199, 200]

When added to human neonatal leukocytes in vitro, recombinant GM-CSF enhances several PMN functions.[201, 202] To date, clinical studies of recombinant myeloid growth factors given to human neonates are limited. In a controlled study,[203] 42 neonates with presumed bacterial sepsis, recognized within the first 3 days of life, were randomly designated to receive three doses of either G-CSF or a placebo. Although the outcome of sepsis was not reported, G-CSF induced a significant increase in the blood PMN count, an increase in the marrow PMN storage pool, and an increase in PMN membrane C3bi expression, the last being an indication of enhanced functional capability.[203] In another study, G-CSF increased blood PMN counts of neutropenic neonates born to mothers with preeclampsia.[204]

In a controlled study of GM-CSF,[205] 20 premature neonates were designated within 72 hours of birth to receive either GM-CSF or a placebo for 7 days. GM-CSF increased the blood PMN count, the marrow PMN storage pool, and C3bi receptor expression. In addition, neonates receiving GM-CSF exhibited an increase in blood monocyte and platelet counts. The study was not designed to assess efficacy in the prevention or treatment of infections, and additional clinical trials are needed to define the role and to identify possible adverse effects before myeloid growth factors should be routinely prescribed to human neonates.

ACKNOWLEDGMENT

Supported by PO1 HL46925 from the National Institutes of Health.

REFERENCES

1. Wegman ME. Annual summary of vital statistics—1988. Pediatrics 1989; 84:943.
2. Guyer B, Wallach LA, Rosen SL. Birth-weight-standardized neonatal mortality rates and the prevention of low birth weight: how does Massachusetts compare with Sweden? N Engl J Med 1982; 306:1230.
3. Sacher RA, Luban NLC, Strauss RG. Current practice and guidelines for the transfusion of cellular blood components in the newborn. Transfus Med Rev 1989; 3:39.
4. Floss AM, Strauss RG, Goeken N, et al. Multiple transfusions fail to provoke antibodies against blood cell antigens in human infants. Transfusion 1986; 26:419.
5. Widness JA, Seward VJ, Kromer IJ, et al. Changing patterns of red blood cell transfusion in very low birth weight infants. J Pediatr 1996; 129:680.
6. Rogers MF, Thomas PA, Starcher ET, et al. Acquired immunodeficiency syndrome in children: report of the Centers for Disease Control national surveillance, 1982 to 1985. Pediatrics 1987; 79:1008.
7. Aubuchon JP, Birkmeyer JD, Busch MP. Safety of the blood supply in the United States: opportunities and controversies. Ann Intern Med 1997; 127:904.
8. Bertolli J, Caldwell B, Lindegren ML, et al. Epidemiology of HIV disease in children. Immunol Allergy Clin North Am 1995; 15:193.
9. European Collaborative Study Group. Natural history of vertically acquired human immunodeficiency virus-1 infection. Pediatrics 1994; 94:815.
10. Blajchman MA, Sheridan D, Rawls WE. Risks associated with blood transfusion in newborn infants. Clin Perinatol 1984; 2:403.
11. Alter HJ, Purcell RH, Shih JW, et al. Detection of antibody to hepatitis C virus in prospectively followed transfusion recipients with acute and chronic non-A, non-B hepatitis. N Engl J Med 1989; 321:1494.
12. Tegtmeier GE. The use of cytomegalovirus-screened blood in neonates. Transfusion 1988; 28:201.
13. Preiksaitis JK, Brown L, McKenzie M. Transfusion-acquired cytomegalovirus infection in neonates: a prospective study. Transfusion 1988; 28:205.
14. Griffin MP, O'Shea M, Brazy JE, et al. Cytomegalovirus infection in a neonatal intensive care unit. Am J Dis Child 1988; 142:1188.
15. Adler SP. Transfusion-acquired CMV infection in premature infants [Letter]. Transfusion 1989; 29:278.
16. Hillyer CD, Snydman DR, Berkman EM. The risk of cytomegalovirus infection in solid organ and bone marrow transplant recipients: transfusion of blood products. Transfusion 1990; 30:659.
17. Verdonck LF, deGraan-Hentzen YCE, Dekker AW, et al. Cytomegalovirus seronegative platelets and leukocyte-poor red blood cells from random donors can prevent primary cytomegalovirus infection after bone marrow transplantation. Bone Marrow Transplant 1987; 2:73.
18. MacKinnon S, Burnett AK, Crawford RJ, et al. Seronegative blood products prevent primary cytomegalovirus infection after bone marrow transplantation. J Clin Pathol 1988; 41:948.
19. Strauss RG. Selection of white cell-reduced blood components for transfusions during early infancy. Transfusion 1993; 33:352.
20. American Association of Blood Banks Association. Leukocyte reduction to prevent transfusion-transmitted cytomegalovirus [Bulletin No. 97-2]. Bethesda, MD: AABB Press, 1997.
21. Brady MT, Milam JD, Anderson DC, et al. Use of deglycerolized red blood cells to prevent posttransfusion infection with cytomegalovirus in neonates. J Infect Dis 1984; 150:334.
22. Gilbert GL, Hayes K, Hudson IL, et al. Prevention of transfusion-acquired cytomegalovirus infection in infants by blood filtration to remove leukocytes. Lancet 1989; 1:1228.
23. Bowden R, Sayers M. The risk of transmitting cytomegalovirus infection by fresh frozen plasma. Transfusion 1990; 30:762.
24. Ohto H, Anderson KC. Posttransfusion graft-versus-host disease in Japanese newborns. Transfusion 1996; 36:117.
25. Sanders MR, Graeber JE. Posttransfusion graft-versus-host disease in infancy. J Pediatr 1990; 117:159.
26. Shaw JCL. Iron absorption by the premature infant: the effect of transfusion and iron supplements on the serum ferritin levels. Acta Pediatr Scand 1982; 299 (suppl):83.
27. Adamkin DH, Shott RJ, Cook LN, et al. Nonhyperoxic retrolental fibroplasia. Pediatrics 1977; 60:828.
28. Sjoberg POJ, Bondesson UG, Sedin EG, et al. Exposure of newborn infants to plasticizers. Transfusion 1985; 25:424.
29. Williams RA, Brown EF, Hurst D, et al. Transfusion of infants with activation of erythrocyte T antigen. J Pediatr 1989; 115:949.
30. Pahwa S, Sia C, Harper R, et al. T lymphocyte subpopulations in high-risk infants: influence of age and blood transfusions. Pediatrics 1985; 76:914.

31. Ringer SA, Richardson DK, Sacher RA, et al. Variations in transfusion practice in neonatal intensive care. Pediatrics 1998; 101:194.
32. Strauss RG. Red blood cell transfusion practices in the neonate. Clin Perinatol 1995; 22:641.
33. Strauss RG, Sacher RA, Blazina JF, et al. Commentary on small-volume red cell transfusions for neonatal patients. Transfusion 1990; 30:565.
34. Stockman JA. Anemia of prematurity: current concepts in the issue of when to transfuse. Pediatr Clin North Am 1986; 33:111.
35. Wardrop CAJ, Holland BM, Beale KEA, et al. Nonphysical anaemia of prematurity. Arch Dis Child 1978; 53:855.
36. Holland BM, Jones JG, Wardrop CAJ. Lessons from the anemia of prematurity. Hematol Oncol Clin North Am 1987; 1:355.
37. Stockman JA III, Garcia JF, Oski FA. The anemia of prematurity. Factors governing the erythropoietin response. N Engl J Med 1977; 296:647.
38. Brown MS, Phibbs RH, Garcia JF, et al. Postnatal changes in erythropoietin levels in untransfused premature infants. J Pediatr 1983; 103:612.
39. Stockman JA III, Graeber JE, Clark DA, et al. Anemia of prematurity: determinants of the erythropoietin response. J Pediatr 1984; 105:786.
40. Brown MS, Garcia JF, Phibbs RH, et al. Decreased response of plasma immunoreactive erythropoietin to "available oxygen" in anemia of prematurity. J Pediatr 1984; 105:793.
41. Shannon KM, Naylor GS, Tordildson JC, et al. Circulating erythroid progenitors in the anemia of prematurity. N Engl J Med 1987; 317:728.
42. Rhondeau SM, Christensen RD, Ross MP, et al. Responsiveness to recombinant human erythropoietin of marrow erythroid progenitors from infants with the "anemia of prematurity." J Pediatr 1988; 112:935.
43. Zanjani ED, Ascensao JL, McGlave PB, et al. Studies in the liver-to-kidney switch of erythropoietin production. J Clin Invest 1981; 67:1183.
44. Widness JA, Susa JB, Garcia JF, et al. Increased erythropoiesis and elevated erythropoietin in infants born to diabetic mothers and in hyperinsulinemic rhesus fetuses. J Clin Invest 1981; 67:637.
45. Snijders RJM, Abbas A, Melby O, et al. Fetal plasma erythropoietin concentration in severe growth retardation. Am J Obstet Gynecol 1993; 168:615.
46. Ohls RK, Yan LI, Trautman MS, et al. Erythropoietin production by macrophages from preterm infants: implications regarding the cause of the anemia in prematurity. Pediatr Res 1994; 35:169.
47. Widness JA, Veng-Pedersen P, Peters C, et al. Erythropoietin pharmacokinetics in premature infants: developmental, nonlinearity, and treatment effects. J Appl Physiol 1996; 80:140.
48. Ruth V, Widness JA, Raivio KO. Postnatal changes in serum Epo in relation to hypoxia before and after birth. J Pediatr 1990; 116:950.
49. George JW, Bracco C, Shannon K, et al. Response of rhesus monkeys to recombinant human erythropoietin: comparison of adults and infants [Abstract]. Pediatr Res 1989; 25:269A.
50. Stockman JA III. Physical properties of the neonatal red blood cell. *In* Stockman JA III, Pochedly C (eds): Developmental and Neonatal Hematology. New York: Raven Press, 1988, pp 297–323.
51. Oski FA, Komazawa M. Metabolism of the erythrocytes of the newborn infant. Semin Hematol 1975; 12:209.
52. Nexo E, Christensen NC, Olesen H. Volume of blood removed for analytical purposes during hospitalization of low-birthweight infants. Clin Chem 1981; 27:759.
53. Obladen M, Sachsenweger M, Stahnke M. Blood sampling in very low birth weight infants receiving different levels of intensive care. Eur J Pediatr 1988; 147:399.
54. Blanchette VS, Hume HA, Levy GJ, et al. Guidelines for auditing pediatric blood transfusion practices. Am J Dis Child 1991; 145:787.
55. Alverson DC, Isken VH, Cohen RS. Effect of booster blood transfusions on oxygen utilization in infants with bronchopulmonary dysplasia. J Pediatr 1988; 113:722.
56. Lister G, Hellenbrand WE, Kleinman CS, et al. Physiologic effects of increasing hemoglobin concentration in left-to-right shunting in infants with ventricular septal defects. N Engl J Med 1982; 306:502.
57. Rosenthal A. Hemodynamics in physiologic anemia of infancy [Editorial]. N Engl J Med 1982; 306:538.
58. Kattwinkel J. Neonatal apnea: pathogenesis and therapy. J Pediatr 1977; 90:342.
59. Joshi A, Gerhardt T, Shandloff P, et al. Blood transfusion effect on the respiratory pattern of preterm infants. Pediatr 1987; 80:79.
60. Keyes WG, Donohue PK, Spivak JL, et al. Assessing the need for transfusion of premature infants and role of hematocrit, clinical signs, and erythropoietin level. Pediatr 1989; 84:412.
61. Stockman JA, Clark DA. Weight gain: a response to transfusion in selected preterm infants. Am J Dis Child 1984; 138:828.
62. Blank JP, Sheagren TG, Cajaria J, et al. The role of RBC transfusion in the premature infant. Am J Dis Child 1984; 138:831.
63. Phillips HM, Holland BM, Abdel-Moiz A, et al. Determination of red cell mass in assessment and management of anaemia in babies needing blood transfusion. Lancet 1986; 1:882.
64. Jones JG, Holland BM, Veale KEA, et al. "Available oxygen," a realistic expression of the ability of the blood to supply oxygen to tissues. Scand J Haematol 1979; 22:77.
65. Gould SA, Rice CL, Moss GS. The physiologic basis of the use of blood and blood products. Surg Annu 1984; 16:13.
66. Levine E, Rosen A, Sehgal L, et al. Physiologic effects of acute anemia: implications for a reduced transfusion trigger. Transfusion 1990; 30:11.
67. McCormick M, Feustel PJ, Newell JC, et al. Effect of cardiac index and hematocrit changes on oxygen consumption in resuscitated patients. J Surg Res 1988; 44:499.
68. Bland RD, Shoemaker WC, Abraham E, et al. Hemodynamic and oxygen transport patterns in surviving and nonsurviving postoperative patients. Crit Care Med 1985; 13:85.
69. Weiskopf RB, Viele MK, Feiner J, et al. Human cardiovascular and metabolic response to acute, severe isovolemic anemia. JAMA 1998; 279:217.
70. Fan FC, Chen RYZ, Schuessler GB, et al. Effects of hematocrit variations on regional hemodynamics and oxygen transport in the dog. Am J Physiol 1980; 238:H545.
71. Holzman IR, Tabata B, Edelstone DI. Blood flow and oxygen delivery to the organs of the neonatal lambs as a function of hematocrit. Pediatr Res 1986; 20:1274.
72. Bernstein D, Teitel DF, Rudolph AM. Chronic anemia in the newborn lamb: cardiovascular adaptations and comparison to chronic hypoxemia. Pediatr Res 1988; 23:621.
73. Wilkerson DK, Rosen AL, Sehgal LR, et al. Limits of cardiac compensation in anemic baboons. Surgery 1988; 103:665.
74. Hudak ML, Koehler RC, Rosenberg AA, et al. Effect of hematocrit on cerebral blood flow. Am J Physiol 1986; 251:H63.
75. Holzman IR, Tabata B, Edelstone DI. Effects of varying hematocrit on intestinal oxygen uptake in neonatal lambs. Am J Physiol 1985; 248:G432.
76. Edelstone DI, Darby MJ, Bass K, et al. Effects of reductions in hemoglobin-oxygen affinity and hematocrit on oxygen consumption and acid-base state in fetal lambs. Am J Obstet Gynecol 1989; 160:820.
77. Hudson IR, Cavill IA, Cooke AD, et al. Biotin labeling of red cells in the measurement of red cell volume in preterm infants. Pediatr Res 1990; 28:199.
78. Hudson I, Cooke A, Holland B, et al. Red cell volume and cardiac output in anaemic preterm infants. Arch Dis Child 1990; 65:672.
79. Mock DM, Lankford GL, Widness JA, et al. Measurement of circulating red blood cell volume by a non-radioactive, biotin method: validation against ^{51}Cr. Transfusion, in press.
80. Liu EA, Mannino FL, Lane TA. Prospective, randomized trial of the safety and efficacy of a limited donor exposure transfusion program for premature neonates. J Pediatr 1994; 125:92.
81. Lee DA, Slagle TA, Jackson TM, et al. Reducing blood donor exposures in low birth weight infants by the use of older, unwashed packed red blood cells. J Pediatr 1995; 125:92.
82. Wood A, Wilson N, Skacl P, et al. Reducing donor exposure in preterm infants requiring blood transfusions. Arch Dis Child 1995; 72:F29.
83. Strauss RG, Burmeister LF, Johnson K, et al. AS-1 red blood cells for neonatal transfusions: a randomized trial assessing donor exposure and safety. Transfusion 1996; 36:873.
84. Strauss RG. Recombinant erythropoietin for the anemia of prematurity: still a promise, not a panacea. J Pediatr 1997; 131:653.
85. Strauss RG. Erythropoietin in the pathogenesis and treatment of neonatal anemia. Transfusion 1995; 35:68.

86. Shannon KM, Keith JF, Mentzer WC, et al. Recombinant human erythropoietin stimulates erythropoiesis and reduces erythrocyte transfusions in very-low-birth-weight preterm infants. Pediatrics 1995; 95:1.
87. Ohls RK, Veerman MW, Christensen RD. Pharmacokinetics and effectiveness of recombinant erythropoietin administered to preterm infants by continuous infusion in total parenteral nutrition solution. J Pediatr 1996; 128:518.
88. Ohls RK, Harcum J, Schibler KR, et al. The effect of erythropoietin on the transfusion requirements of preterm infants weighing 750 grams or less: a randomized, double-blind, placebo-controlled study. J Pediatr 1997; 131:661.
89. Anderson A, Fangman J, Wager G, et al. Retrieval of placental blood from the umbilical vein to determine volume, sterility, and presence of clot formation. Am J Dis Child 1992; 146:36.
90. Bifano EM, Dracker RA, Lorah K, et al. Collection and 28-day storage of human placental blood. Pediatr Res 1994; 36:90.
91. Strauss RG. Autologous transfusions for neonates using placental blood. A cautionary note. Am J Dis Child 1992; 146:21.
92. Kinmond S, Aitchison TC, Holand BM, et al. Umbilical cord clamping and preterm infants: A randomized trial. BMJ 1993; 306:172.
93. Andrew A, Brooker LA. Hemorrhagic complications in newborns. *In* Petz LD, Swisher SN, Kleinman S, et al (eds): Clinical Practice of Transfusion Medicine, 3rd ed. New York: Churchill Livingstone, 1995, pp 647–684.
94. Ludomirsk A, Weiner S, Ashmead CG, et al. Percutaneous fetal umbilical blood sampling: procedure safety and normal fetal hematologic indices. Am J Perinatol 1988; 5:264.
95. Sell EJ, Corrigan JJ Jr. Platelet counts, fibrinogen concentrations, and factor V and factor VIII levels in healthy infants according to gestational age. J Pediatr 1973; 82:1028.
96. Aballi AJ, Puapondh Y, Desposito F. Platelet counts in thriving premature infants. Pediatrics 1968; 42:685.
97. Hemta P, Vasa R, Neumann L, et al. Thrombocytopenia in the high-risk infant. J Pediatr 1980; 97:791.
98. Andrew M, Vegh P, Caco C, et al. A randomized trial of platelet transfusions in thrombocytopenic premature infants. J Pediatr 1993; 123:285.
99. Scheifele DW, Olsen EM, Pendray MR. Endotoxinemia and thrombocytopenia during neonatal necrotizing enterocolitis. Am J Clin Pathol 1985; 83:227.
100. Castle V, Andrew M, Kelton J, et al. Frequency and mechanism of neonatal thrombocytopenia. J Pediatr 1986; 108:749.
101. Andrew M, Castle V, Saigal S, et al. Clinical impact of neonatal thrombocytopenia. J Pediatr 1987; 110:457.
102. Castle V, Coates G, Kelton JG, et al. In-oxine platelet survivals in thrombocytopenic infants. Blood 1987; 70:652.
103. Murray NA, Roberts IAG. Circulating megakaryocytes and their progenitors in early thrombocytopenia in preterm neonates. Pediatr Res 1996; 40:112.
104. Murray NA, Watts TL, Roberts IAG. Endogenous thrombopoietin levels and effect of recombinant human thrombopoietin on megakaryocyte precursors in term and preterm babies. Pediatr Res 1998; 43:148.
105. Whaun JM. Platelet function in the neonate: including qualitative platelet abnormalities associated with bleeding. *In* Stockman JA III, Pochedly C (eds): Developmental and Neonatal Hematology. New York: Raven Press, 1988, pp 131–144.
106. Ts'ao CH, Green D, Schultz K. Function and ultrastructure of platelets of neonates: enhanced ristocetin aggregation of neonatal platelets. Br J Haematol 1976; 32:225.
107. Suarez CR, Gonzalez J, Menendez C, et al. Neonatal and maternal platelets: activation at time of birth. Am J Hematol 1988; 29:18.
108. Stuart MJ, Gross SJ, Elrad H, et al. Effects of acetylsalicylic-acid ingestion on maternal and neonatal hemostasis. N Engl J Med 1982; 307:900.
109. Corazza MS, Davis RF, Merritt TA, et al. Prolonged bleeding time in preterm infants receiving indomethacin for patient ductus arteriosus. J Pediatr 1984; 105:292.
110. Feusner JH. Normal and abnormal bleeding times in neonates and young children utilizing a fully standardized template technic. Am J Clin Pathol 1980; 74:73.
111. Andrew M, Castle V, Mitchell L, et al. Modified bleeding time in the infant. Am J Hematol 1989; 30:190.
112. Blanchette VS, Sacher RA, Ballem PJ, et al. Commentary on the management of autoimmune thrombocytopenia during pregnancy and in the neonatal period. Blut 1989; 59:121.
113. Mueller-Eckhardt C, Kiefel V, Grubert A, et al. 348 cases of suspected neonatal alloimmune thrombocytopenia. Lancet 1989; 1:363.
114. Panzer S, Auerbach L, Cechova E, et al. Maternal alloimmunization against fetal platelet antigens: a prospective study. Br J Haematol 1995; 90:655.
115. Bussel JB, McFarland JG, Berkowitz RL. Antenatal management of fetal alloimmune and autoimmune thrombocytopenia. Transfus Med Rev 1990; 4:149.
116. Burrows RF, Kelton JG. Fetal thrombocytopenia and its relation to maternal thrombocytopenia. N Engl J Med 1993; 329:1463.
117. Strauss RG. The risks of thrombocytopenia and the standard uses of platelet transfusions. Plasma Ther Transfus Technol 1986; 7:279.
118. Gibson B. Neonatal haemostasis. Arch Dis Child 1989; 64:503.
119. Lupton BA, Hill A, Whitfield MR, et al. Reduced platelet count as a risk factor for intraventricular hemorrhage. Am J Dis Child 1988; 142:1222.
120. Moroff G, Friendman A, Robkin-Kline L, et al. Reduction of the volume of stored platelet concentrates for use in neonatal patients. Transfusion 1984; 24:144.
121. Simon TL, Sierra ER. Concentration of platelet units into small volumes. Transfusion 1984; 24:173.
122. Strauss RG. Granulopoiesis and neutrophil function in the neonate. *In* Stockman JA III, Pochedly C (eds): Developmental and Neonatal Hematology. New York: Raven Press, 1988, pp 88–101.
123. Rosenthal J, Cairo MS. Neonatal myelopoiesis and immunomodulation of host defenses. *In* Petz LD, Swisher SN, Kleinman S, et al (eds): Clinical Practice of Transfusion Medicine, 3rd ed. New York: Churchill Livingstone, 1995, pp 685–704.
124. Christensen D, Rothstein G, Anstall HB, et al. Granulocyte transfusions in neonates with bacterial infection, neutropenia and depletion of mature marrow neutrophils. Pediatrics 1982; 70:1.
125. Christensen RD, McFarlane JL, Taylor NL, et al. Blood and marrow neutrophils during experimental group B streptococcal infection: quantification of the stem cell, proliferative, storage and circulating pools. Pediatr Res 1982; 16:549.
126. Erdman SH, Christensen RD, Bradley PP, et al. Supply and release of storage neutrophils. Biol Neonate 1982; 41:132.
127. Christensen RD, Harper TE, Rothstein G. Granulocyte-macrophage progenitor cells in term and preterm neonates. J Pediatr 1986; 109:1047.
128. Nunoi H, Endo F, Chikazawa I, et al. Regulation of receptors and digestive activity toward synthesized formyl-chemotactic peptide in human polymorphonuclear leukocytes. Blood 1985; 66:106.
129. Strauss RG, Snyder EL. Chemotactic peptide binding by intact neutrophils from human neonates. Pediatr Res 1984; 18:63.
130. Anderson DC, Hughes BJ, Smith CW. Abnormal mobility of neonatal polymorphonuclear leukocytes: relationship to impaired redistribution of surface adhesion sites by chemotactic factor or colchicine. J Clin Invest 1984; 68:863.
131. Ambruso DR, Brentwood B, Henson PM, et al. Oxidative metabolism of cord blood neutrophils: relationship of content and degranulation of cytoplasmic granules. J Pediatr 1984; 18:1148.
132. Bruce MC, Baley JE, Medvik KA, et al. Impaired surface membrane expression of C3bi but not C3b receptors on neonatal neutrophils. Pediatr Res 1987; 21:306.
133. Mease AD, Burgess DP, Thomas PJ. Irreversible neutrophil aggregation. Am J Pathol 1981; 104:98.
134. Olson TA, Ruymann FR, Cook BA, et al. Newborn polymorphonuclear leukocyte aggregation: a study of physical properties and ultrastructure using chemotactic peptides. Pediatr Res 1983; 17:993.
135. Rochon YP, Frojmovic MM, Mills EL. Comparative studies of microscopically determined aggregation, degranulation and light-transmission after chemotactic activation of adult and newborn neutrophils. Blood 1990; 75:2053.
136. Anderson DC, Hughes BJ, Wible LJ, et al. Impaired motility of neonatal PMN leukocytes: relationship to abnormalities of cell orientation and assembly of microtubules in chemotactic gradients. J Leuk Biol 1984; 36:1.
137. Strauss RG, Hart MJ. Spontaneous and drug-induced concanavalin A capping of neutrophils from human infants and their mothers. Pediatr Res 1981; 15:1314.

138. Kimura GM, Miller ME, Leake RD, et al. Reduced concanavalin A capping of neonatal polymorphonuclear leukocytes (PMNs). Pediatr Res 1981; 15:1271.
139. Hilmo A, Howard TH. F-actin content of neonate and adult neutrophils. Blood 1987; 69:945.
140. Strauss RG, Snyder EL. Activation and activity of the superoxide-generating system of neutrophils from human infants. Pediatr Res 1983; 17:662.
141. Strauss RG, Snyder EL. Neutrophils from human infants exhibit decreased viability. Pediatr Res 1981; 15:794.
142. Strauss RG, Rosenberger TG, Wallace PD. Neutrophil chemiluminescence during the first month of life. Acta Haematol 1980; 63:326.
143. Van Epps, ED, Goodwin JS, Murphy S. Age-dependent variations in polymorphonuclear leukocyte chemiluminescence. Infect Immun 1978; 22:57.
144. Strauss RG, Snyder EL, Wallace RD, et al. Oxygen-detoxifying enzymes in neutrophils of infants and their mothers. J Lab Clin Med 1980; 95:897.
145. Strauss RG, Snyder EL. Glutathione in neutrophils from human infants. Acta Haematol 1983; 69:9.
146. Laurenti F, Ferro R, Isacchi G, et al. Polymorphonuclear leukocyte transfusion for the treatment of sepsis in the newborn infants. J Pediatr 1981; 98:118.
147. Cairo MS, Rucker R, Bennetts GA, et al. Improved survival of newborns receiving leukocyte transfusions for sepsis. Pediatrics 1984; 74:887.
148. Cairo MS, Worcester C, Rucker R, et al. Role of circulating complement and polymorphonuclear leukocyte transfusion in treatment and outcome in critically ill neonates with sepsis. J Pediatr 1987; 110:935.
149. DeCurtis M, Romano G, Scarpato N, et al. Transfusions of polymorphonuclear leukocytes (PMN) in an infant with necrotizing enterocolitis (NEC) and a defect of phagocytosis. J Pediatr 1981; 99:665.
150. Christensen RD, Anstall H, Rothstein G. Neutrophil transfusion in septic neutropenic neonates. Transfusion 1992; 22:151.
151. Laing IA, Boulton FE, Hume R. Polymorphonuclear leukocyte transfusion in neonatal septicemia. Arch Dis Child 1983; 58:1003.
152. Laurenti F, LaGreca G, Ferro R, et al. Transfusion of polymorphonuclear neutrophils in premature infant with *Klebsiella* sepsis. Lancet 1978; 2:111.
153. Baley JE, Stork EK, Warkentin PI, et al. Buffy coat transfusions in neutropenic neonates with presumed sepsis: a prospective, randomized trial. Pediatrics 1987; 80:712.
154. Wheeler JC, Chauvenet AR, Johnson CA, et al. Buffy coat transfusions in neonates with sepsis and neutrophil storage pool depletion. Pediatrics 1987; 97:422.
155. Newman RS, Waffarn F, Simmons GE, et al. Questionable value of saline prepared granulocytes in the treatment of neonatal septicemia. Transfusion 1988; 28:196.
156. Strauss RG. Current status of granulocyte transfusions to treat neonatal sepsis. J Clin Apheresis 1989; 5:25.
157. Christensen RD, Rothstein G, Hill HR, et al. The effect of hybridoma antibody administration upon neutrophil kinetics during experimental type III group B streptococcal sepsis. Pediatr Res 1983; 17:795.
158. Kim KS. Efficacy of human immunoglobulin and penicillin G in treatment of experimental group B streptococcal infection. Pediatr Res 1987; 21:289.
159. Harper TE, Christensen RD, Rothstein G. The effect of administration of immunoglobulin to newborn rats with *Escherichia coli* sepsis and meningitis. Pediatr Res 1987; 22:455.
160. Harper TE, Christensen RD, Rothstein G, et al. Effect of intravenous immunoglobulin G on neutrophil kinetics during experimental group B streptococcal infection in neonatal rats. Rev Infect Dis 1986; 8:S401.
161. Redd H, Christensen RD, Fischer GW. Circulating and storage neutrophils in septic neonatal rats treated with immune globulin. J Infect Dis 1988; 157:705.
162. Haque KN, Zaidi MN, Haque SK, et al. Intravenous immunoglobulin for prevention of sepsis in preterm and low birth weight infants. Pediatr Infect Dis 1986; 5:622.
163. Chirico G, Rondini G, Plebani A, et al. Intravenous gammaglobulin therapy for prophylaxis of infection in high-risk neonates. J Pediatr 1987; 110:437.
164. Clapp DW, Kliegman RM, Baley JE, et al. Use of intravenously administered immune globulin to prevent nosocomial sepsis in low birth weight infants: report of a pilot study. J Pediatr 1989; 115:973.
165. Conway S, Ng P, Howel D, et al. Prophylactic intravenous immunoglobulin in preterm infants: a controlled trial. Vox Sang 1990; 59:6.
166. Stabile A, Sopo SM, Romanelli V, et al. Intravenous immunoglobulin for prophylaxis of neonatal sepsis in premature infants. Arch Dis Child 1988; 63:441.
167. Magny JF, Bremard-Oury C, Brault D, et al. Intravenous immunoglobulin therapy for prevention in high-risk premature infants: report of a multicenter, double-blind study. Pediatrics 1991; 88:437.
168. Baker CJ, Melish ME, Hall RT, et al. Intravenous immune globulin for the prevention of nosocomial infection in low-birth-weight neonates. N Engl J Med 1992; 327:213.
169. Bussel JB. Intravenous gammaglobulin in the prophylaxis of late sepsis in very-low-birth-weight infants: preliminary results of a randomized, double-blind, placebo-controlled trial. Rev Infect Dis 1990; 12:S457.
170. Fanaroff AA, Korones SB, Wright LL, et al. A controlled trial of intravenous immune globulin to reduce nosocomial infections in very-low-birth-weight infants. N Engl J Med 1994; 330:1107.
171. van Overmeire B, Bleyaert S, van Reempts PJ, et al. The use of intravenously administered immunoglobulins in the prevention of severe infection in very low birth weight neonates. Biol Neonate 1993; 64:110.
172. Weisman LE, Stoll BJ, Kueser TJ, et al. Intravenous immune globulin prophylaxis of late-onset sepsis in premature neonates. J Pediatr 1994; 125:922.
173. Christensen RD, Hardman T, Thornton J, et al. A randomized, double-blind, placebo-controlled investigation of the safety of intravenous immune globulin administration to preterm neonates. J Perinatol 1988; 9:126.
174. Sidiropoulos D, Boehme U, von Muralt G, et al. Immunoglobulin supplementation in prevention or treatment of neonatal sepsis. Pediatr Infect Dis J 1986; 5:S193.
175. Haque KN, Zaidi MH, Bahakim H. IgM-enriched intravenous immunoglobulin therapy in neonatal sepsis. Am J Dis Child 1988; 142:1293.
176. Friedman CA, Wender DG, Temple DM, et al. Intravenous gamma globulin as adjunct therapy for severe group B streptococcal disease in the newborn. Am J Perinatol 1989; 6:453.
177. Weisman LE, Stoll BJ, Kueser TJ, et al. Intravenous immune globulin therapy for early-onset sepsis in premature neonates. J Pediatr 1992; 121:434.
178. Christensen RD, Brown MS, Hall DC, et al. Effect on neutrophil kinetics and serum opsonic capacity of intravenous administration of immune globulin to neonates with clinical signs of early-onset sepsis. J Pediatr 1991; 118:606.
179. Cairo MS, Worcester CC, Rucker RW, et al. Randomized trial of granulocyte transfusions versus intravenous immune globulin therapy for neonatal neutropenia and sepsis. J Pediatr 1992; 120:281.
180. Haque KN, Remo C, Bahakim H. Comparison of two types of intravenous immunoglobulins in the treatment of neonatal sepsis. Clin Exp Immunol 1995; 101:328.
181. Cross AS, Siegel G, Byrne WR, et al. Intravenous immune globulin impairs anti-bacterial defenses of a cyclophosphamide-treated host. Clin Exp Immunol 1989; 76:159.
182. Weisman LE, Weisman E, Lorenzetti PM. High intravenous doses of human immune globulin suppress neonatal group B streptococcal immunity in rats. J Pediatr 1989; 115:445.
183. Cross AS, Alving BM, Sadoff JC, et al. Intravenous immune globulin: a cautionary note. Lancet 1984; 1:912.
184. Cairo MS. The use of granulocyte transfusions in neonatal sepsis. Transfus Med Rev 1990; 4:14.
185. Magny JF, Bremard-Oury C, Brault D, et al. Intravenous immunoglobulin therapy for prevention of infection in high-risk premature infants: report of a multicenter, double-blood study. Pediatrics 1991; 88:437.
186. Bailie KEM, Irvine AE, Bridges JM, et al. Granulocyte and granulocyte-macrophage colony-stimulating factors in cord and maternal serum at delivery. Pediatr Res 1994; 35:164.
187. Bedford Russel AR, Davies EG, McGuigan S, et al. Plasma granu-

locyte colony-stimulating factor concentrations (G-CSF) in the early neonatal period. Br J Haematol 1994; 86:642.
188. Gessler P, Kirchmann N, Kientsch-Engel R, et al. Serum concentrations of granulocyte colony-stimulating factor in healthy term and preterm neonates and in those with various diseases including bacterial infections. Blood 1993; 82:3177.
189. Ohls RK, Li Y, Abdel-Mageed A, et al. Neutrophil pool sizes and granulocyte colony-stimulating factor production in human midtrimester fetuses. Pediatr Res 1995; 37:806.
190. Schibler KR, Liechty KW, White W, et al. Production of granulocyte colony-stimulating factor in vitro by monocytes from preterm and term neonates. Blood 1993; 82:2478.
191. Lee S, Knoppel E, van de Ven C, et al. Transcriptional rates of granulocyte-macrophage colony-stimulating factor, interleukin-3, and macrophage colony-stimulating factor genes in activated cord versus adult mononuclear cells: alteration in cytokine expression may be secondary to posttranscriptional instability. Pediatr Res 1993; 34:560.
192. English BK, Hammond WP, Lewis DB, et al. Decreased granulocyte-macrophage colony-stimulating factor production by human neonatal blood mononuclear cells and T cells. Pediatr Res 1992; 31:211.
193. Cairo MS, Suen Y, Knoppel E, et al. Decreased stimulated GM-CSF production and GM-CSF gene expression but normal numbers of GM-CSF receptors in human term newborns compared with adults. Pediatr Res 1991; 30:362.
194. Frenck RW, Sarman G, Harper TE, et al. The ability of recombinant murine granulocyte-macrophage colony-stimulating factor to protect neonatal rats from septic death due to *Staphylococcus aureus.* J Infect Dis 1990; 162:109.
195. Cairo MS, Mauss D, Kommareddy S, et al. Prophylactic or simultaneous administration of recombinant human granulocyte colony-stimulating factor in the treatment of group B streptococcal sepsis in neonatal rats. Pediatr Res 1990; 27:612.
196. Cairo MS, Plunkett JM, Mauss D, et al. Seven-day administration of recombinant human granulocyte colony-stimulating factor to newborn rats: modulation of neonatal neutrophilia, myelopoiesis, and group B *Streptococcus* sepsis. Blood 1990; 75:1788.
197. Cairo MS, Plunkett JM, Nguyen A, et al. Effect of stem cell factor with and without granulocyte colony-stimulating factor on neonatal hematopoiesis: in vivo induction of newborn myelopoiesis and reduction of mortality during experimental group B streptococcal sepsis. Blood 1992; 80:96.
198. Cairo MS, Plunkett JM, Nguyen A, et al. Sequential administration of interleukin-6 and granulocyte colony-stimulating factor in newborn rats: modulation of newborn granulopoiesis and thrombopoiesis. Pediatr Res 1991; 30:554.
199. Medlock ES, Kaplan DL, Cecchini M, et al. Granulocyte colony-stimulating factor crosses the placenta and stimulates fetal rat granulopoiesis. Blood 1993; 81:916.
200. Novales JS, Salva AM, Modanlou HD, et al. Maternal administration of granulocyte colony-stimulating factor improves neonatal rat survival after a lethal group B streptococcal infection. Blood 1993; 81:923.
201. Jaswon MS, Jones HM, Linch DC. The effects of recombinant human granulocyte-macrophage colony-stimulating factor on the neutrophil respiratory burst in the term and preterm infant when studied in whole blood. Pediatr Res 1994; 36:623.
202. Frenck RW Jr, Buescher ES, Vandhan-Raj S. The effects of recombinant human granulocyte-macrophage colony-stimulating factor on in vitro cord blood granulocyte function. Pediatr Res 1989; 26:43.
203. Gillan ER, Christensen RD, Suen Y, et al. A randomized, placebo-controlled trial of recombinant human granulocyte colony-stimulating factor administration in newborn infants with presumed sepsis: significant induction of peripheral and bone marrow neutrophilia. Blood 1994; 84:1427.
204. Makhlouf RA, Doron MW, Bose CL, et al. Administration of granulocyte colony-stimulating factor to neutropenic low birth weight infants of mothers with preeclampsia. J Pediatr 1995; 126:454.
205. Cairo MS, Christensen R, Sender LS, et al. Results of a phase I/II trial of recombinant human granulocyte-macrophage colony-stimulating factor in very low birthweight neonates: significant induction of circulatory neutrophils, monocytes, platelets, and bone marrow neutrophils. Blood 1995; 86:2509.

CHAPTER 21

Alloimmunization in Neonates

Louis DePalma

The interaction of molecular and cellular events that take place during an immune response to alloantigens is quite complex. Indeed, many aspects of this response are still only partially understood. In the context of red cell transfusion, immunohematologists have established laboratory methods to ensure that blood component therapy for the transfusion recipient is as safe as possible. Historically, *safe* has meant that both the donor and the recipient are immunologically compatible with respect to the major red cell antigen groups A, B, and O. In addition, screening of the recipient serum with reagent red cells, as well as the crossmatch between recipient serum and prospective blood donor red cells, has been used to detect clinically significant recipient red cell alloantibodies. Hemolytic transfusion reactions, which may be associated with significant patient morbidity as well as mortality, are thereby largely avoided.

Although actively formed red cell alloantibodies are commonly detected in the general patient population (see later discussion), such a phenomenon in neonates (younger than 1 month old) and infants (younger than 4 months old) is quite rare. In fact, crossmatching is not performed in this patient population unless there is evidence of passively acquired maternal red cell alloantibodies. The neonatal immune response to an antigenic challenge such as blood transfusion is qualitatively and quantitatively different from that of older infants, children, and adults. Great strides have been made in the elucidation of neonatal immunobiology. We are now beginning to understand the biological basis of this apparent clinical lack of alloantibody formation. In addition, we are learning that in certain clinical situations, neonates and infants may produce clinically significant red cell alloantibodies.

The complex array of cellular and extracellular antigenic exposures that occur in blood transfusion serves as an important experimental model to gain further insights into the nature of the neonatal immune system. This chapter summarizes the current state of knowledge of the neonatal immune response, as well as studies describing its interactions with transfused allogeneic red cells. This knowledge is contrasted with what we know of the adult immune response to blood transfusion, to highlight the marked differences between these two periods.

ADULT IMMUNE RESPONSE TO BLOOD TRANSFUSION

Alloantibody Formation

The reported frequency of clinically significant red cell alloantibodies, as detected by pretransfusion antibody screening in a hospital transfusion service, ranges from 0.7% to 1.6%.[1–4] Giblett[5] estimated that the theoretical incidence of alloimmunization to red blood cell antigens (excluding D) is approximately 1% per unit transfused. Another study observed a frequency of alloimmunization of 0.4% per unit in multitransfused patients.[6] Adult recipients do not appear to lose their ability to form red cell alloantibodies as they age.[7] In addition, although discordant viewpoints exist, several workers found no difference between males and females in their ability to form red cell alloantibodies.[8, 9]

When analyzing data on the frequency of red blood cell alloantibody formation, one must take into account several factors. The demographic profile of patients being evaluated may be important in relating the data from one institution to those from another. In addition, because alloimmunization is detected by conventional red cell agglutination techniques, several causes of decreased sensitivity are possible: the serum antibody titer may be below the critical concentration for detection, the test conditions may not be ideal, or the target red cells may not possess the specific antigen in question.[10]

Alloimmunization due to donor white blood cells (neutrophil-specific antigens, as well as human leukocyte antigens [HLAs]), platelets (platelet-specific antigens and HLAs), and serum proteins also occurs with blood transfusion. Such events are clinically relevant because these alloantibodies are responsible for adverse outcomes. Furthermore, alloantibody formation can significantly complicate the management of very ill patients.[11] Some investigators have advocated the use of autologous blood transfusion when compatible blood cannot be readily obtained.[12] Examples of adverse outcomes attributable to recipient alloantibodies include febrile nonhemolytic reactions (anti–neutrophil-specific and anti-HLA antibodies), allergic reactions (anti–serum protein antibodies), platelet immune refractoriness (anti–platelet-specific and anti-HLA antibodies), and anaphylaxis (anti–immunoglobulin A [IgA] antibody in IgA-deficient hosts).[13] The incidence of post-transfusion HLA alloimmunization depends on the type of blood component, the frequency of transfusion, and the disparity between donor and recipient HLA haplotypes. Sixty percent of patients receiving massive homologous transfusions will make anti-HLA antibodies.[14]

HLA alloimmunization appears to be minimized if transfused components are leukodepleted.[15] In fact, donor HLA class II–expressing cells appear to be necessary for recipient anti–HLA class I antibody formation.[16–18] It is unclear whether leukodepletion of cells expressing HLA class II antigens before transfusion can decrease recipient allosensitization to non-HLA cellular antigens. Because the relevant HLA class II–expressing cells are most likely allogeneic antigen-presenting cells (APCs), such depletion may be useful in decreasing or preventing the formation of recipient alloantibodies to numerous donor cellular and extracellular antigens. Additional investigations are needed to answer this question as well as to evaluate the effect of APC depletion on the cell-mediated immune response to alloantigens.

Cell-Mediated Immune Response

T cytotoxic, T suppressor, and natural killer (NK) lymphocytes constitute the principal effector cells of cell-mediated immunity. Owing to the complex biochemical nature of the cellular and extracellular antigenic determinants, a T cell–dependent cell-mediated immune response to blood transfusion occurs.

Insight into the nature of this type of immune response was gained by the emergence of the immunosuppressive effect of transfusion in the context of solid organ transplantation. Much to the surprise of many investigators, preoperative donor-specific or third-party blood transfusion appeared to enhance the survival of renal allografts.[19] The mechanisms by which blood transfusions lead to allograft survival are not clear, although it is generally believed to be secondary to specific and nonspecific immunosuppression of the host immune system. Opelz and Terasaki[19] suggested that an active induction of immune unresponsiveness was critical. Increasing the number of pretransplant transfusions was shown to decrease the probability of rejection, with 5 units exerting a near-maximal effect.[20] Post-transfusion decrements in in vitro proliferative activity to alloantigens in the mixed lymphocyte reaction assay and to other mitogens have been described.[21, 22] Several studies have demonstrated an increase in arachidonic acid metabolism after transfusion, suggesting that the family of prostaglandin E (PGE) compounds is the principal mediator of transfusion-induced immunosuppression.[23, 24] Other investigations have emphasized the importance of anti-idiotypic antibodies for the transfusion effect. This proposal remains somewhat controversial, because a correlation between graft outcome and anti-idiotypic antibodies has not been uniformly reported.[25, 26] Most studies have used inhibition of the mixed lymphocyte reaction by post-transfusion sera as evidence for the development of anti-idiotypic antibodies. Formation of anti-idiotypic antibodies to anti-HLA after blood transfusions has also been described.[27] However, their importance is not yet known. According to Jerne's idiotype network theory, successive phases of anti-idiotypic antibody synthesis may occur. These blocking antibodies may bind to antigen-specific T cell receptors at the time of transplantation, thereby enhancing allograft survival.

Selected aspects of transfusion-induced cell-mediated immunity have been described in patients other than transplant recipients. For example, patients with renal failure, hemophilia, von Willebrand's disease, and hemoglobinopathies have altered in vitro responses to allogeneic lymphocytes and mitogens, cell-mediated cytotoxicity, and NK cell activity.[28] One large study documented increased expression of HLA-DR antigen on T cells, as well as decreased NK cell activity, in patients who had received multiple transfusions.[29] In addition, increases in the risk of bacterial infection and cancer recurrence after perioperative blood transfusion have been reported.[30]

Early Events

Of significant value to investigators attempting to understand the early effects of blood transfusion on the immune system are a number of studies, which are summarized in Table 21–1. It has been known for some time that atypical lymphocytes appear in the peripheral blood and that increases in DNA synthesis by peripheral lymphocytes can occur as soon as 5 to 7 days after blood transfusion.[31–33]

Researchers from Hungary reported recipient lymphocyte activation after transfusion of several types of modified blood components.[34–36] Previously untransfused male volunteers received allogeneic blood components and were evaluated by serial blood sampling in the immediate post-transfusion period. In one study, subjects received either a buffy coat transfusion derived from a unit of whole blood or a unit of platelets. The platelets were processed by repeated centrifugation before transfusion, resulting in a total platelet transfusion volume of 100 mL containing approximately 8×10^{10} platelets and only 0 to 1×10^5 leukocytes. The recipients were "immunized" intravenously one to four times at 6-week intervals. All donor-recipient pairs were mismatched for one to four class I HLA antigens and one HLA-DR antigen. Two to 3 days after primary antigen exposure, the buffy coat recipients had significant increases in peripheral blood lymphocytes expressing interleukin-2 (IL-2) and HLA-DR, in association with significant increases in γ-interferon, neopterin, and β_2-microglobulin levels. Recipients of leukodepleted platelet concentrates did not demonstrate any changes in the various markers studied. These findings are in agreement with previous data confirming an increase in IL-2– and HLA-DR–expressing lymphocytes, as well as neopterin and γ-interferon, after an antigenic stimulus.[37–39]

T cell activation appears to consist of a sequential expression of the IL-2 receptor within 12 hours and HLA-DR within 24 to 48 hours of a secondary immune response. When the subjects were rechallenged with a second buffy coat transfusion, IL-2 and HLA-DR appeared earlier than after the initial transfusion. Surprisingly, the number of leukocytes contained in the two different types of transfusions did not influence the presence of FcR-blocking antibody production. Repeated alloimmunization with either buffy coat or platelets stimulated a progressive increase in blocking activity on erythrocyte antibody rosette formation.

In a follow-up study, this group documented an increase in IL-2R, dipeptidyl-peptidase (CD26), activation-inducer molecule (CD69), and transferrin receptors (CD71) on day 3 after transfusion of leukodepleted platelets to previously untransfused male volunteer subjects.[35]

Table 21–1. Early Immune Response to Blood Transfusion in Adults

Transfused Component	Marker	Trend	Subject Population	References
Red blood cells	Atypical lymphocytes	Increase	Medical and surgical patients	31–33
Red blood cells, plasma, platelets, buffy coats	IL-2	Increase	Healthy volunteers, surgical patients	34, 35, 41
Buffy coats	HLA-DR	Increase	Healthy volunteers	34, 35
Buffy coats	γ-interferon, neopterin, and β_2-microglobulin	Increase	Healthy volunteers	34–36
Buffy coats, leukodepleted platelets	FcR-blocking antibody	Increase	Healthy volunteers	34
Leukodepleted platelets	Dipeptydilpeptidase (CD26), activation-inducer molecule (CD69), transferrin receptor (CD71), and UCHL-1	Increase	Healthy volunteers	35
Leukodepleted platelets	CD45-RA	Decrease	Healthy volunteers	35
Leukodepleted platelets	CD30, ICAM-1, CDw70	No change	Healthy volunteers	35, 36
Whole blood	IL-2, TNF, γ-interferon, CSF-2	Decrease (at 2 weeks)	Chronic renal failure patients	40
Whole blood	Prostaglandin E_2	Increase	Chronic renal failure patients	40

A significant increase in UCHL1 and a decrease in CD45-RA antigen expression were detected on recipient peripheral lymphocytes on day 7 or 14, suggestive of T cell priming. No changes in other activation molecules (CD30, intercellular adhesion molecule-1, CDw70) nor the presence of cytotoxic anti-HLA antibody was noted. It is unclear why activation occurred in this study and not in the subjects who received a similar type of platelet transfusion in the first study. Although suggestive that lymphocyte activation can be triggered in vivo by primary exposure to major histocompatibility complex (MHC) class I antigens in the absence of MHC class II antigens, this discrepancy requires explanation. Of note, the degree of MHC class I and II mismatching was not reported in this second study. A well-conducted study from Israel, however, documented the effect of a single whole blood transfusion on cytokine secretion in patients with chronic renal failure.[40] Although no significant changes were observed in the secretion of IL-2, colony-stimulating factor 1 (CSF-1), tumor necrosis factor (TNF), and γ-interferon 1 week after blood transfusion, decreases were seen in week 2. A decrease of about 70% was observed in IL-2, TNF, and γ-interferon, along with a 30% decrease in CSF-1. A sharp increase in PGE_2 was also noted. The results of this study, although confirmatory of the immunosuppressive effect of transfusion-induced PGE_2 secretion, are in contrast with those of other studies documenting an increase in parameters of lymphocyte activation. Perhaps the degree of MHC matching and the immunocompetence of these transfusion recipients were different from those of subjects in the previously described studies.

Finally, other investigations have documented early changes in the immune response to blood transfusion in adults undergoing cardiopulmonary bypass (CPB) procedures.[41, 42] Concern over CPB-induced immunosuppression and its role in increasing the risk of post-transfusion graft-versus-host disease as well as in determining depressed humoral and cell-mediated immune function prompted my colleagues and me to study these patients.[41] We documented T cell activation by an increase in IL-2R– and HLA-DR–expressing T helper cells 5 to 7 days after surgery and concomitant transfusion in two massively transfused individuals undergoing CPB. With one exception, only those patients receiving numerous allogeneic donor exposures showed any sign of lymphocyte activation. Of note, we could not exclude the possibility that the activated lymphocytes could have represented transfused allogeneic lymphocytes and a subclinical form of post-transfusion graft-versus-host disease. All patients had uneventful postoperative outcomes.

In summary, evidence for both an immunosuppressive and a lymphocyte-activating effect has been reported by different investigators. This is not surprising, because the immune response to an alloantigenic challenge requires the combination of both pathways, each regulating the other. It is likely that the nature of the net response is secondary to the predominance of one pathway over the other. This, in turn, is determined by host factors (TH1 versus TH2) as well as the biochemical nature of the antigens.

NEONATAL IMMUNOBIOLOGY

This section provides a detailed summary of the maturation events of the principal lymphocyte populations (Table 21–2). Interested readers wishing to learn more can consult recent reviews on the subject.[43, 44] B and T cell–mediated immunity, NK cell function, and APC biology are described.

B Cell–Mediated Immunity

Immunoglobulin production by neonatal B cells is mainly restricted to the IgM isotype. There is a relatively slow progression from IgM to IgG production, and IgA responses are the last to mature.[45] This delay does not appear to be due to a lack of precursor B cells, because the peripheral blood of newborns has large numbers of

Table 21-2. Neonatal Immunobiology

B cell–mediated immunity	IgM-restricted synthesis Defective membrane signal transduction Ineffective early B cell activation events Poor cell-cell interaction Deficient T helper activation
T cell–mediated immunity	Predominant CD4/CD45-RA suppressor activity Defective γ-interferon mRNA production
Natural killer cell function	Poor cell-cell interaction Reduced CD16/CD56 cells in selected neonates
Antigen-presenting cell function	Defective antigen presentation in infants Low HLA class II expression
Cytokines	Deficient production of IL-2, IL-4, and IL-6

circulating B cells expressing surface IgM, IgG, and IgA. The mechanisms accounting for the failure of neonatal B cells to differentiate are not understood. Various aspects of the neonatal B cell response may be involved. Early B cell activation, including the capability of cooperating effectively with neonatal T cells, and surface membrane signal transduction are suspected. In fact, regulatory imbalances between T cell–mediated help and suppression, as well as intrinsic B cell immaturity, may be responsible for both poor antibody production and isotype restriction.

Interesting mixing experiments have provided additional clues about neonatal B cell immaturity.[46] Studies performed with pokeweed mitogen (PWM)–stimulated cord blood mononuclear cells showed minimal immunoglobulin production despite a strong proliferative response. The in vitro immunoglobulin production is principally IgM, and it is approximately 25% of that seen in cultures from adult peripheral blood mononuclear cells. The addition of adult T cells to the PWM-stimulated neonatal B cells enhances IgM production considerably. Interestingly, IgG and IgA plasma cell responses remain deficient. Further evidence that neonatal helper T cell function is deficient is provided by the fact that less than 5% of cord blood T cells express HLA-D antigens as an activation marker after PWM culture.[47] Additional data suggest that enhanced neonatal T cell suppressor activity and deficient helper T cell function may be responsible for poor B cell responses.

Clonal expansion of activated B cells or terminal differentiation may also be ineffective in neonates. Studies indicate that lower cytokine receptor expression and deficient production of cytokines such as IL-2, IL-4, and IL-6 are likely to contribute to the decreased capacity of neonatal lymphocytes to generate any IgG response.[48, 49] In fact, when neonatal lymphocytes are stimulated with immobilized monoclonal antibody to CD3 and supplemented with IL-2, IL-4, or IL-6, all immunoglobulin isotypes are secreted. It has also been shown that fetal and newborn B cells exhibit a unique phenotype, characterized by the expression of the CD5 and CD1c molecule.[50] Many of these cells coexpress activation markers such as 4F2 and IL-2R and can proliferate in the presence of rIL-2, rIL-4, and low-molecular-weight B cell growth factor , indicating at least partial B cell competence. Additional investigations are necessary to establish their function.

T Cell–Mediated Immunity

The enumeration of neonatal T cell subsets on the basis of surface marker antigens has disclosed some differences with respect to older individuals. Whereas the percentage of CD4-positive cells is similar in neonates and adults, the proportion of CD8-positive cells is significantly higher in neonates.[51] In fact, a subset of CD8-positive circulating lymphocytes has been described that is negative for CD3 and CD4.[52] Other researchers have observed cord blood lymphocytes that coexpress both CD4 and CD8, and some believe that this population may represent a unique activation state owing to premature release from the thymus.[53] Suppression is very active in neonates, a finding that may be important for in vivo inhibition of maternal cell proliferation and rejection of the fetus.[54]

The subsets of T cells identified by CD45-RA (2H4), CD45-RO (CDw29 or 4B4), and UCHL-1 represent naive and memory (previously activated) T lymphocytes. CD45-RA expression on naive CD4 lymphocytes (suppressor-inducer) undergoes downregulation shortly after antigenic stimulation, whereas cell surface expression of CD45-RO (helper-inducer) and UCHL-1 increases.[54] Reference levels of these subpopulations in neonates indicate that contrary to what is seen in adults, there is a predominance of naive T lymphocytes and a decrease in the number of memory T cells.[55–58] Interestingly, cord lymphocytes, just like adult lymphocytes, exhibit increased expression of CD45-RO and UCHL-1 as well as three cell adhesion molecules—leukocyte function antigen-3 (LFA-3), CD-2, and LFA-1—and downregulation of CD45-RA after mitogen stimulation.[59]

Some investigators have associated the lack of neonatal helper cell function to the presence of CD4-positive suppressor cells in cord blood.[60, 61] One group showed that the dominant immunoregulatory function of cord blood CD4-positive cells is suppression mediated by CD4-positive, CD45-RA–positive cells.[62] This subset, unlike its adult counterpart, also expresses CD38, a membrane molecule characteristic of immature lymphoid cells that is infrequently expressed by adult CD4-positive cells. The mechanism by which cord blood CD4-positive, CD45-RA–positive cells suppress immunoglobulin production is currently unknown. However, some have found that various prostaglandin synthetase inhibitors reduce or abrogate cord blood mononuclear suppression.[63, 64] Prostaglandins, particularly PGE_2, appear to be major mediators of cord blood suppressive activity.[65]

Additional data regarding neonatal T cell activation have contributed significantly to our attempt to evaluate the effectiveness of the neonatal immune response to antigenic challenge. T cell activation by mitogens results in the accumulation of IL-2, IL-2R, and γ-interferon mRNA. In neonates, T cell IL-2 production and IL-2R surface antigen density are comparable to those in adult cells, but γ-interferon production is markedly lower.[66] Gamma-interferon–induced production of specific mRNA in stimulated neonatal T cells is reduced compared with the accumulation of γ-interferon–induced mRNA in adults.[67] However, neonatal T cells can be induced in vitro to express the lymphokine gene repertoire characteristic for adult T cells.[68]

NK Cell Cytotoxicity and APC Function

Defined as non–MHC-restricted cytotoxic lymphocytes, NK cells express CD16 (FcR-γ) and CD56 (natural killer histoantigen-1 [NKH-1], isoform of neural cellular adhesion molecule [N-CAM]) differentiation antigens, but not T cell receptor–CD3 complexes.[69, 70] Both IL-2 and γ-interferon can increase NK cell activity. Previous investigations reported contradictory results regarding cord blood NK activity. NK activity was reported as either lower than or similar to that in healthy adult control subjects.[71, 72] A Japanese group documented extremely low NK activity in the neonatal period, with sharp increases to the adult level between 1 and 5 months of age.[73] IL-2 enhancement was prominent, especially in the neonatal period. One recent report indicates that IL-2, IL-12, and IL-15 induce functional and phenotypic maturation of cord blood NK cell subsets.[74] Culture of cord blood NK cells with IL-2 or IL-15 led to the appearance of a $CD16^+CD56^+$ phenotype, whereas culture with IL-12 led to acquisition of both $CD16^+CD56^+$ and $CD16^-CD56^+$ phenotypes.

T cells invariably recognize antigens on the surface of other cells and carry out many of their functions by interacting with APCs. Although B cells may act as APCs, numerous investigations have focused on a family of bone marrow–derived cells with a prominent antigen-presenting function. At first, it was believed that the principal APCs among peripheral blood mononuclear cells were monocytes. In addition, it was thought that tissue-based macrophages were critical for antigen presentation to occur in secondary lymphoid organs. We now know that APC function is mainly due to a heterogeneous family of cells known collectively as dendritic cells. In fact, cells with dendritic morphology are critical in providing functions such as antigen processing, antigen retention on the cell surface, antigen transport to lymphatic tissues and presentation to T lymphocytes, and induction of T cells to secrete lymphokines such as those involved in B cell activation and antibody secretion.[75, 76] As mentioned previously, APCs express MHC class II molecules and interact with the T cell receptor–CD3 complex on helper T cells. Alloantigen is associated with the APC class II molecule after having been processed in the intracellular lysosomal compartment and transported through the endoplasmic reticulum to the cell surface.[77] Separate antigenic determinants of the processed alloantigen are associated with separate APC HLA class II molecules. Alloantigen associated with MHC class I cells is presented to cytotoxic T cells in a similar process.[78, 79]

Our group has evaluated the function of neonatal and infant APCs.[80] We noted a specific maturation sequence in the presentation of alloantigen by neonatal and infant APCs to self-helper T cells. In fact, samples from subjects younger than 2 years of age showed an inability to respond in vitro to irradiated stimulator cells (APC-depleted allogeneic adult lymphocytes), as measured by the ability of mixed lymphocyte culture (MLC) supernatants to support an IL-2–dependent cytologic T lymphocyte line. At this time, the specific cause of this reduced function is unclear. Neonates are known to synthesize little specific mRNA γ-interferon, a powerful inducer of class II expression on APCs. Additional costimulatory, accessory molecules are essential in optimal APC function and may be defective in neonates and infants. Regardless of the cause, the finding of poor APC function in this age group helps explain the poor B cell responses as well as T cell responses to various allogeneic challenges previously described.

NEONATAL IMMUNE RESPONSE TO BLOOD TRANSFUSION

Red cell compatibility testing for infants younger than 4 months is routinely omitted, provided that initial antibody screening methods reveal no alloantibodies.[81] One group proposed that neonates do not form red cell alloantibodies owing to an immature immune system,[82] whereas another investigator suggested that transfusion early in life prevented alloimmunization by an acquired tolerance mechanism.[83] Much has been learned about neonatal immunobiology since the appearance of these two reports, and it is clear that numerous factors may be responsible for this poor alloantibody response. One group documented long-term survival of lymphocytes transfused from mothers to their babies, a finding consistent with the acquired tolerance theory.[84] In this study, cytogenetic analysis was performed on the peripheral blood of 14 male infants who had received fetal transfusions of maternal blood, compared with nonrelated, sex-mismatched transfusions in a control group of neonates. Maternal lymphocytes persisted for longer than 2 years in the peripheral blood of four infants who had received fetal transfusions. Even greater long-term effects of neonatal transfusion were documented in another investigation.[85] In a group of women who had been transfused as neonates, there was significantly suppressed MLC with autologous plasma as long as 20 years after the transfusion event.

Two serological reports documented the lack of alloantibody formation against red cell antigens in neonates and infants.[86, 87] A total of 143 infants, each having received numerous donor exposures and red cell transfusions, were followed for up to 30 months. In no case were red cell alloantibodies detected. These studies, however, did not investigate possible mechanisms responsible for the lack of alloantibody formation. Another group documented long-term transfusion effects on the CD4-CD8 ratio in infants between 2 and 12 weeks of age.[88] They found a significant inverse relationship between the number of blood transfusions and the CD4-CD8 ratio but offered no insights into the mechanisms responsible for this influence on the T cell subset distribution.

A series of studies, principally from our laboratory, delineated several important characteristics of the neonatal early immune response to blood transfusion (Table 21–3). Romano and associates[89] evaluated the expression of Ia-like (i.e., I region–associated) antigens and IL-2 receptors on peripheral blood T lymphocytes from newborns receiving postnatal total blood exchange. Patient groups were divided according to whether the whole blood was transfused unmanipulated, irradiated, or leukodepleted.

Table 21–3. Early Immune Response to Blood Transfusion in Neonates

Transfused Component	Marker	Trend	Treatment	Reference
Whole blood	IL-2R, HLA-DR	Increase	Exchange transfusions	89
Washed, irradiated packed red cells	IL-2R, HLA-DR, CD45-RA, CDw29, UCHL-1, neopterin, γ-interferon	No change	10 mL/kg transfusions	90
Washed, irradiated, packed red cells; plasma; platelets	Red cell alloantibody, anti-E	Synthesis	Massive transfusions*	93

*One male infant.

Unfortunately, details regarding irradiation dose, leukodepletion method, and final concentration of white cells in the various transfusions were not reported. A significant increase in Ia- and IL-2R–expressing T cells was seen 2 days after transfusion in those neonates receiving unmanipulated whole blood exchanges. No significant changes were seen in the other groups, except for a modest increase in Ia-expressing T cells 5 days after exchange transfusion with leukodepleted blood. Although it is unclear from this study why no lymphocyte activation was seen in patients receiving irradiated blood or in most recipients of leukodepleted blood, Romano and associates established that neonates appear to respond immunologically to allogeneic blood transfusion. In fact, they were able to show definitively, on the basis of sex-mismatched transfusions and cytogenetic analysis, that the neonatal lymphocyte population expresses the activated antigens.

We evaluated neonates undergoing extracorporeal membrane oxygenation (ECMO), a modified CPB procedure for patients requiring cardiac and respiratory support.[90] All neonates undergoing ECMO received a priming volume of 2 units of red blood cells on the day of the procedure, equivalent to at least a two-volume exchange transfusion. Blood samples obtained on day 1 after the procedure, and those obtained up to 7 days after the first blood transfusion, failed to show an increase in either IL-2R– or HLA-DR–expressing T cells or an increase in B cells. A control group of neonates receiving 10 mL/kg–aliquot blood transfusions of washed, irradiated red cells also failed to show any increase in lymphocyte activation markers on flow cytometric analysis. In fact, no changes were seen in CD3, CD4, CD8, CD19, or NK cell numbers.

In a follow-up study, we evaluated an additional cohort of neonates using flow cytometric analysis of additional lymphocyte subpopulations and serum cytokine determinations.[91] These neonates also received irradiated, washed red blood cell transfusions at a dose of 10 mL/kg with an average white cell concentration of 2×10^7 cells per transfusion. The blood was irradiated with 2800 cGy, and the mean number of donor exposures was 2 ± 1.5. No changes in helper T cells expressing CD45-RA, CDw29, or UCHL-1 antigens, indicative of a shift from naive to memory cells, were noted after transfusion. Mean channel fluorescence intensity was also evaluated for each antigen by overlay-histogram analysis. No shift in fluorescence signal was seen, a finding also indicative of a lack of cellular activation (Table 21–4). Post-transfusion γ-interferon levels as well as neopterin levels were essentially unchanged. The failure to observe lymphocyte activation, although possibly due in part to the low number of donor white blood cells, was principally caused by a lack of recipient recognition of the transfused donor allogeneic blood cell antigens.

Our attention focused next on the ability of neonatal and infant APCs to prime self-helper T cells effectively. This aspect of the afferent immune arm of alloantigen stimulation is essential for an immune response to T cell–dependent antigens, such as those expressed both cellularly and extracellularly in transfused blood. As previously mentioned, we have observed a specific maturation sequence in APCs from birth through infancy into childhood and adulthood. Lymphocytes from subjects 24 months of age or younger were incapable of responding to irradiated APC-depleted allogeneic stimulator lymphocytes.[80] It was also noted that an infant's T helper lymphocytes could use allogeneic APCs for an in vitro response in a one-way MLC. Therefore, it may be possible to observe synthesis of red cell alloantibodies by a neonate or older infant after stimulation by a critical number of allogeneic APCs. It has been established that helper T cell pathways can use both self- and allogeneic APCs; therefore, the presence of immature self-APCs does not exclude the possibility of a helper T cell–mediated response.[92] We described the first well-documented case of a massively transfused infant forming an alloantibody.[93] The baby had received a significant exposure to donor allogeneic APCs as a neonate. The investigation documents the presence of the red cell alloantibody anti-E in an 11-week-old infant in a definitive manner with additional follow-up studies. It still remains to be ascertained whether there is a threshold concentration of allogeneic APCs that may overcome an immature T cell–priming circuit or whether additional costimulatory factors are responsible for alloantibody formation. Additional costimulatory pathways for T cell activation were recently described in both adult and neonatal lymphocytes. One of the most studied costimulatory molecules is CD28,

Table 21–4. Mean Channel Fluorescence Intensity of Lymphocyte Activation Markers in 10 Neonates

Sample*	CD4+/ CD45-RA+	CD4+/ CDw29+	CD4+/ UCHL-1+
0	241 ± 102	167 ± 52	0†
1	275 ± 101	281 ± 93	0
2	317 ± 121	285 ± 158	0
3	343 ± 106	222 ± 88	0

*Samples were obtained approximately every 3 days (3 ± 2) following blood transfusion.

†Only background fluorescence was detected.

a 44-kD glycoprotein member of the immunoglobulin superfamily.[94] Signaling via CD28 of human naive neonatal T lymphocytes appeared to be suboptimal, in that T cell IL-2 production was lower than adult levels after anti-CD2 stimulation.[95] An additional pathway via CD40 ligand contributes to T cell–mediated macrophage activation.[96] Under some experimental conditions, neonatal T cells express much less CD40 ligand than do adult T cells.[97] In another study, there appeared to be no differences.[98] In comparing neonatal to adult T cell activation, it is important to refer to the methods used. When using a mitogen such as phytohemagglutinin or anti-CD3, differences were noted in cord versus adult lymphocyte proliferation but not at the molecular level with respect to c-fos and c-jun mRNA signal.[99] Additional well-designed studies are required to more fully evaluate post-transfusion lymphocyte activation and alloantibody synthesis in neonates.

FUTURE DIRECTIONS

To more fully understand the neonatal immune response to blood transfusions, highly sophisticated techniques need to be used. The molecular aspects of APC function as well as T cell–B cell interactions require further elucidation. Recent reports evaluating the fetal and cord blood T cell repertoire suggest that the subjects' immune system, although naive, is fully constituted and can respond by establishing memory T cells even after intrauterine transfusion.[100, 101] Information derived from such studies will lead us to a more complete understanding of the infant's response to blood transfusion and help us gain insights into developmental immunobiology. Additional dividends from such an approach may be clarification of graft-versus-host disease, acquired tolerance, and autoimmunity.

REFERENCES

1. Spielmann W, Seidl S. Prevalence of irregular red cell antibodies and their significance in blood transfusion and antenatal care. Vox Sang 1974; 26:551.
2. Giblett ER. Blood group alloantibodies: an assessment of some laboratory practices. Transfusion 1977; 17:299.
3. Boral LI, Henry JB. The type and screen: a safe alternative and supplement in selected surgical procedures. Transfusion 1977; 17:163.
4. Heisto H. Pretransfusion blood group serology: limited value of the antiglobulin phase of the crossmatch when a careful screening test for unexpected antibodies is performed. Transfusion 1979; 19:761.
5. Giblett ER. A critique of the theoretical hazard of intra vs. interracial transfusion. Transfusion 1961; 1:233.
6. Lostumbo MM, Holland PV, Schmidt PJ. Isoimmunization after multiple transfusions. N Engl J Med 1966; 275:141.
7. Dzik WH. Age and erythrocyte alloimmunization. Vox Sang 1986; 51:73.
8. Sarnaik S, Schornack J, Lusher JM. The incidence of development of irregular antibodies in patients with sickle cell anemia. Transfusion 1986; 26:249.
9. Brantley SG, Ramsey G. Red cell alloimmunization in multitransfused HLA typed patients. Transfusion 1988; 28:463.
10. Walker RH, Dong-Tsamn L, Hartrick MB. Alloimmunization following blood transfusion. Arch Pathol Lab Med 1989; 113:254.
11. DePalma L, Leitman SF, Carter CS, Gallin JI. Granulocyte transfusion therapy in a child with chronic granulomatous disease and multiple red cell alloantibodies. Transfusion 1989; 29:421.
12. DePalma L, Palmer R, Leitman SF, et al. Utilization patterns in frozen autologous red blood cells: experience in a referral center and a community hospital. Arch Pathol Lab Med 1990; 114:516.
13. Mollison PL, Engelfreit CP, Contreras M. Blood Transfusion in Clinical Medicine, 10th ed. Boston: Blackwell Scientific Publications, 1997, pp 489–499.
14. Gleichmann H, Breininger J. Over 95% sensitization against allogeneic leukocytes following single massive blood transfusion. Vox Sang 1975; 28:66.
15. The TRAP study group. Leukocyte reduction and ultraviolet B irradiation of platelets to prevent alloimmunization and refractoriness to platelet transfusions. N Engl J Med 1997; 337:1861.
16. Welsh KI, Burgos H, Batchelor JR. The immune response to allogeneic rat platelets: Ag-B antigens in matrix form lacking Ia. Eur J Immunol 1977; 7:267.
17. Eernisse JG, Brand A. Prevention of platelet refractioness due to HLA antibodies by administration of leukocyte-poor blood components. Exp Hematol 1981; 9:77.
18. Claas FHJ, Smeenk RJT, Schmidt R, et al. Alloimmunization against the MHC antigens after platelet transfusions is due to contaminating leukocytes in the platelet suspension. Exp Hematol 1981; 9:84.
19. Opelz G, Terasaki P. Improvement of kidney-graft survival with increased numbers of blood transfusions. N Engl J Med 1978; 299:799.
20. Briggs JD, Canavan JSF, Dick HM, et al. Influence of HLA matching and blood transfusion on renal allograft survival. Transplantation 1978; 25:80.
21. Burlingham W, Sparks-Mackety E, Wendell T, et al. Beneficial effect of pretransplant donor-specific transfusions: evidence for an idiotype-network mechanism. Transplant Proc 1985; 17:2376.
22. Lenhard V, Maassen G, Grosse-Wilde H, et al. Effect of blood transfusions on immunoregulatory mononuclear cells in prospective transplant recipients. Transplant Proc 1983; 15:1011.
23. Shelby J, Marushack MM, Nelson EW. Prostaglandin production and suppressor cell induction in transfusion-induced immune suppression. Transplantation 1987; 43:117.
24. Lenhard V, Gemsa D, Opelz G. Transfusion-induced release of prostaglandin E_2 and its role in activation of suppressor cells. Transplant Proc 1985; 17:2380.
25. Pohanka E, Manfro RC, Oto C, et al. Anti-idiotypic antibodies to HLA after donor-specific blood transfusion. Transplant Proc 1989; 21:1806.
26. Okazaki H, Takahashi H, Jimbo M, et al. Transplant outcome with donor-specific buffy coat and lymphocyte-transfused patients. Transplant Proc 1989; 21:1832.
27. Barkley SC, Sakai RS, Ettenger RB, et al. Determination of anti-idiotypic antibodies to anti-HLA IgG following blood transfusions. Transplantation 1987; 44:30.
28. Blumberg N, Heal JM. Transfusion and recipient immune function. Arch Pathol Lab Med 1989; 113:246.
29. Gascon P, Zoumbous NC, Young NS. Immunologic abnormalities in patients receiving multiple blood transfusions. Ann Intern Med 1984; 100:173.
30. Vamvakes EC. Transfusion-associated cancer recurrence and post-operative infection: meta-analysis of randomized, controlled clinical trials. Transfusion 1996; 36:175.
31. Schechter GP, Suehnlen F, McFarland W. Lymphocyte response to blood transfusion in man. N Engl J Med 1972; 287:1169.
32. Hutchinson RM, Sejeny SA, Fraser ID, et al. Lymphocyte response to blood transfusion in man: a comparison of different preparations of blood. Br J Haematol 1976; 33:105.
33. Shimizu K, Kitoh S. Increase in the number of lymphocytes secreting IgG following blood transfusion. Blood 1982; 60:312.
34. Kotlan B, Gyodi E, Szabo T, et al. Comparative study of alloimmune reactions induced by leukocyte and platelet transfusions in humans. Hum Immunol 1988; 22:19.
35. Pocsik E, Mihalik R, Gyodi E, et al. Activation of lymphocytes after platelet allotransfusion possessing only class I MHC product. Clin Exp Immunol 1990; 82:102.
36. Pocsic E, Mihalik R, Reti M, et al. Differences in non-MHC restricted cytotoxic activities of human peripheral blood lympho-

cytes after transfusion with allogeneic leukocytes or platelets possessing class I and/or class II MHC molecules. Immunobiology 1990; 182:22.
37. Yachie A, Miyawaki T, Uwadana N, et al. Sequential expression of T cell activation (TAC) antigen and Ia determinants on circulating human T cells after immunization with tetanus toxoid. J Immunol 1983; 131:731.
38. Huber CH, Fuchs D, Hauser A, et al. Pteridines as a new marker to detect human T cells activated by allogeneic or modified self MHC determinants. J Immunol 1983; 130:1047.
39. Huber CH, Batchelor JR, Fuchs D, et al. Immune response–associated production of neopterin: release from macrophages primarily under control of interferon-gamma. J Exp Med 1984; 160:310.
40. Kalechman Y, Gafter U, Sobelman D, Sredni B. The effect of a single whole blood transfusion on cytokine secretion. J Clin Immunol 1990; 10:99.
41. DePalma L, Yu M, McIntosh CL, et al. Changes in lymphocyte subpopulations as a result of cardiopulmonary bypass: the effect of blood transfusion. J Thorac Cardiovasc Surg 1991; 101:240.
42. Ryhanen P, Ilonen J, Sufal H, et al. Characterization of in vivo activated lymphocytes found in the peripheral blood of patients undergoing cardiac operation. J Thorac Cardiovasc Surg 1987; 93:109.
43. Lewis DB, Wilson CB. Developmental immunology and role of host defenses in neonatal susceptibility to infection. *In* Remington JS, Klein JO (eds): Infectious Diseases of the Fetus and Newborn Infant, 4th ed. Philadelphia: WB Saunders, 1996, pp 20–98.
44. Lawton AR, Cooper MD. Development and function of the immune system. *In* Stiehm ER (ed): Immunologic Disorders in Infants and Children, 4th ed. Philadelphia: WB Saunders, 1996, pp 1–13.
45. Andersson U. Development of B lymphocyte function in childhood. Acta Paediatr Scand 1985; 74:568.
46. Tosato G, Magrath IT, Koski IR, et al. B cell differentiation and immunoregulatory T cell function in human cord blood lymphocytes. J Clin Invest 1980; 66:383.
47. Miyawaki T, Yachie A, Nagaoki T, et al. Expression ability of Ia antigens on T cell subsets defined by monoclonal antibodies on pokeweed mitogen stimulation in early human life. J Immunol 1982; 128:11.
48. Zola H, Fusco M, Macardle PJ, et al. Expression of cytokine receptors by human cord blood lymphocytes: comparison with adult blood lymphocytes. Pediatr Res 1995; 38:397.
49. Splawski JB, Lipsky PE. Cytokine regulation of immunoglobulin secretion by neonatal lymphocytes. J Clin Invest 1991; 88:967.
50. Durandy A, Thuillier L, Forveille M, Fischer A. Phenotypic and functional characteristics of human newborns' B lymphocytes. J Immunol 1990; 144:60.
51. Maccario R, Nespoli L, Mingrat G, et al. Lymphocyte subpopulations in the neonate: identification of an immature subset of OKT8-positive, OKT3-negative cells. J Immunol 1983; 130:1129.
52. Vitiello A, Maccario R, Montagna D, et al. Lymphocyte subpopulations in the neonate: a subset of HNK-1−, OKT3−, OKT8+ lymphocytes displays natural killer activity. Cell Immunol 1984; 85:252.
53. Solinger AM. Immature T lymphocytes in human neonatal blood. Cell Immunol 1985; 92:115.
54. Akbar AN, Terry L, Timms A, et al. Loss of CD45R and gain of UCHL1 reactivity is a feature of primed T cells. J Immunol 1988; 140:2171.
55. Pirruccello SJ, Collins M, Wilson JE, McManus BM. Age-related changes in naive and memory CD4+ T cells in healthy human children. Clin Immunol Immunopathol 1989; 52:341.
56. Bradley LM, Bradley JS, Ching DL, Shiigi SM. Predominance of T cells that express CD45R in the CD4+ helper/inducer lymphocyte subset of neonates. Clin Immunol Immunopathol 1989; 51:426.
57. Landesberg R, Fallon M, Insel R. Alterations in helper-inducer and suppressor-inducer T cell subsets in human neonatal blood. Immunology 1988; 65:323.
58. Notarangelo LD, Panina P, Imberti L, et al. Neonatal T4+ lymphocytes: analysis of the expression of 4B4 and 2H4 antigens. Clin Immunol Immunopathol 1988; 46:61.
59. Sanders ME, Makgoba MW, Sharron SO, et al. Human memory T lymphocytes express increased levels of three cell adhesion molecules (LFA-3, CD-2 and LFA-1) and have enhanced IFN-gamma production. J Immunol 1988; 140:1401.
60. Yachie AT, Miyawaki T, Nagaoki T, et al. Regulation of B cell differentiation by T cell subsets defined with OKT4 and OKT4 Ab in human cord blood. J Immunol 1981; 127:1314.
61. Jacoby DR, Oldstone MBA. Delineation of suppressor and helper activity within the OKT4-defined T lymphocyte subset in human newborns. J Immunol 1983; 131:1765.
62. Clement LT, Vink PE, Bradley GE. Novel immunoregulatory functions of phenotypically distinct subpopulations of CD4+ cells in the human neonate. J Immunol 1990; 145:102.
63. Papadogiannakis N, Johnsen S-A, Olding LB. Strong prostaglandin associated suppression of the proliferation of human maternal lymphocytes by neonatal lymphocytes linked to T versus T cell interactions and differential PGE_2 sensitivity. Clin Exp Immunol 1985; 61:125.
64. Johnsen S-A, Olding LB, Westberg NG, Wilhelmsson L. Strong suppression by mononuclear leukocytes from human newborns on maternal leukocytes: mediation by prostaglandins. Clin Immunol Immunopathol 1982; 23:606.
65. Papadogiannakis N, Johnsen S-A, Olding LB. A prostaglandin mediated suppressive activity of cord as compared to maternal or other adult adherent cells in OKT3 antibody induced proliferation. Cell Immunol 1986; 51:101.
66. Wilson CB, Westall J, Johnston DB, et al. Decreased production of interferon gamma by human neonatal cells: intrinsic and regulatory deficiencies. J Clin Invest 1986; 77:860.
67. Lewis DB, Larsen A, Wilson CB. Reduced interferon-gamma mRNA levels in human neonates. J Exp Med 1986; 163:1018.
68. Ehlers S, Smith KA. Differentiation of T cell lymphokine gene expression: the in vitro acquisition of T cell memory. J Exp Med 1991; 173:25.
69. Abo T, Miller CA, Balch CM. Characterization of human granular lymphocyte subpopulations expressing HNK-1 (leu-7) and Leu-11 antigens in the blood and lymphoid tissues from fetuses, neonates and adults. Eur J Immunol 1984; 14:616.
70. Ales-Martinez JE, Alvarez-Mon M, Merino F, et al. Decreased TcR-CD3+ T cell numbers in healthy aged humans. Eur J Immunol 1988; 18:1827.
71. Sancho L, Martinez AC, Nogales A, et al. Reconstitution of natural killer cell activity in the newborn by interleukin-2. N Engl J Med 1986; 314:57.
72. Bailey JE, Schacter BZ. Mechanisms of diminished natural killer cell activity in pregnant women and neonates. J Immunol 1985; 134:3042.
73. Yabuhara A, Kawai H, Kohiyama A. Development of natural killer cytotoxicity during childhood: marked increases in number of natural killer cells with adequate cytotoxic abilities during infancy to early childhood. Pediatr Res 1990; 28:316.
74. Gaddy J, Broxmeyer HE. Cord blood CD16+ 56− cells with low lytic activity are possible precursors of mature natural killer cells. Cell Immunol 1997; 180:132.
75. Spalding DM, Griffen JA. Different pathways of differentiation of pre-B cell lines are induced by dendritic cells and T cells from different lymphoid tissues. Cell 1986; 44:507.
76. Inaba K, Granelli-Piperno A, Steinman RM. Dendritic cells induce T lymphocytes to release B cell–stimulating factors by an interleukin-2 dependent mechanism. J Exp Med 1983; 158:2040.
77. Harding CV, Unanue ER. Antigen processing and intracellular Ia: possible roles of endocytosis and protein synthesis in Ia function. J Immunol 1989; 142:12.
78. Singer A, Munitz TI, Golding H, et al. Recognition requirements for the activation, differentiation and function of T helper cells specific for class I MHC alloantigens. Immunol Rev 1987; 98: 143.
79. Cox JH, Yewdell JW, Eisenlohr LC, et al. Antigen presentation requires transport of MHC class I molecules from the endoplasmic reticulum. Science 1990; 247:715.
80. Clerici M, DePalma L, Roilides E, et al. Analysis of T helper and antigen presenting cell functions in cord blood and peripheral blood leukocytes from healthy children of different ages. J Clin Invest 1993; 91:2829.
81. Widmann F (ed). Standards for Blood Banks and Transfusion Services, 13th ed. Arlington, VA: American Association of Blood Banks, 1991.

82. Lucivero G, Osso AD, Iannone A, et al. Phenotypic immaturity of T and B lymphocytes in cord blood of full-term normal neonates. Biol Neonate 1983; 44:303.
83. Diamond LK, Allen DM, Magill FB. Congenital (erythroid) hypoplastic anemia. Am J Dis Child 1961; 102:403.
84. Hutchinson DL, Turner JH, Schlesinger ER. Persistence of donor cells in neonates after fetal and exchange transfusion. Am J Obstet Gynecol 1971; 109:281.
85. Beck I, Scott JS, Pepper M, Speck EH. The effect of neonatal exchange and later blood transfusion on lymphocyte cultures. Am J Reprod Immunol 1981; 1:224.
86. Ludvigsen CW, Swanson JL, Thompson TR, McCullough J. The failure of neonates to form red blood cell alloantibodies in response to multiple transfusions. Am J Clin Pathol 1987; 87:250.
87. Floss Am, Strauss RG, Gocken N, Knox L. Multiple transfusions fail to provoke antibodies against blood cell antigens in human infants. Transfusion 1986; 26:419.
88. Pahwa S, Sia C, Harper R, Pahwa R. T lymphocyte subpopulations in high-risk infants: influence of age and blood transfusions. Pediatrics 1985; 76:914.
89. Romano M, El Marsafy A, Marseglia GL, et al. Increased percentage of activated Ia+ T lymphocytes in peripheral blood of neonates following exchange blood transfusion. Clin Immunol Immunopathol 1987; 43:301.
90. DePalma L, Short BL, Van Meurs K, Luban NLC. A flow cytometric analysis of lymphocyte subpopulations in neonates undergoing extracorporeal membrane oxygenation. J Pediatr 1991; 118:117.
91. DePalma L, Duncan B, Chan MM, Luban NLC. The neonatal immune response to washed and irradiated red blood cells: lack of evidence of lymphocyte activation. Transfusion 1991; 31:737.
92. Via CS, Tsokos GC, Stocks NI, et al. Human in vitro allogeneic responses: demonstrations of three pathways of T helper cell activation. J Immunol 1990; 144:2524.
93. DePalma L, Criss VR, Roseff S, Luban NLC. Presence of the red cell alloantibody anti-E in an 11-week old infant. Transfusion 1992; 32:177.
94. June CH, Ledbetter JA, Linsley PS, Thompson CD. Role of CD28 receptor in T cell activation. Immunol Today 1990; 11:211.
95. Hassan J, O'Neill S, O'Neill AJ, et al. Signalling via CD28 of human naive neonatal T lymphocytes. Clin Exp Immunol 1995; 102:192.
96. Noelle RJ. CD40 and its ligand in host defense. Immunity 1996; 4:415.
97. Nonoyama S, Penix LA, Edwards CE, et al. Diminished expression of CD40 ligand by activated neonatal T cells. J Clin Invest 1995; 95:66.
98. Splawalski JB, Nishioka J, Nishioka Y. CD40 ligand is expressed and functional on activated neonatal T cells. J Immunol 1996; 156:119.
99. DePalma L, Brown E, Baker R. C-fos and c-jun mRNA expression in activated cord and adult lymphocytes: an analysis by Northern hybridization. Vox Sang 1998; 75:134.
100. Vietor HE, Hawes GE, vanden Oever C, et al. Intrauterine transfusions affect fetal T-cell immunity. Blood 1997; 90:2492.
101. Garderet L, Dulphy N, Douay C, et al. The umbilical cord blood αβ T-cell repertoire: characteristics of a polyclonal and naive but completely formed repertoire. Blood 1998; 91:340.

SECTION VIII Transplantation

CHAPTER 22

Transplantation Immunology

Herbert A. Perkins
F. Carl Grumet

Transplantation of organs and tissues confronts a serious obstacle. The recipient is programmed during development to distinguish self elements from non-self elements and to mount an immune response against non-self elements with the goal of destroying (rejecting) the invader. This program works to the patient's advantage in terms of survival when the invader is a microorganism that can cause disease; it works against the patient in the implantation of foreign organs or tissues. The obstacle is largely avoided when the organ donor is an identical twin (syngeneic), although the ability to tolerate self elements is not always perfect. The greater the differences between organ donor and organ recipient are, the more vigorous the rejection response is. Organs from the same species (allogeneic) may be tolerated if the differences are not too great and the immune response is suppressed. Transplantation of organs from other xenogenic species has not been successful to date.

Despite these problems, transplantation has become an established method of treatment in the past several decades for end-stage failure of many organs. Successful kidney transplantation was first accomplished by Murray and coworkers[1] in the mid-1950s, starting with identical twins; the use of nonidentical, living, related donors followed. Subsequently, kidney transplantation has depended to a large extent on the availability of organs from cadaver donors. Heart transplantation became an effective form of therapy after the studies by Shumway and colleagues.[2] Liver transplantation is now also widely employed, from the example of Starzl and associates,[3] and pancreatic transplantation for diabetes is now accepted. Transplantation of the heart and lungs together is also possible, and the list of transplantable organs is constantly being expanded. Each organ differs in its ability to resist rejection by the recipient. A liver graft may be tolerated under conditions that would lead to rejection of a kidney. Transplantation of bone marrow has unique problems and is discussed separately.

The successes of today's transplantations are based on the contributions of numerous investigators in widely disparate fields. They include recognition of the major genetic factors responsible for organ rejection and the development of techniques to detect immune responses directed against them, better preservation of organs outside the body, advanced techniques of immunosuppression, the ability to recognize rejection and treat it in the early stages, enhanced surgical techniques, and better supportive care of the patient.

MAJOR HISTOCOMPATIBILITY COMPLEX

Graft rejection is largely accomplished by immune responses directed against products of a single, tightly linked series of genes, the major histocompatibility complex (MHC). The products of these genes in humans, known as human leukocyte antigens (HLAs), were discovered during investigations of alloantibodies to leukocytes in the sera of patients suffering chill-fever reactions to blood transfusions. After the initial report by Dausset,[4] both Payne and colleagues[5] and van Rood and van Leeuwen[6] began to classify the products of the MHC genes. Van Rood and Dausset recognized at the beginning that these products were likely to be transplantation antigens because they were detected on all nucleated cells of the body. They proved that hypothesis with skin transplant experiments.

The HLA system is immensely polymorphic, far beyond any other genetic system known in humans. The rapid identification of new gene products led to an explosion of new information that continues today. Much of the rapid progress can be attributed to a series of international histocompatibility workshops in which a remarkable degree of collaboration by the principal investigators in the field led to rapid agreement on new HLAs, agreement that was formalized each time by a Nomenclature Committee sponsored by the World Health Organization. It is not possible to give credit to all the great scientists who played a major role in these developments, but mention must be made of Bernard Amos, who organized the first histocompatibility workshop; Ruggiero Ceppellini, who organized the third workshop; and Paul Terasaki, who developed the microtechniques that made practical the

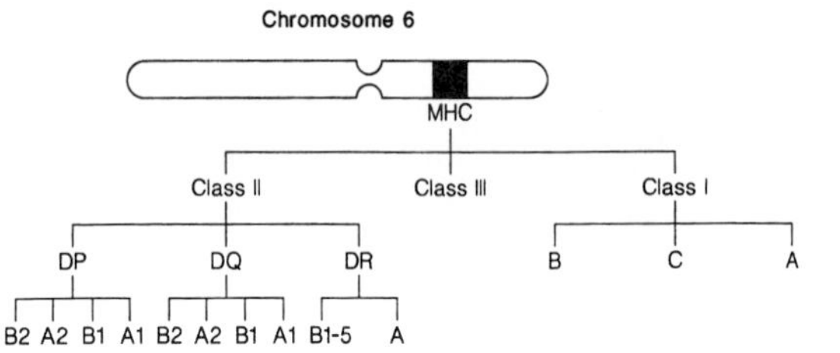

Figure 22–1. Schematic representation of HLA genes.

use of the required large numbers of typing sera, almost all of which are in relatively short supply.

The MHC consists of a large number of genes closely linked on the short arm of chromosome 6 (Fig. 22–1). The genes can be divided into three classes. Class I includes the long-recognized loci for HLA-A, HLA-B, and HLA-C. Class II genes include loci for the DR, DQ, and DP series. Class III genes, located between class I and class II genes, include loci for several of the complement components, the tumor necrosis factor family, and other products that do not appear to be involved in histocompatibility. Table 22–1 lists the class I and II genes and their products recognized by the Nomenclature Committee in 1996.[7] This list is constantly growing as new genes and alleles are discovered, and updated versions are published regularly.

The MHC genes carried on a single chromosome are called a *haplotype* (half of the genotype). In general, all genes of an MHC haplotype are inherited together. However, distances between the loci are sufficient to permit some chance of recombination, which varies according to the distances between loci and the occurrence of recombinant "hot spots." Certain combinations of genes in a haplotype occur more commonly than would be expected on the basis of the genes' frequency in the population. This distortion is called *linkage disequilibrium.* Certain haplotype combinations may confer a survival advantage or may reflect a relative structural bias against recombination, accounting for the persistence of the linkage disequilibrium.

The class I HLA product is a 44-kD glycoprotein chain with three extracellular domains—α_1, α_2, and α_3—plus a transmembrane and a cytoplasmic domain (Fig. 22–2). This chain is joined by noncovalent bonds to a monomorphic molecule of β_2-microglobulin, a product of an unrelated gene on chromosome 15. β_2-microglobulin is required for the tertiary structure of the molecule and is essential for HLA expression and function. The α_1 and α_2 domains are the sites of the significant polymorphisms that define the different HLA class I alleles and their functions. The α_3 domain resembles immunoglobulin in its structure; this portion is closest to the cell surface and binds β_2-microglobulin.

Class II molecules are glycoprotein heterodimers consisting of a 34-kD α chain and a 29-kD β chain (see Fig. 22–2), each produced by its corresponding gene within the appropriate class II region (see Table 22–1). The DRα chain has limited variability, with only two known alleles. The β chains are polymorphic, and there are multiple genes. DRB1 has by far the largest number of recognized alleles and appears to be most important for histocompatibility. DQ and DP products demonstrate polymorphism in both their α and their β chains. Unlike class I genes, which express themselves on almost all cells of the body, class II gene products have a limited distribution. They are on B lymphocytes, macrophages, dendritic cells, and some others. Cells with class II antigens are capable of presenting peptides, derived from both foreign and self-antigens, to T lymphocytes for the recognition phase of the immune response. Class II antigens also appear on T lymphocytes and some other cells, but only when the cells have been activated in an immune response or inflammation. Transfusion of blood platelets, which manifest class I HLA but not class II antigens, readily induces HLA class I alloantibodies, presumably

Table 22–1. HLA Class I and Class II Genes and Their Products

Class	Gene	Product
I	HLA-A	HLA-A alleles
	HLA-B	HLA-B alleles
	HLA-C	HLA-C alleles
	HLA-E, -F, and -G	Products associated with a class I fragment
	HLA-H, -J, -K, and -L	Pseudogenes (not expressed)
II	HLA-DRA	HLA-DR alleles
	HLA-DRB1	HLA-DR alleles
	HLA-DRB3	HLA-DR52
	HLA-DRB4	HLA-DR53
	HLA-DRB5	HLA-DR51
	HLA-DQA1	HLA-DQ alleles
	HLA-DQB1	HLA-DQ alleles
	HLA-DPA1	HLA-DP alleles
	HLA-DPA2	HLA-DP alleles
	HLA-DOB	DOβ chain
	HLA-DMA	DMα chain
	HLA-DMB	DMβ chain
	HLA-DNA	DNα chain
	HLA-DRB2, 6, 7, 8, and 9	Pseudogenes
	HLA-DQA2, B2, and B3	Not proven expressed
	HLA-DPA2 and B2	Pseudogenes
	TAP 1 and 2	Transporter proteins
	LMP 2 and 7	Proteasome-related sequence

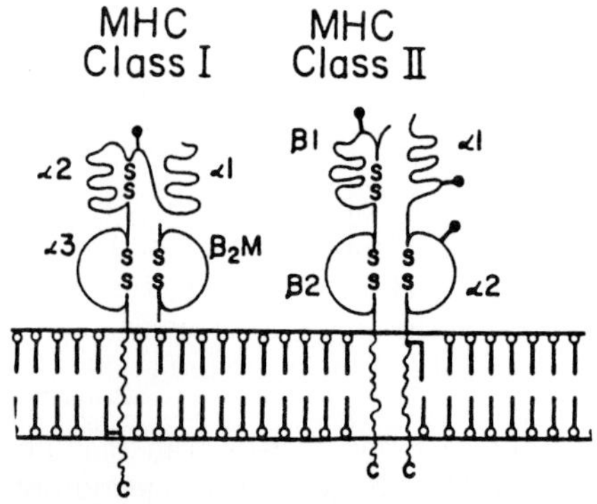

Figure 22–2. Schematic representation of the domains of HLA class I and class II gene products and their relation to the cell membrane. (Modified from Strominger JL. Human histocompatibility antigens: genes and proteins. *In* Pernis B, Vogel HJ [eds]: Cell Biology of the Major Histocompatibility Complex. Orlando, FL: Academic Press, 1985, pp 17–25.)

Table 22–2. Number of Alleles at Each Locus as Defined by Serotyping

Locus	No. of Alleles
HLA-A	28
HLA-B	61
HLA-C	10
HLA-D	26
HLA-DR	24
HLA-DQ	9
HLA-DP	6
Total	164*

*Excludes HLA-D, which sums the effect of all class II differences.

because of the presence of immunogenic contaminating leukocytes bearing both class I and class II. Matching donor and recipient for HLA class I compatibility has become a practical approach to successful transfusion support for thrombocytopenic patients refractory to random donor platelet transfusions because of alloimmunization.

Table 22–2 documents the extensive polymorphism of the HLA genes, quantifying for each locus the serologically defined allelic antigens recognized in 1996.[7] The HLA-A, HLA-B, HLA-C, HLA-DR, and HLA-DQ alloantigens were initially defined by clusters of human antisera or monoclonal antibodies that appear to recognize the same or very similar epitopes. Because each alloantigen molecule has multiple epitopes, the classification has depended on which epitope was first recognized and how that recognition could be related to other known specificities. Thus, previously defined antigens have been "split" as new sera defining narrower subtypes have become available. In other instances, more broadly reacting or "supertypic" sera define an epitope shared by multiple narrower specificities. The best known supertypic specificities are Bw4 and Bw6; one or the other is present on every HLA-B molecule. Reference to cross-reactivity of sera or antigens is common in the HLA literature. How often this antibody cross-reactivity is the result of shared epitopes rather than nonidentical but immunologically similar epitopes is not known.

HLA molecules can be distinguished by other than serological techniques. A second approach uses cellular immune reactions. The mixed lymphocyte culture (MLC) is a test that incubates cells of the donor and recipient together so that the degree of resulting in vitro immune response can be quantified. In one-way MLC, the donor cells are treated to prevent proliferation; these are the *stimulator cells*. The recipient cells are the *responder cells*, and the degree of their response is usually quantified as DNA proliferation by measuring the amount of radioactive tritium incorporated into DNA. DNA production peaks at 5 to 7 days and is followed by the appearance of T cells cytotoxic to the stimulating cells or other cells sharing one or more of the stimulator's HLAs. These cytotoxic cells can be identified in vitro by the killing of their specific targets, through a technique known as cell-mediated lymphocytolysis (CML). The initial response of the responder cell in the MLC is to HLA class II differences in the stimulating cell. This reaction can be modified for typing purposes by using a stimulating cell that is homozygous in the class II region. Then, any cell that fails to be appropriately stimulated can be assumed to share the same class II genes. In this manner, the HLA-D series was defined by homozygous typing cells[8] (see Table 22–2).

Yet another cellular approach was promoted by Sheehy and associates,[9] who observed that cells in MLC, if allowed to incubate past the point of maximal reaction, became quiescent but responded very quickly if reexposed to the original stimulating cell. They called this the *primed lymphocyte typing test*. Shaw and colleagues[10] used this approach for the first definition of alleles of the DP system.

The latest method to define HLA polymorphisms identifies the genes directly. Cellular genomic DNA is extracted, and then, employing the polymerase chain reaction (PCR) or other amplification procedures, the DNA sequences of interest are amplified to a detectable level. Specificity is established by selectivity of the amplification primers used (sequence-specific priming [SSP]), by subsequent hybridization with specific labeled oligonucleotides[11] (sequence-specific oligomer probing [SSOP]), direct genomic sequencing (sequence-based typing [SBT]), or other molecular methods. These approaches have resulted in the definition of many more alleles (splits) of previously defined antigens. As each new allele is defined, it can be sequenced. Such an approach has shown that differences between alleles as small as a single amino acid substitution can be recognized. Fleischhauer and coworkers[12] indicated that a marrow transplant may have been rejected because of such a single amino acid difference.

Table 22–3 enumerates the accepted alleles defined by DNA typing methods as of 1996.[7] For some of the serological antigens, only a single DNA sequence has been identified, but for most antigens, much more polymorphism has been identified by DNA typing; for example, at the time of the last complete report of the Nomenclature Committee,[7] 25 distinct alleles of HLA-A2 were included, as were 26 alleles of HLA-DR4. At the molecular level, it is obvious that the polymorphism of the HLA system will be found to be far more extensive; however, it is not known which of the DNA polymorphisms will be recognizable immunologically or will be clinically significant.

Table 22–3. Number of Alleles at Each Locus Defined by DNA Typing

Locus	No. of Alleles
HLA-A	83
HLA-B	186
HLA-C	42
HLA-DRA1	2
HLA-DRB1	184
HLA-DRB3	11
HLA-DRB4	9
HLA-DRB5	12
HLA-DQA1	18
HLA-DQB1	31
HLA-DPA1	10
HLA-DPB1	77
Total	665

Given this exceedingly complex system, the nomenclature has evolved in a way that attempts to reconcile historical, immunological, and molecular genetic considerations. All HLA class I and class II genes, gene products, and immunological specificities are identified by the prefix "HLA-" to designate the HLA region of chromosome 6. Each (serologically determined) antigen or (molecularly determined) allele is designated by an uppercase letter (or letters) identifying its locus and is assigned a number in the order of its discovery. For example, at the A locus, HLA-A2 was discovered before A28 (the "HLA-" prefix is implied and for convenience may be dropped here); at the B locus, B7 was discovered before B21; and at the DR locus, DR3 was discovered before DR10. Whenever new antisera split an antigen, the new splits get their own numbers, but a link to the original parent antigen is indicated by a trailing parenthesis. Thus, when new sera were found splitting A28, the new antigens were designated A68(28) and A69(28). In like fashion, as new molecularly defined alleles are found, their link to the original serological group is shown by the first two digits of their name and their order of discovery by the second two digits. If a fifth digit or character ("N") is present, it represents a noncoding or nonexpressed variant. For example, the first A68 allele sequenced is called HLA-A*6801, the second is A*6802, and so forth; and the first A69 allele is A*6901 (the "*" denotes an allele defined at the molecular level). In the same way for class II, the first β chain allele at the DRB1 locus sequenced from a DR3 serotyped donor is called HLA-DRB1*0301, the second is DRB1*0302, and so forth.

FUNCTION OF THE MHC IN THE IMMUNE RESPONSE

The importance of MHC polymorphism becomes obvious when its participation in the immune response is understood. The T cell receptor–CD3 complex reacts with a foreign antigen in most instances only when that antigen is presented by an HLA molecule that it recognizes (normally its own). Foreign materials are ingested by macrophages, and a resulting derivative peptide is ultimately bound in the presenting surface of an HLA class II molecule. The T cell receptor recognizes the specific class II molecule and the inserted peptide simultaneously and binds to them. Accessory molecules, including CD4, assist the union. This interaction initiates the *recognition phase* of the immune response.

In the *effector (killing) phase* of the immune response, the recognition process is similar, but peptide presentation is by the class I HLAs, and CD8 is the accessory molecule in place of CD4.

All these concepts were understood before the structure of the HLA molecule was known through the work of Strominger and colleagues. Bjorkman and associates[13] established the structure of the class I molecule shown in Figure 22–3. The molecule is remarkably adapted to fill the functions described. The peptide-binding cleft is formed of two α helical coils on either side of a floor of β plates. The changes in amino acid sequences of the HLA molecules that have been shown to be of physiological importance are all located in the region surrounding the bound peptide and determine which peptides will bind. The class II molecule's structure is similar.

Because the sequence of each HLA allele determines which peptides will be bound and therefore also determines the immune response to specific antigens, it is not surprising that a correlation has been demonstrated between some HLA alleles and the occurrence of certain diseases. The correlation is sufficiently high in some instances that HLA typing can be used to confirm a diagnosis (e.g., HLA-B27 and ankylosing spondylitis). Definition of the exact sequence of alleles associated with a disease

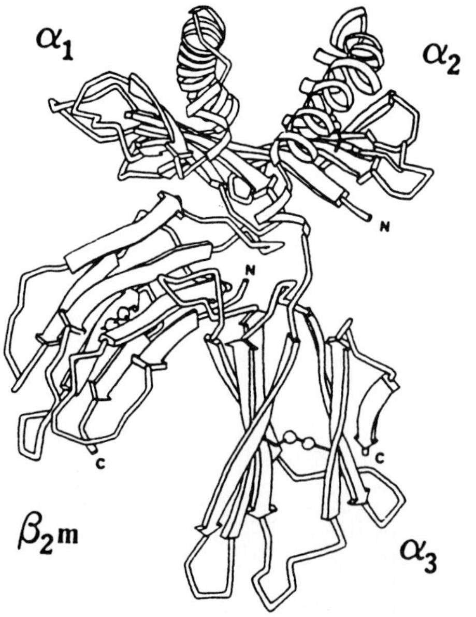

A

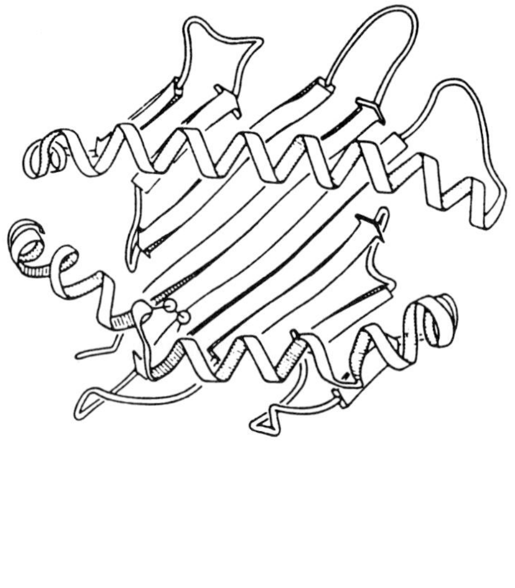

B

Figure 22–3. *A*, The structure of the HLA class I molecule. *B*, View of the HLA molecule looking down into the peptide binding cleft, showing the β plates enclosed by two α helices. (Modified from Bjorkman PJ, Saper MA, Samraoui B, et al. Structure of the human class I histocompatibility antigen, HLA-A2. Nature 1987; 329:506.)

may provide an important clue to understanding the pathogenesis of that disease and ways to avoid its clinical manifestations.

HLA MATCHING FOR TRANSPLANTATION

The importance of HLA matching was recognized in the early stages of kidney transplantation. Graft survival has always been best when the donor (excluding identical twins) is an HLA-identical sibling of the recipient. The chance that two siblings have the same two HLA haplotypes is 25%. Kidneys from donors who share one haplotype with recipients have the next lowest rejection rate and are the second choice. Such matches occur with all parents and their children and with 50% of siblings. Twenty-five percent of sibling pairs differ in both haplotypes, and transplants from these completely unmatched siblings have greater rejection rates. There must also exist histocompatibility antigens that are unrelated to HLA, because even HLA-identical kidneys occasionally get rejected. These non-HLA antigens are called minor histocompatibility antigens and are not yet well identified.

Most renal transplants now come from cadaver donors. The HLA match in this situation is most likely not as good, even when donor and recipient have identical HLA phenotypes. The difference is that unrelated matches are matched only at those polymorphisms we can identify, whereas related donors who share haplotypes have *exactly* the same genes in those haplotypes, including genes whose products cannot be typed. Factors other than histocompatibility, such as age, race, and previous transfusions, also affect subsequent graft survival.

There is little question that the better the HLA match, the better the survival of cadaver grafts. Currently, however, there remains considerable controversy over the practical importance of HLA matching in cadaver kidney transplantation. Results have become progressively better, especially with poorly matched kidneys, as immunosuppression has improved, beginning with the availability of cyclosporine. Even with the newest drug therapies, however, the rank order of better outcomes with better matches persists. Opponents of HLA matching argue that the improvement conferred by matching is a small effect and is theoretically offset by the longer waiting time patients may experience and the longer cold storage time for shipped kidneys (which may affect graft survival), arguments that are very controversial in the literature. Currently, the national kidney-sharing program of the United Network for Organ Sharing (UNOS) requires that organs be shipped to recipients who match all defined donor HLA-A, -B and -DR antigens, but not otherwise.

The data thus far demonstrate the superiority of six-antigen (HLA-A, -B, and -DR) matches,[14] and in large multicenter studies, graft survival is progressively worse as more HLA antigens are mismatched.[15, 16] The beneficial effect of HLA matching seems more obvious after longer periods of observation and also in previously sensitized or retransplanted recipients.[17, 18] Mismatching for HLA-DR may be more important, particularly for early graft loss; mismatching for HLA-B appears to be next in importance, with class I mismatches affecting both early and late graft loss.[18–20] By using DNA typing methods to identify allelic differences not demonstrable by serology, HLA-DPB mismatching and DRB1 high-resolution mismatching are also reported to have an adverse impact, albeit only in retransplantations.[17, 21] HLA-C mismatches have generally been ignored, in part because of their strong linkage disequilibrium with HLA-B, and also because HLA-C antigens are weakly expressed and are weak stimulators of antibody. Serological typing for HLA-C has been impaired by weak and unavailable antisera. DQ and DP matching is generally ignored at present. There is considerable linkage disequilibrium between DR and DQ, which means that matching for DR has a good chance of matching for DQ. DP is considerably more distant from DR and DQ, and linkage disequilibrium is weak.

Because most other solid organs cannot be preserved out of the body as long as the kidney can be, time does not usually permit HLA typing and matching. Retrospective data indicate that there would be some advantage to matching for cardiac transplants[22] and corneal transplants,[23, 24] but this process cannot be implemented for hearts because of the combination of severely limited preservation time and short, acute recipient lists. For bone marrow transplants, the donor must match the recipient's HLA type far more closely than is required for solid organ transplants (see later discussion).

Another consideration in determining the value of better HLA matching for donor organs is a possible effect on the 50- to 100-fold increased (above expected) frequency of non-Hodgkin's lymphoma (NHL) seen in transplant recipients. NHL risk appears to be related to the aggressiveness of immunosuppression,[25] and our own analysis of local and UNOS data shows that better-matched transplants suffer fewer rejection episodes and therefore fewer interventions with aggressive immunosuppression. Further, Opelz and colleagues in the Collaborative Transplant Study[25] presented preliminary data showing that cadaver renal graft recipients have an incidence of NHL that correlates with the number of HLA antigens mismatched, lending further support to the argument for providing better-matched organs for transplantation.

HUMORAL REJECTION

Early in the experience with kidney transplantation, cases were encountered in which the kidney was rejected within hours of implantation, sometimes so rapidly that the rejection could be recognized by the transplantation surgeon before the incision was closed. One cause of this phenomenon was an antibody of the ABO blood group system; this observation led to the recommendation that kidney donors should not have A or B antigens on their cells if the recipient has an ABO type with the corresponding antibody. More recently, it has been shown that ABO mismatches can sometimes be ignored if the donor carries a weak subgroup of A or the recipient has weak antibodies.

More important was the recognition by Kissmeyer-Nielsen and associates[26] and then by Patel and Terasaki[27] that high-titer preexisting antibodies reacting with the HLA class I antigens of the donor were the major cause of such hyperacute rejection. These antibodies had been induced by prior blood transfusions, pregnancies, or organ transplants. The immediate practical effect was the requirement to perform a cytotoxic crossmatch between the serum of the intended recipient and the mononuclear cells of the intended donor. Although the practice of restricting transplantation to situations in which the cytotoxic crossmatch was negative eliminated almost all hyperacute rejections, rejections within the first days or weeks still occurred on occasion, raising the possibility that antibodies undetected in the crossmatch might be responsible. This problem led to application of more sensitive crossmatch techniques: extended incubation, a wash step to eliminate serum anticomplementary activity, or addition of antiglobulin reagent. There is little agreement on which technique is best, but there is general agreement that one of these more sensitive approaches should be used.

Garavoy and colleagues[28] raised the crossmatch to a higher level of sensitivity by using a flow cytometer. There is much controversy over whether this approach adds a measure of safety or complicates the situation with many false-positive readings. Yet another controversy is whether one should crossmatch with B lymphocytes in addition to mixed mononuclear cells (primarily T lymphocytes),[29] because B lymphocytes are more sensitive to the cytotoxic action of class I antibodies and express class II antigens as well. There is much disagreement about the clinical significance of antibodies to class II antigens. Some of the confusion results from the not uncommon presence of autoantibodies in the serum of patients. These may react with the T cells and, even more commonly, with the B cells of all donors. Such autoantibodies do not affect graft survival but must be distinguished from alloantibodies, which may or may not be present. Another cause for discrepant conclusions is a difference in the immunoglobulin class of the antibodies. Clearly, the most important antibodies to detect in the crossmatch are immunoglobulin G alloantibodies directed against HLA class I antigens.

Monitoring the sera of patients waiting for renal transplants provided an opportunity to show that, as expected, antibodies may disappear without further stimulation. It was initially assumed, however, that exposure to the same antigen a second time in the form of a transplanted kidney would cause rapid rebound of antibody (secondary response), resulting in kidney rejection. This assumption led to the practice of requiring monthly serum samples from waiting patients. Each monthly sample was screened for antibodies against a large cell panel. The resulting serum reactivity was recorded as the percentage of cells in the panel with which the serum reacted, referred to by convention as the panel reactive antibody (PRA). Serum samples with the highest reactivity (peak positive) were saved and were then crossmatched with intended donor cells, along with a fresh serum sample.

At first, there was a general requirement that all the crossmatches be nonreactive. Later, however, some groups showed that a reactive peak-positive sample can be ignored and that the outcome of a transplantation done with a nonreactive fresh serum sample is not affected by whether the peak-positive sample is reactive.[30] Unfortunately, other reports indicated that graft survival in situations of nonreactive fresh samples but reactive peak-positive samples may be somewhat inferior to survival rates when both fresh and peak-positive serum samples are nonreactive on crossmatch.

Because the antibodies that subsequently disappear may be important, some laboratories made a strong effort to determine the specificities of the antibodies in the samples routinely tested. They then recommended that kidneys from donors carrying the corresponding antigens not be used. It was also suggested that, for retransplantation, the second kidney should not share antigens present in the first kidney. However, Opelz and Terasaki[31] showed years ago that the results of a second transplantation are not inferior if the second kidney shares one or more HLAs with the first, as long as the first kidney did not induce antibody to the shared antigen. More problematic than a patient with declining PRA is a patient who is crossmatch-positive with almost all donors because of a persistently high PRA. Reports indicate that aggressive therapies such as plasma immunoadsorption or administration of intravenous immunoglobulin can convert many of these patients to a generally negative crossmatch state with a subsequent good transplantation outcome.[32, 33]

A crossmatch is generally done for transplantation of all other solid organs. In general, a positive crossmatch is a contraindication to transplantation. The liver, however, seems unusually resistant to rejection, and positive crossmatches are sometimes ignored in liver transplantation.

CELLULAR REJECTION

The primary problem with the crossmatch test is that it cannot detect a situation in which the patient has made a cellular immune response against an antigen without producing a detectable antibody.[34] There is little doubt that most nonhyperacute rejections are caused partly, if not entirely, by cellular immunity. Transplanted kidneys show donor mononuclear cell infiltrations, even in well-functioning HLA-identical kidneys. With rejection episodes, the amount of cellular infiltrate increases. Infiltrating cells include $CD8^+$ cells, $CD4^+$ cells, and cells with the markers of natural killer cells. It is possible to clone cells from these infiltrates and show that they include recipient cytotoxic cells specific for HLAs of the donor.[35] It would be too time-consuming, immediately before cadaver organ transplantation, to evaluate recipient cytotoxic cells for antidonor activity, but it is theoretically possible (given the time and the money) to determine whether the recipient has circulating cytotoxic cells and the antigens for which they are specific. This procedure is far too complex to be practical on a routine basis, however.

MECHANISMS OF GRAFT ACCEPTANCE

If we could determine the mechanisms that prevent graft rejection, we could improve on them and make them more specific. Currently, we rely on broad immunosuppression by combinations of corticosteroids, azathioprine, antilymphocyte globulin, cyclosporine, tacrolimus, mycophenolate mofetil, monoclonal antibodies to specific T lymphocyte subsets, and, in some cases, total nodal irradiation. All these approaches have serious side effects and depress all immune responses. They leave the patient more susceptible to infections and play a role in the higher frequency of malignancies in patients who have received transplants.

A number of mechanisms could come into play to help the patient retain a graft. Deletion of the clones that can mount an immune response against donor antigens would be a more specific approach. Although clonal deletion in the thymus is the primary mechanism for developing self-tolerance,[36] it occurs early in development, and the thymus becomes progressively involuted after childhood. Clonal anergy can be induced peripherally in some instances; the clones remain but do not respond.[37] In any case, it is likely that responding clones are deleted early after transplantation. Immunosuppression with cytotoxic drugs is at its peak in the early post-transplantation period, and the most susceptible cells would be those proliferating in response to the newly introduced donor antigens. Clonal deletion by this mechanism, however, is clearly never complete, because host cells can be found infiltrating the most successful grafts.

The immune response is controlled by a series of opposing systems. Along with cytotoxic CD8 cells, there are suppressor CD8 cells; helper CD4 cells have antithetical suppressor-inducer CD4 cells. One mechanism for protection of the graft is increased activity of suppressor cells. Clearly, this enhancement can happen under some conditions. MLC reactions between donor and recipient are sometimes suppressed after transplantation, the suppression being caused actively by suppressor cells.[38] Increased suppressor cell activity after transplantation may be specific for donor antigens or it may be nonspecific, suppressing reaction to third-party cells that do not share donor antigens. Unfortunately, there are no consistent patterns within a single study nor agreement between investigators from different institutions.

Cells can be isolated from the peripheral blood or from the graft that show cytotoxic activity against HLA class I antigens of the graft. In successful grafts, hyporesponsiveness of cytotoxic T cells to donor antigens may be found. According to one report, this hyporesponsiveness is caused by a helper-cell defect, not a deficiency of cytotoxic precursor cells.[39]

Humoral factors also play an important role in opposing the recipient's attempts to reject the graft. The concept of an anti-idiotype network to control immune responses was originally proposed by Jerne.[40] The *idiotype* is the unique configuration of that portion of an antibody molecule that confers its specificity. Each idiotype is theoretically capable of acting as an antigenic epitope and stimulating production of an anti-idiotype. The original antibody is often referred to as AB1, the anti-idiotype as AB2. AB2 is identified by its ability to block AB1 when added to it. The most convincing evidence that anti-idiotypic antibodies (AB2) may develop after organ transplantation and that they protect the graft is in the report from Suciu-Foca and colleagues.[41]

Humoral factors may also play a role in the cellular response. The reaction of responding cells in MLC can often be blocked by serum from patients who have accepted grafts. The responsible factor (? antibody) is believed to react with the T cell receptor.

MARROW TRANSPLANTATION

The transplantation of bone marrow results in immunological problems considerably more complex than those affecting solid organ grafts. There are two major differences. The first is the fact that marrow grafts are rejected unless the HLA match is very close, despite the use of far more intensive immunosuppression than is required for solid organ transplants. The second difference is that the marrow graft itself contains immunocompetent cells that can recognize the host as foreign and reject it, producing graft-versus-host disease (GVHD).[42]

Originally, these considerations limited the choice of marrow donors to HLA-identical siblings who had the same two HLA haplotypes and were identical for all products of genes in the MHC, whether or not they had been defined exactly. Even with that degree of matching, failure to engraft or (more rarely) subsequent graft failure could occur. Failure to engraft is related to prior minor histocompatibility antigen exposures of the recipient and to the potency of immunosuppression in the preparative regimen. Patients with leukemia, who are conditioned with a lethal dose of total body irradiation, are far less likely to reject the donor marrow than are patients undergoing transplantation for aplastic anemia, who frequently receive only cytotoxic medications.

An aplastic anemia patient who has been supported by the transfusion of blood components from family members is far more likely to have failure to engraft than a leukemia patient in a similar situation. Family donors of blood components should be avoided in patients with nonmalignant diseases who may require a marrow transplant. Even blood components from unrelated individuals reduce the chances for a successful graft in aplastic anemia patients; patients with severe aplastic anemia should undergo marrow transplantation as early as possible, ideally before they need blood component support.

Graft failure is also more likely to occur if the donor marrow has been depleted of T lymphocytes (see later) before infusion. The harmful effect of T cell depletion may result from removal of accessory cells important to marrow engraftment or from loss of additional stem cells.

The fact that failure to engraft and GVHD can occur when the donor and recipient are HLA-identical proves the clinical relevance of products of non-HLA, minor histocompatibility factors. These minor histocompatibility antigens are just beginning to be defined in the bone marrow transplantation setting.[43, 44]

Finally, there is the possibility that, in appropriate circumstances, the patient can reject a transplant that carries identical genes. Marrow transplants from identical twins may be rejected if immunosuppression is not used. It is possible that self-antigenic determinants are somewhat altered in the process of collecting, processing, and infusing the marrow, promoting an immune response that cross-reacts with self-antigens. Autoimmunity clearly plays a major role in chronic GVHD (see later).

Acute GVHD develops in 30% to 40% of recipients of HLA-identical sibling marrow transplants within 1 to 2 months after transplantation. The organs affected are primarily the skin, liver, and intestinal tract. Mild GVHD is characterized by a pruritic, maculopapular rash, with or without mild liver dysfunction. It is generally easy to control. GVHD can progress in severity to exfoliating skin lesions with massive diarrhea, severe liver failure, and involvement of other organs. Concomitant immunological dysfunction leads to infections that profoundly affect prognosis, a major one being cytomegalovirus pneumonia. The most severe forms of GVHD are 100% fatal.

The therapy of acute GVHD uses various immunosuppressive reagents, and there is increasing interest in the use of monoclonal antibodies, which attack the cells believed to be responsible for the pathology. The likelihood of severe GVHD increases with the age of the patient. This factor is the primary explanation for the superior results of marrow transplantation in children compared with young adults and for the usual hesitancy to perform transplantation in patients older than 50 years.

GVHD can be avoided or markedly minimized if T lymphocytes are removed from the marrow before it is infused. Unfortunately, this depletion also results in a greater chance of graft failure. To date, patient survival rates appear similar with or without T cell depletion, but controlled studies have not yet been completed.

Chronic GVHD[45] affects 30% to 50% of marrow transplant recipients who live 6 months or more. The median time of onset after transplantation is 3 to 4 months. Clinically, chronic GVHD bears some resemblance to collagen vascular diseases, and it is generally accepted that an autoimmune basis is likely. Scleroderma-like changes in the skin and a sicca syndrome are characteristic, and esophageal involvement may cause difficulty in swallowing. Antiglobulin-positive red blood cells are common, and hemolytic anemia has been known to occur. Thrombocytopenia is another manifestation of dysfunction of the immune system.

The problems of marrow transplantation must be considered in relation to the fact that a successful marrow graft can mean a cure for an otherwise lethal disease. Success rates vary with the disease and its stages. A patient with aplastic anemia who has never received a transfusion may have an 80% chance of a cure with marrow transplantation. A patient with chronic granulocytic leukemia who receives a marrow transplant in the first year of the chronic phase may have a 60% chance of a cure. In contrast, patients with acute leukemia in their third relapse have a low success rate.

Increasing rates of success with marrow transplantation have directed attention to the relatively small number of patients with appropriate indications who have suitable donors. The chance that any sibling is HLA-identical with another is only 25%. Because American families are usually small, an average of only 30% of patients have HLA-identical sibling donors. These facts are now leading to a careful exploration of the possibility of transplantation despite minor mismatches. Studies have also been done with family donors who share one haplotype with the recipient. The second haplotype may (by chance) have the same HLA-A, HLA-B, and HLA-DR antigens as the recipient's second haplotype, or it may differ in one, two, or all three antigens. Experience to date suggests that if the donor shares one haplotype and has no more than one antigen of the second haplotype different from the patient's, patient survival is close to that attained with HLA-identical donors, but graft loss is greater and GVHD is more frequent and severe.[46, 47]

Using HLA-nonidentical relatives mismatched for a single antigen increases the likelihood of finding an acceptable donor from 30% to only 35%. Thus, 65% of potentially curable patients would be denied that chance if family donors were the only source of marrow transplants. The logical next step was to try donors who were completely unrelated but who shared, by chance, the HLA antigens of the recipient. It was recognized from the beginning that the extreme polymorphism of the HLA system required establishment of a very large registry of volunteers who were willing to donate marrow for a stranger. Such registries have now been established in many countries. The largest, the National Marrow Donor Program (NMDP), was established in the United States by acts of Congress.[48]

Patients with the most common HLA haplotypes are the ones most likely to find matches, even in a very large registry. A majority of patients have phenotypes that are unique, but most of them could be provided with a donor if one antigen mismatch is accepted. The chances of finding a compatible donor are much reduced for many ethnic minorities, because most of those volunteering to be donors thus far have been white. In addition, African-Americans have considerably more phenotype heterogeneity than other groups. Intensive efforts to recruit donors from nonwhite ethnic groups are under way.

By the end of 1997, the NMDP had a registry of more than 3 million HLA-A– and HLA-B–typed potential donors in its computer, and over 6000 transplantations had been accomplished. The program employs an electronic network that speeds identification, recall, and further testing of compatible donors. Early consensus led to the ruling that NMDP donors would be made available to patients for whom they were HLA-A–, HLA-B–, and HLA-DR–identical at the level of serological typing and also, if the patient and the transplantation team were willing, if there was a single antigen mismatch.

As anticipated, recipients of marrow from unrelated donors have had more problems with GVHD than those with HLA-identical sibling donors, but this is balanced, in the case of malignant disease, by a lower likelihood of relapse. The initial report of results with NMDP donors[49] demonstrated a 2-year disease-free survival of 40% among good-risk patients and 20% among poor-risk patients. More recently, better patient management and prevention of cytomegalovirus disease have improved results to a level close to that obtainable with HLA-identical sibling donors.[50]

With standard serological techniques, it is difficult to be certain that two unrelated individuals with the same phenotype are completely identical. Although there are relatively common HLA haplotypes that may be identical in unrelated individuals, complete identity is obviously less certain. The ability to define specific alleles through DNA typing techniques, and to identify individual amino acid differences by sequencing them, makes it possible to determine on a retrospective basis just how close these matches have been. Recognizing the importance of such a study, the NMDP established a repository where cells of each donor and recipient are stored and converted to B lymphoblastoid lines to provide unlimited quantities for future study. Currently, all prospective class II typing for the NMDP uses DNA techniques. Class I DNA typing is a bit more complicated but is in the process of becoming routine.

According to reports from the Fred Hutchinson Cancer Research Institute, matching at the allelic level improves transplantation results. Patients matched for HLA-DRB1 alleles did better than those matched for DR by serology but with allelic differences.[51] Molecular typing also established that matching for HLA-DQ alleles results in a significantly lower rate of GVHD.[52] Unexpectedly, matching for HLA-C alleles appears to be as important, or more so, than matching for HLA-A or HLA-B.[53] HLA-C was largely ignored in the past because the HLA-C antigens appear to be poor stimulators of antibody formation. In contrast to the results just outlined, mismatches for HLA-DP alleles appear to have little effect.[54]

CONCLUSIONS

Increased success in organ transplantation clearly depends on control of the immune response of the recipient. Ideally, the host immune system should be suppressed only to the specific antigenic differences of the donor. Although rejection may occur because of a single amino acid difference, the evidence is clear that the closer the match, the less likely it is that rejection will occur. Additional factors determining whether rejection will occur are the number of incompatibilities,[55] the specific antigens involved, the ability of the patient to mount an immune response, and the effect of the immunosuppressive agents administered.

Creation of specific tolerance to donor antigens is the ideal solution. Although this goal may seem rather utopian, marrow transplantation results in complete tolerance to donor antigens as host immunocompetent cells are replaced by cells of the donor and immunosuppression is discontinued. Tolerance seems to occur with graft acceptance, even though, in some cases, remaining recipient cells in the blood indicate chimerism.[56] Unlike solid organ transplants, marrow transplants do not require indefinite immunosuppression. If it ever becomes possible to perform marrow transplantation with minimal risk, marrow transplantation could be a means of achieving tolerance to a subsequent solid organ transplant.

REFERENCES

1. Merrill JP, Murray JE, Harrison JH, et al. Successful homotransplantation of the human kidney between identical twins. JAMA 1956; 160:277.
2. Lower RR, Priestley JT, Shumway NE. Homovital transplantation of the heart. J Thorac Cardiovasc Surg 1961; 41:196.
3. Starzl TE, Marchioro TL, Huntley RT, et al. Experimental and clinical homotransplantation of the liver. Ann N Y Acad Sci 1964; 120:739.
4. Dausset J. Iso-leuco-anticorps. Acta Haematol 1958; 20:156.
5. Payne R, Tripp M, Weigle J, et al. A new leukocyte isoantigen system in man. Cold Spring Harb Symp Quant Biol 1964; 29:285.
6. van Rood JJ, van Leeuwen A. Leucocyte grouping: a method and its application. J Clin Invest 1963; 42:1382.
7. Bodmer JG, Marsh SGE, Albert ED, et al. Nomenclature for factors of the HLA system, 1996. Tissue Antigens 1997; 49:297.
8. Dupont B, Jersild C, Hansen GS, et al. Typing for MLC-determinants by means of LD-homozygote and LD-heterozygote test cells. Transplant Proc 1973; 5:1543.
9. Sheehy MJ, Sondel PM, Bach FH, et al. Rapid detection of LD determinants: the PLT assay. *In* Kissmeyer-Nielsen F (ed): Histocompatibility Testing 1975. Copenhagen: Munksgaard, 1975, pp 569–575.
10. Shaw S, Johnson AH, Shearer GM. Evidence for a new segregant series of B cell antigens that are encoded in the HLA-D region and that stimulate secondary allogeneic proliferative and cytotoxic responses. J Exp Med 1980; 152:565.
11. Scharf SJ, Griffith RL, Erlich HA. Rapid typing of DNA sequence polymorphism at the HLA-DRB1 locus using the polymerase chain reaction and nonradioactive oligonucleotide probes. Hum Immunol 1991; 30:190.
12. Fleischhauer K, Kernan NA, O'Reilly RJ, et al. Bone marrow allograft rejection by T lymphocytes recognizing a single amino acid difference in HLA-B44. N Engl J Med 1990; 323:1818.
13. Bjorkman PJ, Saper MA, Samraoui B, et al. Structure of the human class I histocompatibility antigen, HLA-A2. Nature 1987; 329:506.
14. Takemoto S, Camahan E, Terasaki PI. A report of 504 six antigen-matched transplants. Transplant Proc 1991; 23:1318.
15. Opelz G. HLA matching should be utilized for improving kidney transplant success rate. Transplant Proc 1991; 23:46.
16. Terasaki PI, Cecka JM, Cho Y, et al. A report from the UNOS scientific renal transplant registry. Transplant Proc 1991; 23:53.
17. Opelz G, Scherer S, Mytilineous J. Analysis of HLA-DR split-specificity matching in cadaver kidney transplantation. Transplantation 1997; 63:57.
18. Cecka JM. The role of HLA in renal transplantation. Hum Immunol 1997; 56:6.
19. Gjertson DW. A multi-factor analysis of kidney graft outcomes at one and five years post-transplantation: 1996 UNOS update. *In* Cecka JM, Terasaki PI (eds): Clinical Transplants 1996. Los Angeles: UCLA Tissue Typing Laboratory, 1997, pp 343–360.
20. Pirsch JD, Ploeg RJ, Gange S, et al. Determinants of graft survival after renal transplantation. Transplantation 1996; 61:1581.
21. Mytilineous J, Deufel A, Opelz G. Clinical relevance of HLA-DPB locus matching for cadaver kidney retransplants: a report of the Collaborative Transplant Study. Transplantation 1997; 63:1351.
22. Opelz G, Wujciak T. The influence of HLA compatibility on graft survival after heart transplant: the Collaborative Transplant Study. N Engl J Med 1994; 330:816.
23. Gore SM, Vail A, Bradley BA, et al. HLA-DR matching in corneal transplantation: systematic review of published evidence. Transplantation 1995; 60:1033.
24. Muhkhbat B, Hagihara M, Sato T, et al. Association between HLA-DPB1 matching and 1-year rejection-free graft survival in high risk corneal transplantation. Transplantation 1997; 63:1011.
25. Opelz G, Henderson R, for the Collaborative Transplant Study. Incidence of non-Hodgkin lymphoma in kidney and heart transplant recipients. Lancet 1993; 342:1514.
26. Kissmeyer-Nielsen F, Olsen S, Petersen VP, et al. Hyperacute rejection of kidney allografts, associated with pre-existing humoral antibodies against donor cells. Lancet 1966; 1:662.
27. Patel R, Terasaki PI. Significance of the positive crossmatch test in kidney transplantation. N Engl J Med 1969; 280:735.
28. Garavoy MR, Rheinschmidt MA, Bigos M, et al. Flow cytometry analysis: a high technology crossmatch technique facilitating transplantation. Transplant Proc 1983; 15:1939.
29. Taylor CJ, Chapman JR, Ting A, Morris PJ. Characterization of lymphocytotoxic antibodies causing a positive crossmatch in renal transplantation. Transplantation 1989; 48:953.

30. Cardella CJ, Falk JA, Nicholson MJ, et al. Successful renal transplantation in patients with T-cell reactivity to donor. Lancet 1982; 2:1240.
31. Opelz G, Terasaki PI. Absence of immunization effect in human-kidney retransplantation. N Engl J Med 1978; 299:369.
32. Higgins RM, Bevan DJ, Carey BS, et al. Prevention of hyperacute rejection by removal of antibodies to HLA immediately before renal transplantation. Lancet 1996; 348:208.
33. Tyan DB, Li VA, Czer L, et al. Intravenous immunoglobulin suppression of HLA alloantibody in highly sensitized transplant candidates on transplantation with a histoincompatible organ. Transplantation 1994; 57:5553.
34. Zhang L, van Bree S, Gijbels Y, et al. Comparison of the humoral and cytotoxic T-lymphocyte response to individual HLA class I alloantigens in highly immunized patients. Hum Immunol 1991; 30:156.
35. Soulillou J-P, Moreau J-F (eds). International symposium on functional characteristics of cells invading rejected allografts. Transplant Proc 1988; 20:143.
36. Kappler JW, Roehm N, Marrack P. T cell tolerance by clonal elimination in the thymus. Cell 1987; 49:273.
37. Bretscher P, Cohn M. A theory of self-nonself discrimination. Science 1970; 169:1042.
38. Agostino GJ, Kahan BD, Kerman RH. Suppression of mixed leukocyte culture using leukocytes from normal individuals, uremic patients and allograft recipients. Transplantation 1982; 34:367.
39. Grailer AP, Sollinger HW, Kawamura T, Burlingham WJ. Donor-specific cytotoxic T lymphocyte hyporesponsiveness following renal transplantation in patients pretreated with donor-specific transfusions. Transplantation 1991; 51:320.
40. Jerne NK. The immune system (network theory). Sci Am 1973; 229:52.
41. Suciu-Foca N, Reed E, D'Agati VD, et al. Soluble HLA antigens, anti-HLA antibodies, and antiidiotypic antibodies in the circulation of renal transplant recipients. Transplantation 1991; 51:593.
42. Ferrara JLM, Deeg HJ. Graft-versus-host disease. N Engl J Med 1991; 324:667.
43. Goulmy E. Minor histocompatibility antigens: from T cell recognition to peptide identification. Hum Immunol 1997; 54:8.
44. Behar E, Chao NJ, Hiraki DD, et al. Polymorphism of adhesion molecule CD31 and its role in acute graft vs. host disease. N Engl J Med 1996; 334:286.
45. Atkinson K. Chronic graft-versus-host disease. Bone Marrow Transplant 1990; 5:69.
46. Anasetti C, Hansen JA. Bone marrow transplantation from HLA partially matched related donors and unrelated volunteer donors. *In* Forman SJ, Blume KG, Thomas ED (eds): Bone Marrow Transplantation. Boston: Blackwell Scientific Publications, 1994, p 665.
47. Beelen DW, Ottinger HD, Elmaagacli A, et al. Transplantation of filgrastim-mobilized peripheral blood stem cells from HLA-identical sibling or alternative family donors in patients with hematologic malignancies: a prospective comparison on clinical outcome, immune reconstitution, and hematopoietic chimerism. Blood 1997; 90:4725.
48. McCullough J, Hansen J, Perkins H, et al. The National Marrow Donor Program: how it works, accomplishments to date. Oncology 1989; 3:63.
49. Kernan NA, Bartsch G, Ash RC, et al. Analysis of 462 transplantations from unrelated donors facilitated by the National Marrow Donor Program. N Engl J Med 1993; 328:593.
50. Hansen JA, Petersdorf E, Martin PJ, Anasetti C. Hematopoietic stem cell transplants from unrelated donors. Immunol Rev 1997; 157:141.
51. Petersdorf E, Longton GM, Anasetti C, et al. The significance of HLA-DRB1 matching on clinical outcome after HLA-A, B, DR identical unrelated donor marrow transplantation. Blood 1995; 86:1606.
52. Petersdorf EW, Longton GM, Anasetti C, et al. Definition of HLA-DQ as a transplantation antigen. Proc Natl Acad Sci U S A 1996; 93:15358.
53. Petersdorf EW, Longton GM, Anasetti C, et al. Association of HLA-C disparity with graft failure after marrow transplantation from unrelated donors. Blood 1997; 89:1818.
54. Petersdorf EW, Smith AG, Mickelson EM, et al. The role of HLA-DPB1 disparity in the development of acute graft-versus-host disease following unrelated donor marrow transplantation. Blood 1993; 81:1923.
55. Lienert-Weidenbach K, Valiante NM, Brown C, et al. Mismatches for two major and one minor histocompatibility antigen correlate with a patient's rejection of a bone marrow from a serologically HLA-identical sibling. Biol Blood Marrow Transplant 1997; 3:255.
56. Monaco AP, Wood ML, Maki T, et al. The use of donor-specific antigen for the induction of immunologic unresponsiveness to experimental and clinical allografts. Transplant Proc 1988; 20(suppl 1):122.

CHAPTER 23

Bone Marrow Stem Cells

Scott D. Rowley

The number of patients undergoing autologous or allogeneic hematopoietic stem cell (HSC) transplantation has grown rapidly since the 1970s. Registries have collected data on more than 65,000 transplantations, but this number is believed to represent fewer than 50% of all transplantations performed.[1] In Europe alone, more than 12,000 marrow and peripheral blood stem cell (PBSC) transplantations are performed annually.[2] Much of this increased activity derives from the widespread adoption of PBSC transplantation, especially for autologous use. Also, interest in high-dose therapy with stem cell rescue has increased because of apparent success of dose-intensive therapy in achieving durable remissions in common dose-responsive malignancies such as breast cancer. Treatment of breast cancer is now the most frequent indication for autologous transplantation.[3]

Since the discovery in the late 1950s that cellular elements of the bone marrow protect against lethal irradiation,[4] transplantation science has been notable for the following advances: the continued deciphering of the human leukocyte antigen (HLA) system, including HLA-C and HLA-DQ[5–8]; the development of immunosuppressive and antineoplastic conditioning regimens achieving effective tumor cell killing while allowing stable hematopoietic chimerism to occur; the definition of immunosuppressive regimens to treat graft-versus-host disease (GVHD); and the development of cryopreservation and ex vivo purging techniques facilitating autologous bone marrow transplantation. The availability of hematopoietic growth factors and improved techniques for collection of hematopoietic progenitor and stem cells have decreased both the period of intensive medical support and regimen-related toxicity, thereby decreasing the morbidity and overall cost of transplantation for individual patients. An understanding of the hematopoietic and immunological systems has continued to develop, so that enriched populations of HSC or immunological effector cells may be isolated and manipulated ex vivo to generate somatic cell therapy products that differ in function from native bone marrow cells.

Despite these advances in transplantation science, this therapy is successful for only a minority of patients. Post-transplantation relapse, although reduced through better selection of patients whose diseases remain responsive to chemotherapy, is a major cause of therapy failure. GVHD is a continuing problem after allogeneic transplantation, especially with the increasing use of nonsibling, mismatched, or unrelated marrow donors to extend the availability of allogeneic transplantation to patients who lack HLA-identical sibling donors.[9–12] Bone marrow is a complex mixture of cells, including primitive pluripotent stem cells, which are capable of stable, long-term engraftment; mature hematopoietic progenitor cells, which may contribute to hematological recovery; and lymphoid cells, which enhance engraftment and decrease the risk for subsequent relapse but also cause GVHD. Much effort is currently being devoted to determine whether modifications of pretransplantation conditioning regimens, choice of HSC source, ex vivo processing, or supplementation of the cell inoculum with other myeloid or lymphoid cells can affect engraftment kinetics or immunological reconstitution and thereby enhance the therapeutic value of marrow transplantation.

HEMATOPOIESIS AND BONE MARROW TRANSPLANTATION

Regulation and Heterogeneity of Hematopoietic Cell Populations

Advancements in bone marrow transplantation have occurred concurrently with improvements in the understanding of hematopoiesis. Numerous in vitro assays representative of hematopoietic progenitor cells have been developed. Work with these assays, as well as work in human and animal transplantation trials, led to the current, widely accepted model of hematopoiesis, according to which all mature blood cells ultimately arise from totipotential HSC capable of self-proliferation (self-renewal) and maturation along myeloid or lymphoid lineages. Two broad aspects of hematopoiesis—(1) regulation of proliferation and differentiation and (2) the heterogeneity of hematopoietic precursors—are important to the understanding of hematological and immunological recoveries after marrow-lethal therapy, as well as to the understanding of the capabilities and limits of ex vivo graft engineering to affect both hematological and immunological reconstitution.

Hematopoietic regulatory processes controlling the proliferation and differentiation of hematopoietic cells provide for renewal of the primitive stem cells, for maturation of these cells to achieve adequate numbers of circulating mature blood cells, and for expansion of specific cell lineages in response to disease states such as infection and blood loss. Blood cells arise from totipotential stem cells. These are rare, quiescent cells that constitute a distinct subpopulation of hematopoietic cells with proliferative capacity. Daughter cells further along the maturational pathways are more limited in self-renewal potential but are more likely to be proliferative (in active cell cycle). Various descriptions of hematopoietic regulation have been proposed, ranging from random (stochastic) to strict control of proliferation and differentiation (e.g., either by cell-cell interaction with HSC or lymphocytes[13] or by humoral growth stimulatory or inhibitory factors[14]). A theory combining all these ideas is that the response of any particular hematopoietic progenitor cell to regulatory influence is restricted by previous events of cell maturation that the cell has already experienced and can be predicted by probability theory.[15] Thus, different regulatory controls may be operative for different levels of cell maturity. At present, however, the maturational stages at which these regulatory processes may occur, as well as the relative roles of competing (or synergistic) humoral or cellular regulatory factors at any particular stage of hematopoietic cell maturation, are incompletely described.

In particular, little is known about the specific regulatory effects of cellular elements on engraftment of transplanted marrow, although interactions between these cells and hematopoietic progenitors appear to be important in maintaining hematopoiesis. The hematopoietic microenvironment is a complex mixture of cells, possibly of both host and donor origin.[16] Hematopoietic progenitor cells are preferentially maintained in the adherent stromal cell layer of in vitro long-term marrow cultures,[17] and the adherent cells are important in the regulation of hematopoiesis in these cultures.[18, 19] Investigators from the Seattle transplant program have noted that poor granulocyte recovery after allogeneic marrow transplantation is correlated with the inability of cultured host stromal cells to produce granulocyte colony-stimulating factor (G-CSF) in vitro.[20] This group also reported that severe myelofibrosis in the allogeneic transplant recipient results in a delay of platelet engraftment of up to 7 days in comparison to patients without this finding, but does not affect granulocyte engraftment, risk of engraftment failure, or overall survival.[21]

Inherent in the stem cell model is the existence of a hierarchical heterogeneity of hematopoietic progenitors. The more mature hematopoietic progenitor cells may be cloned in vitro, giving rise to colonies composed of cells of single or multiple lineages, depending on the maturational potential of the original progenitor cell. The terms used to describe the progenitor cells by the colonies formed—such as granulocyte-monocyte (macrophage) colony-forming unit (CFU-GM), erythroid burst-forming unit (BFU-E), granulocyte-erythrocyte-macrophage-megakaryocyte colony-forming unit (CFU-GEMM)—unfortunately convey the impression that hematopoiesis occurs in discrete stages. A more rigorous understanding of hematopoiesis depicts these colony-forming cells as a continuum from stem cell to late progenitor cell and, ultimately, mature blood cell; hence a class of progenitor cells defined by certain characteristics (e.g., growth in vitro, cell surface antigens) may actually contain a heterogeneous population.

The relative contributions of cells of delineated hematopoietic potential for hematological recovery after marrow transplantation is not defined for human transplantation, because infusion of purified populations enriched with or depleted of hematopoietic progenitor cells of various maturational stages has not been performed. Rather, bone marrow containing a mixture of hematopoietic cells of varying potentials, as obtained from a healthy donor, is usually infused. Presumably, cells at all stages of maturation contribute to the hematological recovery of the recipient, although engraftment and survival of adequate numbers of pluripotent stem cells are necessary for sustained production of donor-derived cells. The differences, in relative proportions of more mature to primitive hematopoietic progenitor cells, between bone marrow and other sources of hematopoietic cells, such as peripheral blood, may explain both the rapid hematological recovery usually observed after infusion of the latter and the concomitant risk of delayed graft failure if adequate quantities of those cells are not administered.[22] Transplantation of bone marrow supplemented with blood-derived mature hematopoietic progenitors is a clinical technique for shortening post-transplantation aplasia.[23]

Modulation of Engraftment Kinetics

The concepts of regulation and hierarchy are fundamental to our ability to manipulate hematological and immunological recoveries by administering hematopoietic growth factors (cytokines) or by modifying the lymphohematopoietic cell populations infused. Bone marrow engraftment encompasses two concepts: (1) recovery of hematopoietic and immunological function of the bone marrow and (2) the rate at which this recovery occurs. The risk of engraftment failure is proportional to the disparity between donor and recipient for HLA and minor transplant antigens, occurring more commonly in unrelated donor transplantation than in sibling donor transplantation. The risk of engraftment failure is also increased by the removal of T lymphocytes from the marrow inoculum because of the loss of the graft-versus-host effect. This effect suppresses the host-versus-graft reactivity that is a component of graft rejection for some patients. This risk can be reduced by increasing host immunosuppression,[24] but this entails increased regimen-related toxicity as well and, if pushed to even more intensive levels, an eventual decrease in patient survival. The host-versus-graft reaction can also be overcome by increasing the quantity of cells in the inoculum, a technique made feasible for human transplantation by the availability of PBSC used in conjunction with marrow cells.[25] Engraftment failure after allogeneic transplantation may relate to immune-mediated rejection of the donor cells, inadequate stem or accessory cells in the marrow inoculum, or post-transplantation events such as infections, administration of marrow-toxic medications, and GVHD. Engraftment failure after either allogeneic or autologous transplantation may possibly also result from inability of the recipient to support the donor marrow because of stromal defects. Patients who fail to engraft may recover hematopoietic function from their own residual marrow elements that have survived the pretransplantation conditioning regimen. Attempts at retransplantation early in the course (usually within 4 to 8 weeks of the initial transplant) are complicated by the frequently severe regimen-related toxic effects of the additional immunosuppression required to achieve successful engraftment.

The other aspect of engraftment is the rate of hematological and immunological recovery. Delayed recovery increases the risk and cost of transplantation. Autologous bone marrow is usually harvested from patients who have previously received marrow-toxic chemotherapy, and these marrow specimens may then undergo a variety of ex vivo manipulations, including cryopreservation. Autologous marrow recipients frequently experience delayed engraftment in comparison with similar patients undergoing allogeneic or syngeneic transplantation, although the relative kinetics of engraftment after autologous or allogeneic transplantation depend on various factors, including patient selection, diagnosis, and ex vivo marrow processing. For example, Kersey and associates[26] reported faster engraftment for autograft recipients than for allograft recipients being treated for acute lymphoblastic leukemia (ALL); the median times to achieve a white blood cell count of 1000/μL or higher were 24 and 31 days, respectively. In contrast, Lowenburg and coworkers reported faster engraftment for allograft recipients with acute myelogenous leukemia (AML)[27]; median times to achieve a granulocyte count of 500/μL or greater were 21 and 39 days, respectively. Jones and colleagues reported a median time to a granulocyte count of 500/μL of 32.5 days for patients with Hodgkin's disease who received autografts treated with 4-hydroperoxycyclophosphamide (4-HC), in comparison with 14 days for recipients of unmanipulated allografts.[28]

The predictive value of patient diagnosis for engraftment speed can be easily discerned in autologous transplantation trials. Douay and associates reported slower engraftment kinetics for patients being treated for AML than for those being treated for ALL.[29] Investigators at Johns Hopkins Oncology Center similarly reported the predictive value of diagnosis for engraftment kinetics for recipients of 4-HC–purged marrow specimens; engrafting was slowest in patients treated for AML.[30] The differing engraftment kinetics observed probably resulted from previous chemotherapy administered to these patients, although a direct effect of the malignancy on the hematopoietic capacity of the bone marrow was possible. Markedly prolonged periods of aplasia (longer than 40 days to achieve a granulocyte count of 500/μL) are not uncommon after transplantation with marrow specimens purged ex vivo with 4-HC. It is conceivable that hematopoietic recovery for some of these patients may result from residual marrow cells' surviving the conditioning regimen; however, in the absence of markers, it is impossible to evaluate the occurrence or frequency of this event.

Administration of hematopoietic growth factors may speed engraftment after allogeneic or autologous transplantation. A variety of growth factors are available. Randomized studies of granulocyte-macrophage colony-stimulating factor (GM-CSF) or G-CSF administration after autologous transplantation demonstrated that these hematopoietic cytokines speed granulocyte recovery, may decrease the morbidity of the transplantation procedure, and may be associated with a lower probability of relapse.[31–33] Hematological recovery after allogeneic transplantation is similarly hastened,[34] but this fact has not consistently translated into earlier hospital discharge or reduced cost of transplantation. Administration of cytokines that stimulate primarily the proliferation of mature hematopoietic progenitor cells may not affect the time to initial hematopoietic recovery after transplantation; however, the subsequent rate of rise in peripheral blood counts is notably enhanced, which suggests that adequate numbers of cells at the appropriate maturational stage must be present before growth-regulatory effects from these cytokines can be obtained.[35] For example, autologous marrow specimens effectively depleted of mature progenitor cells by purging ex vivo with 4-HC may not respond to GM-CSF.[36] Thus G-CSF or GM-CSF alone may minimally affect the early initial morbidity of transplantation and may have minimal impact on the duration of hospitalization.

Pretreatment of a healthy donor or an autologous transplant recipient with any of the available cytokines has enabled the widespread use of PBSC as a source of stem cells for transplantation.[37, 38] Similarly, the pretreatment of the marrow donor with either GM-CSF or G-CSF may increase the number of myeloid progenitor cells harvested and may decrease the period of post-transplantation aplasia.[39, 40]

Predictors of Engraftment Kinetics

No tests are available to predict engraftment failure after transplantation of "adequate" numbers of viable marrow cells. Many investigators have attempted to predict the speed of hematological recovery. The predictive tests most commonly investigated have been based on enumeration of hematopoietic progenitor cells in the marrow infused. CFU-GM (colony-forming units in culture [CFU-C]),[30, 41, 42] BFU-E,[30] and CFU-GEMM[30] progenitor quantities have all been found to be predictive in various clinical settings (predominantly after autologous transplantation). These correlations were either continuous (exponential)[30, 42] or dichotomous.[41] In both situations, recipients of marrow specimens with higher progenitor cell contents generally experienced shorter periods of aplasia.

Other researchers have been unable to discover a correlation between progenitor cell quantity and speed of marrow recovery.[43, 44] The lack of a correlation may result from a true uncoupling of progenitor cell content and the cells responsible for achieving engraftment, incurred as a complication of ex vivo marrow processing. Post-transplantation events such as viral infections or the administration of marrow-suppressive medications may obscure a correlation. A lack of correlation more likely results from (1) inadequate (for statistical analysis) interpatient differences in either progenitor cell contents or time to achieving engraftment; (2) use of a non–marrow-lethal conditioning regimen, with actual recovery resulting from residual cells in the host; or (3) an inadequate assay for progenitor cell content. Correlations found by enumeration of progenitor cells do not prove a role for those cells in hematological recovery (CFU-GM content may also predict platelet and red cell recoveries). Rather, progenitor cell quantities, like patient diagnosis and other characteristics that predict engraftment, may reflect marrow quality and are of most value in the setting of ex vivo marrow manipulation.

Immunological Recovery

Much of the emphasis in transplantation has been on myeloid engraftment, because initial patient survival depends on recovery of phagocytes and, to a lesser extent, platelets. Severe immunosuppression is a consequence of both allogeneic and autologous bone marrow transplantation, although to less of an extent in the latter. It results from damage to normal barriers such as skin and mucosal linings, loss of phagocytic cells, loss of lymphoid function, and the use of immunosuppressive regimens to prevent or treat GVHD. Lymphoid reconstitution may take months, and even longer, if GVHD occurs. Recoveries of both B and T lymphoid function appear to recapitulate ontogeny, with lymphoid subpopulations recovering at different rates.[45–48] Recovery of lymphoid populations (in the absence of GVHD) is similar in allogeneic, syngeneic, and autologous transplantation, although ex vivo purging of T or B cells can delay recovery of specific subpopulations removed by the purge procedure.[49–51] Opportunistic infections occur commonly until host immunity is recovered. Infections are an especially common cause of both morbidity and mortality for transplant recipients whose condition is complicated by GVHD because of the delay in recovery of immune function caused by this disease and its treatment. Fungal and viral infections commonly occur in association with acute GVHD and its treatment; sinusitis, otitis, and pneumonia are common complications of chronic GVHD.[52] Administration of immunoglobulin G (IgG) supplementation to patients with low IgG levels can prevent some of these infectious complications.[53]

Donor immunity can be transferred at least transiently to the host, as demonstrated by delayed-type transfusion reactions to host red blood cells mediated by donor lymphocytes transfused along with the marrow. Adoptive transfer of donor immunity against specific targets can be achieved, but its persistence requires immunization of both the donor and the recipient.[54, 55] A clinical use for such manipulation of the immune system has not yet been demonstrated but is clearly of interest as a technique for preventing post-transplantation infections or, possibly, relapse.

Immunomodulatory Effects of Allogeneic Transplantation

The ability to cure disease may be dependent on the chemoradiotherapy pretransplantation conditioning regimen and/or the immunological effects of the graft-versus-host reaction. The chemoradiotherapy regimen used for the treatment of patients is intended to cure the underlying disease, with the HSC infused merely to rescue the patient from the marrow-lethal toxicity of the regimen. However, it became evident very early in the history of marrow transplantation that patients who experienced acute or chronic GVHD had a much lower risk of relapse after transplantation than those without these complications. Attempts to increase the intensity of the conditioning regimen and second transplantation of patients who experienced relapse are complicated by greatly increased regimen-related toxicity and by early post-transplantation morbidity. These facts—that cancer is a disease of the elderly who do not easily tolerate current conditioning regimens and that transplantation may be useful in many diseases for which high-dose conditioning regimens are not necessary (e.g., aplastic anemia, sickle cell anemia, thalassemia)—have led to attempts to harness the graft-versus-leukemia (GVL) effect for the treatment of relapse or for treatment of disease without administration of a marrow-lethal conditioning regimen.

The potential of the GVL effect is demonstrated by the infusion of unmodified peripheral blood mononuclear cells from the marrow donor for the treatment of relapse after allogeneic bone marrow transplantation. Kolb and colleagues reported the administration of donor lymphocytes to 135 patients with chronic and acute leukemias who experienced relapse after allogeneic transplantation.[56] Complete remissions were achieved in 73% of patients with chronic myelocytic leukemia (CML) but in only 29% of patients with AML. None of the patients treated for ALL responded to this treatment, which suggests that this approach is most practical for more indolent diseases. Complications of this therapy include the development of GVHD (41%) and myelosuppression (34%). The number of lymphocytes infused is important in achieving this effect, and it may be possible to induce a GVL effect by using doses of lymphocytes that are less likely to result in GVHD.[57] However, a distinction between the cells responsible for inducing a GVL effect and those causing GVHD has not been found. The delay in response between lymphocyte infusion and the development of a GVL effect suggests that only a minority of the cells infused recognize the tumor cell antigens and must undergo in vivo expansion before a therapeutic effect is achieved. It may be possible to develop cytotoxic lymphocytes in the laboratory, decreasing the delay in effect and possibly increasing the effect in the more rapidly proliferative acute leukemias.[58]

Most malignancies are diseases of the elderly, who are less tolerant of the conditioning regimens used for transplantation. Although the use of PBSC as the source of HSC results in a shorter period of aplasia, the practical application of allogeneic bone marrow transplantation requires less stringent conditioning regimens. Furthermore, some hematological and metabolic diseases that are treatable with marrow transplantation do not necessitate complete replacement of the host marrow. The complications of sickle-cell anemia, for example, can be greatly alleviated by a small increase in normal hemoglobin; the development of microchimerism may alleviate the need for immunosuppression in the setting of solid organ transplantation. Storb and coworkers demonstrated in a dog transplantation model that stable mixed chimerism could be achieved after administration of a sublethal dose of total body irradiation and a short course of cyclosporine and mycophenolate mofetil.[59] This is being explored in clinical transplantation trials. Investigators at the M.D. Anderson Cancer Center reported stable chimerism in three of four evaluable patients treated with purine analogs for suppression of the host-versus-graft reaction.[60]

BONE MARROW HARVESTING

Bone marrow harvesting techniques have changed little during the modern history of marrow transplantation, and most centers harvest marrow from the posterior iliac crests, using the techniques described by Thomas and Storb.[61] The use of other sources of HSC, such as PBSC, cord blood–derived stem cells, and even cadaveric marrow,[62, 63] is at least feasible, if not common. Bone marrow harvesting from healthy donors presents little risk of serious morbidity, thereby permitting the recruitment of unrelated bone marrow donors from the population of blood donors[64] and the use of pediatric donors.[65] Equipment has also changed with the introduction of disposable harvest containers with in-line filters to replace the tissue sieves initially used[66] and specially designed needles to decrease surgeon fatigue.[67, 68]

Bone marrow is typically harvested from the posterior iliac crests with the use of general or regional anesthesia. Other harvest sites, such as the sternum, anterior iliac crests, spinal processes, and even the femur, may be used but entail increased risk of complications from accidental laceration or perforation of contiguous anatomical structures. Because the engraftment failures reported in early trials of marrow transplantation resulted from inadequate host immunosuppression or poor HLA matching, the initial concern about the adequacy of the harvested marrow—at least that harvested from healthy donors—is no longer perceived to be a problem. Extending the harvest to other sites of bone marrow, once regarded as necessary, is now unusual. The use of the anterior iliac crests or the sternum as additional sources of bone marrow decreased from reported rates of 78% for allogeneic donor harvests[67] and 70% for autologous marrow collections[68] in the early 1980s to between 0% and 6% for collections reported in the late 1980s.[69, 70] Although the hematopoietic potential of harvested marrow apparently may be predicted by enumeration of myeloid progenitors in a marrow sample or by marrow scintigraphy,[71] these methods are rarely, if ever, necessary for successful harvesting of autologous or allogeneic marrow. Patients with marrow fibrosis (which would be obvious on pretransplantation marrow evaluation), previous pelvic irradiation, or pelvic tumor involvement may receive autologous transplants of PBSC if concerns arise about the ability to obtain adequate marrow for transplantation.

The quantity of marrow cells necessary for marrow engraftment is not known for either the allogeneic graft recipient or the autograft recipient. The quantity of cells is actually a surrogate for, and only indirectly reflects the quantity of, the hematopoietic progenitor cells infused. Successful engraftment for allogeneic recipients may depend more on other factors causing immune-mediated rejection of the marrow—such as degree of HLA match, prior sensitization to donor antigens, degree of immunosuppression achieved by the conditioning regimen, and ex vivo marrow processing such as T lymphocyte depletion—than upon the marrow cell dose administered. Most centers attempt to obtain at least 3×10^8 nucleated bone marrow cells per kilogram of recipient body weight, on the basis of early reports that smaller quantities increased the risk of engraftment failure.[72, 73] Those reports, however, were of select groups of patients being treated for aplastic anemia, in which engraftment failure is a more common event. In another study of 100 patients who received allogeneic transplantation for the treatment of acute leukemia, cell dose per kilogram of recipient body weight (over the range of 0.5 to 13.0×10^8) did not predict successful engraftment.[74] In a review of a large series of 1270 procedures on 1160 allogeneic donors, the range of cells obtained was between 0.3 and 14.4×10^8/kg of recipient body weight,[67] although the researchers did not correlate cell dose with transplantation outcome. A retrospective review of unrelated donor transplantation for the treatment of acute leukemia found that recipients of higher cell doses experienced faster neutrophil and platelet engraftment, as well as higher probability of leukemia-free survival.[75] This same group reported similar findings for patients undergoing unrelated marrow donor transplantation for the treatment of CML.[11]

Immune-mediated rejection of marrow should not occur with autologous transplantation. Some transplant groups routinely attempt to harvest cell quantities similar to those used for allografting, whereas others performing ex vivo marrow manipulation reported harvesting up to 8×10^8 cells/kg.[76] Many transplant programs have therefore focused upon in vitro measurements of hematopoietic progenitor cells. Several investigators have predicted the kinetics of hematological recovery from the quantity of hematopoietic progenitor cells reinfused in purged or unpurged autologous marrow specimens.[41, 42, 77–79]

Bone marrow harvesting is well tolerated, and may be performed even in the outpatient setting.[70, 80, 81] Major complications occur in about 0.27% of healthy allogeneic donors[67] and in up to 0.97% of autograft patients.[68] These complications include infections at the skin puncture sites, systemic infections, and complications of anesthesia. Severe hematomas and neuralgias rarely occur, but attention to pelvic anatomy is necessary to decrease the risk of damage to vessels and nerves lying under or adjacent to the iliac crest harvest sites. Localized pain is common, may last for several days, and may necessitate moderate analgesia.[82] In a survey of almost 500 donors for unrelated marrow transplantation, Stroncek and colleagues found a mean recovery time of 15.8 days, although 10% of the donors required more than 30 days to complete recovery.[64] PBSC collection is not necessarily less toxic, and comparisons of the experiences of PBSC and marrow donors are currently being conducted in phase III studies.

Anemia is also common, resulting from both the pretransplantation blood loss during donor evaluation and the harvest procedures. The usual volume harvested from healthy donors is about 10 to 15 mL of marrow per kilogram of recipient body weight. Thus the average donor for an adult recipient may lose 800 to 1000 mL of blood. Most donors receive blood transfusions, and the routine use of pretransplantation autologous blood storage decreases the risk of transfusion infections. With proper preharvest blood storage, the use of homologous blood for allogeneic donors should be extremely rare. Donors undergoing a second harvesting shortly after the first are more likely to require homologous blood.[83] The quantity of marrow harvested from autologous marrow recipients may be greater than that harvested from healthy allogeneic donors, reflecting previous chemotherapy given to these patients as well as protocol design (some protocols require larger volumes because of anticipated losses from ex vivo processing). Salvage of red blood cells (which would otherwise be discarded before marrow cryopreservation) from autologous bone marrow grafts has been reported by some centers.[84] No complications were reported for the 25 recipients of red cells salvaged from these autologous marrow specimens in one study, although the risks of marrow bacterial contamination resulting from the open harvest technique,[85] and possibly of fat embolism, require careful consideration.

Prospective donors must be assessed for their risk of anesthesia complications, as well as for their suitability as blood donors. Proper preharvest evaluation of donor anesthesia risk probably accounts for the limited morbidity reported to date for this procedure. All donors must also be evaluated with the criteria currently applied to blood donors.[86] Numerous infectious diseases that would not exclude the donor from blood donation, such as cytomegalovirus, may be transmitted with the allograft.[87] Donors who would otherwise be excluded for health reasons from donating blood for transfusion (e.g., because of previous history of hepatitis) may still be eligible to donate bone marrow if the needs of the recipient outweigh the risks of disease transmission. Abnormalities of the donor's bone marrow also can be transmitted to the recipient, as illustrated by the unusual transplantation of donor leukemia not detected during initial evaluation of the donor.[88]

BONE MARROW INFUSION

The infusion of fresh bone marrow is generally well tolerated if the infusion is slow enough to allow for clearance of cells and microembolic material from the pulmonary microvasculature and for metabolism of the heparin used for anticoagulation. Potential complications from infusion of allogeneic marrow are as follows:

- Volume overload
- Allergic reactions to blood components or marrow additives
- Acute or delayed hemolysis from red blood cell (e.g., ABO) incompatibility
- Excessive anticoagulation
- Pulmonary embolism of fat or particulates from unfiltered marrow

Some complications, such as ABO nonidentity, may be intentional, as in mismatched transplantation, or may result from improper identification of the product or the recipient. Thus it is imperative that the general principles of blood transfusion be followed by marrow transplant services.

Although microemboli have been detected in patients after marrow infusion,[61] their presence does not appear to have clinically significant sequelae. A small but statistically significant decrease in lung volume, but not in diffusion capacity, occurs with marrow infusion.[89] The decrease probably results from trapping of marrow cells or fat globules in the pulmonary vasculature. A large proportion of the fat can be removed by simple centrifugation of the marrow and removal of the plasma before transplantation; this procedure should be considered for marrow specimens containing large volumes of fat. Plasma or red cell depletion may also be necessary to avoid infusion of excessive volumes of marrow into small recipients.

Infusion-related toxic effects are commonly observed during the reinfusion of cells cryopreserved in dimethylsulfoxide (DMSO). The incidence of symptoms is related to the volume reinfused, and symptoms are generally of minor severity. Anaphylaxis and cardiac arrest have been temporally associated with the infusion of cells cryopreserved in DMSO, but these events are extremely rare. The use of an in-line blood filter during infusion prevents the embolism of clumps that may form during the cryopreservation procedure.

BONE MARROW PROCESSING

Isolation of Hematopoietic Progenitor Cells

Bone marrow hematopoietic progenitors can be isolated in the buffy coat fraction of the marrow. This first step in preparing autologous marrow specimens for cryopreservation may also be used to deplete red cells from allogeneic marrow specimens for ABO-mismatched transplantation or to reduce volume or the content of fat. Any of a number of blood cell processors or large-capacity centrifuges commercially available may be adapted for isolation of buffy coat cells (or further purified cell populations) from the marrow with the use of published techniques.[90] The number of nucleated cells recovered depends on the technique used and may range from 40% to more than 80%. Virtually all mononuclear cells and CFU-GM are recovered.

Further purification of hematopoietic progenitor cells may be required for some ex vivo purging techniques. Density-gradient centrifugation can separate hematopoietic progenitors from most of the mature blood elements collected as part of the buffy coat. Separation with Percoll or Ficoll-Hypaque (or similar compounds) results in a product containing fairly uniform cell populations, thus decreasing this source of variability in some purge procedures. Between 25% and 30% of nucleated cells are recovered with use of a gradient with a specific density of 1.077 g/mL. Additional processing beyond buffy coat isolation increases the risk of microbial contamination and loss of product, but these risks appear minimal if good laboratory practices are maintained. Commercial products for isolation of hematopoietic progenitor cells are now available.[91]

HSC express the CD34 antigen.[92, 93] Although the function of this cell surface glycoprotein is not fully defined, its level of expression is inversely correlated with the maturational stage of the cell. Thus, virtually all marrow HSC and most of the committed progenitor cells can be isolated in the approximately 1.5% of the marrow cells expressing this antigen.[92] These cells appear more primitive, as shown by in vitro cultures[94–96] and ability to give rise to committed progenitors in culture.[97–99] Berenson and associates reported the successful transplantation in nonhuman primates, using marrow enriched for CD34$^+$ cells.[100] The primates that received marrow cells depleted of CD34$^+$ cells did not sustain engraftment. Berenson and associates subsequently reported on a series of 10 patients being treated for breast carcinoma who received CD34-enriched marrow specimens.[101] The median of 40 days to achieve a granulocyte count above 500/μL in the peripheral blood probably reflected complications from other steps in the processing, because changes in the cryopreservation technique used shortened the period of aplasia to about 20 days. Cell separation devices are now commercially available. One such device uses the biotin-avidin system developed by Berenson and associates.[102] Others use immunomagnetic techniques.[103, 104]

ABO-Mismatched Transplantation

The inheritance of ABO blood group isoantigens is independent of HLA antigens, so an HLA-matched sibling donor is commonly of a blood group different from that of the recipient. Blood group (and other red cell) determinants are not major histocompatibility antigens. Also, primitive lymphohematopoietic stem cells do not express blood group antigens.[105, 106] Thus, red blood cell incompatibility does not preclude allogeneic transplantation. Appropriate steps must be taken to avoid acute or delayed hemolytic reactions during transplantation involving either major incompatibility (recipient has antibodies directed against donor blood group isoantigens) or minor incompatibility (donor has antibodies directed against host blood group isoantigens).

The most obvious concern arising from major red blood cell incompatibility in transplantation is the risk of a hemolytic transfusion reaction resulting from the infusion of large quantities of red blood cells in the harvested marrow. Because of initial reluctance to manipulate the marrow and thereby possibly to increase the risk of engraftment failure, early ABO-mismatched transplantations were preceded by extensive plasmapheresis of the recipient (with or without infusion of incompatible red cells) to decrease the recipient's isoagglutinin titer.[107–111] This step avoided marrow manipulation and the possible loss or damage of HSC necessary for engraftment, but it could have resulted in delayed hemolysis of the incompatible donor red cells if the isoagglutinin titer rebounded.[112]

Subsequently, sedimentation techniques to deplete the marrow of red blood cells ex vivo were developed and shown to be effective and safe.[113–115] Using a Haemonetics Cell Separator, Braine and colleagues[113] were able to collect buffy coat cells containing an average of about 20 mL of incompatible red cells. The infusions were well tolerated (although their patients were prophylactically medicated in anticipation of hemolytic reactions to the small quantities of red cells infused). The switch from recipient to donor blood type occurs over several weeks and can be monitored by standard laboratory assays; meanwhile, recipients of ABO-incompatible marrow specimens must be transfused with group O red cells to avoid serious hemolysis from either donor-derived or residual recipient isoagglutinin. Recipient isoagglutinin may persist for several weeks to years after ABO-mismatched transplantation.[116–118] Although granulocyte and platelet recoveries are not delayed in ABO-incompatible transplantation, the recovery of reticulocytes is slowed, and patients require more red cell transfusions than do recipients of ABO-matched marrow specimens.[113, 119]

Anti-D and other rhesus antigens also appear late in erythroid differentiation.[120] Therefore, incompatibility for these red cell antigens also does not preclude allogeneic transplantation. Although the donor marrow must be depleted of red cells if the recipient has detectable antibodies directed against donor red blood cell antigens,[121] the delayed-type hemolytic reaction seen with minor ABO incompatibility does not appear to occur in the setting of rhesus antibody (Rh) incompatibility. Red cell support may be from Rh-positive or Rh-negative donors when the donor and recipient are not identical for these red blood cell antigens. However, for Rh-negative pairs, it is important to avoid exposure to Rh-positive blood components, especially for young female recipients, who may maintain ovarian function after transplantation.

Minor ABO-mismatched marrow specimens are frequently concentrated (plasma-depleted) to decrease the quantity of donor isoagglutinin infused. If the donor has high isoagglutinin titers, this step may prevent low-grade hemolysis. Affected patients do not have an evident delay in recovery of the erythroid lineage. A delayed hemolytic reaction resulting from the transient production of isoagglutinin by donor lymphocytes infused with the marrow may occur between 7 and 14 days after transplantation.[122] It is essential that recipient type red cell transfusions be avoided, in order to avoid this potentially fatal complication.

The engraftment failures in recipients of ABO-mismatched transplants reported in early trials of allogeneic transplantation probably resulted from the use of inadequate immunosuppressive conditioning regimens, because the risks of engraftment failure were not significantly different in matched and mismatched patients. Currently, neither engraftment failure nor increased risk of GVHD is believed to result from ABO-mismatched transplants,[107, 113, 114, 123, 124] although one group reported a higher incidence of GVHD in recipients of ABO-mismatched marrow specimens (especially for minor ABO-mismatches).[125]

Transfusion support in the setting of red blood cell incompatibility requires attention to recipient and donor isoagglutinins and donor lymphocytes contained in the stem cell inoculum to avoid acute or delayed hemolysis (Table 23–1). Viable lymphocytes in the marrow inoculum are capable of transiently producing donor type antibodies. This usually is clinically important only if third-party red cell infusions of recipient blood type are administered during the first few weeks after transplantation. Because of the potential suppressive effects of isoagglutinins on

Table 23–1. Blood Component Support for ABO-Incompatible Transplantation

Blood Group	Recipient	Donor	Red Blood Cell	Platelets First Choice	Platelets Second Choice	Plasma	Granulocytes
ABO Major	O	A	O*	A	AB	A, AB	O
	O	B	O*	B	AB	B, AB	O
	O	AB	O*	AB	A,* B*	AB	O
	A	AB	A,* O*	AB	A,* B*	AB	A, O
	B	AB	B,* O*	AB	A,* B*	AB	B, O
ABO Minor	A	O	O*	A	AB	A, AB	O
	B	O	O*	B	AB	B, AB	O
	AB	O	O*	AB	A,* B*	AB	O
	AB	A	A,* O*	AB	A,* B*	AB	A, O
	AB	B	B,* O*	AB	A,* B*	AB	B, O
ABO Major and Minor	A	B	O*	AB	A,* B*	AB	O
	B	A	O*	AB	B,* A*	AB	O

*Reduced volume or washed components or components from donors with low isoagglutinin titers.

red cell engraftment, the infusion of plasma-containing blood products with high titers of antibodies directed against donor type red cells should also be avoided.

Somatic Cell Therapy

Somatic cell therapy refers to the processing of cell components to develop a biological therapeutic product that differs from the original cell collection. For example, such products may be genetically manipulated, or contain selectively expanded cells to provide enhanced engraftment or immunological response to malignant or infectious diseases.[126–129] Somatic cell therapies are currently undergoing considerable clinical investigation.

T Lymphocyte Depletion of Allogeneic Marrow

GVHD, in both acute and chronic forms, continues to be a major cause of morbidity and mortality after allogeneic transplantation. Even with the use of prophylactic regimens that include cyclosporine, the incidence of severe, acute GVHD in matched-sibling transplant recipients may exceed 35%.[130, 131] The incidence is higher for mismatched transplantation, rising to more than 75% in haploidentical transplant recipients.[132] The incidence in unrelated donors is higher than for related donors for the same degree of tissue match because of differences in minor transplant antigens not tested for in donor selection. It has been recognized for many years that mature T lymphocytes transferred with the bone marrow are the cause of this complication. Hence, many transplant programs developed T cell–depletion techniques, attempting to reduce the risk of this complication of transplantation.

T cell depletion effectively reduces the risk of severe acute GVHD and probably chronic GVHD, although most techniques have not been studied in randomized trials. Wagner and associates.[133] reported no severe (grade 2 or higher) GVHD for 21 evaluable recipients of marrow specimens with T cells depleted by centrifugal elutriation; Schattenberg and colleagues[134] reported a GVHD incidence of 15% for 75 evaluable patients receiving similarly treated marrow specimens. A 17% actuarial probability of severe GVHD was reported for recipients of T cell–depleted, HLA-matched transplants from unrelated donors,[135] which is lower than that noted in historical experience with similar patients receiving nondepleted marrow specimens. In one randomized study using anti–T cell antibodies and complement, the incidence of GVHD was lower, but a survival advantage was not seen for recipients of the T cell–depleted marrow specimens, because of an increased incidence of engraftment failure and relapse.[136]

It is possible to correlate the occurrence of severe acute GVHD with the number of residual lymphocytes infused with the marrow.[133, 137, 138] Lymphocyte doses of less than 1 to 5 × 10^5/kg of recipient body weight incur less risk of GVHD. An optimal dose of lymphocytes has not been determined, however. The occurrence and severity of GVHD also relate to the degree of compatibility for both HLA and non-HLA antigens. The degree of HLA compatibility may be useful in determining the role for and extent of T cell depletion. Partial depletion of T cells may be adequate to decrease the severity or risk of acute GVHD in matched related patients, whereas more extensive depletion may be necessary for more disparate transplants. Unfortunately, the extent to which T cells need to be removed remains uncertain: although the number of T cells is predictive of GVHD in some studies, there is considerable overlap in the occurrence of this complication. Also, similar correlations of T cell number in infused marrow with the risks of graft failure or disease relapse have not been found.

A variety of approaches have been developed to deplete T cells or T cell subsets (Table 23–2). These involve physical or immunological techniques to separate lymphocytes from hematopoietic progenitor cells capable of depleting 2 to 3 "logs" (99% to 99.9%) of the lymphocytes contained in the marrow inoculum. No approach has been shown to be particularly advantageous with regard to long-term, disease-free survival, although considerable effort has been made to determine the phenotype of the cells that facilitate engraftment without causing GVHD. Depletion of selected T cell subpopulations has been used by some groups in an attempt to attain a lower risk for acute GVHD while avoiding the complications of T cell depletion. In humans, both $CD4^+$ and $CD8^+$ cells

Table 23–2. T Cell–Depletion Techniques

Technique	Selected References
Physical Depletion	
Counterflow elutriation/centrifugation	133, 134
Soybean lectin agglutinin	228
Sheep erythrocyte rosettes	229
Immunological Depletion	
Complement-mediated	135, 150
Immunotoxin	230
Immunomagnetic	231
Enrichment Techniques	
CD34$^+$ cell enrichment	25

may initiate GVHD, in response to differences in class II and class I antigens, respectively.[139] Whether specific subsets of T cells are separately responsible for GVHD, the GVL effect, and the engraftment of marrow remains unknown.

The major complications of T cell–depleted marrow grafts are increased risks of engraftment failure, relapse, B cell neoplasms and infections. The much higher rates of relapse and the slightly higher rates of engraftment failure result in disease-free survival rates comparable to those in studies without T cell depletion. Failure of sustained engraftment of T cell–depleted marrow specimens occurs in 5% to 10% of patients. Murine studies demonstrated that donor T cells prevent rejection by eliminating or inactivating recipient T cells that survive the conditioning regimen.[140, 141] Prevention of engraftment failure depends on the degree of host immunosuppression achieved by the conditioning regimen. In one study using a cocktail of eight monoclonal antibodies and complement, 7 of 11 patients had engraftment failure after conditioning with a regimen that included 12 Gy of total-body irradiation. The failure rate for the same ex vivo treatment in patients conditioned with 15.75 Gy was one of nine patients, which indicates that residual host immunity was responsible at least in part for the higher failure rate observed in some studies.[142] Alternatively, increasing the quantity of HSC infused[25] or the intensity of the post-transplantation immunosuppression may be used.[143] It has been proposed that the infusion of irradiated peripheral blood cells from the marrow donor may decrease the risk of engraftment failure after transplantation of T cell–depleted marrow.[144]

A GVL effect has been associated with the occurrence of GVHD, presumably resulting from T lymphocytes that are infused with the marrow.[145–147] Depletion of T cells increases the risk of relapse, especially for patients treated for CML.[147, 148] Relapse rates may be several times higher than for comparable patients experiencing GVHD. Fixed doses of lymphocytes, as opposed to maximal T cell depletion, may also reduce the risk of graft failure.[149] Again, it is uncertain whether the GVL effect and GVHD can be separated by manipulation of T cell subsets in the marrow inoculum. It is interesting, however, that Champlin and coworkers,[150] using monoclonal antibodies and complement, reduced CD8$^+$ cells from an average of 29% to less than 1% of the infused cells. Although 4 of their 36 patients had failure to engraft or failure to sustain engraftment, none of the 13 patients with CML relapsed. The incidence of severe GVHD was 28%.

Depletion of Tumor Cells From Autologous Marrow

The harvesting and storage of a patient's own bone marrow for subsequent use *(autologous bone marrow transplantation)* is an alternative to allogeneic and syngeneic transplantation for patients lacking appropriate sibling or unrelated donors. The same principles hold for autologous as for allogeneic transplantation for the treatment of malignancy: the cancer being treated must be sensitive in a dose-responsive manner to the therapy being administered. In addition, the source of marrow HSC must be free of disease. For autologous transplantation, these principles are much more problematic, in that many dose-responsive malignancies either are diseases of the bone marrow or involve the bone marrow at some point during their natural course. Contamination of harvested marrow by tumor cells conceivably may result in disseminated relapse of disease when reinfused. This has led to considerable interest in developing techniques of ex vivo marrow manipulation capable of effectively depleting malignant cells from the marrow inoculum.

The necessity for and efficacy of ex vivo tumor cell depletion of autologous bone marrow (purging) are controversial questions. No group has yet reported the results of a randomized trial directly comparing the disease-free survival rates for recipients of purged and unpurged marrow specimens. Instead, the rationale for purging has historically been based on the argument that marrow specimens harvested from patients with incurable diseases involving the marrow (e.g., acute leukemia in second or subsequent remission) invariably contain malignant cells. Other diseases, such as non-Hodgkin's lymphoma and breast cancer, usually involve the bone marrow in their later stages, and so marrow specimens harvested from patients with end-stage disease would also almost certainly contain malignant cells.

The probability that tumor cell contamination of the bone marrow component can contribute to relapse after autologous bone marrow transplantation was demonstrated in studies involving genetically marked marrow cells for patients with AML,[151] neuroblastoma,[152] and CML.[153] In all three series, tumor cells containing the inserted genetic material were found in patients who experienced relapse after transplantation. The level of marked cells detected was very low and these studies cannot conclude that the cell inoculum was the sole source of malignant cells causing the disease relapse. However, the implications of these studies are that the infusion of marrow tumor cells is detrimental to the recipient and that purging, if without undue toxicity, may be beneficial to a subset of patients whose marrow may be contaminated by tumor cells. Techniques for measuring tumor contamination must be capable of detecting minimal levels of contamination. Morphological examination with light microscopy is not adequate for detecting cells that may be present only at levels of 1 cell/10^6 or less. Sensitive immunocytostaining techniques,[154] clonal assays,[155] flow cytometric analysis,[156] and polymerase chain reaction (PCR) amplification of malignant genetic material[157] detect tumor cells in the bone marrow components of many patients with a variety of malignancies. In general, the incidence of contamination (number of patients with positive components) and the level of contamination (number of tumor cells per number of normal cells) is much less for PBSC than for marrow components,[154] although this has not been a consistent finding in all studies.[155] Whether patients with PBSC transplants have a lower relapse rate than do those receiving bone marrow is not known. It will be difficult to design appropriate phase III studies of this question and to enroll patients in them, because of the current general acceptance of PBSC as the component of choice for autologous transplantation.

Evidence demonstrating efficacy and clinical benefit of purging is indirect and sparse. A dose-related response to 4-HC used in the purging of marrow specimens for patients with AML has been suggested.[158] In that study, patients with a greater loss of normal myeloid progenitor cells grown in in vitro cultures (CFU-GM) and longer post-transplantation aplasias were less likely to relapse. The same group also reported that in patients with AML who were in remission and undergoing harvest for autologous transplantation, the probability of post-transplantation relapse was predicted by the sensitivity to 4-HC of leukemia cells cloned in vitro (colony-forming unit for leukemia [CFU-L]) from marrow specimens.[159] Patients whose tumors were sensitive to 4-HC in this in vitro test had a lower probability of relapse after transplantation. A significantly higher probability of disease-free survival was found for recipients of mafosfamide-purged marrow specimens treated for AML if the recipients underwent harvest and transplantation early in first remission.[160] Gribben and associates correlated residual lymphoma cells after immunological purging with subsequent disease relapse.[161]

None of these arguments, however, is conclusive. Malignant cells cloned in vitro from marrow specimens may not represent the tumor cells responsible for disease relapse; moreover, the quantity of malignant cells necessary to cause relapse is unknown. The clinical trials of activated cyclophosphamide purging were not randomized and were possibly subject to patient selection bias. Regardless, it can probably be assumed that ex vivo purging may benefit selected patients undergoing autologous bone marrow transplantation. The challenges are to identify these patients and to develop effective preparative and purging regimens that are adequately cytotoxic to residual disease in both the host and the marrow, respectively.

A variety of techniques have been developed for purging of autologous bone marrow specimens. The criteria for tumor cell purging, the same as those for any marrow processing technique, are as follows:

- Little or nonlimiting HSC toxicity
- Differential effects on desired and undesired cell populations
- Independent of cell cycle
- Purging agent nontoxic for in vivo use or removable from marrow inoculum

In theory, tumor cell–purging techniques should be capable of removing virtually all contaminating tumor cells. Immunological techniques are most commonly employed for the purging of nonmyeloid malignancies. Pharmacological techniques depend on differential effects upon normal and malignant progenitor cells. Physical techniques, such as density separation[162] and cryopreservation,[163, 164] do not discriminate malignant from normal cells adequately enough to be effective.

Monoclonal antibody–based techniques of purging malignant cells are most easily developed for those diseases in which the tumor cells express cell surface antigens not found on HSC. Those cells binding the antibody can then be killed by incubation with complement[165–167] or internalization of a toxin molecule bound to the antibody[168] or can be depleted by binding to magnetic beads.[169] The major difficulty with monoclonal antibody purging is the heterogeneity of antigen expression by the malignant cells.[170] This may be overcome by combining multiple antibodies directed against different antigens and by multiple cycles of treatment.[171, 172] The benefit is selectivity: with proper screening of antibodies and other reagents, normal HSC toxicity should not occur. Ideally, these techniques should spare the hematopoietic progenitors, resulting in little or no delay in marrow recovery.

Immunological techniques may also be used to enrich HSC, possibly thereby achieving a tumor-free inoculum without toxicity to normal hematopoietic progenitors. HSC express the CD34 antigen, and this characteristic can be used to separate normal cells from tumor cells that lack this antigen. The enrichment of $CD34^+$ cells from about 1% to between 70% and 90% of the cells contained in the marrow inoculum results in a considerable, nonspecific depletion of tumor cells. Despite the depletion of more than 99% of the nontarget cells, however, sensitive tumor detection techniques can still demonstrate the presence of malignant cells.[103] The immunomagnetic techniques are ideally suited to combination purging, involving enrichment of $CD34^+$ cells and subsequent depletion of cells expressing tumor cell antigens. For B cell malignancies, this may achieve an additional 10- to 100-fold depletion of tumor cells.[173] The loss of immunologically active cells raises the question of possible loss of any immunity against tumor relapse, as well as a possible increased risk of viral infections after transplantation.[49–51] This effect has not been noted in the limited clinical trials published to date.

Bone marrow may also be purged with pharmacological agents, taking advantage of the difference in sensitivities of malignant and normal HSC. Agents chosen are selected for being nontoxic to stem cells and not cycle specific. Derivatives of cyclophosphamide, active in vitro, have been most commonly used to date. The feasibility of pharmacological purging was first demonstrated with 4-HC in a rat model of leukemia.[174] In that model, increasing doses of 4-HC resulted first in longer periods before death from leukemia, and then, at higher concentrations, in survival of the rat. Investigators at Johns Hopkins Hospital subsequently reported a phase I trial of ex vivo 4-HC purging in which they determined a maximal achievable concentration of 100 μg/mL.[175] A dose-dependent response for duration of aplasia was demonstrated, but the limited numbers of patients with various diagnoses did not allow discovery of a similar relationship for disease-free survival. Such a relationship was later indirectly suggested when these investigators demonstrated that the survival of CFU-GM through the purge technique reflected the cytotoxicity of 4-HC to both normal and leukemic stem cells[77, 158, 176]; this led to a recommendation that incubation of bone marrow with 4-HC be performed under carefully controlled conditions of cell concentration in order to achieve more uniform results.[177]

Mafosfamide is another activated oxazaphosphorine most commonly used in Europe.[160, 178, 179] Phase II studies with both 4-HC and mafosfamide demonstrated the feasibility of treating marrow specimens ex vivo with these agents.[76, 179, 180] Combinations of agents may increase efficacy without increasing the toxicity of the ex vivo purge. Chang and associates, using an in vitro model of tumor and normal hematopoietic cells, suggested that the addition of etoposide would enhance tumor cell cytotoxicity while protecting the normal hematopoietic cells.[181] Vincristine appears to have similar effects.[182] The combination of 4-HC, vincristine, and methylprednisolone sodium succinate was used by the Johns Hopkins group in a phase I study.[183] The addition of vincristine and the corticosteroid did not require a decrease in the 4-HC concentration. They showed no additional cytotoxicity to CFU-GM cloned from these marrow specimens, but they did find a five-log increase in CFU-L killing. Other groups explored two-drug combinations[184] or combinations of 4-HC or other drugs with monoclonal antibodies.[168, 169] Autologous bone marrow transplantation is frequently characterized by a delay in hematological recovery, in comparison with allogeneic transplantation. This is especially true for marrow specimens purged ex vivo with pharmacological agents, and the delay may vary by diagnosis.[30] The median times for granulocyte recovery (500 or more granulocytes/μL) were 39 days for patients with AML receiving marrow specimens purged with 4-HC but 19 days for patients with non-Hodgkin's lymphoma. Numerous patient, marrow, and post-transplantation variables or events can influence the kinetics of engraftment and the probability of engraftment failure.

CRYOPRESERVATION

A fundamental requirement of autologous bone marrow transplantation is the successful storage of adequate numbers of HSC during the administration of the preparative regimen. Cryopreservation of marrow can be successfully achieved, as evidenced by the lack of reports of engraftment failure attributed to proper low-temperature storage of adequate quantities of marrow cells. Cryopreservation of the marrow is not required if the period of storage is less than 7–10 days. However, progressive loss of progenitor cells occurs for marrow specimens stored in vitro, with reported CFU-GM survival rates after 4 days at 4°C ranging from 44% to 97%.[185–188] HSC appear to maintain viability for several days after collection if carefully stored. In a study by Preti and colleagues, the progressive loss of myeloid (CFU-GM) progenitor cells with storage at 4°C did not equal the immediate loss of 33% incurred during cryopreservation and thawing.[188] Cells stored at 4°C showed a progressive, linear loss of total nucleated cells, cell viability, and CFU-GM, but the difference for the myeloid progenitor cells was not significant even after 9 days of refrigerated storage.

Most published reports of noncryopreserved storage describe storage at 4°C. This temperature remains stable, in comparison to storage at ambient temperatures, which can be quite variable. The optimal temperature is not known and will probably depend on such concerns as the source of HSC, prestorage processing, cell concentration, buffering capacity of the solution, and the gas-diffusion capacity of the storage container. One report describes better survival of HSC stored at 37°C and at 25°C than at 4°C.[189] These warmer storage temperatures are comparable to techniques being developed for the in vitro expansion of HSC. None of these studies entailed marrow reconstitution as the experimental end point. The conflicting reports are, therefore, difficult to interpret.

There is limited experience with the autologous transplantation of noncryopreserved HSC. Used primarily in conjunction with high-dose melphalan or cyclophosphamide conditioning,[185, 188, 190–192] refrigerated storage was supplanted by cryopreservation as most transplant centers developed multiday conditioning regimens. In a nonrandomized retrospective analysis by Preti and colleagues, the engraftment kinetics of 54 patients who received cryopreserved marrow cells were compared with those of 45 patients who received refrigerated cells.[188] The refrigerated cells were stored for a median of 4 days (range, 3 to 9). The cryopreserved cells were stored a median of 69 days (range, 5 to 981) at −80°C with a cryoprotectant mixture of DMSO and hydroxyethyl starch (HES). Almost all patients were conditioned with a regimen consisting of bischloroethylnitrosourea (BCNU), etoposide, and cyclophosphamide. Preti and colleagues found no significant difference between engraftment kinetics of these two groups, although a small difference would not have been detected with the limited numbers of patients in this study.

Although cryopreservation results in an immediate loss of some proportion of HSC, the loss is not progressive over storage duration if the storage conditions are appropriate. The other major advantage of cryopreservation is the greater flexibility in timing of transplantation in relation to collection of bone marrow, including the ability to modify or postpone a conditioning regimen already started. Storage conditions for nonfrozen storage have not been tested in an engraftment model, so proper storage conditions are not adequately defined. For laboratories intending to store marrow cells for prolonged periods without freezing, rigorous validation of the storage conditions must be pursued.

Cryopreservation Theory

Glycerol was the first effective cryoprotectant for mammalian cells described[193]; the cryoprotectant properties of DMSO were described 10 years later.[194] Virtually all transplant centers currently use DMSO because glycerol must be removed before marrow infusion, because it is difficult to wash the glycerol from the thawed marrow without excessive cell clumping, and because in vitro studies show better rates of cryosurvival with DMSO.

Both glycerol and DMSO depress the freezing temperature through colligative properties: that is, properties dependent upon the number of molecules in solution. The current understanding of cryobiology is that ice crystal formation during cooling is the primary cause of cell damage.[195] This damage can be classified into two categories: (1) At rapid rates of cooling, intracellular ice crystals may form, resulting in *mechanical* disruption of the cell and immediate cell death. (2) At slower rates of cooling, ice crystal formation preferentially occurs in the extracellular space, resulting in increasing osmolality as free water is incorporated into the growing ice crystals. This loss of free water results in the concentration of extracellular solutes such as sodium that do not freely penetrate the cell membrane, in extreme hyperosmolality, and in *dehydration* injury. For example, the molality of NaCl in a saline solution at −10°C is about 5.3 mol, and at −20°C, about 10.5 mol. Progressive dehydration with concentration of intracellular solutes prevents supercooling of intracellular water and protects the cells from the formation of intracellular ice crystals.

Glycerol and DMSO are colligative cryoprotectants that prevent dehydration injury by moderating the increased concentration of nonpenetrating extracellular solutes during ice formation. *Colligative* refers to properties dependent on the number of particles (solute), not on the composition of the particles. The freezing point of water is depressed by the addition of solute. For any particular mixture of solute and water, there is a defined temperature at which ice crystals can form. Unlike pure water, ice crystal growth in aqueous solutions occurs over a temperature range. The incorporation of water into growing ice crystals results in concentration of the solute and further depression of the freezing temperature of the remaining water, thereby preventing additional ice formation unless further cooling occurs. Temperature defines the equilibrium between ice and the nonfrozen solution. The molality of a solution in equilibrium with ice, therefore, is determined by the temperature of the solution, not the initial concentration of the solute.[196]

A saline solution at −20°C has a NaCl molality of about 10.5 mol. For a three-component system such as DMSO and NaCl in water, both solutes will contribute to the molality of the unfrozen solution in the same relative proportion found in the initial solution. The molality (before freezing) of 10% DMSO (v/v) in normal saline (140 mM) solution is about 1.6 mol, with DMSO contributing about 10 times the molality contributed by NaCl to the medium. At −20°C, this molal ratio between DMSO and NaCl will be maintained. The molality contributed by NaCl will be about 1.05 mol, or about seven times the molality of NaCl in a solution without ice. DMSO freely penetrates the HSC cell membrane so that the intracellular concentration of DMSO will equal the extracellular concentration throughout the temperature range. The addition of a penetrating cryoprotectant to an aqueous saline solution therefore reduces the osmotic stress across the cell membrane at −20°C from about 75 times to about 7 times that of an ice-free solution. According to this theory, colligative cryoprotectants must be capable of permeating the cell and must be nontoxic to the cells at the high concentration required for this effect.

Colligative properties do not explain the cryoprotection achieved by freezing cells in solutions of macromolecules such as HES. Solutions of high-molecular-weight polymeric cryoprotectants contain relatively few particles and, moreover, do not freely penetrate the cell. These cryoprotectants may protect the cell by forming a viscous, glassy shell that retards the movement of water, thereby preventing progressive dehydration as water is incorporated into the extracellular ice crystals.[197]

Macromolecular cryoprotectants may be used as single agents, but the major focus in the study of HSC cryopreservation with extracellular cryoprotectants has been their use in combination with penetrating cryoprotectants. In one early study, the addition of polyvinylpyrrolidone (PVP), another macromolecular cryoprotectant, to glycerol or DMSO improved the cryopreservation of murine cells, in comparison with the use of a penetrating agent alone.[198] Stiff and associates froze human cells in a combination of 5% DMSO, 6% HES, and 4% human serum albumin, and reported improved progenitor cell survival as determined using in vitro cultures.[199] They subsequently used this mixture of cryoprotectants to cryopreserve the marrow of 60 patients successfully.[200] No engraftment failure was attributed to this technique,[200] nor did engraftment failure occur after the similar cryopreservation of peripheral blood-derived HSC.[201] Only one comparative clinical study between DMSO/HES and DMSO alone has been reported.[202] That trial, limited to 12 patients receiving PBSC transplants in each arm of the study, did not detect any difference in the kinetics of engraftment. The small number of patients enrolled, however, limits the power of the study to detect small differences.

Long-Term Storage

Marrow specimens are stored below −120°C in either mechanical freezers or nitrogen refrigerators (either in the vapor phase or by liquid immersion). Whether prolonged storage at these temperatures deleteriously affects engraftment kinetics is not known. The duration of storage may be indefinite if adequate temperatures are maintained and appropriate cryopreservation technique is used. Evidence supporting this premise is found in both laboratory and clinical experience. Parker and coworkers found no loss of CFU-C after storage of human marrow in vapor-phase nitrogen for a median of 42 months.[203] Furthermore, limited numbers of patients have received HSC components stored for prolonged periods of time. One report of experience from multiple centers reported transplantation of cells stored for up to 11 years.[204] In that study of 33 patients, however, the median duration of storage was only 2.8 years, the authors did not correlate duration of storage with engraftment kinetics or other markers of HSC survival, and some components were treated ex vivo with mafosfamide, which is known to delay engraftment. Some patients had markedly prolonged post-transplantation aplasia (up to 119 days), and in two patients, engraftment failed. Another study reported the outcome of transplantation for 36 patients who received marrow stored for 2 to 7.8 years and found, in retrospective comparison with a control group, no differences in success or speed of engraftment.[205] The components in that report were stored either in nitrogen vapor phase refrigerators or mechanical freezers at −135°C.

Engraftment failure has been reported for canine recipients of marrow cells stored in the vapor phase of nitrogen for 18 months.[206] Storage temperatures were not monitored, however, and occasional warming from refrigerator opening or during inventory shifting could have destroyed the marrow specimens. Cells may be repetitively exposed to warming during normal operation of the refrigerator, and this warming may be progressively damaging to the HSC. The temperature gradient in the vapor phase can be minimized by constructing frames from metals with better heat conductivity such as aluminum. Rowley and Byrne found a gradient of only 5.9°C at 22 inches above the liquid when using an aluminum racking system, in comparison with a gradient of 86°C for a similar refrigerator containing a racking system constructed from steel.[207] Stability of temperature is an obvious advantage of storage in liquid nitrogen, although liquid nitrogen may serve as a reservoir for viruses.[208] This was dramatically illustrated by the transmission of hepatitis B infection to at least three patients whose cells were immersed in the same liquid nitrogen refrigerator as those of the index case.[209] Molecular typing of the virus and its isolation from the detritus of the refrigerator on subsequent investigation confirmed this mode of transmission.

Cryopreservation of Marrow for Allogeneic Transplantation

Cryopreserved HSC components are not commonly used in allogeneic transplantation. The availability of a volunteer donor obviates the cost and risks inherent with cryopreservation of cells. When concerns about the availability of the donor arise, however, collection and cryopreservation of cells may be justified. Limited experience in the allogeneic transplantation of cryopreserved marrow from related or unrelated donors has been published.[210–213] The probability and rate of engraftment were similar for recipients of cryopreserved cells and retrospective control groups of patients in the two studies that performed this analysis. Long-term survival rates of these patients also appeared similar. Eckardt and coworkers, however, found a significantly lower incidence of acute GVHD for the recipients of cryopreserved cells.[211] Stockschlader and associates found in a similar study no difference in incidence of either acute or chronic GVHD.[212] Both studies used total body irradiation (TBI) or busulfan-based conditioning regimens, and cyclosporine and methotrexate for prophylaxis against GVHD for most patients. Stockschlader and associates subsequently published their experience with cryopreserved cells from unrelated donors. The incidence of severe acute GVHD for recipients of cryopreserved marrow was 75%,[213] which is similar to the reported experience of transplantation of noncryopreserved cells from unrelated donors at a number of different centers. These data indicate that HSC intended for allogeneic transplantation may be cryopreserved but with the increased costs of the additional processing and the increased risks inherent in the use of cryopreserved cells. A potential benefit from reduced risk of GVHD proposed by one center has not been confirmed by another. For these reasons, it is likely that cryopreservation of cells from allogeneic donors will be limited to specific situations in which the practicality of having cryopreserved cells outweighs these risks.

Cryosurvival of Malignant Cells

Some investigators have suggested that cryopreservation provides a purging mechanism that will reduce the risk of relapse after autologous hematopoietic cell transplantation.[164, 214] In the first study, which used a rat model of acute myelogenous leukemia (AML), Hagenbeek and Martens demonstrated a 30% recovery of normal spleen colony-forming units (CFU-S) but only a 1.4% survival of splenic colonies derived from the leukemic cell line. Allieri and colleagues[164] cloned leukemic progenitor cells (CFU-L) from the peripheral blood of five patients with AML before and after cryopreservation and compared the recovery of these cells with the recovery of CFU-GM and BFU-E from marrow specimens from healthy donors. The percentage recovery of CFU-L was always less than half of the percentage recovery of the normal cells in a series of different cryopreservation experiments. Questions about the relevance of the models can be raised; the question of whether cryopreservation of cells reduces the risk of relapse after autologous transplantation is not answered by these two studies. The more recent demonstration, with genetically marked cells, that cryopreserved marrow components can be a source of relapse in patients treated for AML, neuroblastoma, and CML suggests that cryopreservation is not a highly efficient purging technique.[151–153]

Cryoprotectant Toxicity

A high incidence of generally mild, infusion-related morbidity with the reinfusion of cryopreserved cells has been reported by several centers.[216–218] DMSO itself has a variety of pharmacological effects,[219] which may be compounded by the presence of lysed blood cells, foreign proteins from tumor cell–purging procedures, or contaminants from nonpharmaceutical grades of reagents used in the processing. The amounts of DMSO required to kill 50% of test animals (LD_{50} values) reported for intravenous infusion of DMSO are 3.1 to 9.2 g/kg for mice and 2.5 g/kg for dogs.[220] The acute toxic dose of DMSO for humans has not been determined. If a large amount of cryopreserved material is to be infused, the infusion can be performed over 2 days, to avoid complications from infusion of excessive amounts of DMSO.

DMSO does not need to be washed from the marrow before reinfusion, although the toxicity of this agent must be recognized. The osmolality of thawed marrow (with 10% DMSO) is about 1800 mOsm/kg, so that central venous catheters are the usual route of administration. The incidence of the more common reactions appears to be related to the volume of marrow (and DMSO) infused. The infusion of large quantities of poorly cryopreserved mature blood cells may also cause renal failure.[179] Better fractionation of the marrow decreases the incidence of somatic complaints and physiological changes.

The most dramatic toxic effect is the rare anaphylactic reaction occurring during the initial administration of thawed cells. This appears to be an allergic reaction to DMSO or other components of the solution used for cryopreservation and, after resuscitation of the recipient, the remainder of the cells may be administered cautiously. Nonallergic, profound hypotension may result from the intravenous infusion of DMSO, presumably from histamine-induced vasodilatation.[219] Flushing, dyspnea, abdominal cramping, nausea, and diarrhea, reported to varying degrees after HSC infusion, can also all be attributed to DMSO-induced histamine release. These complaints resolve over a few hours and are treated symptomatically.

DMSO has a variety of cardiovascular effects. In a series of 82 patients who were premedicated with diphenhydramine, Davis and coworkers observed increased blood pressure and decreased heart rate, which were maximal about 1 hour after the completion of the marrow infusion.[216] Other authors have noted cardiac arrest or high-degree heart block occurring during or immediately after the infusion of cryopreserved marrow or PBSC.[221–224] In two series, the incidences of bradycardia (heart rate < 60 beats per minute) were 48.8% and 65%, those of second-degree heart block were 9.7% and 24%, and those of complete (third-degree) heart block were 4.8% and 5.9%.[223, 224] In both reports, the median time of onset was about 3 hours after the completion of the infusion. In one series, the authors noted that the heart block was often episodic, occurring with episodes of emesis.[223] In both series, the cardiac rhythm abnormalities resolved spontaneously within 24 hours of infusion. In contrast, Lopez-Jimenez and associates found no cardiac rhythm changes in a prospective series of 29 patients.[225] A slower overall infusion rate may have accounted for the lack of rhythm changes.

Although headache in up to 70% of recipients of cryopreserved cells has been reported,[218] other central nervous system complications are rare and generally related to the amount of DMSO infused. In two recipients who received HSC components containing a total of 225 mL and 120 mL, respectively, of DMSO, reversible encephalopathy developed.[226] The first patient underwent plasmapheresis and showed prompt improvement in mental status; the second patient recovered over 5 days without specific treatment. The weights of the patients were not cited in this report, but both patients probably received over 2 g of DMSO per kilogram of body weight. The use of DMSO to reduce cerebral edema has been associated with severe hyperosmolality in a patient who received the equivalent of about 10 g of DMSO per kilogram of body weight.[227]

CFU-GM survival rates after marrow cryopreservation have been reported to range from 0% to over 100%. A portion of the loss of CFU-GM may be artifactual, resulting from the steps necessary to remove the cryoprotectants from the thawed cells before culture. Most investigators have found that stepwise dilution to minimize osmolar shock results in better in vitro cultures, although marrow specimens are reinfused into patients without manipulation. Despite these differences, the proportion of CFU-GM surviving the cryopreservation and thaw steps appears to predict engraftment kinetics. Gorin and colleagues[179] suggested that poor cell survival (less than 50% CFU-GM survival) was predictive for delayed or failed engraftment. In studies with 4-HC–purged marrow specimens, CFU-GM survival also predicted engraftment kinetics, although no engraftment failure was reported.[176] Neither team of investigators described patient or marrow features that predicted for poor CFU-GM cryosurvival; the cause of this variability in cryosurvival of hematopoietic progenitor cells therefore remains uncertain. Nonetheless, it is evident that all storage procedures are associated with some hematopoietic progenitor cell loss that could be critical if only borderline quantities of these cells are harvested or survive other aspects of ex vivo processing. It has been suggested (on the basis of experiments using tumor-derived cell lines) that the differences in survival rates of malignant and normal cells with cryopreservation achieves a limited degree of tumor purging.[164, 214]

It has been stated that 10% DMSO is toxic to hematopoietic progenitor cells. In one study, the CFU-C survival rate fell to 76% of control levels after 5 minutes and to 23.5% of control after 60 minutes of exposure to this concentration of DMSO.[232] Later studies using a pharmaceutical grade of DMSO have failed to confirm this toxic effect,[233] which suggests that the loss of progenitor cells was not a direct result of the DMSO.

REFERENCES

1. Horowitz MM, Rowlings PA. An update from the International Bone Marrow Transplant Registry and the Autologous Blood and Marrow Transplant Registry on current activity in hematopoietic stem cell transplantation. Curr Opin Hematol 1997; 4:395.
2. Gratwohl A, Hermans J, Baldomero H. Blood and marrow transplantation activity in Europe 1995. European Group for Blood and Marrow Transplantation. Bone Marrow Transplant 1997; 19:407.
3. Antman KH, Rowlings PA, Vaughan WP, et al. High-dose chemotherapy with autologous hematopoietic stem-cell support for breast cancer in North America. J Clin Oncol 1997; 15:1870.
4. Santos GW. History of bone marrow transplantation. Clin Haematol 1983; 12:611.
5. Hurley CK. Acquisition and use of DNA-based HLA typing data in bone marrow registries. Tissue Antigens 1997; 49:323.
6. Petersdorf EW, Longton GM, Anasetti C, et al. Definition of HLA-DQ as a transplantation antigen. Proc Natl Acad Sci U S A 1996; 93:15358.
7. Nagler A, Brautbar C, Slavin S, Bishara A. Bone marrow transplantation using unrelated and family related donors: the impact of HLA-C disparity. Bone Marrow Transplant 1996; 18:891.
8. Petersdorf EW, Longton GM, Anasetti C, et al. Association of HLA-C disparity with graft failure after marrow transplantation from unrelated donors. Blood 1997; 89:1818.
9. Szydlo R, Goldman JM, Klein JP, et al. Results of allogeneic bone marrow transplants for leukemia using donors other than HLA-identical siblings. J Clin Oncol 1997; 15:1767.
10. Henslee-Downey PJ, Abhyankar SH, Parrish RS, et al. Use of partially mismatched related donors extends access to allogeneic marrow transplant. Blood 1997; 89:3864.
11. Hansen JA, Gooley TA, Martin PJ, et al. Bone marrow transplants from unrelated donors for patients with chronic myeloid leukemia. N Engl J Med 1998; 338:962.
12. Petersdorf E, Anasetti C, Servida P, et al. Effect of HLA matching

on outcome of related and unrelated donor transplantation therapy for chronic myelogenous leukemia. Hematol Oncol Clin North Am 1998; 12:107.
13. Torok-Storb B. Cellular interactions. Blood 1988; 72:373.
14. Tubiana M, Frindel E. Regulation of pluripotent stem cell proliferation and differentiation: the role of long-range humoral factors. J Cell Physiol 1982; 1(suppl 1):13.
15. Ogawa M, Porter PN, Nakahata T. Renewal and commitment to differentiation of hemopoietic stem cells (an interpretive review). Blood 1983; 61:823.
16. Gordon MY. The origin of stromal cells in patients treated by bone marrow transplantation. Bone Marrow Transplant 1988; 3:247.
17. Coulombel L, Eaves AC, Eaves CJ. Enzymatic treatment of long-term human marrow cultures reveals the preferential location of primitive hemopoietic progenitors in the adherent layer. Blood 1983; 62:291.
18. Cashman J, Eaves AC, Eaves CJ. Regulated proliferation of primitive hematopoietic progenitor cells in long-term human marrow cultures. Blood 1985; 66:1002.
19. Rafii S, Shapiro F, Pettengell R, et al. Human bone marrow microvascular endothelial cells support long-term proliferation and differentiation of myeloid and megakaryocytic progenitors. Blood 1995; 86:3353.
20. Migliaccia AR, Migliaccio G, Johnson G, et al. Comparative analysis of hematopoietic growth factors released by stromal cells from normal donors or transplanted patients. Blood 1990; 75:305.
21. Soll E, Massumoto C, Clift RA, et al. Relevance of marrow fibrosis in bone marrow transplantation: a retrospective analysis of engraftment. Blood 1995; 86:4667.
22. Juttner CA, To LB, Haylock DN, et al. Circulating autologous stem cells collected in very early remission from acute non-lymphoblastic leukaemia produce prompt but incomplete haemopoietic reconstitution after high dose melphalan or supralethal chemoradiotherapy. Br J Haematol 1985; 61:739.
23. Lopez M, Mortel O, Pouillart P, et al. Acceleration of hematopoietic recovery after autologous bone marrow transplantation by low doses of peripheral blood stem cells. Bone Marrow Transplant 1991; 7:173.
24. Slattery JT, Clift RA, Buckner CD, et al. Marrow transplantation for chronic myeloid leukemia: the influence of plasma busulfan levels on the outcome of transplantation. Blood 1997; 89:3055.
25. Aversa F, Tabilio A, Terenzi A, et al. Successful engraftment of T-cell–depleted haploidentical "three-loci" incompatible transplants in leukemia patients by addition of recombinant human granulocyte colony-stimulating factor-mobilized peripheral blood progenitor cells to bone marrow inoculum. Blood 1994; 84:3948.
26. Kersey JH, Weisdorf D, Nesbit ME, et al. Comparison of autologous and allogeneic bone marrow transplantation for treatment of high-risk refractory acute lymphoblastic leukemia. N Engl J Med 1987; 317:461.
27. Lowenburg B, Verdonck LJ, Dekker AW, et al. Autologous bone marrow transplantation in acute myeloid leukemia in first remission: results of a Dutch prospective study. J Clin Oncol 1990; 8:287.
28. Jones RJ, Piantadosi S, Mann RB, et al. High dose cytotoxic therapy and bone marrow transplantation for relapsed Hodgkin's disease. J Clin Oncol 1990; 8:527.
29. Douay L, LaPorte JP, Mary JY, et al. Difference in kinetics of haematopoietic reconstitution between ALL and ANLL after autologous bone marrow transplantation with marrow treated in vitro with mafosfamide (Asta Z 7557). Bone Marrow Transplant 1987; 2:33.
30. Rowley SD, Piantadosi S, Marcellus DC, et al. Analysis of factors predicting speed of hematologic recovery after transplantation with 4-hydroperoxycyclophosphamide–purged autologous bone marrow grafts. Bone Marrow Transplant 1991; 7:183.
31. Nemunaitis J, Rabinowe SN, Singer JW, et al. Recombinant granulocyte-macrophage colony-stimulating factor after autologous bone marrow transplantation for lymphoid cancer. N Engl J Med 1991; 324:1773.
32. Gulati SC, Bennett CL. Granulocyte-macrophage colony-stimulating factor (GM-CSF) as adjunct therapy in relapsed Hodgkin disease. Ann Intern Med 1992; 116:177.
33. Advani R, Chao NJ, Horning SJ, et al. Granulocyte-macrophage colony-stimulating factor (GM-CSF) as an adjunct to autologous hemopoietic stem cell transplantation for lymphoma. Ann Intern Med 1992; 116:183.
34. De Witte T, Gratwohl A, Van der Lely N, et al. Recombinant human granulocyte-macrophage colony-stimulating factor accelerates neutrophil and monocyte recovery after allogeneic T-cell–depleted bone marrow transplantation. Blood 1992; 79:1359.
35. Brandt SJ, Peters WP, Atwater SK, et al. Effect of recombinant human granulocyte-macrophage colony-stimulating factor on hematopoietic reconstitution after high dose chemotherapy and autologous bone marrow transplantation. N Engl J Med 1988; 318:869.
36. Blazer BR, Kersey JH, McGlave PB, et al. In vivo administration of recombinant human granulocyte/macrophage colony-stimulating factor in acute lymphoblastic leukemia patients receiving purged autografts. Blood 1989; 73:849.
37. Siena S, Bregni M, Brando B, et al. Circulation of $CD34^+$ hematopoietic stem cells in the peripheral blood of high-dose cyclophosphamide–treated patients: enhancement by intravenous recombinant human granulocyte-macrophage colony-stimulating factor. Blood 1989; 74:1905.
38. Molineux G, Pojda Z, Hampson IN, et al. Transplantation potential of peripheral blood stem cells induced by granulocyte colony-stimulating factor. Blood 1990; 76:2153.
39. Isola LM, Scigliano E, Skerrett D, et al. A pilot study of allogeneic bone marrow transplantation using related donors stimulated with G-CSF. Bone Marrow Transplant 1997; 20:1033.
40. Weisdorf D, Jiller J, Verfaillie C, et al. Cytokine-primed bone marrow stem cells vs. peripheral blood stem cells for autologous transplantation: a randomized comparison of GM-CSF vs. G-CSF. Biol of Blood and Marrow Transplant 1997; 3:217.
41. Douay L, Gorin NC, Mary JY, et al. Recovery of CFU-GM from cryopreserved marrow and in vivo evaluation after autologous bone marrow transplantation are predictive of engraftment. Exp Hematol 1986; 14:358.
42. Spitzer G, Verma DS, Fisher R, et al. The myeloid progenitor cell—its value in predicting hematopoietic recovery after autologous bone marrow transplantation. Blood 1980; 55:317.
43. Torres A, Alonso MC, Gomez-Villagran JLG, et al. No influence of number of donor CFU-GM on granulocyte recovery in bone marrow transplantation for acute leukemia. Blut 1985; 50:89.
44. Atkinson K, Norrie S, Chan P, et al. Lack of correlation between nucleated bone marrow cell dose, marrow CFU-GM dose or marrow CFU-E dose and the rate of HLA-identical sibling marrow engraftment. Br J Haematol 1985; 60:245.
45. Lum LG. The kinetics of immune reconstitution after human marrow transplantation. Blood 1987; 69:369.
46. Witherspoon RP, Lum LG, Storb R. Immunologic reconstitution after human marrow grafting. Semin Hematol 1984; 21:2.
47. Small TN, Keever CA, Weiner-Fedus S, et al. B-cell differentiation following autologous, conventional, or T-cell depleted bone marrow transplantation: a recapitulation of normal B-cell ontogeny. Blood 1990; 76:1647.
48. Atkinson K. Reconstruction of the haemopoietic and immune systems after marrow transplantation. Bone Marrow Transplant 1990; 5:209.
49. Anderson KC, Soiffer R, DeLage R, et al. T-cell–depleted autologous bone marrow transplantation therapy: analysis of immune deficiency and late complications. Blood 1990; 76:235.
50. Pedrazzini A, Freedman AS, Andersen J, et al. Anti–B-cell monoclonal antibody-purged autologous bone marrow transplantation for B-cell non-Hodgkin's lymphoma: phenotypic reconstitution and B-cell function. Blood 1989; 74:2203.
51. Daley JP, Rozans MK, Smith BR, et al. Retarded recovery of functional T cell frequencies in T cell–depleted bone marrow transplant recipients. Blood 1987; 70:960.
52. Ferrara JLM, Deeg HJ. Graft-versus-host disease. N Engl J Med 1991; 324:667.
53. Sullivan KM, Kopecky KJ, Jocom J, et al. Immunomodulatory and antimicrobial efficacy of intravenous immunoglobulin in bone marrow transplantation. N Engl J Med 1990; 323:705.
54. Gottlieb DJ, Cryz SJ, Furer E, et al. Immunity against *Pseudomonas aeruginosa* adoptively transferred to bone marrow transplant recipients. Blood 1990; 76:2470.
55. Donnenberg AD, Hess AD, Duff SC, et al. Regeneration of genetically restricted immune functions after human bone marrow

transplantation: influence of four different strategies for graft-v-host disease prophylaxis. Transplant Proc 1987; 19(suppl 7):144.
56. Kolb H-J, Schattenberg A, Goldman JM, et al. Graft-versus-leukemia effect of donor lymphocyte transfusions in marrow grafted patients. Blood 1995; 86:2041.
57. Mackinnon S, Papadopoulos EB, Carabasi MH, et al. Adoptive immunotherapy evaluating escalating doses of donor leukocytes for relapse of chronic myeloid leukemia after bone marrow transplantation: separation of graft-versus-leukemia responses from graft-versus-host disease. Blood 1995; 86:1261.
58. Choudhury A, Gajewski JL, Liang JC, et al. Use of leukemic dendritic cells for the generation of antileukemic cellular cytotoxicity against Philadelphia chromosome–positive chronic myelogenous leukemia. Blood 1997; 89:1133.
59. Storb R, Yu C, Wagner JL, et al. Stable mixed hematopoietic chimerism in DLA-identical littermate dogs given sublethal total body irradiation before and pharmacological immunosuppression after marrow transplantation. Blood 1997; 89:3048.
60. Giralt S, Estey E, Albitar M, et al. Engraftment of allogeneic hematopoietic progenitor cells with purine analog-containing chemotherapy: harnessing graft-versus-leukemia without myeloablative therapy. Blood 1997; 89:4531.
61. Thomas ED, Storb R: Technique for human marrow grafting. Blood 1970; 36:507.
62. Mugishima H, Teresaki P, Sueyoshi A: Bone marrow from cadaver donors for transplantation. Blood 1985; 65:392.
63. Blazer BR, Lasky LC, Perentesis JP, et al. Successful donor cell engraftment in a recipient of bone marrow from a cadaveric donor. Blood 1986; 67:1655.
64. Stroncek DF, Holland PV, Bartch G, et al. Experiences of the first 493 unrelated marrow donors in the National Marrow Donor Program. Blood 1993; 81:1940.
65. Sanders J, Buckner CD, Bensinger WI, et al. Experience with marrow harvesting from donors less than two years of age. Bone Marrow Transplant 1987; 2:45.
66. Lin A, Carr T, Herzig R, et al. Evaluation of a disposable bone marrow collection and filtration kit. Transfusion 1987; 27:524.
67. Buckner CD, Clift RA, Sanders JE, et al. Marrow harvesting from normal donors. Blood 1984; 64:630.
68. Jin NR, Hill RS, Petersen FB, et al. Marrow harvesting for autologous marrow transplantation. Exp Hematol 1985; 13:879.
69. Kessinger A, Armitage JO. Harvesting marrow for autologous transplantation from patients with malignancies. Bone Marrow Transplant 1987; 2:15.
70. Brandwein JM, Callum J, Rubinger M, et al. An evaluation of outpatient bone marrow harvesting. J Clin Oncol 1989; 7:648.
71. Kucuk O, Gordon LI, Kies MS, et al. Estimation of hemopoietic potential by CFU-C and bone marrow scan in cancer patients. Exp Hematol 1984; 12:101.
72. Storb R, Prentice RL, Thomas ED. Marrow transplantation for treatment of aplastic anemia. N Engl J Med 1977; 296:61.
73. Hows JM, Marsh JCW, Yin JL, et al. Bone marrow transplantation for severe aplastic anaemia using cyclosporin: long-term follow-up. Bone Marrow Transplant 1989; 4:11.
74. Thomas ED, Buckner CD, Benaji M, et al. One hundred patients with acute leukemia treated by chemotherapy, total body irradiation, and allogeneic marrow transplantation. Blood 1977; 49:511.
75. Sierra J, Storer B, Hansen JA, et al. Transplantation of marrow cells from unrelated donors for treatment of high-risk acute leukemia: the effect of leukemic burden, donor HLA–matching, and marrow cell dose. Blood 1997; 89:4226.
76. Rosenfeld C, Shadduck RK, Przepiorka D, et al. Autologous bone marrow transplantation with 4-hydroperoxycyclophosphamide purged marrows for acute nonlymphocytic leukemia in late remission or early relapse. Blood 1989; 74:1159.
77. Rowley SD, Zuehlsdorf M, Braine HG, et al. CFU-GM content of bone marrow graft correlates with time to hematologic reconstitution following autologous bone marrow transplantation with 4-hydroperoxycyclophosphamide–purged bone marrow. Blood 1987; 70:271.
78. Emminger W, Emminger-Schmidmeier W, Hocker P, et al. Myeloid progenitor cells (CFU-GM) predict engraftment kinetics in autologous transplantation in children. Bone Marrow Transplant 1989; 4:415.
79. Arnold R, Schmeiser T, Heit W, et al. Hemopoietic reconstitution after bone marrow transplantation. Exp Hematol 1986; 14:271.
80. Thorne AC, Malbin KF, Jain M, et al. Autologous bone marrow harvesting in outpatients. J Clin Anesthesia 1996; 8:551.
81. Bolwell BJ, Maurer W, Anderson S, et al. Outpatient bone marrow harvest: the Cleveland Clinic experience. Bone Marrow Transplant 1995; 16:703.
82. Hill HF, Chapman CR, Jackson TI, Sullivan KM. Assessment and management of donor pain following marrow harvest for allogeneic bone marrow transplantation. Bone Marrow Transplant 1989; 4:157.
83. Stroncek DF, McGlave P, Ramsay N, McCullogh J. Effects on donors of second bone marrow collections. Transfusion 1991; 31:819.
84. Sonneveld P, De Leeuw CA, Schipperus M, et al. Transfusion of red cells after autologous bone marrow harvest in patients with acute leukemia and malignant lymphoma. Transfusion 1990; 30:310.
85. Rowley SD, Davis J, Dick J, et al. Bacterial contamination of bone marrow grafts intended for autologous and allogeneic bone marrow transplantation: incidence and clinical significance. Transfusion 1988; 28:109.
86. Standards for blood and marrow progenitor cell collection, processing and transplantation. Foundation for the Accreditation of Hematopoietic Cell Therapy, Omaha, NE, 1996.
87. Gottesdiener KM: Transplanted infections: donor to host transmission with the allograft. Ann Intern Med 1989; 110:1001.
88. Niederwieser DW, Appelbaum FR, Gastl G, et al. Inadvertent transmission of a donor's acute myeloid leukemia in bone marrow transplantation for chronic myelocytic leukemia. N Engl J Med 1990; 25:1794.
89. Springmeyer SC, Silvestri RC, Flournoy N, et al. Pulmonary function of marrow transplant patients: I. Effects of marrow infusion, acute graft-versus-host disease, and interstitial pneumonitis. Exp Hematol 1984; 12:805.
90. Gee A (ed). Bone Marrow Processing and Purging. A Practical Guide. Boca Raton, FL: CRC Press, 1991.
91. Przepiorka D, Van Vlasselaer P, Huynh L, et al. Rapid debulking and $CD34^+$ enrichment of filgrastim-mobilized peripheral blood stem cells by semiautomated density gradient centrifugation in a closed system. J Hematother 1996; 5:497.
92. Civin CI, Strauss LC, Brovall C, et al. Antigenic analysis III: a hematopoietic progenitor cell surface antigen defined by a monoclonal antibody raised against KG-1a cells. J Immunol 1984; 133:157.
93. Krause DS, Fackler MJ, Civin CI, May WS. $CD34^+$: structure, biology, and clinical utility. Blood 1996; 87:1.
94. Strauss LC, Rowley SD, Larussa VF, et al. Antigenic Analysis V: characterization of My-10 antigen expression by normal lymphohematopoietic progenitor cells. Exp Hematol 1986; 14:878.
95. Leary AG, Strauss LC, Civin CI, Ogawa M. Disparate differentiation in hemopoietic colonies derived from human paired progenitors. Blood 1985; 66:327.
96. Andrews RG, Singer JW, Bernstein ID. Monoclonal antibody 12-8 recognizes a 115 kD molecule present on both unipotent and multipotent hematopoietic colony-forming cells and their precursors. Blood 1986; 67:842.
97. Bernstein ID, Andrews RG, Zsebo KM. Recombinant human stem cell factor (SCF) enhances the formation of colonies by $CD34^+$ and $CD34^+lin^-$ cells, and the generation of colony-forming cell progeny from $CD34^+lin^-$ cells cultured with IL-3, G-CSF, or GM-CSF. Blood 1991; 77:2316.
98. Andrews RG, Singer JW, Bernstein ID. Precursors of colony-forming cells in humans can be distinguished from colony-forming cells by expression of the CD33 and $CD34^+$ antigens and light scatter properties. J Exp Med 1989; 169:1721.
99. Andrews RG, Singer JW, Bernstein ID. Human hematopoietic precursors in long term culture: single $CD34^+$ cells that lack detectable T cell, B cell, and myeloid antigens produce multiple colony-forming cells when cultured with marrow stromal cells. J Exp Med 1990; 172:355.
100. Berenson RJ, Andrews RG, Bensinger WI, et al. Antigen $CD34^+$ marrow cells engraft lethally irradiated baboons. J Clin Invest 1988; 81:951.
101. Berenson RJ, Bensinger WI, Hill RS, et al. Engraftment after infusion of $CD34^+$ marrow cells in patients with breast cancer or neuroblastoma. Blood 1991; 77:1717.

102. Shpall EJ, Jones RB, Bearman SI, et al: Transplantation of enriched CD34-positive autologous marrow into breast cancer patients following high-dose chemotherapy: influence of CD34-positive peripheral-blood progenitors and growth factors on engraftment. J Clin Oncol 1994; 12:28.
103. Rowley SD, Loken M, Radich J, et al. Isolation of $CD34^+$ cells from blood stem cell components using the Baxter Isolex® system. Bone Marrow Transplant 1998; 21:1253.
104. Krüger W, Grobes M, Hennings S, et al. Purging and haemopoietic progenitor cell selection by $CD34^+$ cell separation. Bone Marrow Transplant 1998; 21:665.
105. Karhi KK, Andersson LC, Vuopio P, Gahmberg CG. Expression of blood group A antigens in human bone marrow cells. Blood 1981; 57:147.
106. Fitchen JH, Foon KA, Cline MJ. The antigenic characteristics of hematopoietic stem cells. N Engl J Med 1981; 305:17.
107. Gale RP, Feig S, Ho W, et al. ABO blood group system and bone marrow transplantation. Blood 1977; 50:185.
108. Buckner CD, Clift RA, Sanders JE, et al. ABO-incompatible marrow transplants. Transplantation 1978; 26:233.
109. Hershko C, Gale RP, Ho W, Fitchen J. ABH antigens and bone marrow transplantation. Br J Haematol 1980; 44:65.
110. Berkman EM, Caplan S, Kim CS. ABO-incompatible bone marrow transplantation: preparation by plasma exchange and in vivo antibody absorption. Transfusion 1978; 18:504.
111. Bensinger WI, Baker DA, Buckner CD, et al. Immunoadsorption for removal of A and B blood-group antibodies. N Engl J Med 1981; 304:160.
112. Warkentin PI, Yomtovian R, Hurd D, et al. Severe delayed hemolytic transfusion reaction complicating an ABO-incompatible bone marrow transplantation. Vox Sang 1983; 45:40.
113. Braine HG, Sensenbrenner LL, Wright SK, et al. Bone marrow transplantation with major ABO blood group incompatibility using erythrocyte depletion of marrow prior to infusion. Blood 1982; 60:420.
114. Dinsmore RE, Reich LM, Kapoor N, et al. ABH incompatible bone marrow transplantation: removal of erythrocytes by starch sedimentation. Br J Haematol 1983; 54:441.
115. Ho WG, Champlin RE, Feig SA, Gale RP. Transplantation of ABH incompatible bone marrow: gravity sedimentation of donor marrow. Br J Haematol 1984; 57:155.
116. Volin L, Ruutu T. Pure red-cell aplasia of long duration after major ABO-incompatible bone marrow transplantation. Acta Haematol 1990; 84:195.
117. Gmur JP, Burger J, Schaffner A, et al. Pure red cell aplasia of long duration complicating major ABO-incompatible bone marrow transplantation. Blood 1990; 75:290.
118. Sniecinski IJ, Petz LD, Blume KG. Immunohematologic consequences of major ABO-mismatched bone marrow transplantation. Transplantation 1988; 45:530.
119. Hows JM, Chipping PM, Palmer S, Gordon-Smith EC. Regeneration of peripheral blood cells following ABO incompatible allogeneic bone marrow transplantation for severe aplastic anaemia. Br J Haematol 1983; 53:145.
120. Rearden A, Masouredis SP. Blood group D antigen content of nucleated red cell precursors. Blood 1977; 50:981.
121. Berkman EM, Caplan SN. Engraftment of Rh-positive marrow in a recipient with Rh antibody. Transplant Proc 1977; 9(suppl 1):215.
122. Hows J, Beddow K, Gordon-Smith E, et al. Donor-derived red blood cell antibodies and immune hemolysis after allogeneic bone marrow transplantation. Blood 1986; 67:177.
123. Peralvo J, Bacigalupo A, Pittaluga PA, et al. Poor graft function associated with graft-versus-host disease after allogeneic marrow transplantation. Bone Marrow Transplant 1987; 2:279.
124. Anasetti C, Amos D, Beatty PG, et al. Effect of HLA compatibility on engraftment of bone marrow transplants in patients with leukemia or lymphoma. N Engl J Med 1989; 320:197.
125. Bacigalupo A, Van Lint MT, Occhini D, et al. ABO compatibility and acute graft-versus-host disease following allogeneic bone marrow transplantation. Transplantation 1988; 45:1091.
126. Dunbar CE. Gene transfer to hematopoietic stem cells: implications for gene therapy of human disease. Annu Rev Med 1996; 47:11.
127. Brugger W, Heimfeld S, Berenson RJ, et al. Reconstitution of hematopoiesis after high-dose chemotherapy by autologous progenitor cells generated ex vivo. New Engl J Med 1995; 333:283.
128. Von Kalle C, Glimm H, Schulz G, et al. New developments in hematopoietic stem cell expansion. Current Opin Hematol 1998; 5:79.
129. Roskrow MA, Suzuki N, Gan YJ, et al. Epstein-Barr virus (EBV)–specific cytotoxic T lymphocytes for the treatment of patients with EBV-positive relapsed Hodgkin's disease. Blood 1998; 91:2925.
130. Storb R, Deeg HJ, Thomas ED, et al. Marrow transplantation for chronic myelocytic leukemia: a controlled trial of cyclosporine versus methotrexate for prophylaxis of graft-versus-host disease. Blood 1985; 66:698.
131. Deeg HJ, Storb R, Thomas ED, et al. Cyclosporine as prophylaxis for graft-versus-host disease: a randomized study in patients undergoing marrow transplantation for acute nonlymphoblastic leukemia. Blood 1985; 65:1325.
132. Beatty PG, Clift RA, Mickelson EM, et al. Marrow transplantation from related donors other than HLA-identical siblings. N Engl J Med 1985; 313:765.
133. Wagner JE, Santos GW, Noga SJ, et al. Bone marrow graft engineering by counterflow centrifugal elutriation: results of a phase I–II clinical trial. Blood 1990; 75:1370.
134. Schattenberg A, De Witte T, Preijers F, et al. Allogeneic bone marrow transplantation for leukemia with marrow grafts depleted of lymphocytes by counterflow centrifugation. Blood 1990; 75:1356.
135. Ash RC, Casper JT, Chitambar CR, et al. Successful allogeneic transplantation of T-cell–depleted bone marrow from closely HLA-matched unrelated donors. N Engl J Med 1990; 322:485.
136. Mitsuyasy RT, Champlin RE, Gale RP, et al. Treatment of donor bone marrow with monoclonal anti–T-cell antibody and complement for the prevention of graft-versus-host disease. A prospective, randomized, double-blind trial. Ann Intern Med 1986; 105:20.
137. Kernan NA, Colins NH, Juliano L, et al. Clonable T lymphocytes in T cell–depleted bone marrow transplants correlate with development of graft-v-host disease. Blood 1986; 68:770.
138. Atkinson K, Farrelly H, Cooley M, et al. Human marrow T cell dose correlates with severity of subsequent acute graft-versus-host disease. Bone Marrow Transplant 1987; 2:51.
139. Ferrara JLM, Deeg HJ. Graft-versus-host disease. N Engl J Med 1991; 324:667.
140. Martin PJ. Donor CD8 cells prevent allogeneic marrow graft rejection in mice: potential implications for marrow transplantation in humans. J Exp Med 1993; 178:703.
141. Martin PJ. Prevention of allogeneic marrow graft rejection by donor T cells that do not recognize recipient alloantigens: potential role of a veto mechanism. Blood 1996; 88:962.
142. Martin PJ, Hansen JA, Buckner CD, et al. Effects of in vitro depletion of T cells in HLA-identical allogeneic marrow grafts. Blood 1985; 66:664.
143. Noga SJ, Wagner JE, Rowley SD, et al. Using elutriation to engineer bone marrow allografts. Prog Clin Biol Res 1990; 333:345.
144. Gratwohl A, Tichelli A, Wursch A, et al. Irradiated donor buffy-coat cells after T cell–depleted bone marrow transplants. Bone Marrow Transplant 1988; 3:577.
145. Butturini A, Bortin MM, Gale RP. Graft-versus-leukemia following bone marrow transplantation. Bone Marrow Transplant 1987; 2:233.
146. Weiden PL, Flournoy N, Thomas ED, et al. Antileukemic effect of graft-versus-host disease in human recipients of allogeneic-marrow grafts. N Engl J Med 1979; 300:1068.
147. Weisdorf DJ, Nesbit ME, Ramsay NKC, et al. Allogeneic bone marrow transplantation for acute lymphoblastic leukemia in remission: prolonged survival associated with acute graft-versus-host disease. J Clin Oncol 1987; 5:1348.
148. Goldman JM, Gale RP, Horowitz MM, et al. Bone marrow transplantation for chronic myelogenous leukemia in chronic phase: increased risk for relapse associated with T-cell depletion. Ann Intern Med 1988; 108:806.
149. Verdonck LF, de Gast GC, van Heugten HG, Dekker AW. A fixed low number of T cells in HLA-identical allogeneic bone marrow transplantation. Blood 1990; 75:776.
150. Champlin R, Ho W, Gajewski J, et al. Selective depletion of $CD8^+$ T lymphocytes for prevention of graft-versus-host disease after allogeneic bone marrow transplantation. Blood 1990; 76:418.
151. Brenner MK, Rill DR, Moen RC, et al. Gene-marking to trace

origin of relapse after autologous bone-marrow transplantation. Lancet 1993; 341:85.
152. Rill DR, Santana VM, Roberts WM et al: Direct demonstration that autologous bone marrow transplantation for solid tumors can return a multiplicity of tumorigenic cells. Blood 1994; 84:380.
153. Deisseroth AB, Zu Z, Claxton D, et al. Genetic marking shows that Ph^+ cells present in autologous transplants of chronic myelogenous leukemia (CML) contribute to relapse after autologous bone marrow in CML. Blood 1994; 83:3068.
154. Ross AA, Cooper BW, Lazarus HM, et al: Detection and viability of tumor cells in peripheral blood stem cell collections from breast cancer patients using immunocytochemical and clonogenic assay techniques. Blood 1993; 82:2605.
155. Moss TJ, Cairo M, Santana VM, et al: Clonogenicity of circulating neuroblastoma cells: implications regarding peripheral blood stem cell transplantation. Blood 1994; 83:3085.
156. Stelzer GT, Shults KE, Wormsley SB, Loken MR. Detection of occult lymphoma cells in bone marrow aspirates by multi-dimensional flow cytometry. Prog Clin Biol Res 1992; 337:629.
157. Negrin RS, Kiem HP, Schmidt-Wolf IGH, et al: Use of the polymerase chain reaction to monitor the effectiveness of ex vivo tumor cell purging. Blood 1991; 77:654.
158. Rowley SD, Jones RJ, Piantadosi S, et al. Efficacy of ex vivo purging for autologous bone marrow transplantation in the treatment of acute nonlymphoblastic leukemia. Blood 1989; 74:501.
159. Miller CB, Zehnbauer BA, Piantadosi S, et al. Correlation of occult clonogenic leukemia drug sensitivity with relapse after autologous bone marrow transplantation. Blood 1991; 78:1125.
160. Gorin NC, Aegerter P, Auvert B, et al. Autologous bone marrow transplantation for acute myelocytic leukemia in first remission: a European survey of the role of marrow purging. Blood 1990; 75:1606.
161. Gribben JG, Freedman AS, Neuberg D, et al. Immunologic purging of marrow assessed by PCR before autologous bone marrow transplantation for B-cell lymphoma. N Engl J Med 1991; 325:1525.
162. Dicke KA, Spitzer G, Peters L, et al. Autologous bone-marrow transplantation in relapsed adult acute leukemia. Lancet 1979; 1:514.
163. Hagenbeek A, Martens ACM. Cryopreservation of autologous marrow grafts in acute leukemia: survival of in vitro clonogenic leukemic cells and normal hemopoietic stem cells. Leukemia 1989; 3:535.
164. Allieri MA, Lopez M, Douay L, et al. Clonogenic leukemic progenitor cells in acute myelocytic leukemia are highly sensitive to cryopreservation: possible purging effect for autologous bone marrow transplantation. Bone Marrow Transplant 1991; 7:101.
165. Ramsay N, LeBien TW, Nesbit M, et al. Autologous bone marrow transplantation for patients with acute lymphoblastic leukemia in second or subsequent remission: results of bone marrow treated with monoclonal antibodies BA-1, BA-2, BA-3 plus complement. Blood 1985; 66:508.
166. Ritz J, Sallan SE, Bast RC Jr, et al. Autologous bone marrow transplantation in CALLA-positive acute lymphoblastic leukemia after in vitro treatment with J5 monoclonal antibody and complement. Lancet 1982; 2:60.
167. Ball ED, Mills LE, Cornwell GG III, et al. Autologous bone marrow transplantation for acute myeloid leukemia using monoclonal antibody-purged bone marrow. Blood 1990; 75:1199.
168. Uckun FM, Kersey JH, Vallera DA, et al. Autologous bone marrow transplantation in high-risk remission T-lineage acute lymphoblastic leukemia using immunotoxins plus 4-hydroperoxycyclophosphamide for marrow purging. Blood 1990; 76:1723.
169. Anderson IC, Shpall EJ, Leslie DS, et al. Elimination of malignant clonogenic breast cancer cells from human bone marrow. Cancer Res 1989; 49:4659.
170. Gee AP, Bruce KM, van Hilten J, et al. Selective loss of expression of a tumor-associated antigen on a human leukemia cell line induced by treatment with monoclonal antibody and complement. J Natl Cancer Inst 1987; 78:29.
171. LeBien TW, Stepan DE, Bartholomew RM, et al. Utilization of a colony assay to assess the variables influencing elimination of leukemic cells from human bone marrow with monoclonal antibodies and complement. Blood 1985; 65:945.
172. Bast RC, De Fabritiis P, Lipton J, et al. Elimination of malignant clonogenic cells from human bone marrow using multiple monoclonal antibodies and complement. Cancer Research 1985; 45:499.
173. Rocca P, Roecklein B, Mills BJ, Rowley SD. Novel double-purging consisting of simultaneous $CD34^+$ cell selection and B-cell depletion versus $CD34^+$ selection alone. Blood 1997;90(suppl 1):959.
174. Sharkis SJ, Santos GW, Colvin OM. Elimination of acute myelogenous leukemic cells from marrow and tumor suspensions in the rat with 4-hydroperoxycyclophosphamide. Blood 1980; 55:521.
175. Kaizer H, Stuart RK, Brookmeyer R, et al. Autologous bone marrow transplantation in acute leukemia: a phase I study of in vitro treatment of marrow with 4-hydroperoxycyclophosphamide to purge tumor cells. Blood 1985; 65:1504.
176. Jones RJ, Zuehlsdorf M, Rowley SD, et al. Variability in 4-hydroperoxycyclophosphamide activity during clinical purging for autologous bone marrow transplantation. Blood 1987; 70:1490.
177. Rowley SD, Davis JM, Piantadosi S, et al: Density-gradient separation of autologous bone marrow grafts before ex vivo purging with 4-hydroperoxycyclophosphamide. Bone Marrow Transplant 1990; 6:321.
178. Williams CD, Goldstone AH, Pearce T, et al. Purging of bone marrow in autologous bone marrow transplantation for non-Hodgkin's lymphoma: a case-matched comparison with unpurged cases by the European Blood and Marrow Transplant Lymphoma Registry. J Clin Oncol 1996; 14:2454.
179. Gorin NC, Douay L, Laporte JP, et al. Autologous bone marrow transplantation using marrow incubated with Asta Z 7557 in adult acute leukemia. Blood 1986; 67:1367.
180. Yeager AM, Kaizer H, Santos GW, et al. Autologous bone marrow transplantation in patients with acute nonlymphocytic leukemia, using ex vivo marrow treatment with 4-hydroperoxycyclophosphamide. N Engl J Med 1986; 315:141.
181. Chang TT, Gulati SC, Chou TC, et al. Synergistic effect of 4-hydroperoxycyclophosphamide and etoposide on a human promyelocytic leukemia cell line (HL-60) demonstrated by computer analysis. Cancer Res 1985; 45:2434.
182. Jones RJ, Miller CB, Zehnbauer BA, et al. In vitro evaluation of combination drug purging for autologous bone marrow transplantation. Bone Marrow Transplant 1990; 5:301.
183. Rowley SD, Miller CB, Piantadosi S, et al. Phase I study of combination drug purging for autologous bone marrow transplantation. J Clin Oncol 1991; 9:2210.
184. Gulati SC, Shank B, Sarris A, et al. Autologous bone marrow transplant using 4-HC, VP-16 purged bone marrow for acute nonlymphoblastic leukemia. Bone Marrow Transplant 1989; 4:116.
185. Burnett AK, Tansey P, Hills C, et al. Haematological reconstitution following high dose and supralethal chemo-radiotherapy using stored, non-cryopreserved autologous bone marrow. Brit J Haematol 1983; 54:309.
186. Kohsake M, Yanes B, Ungerleider JS, Murphy MJ. Non-frozen preservation of committed hematopoietic stem cells from normal human bone marrow. Stem Cells 1981; 1:111.
187. Delforge A, Ronge-Collard E, Stryckmans P, et al. Granulocyte-macrophage progenitor cell preservation at 4°C. Brit J Haematol 1983; 53:49.
188. Preti RA, Razis E, Ciavarella D, et al. Clinical and laboratory comparison study of refrigerated and cryopreserved bone marrow for transplantation. Bone Marrow Transplant 1994; 13:253.
189. Niskanen E. Preservation of human granulopoietic precursors following storage in the nonfrozen state. Transplantation 1983; 36:341.
190. Sierra J, Conde E, Iriondo A, et al. Frozen vs. nonfrozen bone marrow for autologous transplantation in lymphomas: a report from the Spanish GEL/TAMO Cooperative Group. Ann Hematol 1993; 67:111.
191. Ruiz-Arguelles GJ, Ruiz-Arguelles A, Perez-Romano B, et al. Filgrastim-mobilized peripheral blood stem cells can be stored at 4 degrees and used in autografts to rescue high-dose chemotherapy. Am J Hematol 1995; 48:100.
192. Seymour LK, Dansey RD, Bezwoda WR. Single high-dose etoposide and melphalan with non-cryopreserved autologous marrow rescue as primary therapy for relapsed, refractory and poor-prognosis Hodgkin's disease. Br J Cancer 1994; 70:526.
193. Polge C, Smith AU, Parkes AS. Revival of spermatozoa after vitrification and dehydration at low temperatures. Nature 1949; 164:666.

194. Lovelock JE, Bishop MWH. Prevention of freezing damage to living cells by dimethylsulphoxide. Nature 1959; 183:1394.
195. Karow AM, Webb WR. Tissue freezing. A theory for injury and survival. Cryobiology 1965; 2:99.
196. Mazur P. Cryobiology: The freezing of biological systems. Science 1970; 168:939.
197. Takahashi T, Hirsh A, Erbe E, Williams RJ. Mechanism of cryoprotection by extracellular polymeric solutes. Biophys J 1988; 54:509.
198. van Putten LM. Monkey and mouse bone marrow preservation and the choice of technique for human application. *In* Proceedings of the 11th Congress of the International Society for Blood Transfusion, Sidney, Australia, 1968, pp 797–801.
199. Stiff PJ, Murgo AJ, Zaroulis CG, et al. Unfractionated human marrow cell cryopreservation using dimethylsulfoxide and hydroxyethyl starch. Cryobiology 1983; 20:17.
200. Stiff PJ, Koester AR, Weidner MK, et al. Autologous bone marrow transplantation using unfractionated cells cryopreserved in dimethylsulfoxide and hydroxyethyl starch without controlled-rate freezing. Blood 1987; 70:974.
201. Makino S, Harada M, Akashi K, et al. A simplified method for cryopreservation of peripheral blood stem cells at −80°C without rate-controlled freezing. Bone Marrow Transplant 1991; 8:239.
202. Takaue Y, Abe T, Kawano Y, et al. Comparative analysis of engraftment after cryopreservation of peripheral blood stem cell autografts by controlled- versus uncontrolled-rate methods. Bone Marrow Transplant 1994; 13:801.
203. Parker LM, Binder N, Gelman R, et al. Prolonged cryopreservation of human bone marrow. Transplantation 1981; 31:454.
204. Aird W, Labopin M, Gorin NC, Antin JH. Long-term cryopreservation of human stem cells. Bone Marrow Transplant 1992; 9:487.
205. Attarian H, Feng Z, Buckner CD, et al. Long-term cryopreservation of bone marrow for autologous transplantation. Bone Marrow Transplant 1996; 17:425.
206. Appelbaum FR, Herzig GP, Graw RG, et al. Study of cell dose and storage time on engraftment of cryopreserved autologous bone marrow in a canine model. Transplantation 1976; 26:245.
207. Rowley SD, Byrne DV. Low-temperature storage of bone marrow in nitrogen vapor-phase refrigerators: decreased temperature gradients using aluminum racking systems. Transfusion 1992; 32:750.
208. Schafer TW, Everett J, Silver GH, Came PE. Biohazard—virus contaminated liquid nitrogen (letter). Science 1976; 191:24.
209. Tedder RS, Zuckerman MA, Goldstone AH, et al. Hepatitis B transmission from contaminated cryopreservation tank. Lancet 1995; 346:137.
210. Lasky LC, Van Buren N, Weisdorf DJ, et al. Successful allogeneic cryopreserved marrow transplantation. Transfusion 1989; 29:182.
211. Eckardt JR, Roodman GD, Boldt DH, et al. Comparison of engraftment and acute GVHD in patients undergoing cryopreserved or fresh allogeneic BMT. Bone Marrow Transplant 1993; 11:125.
212. Stockschlader M, Kruger W, Kroschke G, et al. Use of cryopreserved bone marrow in allogeneic bone marrow transplantation. Bone Marrow Transplant 1995; 15:569.
213. Stockschlader M, Kruger W, tom Dieck A, et al. Use of cryopreserved bone marrow in unrelated allogeneic transplantation. Bone Marrow Transplant 1996; 17:197.
214. Hagenbeek A, Martens ACM. Cryopreservation of autologous marrow grafts in acute leukemia: survival of in vivo clonogenic leukemic cells and normal hemopoietic stem cells. Leukemia 1989; 3:535.
215. Kessinger A, Schmit-Pokorny K, Smith D, Armitage J. Cryopreservation and infusion of autologous peripheral blood stem cells. Bone Marrow Transplant 1990; 5(suppl 1):25.
216. Davis JM, Rowley SD, Braine HG, et al. Clinical toxicity of cryopreserved bone marrow graft infusion. Blood 1990; 75:781.
217. Stroncek DF, Fautsch SK, Lasky LC, et al. Adverse reactions in patients transfused with cryopreserved marrow. Transfusion 1991; 31:521.
218. Okamoto Y, Takaue Y, Saito S, et al. Toxicities associated with cryopreserved and thawed peripheral blood stem cell autografts in children with active cancer. Transfusion 1993; 33:578.
219. David NA. The pharmacology of dimethyl sulfoxide 6544. Annu Rev Pharmacol 1972; 12:353.
220. Willhite CC, Katz PI. Dimethyl sulfoxide. J Appl Toxicol 1984; 4:155.
221. Vriesendorp R, Aalders JG, Sleijfer DT, et al. Effective high-dose chemotherapy with autologous bone marrow infusion in resistant ovarian cancer. Gynecol Oncol 1984; 17:271.
222. Rapoport AP, Rowe JM, Packman CH, Ginsberg SJ. Cardiac arrest after autologous marrow infusion. Bone Marrow Transplant 1991; 7:401.
223. Styler MJ, Topolsky DL, Crilley PA, et al. Transient high grade heart block following autologous bone marrow infusion. Bone Marrow Transplant 1992; 10:435.
224. Keung Y-K, Lau S, Elkayam U, et al. Cardiac arrhythmia after infusion of cryopreserved stem cells. Bone Marrow Transplant 1994; 14:363.
225. Lopez-Jimenez J, Cervero C, Munoz A, et al. Cardiovascular toxicities related to the infusion of cryopreserved grafts: results of a controlled study. Bone Marrow Transplant 1994; 13:789.
226. Dhodapkar M, Goldberg SL, Tefferi A, Gertz MA. Reversible encephalopathy after cryopreserved peripheral blood stem cell infusion. Am J Hematol 1994; 45:187.
227. Runckel DN, Swanson JR. Effect of dimethyl sulfoxide on serum osmolality. Clin Chem 1980; 26:1745.
228. Reisner Y, Kapoor N, Kirkpatrick D, et al. Transplantation for severe combined immunodeficiency with HLA-A,B,D,Dr incompatible parental marrow cells fractionated by soybean agglutinin and sheep red blood cells. Blood 1983; 61:341.
229. Fischer A, Durandy A, De Villartay JP, et al. HLA-haploidentical bone marrow processing for severe combined immunodeficiency using E rosette fractionation and cyclosporine. Blood 1986; 67:444.
230. Filipovich AH, Vallera DA, Youle RJ, et al. Ex-vivo treatment of donor bone marrow with anti–T-cell immunotoxins for prevention of graft-versus-host disease. Lancet 1984; 1:469.
231. Gee AP, Lee C, Sleasman JW, et al. T-lymphocyte depletion of human peripheral blood and bone marrow using monoclonal antibodies and magnetic microspheres. Bone Marrow Transplantation 1987; 2:155.
232. Dovay L, Gorin NC, David R, et al. Study of granulocyte-macrophage progenitor (CFU_C) preservation after slow freezing in the gas phase of liquid nitrogen. Exp Hematol 1982; 10:360.
233. Rowley SD, Anderson GL. Effect of DMSO exposure without cryopreservation on hematopoietic progenitor cells. Bone Marrow Transplant 1993; 11:389.

CHAPTER 24

Peripheral Blood Stem Cells

Anne Kessinger

QUANTITATIVE AND QUALITATIVE CHARACTERISTICS OF PERIPHERAL BLOOD STEM CELLS

The predictable consequences of the discovery that hematopoietic progenitors (stem cells) known to reside in bone marrow routinely circulate in peripheral blood[1–3] were studies to characterize these cells and to compare the functional capacities of stem cells from each source. Investigators found that the number of circulating stem cells varies not only from one species to another[4] but also between individuals of the same species.[5] In humans, males have a higher number of these circulating cells than females.[5, 6] For patients with chemotherapy-treated malignancies, however, the number of stem cells present in a given circulating mononuclear cell population is approximately the same for males and females.[7] The levels of colony-forming unit for granulocytes and macrophages (CFU-GM) in human umbilical cord blood are 30- to 1200-fold higher than in adult blood.[8, 9] In addition, the number of circulating stem cells within an individual varies throughout the day[10] and month.[9] However, the frequency of hematopoietic stem cells among mononuclear cells in every studied species is greater in the bone marrow than in the blood.[11–15]

The potential of autologous and allogeneic circulating stem cells to restore myelopoiesis after marrow ablation was demonstrated in a number of early studies with animal models.[15–18] In addition, peripheral blood stem cells (PBSCs) differ in some ways from their bone marrow counterparts. For example, in a murine system, circulating hematopoietic progenitors are less radiosensitive than marrow progenitors and have a higher seeding efficiency.[19] In humans, the proportions of lineage-specific progenitors are different in blood versus bone marrow[20]: in cell culture studies, a higher percentage of eosinophils are present in peripheral blood–derived CFU-GM colonies than in bone marrow–derived CFU-GM colonies.[21] When human circulating progenitors collected from patients with malignancies are placed in long-term liquid culture, an additional difference from bone marrow stem cells becomes evident. Even when the cultures are maintained for up to 8 weeks, a stromal adherent layer does not develop, suggesting that the blood-derived nonadherent cell population is a self-sustaining population.[22] In contrast, long-term liquid cultures of bone marrow stem cells routinely develop a stromal adherent layer from which CFU-GM are released.[23]

PBSC transplants are referred to in the literature as blood stem cell transplants, peripheral blood progenitor cell transplants, blood cell transplants, circulating blood stem cell transplants, and blood progenitor cell transplants. Occasionally they are simply called stem cell transplants. In the interest of clarity, all such transplants are referred to as PBSC transplants in this chapter.

After successful PBSC transplantation was reported for laboratory animals, attempts to transfer the technique to the clinical arena began. The early clinical efforts brought both victories and defeats but also identified the problems that required solutions before clinical transplantation could become routine. Allogeneic PBSC transplantation is discussed later in this chapter, but issues identified early on essentially eliminated allogeneic transplantation from initial clinical trials. The first large series of autologous PBSC transplantation began in the late 1970s and involved patients with chronic myelogenous leukemia (CML).[24] PBSCs were collected from the patients, cryopreserved, and stored while their disease was in the chronic phase. Because CML was considered a disease of the most primitive stem cell, these collected stem cells were acknowledged to contain the chronic phase of CML. When the patients' disease eventually entered a more aggressive phase, they were treated with marrow-ablative therapy followed by autologous PBSC transplantation. Forty-seven of 50 patients recovered myelopoietic function, which included restoration of the chronic phase of the disease, suggesting that the PBSCs were responsible for the recovery of marrow function.[15] In 1979 and 1980, two reports of the failure of syngeneic PBSC transplants to restore marrow function led to admonitions regarding the ability of nonleukemic peripheral stem cells to provide a clinically useful graft product.[25, 26] The reason for the failure of these two attempts now seems obvious. In an effort to avoid fluid overload from reinfusion of large volumes of stem cell products, the cells were infused intermittently over a 1- to 2-week period rather than all at once, as is the current practice. In 1986, six separate reports of successful autologous PBSC transplantation from centers in various parts of the world appeared. Since that time, the number of PBSC transplantations has surpassed the number of autologous bone marrow transplantations performed.

COLLECTION OF PBSCs

The adequacy of an autologous bone marrow collection for transplantation is determined by the number of nucleated cells in the product.[27] A typical bone marrow harvest from a 70-kg individual contains about 1.4×10^{10} nucleated cells in approximately 750 mL of marrow. Because the peripheral blood contains fewer stem cells per mononuclear cell than does the bone marrow,[15] collection of a sufficient number of PBSCs to perform a successful transplantation requires the removal of much more than an equivalent volume of blood. Approximately 4.9×10^{10} mononuclear cells harvested from 45 to 60 L of blood while marrow function is in steady state result in a product suitable for transplantation.[28] The most efficient and the only practical way to remove progenitors from such a large volume of peripheral blood is with apheresis.

Every commercially available blood cell separator has been used to harvest human peripheral stem cells for transplantation. The machine is programmed to collect lymphocytes or low-density mononuclear cells. A single collection occasionally involves apheresis for a specific time (e.g., 4 hours),[28] but more commonly for a specific volume of blood (e.g., 10 L).[29] The collection procedure can be repeated on a daily basis until the targeted number of cells is obtained.

Venous access for stem cell apheresis can be problematical, especially in heavily pretreated cancer patients, about 60% of whom will need a central venous catheter to complete the collection process.[30] Apheresis catheters placed via the subclavian vein into or near the right atrium are commonly used to collect peripheral stem cells,[31, 32] and they are occasionally involved in thrombotic complications.[33] Should the patient have such a complication, or if venous access to the right atrium has been compromised by earlier surgical procedures, the catheter can be placed in the inferior vena cava.[30] Arrhythmias have been reported when citrate-anticoagulated blood is reinfused near the right atrium,[34] but this complication has not been observed with right atrial catheters during PBSC harvesting.

PROCESSING PBSC GRAFT PRODUCTS

The PBSC graft product can be removed from the apheresis machine and immediately cryopreserved, but most centers remove many of the contaminating red cells and granulocytes, and occasionally platelets, before cryopreservation. Even though the presence of platelets in the cryopreserved product at the time of transplantation has no known adverse clinical significance, platelets removed with a "soft spin" centrifugation just after collection can be returned to the patient, thereby minimizing the thrombocytopenia that can result from frequent apheresis procedures.[35] Removal of red cells and granulocytes may be of greater importance,[36, 37] because they usually do not survive the freeze-thaw process intact, and either the hemoglobin released by lysed red cells or clumps of DNA released by lysed granulocytes may produce renal and respiratory dysfunction in the recipient. A number of purification methods, including density gradients,[38] counterflow centrifugation,[39] and repeat apheresis,[28] have been used to eliminate these high-density cells from the collections. Caution must be exercised when choosing a particular purification technique to be certain that the quality of the graft is not affected.[37]

CRYOPRESERVATION

Two cryopreservation methods, sometimes with minor modifications, have been used to ensure the long-term viability of stored PBSCs. Both techniques have also been employed to cryopreserve autologous bone marrow. The original protocol for cryopreservation used the cryoprotectant dimethylsulfoxide (DMSO) at a final concentration of 10% by volume. The cellular concentration of the product is usually adjusted by the removal (or, less often, the addition) of autologous plasma to approximately 1 to 2×10^8 cells/cm^3. The cryopreservation bag containing the product is placed in an aluminum cassette and transferred to a controlled-rate freezer, where it is cooled to approximately −85°C. Then the cassette is stored in a liquid nitrogen freezer.[40] The second protocol differs in essentially two aspects. First, the final concentration of DMSO is 5% by volume, and hydroxyethyl starch is added to the freezing media. Second, the cells are not cooled in a controlled-rate freezer but are placed directly in a −80°C freezer, where they are both cooled and stored.[41] Each of the two methods has been used clinically, and there is no evidence that one is superior to the other in terms of the quality of the transplanted product. However, the 5% DMSO method of cryopreservation is often reserved for instances when storage time is anticipated to be 4 to 6 months or less.[41, 42]

MOBILIZATION OF PBSCs

Hematopoietic progenitors are present in fewer numbers in the peripheral blood than in the marrow. For example, 1 of every 1000 mononuclear cells in the bone marrow is a CFU-GM, whereas only 1 of every 100,000 mononuclear cells in the peripheral blood is a CFU-GM.[15] If the numbers of circulating CFU-GM were increased, the time required to collect an adequate number for transplantation would be reduced. Several reported methods rapidly mobilize large numbers of hematopoietic progenitors into the circulation, thereby suggesting that extravascular storage areas of progenitor cells exist. The lymphatic system is not considered a potential extravascular storage site, because transfusions of thoracic duct–derived mononuclear cells to lethally irradiated laboratory animals have usually failed to restore myelopoiesis.[43] In humans, the administration of agents such as endotoxin,[44] epinephrine,[45] hydrocortisone,[46] corticotropin (ACTH),[47] and recombinant human erythropoietin[48] has resulted in higher numbers of circulating stem cells, although these agents have rarely been used clinically to facilitate the collection of PBSCs. Exercise can also increase the number of circulating progenitors,[47] but because the effect lasts only 15 minutes, it cannot be used for peripheral stem cell collections. Some methods produce a less rapid but equally profound mobilization effect, supporting the view that the hematopoietic system may be capable of a proliferative response to demands for circulating stem cells. For example, the performance of leukapheresis per se causes an increase in the number of circulating CFU-GM approximately 1 week after the procedure.[49]

Three mobilization methods have been used clinically to facilitate the collection of PBSCs: chemotherapy-induced mobilization, cytokine-induced mobilization, and a combination of the two. Currently, only two of these methods are in use. The first method ever utilized clinically, and since abandoned, involved administration of chemotherapy. The phenomenon of chemotherapy-induced mobilization was first described in 1976.[50] Mobilization occurs after the administration of a sufficient dose of cytotoxic drugs to produce a profound but not excessively prolonged period of leukopenia.[51] The apheresis procedures were performed at the peak of the mobilization effect, approximately 2 weeks after the chemotherapy was given, while the patient was in the recovery phase from leukopenia.[52] When cytokines, specifically granulocyte-macrophage colony-stimulating factor (GM-CSF) and granulocyte colony-stimulating factor (G-CSF), were found to routinely mobilize hematopoietic precursors into the circulation,[53, 54] these growth factors were quickly incorporated into mobilization strategies. GM-CSF[55] and more often G-CSF[56] have been used as single agents to mobilize PBSCs. About 5 days after initiating daily administration of either cytokine, the circulating progenitors reach a maximal number and the collections begin. Reports describing administration of myelotoxic chemotherapy plus a cytokine for mobilization[57, 58] have suggested that the combination produces a greater number of progenitors in the circulation than either method alone, again indicating that more than one mechanism may be capable of producing mobilization. Because the combination is more effective than chemotherapy alone, the latter mobilization technique has fallen into disuse.

Clearly, the process of PBSC collection not only is more time efficient when mobilization techniques are used but also requires the expenditure of fewer medical resources. However, the advantage of mobilization extends beyond the procurement of cells. When mobilized PBSCs are transplanted, hematopoietic recovery occurs sooner.[59] With a shorter period of aplasia, the duration of aplasia-associated morbidity decreases, along with the financial costs of the procedure.[60] Some centers added mobilized autologous PBSCs to autologous marrow for transplantation, so that more rapid recovery would occur and pluripotent stem cells collected from the marrow were certain to be included in the graft product.[61, 62] The use of two sources of autologous cells added expense, and as data accumulated regarding the reliability of peripheral blood progenitor cells alone in restoring marrow function, the practice faded. The optimal use of growth factors during autologous bone marrow transplantation has not decreased the period of aplasia to an equivalent or greater degree than mobilized PBSC transplantation.[60]

An issue associated with mobilized peripheral stem cell collection is determining when an adequate transplantation product has been harvested. For nonmobilized peripheral stem cell grafts, a product containing at least 6.5×10^8 mononuclear cells per kilogram of patient weight was usually sufficient to restore marrow function after transplantation.[28] However, nonmobilized PBSC transplantation is no longer used clinically, and for mobilized peripheral stem cell collections, the number of CFU-GM collected appears to be more predictive of an effective graft than the number of harvested mononuclear cells.[51] Because CFU-GM culture assays require 2 weeks to complete, one can only estimate the number of apheresis procedures an individual patient will require in order to gather the target number of CFU-GM.

Early hematopoietic progenitor cells manifest the CD34 cell surface antigen. Assays for $CD34^+$ cells are not entirely reproducible among different laboratories,[63] but in an individual center, a specified number of $CD34^+$ cells can be identified that correlates with the number of CFU-GM in the product and predicts reliable and rapid engraftment. The assay can be completed in a few hours with flow cytometric techniques, allowing a timely and accurate determination of the number of apheresis procedures required for an individual patient.[64] In general, the number of $CD34^+$ cells targeted ranges between 2 and 5×10^4/kg body weight of the recipient.

Although not observed in every cancer patient who received mobilizing therapy before PBSC collection, mobilization of tumor cells along with the hematopoietic progenitors has occurred.[65, 66] The biological potential of these mobilized tumor cells when included in the apheresis products and infused with the graft is unknown, but concerns about their role in tumor relapse after high-dose therapy seem prudent. The phenomenon has been observed in patients with breast cancer,[65] myeloma,[66, 67] and non-Hodgkin's lymphoma.[68] Mobilization of tumor cells has occurred after the use of chemotherapy plus cytokine[65, 66] or cytokine alone.[67] As investigators continue to search for better mobilization strategies, this issue must be taken into account, along with the vigor of hematopoietic progenitor mobilization.

Some donors do not respond to mobilization therapies. In the autologous setting, patients who have received several prior chemotherapy cycles,[69] have undergone previous radiation therapy to a significant percentage of their marrow volume,[70] or have overt marrow metastases may have inadequate responses.[71] However, patients with these characteristics may also respond well to mobilization attempts, and autologous donors with none of these risk factors may fail to mobilize. Even normal donors of allogeneic PBSC graft products have occasionally been refractory to mobilization attempts with cytokines.[72] Therefore, a damaged stem cell pool is not the only cause for mobilization failure. Genetic factors may play a role,[73] and the presence of a circulating factor that suppresses the mobilization response has been suggested as another causative factor.[74]

Efforts to identify more effective mobilizing strategies are ongoing, and a number of other cytokines are being investigated, including interleukin-3,[75] erythropoietin,[76] and stem cell factor.[77] Many new cytokines are currently under development, and these will undoubtedly be studied for their mobilizing potential as well.

INFUSION OF PBSCs

Just before transplantation begins, intravenous hydration is usually given to optimize renal function.[37] The cryopreserved cells are removed from the storage freezer and moved to the patient's bedside or to the processing laboratory. In the processing laboratory, they may be thawed and then diluted with autologous plasma[78] or washed with a mixture of saline, albumin, and acid-citrate-dextrose[79] just before reinfusion. More often, however, the cells are thawed in a 37°C water bath at the patient's bedside and immediately infused unfiltered through a central venous line. If the volume of the infusate is especially large, half the cells can be given on 2 consecutive days, but this would be unusual; generally the entire transplantation occurs in a 1- to 4-hour time frame.[80]

A number of toxicities can occur during PBSC transplantation.[36, 81, 82] The likelihood of side effects depends to some degree on whether a purification step was used during processing.[37] Hemoglobinuria during the infusion is nearly universal but disappears within 24 hours without specific therapy. Other commonly observed side effects include nausea, blood pressure elevation, fever, chills, vomiting, and increased pulse rate. Less common toxicities include increased respiratory rate, elevated serum bilirubin, cough, diarrhea, elevated serum creatinine, and headache. Generally, larger volumes of stem cell infusates and a larger proportion of red cells in the infusate are correlated with a greater number of side effects.[36] Patients have been given diphenhydramine hydrochloride and meperidine hydrochloride before the transplantation in an effort to prevent or decrease the severity of these side effects.

ALLOGENEIC PBSC TRANSPLANTATION

The emergence of PBSC transplantation in the allogeneic setting was delayed for several years after autologous PBSC transplantation became an accepted procedure for three reasons. First was the concern that circulating pluripotent stem cells might not be present in humans (a successful allogeneic PBSC transplantation requires the effective transplantation of pluripotent stem cells). Although no assay was available for this cell, so that its presence could not be verified in the human circulation, allogeneic PBSC transplantation had been reported to successfully restore and sustain marrow function after marrow-ablative radiation in mice[83] and dogs.[84] Nonetheless, investigators hesitated to use blood as an allograft source because marrow had served the purpose reliably for decades, no particular advantage of using blood rather than marrow could be envisioned, and the danger of transplanting a product that might not contain pluripotent stem cells could not be justified. The autologous PBSC transplantation successes in the 1980s and early 1990s did not prove that the human pluripotent stem cell had been transplanted, because no marker existed to distinguish transplanted autologous PBSC short- or long-term progeny from autochthonous marrow stem cell progeny. Specifically, committed progenitors could have been responsible for restoring early marrow function, thereby allowing sufficient time for autochthonous pluripotent stem cells in the marrow to recover, which subsequently provided durable marrow function. The human pluripotent stem cell was known to have the capacity to recover from total body irradiation (TBI), because some allogeneic bone marrow transplant recipients subsequently developed permanent chimerism.[85] Therefore, the use of TBI before autologous PBSC transplantation was no guarantee that permanent marrow ablation had occurred. Successful allogeneic transplantation in which cord blood is the source of stem cells had also been reported,[86] but the progenitor cell composition of cord blood is quite different from that in circulating blood in both children and adults.[8, 9, 87] Therefore, successful cord blood allografts did not establish that pluripotent stem cells circulate in humans. Two children with severe combined immunodeficiency syndrome had received allogeneic peripheral mononuclear cell transplants in the early 1980s and experienced production of allogeneic lymphoid cells, but no evidence of myeloid engraftment was seen,[88, 89] so there was no evidence that a pluripotent stem cell had been transplanted.

Second, investigators were reluctant to administer cytokines to normal donors to stimulate mobilization. Although cytokines had been given to patients for prolonged periods with no obvious ill effects, the risk of delayed or late-appearing toxicities was unknown. The use of nonmobilized peripheral stem cells was not considered, because the number of apheresis procedures required would have been unwieldy to the point that marrow harvesting would be more efficient and less morbid.

The third reason was the increased numbers of T cells in blood versus marrow graft products. Approximately 60% of peripheral blood mononuclear cells,[90] but only 8.5% to 30% of bone marrow cells, are T lymphocytes.[91–93] T lymphocytes are considered responsible for graft-versus-host disease (GVHD),[94] a morbid and often fatal complication of allogeneic transplantation that compromises hepatic, gastrointestinal, and cutaneous structure and function. Although depletion of T cells from marrow graft products is associated with a decrease in the incidence and severity of GVHD, it is also associated with an increased incidence of malignant relapse[95] and graft failure.[96, 97] Eventually, these three obstacles to allogeneic PBSC transplantation were reconciled.

The first attempted clinical allogeneic PBSC transplantation occurred in 1988.[98] The PBSC donor, a human leukocyte antigen (HLA)–matched sibling, was unwilling to donate marrow. Mobilizing cytokines were not available and the use of chemotherapy to mobilize a normal donor was unthinkable, so nonmobilized cells were collected. The T cell content of the graft product was reduced to the approximate number of T cells in a marrow harvest in an effort to prevent excessive GVHD. Circulating granulocytes quickly appeared after transplantation, and mild GVHD was localized to the skin and responded to treatment, but the patient died of a fungal infection 32 days after transplantation. Although all marrow cells (which demonstrated complete trilineage engraftment) and peripheral blood cells assayed from the patient after transplantation were of donor origin, the patient did not survive long enough to ensure that the graft was durable.

In 1993, two more allogeneic PBSC transplantations were reported.[99, 100] Allogeneic marrow had failed to engraft in the first patient after two attempts, and the second patient's donor was an anesthetic risk. Both donors received G-CSF as a mobilizing agent, neither graft product was manipulated to alter T cell content, the engraftment was rapid, and GVHD was mild and easily managed. Donor cells were documented as responsible for sustained marrow function after transplantation.

Since then, hundreds of allogeneic PBSC transplantations have been reported in the literature. Many questions remain, but preliminary agreement has been reached on a few issues. Hematopoietic recovery appears to be more rapid after allogeneic PBSC transplantation than after bone marrow transplantation.[101, 102] The short-term safety of cytokine administration to normal donors for mobilization seems acceptable, but the long-term safety cannot be assessed without additional follow-up.[103] The sustained engraftment of allogeneic PBSCs, as evidenced by long-term (>21 months after transplantation) evidence of donor-origin cells in allograft recipients,[104] provides verification that human pluripotent stem cells are present in the circulation. Most investigators have found that the incidence and severity of acute GVHD after allogeneic PBSC transplantation are similar to those found after allogeneic marrow transplantation, even though the number of T lymphocytes in the PBSC graft is a lot greater than that in the marrow graft.[102, 105] However, the risk of chronic GVHD after allogeneic PBSC transplantation is not yet defined. Some investigators who initially identified no differences in chronic GVHD between marrow and PBSC allograft recipients[102] have now expressed concern that excessive chronic GVHD may be a characteristic of allogeneic PBSC transplantation.[106] An important study that is now under way by the European Group for Blood and Marrow Transplantation compares blood and marrow stem cells for sibling allografting and may provide some answers to these daunting issues.

ADVANTAGES AND PROBLEMS, PRESENT AND FUTURE

What are the reasons for considering PBSCs rather than marrow for patients who are candidates for high-dose therapy and need an autologous transplant? First, the peripheral blood can serve as an alternative source of hematopoietic progenitors for patients with bone marrow that is unsuitable for transplantation. Generally, these are patients who have hypocellular pelvic marrow owing to prior radiation therapy,[29] chemotherapy,[28] or metastatic disease in the marrow.[107] A second reason is that transplantation of mobilized peripheral stem cells results in a quicker recovery of marrow function than does autologous bone marrow transplantation,[62, 63] thereby decreasing the morbidity associated with prolonged pancytopenia and reducing the cost of the transplantation procedure.[60, 108]

Several potential advantages of PBSC over bone marrow transplantation have been hypothesized or contemplated, although studies to support them are at present formative, incomplete, or inconclusive. One possible advantage is a more rapid reconstitution of immune function after transplantation. Because the lymphocyte fraction of mononuclear cells in a peripheral stem cell collection is larger than in a bone marrow collection, a considerable number of immunocompetent cells are infused with PBSC transplantation. A faster recovery of total lymphocyte count after mobilized PBSC transplantation has been described,[109] and faster and more complete immune reconstitution after PBSC compared with marrow transplantation in both autologous and allogeneic settings has been reported.[110, 111] Whether this difference in immune reconstitution translates into a clinical advantage is not clear. More rapid immune reconstitution could result in fewer infections after hematopoietic recovery or fewer relapses. A lower rate of disease relapse after PBSC compared with marrow autografting has been suggested[28] but awaits confirmation.

Autologous PBSC collections from patients with histopathological evidence of tumor in the bone marrow are less likely to contain occult malignancy, as determined by long-term cell culture assays, than are histopathologically normal autologous bone marrow harvests.[112] Therefore, peripheral stem cell collections may be an alternative or an adjunct to bone marrow purging. Whether reinfusion of occult circulating tumor cells at the time of transplantation has clinical significance remains unclear.

Challenges ahead include the optimization of mobilization techniques and the potential manipulation of grafts to provide the best immunological recovery after transplantation. The field of allogeneic PBSC transplantation is just opening, and the future of this technique is still being debated.

REFERENCES

1. Brecher G, Cronkite RP. Postradiation parabiosis and survival in rats. Proc Soc Exp Biol Med 1951; 77:292.
2. Goodman JW, Hodgson GS. Evidence for stem cells in the peripheral blood of mice. Blood 1962; 19:702.
3. Barr RD, Whang-Peng J, Perry S. Hemopoietic stem cells in human peripheral blood. Science 1975; 190:284.
4. Fliedner TM, Calvo W, Korbling M, et al. Hematopoietic stem cells in blood: characteristics and potentials. *In* Golde DW, Cline MJ, Metcalf D (eds): Hematopoietic Cell Differentiation. New York: Academic Press, 1978, p 193.
5. Rubin SH, Cowan DH. Assay of granulocytic progenitor cells in human peripheral blood. Exp Hematol 1973; 1:127.
6. Barrett AJ, Faille A, Ketels F. Variation in granulocyte colony forming cell numbers in adult blood. Br J Haematol 1979; 42:337.
7. Kessinger A. Quantitative aspects, mobilization, enrichment, and purification of blood stem cells: an overview. *In* The Hematopoietic Stem Cell. Ulm: Universitatsverlag Ulm GmbH, 1990, p 57.
8. Ueno Y, Koizumi S, Yamagami M, et al. Characterization of hemopoietic stem cells (CFU-C) in cord blood. Exp Hematol 1981; 9:717.
9. Knudtzon S. In vitro growth of granulocyte colonies from circulating cells in human cord blood. Blood 1974; 43:357.
10. Verma DS, Fisher R, Spitzer G, et al. Diurnal changes in circulating myeloid progenitor cells in man. Am J Hematol 1980; 9:185.
11. Trobaugh FE, Lewis JP. Repopulating potential of blood and marrow. J Clin Invest 1964; 43:1306.
12. Bradley TR, Telfer PA, Fry P. The effect of erythrocytes on mouse bone marrow colony development in vitro. Blood 1971; 38:353.
13. Erickson V, Torok-Storb B. Erythroid burst forming units (BFU-E) grown from canine marrow and peripheral blood. Exp Hematol 1981; 9:468.
14. Kovacs P, Bruch C, Fliedner TM. Colony formation by canine hemopoietic cells in vitro: inhibition by polymorphonuclear leukocytes. Acta Haematol 1976; 56:107.
15. McCarthy DM, Goldman JM. Transfusion of circulating stem cells. Crit Rev Clin Lab Sci 1984; 20:1.
16. Korbling M, Fliedner TM, Calvo W, et al. Albumin density gradient purification of canine hemopoietic blood stem cells: long-term allogeneic engraftment without GVH-reaction. Exp Hematol 1979; 7:277.
17. Scarpel SC, Zander AR, Harvath L, et al. The collection, preservation and function of peripheral blood hematopoietic cells in dogs. Exp Hematol 1979; 7:113.

18. Storb R, Graham TC, Epstein RB, et al. Demonstration of hemopoietic stem cells in the peripheral blood of baboons by cross circulation. Blood 1977; 50:537.
19. Gidali J, Feher J, Antal S. Some properties of the circulating hemopoietic stem cells. Blood 1974; 43:573.
20. Lasky LC, Kaliszewski SD, Dettick RA, et al. In vitro treatment of peripheral blood stem cells to increase committed progenitor content. Exp Hematol 1989; 17:587.
21. Verma DS, Spitzer G, Zander AR, et al. The myeloid progenitor cell: a parallel study of subpopulations in human marrow and peripheral blood. Exp Hematol 1980; 8:32.
22. Douay L, Lefrancois G, Castaigne S, et al. Long-term human blood cultures: application to circulating progenitor cell autografting. Bone Marrow Transplant 1987; 2:67.
23. Slovick FT, Abboud CM, Brennan JK, et al. Survival of granulocytic progenitors in the nonadherent and adherent compartments of human long-term marrow cultures. Exp Hematol 1984; 3:32.
24. Goldman JM, Johnson SM, Islam A, et al. Haematological reconstitution after autografting for chromic granulocytic leukaemia in transformation: the influence of previous splenectomy. Br J Haematol 1980; 45:223.
25. Hershko C, Gale RP, Ho WG, et al. Cure of aplastic anaemia in paroxysmal nocturnal haemoglobinuria by marrow transfusion from identical twin: failure of peripheral-leukocyte transfusion to correct marrow aplasia. Lancet 1979; 1:945.
26. Abrams RA, Glaubiger D, Appelbaum FR, et al. Result of attempted hematopoietic reconstitution using isologous, peripheral blood mononuclear cells: a case report. Blood 1980; 56:516.
27. Kessinger A, Armitage JO. Harvesting marrow for autologous transplantation from patients with malignancies. Bone Marrow Transplant 1987; 2:15.
28. Kessinger A, Bierman PJ, Vose JM, et al. High-dose cyclophosphamide, carmustine, and etoposide followed by autologous peripheral stem cell transplantation for patients with relapsed Hodgkin's disease. Blood 1991; 77:2322.
29. Korbling M, Holle R, Haas R, et al. Autologous blood stem-cell transplantation in patients with advanced Hodgkin's disease and prior radiation to the pelvic site. J Clin Oncol 1990; 8:978.
30. Haire WD, Lieberman RP, Lund GB, et al. Translumbar inferior vena cava catheters: experience with 58 catheters in peripheral stem cell collection and transplantation. Transfus Sci 1990; 11:195.
31. Williams SF, Bitran JD, Richards PJ, et al. Peripheral blood-derived stem cell collections for use in autologous transplantation after high dose chemotherapy: an alternative approach. Bone Marrow Transplant 1990; 5:129.
32. Lasky LC, Hurd DD, Smith JA, et al. Clinical collection and use of peripheral blood stem cells in pediatric patients. Transplantation 1989; 47:613.
33. Haire WD, Edney JA, Landmark JD, et al. Thrombotic complications of subclavian apheresis catheters in cancer patients: prevention with heparin infusion. J Clin Apheresis 1990; 5:188.
34. Sutton DMC, Cardella CJ, Uldall PR, et al. Complications of intensive plasma exchange. Plasma Ther 1981; 2:19.
35. Lasky LC, Bostrom B, Smith J, et al. Clinical collection and use of peripheral blood stem cells in pediatric patients. Transplantation 1989; 47:613.
36. Kessinger A, Schmit-Pokorny K. Toxicities associated with cryopreserved autologous peripheral stem cell infusions: influence of purification methods. J Clin Apheresis 1990; 5:156.
37. Kessinger A, Schmit-Pokorny K, Smith D, et al. Cryopreservation and infusion of autologous peripheral blood stem cells. Bone Marrow Transplant 1990; 5(suppl 1):25.
38. Juttner CA, To HO, Ho JQK, et al. Early lympho-hemopoietic recovery after autografting using peripheral blood stem cells in acute non-lymphoblastic leukemia. Transplant Proc 1988; 20:40.
39. Schouten HC, Kessinger A, Smith DM, et al. Counterflow centrifugation apheresis for the collection of autologous peripheral blood stem cells from patients with malignancies: a comparison with a standard centrifugation apheresis procedure. J Clin Apheresis 1990; 5:140.
40. Smith DM, Kessinger A, Lobo F, et al. Peripheral blood stem cell collection and toxicity. *In* Dicke KA, Spitzer G, Jagannath S, et al. (eds): Autologous Bone Marrow Transplantation. Proceedings of the Fourth International Symposium. Houston: University of Texas MD Anderson Cancer Center, 1989, p 697.
41. Stiff PJ, Koester AR, Weidner MK, et al. Autologous bone marrow transplantation using unfractionated cells cryopreserved in dimethyl sulfoxide and hydroxy ethyl starch without controlled-rate freezing. Blood 1987; 70:974.
42. Watts M, Sullivan A, Ings S, et al. Storage of PBSC at −80°C. Bone Marrow Transplant 1998; 21:111.
43. Gesner GM, Gowens JL. The fate of lethally irradiated mice given isologous and heterologous thoracic duct lymphocytes. Br J Exp Pathol 1962; 43:431.
44. Cline MJ, Golde DW. Mobilization of haematopoietic stem cells (CFU-C) into the peripheral blood of man by endotoxin. Exp Hematol 1977; 5:186.
45. Morra L, Ponassi A, Caristo G, et al. Comparison between diurnal changes and changes induced by hydrocortisone and epinephrine in circulating human hemopoietic progenitor cells (CFU-GM) in man. Biomed Pharmacother 1984; 38:167.
46. Morra L, Ponassi A, Parodi CB, et al. Mobilization of colony-forming cells (CFU-C) into the peripheral blood of man by hydrocortisone. Biomedicine 1981; 35:87.
47. Barrett AJ, Longhurst P, Sneath P, et al. Mobilisation of CFU-C by exercise and ACTH induced stress in man. Exp Hematol 1978; 6:590.
48. Ganser A, Bergmann M, Volkers B, et al. In vivo effects of recombinant human erythropoietin on circulating human hemopoietic progenitor cells. Exp Hematol 1989; 17:433.
49. Hillyer CD, Tiegerman KO, Berkman EM. Increase in circulating colony-forming units–granulocyte-macrophage during large-volume leukapheresis: evaluation of a new cell separator. Transfusion 1991; 31:327.
50. Richman CM, Weiner RS, Yankee RA. Increase in circulating stem cells following chemotherapy in man. Blood 1976; 47:1013.
51. To LB, Shepperd KM, Haylock DN, et al. Single high doses of cyclophosphamide enable the collection of high numbers of hemopoietic stem cells from the peripheral blood. Exp Hematol 1990; 18:442.
52. To LB, Haylock DN, Kimber RJ, et al. High levels of circulating haemopoietic stem cells in very early remission from acute non-lymphoblastic leukaemia and their collection and cryopreservation. Br J Haematol 1984; 58:399.
53. Socinski MA, Cannistra SA, Elias A, et al. Granulocyte-macrophage colony stimulating factor expands the circulating haemopoietic progenitor cell compartment in man. Lancet 1988; 1:1194.
54. Duhrsen U, Villeval JL, Boyd J, et al. Effects of recombinant human granulocyte colony-stimulating factor on hematopoietic progenitor cells in cancer patients. Blood 1988; 72:2074.
55. Haas R, Ho AD, Bredthauer U, et al. Successful autologous transplantation of blood stem cells mobilized with recombinant human granulocyte-macrophage colony-stimulating factor. Exp Hematol 1990; 18:94.
56. Molineux G, Podjda Z, Hampson IN, et al. Transplantation potential of peripheral blood stem cells induced by granulocyte colony-stimulating factor. Blood 1990; 76:2153.
57. Siena S, Bregni M, Brando B, et al. Circulation of $CD34^+$ hematopoietic stem cells in the peripheral blood of high-dose cyclophosphamide treated patients: enhancement by intravenous recombinant human granulocyte-macrophage colony-stimulating factor. Blood 1989; 74:1905.
58. Elias A, Mazanet R, Wheeler C, et al. Peripheral blood progenitor cells: two protocols using GM-CSF potentiated progenitor cell collection. *In* Dicke KA, Armitage JO, Dicke-Evinger MJ (eds): Autologous Bone Marrow Transplantation. Proceedings of the Fifth International Symposium. Omaha: University of Nebraska Medical Center, 1991, p 875.
59. To LB, Haylock DN, Thorp D, et al. The optimization of collection of peripheral blood stem cells for autotransplantation in acute myeloid leukaemia. Bone Marrow Transplant 1989; 4:41.
60. Hartmann O, LeCorroller AG, Blaise D, et al. Peripheral blood stem cell and bone marrow transplantation for solid tumors and lymphomas: hematologic recovery and costs. Ann Intern Med 1997; 126:600.
61. Gianni AM, Siena S, Bregni M, et al. Granulocyte-macrophage colony-stimulating factor to harvest circulating haemopoietic stem cells for autotransplantation. Lancet 1989; 2:580.
62. Lopez M, Mortel O, Pouillart P, et al. Acceleration of hemopoietic recovery after autologous bone marrow transplantation by low

doses of peripheral blood stem cells. Bone Marrow Transplant 1991; 7:173.
63. Brecher ME, Sims L, Schmitz J, et al. North American multicenter study on flow cytometric enumeration of CD34+ hematopoietic stem cells. J Hematother 1996; 5:227.
64. Siena S, Bregni M, Brando B, et al. Flow cytometry for clinical estimation of circulating hematopoietic progenitors for autologous transplantation in cancer patients. Blood 1991; 77:400.
65. Brugger W, Bross JK, Glatt M, et al. Mobilization of tumor cells and hematopoietic progenitor cells into peripheral blood of patients with solid tumors. Blood 1994; 83:636.
66. Lemoli RM, Fortuna A, Motta MR, et al. Concomitant mobilization of plasma cells and hematopoietic progenitors into peripheral blood of multiple myeloma patients: positive selection and transplantation of enriched CD34+ cells to remove circulating tumor cells. Blood 1996; 87:1625.
67. Vora AJ, Toh CH, Peel J, et al. Use of granulocyte colony-stimulating factor (G-CSF) for mobilizing peripheral blood stem cells: risk of mobilizing clonal myeloma cells in patients with bone marrow infiltration. Br J Haematol 1994; 86:180.
68. Sharp JG, Chan W, Wu G, et al. Comparison of culture versus molecular detection of lymphoma in the context of a randomized prospective trial of blood versus marrow for reconstitution after high-dose therapy: an interim analysis. *In* Dicke KA, Keating A (eds): Autologous Bone Marrow Transplantation. Proceedings of the Eighth International Symposium. Charlottesville, VA: Carden Jennings (in press).
69. Brugger W, Bross K, Frisch J, et al. Mobilization of peripheral blood progenitor cells by sequential administration of interleukin-3 and granulocyte-macrophage colony-stimulating factor following polychemotherapy with etoposide, ifosfamide and cisplatin. Blood 1992; 79:1193.
70. Haas R, Mohle R, Fruhauf S, et al. Patient characteristics associated with successful mobilizing and autografting of peripheral blood progenitor cells in malignant lymphoma. Blood 1994; 83:3787.
71. Bensinger W, Appelbaum F, Rowley S, et al. Factors that influence collection and engraftment of autologous peripheral-blood stem cells. J Clin Oncol 1995; 13:2547.
72. Bensinger WI, Clift RA, Anasetti C, et al. Transplantation of allogeneic peripheral blood stem cells mobilized by recombinant human granulocyte colony stimulating factor. Stem Cells 1996; 14:90.
73. Roberts AW, Foote S, Alexander WS, et al. Genetic influences determining progenitor cell mobilization and leukocytosis induced by granulocyte colony-stimulating factor. Blood 1997; 89:2736.
74. Sharp JG, Kessinger A, Clausen SR, et al. Concurrent partial body radiation prevents cytokine mobilization of blood progenitor cells: an effect mediated by a circulating factor. J Hematother (in press).
75. Geissler K, Peschel C, Niederwieser D, et al. Potentiation of granulocyte colony-stimulating factor–induced mobilization of circulating progenitor cells by seven-day pretreatment with interleukin-3. Blood 1996; 87:2732.
76. Oliveri A, Offidani M, Cantori I, et al. Addition of erythropoietin to granulocyte colony-stimulating factor after priming chemotherapy enhances hemopoietic progenitor mobilization. Bone Marrow Transplant 1995; 16:765.
77. Weaver A, Ryder D, Crowther D, et al. Increased numbers of long-term culture-initiating cells in the apheresis product of patients randomized to receive increasing doses of stem cell factor administered in combination with chemotherapy and a standard dose of granulocyte colony-stimulating factor. Blood 1996; 88:3323.
78. Reiffers J, Bernard P, David B, et al. Successful autologous transplantation with peripheral blood hemopoietic cells in a patient with acute leukemia. Exp Hematol 1986; 14:312.
79. Tilly H, Bastit D, Lucet J-C, et al. Haemopoietic reconstitution after autologous peripheral blood stem cell transplantation in acute leukaemia. Lancet 1986; 2:154.
80. Kessinger A, Armitage JO, Landmark JD, et al. Autologous peripheral hematopoietic stem cell transplantation restores hematopoietic function following marrow ablative therapy. Blood 1988; 71:723.
81. Korbling M, Martin H. Transplantation of hemapheresis-derived hemopoietic stem cells: a new concept in the treatment of patients with malignant lymphohemopoietic disorders. Plasma Ther Transfus Technol 1988; 9:119.
82. Zander AR, Cockerill KJ. Autologous transplantation with circulating hemopoietic stem cells. J Clin Apheresis 1987; 3:191.
83. Goodman JW, Hodgson GS. Evidence for stem cells in the peripheral blood of mice. Blood 1962; 19:702.
84. Korbling M, Fliedner TM, Calvo W, et al. Albumin density gradient purification of canine hemopoietic blood stem cells: long-term allogeneic engraftment without GVH-reaction. Exp Hematol 1979; 7:277.
85. Branch DR, Gallagher MT, Forman SJ, et al. Endogenous stem cell repopulation resulting in mixed hematopoietic chimerism following total body irradiation and marrow transplantation for acute leukemia. Transplantation 1982; 34:226.
86. Gluckman E, Broxmeyer HE, Auerbach A, et al. Hematopoietic reconstitution in a patient with Fanconi's anemia by means of umbilical-cord blood from an HLA-identical sibling. N Engl J Med 1989; 321:1174.
87. Broxmeyer HE, Douglas GW, Hangoc G, et al. Human umbilical cord blood as a potential source of transplantable hematopoietic stem/progenitor cells. Proc Natl Acad Sci U S A 1989; 86:3828.
88. Rich KC, Richman CM, Mejias E, et al. Immunoreconstitution by peripheral blood leukocytes in adenosine deaminase–deficient severe combined immunodeficiency. J Clin Invest 1980; 66:518.
89. Polmar SH, Schacter BZ, Sorenson RU. Long-term immunological reconstitution by peripheral blood leucocytes in severe combined immune deficiency disease: implications for the role of mature lymphocytes in histocompatible bone marrow transplantation. Clin Exp Immunol 1986; 64:518.
90. Ohta Y, Fujiwara K, Nishi T, et al. Normal values of peripheral lymphocytes and T cell subsets at a fixed time of day: a flow cytometric analysis with monoclonal antibodies in 210 healthy adults. Clin Exp Immunol 1986; 64:146.
91. Blazar BR, Quinones RR, Heintz KJ, et al. Comparison of three techniques for the ex vivo elimination of T cells from human bone marrow. Exp Hematol 1985; 13:123.
92. DeWitte T, Hoogenhout J, DePauw B, et al. Depletion of donor lymphocytes by counterflow centrifugation successfully prevents acute graft versus host disease in matched allogeneic marrow transplantation. Blood 1986; 67:1320.
93. Trigg ME, Peterson A, Erickson C, et al. Depletion of T cells from bone marrow for allogeneic transplantation: method for treatment of bone marrow in bulk. Exp Hematol 1986; 14:21.
94. Ferrera JLM, Deeg HJ. Graft-versus-host disease. N Engl J Med 1991; 324:667.
95. Champlin R. T-cell depletion for allogeneic bone marrow transplantation: impact on graft-versus-host disease, engraftment and graft-versus leukemia. J Hematother 1993; 2:27.
96. Kernan NA, Flomenberg N, DuPont B, O'Reilly RJ. Graft rejection in recipients of T cell–depleted HLA-nonidentical marrow transplants for leukemia. Transplantation 1987; 43:842.
97. Mitsuyasu RT, Champlin RE, Gale RP, et al. Treatment of donor bone marrow with monoclonal anti-T-cell antibody and complement for the prevention of graft-versus-host disease. Ann Intern Med 1986; 105:20.
98. Kessinger A, Smith DM, Strandjord SE, et al. Allogeneic transplantation of blood-derived, T cell–depleted hemopoietic stem cells after myeloablative treatment in a patient with acute lymphoblastic leukemia. Bone Marrow Transplant 1989; 4:643.
99. Dreger P, Suttorp M, Haverlach T, et al. Allogeneic granulocyte colony-stimulating factor–mobilized peripheral blood progenitor cells for treatment of engraftment failure after bone marrow transplantation. Blood 1993; 81:1404.
100. Russell NH, Hunter A, Rogers S, et al. Peripheral blood stem cells as an alternative to marrow for allogeneic transplantation. Lancet 1993; 341:1482.
101. Pavletic ZS, Bishop MR, Tarantolo SR, et al. Hematopoietic recovery after allogeneic blood stem cell transplantation in patients with hematologic malignancies. J Clin Oncol 1997; 15:1608.
102. Bensinger WI, Clift R, Martin P, et al. Allogeneic peripheral blood stem cell transplantation in patients with advanced hematologic malignancies: a retrospective comparison with marrow transplantation. Blood 1996; 88:2794.
103. Anderlini P, Korbling M, Dale D, et al. Allogeneic blood stem cell transplantation: consideration for donors. Blood 1997; 90:903.
104. Briones J, Urbano-Ispizua A, Orafo A, et al. Demonstration of donor origin of CD34+ HLA-DR-bone marrow cells after alloge-

neic peripheral blood transplantation with a long follow-up. Bone Marrow Transplant 1998; 21:189.
105. Przepiorka D, Anderlini P, Ippoliti C, et al. Allogeneic blood stem cell transplantation in advanced hematologic cancers. Bone Marrow Transplant 1997; 19:455.
106. Storek J, Gooley T, Siadak M, et al. Allogeneic peripheral blood stem cell transplantation may be associated with a high risk of chronic graft-versus-host disease. Blood 1997; 90:4705.
107. Kessinger A, Vose JM, Bierman PJ, et al. High dose therapy and autologous peripheral stem cell transplantation for patients with relapsed lymphomas and bone marrow metastases. *In* Dicke KA, Armitage JO, Dicke-Evinger MJ (eds): Autologous Bone Marrow Transplantation. Proceedings of the Fifth International Symposium. Omaha: University of Nebraska Medical Center, 1991, p 837.
108. Woronoff-Lemsi MC, Arveux P, Limat S, et al. Cost comparative study of autologous peripheral blood progenitor cells (PBPC) and bone marrow (ABM) transplantations for non-Hodgkin's lymphoma patients. Bone Marrow Transplant 1997; 20:975.
109. To LB, Juttner CA. Peripheral blood stem cell autografting: a new therapeutic option for AML? Br J Haematol 1987; 66:285.
110. Ottinger HD, Beelen DW, Scheulen B, et al. Improved immune reconstitution after allotransplantation of peripheral blood stem cells instead of bone marrow. Blood 1996; 88:2775.
111. Talmadge JE, Reed E, Ino K, et al. Rapid immunologic reconstitution following transplantation with mobilized peripheral blood stem cells as compared to bone marrow. Bone Marrow Transplant 1997; 19:161.
112. Sharp JG, Kessinger MA, Pirruccello SJ, et al. Frequency of detection of suspected lymphoma cells in peripheral blood stem cell collections. *In* Dicke KA, Armitage JO, Dicke-Evinger MJ (eds): Autologous Bone Marrow Transplantation. Proceedings of the Fifth International Symposium. Omaha: University of Nebraska Medical Center, 1991, p 801.

CHAPTER 25

Cord Blood Stem and Progenitor Cells for Transplantation

Hal E. Broxmeyer

Hematopoietic cells circulating in blood and found in other tissue areas are produced by stem and progenitor cells[1–4] and are under the regulatory control of cytokine and accessory–stromal cell interactions.[5] In adults, the primary source of hematopoietic stem and progenitor cells is the bone marrow,[1–5] which is currently the most common choice for hematopoietic reconstitution in an autologous or major histocompatibility complex (MHC)–matched allogeneic setting.[6] Adult peripheral blood has increasingly been used in autologous and, more recently, allogeneic settings as an alternative source of transplantable cells.[7] The movement of stem and progenitor cells from organ to organ during embryogenesis and fetal development is a poorly understood phenomenon. Ontologically, stem and progenitor cells are found first in the aorta-gonad-mesonephros and intraembryonic splanchnopleural regions and the yolk sac, later in fetal liver and spleen, and then in fetal bone marrow.[8–15] Fetal liver has been used in a limited setting for clinical transplantation to correct human hematopoietic deficiencies in children as well as fetuses,[16, 17] but this material is not easily attainable for large-scale use, cannot usually be used in a human leukocyte antigen (HLA)–matched setting, and is now considered mainly in the context of in utero transplantation.

We are just beginning to ascertain how stem and progenitor cells migrate. In part, this appears to reflect the actions of cytokines with chemotactic activities, including members of the chemokine family of molecules, such as stromal cell–derived factor (SDF)-1 and CKb-11, along with Steel factor and other unknown cytokines.[18–21] Specific chemokine receptors such as CXCR2, which binds interleukin-8 (IL-8) along with other CXC chemokines, and CCR1, which binds MIP-1a and other CC chemokines, have also been implicated in stem and progenitor cell movement.[22, 23] In addition, adhesion molecules such as integrins[24–31] are no doubt involved. Regardless of our understanding of stem and progenitor cell movement, clinical medicine is already the beneficiary of this process. Human umbilical cord blood is a viable alternative to bone marrow as a source of hematopoietic stem and progenitor cells, which was, until 1988, typically discarded.[32] Cord blood contains the following cells in relatively high frequency as assessed by in vitro colony assays[32–46]: stem cells; progenitor cells such as the colony-forming unit for granulocytes and macrophages (CFU-GM) and for megakaryocytes (CFU-Meg); the multipotential progenitor cell, the colony-forming unit for granulocytes, erythroid cells, macrophages, and megakaryocytes (CFU-GEMM); and the erythroid burst-forming unit (BFU-E) and erythroid colony-forming unit (CFU-E), or proerythroblast. Although the concentrations of myeloid progenitor cells (MPCs) are higher in the blood of newborns for weeks after birth than in adult blood,[34, 43, 47] by 1 day after birth, the circulating concentrations of MPCs per milliliter are only 22% to 49% of those found in the cord blood of the same infants.[47] During the first month of life, CFU-GM are reduced on average about 10-fold compared with levels in cord blood but remain about fivefold higher than levels in adult blood.[43] Concentrations of spleen colony-forming cells (CFU-S), which are more mature pluripotential stem cells lacking repopulating capability,[3, 4] are higher in the blood of fetal and neonatal mice than they are after birth.[48, 49]

A number of reports[50, 51] that human umbilical cord blood could be maintained for many weeks in "long-term" culture—at least as long as bone marrow, and perhaps even longer[50]—suggested that progenitors are produced in cord blood from more primitive cells. These observations led us to evaluate the possible use of human cord blood as a source of hematopoietic reconstituting cells. Using congenic mice, we obtained evidence that blood from histocompatible near-term hybrid mouse embryos and newborns (less than 24 hours old) could successfully reconstitute the hematopoietic system of lethally irradiated mice.[52] As part of a national multi-institutional study evaluating the harvest, transport, content, cryopreservation, and thawing of human hematopoietic progenitors in over 100 cord blood collections, we estimated that there were sufficient stem and progenitor cells in single cord blood collections for clinical transplantation and hematopoietic reconstitution.[32]

The studies broadened into a wider national and international multi-institutional study coordinated in major part at Indiana University, where cord blood from an infant was tested, frozen, and later transplanted into an HLA-matched sibling with Fanconi anemia by Dr. Elaine Gluckman in Paris.[53] Complete engraftment of the myeloid system with donor cells was evidenced by cytogenetics, ABO typing, DNA polymorphisms, and normal cellular resistance to cytotoxic agents that reveal the fragility of Fanconi anemia cells. Although the blood contained residual host lymphocytes exhibiting chromosome damage, the lymphoid system was 98% or more of donor

Table 25–1. HLA-Matched Sibling Cord Blood Transplants Done With Cells Frozen at Indiana University

	Patient 1	Patient 2	Patient 3	Patient 4	Patient 5
Disease	*Fanconi anemia*	*Fanconi anemia*	*Fanconi anemia*	*Juvenile chronic myelogenous leukemia*	*Fanconi anemia*
Age at time of transplant (years)	5	4	7	4	8
Sex (donor/recipient)	F/M	F/F	M/M	F/M	M/F
Volume cord blood collected (mL)	160	150	75	89	282
Total nucleated cells infused (10^{-8} per kg body weight)	0.4	0.8	0.2	0.5	1.1
Engraftment?	Yes	Yes	Yes	Yes*	No†
Time since transplant (months)‡	124	107	105	9*	—

*Patient relapsed at about 9 months.
†Not clear whether this was lack of engraftment or rejection.
‡As of February 1999.

origin at 1 year after transplantation.[52–54] By early 1993, three patients with Fanconi anemia had been successfully transplanted with umbilical cord blood that was cryopreserved, stored, and assessed for progenitor cells at Indiana University. The first two transplantations were performed in Paris, and the recipients are doing well approximately 10 and 9 years after transplantation. A third transplantation was performed in Cincinnati, and the recipient is doing well about 8.5 years after transplantation. A fourth transplantation for Fanconi anemia was not successful.

In addition, engraftment was obtained with HLA-matched sibling cord blood stored at Indiana and transplanted in a patient with juvenile chronic myelogenous leukemia.[55] Engraftment in this case was substantiated by restriction fragment length polymorphism, polymerase chain reaction, and cytogenetic analysis of the bone marrow and peripheral blood of the recipient after transplantation. Unfortunately, this patient had a relapse after about 9 months. However, this patient underwent transplantation with bone marrow from the donor whose cord blood had previously been used and achieved remission. Graft-versus-host disease has been slight in the four patients receiving HLA-matched sibling cord blood. Table 25–1 summarizes the clinical outcome for these initial five transplant recipients. The historical background for the laboratory and clinical studies is described elsewhere.[52, 54, 56]

CORD BLOOD MPCs AS INDICATORS OF THE REPOPULATING CONTENTS OF SINGLE CORD BLOOD COLLECTIONS

Although no direct quantitative assay for human hematopoietic repopulating cells is available, MPCs, particularly CFU-GM, have been used as an indicator of marrow engrafting capability in humans[57–61] and in mice.[62] After determining that CFU-GM, BFU-E, and CFU-GEMM remain functionally viable in cord blood for 3 days both at 4°C and at room temperature and could be transported by overnight mail, we[32] analyzed over 100 cord blood samples. The number of progenitors present in the low-density fraction (<1.077 g/mL) after Ficoll-Hypaque separation was within the lower range required for successful engraftment with bone marrow cells. However, standard procedures to remove erythrocytes or granulocytes before freezing, as well as washing of thawed cells before plating, resulted in large losses of progenitors. Nonetheless, calculation of the number of MPCs in unseparated cord blood suggested that there would be enough cells for clinical transplantation,[32] and we therefore recommended that cord blood cells be frozen without any attempt at separation and infused into recipients without washing. As mentioned earlier, this procedure resulted in the first four successful cord blood transplantations in children.[52–55]

It should be noted that culture conditions used in various laboratories (Table 25–2) make it difficult to compare progenitor cell values, unless it is clearly stated exactly what assays are used and how they are done.[52, 63]

A critical question was whether single collections of cord blood also contained sufficient numbers of immature cells to engraft the hematopoietic system in adults. When collections of bone marrow cells are made for autologous or allogeneic transplantation, it is usual to collect as many cells as possible. In contrast, what is collected from the cord blood is limited by what is present.

Table 25–2. Potential Areas of Variability Among Laboratories in the Calculation of Myeloid Progenitor Cells

Semisolid Support Medium
Agar, methylcellulose, plasma clot, fibrin clot, agarose

Incubation Conditions
Ambient (20%) vs. lowered (5%) oxygen tension

Culture Ingredients
McCoy's medium, Iscove's medium, supplementation with essential and nonessential amino acids, etc.

Growth Factors
Medium conditioned by different cell types that could contain different combinations and concentrations of CSFs and interleukins: purified CSFs (GM-CSF, G-CSF, IL-3, IL-5, EPO); SLF; interleukins that do not have CSF activity but can modify CSF actions (e.g., IL-1, IL-2, IL-4, IL-6, IL-7, IL-8, IL-9, IL-10, IL-11)

Cell Populations Assessed
Unseparated vs. fractionated cells (e.g., low density, nonadherent, T cell depleted, CD34 enriched)

Scoring Criteria
Day scored; criteria to distinguish a colony

CSF, colony-stimulating factor; EPO, erythropoietin; G, granulocyte; GM, granulocyte-macrophage; IL, interleukin; SLF, Steel factor.

Our original calculations of MPCs in blood were estimated by using either recombinant human granulocyte-macrophage colony-stimulating factor (GM-CSF) or a medium conditioned by the urinary bladder carcinoma cell line 5637 (5637 CM, a source of GM-CSF and other CSFs and interleukins) to stimulate colony formation of CFU-GM.[32] Erythropoietin (EPO) plus either 5637 CM or interleukin-3 (IL-3) was used to stimulate colony formation of CFU-GEMM, and EPO (with or without 5637 CM or IL-3) was used to stimulate colony formation of BFU-E. It is now known that a number of other cytokines either directly or indirectly stimulate or enhance colony formation of MPCs in a synergistic manner,[1, 5, 64] suggesting that we had probably underestimated the number of MPCs in cord blood collections.

One of the newly identified growth factors at that time was the potent costimulating cytokine Steel factor (SLF),[65] which has also been termed mast cell growth factor,[66–69] stem cell factor,[70–72] and *kit* ligand.[73–75] The "Sl" locus on mouse chromosome 12q22–24[76] encodes SLF. SLF is the ligand[66–75] for the protein tyrosine kinase receptor expressed by the *c-kit* proto-oncogene, which is encoded by the "W" locus on mouse chromosome 5.[77–79] SLF mediates its actions intracellularly via protein phosphorylation.[80–82]

Using SLF in combination with CSFs, we reevaluated the number of MPCs in cord blood.[47] SLF plus GM-CSF detected 8- to 11-fold more CFU-GM than did GM-CSF or 5637 CM. When SLF was used along with EPO plus IL-3, 15-fold more CFU-GEMM were detected than when cells were stimulated with EPO plus either IL-3 or 5637 CM. Table 25–3 lists progenitor cell values in complete collections of cord blood detected in the absence and presence of SLF. Because SLF is an early-acting cytokine, its use probably facilitated the detection of early subpopulations of MPCs. A comparative analysis assessing the effects of SLF on bone marrow cells showed that it also permitted detection of bone marrow CFU-GM and CFU-GEMM, but to a lesser extent than seen with cord blood. SLF plus GM-CSF and SLF plus EPO and IL-3 resulted in increases of only two- to fourfold for bone marrow CFU-GM and six- to eightfold for bone marrow CFU-GEMM. The use of other potent costimulating factors, such as the Flt-3 ligand, in combination with CSFs also allowed detection of enhanced numbers of progenitors in cord blood collections.[83]

The quality of stem and progenitor cells is as important as the quantity. In this regard, it is of interest that enhanced detection of cord blood CFU-GEMM with SLF and EPO was directly related to decreased detection of BFU-E.[47] When detection of CFU-GEMM was further enhanced by the addition of IL-3 to the combination of SLF and EPO, even greater decreases were noted in the detection of BFU-E. The immature nature of cord blood BFU-E, which may really be CFU-GEMM, is the most likely explanation. This is not the case for bone marrow BFU-E, because SLF plus EPO enhances the detection of bone marrow BFU-E and CFU-GEMM; detection of both progenitor cell populations is enhanced when IL-3 is added to SLF plus EPO.[47]

Further information suggesting a more immature profile of early cells in cord blood than in bone marrow is based on the comparative replating capacities of CFU-GEMM in cord blood and in bone marrow.[84–86] Self-renewal, the ability of a stem cell to duplicate itself, is extremely important to the maintenance of blood cell production but is a poorly understood event.[87] The murine CFU-S assay in vivo has been used to measure stem cell self-renewal and the multipotential nature of the cells.[88, 89] Its in vitro counterpart may be the stem cell assay, in which the ability of single stem cell colonies to be replated into secondary cultures with resultant multipotential and lineage-restricted colonies reflects the self-renewable nature of stem cells.[90, 91] Murine[90, 91] and, to a lesser extent, human[40, 42, 45, 92, 93] stem cells thus have been considered to have self-renewal capabilities on the basis of colony replating studies. Because CFU-GEMM, BFU-E, and CFU-GM appeared to have little or no ability to be replated,[94–96] they had been considered to have little or no self-renewal capacity.

We reanalyzed the capacity of CFU-GEMM from both cord blood and bone marrow to be replated in vitro, using SLF.[84] Primary cultures were established in methylcellulose culture medium with EPO, EPO plus IL-3, or EPO plus SLF. Single CFU-GEMM colonies were removed after 14 days of incubation, washed, and plated in secondary methylcellulose cultures containing EPO plus SLF plus GM-CSF. The number of secondary cultures giving rise to one or more colonies was calculated after another 14 days of incubation. A high replating efficiency of both cord blood and bone marrow CFU-GEMM was apparent from cells growing in primary cultures with EPO plus SLF. The numbers were greater than those seen without SLF in the primary cultures. Most pertinent to CFU-GEMM quality was the finding that replated cord blood CFU-GEMM gave rise to CFU-GM, BFU-E, and CFU-GEMM colonies in secondary cultures, whereas bone marrow CFU-GEMM gave rise almost entirely to CFU-GM colonies.[84]

A strict definition of self-renewal would be division of cells that give rise to daughter cells with the same

Table 25–3. Cellular Contents of Umbilical Cord Blood Collections*

Volume (mL)	110 ± 47
Nucleated cellularity (10^{-8})	14.3 ± 1.0
CFU-GM	
Responsive to GM-CSF	24.3 ± 27.0
Responsive to GM-CSF + SLF	93.8 ± 9.8
BFU-E	
Responsive to EPO + IL-3	94.5 ± 99.4
CFU-GEMM	
Responsive to EPO + SLF	112.6 ± 127.7

*These data represent average results of the first 65 consecutive collections for possible use in sibling transplant. Growth factors were used at the following concentrations: recombinant human (rhu) GM-CSF, 100 U/mL; rhuSLF, 50 ng/mL; rhuEPO, 1 U/mL; rhuIL-3, 100 U/mL. CFU-GM assays were set up in 0.3% agar culture medium with 10% heat-inactivated fetal bovine serum (FBS), and BFU-E and CFU-GEMM assays were set up in 0.8% methylcellulose culture medium with 30% non–heat-inactivated FBS. Cultures were scored after 14 days' incubation at 5% CO_2 and 5% O_2 in a humidified chamber.[63]

BFU-E, erythroid burst-forming unit; CFU-GEMM, colony-forming unit for granulocytes, erythroid cells, macrophages, and megakaryocytes; CFU-GM, colony-forming unit for granulocytes and macrophages; EPO, erythropoietin; GM-CSF, granulocyte-macrophage colony-stimulating factor; IL, interleukin; SLF, Steel factor.

capacity for proliferation and differentiation as the parent cell. Although the multipotential nature of the replated colonies was verified, the CFU-GEMM colonies formed in the secondary cultures were smaller than those colonies in the primary cultures. Thus we could not be absolutely sure that we had measured self-renewal. Further studies using additional growth factors found in cord blood plasma have identified secondary cord blood CFU-GEMM colonies that are as large as the primary CFU-GEMM colonies from which they were derived.[85] Thus, cord blood CFU-GEMM have at least some self-renewal capacity. We also found that high proliferative potential colony-forming cells from cord blood have extensive self-renewal capacity.[86]

In addition to the qualitative differences between cord blood and marrow cells (most cord blood BFU-E apparently being CFU-GEMM with self-renewal capacity), we compared the numbers of MPCs in single collections of cord blood and in collections of bone marrow associated with successful engraftment after autologous transplantation.[47] Although the nucleated cellularity of cord blood collections was only 14.1% of that found in the autologous marrow collections, the percentages of CFU-GM, BFU-E, and CFU-GEMM in freshly collected cord blood averaged 46% to 98%, 30%, and 23% to 24%, respectively, of the numbers of these progenitors found in the marrow samples. There was considerable overlap in total numbers of MPCs found between individual collections of cord blood and marrow; however, the numbers of CFU-GM that were responsive to GM-CSF plus SLF were higher in all the cord blood samples than in the successfully engrafting marrow sample with the fewest number of these cells. CFU-GM numbers seem to correlate best with engrafting potential in marrow samples.[57–61]

Recent studies on the use of mice with severe combined immunodeficiency (SCID) as recipients for human cell engraftment have demonstrated that cord blood appears to have a higher engrafting capability than cells from adult bone marrow.[97–101] It is possible that the SCID-mouse repopulating cell is detecting a very early number of the stem cell series not detected by current in vitro assays.[101–104]

Taken together, this information suggested to us that single collections of cord blood would most likely contain enough cells to engraft not only the hematopoietic systems of children but also those of adults. There have now been over 700 cord blood transplantations in either a sibling or unrelated allogeneic setting, although many of these cases have not yet been reported in detail in a refereed paper.[53–55, 105–112] The success rate has been encouraging, with engraftment noted in 80% to 90% of recipients. In addition, the incidence of graft-versus-host disease has been relatively low, even in partial HLA-matched, unrelated cord blood transplantation. Adults have been successfully engrafted with cord blood, but the majority of experience has been with children.

EXPANSION OF STEM AND PROGENITOR CELLS

Being able to expand the number of stem and progenitor cells in vitro would be a tremendous advancement. Unfortunately, no assay is yet available to characterize and quantitate the human marrow repopulating cells, although the human-SCID mouse assay may be helpful here. Efforts to expand cells have relied for the most part on quantitation of MPCs. MPC values may indeed be found to reflect the levels of repopulating cells, but extreme caution is still warranted in using such a correlation. It is known that the number of human marrow MPCs can be expanded in short-term suspension cultures in vitro.[113, 114] Combinations of cytokines allow detection of MPCs in primary semisolid cultures, which is not possible with the use of single cytokines[1, 15, 115, 116]; when four or five cytokines are used in combination, each additional cytokine allows detection of a larger number of MPCs.[115, 116] This relationship is apparent even at the single cell level,[116] suggesting that at least some MPCs have receptors for and respond to the actions of a number of different cytokines.

Combinations of cytokines also allow for expansion of MPCs in suspension culture, and SLF is active in these effects.[117–120] We found that SLF allows expansion of cord blood MPCs in culture, and that addition of a second cytokine, such as GM-CSF, granuloctye colony-stimulating factor (G-CSF), IL-3, or EPO, to the suspension culture enhances this expansion.[47] Incubation of low-density or unseparated cord blood cells in suspension with SLF for 7 days was found to result in increases of 7.9-fold for CFU-GM, 2.2-fold for BFU-E, and 2.7-fold for CFU-GEMM; the addition of a second cytokine enhanced these expansions to 12.5-fold, 3.6-fold, and 3.5-fold, respectively. These results are similar to the expansion of MPCs noted with bone marrow cells. As with mouse marrow cell suspension cultures,[118] expansion of human MPCs can be enhanced by additional cytokines. It is not yet clear that SLF is a self-renewal factor,[84, 85] but the elucidation of such a factor, along with the development of an assay for the human marrow repopulating cell, would be of obvious advantage for expansion of the important cells needed for transplantation. There have now been numerous studies published on attempts to expand stem and progenitor cells ex vivo.[5, 121]

Alternatively, cells could be expanded in vivo by giving SLF, CSFs, or interleukins to patients who have received cord blood transplants. Expansion of cells in vivo might be more practical, because the number of centers that could expand cells in vitro would probably be limited, whereas in vivo cytokine trials are being performed in increasing numbers of clinical centers.[5, 122, 123]

FUTURE DIRECTIONS

The use of umbilical cord blood has been shown to be efficacious in the setting of transplanting fully or partially HLA-matched sibling and unrelated allogeneic stem and progenitor cells in children and in some adults.[53–55, 105–112] It is of interest that a relatively low incidence of graft-versus-host disease has been noted in the recipients of cord blood transplants, perhaps reflecting the immature or tolerant nature of cord blood immune cells, as has been suggested in a number of publications.[124–131] The extent of the suitability of cord blood as a source of transplantable cells remains to be defined, especially in the context of controlled clinical trials.[112] Cord blood banks have allowed access to stored samples of HLA-typed cells not currently available through the bone marrow registry. There are a number of regulatory and ethical issues[112] that need to be better defined in a peer-reviewed setting, such as public versus private cord blood banking and the issues of ownership of cord blood and eventual allocation of the units. Further research into characterization of the earliest cells in cord blood is needed, as is research on the expansion of these cells and the immunological reactivity inherent in cells within cord blood collections. In addition, with regard to cord blood banking, it is still not known how long one can store cord blood in a cryopreserved state. Theoretically, this should be for at least the lifetime of an individual. Practically, the longest time cord blood has been stored and used successfully for transplantation has been about 4 years; however, viable stem and progenitor cells with extensive capacity for proliferation have been retrieved after 10 years in storage.[132] The use of cord blood for gene transfer and gene therapy is also an exciting possibility. Cord blood stem and progenitor cells have served as good vehicles for newly introduced genes in an in vitro setting[133–140] and in the context of a preliminary clinical study.[141, 142] However, it is still not clear how efficiently genes can be inserted into the earliest stem cell populations with long-term marrow repopulating capability, which are usually noncycling in G_1 or G_0 phases of the cell cycle. Thus far, retroviral vectors have not been able to efficiently transduce these slow or noncycling cells. Other viruses, such as adeno-associated viruses (AAVs), may be useful in this context,[143, 144] but there are still a number of problems with the use of AAVs that need to be overcome including the inability of AAV to transduce CD34$^+$ stem and progenitor cells from all donors.[145] The discovery of co-receptors for AAV[146] and tyrosine phosphorylation of a protein involved in AAV mediated transgene expression[147] may be of help here. The search for the appropriate vectors for gene therapy is ongoing at a number of centers, and this includes use of HIV-based lentiviruses.[148]

REFERENCES

1. Broxmeyer HE, Williams DE. The production of myeloid blood cells and their regulation during health and disease. Crit Rev Oncol Hematol 1988; 8:173.
2. Broxmeyer HE. Hematopoietic stem cells. *In* Trubowitz S, Davis E (eds): Human Bone Marrow. Boca Raton, FL: CRC Press, 1982, pp 77–123.
3. Broxmeyer HE. Colony assays of hematopoietic progenitor cells and correlations to clinical situations. Crit Rev Oncol Hematol 1983; 1:227.
4. Williams DE, Lu L, Broxmeyer HE. Characterization of hematopoietic stem and progenitor cells. Surv Immunol Rev 1987; 6:294.
5. Broxmeyer HE. The hematopoietic system: principles of therapy with hematopoietically active cytokines. *In* Ganser A, Hoelzer D (eds): Cytokines in the Treatment of Hematopoietic Failure. New York: Marcel Dekker, 1999, pp 1–37.
6. Thomas ED. Frontiers in bone marrow transplantation. Blood Cells 1991; 17:259.
7. To LB, Haylock DN, Simmons PJ, Juttner CA. The biology and clinical uses of blood stem cells. Blood 1997; 89:2233.
8. Medvinsky A, Dzierzak E. Definitive hematopoiesis is autonomously initiated by the GM region. Cell 1996; 86:897.
9. Cumano A, Dieterlen-Lievre F, Godin I. Lymphoid potential, probed before circulation in mouse, is restricted to caudal intraembryonic splanchnopleura. Cell 1996; 86:907.
10. Yoder MC, Hiatt K. Engraftment of embryonic hematopoietic cells in conditioned newborn recipients. Blood 1997; 89:2176.
11. Tavassoli M. Embryonic and fetal hematopoiesis: an overview. Blood Cells 1991; 17:269.
12. Moore MAS, Metcalf D. Ontogeny of the haematopoietic system: yolk sac origin of in vivo and in vitro colony forming cells in the developing mouse embryo. Br J Haematol 1970; 18:279.
13. Johnson GR, Moore MAS. Role of stem cell migration in initiation of mouse fetal liver haematopoiesis. Nature 1975; 258:726.
14. Wong PMC, Chung SW, Chill DKH, Eaves CJ. Properties of the earliest clonogenic hemopoietic precursors to appear in the developing murine yolk sac to liver transition. Proc Natl Acad Sci U S A 1986; 83:3851.
15. Migliaccio G, Migliaccio AR, Petti S, et al. Human embryonic hemopoiesis: kinetics of progenitors and precursors underlying the yolk sac to liver transition. J Clin Invest 1986; 78:51.
16. Gale RP, Touraine JL, Lucarelli G. Fetal Liver Transplantation. New York: Alan R. Liss, 1985, pp 237–342.
17. Touraine JL. In utero transplantation of fetal liver stem cells in humans. Blood Cells 1991; 17:379.
18. Aiuti A, Webb IJ, Bleul C, et al. The chemokine SDF-1 is a chemoattractant for human CD34$^+$ hematopoietic progenitor cells and provides a new mechanism to explain the mobilization of CD34$^+$ progenitors to peripheral blood. J Exp Med 1997; 185:111.
19. Kim CH, Broxmeyer HE. In vitro behavior of hematopoietic progenitor cells under the influence of chemoattractants: SDF-1, Steel factor and the bone marrow environment. Blood 1998; 91:100.
20. Nagasawa T, Hirota S, Tachibana K, et al. Defects of B-cell lymphopoiesis and bone-marrow myelopoiesis in mice lacking the CXC chemokine PBSF/SDF-1. Nature 1996; 382:635.
21. Kim CH, Pelus LM, White JR, et al. CKβ-11/MIP-3β/ELC, a CC chemokine is a chemoattractant for myeloid progenitor cells with a specificity for macrophage progenitors among myeloid progenitor cells. J Immunol 1998; 161:2580.
22. Broxmeyer HE, Cooper S, Cacalano G, et al. Interleukin-8 receptor is involved in negative regulation of myeloid progenitor cells in vivo: evidence from mice lacking the murine IL-8 receptor homolog. J Exp Med 1996; 184:1825.
23. Gao JL, Wynn TA, Chang Y, et al. Impaired host defense, hematopoiesis, granulomatous inflammation and type 1/type 2 cytokine balance in mice lacking cc chemokine receptor 1. J Exp Med 1997; 185:1959.
24. Hynes RO. Integrins: versatility, modulation and signaling in cell adhesion. Cell 1992; 69:11.
25. Williams DA, Rios M, Stephens C, Patel VP. Fibronectin and VLA-4 in haematopoietic stem cell-microenvironment interactions. Nature 1991; 352:438.
26. Verfaillie CM, McCarthy JB, McGlave PB. Differentiation of primitive human multipotential hematopoietic progenitors into single lineage clonogenic progenitors is accomplished by alteration in their interaction with fibronectin. J Exp Med 1991; 174:693.
27. Simmons PJ, Zannettino A, Gronthos A, Leavesley D. Potential adhesion mechanisms for localization of haematopoietic progenitors to bone marrow stroma. Leuk Lymphoma 1994; 12:353.
28. Levesque JP, Leavesley DI, Niutta S, et al. Cytokines increase human hematopoietic cell adhesiveness by activation of very late antigen (VLA)-4 and VLA-5 integrins. J Exp Med 1995; 181:1805.
29. Takahira H, Gotoh A, Ritchie A, Broxmeyer HE. Steel factor enhances integrin-mediated tyrosine phosphorylation of focal adhesion kinase (pp125^{FAK}) and paxillin. Blood 1997; 89:1574.
30. Gotoh A, Takahira H, Geahlen RL, Broxmeyer HE. Cross-linking of integrins induces tyrosine kinase Syk in a human factor-dependent myeloid cell line. Cell Growth Differ 1997; 8:721.
31. Gotoh A, Ritchie A, Takahira H, Broxmeyer HE. Thrombopoietin and erythropoietin activate inside-out signal of integrin and enhance adhesion to immobilized fibronectin in human growth-factor-dependent hematopoietic cell. Ann Hematol 1997; 75:207.
32. Broxmeyer HD, Douglas GW, Hangoc G, et al. Human umbilical cord blood as a potential source of transplantable hematopoietic stem/progenitor cells. Proc Natl Acad Sci U S A 1989; 86:3828.
33. Knudtzon S. In vitro growth of granulocyte colonies from circulating cells in human cord blood. Blood 1974; 43:357.

34. Gabutti V, Foa R, Mussa F, Aglietta M. Behavior of human haematopoietic stem cells in cord and neonatal blood. Haematologica 1975; 60:492.
35. Fauser AA, Messner HA. Granuloerythropoietic colonies in human bone marrow, peripheral blood and cord blood. Blood 1978; 52:1243.
36. Prindull G, Prindull P, Meulen N. Haematopoietic stem cells (CFUc) in human cord blood. Acta Paediatr Scand 1978; 67:413.
37. Vainchenker W, Gruchard J, Breton-Gorius J. Growth of human megakaryocyte colonies in culture from fetal, neonatal and adult peripheral blood cells: ultrastructural analysis. Blood Cells 1979; 5:25.
38. Hasson MW, Lutton JD, Levere RD, et al. In vitro culture of erythroid colonies from human fetal liver and umbilical cord blood. Br J Haematol 1979; 41:477.
39. Tchernia G, Mielot F, Coulombel L, Mohandas N. Characteristics of circulating erythroid progenitor cells in human newborn infants. J Lab Clin Med 1981; 97:322.
40. Nakahata T, Ogawa M. Hemopoietic colony-forming cells in umbilical cord blood with extensive capability to generate mono- and multipotential hemopoietic progenitors. J Clin Invest 1982; 70:1324.
41. Lynch DC, Knott LY, Rodek CH, Huehns ER. Studies of circulating hemopoietic progenitor cells in human fetal blood. Blood 1982; 59:976.
42. Leary AG, Ogawa M, Strauss LC, Civin CI. Single cell origin of multilineage colonies in culture. J Clin Invest 1984; 74:2193.
43. Geissler K, Geissler W, Hinterberger W, et al. Circulating committed and pluripotential haemopoietic progenitor cells in infants. Acta Haematol 1986; 75:18.
44. Bodger MP. Isolation of hemopoietic progenitor cells from human umbilical cord blood. Exp Hematol 1987; 15:869.
45. Leary AG, Ogawa M. Blast cell colony assay for umbilical cord blood and adult bone marrow progenitors. Blood 1987; 69:953.
46. Koizumi S, Yamagami M, Miura M. Expression of Ia-like antigens defined by monoclonal OKIa 1 antibody on hematopoietic progenitor cells in cord blood: a comparison with human bone marrow. Blood 1982; 60:1046.
47. Broxmeyer HE, Hangoc G, Cooper S, et al. Growth characteristics and expansion of human umbilical cord blood and estimation of its potential for transplantation of adults. Proc Natl Acad Sci U S A 1992; 89:4109.
48. Barnes DWH, Ford CE, Loutit JF. Haemopoietic stem-cells. Lancet 1964; 1:1395.
49. Barker JE. Embryonic mouse peripheral blood colony forming units. Nature 1970; 228:1305.
50. Salahuddin SZ, Markham PD, Ruscetti FW, Gallo RC. Long-term suspension culture of human cord blood myeloid cells. Blood 1981; 58:931.
51. Smith S, Broxmeyer HE. The influence of oxygen tension on the long term growth in vitro of haematopoietic progenitor cells from human cord blood. Br J Haematol 1986; 53:29.
52. Broxmeyer HE, Kurtzberg J, Gluckman E, et al. Umbilical cord blood hematopoietic stem and repopulating cells in human clinical transplantation. Blood Cells 1991; 17:313.
53. Gluckman E, Broxmeyer HE, Auerbach AD, et al. Hematopoietic reconstitution in a patient with Fanconi's anemia by means of umbilical-cord blood from an HLA-identical sibling. N Engl J Med 1989; 321:1174.
54. Broxmeyer HE, Gluckman E, Auerbach A, et al. Human umbilical cord blood: a clinically useful source of transplantable hematopoietic stem/progenitor cells. Int J Cell Cloning 1990; 8:76.
55. Wagner JE, Broxmeyer HE, Byrd RL, et al. Transplantation of umbilical cord blood after myeloablative therapy: analysis of engraftment. Blood 1992; 79:1874.
56. Broxmeyer HE. Introduction: the past, present and future of cord blood transplantation. *In* Broxmeyer HE (ed): Cellular Characteristics of Cord Blood and Cord Blood Transplantation. Bethesda, MD: AABB Press, 1998, pp 1–9.
57. Spitzer G, Verma DS, Fisher R, et al. The myeloid progenitor cell: its value in predicting hematopoietic recovery after autologous bone marrow transplantation. Blood 1980; 55:317.
58. Faille A, Maraninchi D, Gluckman E, et al. Granulocyte progenitor compartments after allogeneic bone marrow grafts. Scand J Haematol 1981; 26:202.
59. Douay L, Gorin NC, Mary JY, et al. Recovery of CFU-GM from cryopreserved marrow and in vivo evaluation after autologous bone marrow transplantation are predictive of engraftment. Exp Hematol 1986; 14:358.
60. Ma DDF, Varga DE, Biggs JC. Donor marrow progenitors (CFU-mix, BFU-E and CFU-GM) and haemopoietic engraftment following HLA matched sibling bone marrow transplantation. Leuk Res 1987; 11:141.
61. Rowley SD, Zuehlsdorf M, Braine HG, et al. CFU-GM content of bone marrow graft correlates with time to hematologic reconstitution following autologous bone marrow transplantation with 4-hyperoxyclophosphamide-purged bone marrow. Blood 1987; 70:271.
62. Jones RJ, Sharkis SJ, Celano P, et al. Progenitor cell assays predict hematopoietic reconstitution after synergeneic transplantation in mice. Blood 1987; 70:1186.
63. Cooper S, Broxmeyer HE. Clonogenic methods in vitro for the enumeration of granulocyte-macrophage progenitor cells (CFU-GM) in human bone marrow and mouse bone marrow and spleen. J Tissue Culture Methods 1991; 13:77.
64. Broxmeyer HE. The interacting effects of cytokines on hematopoietic stem and progenitor cells. *In* Mertelsmann R, Herrmann F (eds): Hematopoietic Growth Factors in Clinical Application. New York: Marcel Dekker, 1990, pp 3–24.
65. Broxmeyer HE, Maze R, Miyazawa K, et al. The *kit* receptor and its ligand, Steel factor, as regulators of hemopoiesis. Cancer Cells 1991; 3:480.
66. Boswell HS, Mochizuki DY, Burgess GS, et al. A novel mast cell growth factor (MCGF-3) produced by marrow-adherent cells that synergizes with interleukin 3 and interleukin 4. Exp Hematol 1990; 18:794.
67. Williams DE, Eisenman J, Baird A, et al. Identification of a ligand for the *c-kit* proto-oncogene. Cell 1990; 63:167.
68. Copeland NG, Gilbert DH, Cho BC, et al. Mast cell growth factor maps near the Steel locus on mouse chromosome 10 and is deleted in a number of Steel alleles. Cell 1990; 63:175.
69. Anderson DM, Lyman SD, Baird A, et al. Molecular cloning of mast cell growth factor, a hematopoietin that is active in both membrane bound and soluble forms. Cell 1990; 63:234.
70. Zsebo KM, Wypych J, McNiece IK, et al. Identification, purification, and biological characterization of hematopoietic stem cell factor from buffalo rat liver-conditioned medium. Cell 1990; 63:195.
71. Martin FH, Suggs SV, Langley KE, et al. Primary structure and functional expression of rat and human stem cell factor DNAs. Cell 1990; 63:203.
72. Zsebo KM, Williams DA, Geissler EN, et al. Stem cell factor is encoded at the S1 locus of the mouse and is the ligand for the *c-kit* tyrosine kinase receptor. Cell 1990; 63:213.
73. Nocka K, Buck J, Levi E, Besmer P. Candidate ligand for the *c-kit* transmembrane kinase receptor: KL, a fibroblast derived growth factor stimulates mast cells and erythroid progenitors. EMBO J 1990; 9:3287.
74. Huang E, Nocka E, Beier DR, et al. The hematopoietic growth factor KL is encoded by the Sl locus and is the ligand for the *c-kit* receptor, the gene product of the W locus. Cell 1990; 63:225.
75. Flanagan JG, Leder P. The *kit* ligand: a cell surface molecule altered in Steel mutant fibroblasts. Cell 1990; 63:185.
76. Anderson DM, Williams DE, Tushinski R, et al. Alternative splicing of mRNA encoding human mast cell growth factor and localization of the gene to chromosome 12q22–24. Cell Growth Differ 1991; 2:373.
77. Chabot B, Stephenson DA, Chapman VM, et al. The proto-oncogene *c-kit* encoding a transmembrane tyrosine kinase receptor maps to the mouse W locus. Nature 1988; 355:88.
78. Geissler EN, Ryan MA, Houseman DE. The dominant-white spotting (W) locus of the mouse encodes the *c-kit* proto-oncogene. Cell 1988; 55:185.
79. Yarden Y, Kuang W, Yang-Feng T, Ullrich A. Human proto-oncogene *c-kit*: a new cell surface receptor tyrosine kinase for an unidentified ligand. EMBO J 1987; 6:3341.
80. Rottapel R, Reedijk M, Williams DE, et al. The Steel/W transduction pathway: *kit* autophosphorylation and its association with a unique subset of cytoplasmic signaling proteins is induced by the Steel factor. Mol Cell Biol 1991; 11:3043.

81. Miyazawa K, Hendrie PC, Mantel C, et al. Comparative analysis of signaling pathways between mast cell growth factor (*c-kit* ligand) and granulocyte-macrophage colony stimulating factor in a human factor-dependent myeloid cell line involves phosphorylation of RAF-1, GTPase-activating protein and mitogen activated protein kinase. Exp Hematol 1991; 19:1110.
82. Reith AD, Ellis C, Lyman SD, et al. Signal transduction by normal isoforms and W mutant variants of the *kit* receptor tyrosine kinase. EMBO J 1991; 10:2451.
83. Broxmeyer HE, Lu L, Cooper S, et al. Flt-3-ligand stimulates/co-stimulates the growth of myeloid stem/progenitor cells. Exp Hematol 1995; 23:1121.
84. Carow CE, Hangoc G, Cooper SH, et al. Mast cell growth factor (*c-kit* ligand) supports the growth of human multipotential (CFU-GEMM) progenitor cells with a high replating potential. Blood 1991; 78:2216.
85. Carow CE, Hangoc G, Broxmeyer HE. Human multipotential progenitor cells (CFU-GEMM) have extensive replating capacity for secondary CFU-GEMM: an effect enhanced by cord blood plasma. Blood 1993; 81:942.
86. Lu L, Xiao M, Shen RN, et al. Enrichment, characterization and responsiveness of single primitive $CD34^{+++}$ human umbilical cord blood hematopoietic progenitor cells with high proliferative and replating potential. Blood 1993; 81:41.
87. Broxmeyer HE. Self-renewal and migration of stem cells during embryonic and fetal hematopoiesis: important but poorly understood event. Blood Cells 1991; 17:282.
88. Till JE, McCulloch EA. A direct measurement of the radiation sensitivity of normal mouse bone marrow cells. Radiat Res 1961; 14:213.
89. Siminovitch L, McCulloch EA, Till JE. The distribution of colony-forming cells among spleen colonies. J Cell Comp Physiol 1963; 62:327.
90. Nakahata T, Ogawa M. Identification of a class of hematopoietic colony-forming units with extensive capability to self-renew and generate multipotential hemopoietic colonies. Proc Natl Acad Sci U S A 1982; 79:3843.
91. Williams DE, Boswell HS, Floyd AD, Broxmeyer HE. Pluripotential stem cells in post 5-fluorouracil murine bone marrow express the Thy-1 antigen. J Immunol 1985; 135:1004.
92. Rowley SD, Sharkis SJ, Hattenburg C, Sensenbrenner LL. Culture from human bone marrow of blast progenitor cells with an extensive proliferative capacity. Blood 1987; 69:804.
93. Brandt JE, Baird N, Lu L, et al. Characterization of a human hematopoietic progenitor cell capable of forming blast cell containing colonies in vitro. J Clin Invest 1988; 82:1017.
94. Metcalf D, Johnson GR, Mandel TE. Colony formation in agar by multipotential hemopoietic cells. J Cell Physiol 1979; 98:401.
95. Messner HA, Fauser AA. Human pluripotent hemopoietic progenitors (CFU-GEMM) in culture. *In* Levine AS (ed): Proceedings of the Conference on Aplastic Anemia: A Stem Cell Disease. Bethesda, MD: National Institutes of Health, 1981, pp 67–75.
96. Ash RC, Detrick RA, Zanjana ED. Studies of human pluripotential hemopoietic stem cells (CFU-GEMM) in vitro. Blood 1981; 58:309.
97. Vormoor J, Lapidot T, Pflumio F, et al. Immature human cord blood progenitors engraft and proliferate to high levels in immune-deficient SCID mice. Blood 1994; 83:2489.
98. Orazi A, Braun SE, Broxmeyer HE. Immunohistochemistry represents a useful tool to study human cell engraftment in SCID mice transplantation models. Blood Cells 1994; 20:323.
99. Bock TA, Orlic D, Dunbar CE, et al. Improved engraftment of human hematopoietic cells in severe combined immunodeficient (SCID) mice carrying human cytokine transgenes. J Exp Med 1995; 182:2037.
100. Lowry PA, Scultz LD, Greiner DL, et al. Improved engraftment of human cord blood stem cells in NOD/LtSz-scid/scid mice after irradiation or multiple-day injections into unirradiated patients. Bone Marrow Transplant 1996; 2:15.
101. Larochelle A, Vormoor J, Hanenberg H, et al. Identification of primitive human hematopoietic cells capable of repopulating NON/SCID mouse bone marrow: implications for gene therapy. Nat Med 1996; 2:1329.
102. Bhatia M, Wang JCY, Kapp U, et al. Purification of primitive human hematopoietic cells capable of repopulating immune-deficient mice. Proc Natl Acad Sci U S A 1997; 94:5320.
103. Hogan CJ, Shpall EJ, McNulty O, et al. Engraftment and development of human $CD34^{+}$-enriched cells from umbilical cord blood in NOD/LtSz-scid/scid mice. Blood 1997; 90:85.
104. Wang JCY, Doedens M, Dick JE. Primitive human hematopoietic cells are enriched in cord blood compared with adult bone marrow or mobilized peripheral blood as measured by the quantitative in vivo SCID-repopulating cell assay. Blood 1997; 89:3919.
105. Wagner JE, Broxmeyer HE, Byrd RL, et al. Transplantation of umbilical cord blood after myeloblative therapy: analysis of engraftment. Blood 1992; 79:1874.
106. Kurtzberg J, Laughlin M, Graham ML, et al. Placental blood as a source of hematopoietic stem cells for transplantation into unrelated recipients. N Engl J Med 1996; 335:157.
107. Wagner JE, Rosenthal J, Sweetman R, et al. Successful transplantation of HLA-matched and HLA-mismatched umbilical cord blood from unrelated donors: analysis of engraftment and acute graft-versus-host disease. Blood 1996; 88:795.
108. Gluckman E, Rocha V, Boyer-Chammard A, et al. Outcome of cord blood transplantation from related and unrelated donors. N Engl J Med 1997; 337:373.
109. Kohli-Kumar M, Shahidi NT, Broxmeyer HE, et al. Haematopoietic stem/progenitor cell transplant in Fanconi anemia using HLA-matched sibling umbilical cord blood cells. Br J Haematol 1993; 85:419.
110. Smith FO, Robertson KA, Lucas KG, et al. Umbilical cord blood transplantation from HLA-mismatched unrelated donors: the Indiana University experience [Abstract]. Blood 1996; 88(suppl 1):266a.
111. Rubinstein P, Carrier C, Scaradavou A, et al. Outcomes among 562 recipients of placental-blood transplants from unrelated donors. N Engl J Med 1998; 339:1565.
112. Broxmeyer HE, Smith FO. Cord blood stem cell transplantation. *In* Forman SI, Blume KG, Thomas ED (eds): Stem Cell Transplantation. Cambridge, MA: Blackwell Scientific Publications, 1998, pp 431–443.
113. Jacobsen N, Broxmeyer HE, Grossbard E, Moore MAS. Colony forming units in diffusion chambers (CFU-D) and colony forming units in agar culture (CFU-C) obtained from human bone marrow: a possible parent progeny relationship. Cell Tissue Kinet 1979; 12:213.
114. Moore MAS, Broxmeyer HE, Sheridan APC, et al. Continuous human bone marrow culture: Ia antigen characterization of probable pluripotential stem cells. Blood 1980; 55:6820.
115. Lowry PA, Zsebo KM, Deacon DH, et al. Effects of rrSCF on multiple cytokine responsive HPP-CFC generated from $SCA^{+}Lin^{-}$ murine hematopoietic progenitors. Exp Hematol 1991; 19:994.
116. Xiao M, Leemhuis T, Broxmeyer HE, Lu L. Influence of combinations of cytokines on proliferation of isolated single cell-sorted human bone marrow hematopoietic progenitor cells in the absence and presence of serum. Exp Hematol 1992; 20:276.
117. de Vries P, Brasel KA, Eisenman JR, et al. The effect of recombinant mast cell growth factor on purified murine hematopoietic stem cells. J Exp Med 1991; 173:1205.
118. Moore MAS. Clinical implications of positive and negative hematopoietic stem cell regulators. Blood 1991; 78:1.
119. Migliaccio G, Migliaccio AR, Valinsky J, et al. Stem cell factor induces proliferation and differentiation of highly enriched murine hematopoietic cells. Proc Natl Acad Sci U S A 1991; 88:7420.
120. Bernstein ID, Andrews RG, Zsebo KM. Recombinant human stem cell factor enhances the formation of colonies by $CD34^{+}$ and $CD34^{+}lin^{-}$ cells, and the generation of colony forming cell progeny from $CD34^{+}lin^{-}$ cells cultured with interleukin-3, granulocyte colony-stimulating factor, or granulocyte-macrophage colony-stimulating factor. Blood 1991; 77:2316.
121. Broxmeyer HE. Phenotypic and proliferative characteristics of cord blood hematopoietic stem and progenitor cells and gene transfer. *In* Broxmeyer HE (ed): Cellular Characteristics of Cord Blood and Cord Blood Transplantation. Bethesda, MD: AABB Press, 1998, pp 11–43.
122. Broxmeyer HE, Vadhan-Raj S. Preclinical and clinical studies with the hematopoietic colony stimulating factors and related interleukins. Immunol Res 1989; 8:185.
123. Broxmeyer HE, Lu L, Vadhan-Raj S, Shen RN. Hematopoietically active cytokines: their effects on tumor growth and potential roles

for therapy of malignant disease. *In* Brenner MK, Hoffbrand AV (eds): Recent Advances in Hematology. London: Churchill Livingstone, 1991, pp 193–205.
124. Risdon G, Gaddy J, Stehman FB, Broxmeyer HE. Proliferative and cytotoxic responses of human cord blood T-lymphocytes following allogeneic stimulation. Cell Immunol 1994; 154:14.
125. Risdon G, Gaddy J, Broxmeyer HE. Allogeneic responses of human umbilical cord blood. Blood Cells 1994; 20:566.
126. Risdon G, Gaddy J, Horie M, Broxmeyer HE. Alloantigen priming induces a state of unresponsiveness in human cord blood T cells. Proc Natl Acad Sci U S A 1995; 92:2413.
127. Porcu P, Gaddy J, Broxmeyer HE. Alloantigen-induced unresponsiveness in cord blood T-lymphocytes is associated with defective activation of *ras*. Proc Natl Acad Sci U S A 1998; 95:4538.
128. Roncarolo MG, Vaccarinom E, Caracco P, et al. Immunologic properties of cord blood. *In* Broxmeyer HE (ed): Cellular Characteristics of Cord Blood and Cord Blood Transplantation. Bethesda, MD: AABB Press, 1998, pp 67–81.
129. Gaddy J, Broxmeyer HE. Cord blood natural killer cells: implications for cord blood transplantation and insights into natural killer cell differentiation. *In* Broxmeyer HE (ed): Cellular Characteristics of Cord Blood and Cord Blood Transplantation. Bethesda, MD: AABB Press, 1998, pp 83–111.
130. Gaddy J, Risdon C, Broxmeyer HE. Cord blood natural killer cells are functionally and phenotypically immature but readily respond to IL-2 and IL-12. J Interferon Cytokine Res 1995; 15:527.
131. Gaddy J, Broxmeyer HE. Cord blood $CD16^+56^-$ natural killer cells with low lytic activity are possible precursors of mature natural killer cells. Cell Immunol 1997; 180:132.
132. Broxmeyer HE, Cooper S. High efficiency recovery of immature hematopoietic progenitor cells with extensive proliferative capacity from human cord blood cryopreserved for ten years. Clin Exp Immunol 1997; 107:45.
133. Moritz T, Keller DC, Williams DA. Human cord blood cells as targets for gene transfer: potential use in genetic therapies of severe combined immunodeficiency disease. J Exp Med 1993; 178:529.
134. Lu L, Xiao M, Clapp DW, et al. High efficiency retroviral-mediated gene transfer into single isolated immature and replatable $CD34^{+++}$ hematopoietic stem/progenitor cells from human umbilical cord blood. J Exp Med 1993; 178:2089.
135. Lu L, Xiao M, Clapp DW, et al. Stable integration of retrovirally transduced genes into human umbilical cord blood high proliferative potential colony forming cells (HPP-CFC) as assessed after multiple HPP-CFC colony replatings in vitro. Blood Cells 1994; 20:525.
136. Lu L, Ge Y, Li ZH, et al. Influence of retroviral-mediated gene transduction of recombinant human erythropoietin receptor gene into single hematopoietic stem/progenitor cells from human cord blood on the growth of these cells. Blood 1996; 87:525.
137. Xiao M, Yang YC, Lang L, et al. Transduction of human interleukin-9 receptor gene into human cord blood erythroid progenitor increases the number of erythropoietin-dependent erythroid colonies. Bone Marrow Transplant 1996; 18:1103.
138. Lu L, Li ZH, Xiao M, Broxmeyer HE. Influence of retroviral mediated gene transduction of both the recombinant human erythropoietin receptor and interleukin-9 receptor genes into single $CD34^{+++}CD33^{-\text{ or low}}$ cord blood cells on cytokine stimulated erythroid colony formation. Exp Hematol 1996; 24:347.
139. Li ZH, Broxmeyer HE, Lu L. Cryopreserved cord blood myeloid progenitor cells can serve as targets for retroviral-mediated gene transduction and gene-transduced progenitors can be cryopreserved and recovered. Leukemia 1995; 9:S12.
140. Lu L, Ge Y, Li ZH, et al. $CD34^{+++}$ stem/progenitor cells purified from cryopreserved normal cord blood can be transduced with high efficiency by a retroviral vector and expanded ex vivo with stable integration and expression of Fanconi anemia complementation C gene. Cell Transplant 1995; 4:493.
141. Kohn DB, Weinberg KI, Nolta JA, et al. Engraftment of gene-modified umbilical cord blood cells in neonates with adenosine deaminase deficiency. Nat Med 1995; 10:1.
142. Kohn DB, Hershfield MS, Carbonaro D, et al. T lymphocytes with a normal ADA gene accumulate after transplantation of transduced autologous umbilical cord blood $CD34^+$ cells in ADA-deficient SCID neonates. Nature Med 1998; 7:775.
143. Zhou SZ, Broxmeyer HE, Cooper S, et al. Adeno-associated virus 2–mediated gene transfer in murine hematopoietic progenitor cells. Exp Hematol 1993; 21:928.
144. Zhou SZ, Cooper S, Kang LY, et al. Adeno-associated virus 2–mediated high efficiency gene transfer into immature and mature subsets of hematopoietic progenitor cells in human umbilical cord blood. J Exp Med 1994; 179:1867.
145. Ponnazhagan S, Mukherjee P, Wang X-S, et al. Adeno-associated virus type 2-mediated transduction in primary human bone marrow-derived $CD34^+$ hematopoietic progenitor cells: Donor variation and correlation of transgene expression with cellular differentiation. J Virol 1997; 71:8262.
146. Qing K, Mah C, Hansen J, et al. Human fibroblast growth factor receptor 1 is a co-receptor for infection by adeno-associated virus 2. Nature Med 1999; 5:71.
147. Qing K, Wang X-U, Kube DM, et al. Role of tyrosine phosphorylation of a cellular protein in adeno-associated virus 2–mediated transgene expression. Proc Natl Acad Sci U S A 1997; 94:10879.
148. Miyoshi H, Smith KA, Mosier DF, et al. Transduction of human $CD34^+$ cells that mediate long-term engraftment of NOD/SCID mice by HIV vectors. Science 1999; 283:682.

SECTION

IX Immune Effects of Transfusion

CHAPTER 26

Alloimmunization to Blood Group Antigens

R. Sue Shirey
Karen E. King

The immune system in humans exists primarily as a defense mechanism against disease-causing microorganisms. When a foreign agent (antigen) invades the host and triggers the immune response, a complex series of events occurs involving the proliferation, interaction, and cooperation of T and B lymphocytes and accessory or antigen-presenting cells.[1–3] T lymphocytes are generally responsible for cell-mediated immunity, and B lymphocytes provide humoral immunity by synthesizing and secreting antibody into the blood and tissue fluids.

Unfortunately, the immune system is often unable to discriminate between foreign antigens borne on potentially harmful bacteria and those present on human blood cells and tissue. Thus, individuals exposed to foreign blood group antigens through transfusion, pregnancy, or tissue transplantation may produce antibodies. The nature of the immune response to blood group antigens, or whether it occurs at all in a given individual, depends on several factors, including the immunogenicity of the antigen, the dose and route of administration, and the apparent genetic disposition of the host.[4–7]

PRIMARY AND SECONDARY IMMUNE RESPONSES

When an individual is first exposed to a foreign blood group antigen, the immune response is relatively slow. Antibody may not be serologically detectable for 4 weeks or even several months after transfusion.[8, 9] This primary immune response usually results in low levels of immunoglobulin M (IgM) antibody that gradually decline. After a second exposure to antigen, the immune response is rapid, with antibody titers rising as early as 48 hours after injection. This secondary or anamnestic immune response is generally characterized by increased production of IgG antibody that may peak as early as 6 days after injection.[4–7] The dose of antigen needed to provoke an optimal secondary immune response is relatively small compared with the dose needed to stimulate primary immunization.[4]

It is not clear whether alloantibody production to red cell antigens always proceeds through an IgM stage, because only IgG antibody is detected in many cases. This observation may be due either to the inability of routine serological tests to detect low levels of IgM antibody or to the rapid conversion from IgM to IgG antibody production.[5] The persistence of serologically detectable antibody after antigen exposure may also vary considerably among different individuals.[10–12] In general, IgM antibodies are more transient than antibodies of the IgG class. Indeed, IgG antibodies, such as anti-D, may persist for 30 or more years after the stimulating event.[10–12]

IMMUNOGENICITY OF BLOOD GROUP ANTIGENS

Immunogenicity refers to the ability of an antigen to stimulate an immune response or antibody production. Fortunately, most blood group antigens are poor immunogens. In fact, of all patients transfused with allogeneic red cells, probably less than 1% form blood group antibodies.[5] The factors responsible for the apparent differences in immunogenicity among blood group antigens have not been clearly explained. The experimental work by Sela[13] with polypeptide antigens suggests that such factors as molecular weight, number of aromatic amino acid residues, and net molecular charge may influence the host's immune response.

Clearly, the most immunogenic blood group antigens are A and B, because antibodies to these antigens occur in virtually all individuals lacking the corresponding antigen, regardless of exposure to blood products. It is generally accepted that anti-A and anti-B are stimulated by substances that are ubiquitous in nature, such as bacteria, which possess chemical substances similar to human A and B antigens. Considerable evidence supports this mechanism for the origin of ABO antibodies. Springer and associates,[14] for example, demonstrated that White Leghorn chicks raised in a germ-free environment did not make anti-B, whereas chicks raised under normal conditions developed a high titer of anti-B. The ability of bacteria to stimulate ABO antibodies in humans through ingestion or inhalation has also been shown in a series of experiments.[15] In one study, killed *Escherichia coli* O_{86} with blood group B specificity caused a significant in-

Table 26–1. Alloantibody Frequency and Relative Antigen Immunogenicity

Blood Group System	Relative Frequency of Antibody (%)	Relative Immunogenicity†
Rh*	55.1	0.7
Kell	28.7	1.0
Duffy	11.2	0.14
Kidd	4.3	0.06
Other	0.7	Negligible

*Excluding anti-D.
†Relative immunogenicity compared with that of K antigen.

crease in anti-B titers in 11 of 16 infants with diarrhea, whereas only 1 of 7 healthy infants had an increased anti-B titer.[15] The same bacteria administered by nasal spray to adults induced increases in anti-B production in 4 of 12 subjects. ABO antibodies are usually IgM, or combinations of IgM and IgG, and can generally be demonstrated in the sera of infants at 3 to 6 months of age.[4, 5]

Anti-A and anti-B have been called "naturally occurring" antibodies because they develop without an allogeneic red cell stimulus. There are many other blood group alloantibodies that may be "naturally occurring," such as anti-M, anti-N, and anti-P_1.[4, 5] Cold-reactive, IgM agglutinins occurring in individuals with no known exposure to foreign red cells might represent T cell–independent responses.[7] The demonstration in animals that IgM antibody responses to some antigens, particularly polysaccharides, do not appear to require helper T cells supports this view.[7]

Antibodies stimulated by exposure to foreign red cells are usually of the IgG class and are called "immune" alloantibodies. The D antigen of the Rh system appears to be the most immunogenic of blood group antigens. On the basis of biochemical studies, it appears that the immunogenic D epitope is not a simple peptide sequence but probably involves a precise surface conformation that results from the cooperative interactions of at least one of the Rh polypeptides with surrounding glycoproteins and may also require a specific exofacial free sulfhydryl and certain adjacent lipid structures in the red cell membrane.[16]

The D antigen is significantly more immunogenic than any other Rh system antigen. It is presumed that the explanation for the immunogenicity of D is related to the genetic basis and organization of the Rh system.[5] It is now understood that the Rh system is encoded by two separate genes: *RHD* encodes D antigen and *RHCE* encodes the C, c, E, and e antigens. Although exceptions have been described, most D-positive individuals have the *RHD* gene, leading to the production of D antigen, and most D-negative individuals have deletion of the *RHD* gene, so that no D antigen, not even an altered form, is produced.[16–18] The antigens encoded by the *RHCE* gene show significant homology, such that C and c differ by only four amino acids with potentially only one significant amino acid change, and there is only a single amino acid change between E and e. Thus, a D-negative recipient of D-positive red cells will recognize an entirely foreign antigen, whereas the E-negative recipient of E-positive red cells will have to recognize a single amino acid difference to see the antigen as foreign, leading to an immune response. It is because of the exceptional immunogenicity of the D antigen that we routinely prophylactically match for D-negative status, which we do for no other antigen.

The relative immunogenicity of other (non-D) blood group antigens is based partially on the frequency with which the blood group antibodies are encountered. Rh antibodies other than D account for more than half of the immune alloantibodies that are found in pregnancy and transfusion (Table 26–1).[19] Anti-K and anti-Fy^a constitute about 40% of the total, leaving only about 5% for all other immune alloantibodies.

To determine the relative immunogenicity (RI) or potency of different red cell antigens, the actual frequency with which particular alloantibodies are encountered can be compared with the calculated frequency of the probability of exposure or opportunity for immunization (Table 26–2).[20] For example, the relative immunogenicity of Fy^a and that of K can be compared as follows: The opportunity for immunization (OI) to Fy^a and K can be calculated by comparing the frequency of the combination of an Fy(a+) donor and an Fy(a−) recipient ($0.67 \times 0.33 = 0.22$) with the frequency of the combination of a K-positive donor and K-negative recipient ($0.09 \times 0.91 = 0.08$). Thus, the OI to Fy^a is about 3 times that for K. Although OI to Fy^a is 3 times greater than the OI to K, the observed frequency of Fy^a antibody is actually one-third that of K antibody. Thus, K is approximately 9 times more immunogenic than Fy^a. Giblett[20] calculated that K is 25 times more potent than Fy^a and 3 times more immunogenic than Rh antigens other than D. Although the relative immunogenicity may vary considerably, depending on the frequency of observed alloantibodies, studies have consistently shown that the relative likelihoods of blood group antibody formation are as follows: $D > K > E > Fy^a > Jk^a$.[4–6]

DOSE AND ROUTE OF ADMINISTRATION

Although the immunogenicity of blood group antigens probably is the major determinant of whether an antibody response occurs, the dose of antigen administered is also an important factor in alloimmunization. This factor is best illustrated by the disparity in immunization rates observed in transfusion and in pregnancy. An individual is far more likely to develop an antibody from a single transfusion of red cells possessing a foreign antigen than from pregnancy with a fetus whose red cells possess the same immunogen. Presumably, the volume of transpla-

Table 26–2. Calculating the Relative Immunogenicity (RI) of Blood Group Antigens

$$RI = OI\ (ag1)/OI\ (ag2) \times F(ab2)/F(ab1)$$

where
OI (ag1) = opportunity for immunization to antigen 1
OI (ag2) = opportunity for immunization to antigen 2
F(ab1) = frequency of antibody 1
F(ab2) = frequency of antibody 2

cental hemorrhage in most pregnancies is not sufficient for primary immunization.[4] Because a secondary immune response generally requires less antigenic stimulus, women who become alloimmunized during pregnancy often have a history of previous exposure to foreign red cells by transfusion.

The fact that many individuals fail to produce blood group antibodies after multiple red cell transfusions may also be related to dosage. Because an immune response probably can occur only when the red cell antigens have been processed by macrophages, the small volume of senescent transfused cells removed by splenic sequestration each day (about 1%) may not be sufficient to elicit a primary immune response.[5, 6] Undoubtedly, the minimum dose, the number of doses, and the interval between doses that effectively stimulate immunization varies among alloantigen specificities.

Virtually all blood group antibodies arise from intravenous exposure to foreign red cells, although Shepherd and colleagues[21] reported that a male volunteer developed anti-Xg^a after weekly intradermal injections of mixed leukocytes and red cells.

Of note, there have been several reports of alloimmunization related to incompatible bone allografts.[22–26] Although many of the resultant alloantibodies have been anti-D,[22, 26] other Rh system antibodies (including anti-C, -E, and -G)[24, 25] and red cell antibodies with non–Rh system specificities (anti-Fy^a and anti-Jk^a)[23] have been reported. Furthermore, incompatible bone allografts have been implicated in both primary and secondary alloimmunization.[22–26] This setting of red cell alloimmunization by bone allograft exposure raises the issue of immunogenicity of red cell stroma as compared with intact red cells. Because bone allografts are extensively processed, it is most likely that red cell stroma, not intact red cells, is responsible for the alloimmunization associated with bone allografts. Schneider and Preisler[27] compared the rates of Rh alloimmunization using intact red cells versus lysed red cells. Their data show that red cell stroma can induce Rh immunization, although the rate of antibody production is much lower than when intact Rh positive red cells are used.

GENETIC FACTORS

The immune system is not fully developed at birth; several lymphocyte and monocyte functions have not reached maturity in neonates.[28, 29] Apparently owing to this incomplete immune constitution, infants younger than 4 months of age seem to be incapable of producing antibodies in response to multiple transfusions.[30, 31] Although there is considerable variation among adults in the response to alloantigens, the ability to respond to transfusions by forming red cell antibodies, once developed, does not appear to decline with age.[32]

Immune responsiveness is determined, at least in part, by the products of the major histocompatibility complex (MHC) genes, particularly HLA-DR genes.[2, 3, 33, 34] Several studies have sought to associate the HLA phenotype and the immune response to various antigens.[35] Although alloimmunization to HPA-1a (Pl^{A1}) platelet antigen has been strongly associated with HLA-B8, HLA-DR3, and HLA-DRw52,[36, 37] immunization to blood group antigens, especially the highly immunogenic D antigen, has not been shown to correlate significantly with HLA type.[38–42] There is one report showing an association between HLA-B35 and alloimmunized sickle cell patients.[43] In this study, HLA-B35–positive sickle cell patients were six times more likely to form red cell alloantibodies than those lacking that HLA antigen. Although there appears to be an association between HLA phenotype and the propensity for blood group alloimmunization, no direct relationship has been demonstrated. Perhaps this inability to show such a relationship is because the immune response is influenced by genes independent of HLA, such as T cell receptor genes.[2, 3]

IMMUNIZATION TO D ANTIGEN

After the A and B antigens, the D antigen is the most immunogenic of blood group antigens and often is clinically significant. Anti-D is almost always an immune antibody produced in response to red cell stimulation, although there are rare reports of "naturally occurring" anti-D.[44] Immunization to D in D-negative volunteers has been studied extensively.[8, 9, 45–49] Approximately 80% of D-negative individuals who receive a single transfusion of 200 mL or more of D-positive red cells develop serologically detectable anti-D within 2 to 5 months.[4, 8, 45] About 20% of D-negative subjects are "nonresponders" who do not develop anti-D even after repeated injections of D-positive red cells. Although small doses of D-positive red cells can provoke primary immunization, the number of individuals who respond is fewer and the titers of anti-D produced are lower than is observed after exposure to larger doses of D-positive cells.[49] For example, according to combined data from three studies (Table 26–3), 30% of D-negative individuals developed anti-D after an initial dose of 1 mL of D-positive red cells, and 51% had anti-D after a second 1-mL dose.[46–49] The rate of primary immunization after the first 1-mL dose is probably higher, but the concentration of anti-D is too low to detect serologically.

In some cases, the presence of anti-D indicating primary immunization may be evidenced only by the finding of accelerated destruction of a second dose of D-positive red cells.[46, 50] In the studies by Mollison and associates,[46] for example, only 2 of 13 transfusion recipi-

Table 26–3. Summary of Data on D Immunization From Three Studies

Study	No. of Subjects	No. of Subjects With Anti-D (%): After Dose No. 1*	After Dose No. 2*
Mollison et al.[46]	13	2 (15%)	4 (31%)
Samson and Mollison[47]	12	5 (42%)	9 (75%)
Contreras and Mollison[48]	12	4 (33%)	6 (50%)
	37	11 (30%)	19 (51%)

*Each dose was 1 mL of D-positive red cells.

ents formed serologically detectable anti-D within 6 months after an initial 1-mL dose of D-positive red cells. However, when a second injection of red cells was given to the 11 apparent nonresponders, 5 showed a significant reduction in the survival of D-positive red cells, confirming that primary immunization had occurred. Four of the 5 had serologically detectable anti-D about 1 month after the second injection (see Table 26–3).

Primary immunization to D without serologically detectable antibody has been termed *sensibilization* and is commonly observed after exposure to small quantities of red cells, as may occur in pregnancy.[51] There is some evidence that the minimum dose of red cells necessary for primary immunization is only 0.03 mL.[49, 52] In individuals who have already been primarily immunized, as little as 0.2 to 2 mL of red cells may be sufficient to cause a secondary antibody response, with maximum production of anti-D within 3 weeks of exposure.[4]

Several workers have noted that responders who produce anti-D are also more likely to produce antibodies directed at other blood group antigens. Issitt[53] found that 5 (12%) of 42 D-negative women with anti-D also made non-D antibodies, whereas only 1 (0.1%) of 877 D-positive women made non-D antibodies. During deliberate immunization studies in D-negative volunteers, Archer and colleagues[54] reported that 14 (19%) of 73 transfused patients who made anti-D antibodies also made other antibodies, yet none of the 48 nonresponders to D made antibodies with other specificities.

This higher incidence of non-D blood group antibodies in responders who have produced anti-D may be related to a "concentration effect." For example, in D-negative subjects who have anti-D antibody, D-positive foreign red cells are rapidly sequestered in the spleen. Other antigens (e.g., Fy^a, Jk^a) that are present on the D-positive cells are also presented to splenic immunocytes in a concentrated form, thereby enhancing or augmenting the immune response.[55, 56] D-positive individuals who are "good responders," that is, with evidence of antibodies to other blood group antigens, do exist; however, D is a strong immunogen compared with other blood group antigens, and it is therefore easier to recognize "good responders" in D-negative subjects.[53]

The question arises as to whether nonresponders to D antigen are also nonresponders to other cell-borne antigens. The data are insufficient to answer this question in regard to red cell antigens.[4] An interesting study by Baldwin and colleagues,[57] however, indicated that nonresponders to D antigen are able to produce antibodies to leukocyte antigens. In this study, 49 D-negative oncology patients who received D-positive platelet transfusions were examined for the development of anti-D and lymphocytotoxic antibodies (LCAs). LCAs were identified in 4 of 9 (44%) patients with anti-D and in 12 of 40 (30%) patients who did not develop anti-D. Because both D and HLA antigens are considered highly immunogenic, the authors concluded that the likelihood of alloimmunization to D appears to be unrelated to alloimmunization to HLA antigens.

SUPPRESSION OF PRIMARY ALLOIMMUNIZATION

Primary alloimmunization of D-negative individuals exposed to D-positive red cells can be prevented by administration of passive IgG anti-D. The mechanism of antibody-mediated immune suppression remains controversial.[58–60] Nevertheless, the routine use of Rh immune globulin prophylaxis in women at risk has nearly eliminated hemolytic disease of the newborn due to anti-D.

Levine[61, 62] noted that immunization to D in pregnancy was less common when the fetus was ABO incompatible with the mother. This observation led Race and Sanger[63] to propose that immune clearance of ABO-incompatible fetal cells in the maternal circulation protects against Rh immunization. It has been theorized that maternal ABO antibodies that are capable of activating complement may cause intravascular hemolysis of ABO-incompatible, D-positive fetal red cells, thereby diverting antigen from antibody-forming cells in the spleen.[58] Although the red cell stroma resulting from intravascular hemolysis is still immunogenic, it is believed that stroma is removed from the circulation predominantly by the liver rather than the spleen.[4] This theory of antigen deviation and clearance could explain the low incidence of alloimmunization observed in this setting and also could elucidate the mechanism of prevention of Rh immunization by passive antibody. Thus, passive anti-D does not activate complement and could result in extravascular phagocytosis and destruction of antigen-bearing cells by lysosomal enzymes, thereby preventing immunization to Rh antigen.[58]

Finn and colleagues[64, 65] found an apparent relationship between the protection against alloimmunization provided by passive anti-D and accelerated clearance of antigen. Although this proposal was correct, the efficacy of antibody-mediated suppression of primary immunization cannot be explained solely on the basis of rapid immune clearance. Indeed, immunization can be prevented even when there is only a slight increase in the rate of red cell clearance.[8, 66] Moreover, because antigen must exit the circulation before immunization can occur, one could argue that the best way to preclude an immune response would be to prevent, rather than enhance, clearance of the antigen-bearing cells.[58]

Another simple mechanism to explain suppression of the primary immune response by passive antibody is that all D antigen epitopes are blocked by antibody and are not available to lymphocyte receptors.[58] However, this concept seems untenable, in view of the fact that F(Ab) or $F(Ab)_2$ antibody fragments are not effective in suppressing in vivo primary immunization.[67–69] Furthermore, it is recognized that only 20 μg of passive anti-D per milliliter of D-positive red cells is suppressive, even though this dose is not sufficient to saturate all of the D antigen sites.

Pollack[58] favors a "central control concept" to explain suppression by passive antibody. In this model, the formation of IgG immune complexes (anti-D and D antigen) in the follicular areas of the lymph nodes and spleen may trigger the release of lymphokines or other negative mediators that effectively suppress the primary immune response. Regardless of the mechanism involved, the suppression of D immunization by passive anti-D appears to be antigen specific, because passive IgG anti-D does not seem to suppress immunization to other blood group antigens that may be present on D-positive red cells.[58]

AUGMENTATION OF PRIMARY ALLOIMMUNIZATION

Augmentation of the immune response by passive antibody remains the subject of much controversy. In humans, *augmentation* generally refers to an enhancement or increase in the primary immune response, as measured by (1) an earlier appearance of antibody, (2) an increase in antibody production, or (3) an increase in the probability of responding to a given dose of antigen.[4, 49]

Evidence of augmentation caused by low doses of passively administered anti-D was first reported by Pollack and associates.[66] D-negative subjects were given approximately 2.3 mL of D-positive red cells; 3 days later, various amounts of IgG anti-D were injected. Eighty-four days after injection, 8 of 11 (72.7%) subjects who received red cells plus 10 μg of antibody developed anti-D; only 1 of 6 (16.7%) in the control group, which received red cells alone, formed anti-D. In this as well as other series, small amounts of passive IgG anti-D produced an apparent increase in the proportion of individuals developing a primary immune response, compared with the number of subjects immunized by antigen stimulation alone.[49, 66, 70] No difference was found between test and control subjects in the time at which antibody was first detected or in the amount of antibody produced.[70] The cumulative data suggest that augmentation may occur in humans, because a seemingly ineffective dose of antigen becomes effective in stimulating a primary response when small amounts of passive IgG antibody are given concurrently. Whether or not IgM antibody can augment primary alloimmunization is still unclear, but at least one experiment with purified IgM anti-D showed no evidence of augmentation.[71]

It appears that the ratio of IgG antibody to antigen-bearing red cells is the major factor determining whether there is a primary immune response suppressed or augmented. Whereas a dose of 20 μg of IgG anti-D per milliliter of red cells suppresses a primary response, an estimated dose of 0.5 to 2 μg/mL of D-positive red cells may promote augmentation or increase the likelihood of primary immunization.[49] Applying Pollack's central control model,[58] it would appear that augmentation of the immune response would occur when antibody was sufficient to cause trapping within the spleen but was insufficient to result in Fc binding and inhibition of the immune response. In clinical practice, there is no convincing evidence that augmentation of immunization in Rh prophylactic therapy actually occurs.

Rh IMMUNE GLOBULIN (RhIG)

A dose of 20 μg of IgG anti-D is sufficient to suppress the primary immunizing ability of 1 mL of D-positive red cells. A single dose of RhIG consists of 300 μg of concentrated IgG anti-D and is used primarily for the prevention of Rh immunization in pregnancy, or to suppress the development of anti-D in D-negative patients who have been transfused with D-positive blood components. Postpartum administration of RhIG to D-negative women delivered of D-positive infants reduces the rate of immunization from 8% to 1%; the implementation of antepartum RhIG at 28 weeks of gestation to women at risk has decreased the immunization rate to only 0.1%.[72–74]

Antepartum RhIG prophylaxis was based on the studies by Bowman and coworkers[72] in which 300 μg of RhIG was administered at 28 to 34 weeks of gestation to 1204 D-negative women who subsequently were delivered of D-positive infants. None of the women became immunized, although historically 21 would have been expected to develop anti-D had they received only postpartum prophylaxis. On the basis of the half-life of IgG, Bowman and coworkers[72] predicted that a single dose of 300 μg of RhIG at 28 weeks would be protective for 12 weeks (84 days), or throughout the third trimester of pregnancy. Given that the half-life of IgG is 22 days, a 300-μg dose of RhIG should result in a residual dose of 20 μg 12 weeks after injection. Studies on the postinjection kinetics of RhIG given antepartum have shown, however, that 5 of 10 patients did not have serologically detectable anti-D 8 to 29 days before delivery, suggesting that these women may not have been protected from immunization for as long as 1 month of the pregnancy.[75] Furthermore, at least theoretically, low or serologically undetectable levels of passive antibody may actually cause augmentation of the immune response from a fetal-maternal hemorrhage in the late third trimester.[4, 49, 76]

Passive anti-D due to administration of antepartum RhIG may be serologically indistinguishable from anti-D owing to active immunization. In general, passive anti-D (RhIG) reacts only at the indirect antiglobulin phase and does not exceed a titer of 4.[73, 75] D-positive infants delivered of D-negative mothers may have a positive direct antiglobulin test, owing to sensitization with maternal RhIG; however, antepartum RhIG does not cause hemolytic disease of the newborn, nor is it harmful to the developing fetus.[72] It should be emphasized that RhIG can prevent primary but not secondary immunization. RhIG given to immunized patients who have only low concentrations of anti-D fails to suppress an anamnestic response to D-positive red cells.[56, 77]

ALLOIMMUNIZATION AND DISEASE

There is some evidence that the immune response to blood group antigens may be different in patients with certain diseases. Several studies have been performed to determine the rates of alloimmunization in various disorders in which the patients generally require chronic transfusion therapy (Table 26–4).[78–89] Blumberg and colleagues[79] and Fluitt and associates[80] found that patients with acute lymphocytic leukemia were unlikely to form alloantibodies even after multiple red cell transfusions; 5.7% to 16% of patients with myelogenous leukemia or aplastic anemia developed red cell antibodies, often before the 10th transfusion. This immune unresponsiveness in acute lymphocytic leukemia could be related to the disease's pathophysiology or chemotherapy, both of which may have an immunosuppressive effect.[90, 91] As might be expected, patients with diseases that result in hypogam-

Table 26–4. Reported Frequencies of Alloantibodies in Various Diagnostic Groups

Diagnostic Group	Frequency (%)
Transfusion recipients†[5, 78]	<1.0
Diagnostic groups‡	
Myelogenous leukemia[79–81]	5.7–16.0
Lymphocytic leukemia[79–81]	0.0
Aplastic anemia[79, 81]	11.0
Multiple myeloma[79, 81]	11.8
Sickle cell anemia[82–88]	17.6–36
Thalassemia[88, 89]	5.2–11.0

*Chapter references.
†Patients who have received at least one allogeneic red cell transfusion.
‡Patients who generally require chronic red cell transfusions.

maglobulinemia also have a greatly diminished capacity to produce red cell antibodies.

Although it is difficult to consolidate the data because of a number of variables that are not consistently considered in all studies, rates of alloimmunization in sickle cell disease appear to be high (see Table 26–4). However, it is not clear whether patients with sickle cell anemia differ from other chronically transfused African-American patients in their tendency to alloimmunization.[92] In part, this high rate of immunization appears to be due to racial differences between the blood donor and recipient populations.[82] Some investigators [82, 93–96] have advocated providing sickle cell patients with blood phenotypically matched for major blood group antigens in the Rh, Kell, Duffy, and Kidd systems to prevent alloimmunization.[71] This approach may be most justified in patients with one or more alloantibodies, who are more susceptible to delayed hemolytic transfusion reactions.[86, 95–98]

Orthotopic liver transplant patients, although not generally chronically transfused, often require large amounts of red cell products at the time of transplantation and in the perioperative period. Casanueva and associates[99] found no alloimmunization directed against D antigen in a group of 17 D-negative orthotopic liver transplant patients who received 5 to 41 units of D-positive red cells during surgery. These patients are routinely immunosuppressed to prevent rejection of their liver allografts, and it is hypothesized that the immunosuppressive regimen, including cyclosporin A, inhibits lymphocyte activation, leading to prevention of the primary immune response.

CONCLUSION

Our current understanding of blood group alloimmunization is based predominantly on empirical data. Major advances have been made in the identification of blood group antibodies and suppression of Rh alloimmunization, but the mechanisms of the human immune response are still unclear. An individual's immune response to alloantigens is probably genetically determined. With the advent of newer technologies, such as DNA hybridization, monoclonal antibody production, and gene cloning, the structure, function, and products of genes involved in blood group alloimmunization may be elucidated. Specific methods for assessing the immunological functions of lymphocytes and monocytes are now being used to evaluate responses to blood transfusions. Ideally, in the future, an in vitro test to distinguish responders from nonresponders prospectively will be available. Perhaps the use of specific immunoglobulins, induction of specific tolerance, or other immunosuppressive methods will markedly abrogate red cell alloimmunization.

REFERENCES

1. Janaway CA Jr, Travers P. Immunobiology: The Immune System in Health and Disease, 3rd ed. New York: Garland Publishing, 1997.
2. Stites DP, Stobo JD, Wells JV (eds). Basic and Clinical Immunology, 6th ed. Norwalk, CT: Appleton & Lange, 1987.
3. Tregellas WM, Keating LJ (eds). Immunology. Arlington, VA: American Association of Blood Banks, 1985.
4. Mollison PL, Engelfriet CP, Contreras M. Blood Transfusions in Clinical Medicine, 10th ed. Oxford: Blackwell, 1997.
5. Issitt PD, Anstee DJ. Applied Blood Group Serology, 4th ed. Miami, FL: Montgomery Scientific, 1998.
6. Case J. The immune response. *In* Dawson RB (ed): Blood Bank Immunology: A Technical Workshop. Washington, DC: American Association of Blood Banks, 1977, pp 87–96.
7. Silberstein LE. The antibody response to antigen. *In* Nance ST (ed): Alloimmunity: 1993 and Beyond. Bethesda, MD: American Association of Blood Banks, 1993, pp 25–47.
8. Pollack W, Ascari WQ, Crispen JF, et al. Studies on Rh prophylaxis: II. Rh immune prophylaxis after transfusion with Rh-positive blood. Transfusion 1971; 11:340.
9. Gunson HH, Stratton F, Cooper DG. Primary immunization of Rh-negative volunteers. BMJ 1970; 1:593.
10. Ramsey G, Larson P. Loss of red cell alloantibodies over time. Transfusion 1988; 28:162.
11. Hopkins DF. The decline and fall of anti-Rh(D). Br J Haematol 1969; 17:199.
12. Ward HK. The persistence of antibodies in the absence of antigenic stimulus. Aust J Exp Biol Med Sci 1957; 35:499.
13. Sela M. Antigenicity, some molecular aspects. Science 1969; 166:1365.
14. Springer GF, Horton RE, Forbes M. Origin of anti-human blood group B agglutinins in White Leghorn chicks. J Exp Med 1959; 110:221.
15. Springer GF, Horton RE. Blood group isoantibody stimulation in man by feeding blood group-active bacteria. J Clin Invest 1969; 48:1280.
16. Agre P, Cartron JP. Molecular biology of the Rh antigens. Blood 1991; 78:551.
17. Cartron JP, Agre P. Rh blood group antigens: protein and gene structure. Semin Hematol 1993; 30:193.
18. Huang C-H. Molecular insights in the Rh protein family and associated antigens. Curr Opin Hematol 1997; 4:94.
19. Grove-Rasmussen M, Huggins CE. Selected types of frozen blood for patients with multiple blood group antibodies. Transfusion 1973; 13:124.
20. Giblett ER. A critique of the theoretical hazard of inter- versus intra-racial transfusion. Transfusion 1961; 1:233.
21. Shepherd LP, Feingold E, Shanbrom E. An unusual occurrence of anti-Xg_a. Vox Sang 1969; 16:157.
22. Shi PA, Shirey RS, King KE, Ness PM. Primary and secondary Rh alloimmunization induced by bone allografts [Abstract]. Transfusion 1998; 38:68S.
23. Cheek RF, Harmon JF, Stowell CP. Red cell alloimmunization after a bone allograft. Transfusion 1995; 35:507.
24. Johnson CA, Brown BA, Lasky LC. Rh immunization caused by osseous allograft [Letter]. N Engl J Med 1985; 312:121.
25. Jensen TT. Rhesus immunization after bone allografting: a case report. Acta Orthop Scand 1987; 58:584.
26. Muslow CE, Bell RS, Beaudry-Clouatre M. Rh stimulation after bone allografting. Presented at the 15th Annual Meeting of the American Association of Tissue Banks, Clearwater Beach, FL, 1991, p 31.

27. Schneider J, Preisler O. Untersuchungen zur serologischen Prophylaxe der Rh-Sensibilisierung. Blut 1965; 12(1):4.
28. Burgio GR, Ugazio AG, Notarangelo LD. Immunology of the neonate. Curr Opin Immunol 1989; 90(2):770.
29. DePalma L, Duncan B, Chan MM, Luban NLC. The neonatal immune response to washed and irradiated red cells: lack of evidence of lymphocyte activation. Transfusion 1991; 31:737.
30. Floss AM, Strauss RG, Goeken N, Knox L. Multiple transfusions fail to provoke antibodies against blood cell antigens in human infants. Transfusion 1986; 26:419.
31. Ludvigsen CW, Swanson JL, Thompson TR, McCullough J. The failure of neonates to form red blood cell alloantibodies in response to multiple transfusions. Am J Clin Pathol 1987; 57:250.
32. Dzik WH, Medeiros LJ. Age and erythrocyte alloimmunization [Letter]. Vox Sang 1986; 51:73.
33. Benacerraf B. Role of MHC gene products in immune regulation. Science 1981; 212:1229.
34. Marx JL. Histocompatibility restriction explained. Science 1987; 235:843.
35. Tiwari JL, Terasaki PI. HLA and Disease Associations. New York: Springer-Verlag, 1985.
36. de Waal LP, van Dalen CM, Engelfriet CP, von dem Borne AEGK. Alloimmunization against the platelet-specific Zw[a] antigen, resulting in neonatal alloimmune thrombocytopenia or post-transfusion purpura, is associated with the supertypic DRw52 antigen including DR3 and DRw6. Hum Immunol 1986; 17:45.
37. Reznikoff-Etievant MF, Muller JY, Julien F, Patereau C. An immune response gene linked to MHC in man. Tissue Antigens 1983; 22:312.
38. Brantley SG, Ramsey G. Red cell alloimmunization in multi-transfused HLA-typed patients. Transfusion 1988; 28:463.
39. Darke C, Street J, Sargeant C, Dyer PA. HLA-DR antigens and properdin factor B allotypes in responders and non-responders to the Rhesus-D antigen. Tissue Antigens 1983; 21:333.
40. Darke C. HLA types and the immune response to the Rh(D) antigen. Tissue Antigens 1977; 9:171.
41. Brain P, Hammond MG. Association between histocompatibility type and the ability to make anti-Rh antibodies. Eur J Immunol 1974; 4:223.
42. Kruskall MS, Yunis EJ, Watson A, et al. Major histocompatibility complex markers and red cell antibodies to the Rh (D) antigen: absence of association. Transfusion 1990; 30:15.
43. Alarif L, Castro O, Ofosu M, et al. HLA-B35 is associated with red cell alloimmunization in sickle cell disease. Clin Immunol Immunopathol 1986; 38:178.
44. Contreras M, DeSilva M, Teesdale P, Mollison PL. The effect of naturally occurring Rh antibodies on the survival of serologically incompatible red cells. Br J Haematol 1987; 65:475.
45. Urbaniak SJ, Robertson AE. A successful program for immunizing Rh-negative volunteers for anti-D production using frozen/thawed blood. Transfusion 1981; 21:64.
46. Mollison PL, Hughes-Jones NC, Lindsay M, Wesseley J. Suppression of primary Rh immunization by passively-administered antibody: experiments in volunteers. Vox Sang 1969; 16:421.
47. Samson D, Mollison PL. Effect on primary Rh immunization of delayed administration of anti-Rh. Immunology 1975; 28:349.
48. Contreras M, Mollison PL. Failure to augment primary Rh immunization using a small dose of "passive" IgG anti-Rh. Br J Haematol 1981; 49:371.
49. Mollison PL. Some aspects of Rh hemolytic disease and its prevention. *In* Garratty G (ed): Hemolytic Disease of the Newborn. Arlington, VA: American Association of Blood Banks, 1984, pp 1–32.
50. Woodrow JC, Finn R, Krevans JR. Rapid clearance of Rh-positive blood during experimental Rh immunization. Vox Sang 1969; 17:349.
51. Nevanlinna HR. Factors affecting maternal Rh immunization. Ann Med Exp Fenn 1953; 31(suppl 2).
52. Jakobowicz R, Williams L, Silberman F. Immunization of Rh-negative volunteers by repeated injections of very small amounts of Rh-positive blood. Vox Sang 1972; 23:376.
53. Issitt PD. On the incidence of second antibody populations in the sera of women who have developed anti-Rh antibodies. Transfusion 1965; 5:355.
54. Archer GT, Cooke BR, Mitchell K, Parry P. Hyperimmunization of blood donors for the production of anti-Rh(D)-globulin. Bibl Haematol 1971; 38:877.
55. Issitt PD. Serology and Genetics of the Rhesus Blood Group System. Cincinnati, OH: Montgomery Scientific, 1979.
56. Mollison PL. Rh immunization and its suppression. *In* Schmidt PJ (ed): Progress in Transfusion and Transplantation. Washington, DC: American Association of Blood Banks, 1972, p 119.
57. Baldwin ML, Ness PM, Scott D, et al. Alloimmunization to D antigen and HLA in D-negative immunosuppressed oncology patients. Transfusion 1988; 28:330.
58. Pollack W. Mechanisms of Rh immune suppression by Rh immune globulin. *In* Garratty G (ed): Hemolytic Disease of the Newborn. Arlington, VA: American Association of Blood Banks, 1984, pp 53–66.
59. Pollack W, Gorman JG. Rh immune suppression: an immunostat hypothesis. *In* Scientific Symposium: Rh Antibody-Mediated Immunosuppression. Raritan, NJ: Ortho Research Institute of Medical Science, 1975, pp 115–124.
60. Gorman JG. The Role of the Laboratory in Hemolytic Disease of the Newborn. Philadelphia: Lea & Febiger, 1975.
61. Levine P. Serological factors as possible causes in spontaneous abortions. J Hered 1943; 34:71.
62. Levine P. The influence of the ABO system on hemolytic disease. Hum Biol 1958; 30:14.
63. Race RR, Sanger R. Blood Groups in Man. Oxford: Blackwell, 1950, p 290.
64. Finn R, Clarke CA, Donohoe WTA, et al. Experimental studies on the prevention of Rh hemolytic disease. BMJ 1961; 1:1486.
65. Finn R, Krevans JR, Clarke CA. An approach to the prevention of Rh hemolytic disease. J Clin Invest 1962; 41:1358.
66. Pollack W, Gorman JF, Hager HJ, et al. Antibody-mediated immune suppression to the Rh factor: animal models suggesting mechanism of action. Transfusion 1968; 8:134.
67. Lees RK, St. Sinclair NR. Regulation of the immune response: VII. In vitro immunosuppression by F(ab)2 or intact IgG antibodies. Immunology 1973; 24:735.
68. Chang H, Schenck S, Brody NI, et al. Studies on the mechanism of the suppression of active antibody synthesis by passively administered antibody. J Immunol 1969; 102:37.
69. St. Sinclair NR. Regulation of the immune response: I. Reduction inability of specific antibody to inhibit long-lasting IgG immunological priming after removal of the Fc-fragment. J Exp Med 1969; 129:1183.
70. Contreras M, Mollison PL. Rh immunization facilitated by passively-administered anti-Rh? Br J Haematol 1983; 53:153.
71. Holburn AM, Frame M, Hughes-Jones NC, Mollison PL. Some biological effects of IgM anti-Rh(D). Immunology 1971; 20:681.
72. Bowman JM, Chown B, Lewis M, Pollack JM. Rh isoimmunization during pregnancy: antenatal prophylaxis. Can Med Assoc J 1978; 118:623.
73. American College of Obstetrics and Gynecologists. Prevention of D isoimmunization. ACOG Technical Bulletin 147. Washington, DC: ACOG, 1990.
74. Vengelen-Tyler V (ed). Technical Manual, 12th ed. Bethesda, MD: American Association of Blood Banks, 1996.
75. Witter FR, Shirey RS, Nicol SL, Ness PM. Postinjection kinetics of antepartum Rh immune globulin. Am J Obstet Gynecol 1990; 163:784.
76. Bowman JM, Pollack JM. Failures of intravenous Rh immune globulin prophylaxis: an analysis of the reasons for such failures. Trans Med Rev 1987; 1:101.
77. Bowman JM. Suppression of Rh isoimmunization: a review. Obstet Gynecol 1978; 52:385.
78. Spielmann W, Seidl S. Prevalence of irregular antibodies and their significance in blood transfusion and antenatal care. Vox Sang 1974; 26:551.
79. Blumberg N, Peck K, Ross K, Avila E. Immune response to chronic red blood cell transfusion. Vox Sang 1983; 44:212.
80. Fluitt CRMG, Kunst VAJM, Drenthe-Schonk AM. Incidence of red cell antibodies after multiple blood transfusions. Transfusion 1990; 30:532.
81. Blumberg N, Ross K, Avila E, Peck K. Should chronic transfusions be matched for antigens other than ABO and Rho(D)? Vox Sang 1984; 47:205.
82. Vichinsky EP, Earles PNP, Johnson RA, et al. Alloimmunization in sickle cell anemia and transfusion of racially unmatched blood. N Engl J Med 1990; 322:1617.

83. Rosse WF, Gallagher D, Kinney TR, et al. Cooperative Study of Sickle Cell Disease: transfusion and alloimmunization in sickle cell disease. Blood 1990; 76:1431.
84. Ambruso DR, Githens JH, Alcorn R, et al. Experience with donors matched for minor blood group antigens in patients with sickle cell anemia who are receiving chronic transfusion therapy. Transfusion 1987; 27:94.
85. Davies SC, McWilliams AC, Hewitt PE, et al. Red cell alloimmunization in sickle cell disease. Br J Haematol 1986; 63:241.
86. Cox JV, Steane E, Cunningham G, Frenkel EP. Risk of alloimmunization and delayed hemolytic transfusion reactions in patients with sickle cell disease. Arch Intern Med 1988; 148:2485.
87. Orlina AR, Unger PJ, Koshy M. Post-transfusion alloimmunization in patients with sickle cell disease. Am J Hematol 1978; 5:101.
88. Coles SM, Klein HG, Holland PV. Alloimmunization in two multitransfused patient populations. Transfusion 1981; 21:462.
89. Sirchia G, Zanella A, Parravicini A, et al. Red cell alloantibodies in thalassemia major. Transfusion 1985; 25:110.
90. Holohan TV, Terasaki PI, Deisseroth AB. Suppression of transfusion-related alloimmunization in intensely treated cancer patients. Blood 1981; 58:122.
91. Griswold DE, Heppner GH, Calabresi P. Selective suppression of humoral and cellular immunity with cytosine arabinoside. Cancer Res 1972; 32:298.
92. Charache S. Problems in transfusion therapy [Editorial]. N Engl J Med 1990; 322:1666.
93. Tahhan HR, Holbrook CT, Braddy LR, et al. Antigen-matched donor blood in the transfusion of patients with sickle cell disease. Transfusion 1994; 34:562.
94. Tahhan HR, Werner AL, Bergante RA, Harris SC. Antigen-matching in the transfusional management of pediatric patients with sickle cell disease [Abstract]. Transfusion 1995; 35:16S.
95. Ness P. To match or not to match: the question for the chronically transfused patients with sickle cell anemia [Editorial]. Transfusion 1994; 34:558.
96. Rosse WF, Telen M, Ware RE. Transfusion Support for Patients with Sickle Cell Disease. Bethesda, MD: American Association of Blood Banks, 1998.
97. King KE, Shirey RS, Lankiewicz J, et al. Delayed hemolytic transfusion reactions in sickle cell disease: simultaneous destruction of recipients' red cells. Transfusion 1997; 37:376.
98. Petz LD, Calhoun L, Shulman IA, et al. The sickle cell hemolytic transfusion reaction syndrome. Transfusion 1997; 37:382.
99. Casanueva M, Valdes V, Ribera MC. Lack of alloimmunization to D antigen in D-negative immunosuppressed liver transplant recipients. Transfusion 1994; 34:570.

CHAPTER 27

Autoantibodies

Bruce Hug
Leslie E. Silberstein
Don L. Siegel

CLINICAL AND SEROLOGICAL ASPECTS

Autoimmune hemolytic anemia (AIHA) comprises three major clinical disorders characterized by the serological behavior of the associated autoantibodies: warm AIHA, cold AIHA, and paroxysmal cold hemoglobinuria.[1] In warm AIHA, autoantibodies attach to the patient's red cells, optimally at 37°C, and may result in splenic sequestration and extravascular hemolysis. This is the most common form of AIHA, and the production of these autoantibodies may be idiopathic (i.e., unassociated with an underlying disease) or secondary to lymphoproliferative disorders, collagen vascular diseases, immune deficiency syndromes, infections, or drug therapy.[2] The autoantibodies are generally of the immunoglobulin G (IgG) class and appear to bind to antigens common to all normal red cells.

There are two types of AIHA caused by autoantibodies that preferentially bind to a patient's red cells in the cold (typically room temperature and below). In cold AIHA (cold agglutinin disease [CAD]), immunoglobulin M (IgM) autoantibodies, usually directed against the red cell I antigen (also i and Pr), occur spontaneously, during the course of a lymphoproliferative disorder, or as a post-infectious complication of *Mycoplasma* pneumonia or infectious mononucleosis.[3, 4] Patients with this disease may have cold agglutinin titers in the thousands or even millions, in comparison to normal individuals, who may have low titers (<32). Because of the low thermal-binding properties of the IgM autoantibodies, they appear to bind to red cells and fix complement in the peripheral circulation, where temperatures fall below 32°C. As the cells return to warmer parts of the circulation, the IgM dissociates, leaving the cells coated with only complement. Complement activation may lead to intravascular hemolysis.

Paroxysmal cold hemoglobinuria (PCH), like CAD, is caused by cold-reactive autoantibodies that react with red cells in cooler parts of the body and cause irreversible binding of complement to the cells. With warming, elution of the autoantibodies from the erythrocyte surfaces occurs. It has a dramatic clinical presentation: the sudden onset of shaking chills, back and leg pain, abdominal cramps, and high fever, and the passage of black urine. In PCH, the autoantibodies are IgG molecules usually directed at P blood group antigens (Table 27–1)[5] and are present in relatively low titers (<64). Because the presence in serum of these biphasic IgG antibodies may be difficult to detect with standard serological methods, specialized tests in which in vitro hemolysis indicates IgG-induced complement sensitization can be employed (Donath-Landsteiner test).[6] PCH may be idiopathic or secondary to syphilis or viral infection.

COLD-REACTIVE AUTOANTIBODIES

Antigens

i/I Blood Group

The majority of cold-reactive anti–red cell autoantibodies bind to carbohydrate structures on membrane glycolipids or glycoproteins. Most of these autoantibodies are IgMs directed at i/I blood group antigens (Fig. 27–1).[7, 8]

The i/I antigen system consists of two structurally similar oligosaccharide chains expressed at different stages of development. The oligosaccharide chains are composed of repeating *N*-acetylgalactosamine (Gal[β1→4]GlcNac[β1→3]) units linked to ceramide or the membrane glycoproteins band 3 and band 4.5.[9, 10] The best available evidence indicates that the difference between I and i antigens relates to branching of the oligosaccharide chain; anti-i antibodies recognize a linear *N*-acetylgalactosamine oligosaccharide, whereas anti-I antibodies recognize a similar chain that is branched.[11–13]

There appears to be a developmentally regulated transition in expression of the i/I antigens. Fetal and newborn red cells express mostly i antigen, but adult red cells express mostly I antigen. This transition appears to involve the acquisition of a "branching enzyme" ([β1-6]-*N*-acetylglucaminyl transferase).[13, 14]

The expression of i/I antigen is not limited to red blood cells. The oligosaccharide chains are present on

Table 27–1. P Blood Group Antigens

P^k	Gal(α1→4)Gal(ß1→4)Glc-ceramide
P	GalNAc(ß1→3)Gal(α1→4)Gal(ß1→4)Glc-ceramide
P_1	Gal(α1→4)Gal(ß1→4)GlcNAc(ß1→3)Gal(ß1→4)Glc-ceramide

Gal, galactose; Glc, glucose; GalNAc, *N*-acetylgalactosamine; GlcNAc, *N*-acetylglucosamine.

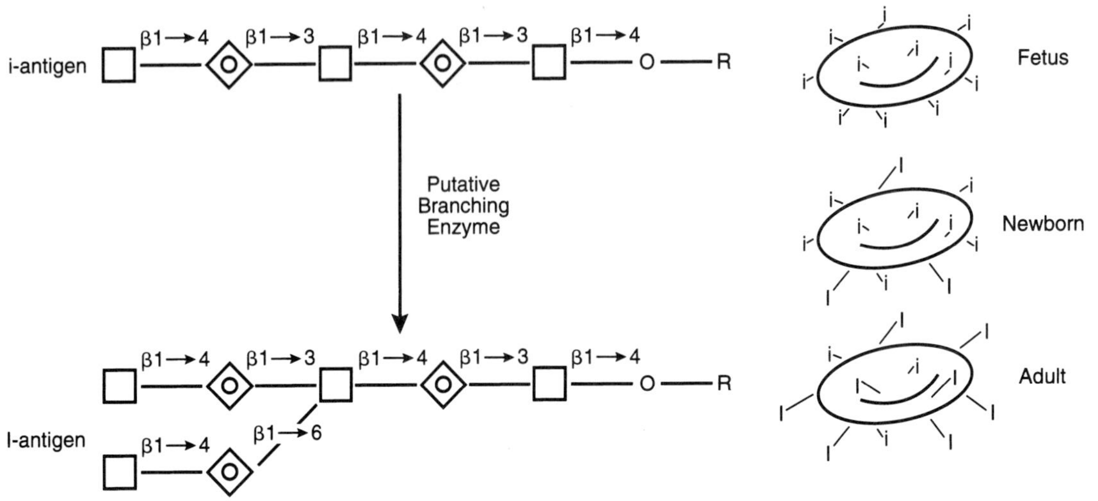

Figure 27–1. Structure and expression of human erythrocyte I/i blood group antigens. R, ceramide or protein. Hollow squares represent galactose. Circles within squares represent *N*-acetylglucosamine.

human granulocytes, macrophages, platelets, and lymphocytes; antibodies to these antigens can be lymphocytotoxic.[2, 15] Also, they are variably expressed on nonhuman red cells and cultured cell lines of several animal species.[16, 17]

Pr and Other Blood Groups

Pr refers to a group of red cell antigens defined serologically to possess the following characteristics: inactivation by proteases, equivalent expression on adult and newborn red cells, and inactivation by neuraminidase.[18, 19] Anti-Pr antibodies were originally divided into the subclasses Pr_1, Pr_2, Pr_3, and Pr_a on the basis of their reactivity with various animal red cells and hemagglutination inhibition experiments with chemically modified human red cell sialoglycoprotein preparations.[20] Although the biochemistry of this blood group system is still not completely understood, the best available evidence indicates that the Pr antigens are O-linked sialated oligosaccharide structures that reside within the N-terminal 26 amino acid residues of glycophorins A and B.[21–23] This conclusion arises in part from the findings that anti-Pr antisera fail to agglutinate neuraminidase-treated human red cells and are inhibited by the O-linked sialotetrasaccharides isolated from red cell sialoglycoprotein preparations. Their putative location on glycophorins A and B (and not glycophorin C) is based on the observation that anti-Pr reactivity is dramatically reduced with En(a–) erythrocytes (which lack glycophorin A) and is totally eliminated with homozygous M^KM^K red cells (which lack glycophorins A and B but have normal amounts of glycophorin C).[24] Like the i/I blood group antigens, Pr antigens have been found on human lymphocytes, granulocytes, and monocytes,[25] as well as on kidney, liver, stomach, pancreas, lung, and brain tissue.[26] The significance of these findings has yet not been reported. Other targets for cold-reactive IgM autoantibodies include Gd (for glycolipid-dependent) gangliosides[27] and other neuraminidase-sensitive or protease-sensitive antigens, referred to as Sa, Lud, Fl, Vo, and Li.[28]

Antibodies

Anti-i/I

The majority of cold agglutinins are IgMs directed against i/I blood group antigens. Antibodies are classified as anti-I or anti-i on the basis of specificity for adult or fetal red blood cells, respectively. Antibodies that react equally with I and i antigens have also been described and are classified as anti-j antibodies.[29] Autoantibodies directed at I and/or i antigens may be present both under normal conditions and in the setting of CAD.

Normal and pathologic anti-i/I autoantibodies differ in clonality, titer, and clinical significance. Almost all human sera contain anti-i/I antibodies. These ubiquitous antibodies are usually polyclonal, typically present at low titers, and seldom hemolytic. They are significant only in that they may produce false-positive results during antiglobulin testing of the involved serum. The pathological anti-i/I autoantibodies causing CAD may be secondary to another disorder such as infection (mycoplasma, Epstein-Barr virus [EBV]) or lymphoproliferative disease (chronic lymphocytic leukemia, Waldenström's macroglobulinemia, lymphoma), or they may be idiopathic. Those anti-i/I autoantibodies secondary to infection, similar to the naturally occurring cold agglutinins, are polyclonal and present at low titers. They occasionally cause CAD. In contrast, anti-i/I autoantibodies associated with lymphoproliferative disorders are monoclonal, present at high titers (>1:10,000), and frequently a cause of CAD.[30] Although CAD may be present without an evident underlying cause, some groups argue that the CAD conventionally classified as idiopathic may in fact be a low-grade lymphoproliferative disorder. Such arguments are based on the high frequency of detection of monoclonal B cell populations when aggressive attempts are made to diagnose abnormal lymphoid processes (flow cytometry, bone marrow biopsy, and so forth).[31] Attempts to understand CAD and cold agglutinins in general have focused on antibody structure.

Initial studies focused on pathological antibodies because the clones producing these antibodies are present in much higher quantities than those B cells producing the naturally occurring cold agglutinins. The early structural studies of these pathological antibodies examined the immunoglobulin molecule constant regions. The composition of nearly all anti-I and anti-i autoantibodies was found to be IgMκ, although IgM cold agglutinins with associated λ light chains were also described.[28] Later attention focused on the structural diversity of the variable regions of these autoantibodies. Diversity results from differences in amino acid sequence in both heavy-chain and light-chain variable regions. Anti-idiotypic antibodies can be used to recognize variable-region determinants within or outside the antigen-combining site. With the use of such anti-idiotypic antisera, cross-reactive idiotypes were found among red cell autoantibodies.[32] This cross-reactivity appeared to be restricted to red cell autoantibodies with similar specificity. For example, anti-idiotypic antibodies raised against anti-Pr cold agglutinins generally did not cross-react with anti-I cold agglutinins, and vice versa. A structural basis for this idiotypic cross-reactivity could not be fully appreciated at the time because of insufficient data on variable-region gene usage, which had been derived from amino acid sequences limited to the first framework region.[33]

Subsequent studies by Stevenson and colleagues[34] described a monoclonal anti-idiotypic antibody termed "9G4," which recognizes an idiotypic determinant present on the heavy chains of both anti-I and anti-i cold agglutinins as well as on neoplastic B cells secreting cold agglutinins. The specificity of the anti-idiotypic 9G4 antibody for anti-i/I autoantibodies has been clearly demonstrated in competitive enzyme-linked immunosorbent assays and hemagglutination inhibition assays. 9G4 was shown to have reactivity with the serum of 66 of 67 patients expressing anti-I, anti-i, or anti-j autoantibodies. Conversely, the antibody did not have reactivity with the serum of 42 patients with cold agglutinins of a variety of non-i/I specificities, including members of the Pr, Sa, Lud, and Sia families.[35] This finding suggests that the heavy-chain variable regions of anti-I and anti-i may share some structural elements.

A structural basis for this cross-reactive idiotype was suggested by Silverman and colleagues,[36] who used primary sequence-dependent polyclonal antibodies to heavy-chain variable-region determinants to show that both anti-I and anti-i cold agglutinins are derived from a distinct subset of V_H4 family genes.[37, 38] The establishment of EBV-transformed B cell lines secreting either anti-I or anti-i autoantibodies has allowed for nucleotide sequence analysis of the entire length of the expressed variable-region genes in order to assess the molecular basis for the autoimmune response.[37, 38] Numerous groups have now demonstrated that almost all anti-i/I autoantibodies associated with CAD are encoded by the V_H4-34(V_H4.21) gene.[37, 39–42]

It appears that the 9G4 anti-idiotype reactivity with anti-I autoantibodies is largely determined by a combination of essential and permissive regions of the V_H4-34(V_H4.21) heavy chain. Several groups have used a baculovirus expression system to interchange domains of V_H4-34(V_H4.21) with domains of other V_H4 family members. These mutant antibodies have been tested for interaction with 9G4 and revealed that the anti-I heavy-chain framework region 1 (FR1) is essential for reactivity with 9G4. In addition, one of a permissive subset of complementarity-determining region 3 (CDR3) sequences must be present for reactivity. CDR1 and CDR2, however, do not appear to affect binding of 9G4 to anti-I, because antibody with appropriate FR1 and CDR3 regions binds regardless of the other CDR sequences.[43, 44] Undoubtedly, continued use of this system will allow further clarification of the sequences essential for cold agglutinin activity of both anti-I and anti-i antibodies.

In contrast to the restriction of variable-region gene use by the anti-i/I heavy chains, the variable-region genes used by the light chains demonstrate limited restriction. Although the anti-I cold agglutinin light chains appear to preferentially derive from the VκIII gene family, the anti-I cold agglutinins use light chains from a number of different Vκ families.[37] To determine whether the anti-i/I light chains that use VκIII might exhibit idiotypic cross-reactivity similar to that observed for the heavy chains, a panel of eight VκIII light-chain–dependent monoclonal anti-idiotypic antibodies was raised against an anti-I autoantibody expressing V_H4 and VκIII genes. Significant idiotypic heterogeneity was observed among VκIII-expressing cold agglutinin light chains. In addition, the idiotypic heterogeneity could be ascribed to the use of at least three different VκIII gene segments, as well as to somatic diversification of the germ line–encoded genes.[45]

The remarkable finding of restriction in the variable-region genes used for the anti-i/I heavy chains, along with diversification in the associated variable-region genes used for light chains, is consistent with the results from baculovirus expression systems. These systems permit the mixing of heavy chains and light chains from different immunoglobulin molecules, and results from such systems indicate that although the V_H4-34(V_H4.21) heavy chain is necessary for binding by anti-idiotypic antibody, it is not sufficient. Binding also requires a compatible light chain. These findings suggest a model for the relative contributions of heavy and light chains to antigen binding. The V_H sequence may be required for the global interaction with the i/I antigen complex, whereas the V_L sequence may confer the fine specificity that distinguishes between these distinct yet related carbohydrate structures.[34]

The expressed variable-region genes have also been examined for the number and pattern of somatic mutations in order to evaluate the potential role of antigen-mediated selection.[37] It was determined that both V_H and V_L genes encoding the anti-i antibody were identical to germ line sequences, whereas numerous base-pair differences were noted in the anti-I response. Compared with its most likely germ line precursor, V_H4-34(V_H4.21), the V_H gene encoding anti-I had only three amino acid differences: two located in FRs and one in a CDR, or region of antigen contact. In contrast, the V_L sequence of anti-I had a relatively high number of amino acid substitutions (relative to the total number of silent mutations) when compared with its likely precursor germ line sequence. These amino acid changes resulted from a nonrandom distribution of replacement mutations in the CDRs.

Taken together, these results provide evidence that positive selection by antigen led to the accumulation of amino acid substitutions in the light chain of the anti-I antibody studied. If this proves to be a universal feature of anti-I cold agglutinins, it may represent a consequence of differential regulation of the immune responses to the related i/I antigens. Perhaps the high expression of i antigen on fetal red cells mediates tolerance to i, either by clonal anergy or by deletion of B cells with anti-i specificity. The expression of I antigen occurs much later in development; immunological tolerance for I may therefore differ from that for i.

The structure of anti-i/I autoantibodies from patients with infectious mononucleosis or *Mycoplasma pneumoniae* has also been examined. Patients develop cold agglutinins that, like those described earlier, preferentially use the V_H4-34(V_H4.21) gene. Chapman and colleagues[46] showed that patients with infectious mononucleosis or *Mycoplasma pneumoniae* had increased serum 9G4 idiotype reactivity compared with controls, although total serum immunoglobulin was normal. To determine the structural features of these idiotype-reactive antibodies, six idiotype-producing hybridomas from four individuals were analyzed. Consistent with the reactivity patterns described earlier, six of six antibodies had anti-i reactivity, and each antibody used the V_H4-34(V_H4.21) heavy-chain gene. Light-chain use, as predicted, varied. This indicates that the antibody structure of cold agglutinins produced during the polyclonal antibody response to infection is the same as the structure of the monoclonal antibodies found in B cell lymphoproliferative disorders.

Naturally occurring anti-i/I cold agglutinins, in contrast to those described earlier, may be encoded by a more diverse repertoire of V_H genes. Jefferies and colleagues[47] found minimal 9G4 idiotype expression in the serum of 15 normal donors. In fact, less than 30% of IgM with anti-i activity and less than 15% of IgM with anti-I activity were reactive with 9G4. Furthermore, inhibition of cold agglutinin activity was achieved more readily with V_H3 neutralization than with V_H4-34(V_H4.21) neutralization. Heavy-chain structural analysis of cold agglutinin–producing hybridomas from normal donors was consistent with this finding. Two clones with anti-I specificity and one clone with anti-i specificity were obtained. Although the anti-i–producing clone used the V_H4-34(V_H4.21) gene, the anti-I–producing clones used the V_H3 gene, demonstrating that naturally occurring cold agglutinins are not limited to using the V_H4-34(V_H4.21) gene associated with pathological cold agglutinins.[47]

Although naturally occurring cold agglutinins are not limited to V_H4-34(V_H4.21) gene expression, V_H4-34(V_H4.21)-encoded autoantibodies are present. Whereas most naturally occurring anti-i/I autoantibodies are of anti-I specificity, most of the naturally occurring V_H4-34(V_H4.21)-encoded cold agglutinins have anti-i specificity. Furthermore, these anti-i autoantibodies express both κ and λ light chains, with most of the κ light chains being Vκ1, Vκ3, and Vκ4. This is consistent with the profile of light-chain expression by pathological anti-i–producing B cells. It is not clear why pathological B cells producing cold agglutinins show V_H4-34(V_H4.21) restriction while other B cells, producing naturally occurring cold agglutinins, do not (Fig. 27–2).[47]

Anti-Pr_2

In contrast to the structural uniformity of anti-I cold agglutinins, substantial structural differences occur in the two anti-Pr_2 cold agglutinins that have been sequenced.[48, 49] In one case of well-characterized anti-Pr_2–specific lymphoma, the heavy-chain variable region was 88% homologous to a V_H1 germ line gene, whereas the light-chain variable region was 97% homologous to a V_κ1 germ line gene.[48] Anti-idiotypic antibodies raised against the anti-

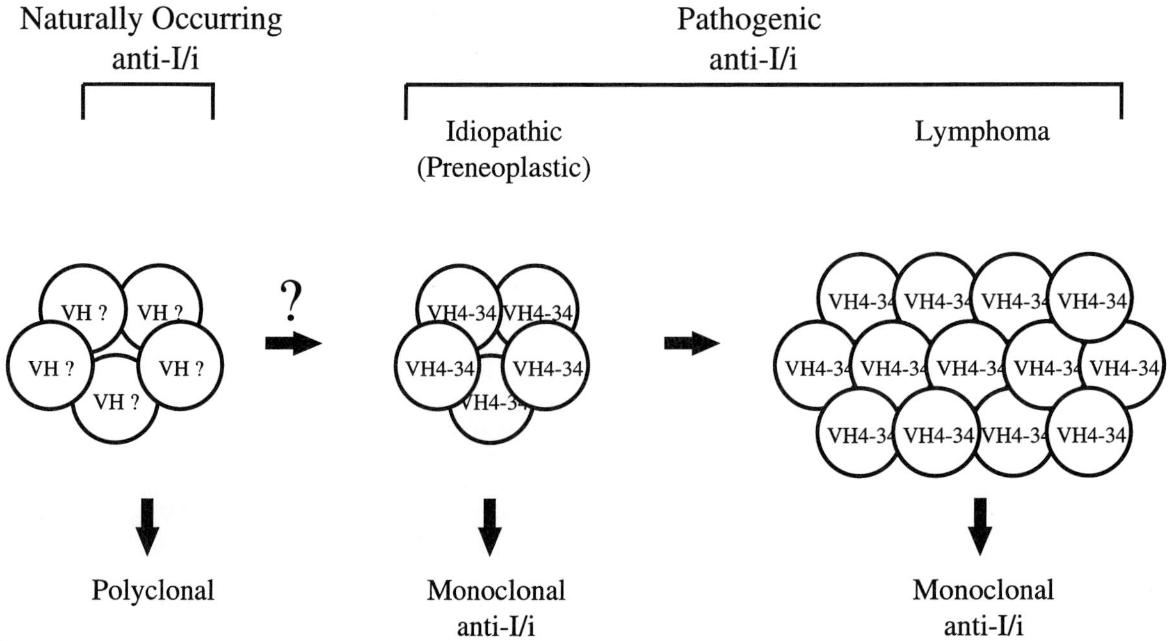

Figure 27–2. Clonality of naturally occurring and pathogenic cold autoantibodies.

Pr_2 cold agglutinins from this patient did not show cross-reactivities with red cell autoantibodies from other individuals with anti-Pr or different specificities and thus were unique to this patient's anti-Pr_2 autoantibody.[50] A longitudinal molecular and idiotypic analysis of the Pr_2-specific response suggested that self-antigen played a role in the pathogenesis of the autoreactive B cell neoplasm.[51]

WARM-REACTIVE AUTOANTIBODIES

Three classes of antigens are the probable targets of most warm-reactive autoantibodies: Rh-related proteins, band 3 protein, and glycophorins. Although some evidence suggests autoanti-K,[52] autoanti-Jk[a],[53] and autoanti–band 4.1[54] may also cause AIHA, these reactivities are not discussed in this chapter.

Antigens

Rh Related

Many serological studies have suggested that warm-reacting autoantibodies may be directed at Rh blood group antigens by virtue of their "pan-reactivity" with all red cell phenotypes except Rh_{null} cells, which lack all Rh components.[55–58] This pattern of reactivity has led to the notion of a common "Rh core" structure to which these antibodies are directed. However, what these serological observations mean in molecular terms is not clear. For example, it is possible that these autoantibodies do not bind to Rh antigens per se but to Rh antigens in combination with some other ubiquitous red cell membrane components.[59, 60] Alternatively, the autoantigens may not be Rh related at all, because Rh_{null} cells, which are misshapen and fragile,[61] have other defects,[62] including membrane transport abnormalities and decreased expression of certain blood group antigens, such as S, s, U, and N.[63] In a small number of cases, a "relative Rh specificity" can be observed, in which antisera are pan-reactive but display greater reactivity against cells possessing certain Rh antigens, such as Rh(e). In still fewer cases, autoantibodies specific for particular Rh antigens have been described.[64, 65] In these situations, red cells that lack the corresponding Rh antigen have been found to survive better in vivo than those that express antigen.

Molecular studies further argue for the Rh specificity of warm autoantibodies.[66, 67] Leddy and colleagues[67] eluted the immunoglobulins adsorbed to the red blood cells of 20 patients with AIHA and used these autoantibodies to immunoprecipitate proteins from red blood cell membranes. Collectively, four proteins were immunoprecipitated, including two Rh-like proteins, p34 and gp37-55. (Band 3 protein and glycophorin A were also isolated and are discussed later.) p34 is a 34-kD protein that was immunoprecipitated by immunoglobulin from 9 of the 20 patients with AIHA examined in this study; gp37-55 is a variably glycosylated glycoprotein of 37 to 55 kD that was immunoprecipitated from the 7 patients with the highest yields of p34. Both proteins are suspected to be Rh family members on the basis of molecular weight and lack of expression in Rh_{null} red blood cells. Of course, molecular weight is not a specific characteristic, and the membrane phenotype of Rh_{null} cells is, likewise, not limited to Rh proteins, as discussed earlier. These findings, therefore, suggest but do not prove that anti-Rh autoantibodies may be present in warm AIHA.

Band 3 Protein

Band 3, the anion transport protein, is present at high levels in the red blood cell membrane. It has been assigned numerous blood group antigens, including Wright (Wr), Diego (Di), Waldner, Redelberger, and Warrior.[68] Autoantibodies of patients with AIHA have been described with anti-Wr[b] and anti-Di[b] specificities.[69, 70] It is therefore not surprising that immunoprecipitation experiments using warm autoantibodies have isolated band 3 from the membranes of red blood cells.

The immunoaffinity isolation performed by Leddy and colleagues[67] demonstrated that the serum of patients with AIHA may contain anti–band 3 antibodies. Band 3 was isolated at levels above background with the use of the eluted immunoglobulin from 18 of 20 patients analyzed in this study. The quantity of protein isolated from Rh_{null} cells was not diminished in comparison to wild type, and the isolated protein was definitively identified by Western blot analysis with anti–band 3 antibodies. Although the antigen specificities (Wr[b], Di[b], and so forth) of these antibodies were not investigated, this finding further implicates band 3 protein as a common target of autoantibodies in warm AIHA.

Glycophorin

Glycophorins, like band 3, are present at high levels in the erythrocyte membrane. Antigens assigned to glycophorin family members include those of the MNSsU, Pr, and Gerbich systems. Furthermore, as discussed later, Wr[b] expression is dependent on glycophorin A expression. Autoantibodies directed against glycophorins (N, S, U, Wr[b], En[a], Pr) have been described in the past.[71, 72] In contrast to band 3, however, warm autoantibodies have not yielded glycophorins alone in immunoprecipitation experiments. Glycophorin A has been isolated only in association with band 3.

In the immunoprecipitations by Leddy and colleagues,[67] half of the eluted immunoglobulin that yielded band 3 also yielded a 41-kD protein identified as glycophorin A by Western blot analysis. Not only was glycophorin A never isolated alone, but the coisolation of glycophorin A with band 3 was not predicted by the quantity of band 3 precipitated. This nonstoichiometric relationship suggests that glycophorin A is not simply coprecipitated, directly or indirectly, by anti–band 3 autoantibodies.

Wr[b]

The discovery of autoantibodies coprecipitating band 3 and glycophorin A raises the possibility that a single antibody is reacting with a single epitope produced by an interaction of the two proteins. If, in the work by Leddy and colleagues,[67] two or more antibodies were responsible for the immunoprecipitation of band 3 and glycophorin A through the recognition of separate epitopes, it is curious that no patients produced pure anti–glycophorin A activity (i.e., anti–glycophorin A activity in the absence of anti–band 3 activity). The finding that the two proteins can be coprecipitated is reminiscent of the coimmunoprecipitation of band 3 and glycophorin by anti-Wr^b monoclonal antibodies.[73, 74] Although monoclonal antibodies directed against either band 3 or glycophorin A fail to coprecipitate the other, anti-Wr^b monoclonal antibodies apparently recognize an epitope dependent on both proteins.

Wr^b is a high-frequency antigen (antithetical to Wr^a) whose formation is dependent on both band 3 and glycophorin A.[75, 76] Bruce and colleagues[76] showed that the Wr^b phenotype segregates with the more common allele of band 3 (in a wild-type glycophorin A background). A rare mutation in band 3 protein (glu658→lys) forms the Wr^a antigen. Interestingly, in a background deficient for glycophorin A (i.e., En[a–], M^K/M^K), Wr^b is not formed even if the glu658 form of band 3 is present, suggesting that the two proteins are necessary for formation of the Wr^b antigen. The interaction is evidently complex, because glycophorin A–glycophorin B hybrids (GPSat) that include the extracellular domain of glycophorin A still fail to reconstitute the Wr^b epitope. Although evidence for direct physical contact between band 3 and glycophorin A is tenuous, the described genetic findings clearly demonstrate that Wr^b is produced by band 3 (glu658) in the appropriate glycophorin A background.[77]

A follow-up study by Leddy and colleagues[78] proved that some autoantibodies coprecipitating glycophorin A and band 3 have anti-Wr^b specificity. Autoantibodies from the six eluates that coimmunoprecipitated glycophorin A and band 3 were tested for reactivity with Wr(a+b–) red blood cells. Three reactivity profiles were observed. One patient's autoantibody failed to react with the Wr(a+b−) cells, suggesting that pure anti-Wr^b is the activity observed. Two patients' autoantibodies showed reduced reactivity with Wr(a+b−) cells, indicating that anti-Wr^b is at least partially responsible for the reactivity in the serum. Finally, the autoantibodies of three patients showed virtually the same reactivity with Wr(a+b−) cells as with Wr(a−b+) cells, demonstrating that these autoantibodies lacked anti-Wr^b activity. This study indicates that although warm autoantibodies may demonstrate anti-Wr^b reactivity, additional epitopes dependent on both glycophorin A and band 3 may be the targets of autoantibodies as well.

Antibodies

With respect to the structure of warm-reacting red cell autoantibodies, few data have been produced in comparison to those describing cold-reacting autoantibodies. This is primarily because of the difficulty in establishing warm autoantibody–producing B cell clones from lymphocytes of patients with AIHA. The identification of antigens recognized by warm autoantibodies and the development of "phage display" technology will likely lead to a clearer understanding of autoantibody heavy- and light-chain structure.

The available structural information is limited to descriptions of the constant regions of the antibodies. Although IgM and immunoglobulin A (IgA) autoantibodies can contribute to immune hemolysis, most warm autoantibodies are of the IgG class, and most warm-reacting autoantibodies that cause immune hemolysis are thought to belong to the IgG1 and IgG3 subclasses.[28]

Because multiple subclasses can exist simultaneously in a patient, the antibodies are considered to be polyclonal. There is evidence, however, that they can be restricted with respect to their Gm allotype and/or light-chain type.[79, 80]

ORIGIN OF ERYTHROCYTE AUTOANTIBODIES

The cellular origin of cold-reactive autoantibodies has been elucidated by model systems of EBV-transformed cell lines secreting anti-i, anti-I, and anti-Pr_2 pathogenic autoantibodies. It was recognized that in approximately 40% of patients, a circulating B cell clone could be readily found with a distinctive karyotypic marker: trisomy 3, trisomy 12, or 48XX,+3,+12. This chromosomal aberrancy was associated with the chronic idiopathic cold agglutinin syndrome, as well as with monoclonal cold agglutinins secondary to a B cell neoplasm. The marker proved useful for demonstrating the close relationship between the EBV-transformed B cell clones and the B cell populations in the peripheral blood of patients. In addition, it could be demonstrated not only that both in vitro and in vivo B cells had the same karyotypic marker and immunoglobulin restriction fragments but also that their secreted monoclonal antibodies had the same serological specificity and isoelectric focusing spectrotype. Collectively, these studies showed that the monoclonal cold agglutinins are derived from the associated (pre)neoplastic B cell populations found in patients.[81, 82]

Virtually nothing is known of the warm-reacting immunoglobulin erythrocyte autoantibodies. It has not been possible to generate relevant, stable, in vitro cell lines that provide a continuous source of homogeneous antibody for antigen-binding and structural analysis. The high association of AIHA of the warm-reacting IgG type with systemic autoimmune disorders such as systemic lupus erythematosus in humans and animal models (NZB mice) has suggested that these antierythrocyte autoantibodies, in contrast to the clonal cold-reactive autoantibodies, might arise from polyclonal activation rather than from activation by specific (self) antigen.[83] Furthermore, several studies indicate that warm-reacting autoantibodies, when associated with a clonal B cell lymphoproliferative disorder such as chronic lymphocytic leukemia, are not secreted by the neoplastic B cell. For example, the pathogenic red blood cell autoantibodies are of a different isotype from the immunoglobulin expressed by the neoplastic B cell (IgM). In addition, when hybridomas are made from the neoplastic chronic lymphocytic leukemia cells, the secreted antibodies do not bind erythrocyte antigens.[84] An alternative etiological mechanism involving the production of warm-reacting IgG-erythrocyte autoantibodies is that they might arise from immunological network interactions involving anti-idiotypes. A transgenic model of AIHA has been established by inserting V_H and V_L genes for an NZB antierythrocytic autoantibody in the germ line of a normal strain of mice.[85] In this model, it was found that not all the anti-self-specific (i.e., erythrocyte-specific) B cells were tolerized and that in many instances these mice could develop autoimmune hemolytic syndromes with similar characteristics as in humans. It is also noteworthy that the $CD5^+$ B cell appeared to be the main source of erythrocyte autoantibodies in the F1 transgenic mice.[85] Moreover, these $CD5^+$ B cells reside predominantly in the peritoneal cavity. The peritoneal fluid contains very few red blood cells, which may explain in part the lack of tolerance (and deletion) of the peritoneal $CD5^+$ B cells to erythrocyte antigens. The observation that erythrocyte-specific B cells may reside in an immunologically privileged site such as the peritoneal cavity may explain why it has been so difficult to isolate and immortalize B cell clones from peripheral blood, bone marrow, or spleens of patients with warm-reactive AIHA.

REFERENCES

1. Siegel D, Silberstein L. Acquired hemolytic anemia. *In* Conn RB (ed): Current Diagnosis. Philadelphia: WB Saunders, 1991, p 559.
2. Pruzanski W, Sumak K. Biologic activity of cold-reacting antibodies. N Engl J Med 1977; 297:538.
3. Janney FA, Lee LT, Howe C. Cold hemagglutinin cross-reactivity with *Mycoplasma pneumoniae*. Infect Immunol 1978; 22:29.
4. Rosenfield R, Schmidt R, Calvo R, McGinniss M. Anti-i, a frequent cold agglutinin in infectious mononucleosis. Vox Sang 1965; 10:631.
5. Worlledge S, Rousso C. Studies on the serology of PCH with special reference to its relationship with the P blood group system. Vox Sang 1965; 10:293.
6. Donath J, Landsteiner K. Über paroxysmale Hämoglobinurie. Munchen Med Wochenschr 1904; 51:1590.
7. Weiner A, Unger L, Cohen L. Type-specific cold autoantibodies as a cause of acquired hemolytic anemia and hemolytic transfusion reactions: biologic test with bovine red cells. Ann Intern Med 1956; 44:221.
8. Dacie J. The Haemolytic Anaemias. Congenital and Acquired. London: Churchill, 1962.
9. Childs RA, Feizi T, Fukuda M. Blood group I activity associated with band 3, the major intrinsic membrane protein of human erythrocytes. J Biol Chem 1978; 173:333.
10. Fukuda M, Fukuda MN, Hakomori S. The developmental change and genetic defect in carbohydrate structures of band 3 glycoprotein of human erythrocyte membranes. J Biol Chem 1979; 254:3700.
11. Feizi T, Childs K, Watanabe K, Hakomori S. Three types of blood group specificities among monoclonal anti-autoantibodies revealed by analogues of a branched erythrocyte glycolipid. J Exp Med 1979; 149:975.
12. Niemann H, Watanabe K, Hakomori S. Blood group i and I activities of "lacto-N-nor-hexaosylceramide" and its analogues: the structural requirements for i-specificities. Biochem Biophys Res Commun 1976; 81:1286.
13. Watanabe K, Hakomori S. Status of blood group carbohydrate chains in autogenesis and oncogenesis. J Biol Chem 1976; 254:3221.
14. Marsh WL. Anti-i: a cold antibody defining the Ii relationship in human red cells. Br J Haematol 1961; 7:200.
15. Dunstan RA, Simpson MB, Borowitz MJ. Heterogeneous distribution of antigens on human platelets demonstrated by fluorescence flow cytometry. Br J Haematol 1985; 61:603.
16. Wiener A, Moore-Janowski J, Gordon E, Davis J. The blood factors i and I in primates including man and in lower species. Am J Phys Anthropol 1965; 23:389.
17. Childs RA, Kapadia A, Feizi T. *In* Schauer R (ed): Glycoconjugates. Stuttgart: Georg Thieme, 1979, pp 518–519.
18. Marsh WL, Jenkins WJ. Anti-Sp1: the recognition of a new cold auto-antibody. Vox Sang 1968; 15:177.
19. Roelcke D. A new serological specificity in cold antibodies of high titer: anti-HD. Vox Sang 1969; 16:76.
20. Roelcke D, Ebert W, Giesen HP. Anti-Pr_3: serological and immunochemical identification of a new anti-Pr subspecificity. Vox Sang 1976; 30:122.
21. Ebert W, Fey J, Gartner C, et al. Isolation and partial characterization of the Pr autoantigen determinants. Mol Immunol 1979; 16:413.
22. Anstee DJ. The blood group MNSs-active sialoglycoprotein. Semin Hematol 1981; 18:13.
23. Uemura K, Roelcke D, Yoshitakia N, Feizi T. The reactivity of human erythrocyte autoantibodies anti-Pr_2, and Gd, Fl, and Sa with gangliosides in a chromatogram binding assay. Biochem J 1984; 219:865.
24. Anstee D. Blood group MNSs-active sialoglycoproteins of the human erythrocyte membrane. *In* Immunobiology of the Erythrocyte. New York: Alan R. Liss, 1980, pp 67–98.
25. Pruzanski W, Roelcke D, Armstrong M, Manly M. Pr and Gd antigens on human B and T lymphocytes and phagocytes. Clin Immunol Immunopathol 1980; 15:631.
26. Romer W, Seelig H, Lenhard W, Roelcke D. The distribution of i/I, Pr, and Gd antigens in mammalian tissues. Invest Cell Pathol 1979; 2:157.
27. Roelcke D, Riesen W, Geisen H, Ebert W. Serological identification of the new cold agglutinin specificity anti-Gd. Vox Sang 1977; 33:304.
28. Mollison P, Engelfreit C, Contreras M. Blood Transfusion in Clinical Medicine, 8th ed. Oxford, UK: Blackwell, 1988.
29. Roelcke D, Kreft H, Hack H, Stevenson F. Anti-j: human cold agglutinins recognizing linear (i) and branched (I) type 2 chains. Vox Sang 1994; 67:216.
30. Schwartz RS, Silberstein LE, Berkman EM. Autoimmune hemolytic anemias. *In* Hoffman R, Benz E, Shattil S, et al (eds): Hematology: Basic Principles and Practice, 2nd ed. New York: Churchill Livingstone, 1995, p 710.
31. Berentsen S, Bo K, Shammas FV, et al. Chronic cold agglutinin disease of the "idiopathic" type is a premalignant or low-grade malignant lymphoproliferative disease. APMIS 1997; 105:354.
32. Williams R, Kunkel H, Capra J. Antigenic specificities related to the cold agglutinin activity of gamma M globulins. Science 1968; 161:379.
33. Gergely J, Wang AC, Fudenberg HH. Chemical analyses of variable regions of heavy and light chains of cold agglutinins. Vox Sang 1973; 24:432.
34. Stevenson F, Smith G, North J, et al. Identification of normal B-cell counterparts of neoplastic CLL's which secrete cold agglutinins of anti-L and anti-i specificity. Br J Haematol 1989; 72:9.
35. Smith G, Spellerberg M, Boulton F, et al. The immunoglobulin V_H gene, V_H4-21, specifically encodes autoanti–red cell antibodies against the I or i antigens. Vox Sang 1995; 68:231.
36. Silverman G, Goni F, Fernandez J. Distinct patterns of heavy chain variable region subgroup use by human monoclonal autoantibodies of different specificity. J Exp Med 1988; 168:2361.
37. Silberstein LE, Jefferies LC, Goldman J, et al. Variable region gene analysis of pathologic human autoantibodies to the related i and I red blood cell antigens. Blood 1991; 73:2372.
38. Pascual V, Vistor K, Leisz D. Nucleotide sequence analysis of the V regions of two IgM cold agglutinins: evidence that the V_H4-21 gene segment is responsible for the major cross reactive idiotype. J Immunol 1991; 146:4385.
39. Pascual V, Victor K, Lelsz D, et al. Nucleotide sequence analysis of the B regions of two IgM cold agglutinins: evidence that the V_H4-21 gene segment is responsible for the major cross-reactive idiotype. J Immunol 1991; 146:4385.
40. Grillot-Courvalin C, Brouet JC, Piller F, et al. An anti–B cell autoantibody from Wiskott-Aldrich syndrome which recognizes I blood group specificity on normal human B cells. Eur J Immunol 1992; 22:1781.
41. Leoni L, Ghiso J, Goni F, Frangione B. The primary structure of the Fab fragment of protein KAU, a monoclonal immunoglobulin M cold agglutinin. J Biol Chem 1991; 266:2836.

42. Pascual V, Victor K, Spellerberg M, et al. VH restriction among human cold agglutinins: the V_H4-21 gene segment is required to encode anti-i and anti-I specificities. J Immunol 1992; 149:2337.
43. Li Y, Spellerberg MB, Stevenson FK, et al. The I binding specificity of human V_H4-34 (V_H4-21) encoded antibodies is determined by both V_H framework region 1 and complementarity determining region 3. J Mol Biol 1996; 256:577.
44. Potter KN, Li YC, Pascual B, et al. Molecular characterization of a cross-reactive idiotype on human immunoglobulins utilizing the V_H4-21 gene segment. J Exp Med 1993; 178:1419.
45. Jefferies LC, Silverman GJ, Carchidi CM, Silberstein LE. Idiotypic heterogeneity of VκIII autoantibodies to red blood cell antigens. Clin Immunol Immunopathol 1992; 65:119.
46. Chapman CH, Spellerberg MB, Smith GA, et al. Autoanti–red cell antibodies synthesized by patients with infectious mononucleosis utilize the V_H4-21 gene segment. J Immunol 1993; 151:1051.
47. Jefferies LC, Carchidi CM, Silberstein LE. Naturally occurring anti-i/I cold agglutinins may be encoded by different V_H3 genes as well as the V_H4.21 gene segment. J Clin Invest 1993; 92:2821.
48. Silberstein LE, Litwin S, Carmack CE. Relationship of variable region genes expressed by a human B-cell lymphoma secreting pathologic anti-Pr_2 erythrocyte autoantibodies. J Exp Med 1989; 169:1631.
49. Wang AC, Fudenberg HH, Wells JV, Roelcke D. A new subgroup of the kappa chain variable region associated with anti-Pr cold agglutinins. Nature 1973; 243:126.
50. Jefferies LC, Stevenson FK, Goldman J, et al. Anti-idiotypic antibodies specific for a pathologic anti-Pr_2 cold agglutinin. Transfusion 1990; 30:495.
51. Friedman DF, Cho EA, Goldman J, et al. The role of clonal selection in the pathogenesis of an autoreactive human B cell lymphoma. J Exp Med 1991; 174:525.
52. Marsh WL, Oyen E, Alicea E. Autoimmune hemolytic anemia and the Kell blood group. Am J Hematol 1979; 7:155.
53. Van Loghem J, Van der Hart M. Varieties of specific auto-antibodies in acquired hemolytic anemia. Vox Sang 1954; 4:2.
54. Wakui H, Imai H, Kobayashi R. Autoantibodies against erythrocyte protein band 4.1 in a patient with autoimmune hemolytic anemia. Blood 1988; 72:408.
55. Weiner W, Vos G. Serology of acquired hemolytic anemia. Blood 1963; 22:606.
56. Petz L, Garratty G. Acquired Hemolytic Anemia. New York: Churchill Livingstone, 1980.
57. Eaton RB, Schneider G, Schur PH. Enzyme immunoassay for antibodies to native DNA. Arthritis Rheum 1983; 26:52.
58. Issit PD, Pavone BG. Critical reexamination of the specificity of auto-anti-Rh antibodies in patients with a positive direct agglutination test. Br J Haematol 1978; 38:63.
59. Agre P, Cartron JP. Molecular biology of the Rh antigens. Blood 1991; 78:551.
60. Victoria E, Pierce S, Branks M, Masouredis S. IgG red blood cell autoantibodies in autoimmune hemolytic anemia bind to epitopes on red blood cell membrane band 3 glycoprotein. J Lab Clin Med 1990; 115:74.
61. Sturgeon P. Hematologic observations on the anemia associated with blood type Rh_{null}. Blood 1970; 36:310.
62. Lauf PK, Joiner CH. Increased potassium transport and oubain binding in human Rh_{null} red blood cells. Blood 1976; 48:457.
63. Dahr W, Kordowicz M, Moulds J. Characterization of the Ss sialoglycoprotein and its antigens in Rh_{null} erythrocytes. Blood 1987; 54:13.
64. Hogman C, Killander J, Sjolin S. A case of idiopathic autoimmune haemolytic anemia due to anti-e. Acta Paediatr Scand 1960; 49:270.
65. Sachs V. Anti-C as a sole autoantibody in autoimmune hemolytic anemia. Transfusion 1985; 25:587.
66. Barker RN, Casswell M, Reid ME, et al. Identification of autoantigens in autoimmune haemolytic anaemia by a non-radioisotope immunoprecipitation method. Br J Haematol 1992; 82:126.
67. Leddy JP, Falany JL, Kissel GE, et al. Erythrocyte membrane proteins reactive with human (warm-reacting) anti–red cell autoantibodies. J Clin Invest 1993; 91:1672.
68. Bruce LJ, Tanner MJA. Structure-function relationships of band 3 variants. Cell Mol Biol 1996; 42:953.
69. Issit PD, Pavone BG, Goldfinger D, et al. Anti-Wr^b, and other autoantibodies responsible for positive direct antiglobulin tests in 150 individuals. Br J Haematol 1976; 34:5.
70. Issit PD, Combs MR, Allen J, Melroy-Carawan H. Anti-Di^b as a red cell autoantibody. Transfusion 1996; 36:802.
71. Roush GR, Rosenthal NS, Gerson SL, et al. An unusual case of autoimmune hemolytic anemia with reticulocytopenia, erythroid dysplasia, and an IgG2 autoanti-U. Transfusion 1996; 36:575.
72. Garratty G, Arndt P, Domen R, et al. Severe autoimmune hemolytic anemia associated with IgM warm autoantibodies directed against determinants on or associated with glycophorin A. Vox Sang 1997; 72:124.
73. Teleri MJ, Chasis JA. Relationship of the human erythrocyte Wr^b antigen to an interaction between glycophorin A and band 3. Blood 1990; 76:842.
74. Ring SM, Tippett P, Swallow DA. Comparative immunochemical analysis of the Wr^a and Wr^b red cell antigens. Vox Sang 1994; 67:226.
75. Wren MR, Issitt PD. Evidence that Wr^a and Wr^b are antithetical. Transfusion 1988; 28:113.
76. Bruce LJ, Ring SM, Anstee DJ, et al. Changes in the blood group Wright antigens are associated with a mutation at amino acid 658 in human erythrocyte band 3: a site of interaction between band 3 and glycophorin A under certain conditions. Blood 1995; 85:541.
77. Huang CH, Reid ME, Xie SS, Blumenfeld OO. Human red blood cell Wright antigens: a genetic and evolutionary perspective on glycophorin A–band 3 interaction. Blood 1996; 87:3942.
78. Leddy JP, Wilkinson SL, Kissel GE, et al. Erythrocyte membrane proteins reactive with IgG (warm-reacting) anti–red blood cell autoantibodies: II. Antibodies coprecipitating band 3 and glycophorin A. Blood 1994; 84:650.
79. Litwin SD, Balaban S, Eyster M. Gm allotype preference in erythrocyte IgG antibodies of patients with autoimmune hemolytic anemia. Blood 1973; 241:6.
80. Leddy JP, Bakemeier RF. Structural aspects of human erythrocyte autoantibodies. J Exp Med 1965; 121:17.
81. Silberstein LE, Goldman J, Kant JA, Spitalnik SL. Comparative biochemical and genetic characterization of clonally related human B-cell lines secreting pathogenic anti-Pr_2 cold agglutinins. Arch Biochem Biophys 1988; 264:244.
82. Silberstein LE, Robertson GA, Hannam Harris AC, et al. Etiologic aspects of cold agglutinin disease: evidence for cytogenetically defined clones of lymphoid cells and the demonstration that an anti-Pr cold autoantibody is derived from a chromosomally aberrant B cell clone. Blood 1986; 67:1705.
83. Theofilopoulos AN, Dixon FJ. Murine models of systemic lupus erythematosus. Adv Immunol 1985; 37:269.
84. Friedman DF, Moore JS, Erikson J, et al. Variable region gene analysis of an isotype-switched (IgA) variant of chronic lymphocytic lymphoma. Blood 1992; 80:2287.
85. Okamoto M, Murakami M, Shimuzu A, et al. A transgenic model of autoimmune hemolytic anemia. J Exp Med 1992; 175:71.

CHAPTER 28

Platelet Alloimmunization

K. J. Kao
Maria Luz del Rosario

Platelet transfusion therapy has allowed the prevention and treatment of hemorrhagic complications associated with thrombocytopenia since the 1960s. Consequently, the use of platelets has increased at an exponential rate. The number of platelet units transfused rose from 2,857,000 in 1980 to 4,688,000 in 1992, and the number of apheresis platelets increased from 56,000 to 638,000 in the same period.[1,2] Because platelet concentrates are immunogenic, increased platelet use has been accompanied by an increase in immunological complications. The most common complication is antibody development to donor human leukocyte antigen (HLA) class I.[3,4] Owing to high concentrations of HLAs on platelets, platelets are susceptible to these antibodies. Many immunized patients become unresponsive to pooled random donor platelets and require apheresis platelets from HLA-matched donors. Unfortunately, only a handful of acceptable donors can be identified from a pool of several thousand HLA-typed donors because of the highly polymorphic nature of HLAs.[5,6] HLA alloimmunization has therefore become a major challenge in platelet transfusion therapy.

Considerable research has been conducted to elucidate the mechanisms responsible for platelet transfusion–induced HLA alloimmunization. These efforts have led to successful application of leukocyte-depleted or leukocyte-inactivated platelet concentrates for the prevention of HLA alloimmunization. Results of these studies have also provided new insights for the development of innovative therapeutic approaches aimed toward the induction of specific immune tolerance of donor HLAs. The goal of this chapter is to review the immunological complications of platelet transfusion therapy and to discuss advances in elucidating the scientific basis of platelet transfusion–induced HLA alloimmunization.

IMMUNOGENIC ELEMENTS IN PLATELET CONCENTRATES

Two types of platelet concentrates—platelets and apheresis platelets—are available for transfusion.[7] Platelets are prepared from donated whole blood by differential centrifugation, and apheresis platelets are harvested from individual donors through apheresis. Although platelets are the predominant cellular component, both products also contain significant amounts of donor red cells, leukocytes, and plasma (Table 28–1). All these blood components in platelet concentrates are immunogenic and can lead to various immunological and clinical consequences in transfusion recipients.

Red Blood Cells

Platelet concentrates prepared from whole blood contain variable amounts of red cells. On average, 0.3 to 0.5 mL of red blood cells is present in platelet concentrates[8–10] prepared from one unit of whole blood. In a unit of apheresis platelets prepared with currently available apheresis equipment, the quantity of contaminating red cells is between 0.5 and 3 mL.[11]

In addition to blood group antigens, HLAs are present on red cells.[12,13] One red cell has between 100 and 200 HLA molecules[13] (Table 28–2); this can be upregulated to a few thousand molecules after patients are treated with interferon.[14] However, red cells that are newly released from bone marrow express increased numbers of HLAs after interferon treatment; peripheral red cells are not similarly affected. Therefore, red cell HLAs are remnants of nucleated normoblasts.[14] Because red cells have only a small number of HLAs, they do not play a significant role in transfusion-induced primary HLA alloimmunization and are not clinically important. Nevertheless, HLAs on red cells could trigger a secondary anamnestic response in patients with prior HLA alloimmunization.[13]

Table 28–1. Contents of Platelet Products

	Apheresis Platelets (One Unit)	Platelets (One Unit)
Platelets		
Minimum	3.0×10^{11}	5.5×10^{10}
Average	4×10^{11}	$6–7 \times 10^{10}$
Leukocytes	$<10^{9}$*	$10^{7}–10^{8}$
Lymphocytes (%)	40–60	80–90
Monocytes (%)	20–30	5–10
Granulocytes (%)	10–20	5
Red Cells (mL)	0.5–3	<0.5
Plasma (mL)	200–300	50

From quality control results from the Lifesouth Community Blood Bank, Gainesville, FL.

*Numbers of leukocytes vary significantly, depending on the type of apheresis instrument and software used for platelet collection.

Table 28–2. Quantitative Distribution of Human Leukocyte Antigens (HLAs) in Blood

	HLA Molecules per Cell	HLA Concentration* μg/mL Whole Blood
Red cell	200†	0.09 (3%)
Granulocyte	NA‡	0.07 (2%)‡
Lymphocyte	3×10^5†	0.07 (2%)
Platelet	1×10^5†	2.37 (70%)
Plasma		0.81 (23%)†

*HLA concentrations were calculated by assuming that the molecular weight of HLA (HLA heavy chain and β_2-microglobulin) is 57 kD and that there are 2.5×10^8, 2.5×10^6, and 5×10^9 platelets, lymphocytes, and red cells, respectively, in 1 mL of whole blood. A hematocrit of 45% was used to determine the amount of plasma HLA in 1 mL of whole blood.

†The numbers were obtained from references 14, 16, and 24.

‡Not available. It was reported that the overall content of HLAs on granulocytes was similar to that of lymphocytes in peripheral blood.[25]

Plasma

During each platelet transfusion, a recipient is exposed to 200 to 300 mL of donor plasma. This volume is equivalent to a unit of fresh frozen plasma. Because many plasma proteins carry polymorphic antigenic epitopes, recipients of platelet concentrates can become immunized to donor plasma proteins. The antibodies formed against plasma proteins can cause immediate-type hypersensitivity reactions with varying degrees of severity.

Plasma also contains approximately 1 μg/mL of HLAs (see Table 28–2), which are present in two to four different molecular-weight forms.[15, 16] These different forms of HLAs are derived from the shedding of intact HLAs from cell membrane,[17, 18] secretion of the alternatively spliced and water-soluble form by circulating leukocytes,[16] and proteolytic degradation of cell surface HLAs.[16] The exact biological function of plasma HLAs is not known and is currently being investigated.[19–21] Although plasma HLAs have been shown to induce low titers of antibodies in some transfusion recipients, they are not very immunogenic and do not play a major role in transfusion-induced HLA alloimmunization. Because plasma HLAs in donor units can neutralize anti-HLA antibodies,[22] these HLAs theoretically could protect the transfused platelets from anti-HLA antibodies in alloimmunized patients. However, this potential benefit in alloimmunized platelet transfusion recipients yet has to be demonstrated.

Leukocytes

The number of contaminating leukocytes in platelet units varies widely, depending on preparation protocols.[23] Because of the similar cellular density between lymphocytes and platelets, the majority of contaminating leukocytes in platelet units are lymphocytes. According to a study on 100 units of platelet concentrates, more than 80% of contaminating leukocytes are lymphocytes, 5% to 10% are monocytes, and the remaining are granulocytes (see Table 28–1). These numbers are similar to those reported previously.[10] For apheresis platelets, the relative number of lymphocytes is somewhat less than for random platelet concentrates (see Table 28–1). On leukocytes there are HLAs and lineage-specific alloantigens. The number of class I HLAs on a leukocyte is between 1×10^5 and 3×10^5 (see Table 28–2).[24, 25] Because there are significantly fewer leukocytes in platelet concentrates than in platelets, the amount of HLAs on all leukocytes in platelet concentrates accounts for less than 1% of total HLAs in platelet units (Table 28–3). The small amount of HLAs on donor leukocytes suggests that they are not likely to be important in blood transfusion–induced HLA alloimmunization. However, all the available studies have shown that these leukocytes are critical for platelet transfusion–induced HLA alloimmunization. Their importance is discussed in detail later in this chapter.

The best-characterized lineage-specific alloantigens on leukocytes are granulocyte-specific antigens. Although these antigens are immunogenic, the development of antibodies to granulocyte-specific antigens usually does not have a direct adverse effect on platelet transfusion. These antibodies are associated with various transfusion reactions such as febrile nonhemolytic reactions and transfusion-associated lung injury.

Platelets

Three major groups of alloantigens are present on platelets: blood group antigens, platelet-specific antigens, and HLAs. Although blood group antigens and HLAs are not platelet specific, these antigens are intrinsic components of platelet membrane.

Blood Group Antigens. Blood group antigens on platelets include ABH, Lewis, Ii, and P antigens.[26–31] These antigens are present in platelet membrane glycoproteins.[28] Portions of ABO and Lewis antigens are acquired from plasma by adsorption.[29–31] Antibodies to ABO, Lewis, and P antigens often develop spontaneously in antigen-negative persons, and antibodies to I antigens are cold-reacting autoantibodies.[32] Because antibodies to these blood group antigens are already present in most patients and do not have a significant negative impact on post-transfusion recovery of antigen-positive platelets, platelet transfusion–induced alloimmunization to these antigens is not clinically important.

The impact of ABO compatibility on post-transfusion platelet recovery, albeit small, has been demonstrated.[33–36] When the average corrected count increments (CCIs) of ABO-compatible and ABO-incompatible platelet transfusions were determined in 40 leukemic patients undergoing induction chemotherapy, they were $14.9 \times 10^3/\mu L$ and $9.5 \times 10^3/\mu L$, respectively ($p < .0007$).[33] Similar effects of ABO compatibility on transfusion responses

Table 28–3. Quantitative Distribution of Human Leukocyte Antigens (HLAs) in a Pool of Six-Unit Platelet Concentrates

	HLAs*
Platelets (3.6×10^{11})	3.4 mg (94%)
Plasma (300 mL)	0.2 mg (5.5%)
Leukocytes (6×10^8)	17 μg (0.5%)

*The amounts of HLAs were calculated using the values shown in Table 28–2.

have been observed in patients who were refractory to random-donor platelets and received HLA-matched single-donor apheresis platelet transfusions.[34] In patients who received HLA-matched apheresis platelets, transfusions of ABO-compatible platelets resulted in average platelet recovery of 73 ± 4% at 1 hour, compared with 55 ± 5% for ABO-incompatible transfusions ($p < .01$). Recoveries at 24 hours after transfusion were 37 ± 3% for ABO-compatible platelets versus 29 ± 4% for ABO-incompatible platelets ($p < .05$). In another study of 51 patients refractory to pooled random-donor platelets who received 316 HLA-selected apheresis transfusions, ABO-compatible platelet transfusions gave average CCIs of 10 $\times$ $10^3/\mu L$, whereas transfusions of platelets incompatible with recipients' plasma anti-A/B antibodies yielded CCIs of 5.9 $\times$ $10^3/\mu L$ ($p < .01$).[35] Despite all these positive results, some investigators have not observed similar adverse effects of ABO incompatibility.[37–40] The discrepant findings indicate that the effect of ABO incompatibility on platelet transfusion is subtle and may be influenced by variable expression of A and/or B antigens on platelets among individuals[41] and varying titers of ABO isoagglutinins in transfusion recipients.[34, 36]

Platelet-Specific Antigens. Platelet membrane glycoproteins contain antigenic epitopes that are not found on other types of blood cells. More than 20 such platelet-specific alloantigens have been identified,[42–44] and many have been well characterized at the molecular level.[43, 44] These platelet-specific alloantigens are present in dimorphic forms, and the allelic frequencies are unequally distributed in a high-frequency public form and a low-frequency private form.[42–45] They can elicit the production of antibodies through transfusion or pregnancy. The development of such antibodies can result in three clinical conditions: neonatal alloimmune thrombocytopenia—mothers become immunized to platelets of fetuses and give birth to thrombocytopenic infants; post-transfusion purpura—patients become immunized to platelet-specific alloantigens after blood transfusion and develop thrombocytopenia; and transfusion-associated alloimmune thrombocytopenia—patients receive multiple platelet transfusions and become refractory to random-donor platelets.[42, 46]

HLAs. HLA class I molecules constitute the third group of platelet alloantigens. These antigens are heterodimeric membrane glycoproteins that consist of a 44-kD highly polymorphic heavy chain and a 12-kD invariant β_2-microglobulin.[47] These two polypeptides are noncovalently associated with each other and are present in varying quantities on most cells in an individual. The genes encoding HLA heavy chains are located at three different loci (A, B, and C) of chromosome 6. Functionally, HLAs play a major role in presenting antigenic peptides to cytotoxic T lymphocytes (CTLs)[48] and are essential for ontogenetic development of $CD8^+$ cytotoxic T cells in the thymus.[49, 50] Clinically, HLA is the primary antigenic system that determines the survival of transplanted allografts. Antibodies to HLAs are responsible for greater than 90% of immune-mediated platelet transfusion refractoriness.[4, 46]

The number of HLAs per platelet varies widely among people, ranging from 50,000 to 180,000 molecules,[15, 51] with an average of 100,000 HLA molecules per platelet.[15] Considering the small size of platelets, the density of HLAs on platelets is the highest among all types of blood cells. Interestingly, approximately 70% of platelet HLAs can be removed by treatment with hypertonic acid chloroquine solution.[15, 51, 52] This loss is due to both denaturation and physical elution.[53] Because platelets had been shown to acquire HLAs from plasma,[54] it was speculated that a significant amount of platelet HLAs might be derived from plasma. When a sensitive and quantitative immunofluorescent flow cytometric method was used to measure HLAs acquired from plasma, it was found that they accounted for a very small fraction of total platelet HLAs.[55] Later, precise quantitative measurement of platelet and plasma HLAs also failed to find any proportional correlation between plasma and total or chloroquine-elutable HLAs on platelets.[15] Therefore, any binding of plasma HLAs to platelets is likely to be of low affinity and nonspecific in nature. Moreover, it has been shown that messenger RNA (mRNA) for class I HLAs is present in platelets and capable of synthesizing class I HLA protein.[56] All these findings indicate that the majority of platelet HLAs are integral membrane proteins and are not derived from plasma.

IMMUNOLOGICAL CONSEQUENCES OF PLATELET TRANSFUSIONS

HLA Alloimmunization

Alloimmunization to donor class I HLAs is a major immunological complication of platelet transfusion. This complication often leads to platelet transfusion refractoriness. According to earlier studies,[57–64] HLA alloimmunization occurred in 30% to 70% of patients who received multiple platelet and red cell transfusions. In patients who did not have significant immunosuppression and had isolated exposure to platelets and red cells during open heart surgery, the incidence of HLA alloimmunization was about 74%.[65]

As mentioned earlier, providing adequate platelet transfusion support to patients who develop alloimmune platelet refractoriness is a continuing clinical challenge. To overcome this obstacle, considerable research has been done on transfusion-induced HLA alloimmunization. Results generated from these studies have not only contributed to the development of effective ways of preventing transfusion-induced HLA alloimmunization but also provided deeper understanding of the unique cellular mechanism responsible for this immunological complication.

Indirect Versus Direct Antigen Presentation. Normally, generation of antibodies to foreign proteins is initiated by host antigen-presenting cells (APCs). The APCs include dendritic cells, macrophages/monocytes, B lymphocytes, and skin Langerhans cells.[66] All these bone marrow–derived host APCs are able to ingest and process foreign proteins into peptides.[67, 68] The processed antigenic peptides are presented on the surface of APCs through binding to the major histocompatibility complex (MHC) class II molecules. These MHC class II molecules with bound antigenic peptides are recognized by host CD4+ helper T lymphocytes via their T cell receptors (TCRs) (Fig. 28–1*A*). Unlike HLA class I molecules, which are expressed on virtually all types of cells,[13, 15, 69] the expression of MHC class II molecules is limited to APCs and activated T lymphocytes.[66] Because foreign proteins have to be ingested and processed before being presented by host APCs, this initial step is referred to as indirect antigen presentation (see Fig. 28–1*A*).

Indirect antigen presentation is the predominant pathway responsible for host immune responses to most foreign antigens, including those present on red cells, platelets, leukocytes, and plasma proteins of donor blood. Nevertheless, this pathway fails to explain the immunogenicity of class I HLAs, despite the highly polymorphic nature of HLAs and their presence in large quantities on platelets. Therefore, HLA alloimmunization is likely mediated through a different antigen presentation mechanism.

In 1978 Batchelor and colleagues,[70] using rat and mouse models, demonstrated that class I MHC antigens per se are poorly immunogenic. Viable and functioning leukocytes are necessary for inducing alloimmunization to foreign class I MHC molecules. The importance of viable donor leukocytes for alloimmunization is further supported by the fact that stored blood has reduced HLA immunogenicity.[71] These findings suggest that direct interaction between functional donor leukocytes and the immune systems of transfusion recipients is critical for the induction of antibody responses to non–self-MHC

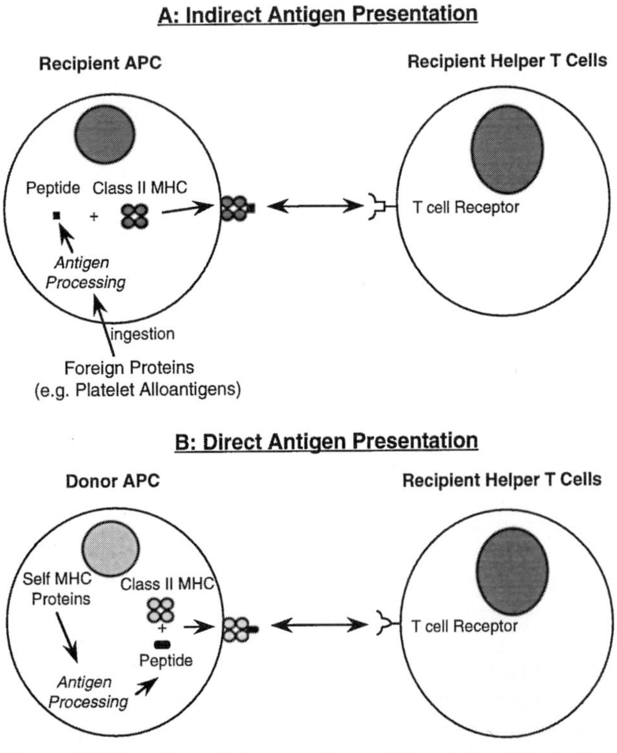

Figure 28–1. Indirect (*A*) versus direct (*B*) antigen presentation. APCs, antigen-presenting cells, which include dendritic cells, macrophages, monocytes, and B cells; MHC, major histocompatibility complex.

antigens within the same species. This conclusion was corroborated by the study by Claas and colleagues,[72] in which they showed that removal of leukocytes can prevent platelet transfusion–induced alloimmunization to donor MHC antigens. The importance of leukocytes in immunizing recipients to donor MHC antigens is also supported by the finding that passenger leukocytes in renal allografts are the primary immunogenic elements causing graft rejection.[73]

Prompted by these intriguing findings, numerous transfusion studies were launched to investigate whether leukocyte-reduced platelet concentrates and red cells could prevent alloimmunization to donor MHC antigens or immune platelet transfusion refractoriness.[74–80] Unfortunately, results generated from these studies were conflicting and inconclusive owing to the heterogeneity of patient populations included in the studies and the technical difficulties associated with preparing high-quality leukocyte-depleted blood components for transfusion. Conclusive demonstration of the effectiveness of using leukocyte-depleted or leukocyte-inactivated platelet concentrates to prevent HLA alloimmunization was finally provided by the completion of a carefully designed multicenter transfusion trial.[4] The results of this trial show that both leukocyte depletion by filtration and leukocyte inactivation by irradiation with medium wavelength ultraviolet B (UVB) light can reduce platelet transfusion–induced HLA alloimmunization by half in patients with acute myelogenous leukemia.

Because the amount of HLAs on leukocytes accounted for less than 1% of total HLAs in a pool of six units of random-donor platelets (see Table 28–3), and because removal of such a small quantity of HLAs is able to reduce the HLA immunogenicity of platelet concentrates, one has to conclude that HLAs by themselves are indeed poorly immunogenic[70] and that indirect antigen presentation is ineffective for initiating an immune response to non–self-MHC antigens. It is most likely that direct antigen presentation by class II–positive donor leukocytes to recipient helper T cells is responsible for transfusion-induced HLA alloimmunization (see Fig. 28–1*B*).

Mechanism of Transfusion-Induced HLA Alloimmunization. Direct antigen presentation (see Fig. 28–1*B*) is most likely responsible for initiating transfusion-induced HLA alloimmunization. Although the primary role of TCRs on host T lymphocytes is to interact with MHC class II molecules on APCs in a self-restricted manner, it is known that TCRs on helper T cells are also able to recognize non-self class II molecules on foreign APCs.[81, 82] The prime example of this alloreactivity of host helper T cells is the classical mixed leukocyte reaction (MLR).[83] In MLR, leukocytes from MHC-disparate persons are cultured together. Class II–positive leukocytes from one person are irradiated with gamma rays and used as stimulatory cells. T cells from the other person are used as responding cells. The responding T cells proliferate and incorporate radiolabeled thymidine in response to the stimulation by foreign class II–positive leukocytes. This interaction is similar to the one between recipient helper T cells and donor APCs during the initial phase of transfusion-induced alloimmune responses. Therefore, HLA alloimmunization is initiated by interaction between non–self-APCs in blood components and host alloreactive helper T lymphocytes (see Fig. 28–1*B*; step I of Fig. 28–2). A study using class II–deficient and class II–depleted leukocytes to determine the immunogenicity of donor leukocytes in a murine transfusion model showed that class II–positive donor leukocytes play a major role in transfusion-induced alloimmunization to donor class I MHC antigens.[84] After initial binding between donor MHC class II molecules and recipient TCRs, this interaction is further stabilized and enhanced through the participation of additional accessory cell adhesion receptors and ligands on APCs and T helper lymphocytes.[85–87] These interactions then result in full activation of APCs.

After activation, APCs begin to secrete interleukin-1 (IL-1), IL-12, and other cytokines and to express CD80 and CD86 costimulatory signals on the cell surface (see step I of Fig. 28–2).[88, 89] The CD80 and CD86 costimulatory signals on the APCs bind to CD28 molecules and further activate T helper cells (see step II of Fig. 28–2).[90, 91] Activation of helper T cells leads to the increased expression of CD40 ligand (CD40L) and IL-2 receptors and the secretion of IL-2, IL-3, IL-4, IL-5, IL-6, IL-10, IL-13, tumor necrosis factor-β, and/or interferon-γ (IFN-γ). CD40L, IL-4, IL-5, IL-10, and IL-13 provide critical T cell help to B lymphocytes for their proliferation, maturation, and antibody production (see step III of Fig. 28–2).[85, 92, 93] The secreted IL-2 further stimulates T cells to proliferate and amplifies T cell help to B cells. At the same time, the class II MHC molecules on B lymphocytes allow their intimate interaction with activated helper T cells in an antigen-specific manner (see Fig. 28–2). All these intricate interactions culminate in the production of antibodies to donor MHC class I antigens.

To investigate the role of costimulatory signals (see step II of Fig. 28–2), we studied the effect of 8-methoxypsoralen (8-MOP) treatment and long-wavelength ultraviolet A (UVA) irradiation on the alloantigenicity of platelet concentrates in a murine transfusion model.[94] The treatment of leukocytes with 8-MOP and UVA irradiation covalently crosslinks two different strands of DNA and inhibits the expression of costimulatory signals by APCs. The results of this study showed that such treatment reduced the alloantigenicity of platelet concentrates. Similar results were obtained when donor APCs in platelet concentrates were inactivated by irradiation with UVB[95] or UVC.[96] Both UVB and UVC are able to inhibit and downregulate the expression of costimulatory signals and adhesion molecules.[95, 97, 98] These findings support the hypothesis that HLA alloimmunization is mediated through direct antigen presentation by donor class II–positive leukocytes as depicted in Figure 28–2. At present, it is not known whether the recipient T helper cells that initially interact with donor class II–positive leukocytes and those that subsequently interact with recipient B cells are the same. Nor is it clear whether MHC class II molecules on the donor APCs have to present antigenic peptides derived from donor MHC class I antigens, or whether MHC class II molecules on the recipient B cells present the same antigenic peptides. Further study is needed to answer these questions.

Although direct antigen presentation is the predominant pathway for transfusion-induced HLA alloimmunization, the indirect antigen presentation pathway is also

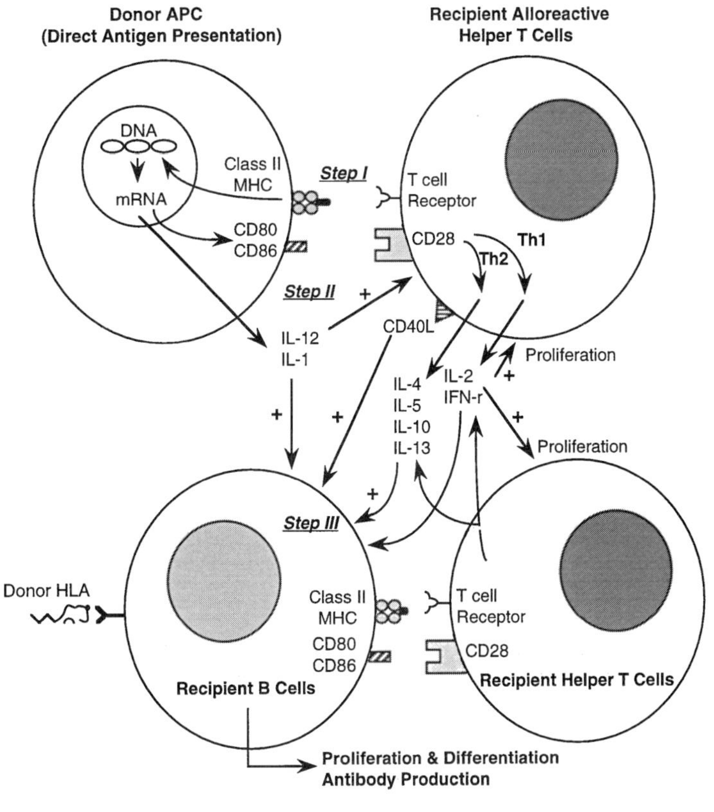

Figure 28–2. Mechanism of transfusion-induced alloimmunization to human leukocyte antigens (HLAs) of blood donors. *Step I*, Initial direct antigen presentation from donor antigen-presenting cells (APCs) to recipient helper T cells. *Step II*, Activation of donor APCs, expression of costimulatory signals and cytokines, and subsequent full activation of recipient helper T cells. *Step III*, Response of recipient B cells to T cell help. IFN, interferon; IL, interleukin; MHC, major histocompatibility complex; Th, helper T cells.

operational, albeit inefficient. With a murine transfusion model, it has been shown that highly purified platelets with little contamination of leukocytes are capable of inducing a humoral immune response to donor MHC class I antigens through the indirect antigen presentation by host APCs.[99] The presence of a functional indirect presentation pathway is also supported by the finding that weak HLA alloimmuization can be induced by plasma in some transfusion recipients.[19] Nonetheless, indirect antigen presentation plays only a minor role in HLA alloimmunization, as demonstrated by studies showing that leukocyte depletion is effective in preventing HLA alloimmunization.[4, 76–80]

Factors Influencing HLA Alloimmunization. Although HLA alloimmunization is the most frequent immunological complication of platelet transfusion, significant numbers of patients receiving multiple platelet and red cell transfusions do not develop anti-HLA antibodies.[57–64] It is therefore of interest to learn which clinical factors influence transfusion-induced HLA alloimmunization. Variables that have been identified include antigenic load, underlying disease, and chemotherapy regimen. Although antigenic load appears to be an influencing factor, the relationship between number of platelet transfusions and HLA alloimmunization remains controversial. Several studies have shown a direct relationship,[40, 100–102] but other investigators have suggested otherwise.[58, 103–105] These conflicting findings are probably due to the heterogeneity of patient populations in terms of underlying disease, immunosuppressive treatment, and prior sensitization to HLAs by transfusions and/or pregnancies.

The effect of underlying disease on HLA alloimmunization differs in patients with different hematological disorders. Patients with aplastic anemia have higher frequencies of HLA alloimmunization (80% to 90%) than do patients with hematological malignancies (40% to 60%).[101] Patients with acute myelogenous leukemia undergoing induction therapy are more likely to develop HLA alloimmunization than are patients with acute lymphoblastic leukemia (44% vs. 18%).[105] The development of HLA antibody also occurs earlier in patients with acute myelogenous leukemia.[61] These differences may be attributed to varying degrees of immunosuppression resulting from the disease process itself or from treatment with immunosuppressive steroids.[105] Genetic predisposition may also play a role, as illustrated by a study conducted in patients undergoing open heart surgery and without significant immunosuppression.[65] In this study, 74% of patients developed cytotoxic anti-HLA antibodies after perioperative platelet and red cell transfusions.

Alloimmunization to Platelet-Specific Antigens

Alloimmunization to platelet-specific alloantigens occurs as a result of pregnancy or blood transfusion and is clinically responsible for neonatal alloimmune thrombocytopenia and post-transfusion thrombocytopenic purpura. However, the role of antibodies to platelet-specific antigens in immune-mediated platelet transfusion refractoriness is uncertain. According to the multicenter Trial to Reduce Alloimmunization to Platelets (TRAP),[4] the development of antibodies to platelet-specific alloantigens was detected in 8% of recipients after multiple platelet transfusions. This finding is consistent with the results of earlier studies.[59, 61, 62, 106] Despite positive detection of platelet-specific alloantibodies by in vitro assays, these antibodies usually do not have a significant impact on platelet transfusion response.[62, 107, 108] Only a few cases of platelet transfusion failure could be attributed to the presence of these alloantibodies.[109–112] The reason for this finding is not clear. Because platelet-specific antigens are present in dimorphic forms and the allelic frequencies are unequally distributed in a high-frequency public form and a low-frequency private form,[43–45] the antiplatelet antibodies are often against platelets from a fraction of blood donors and clinically inconsequential. Some cases appear to be autoantibodies to platelet autoantigens.[62, 108] Refractoriness due to alloimmunization to high-frequency platelet-specific antigens could pose a major challenge in finding compatible donors. However, these cases are rare.[110, 113]

The development of antibodies to platelet-specific alloantigens has been associated with certain HLA class II phenotypes in pregnant women. For instance, a higher incidence of alloimmunization to human platelet antigen (HPA)-1a (Pl^{A1}, Zw^a) is found in persons positive for HLA-DR3 and HLA-DRw52,[113–115] and alloimmunization to HPA-5b (Br^a) is associated with HLA-DRw6.[116] These associations may be related to the ontogenetic selection of helper T cells that preferentially recognize platelet-specific antigenic peptides presented by specific HLA class II molecules. In addition to the MHC class II phenotypes, the nonclassic HLA genes involved in transporting antigenic peptides from cytosol into endoplasmic reticulum have been implicated in influencing alloimmunization against platelet-specific antigens.[117] Because donor platelet-specific alloantigens cannot be presented directly to helper T cells of transfusion recipients, antibody development against platelet alloantigens is mediated through indirect antigen presentation (see Fig. 28–1A).

Another type of humoral immune response against platelet-specific antigens involves people with deficiencies of various platelet glycoproteins.[118] After exposure to normal donor platelets, isoimmunization to the deficient platelet glycoprotein develops. As expected, the developed isoantibodies react to platelets from almost all donors. Consequently, it is difficult to find unrelated compatible platelet donors for these patients; family members can be tested for compatibility. Fortunately, these conditions are limited to rare patients with hereditary deficiency of platelet membrane glycoproteins.

Alloimmunization to Red Cell and Plasma Protein Antigens

Although only small numbers of red cells are present in platelet concentrates (see Table 28–1), these red cells are potentially immunogenic. In a retrospective study of 102 Rh-D–negative and immunosuppressed patients, 7.8% of them developed anti-D antibodies after transfusions of platelets from Rh-D–positive donors.[119] Similarly, 9 of 73 (12%) Rh-D–negative patients with various hematological malignancies became alloimmunized after receiving Rh-D–positive platelet transfusions.[120] The contaminating red cells in platelet units therefore are immunogenic. The incidence of platelet transfusion–induced alloimmunization to other blood group antigens is not known, because patients who need multiple platelet transfusions also require transfusions of red cells, which are not matched for blood group antigens other than ABO and Rh-D antigens. It is therefore difficult to separate the effects of red cell and platelet transfusions on alloimmunization to blood group antigens. For this reason, and because of the absence of any direct impact of red cell alloantibodies on platelet transfusion, platelet transfusion–induced alloimmunization to other blood group antigens has not been investigated.

During each platelet transfusion, 200 to 300 mL of plasma is infused into a recipient, so the development of antibodies to alloantigens in donor plasma proteins is not unexpected. The exact incidence of platelet transfusion–induced alloimmunization to plasma proteins is not known. Nevertheless, results from the multicenter TRAP trial indicate that only 24 of 598 patients with acute myelogenous leukemia undergoing induction chemotherapy experienced 31 episodes of transfusion-associated urticarial reaction, and none had anaphylactic reaction.[121] This finding suggests that alloimmunization to plasma proteins is uncommon and not of major clinical significance.

LABORATORY DETECTION OF PLATELET ALLOIMMUNIZATION

Although platelet alloimmunization often leads to platelet transfusion refractoriness, nonimmune clinical factors are more frequently responsible for poor platelet transfusion responses in thrombocytopenic patients.[37, 107] Because management of patients with immune as opposed to nonimmune platelet transfusion refractoriness is quite different, laboratory testing to correctly identify the underlying cause is important.

The lymphocytotoxicity assay (LCA) is the primary method for detecting HLA antibodies.[122] A patient's serum is incubated with a panel of lymphocytes collected from 20 to 60 different HLA-phenotyped donors, followed by the addition of rabbit complement. The presence of antibodies against target lymphocytes can be detected by assessing complement-dependent killing of target lymphocytes. The detected antibody is then expressed as a percentage of all targets in a panel showing positive killing. This percentage is called the panel reactive antibody (PRA). A high PRA indicates the presence of antibodies to a large number of different HLAs and/or to a few high-frequency HLAs. This assay also provides information regarding the specificity of HLA antibodies. However, the LCA is not always specific for HLA antibodies. Antibodies against other surface antigens on target lymphocytes can also generate positive results. In addition, non–complement-fixing antibodies may be missed by the LCA. To detect non–complement-fixing antibodies, an additional step of incubating target lymphocytes with antibodies to human immunoglobulin (Coombs' reagent) before the addition of complement has been introduced. Although the methodology of LCA is not complex, it requires special preservation of viable target lymphocytes.

Another test for detecting anti-HLA antibodies is immunofluorescent flow cytometry.[123] Again, a patient's serum is incubated with a panel of lymphocytes collected from HLA-phenotyped persons. The presence of antibodies is detected by an anti–human globulin labeled with fluorescent dye. This test is more sensitive than the LCA and can detect non–complement-fixing antibodies. However, like the LCA, this test is not always specific for HLAs. In addition, the instrument required is expensive and complex and is not widely available.

A highly specific and sensitive enzyme-linked immunosorbent assay (ELISA) has become available for the detection of HLA antibodies.[124, 125] This simple test uses HLAs purified from several hundred people to detect HLA antibodies. It is as sensitive as flow cytometry and can be carried out in most hospital and blood center laboratories. The test is able to determine whether a patient has developed HLA alloimunization. However, the ELISA, unlike the LCA, cannot provide information regarding the specificity of anti-HLA antibodies.

For detection of antibodies to platelet-specific alloantigens,[126] two different approaches are commonly used. The first approach is similar to the identification of red cell antibodies. A patient's serum is incubated with a panel of platelets carrying different known platelet-specific alloantigens. The antibodies reacting with platelets are detected by anti–human globulin labeled with different reagents such as enzymes, fluorescent dyes, or radioactive isotopes. One can also use labeled protein A[127] or red cells coated with anti–human immunoglobulin G (IgG)[128] to detect the binding of antibodies to platelets. A test in which red cells coated with anti–human IgG are used to detect platelet antibodies is commercially available. Major problems associated with these methods to detect platelet-specific antibodies include the difficulty of obtaining a complete collection of platelets with known platelet-specific alloantigens and interference by coexisting anti-HLA antibodies in patient's serum, which complicates the identification of antibodies to platelet-specific alloantigens.

The second approach is to use captured or purified platelet antigens for the detection of antiplatelet antibodies. After incubating target platelets with patient serum, the platelets are solubilized with detergents, and murine monoclonal antibodies to various platelet membrane glycoproteins are used to capture complexes of patient antibodies and platelet-specific antigens. The antibodies on the captured antigens are then detected by labeled anti–human immunoglobulin.[129] Another more simplistic and specific approach is to use purified platelet membrane glycoproteins for the direct detection of antibodies to platelet-specific alloantigens by ELISA. Alternative approaches for detecting antibodies to platelet-specific alloantigens include Western blotting and immunoprecipitation of platelet membrane proteins with iodine-125 or other radioactive tags.[126] These approaches are labor intensive and technically demanding.

PREVENTION OF HLA ALLOIMMUNIZATION

Because direct antigen presentation by donor leukocytes is responsible for transfusion-induced HLA alloimmunization, this immunological complication can be easily prevented by depletion or inactivation of donor leukocytes. However, neither approach was feasible until the late 1980s, when high-efficiency filters for removing leukocytes[130–132] and sterile plastic bags with improved UVB transmission for inactivating leukocytes[133, 134] became available. These technological advances allow the preparation of platelet concentrates and red cells containing sufficiently low numbers of leukocytes or fully inactivated leukocytes to prevent primary HLA alloimmunization.[4] Despite the proven effectiveness of both approaches for preventing HLA alloimmunization and immune platelet refractoriness, 10% of patients without prior alloimmunization still became immunized to HLAs after receiving treated blood components.[4] It is not known whether HLA alloimmunizaton in these patients is due to inadvertent exposure to a few untreated blood components, insufficient depletion of leukocytes, or a more active innate indirect antigen presentation pathway (high immune responders). Also unknown is the maximal number of donor leukocytes allowed during each platelet or red cell transfusion. Until answers to these questions become available, it would be prudent to avoid any inadvertent exposure of patients to untreated blood components and to ensure that leukocyte depletion or inactivation meets the highest standard if prevention of HLA alloimmunization is required.

For patients with prior alloimmuization to HLAs, it has been shown that leukocyte-depleted or washed red cells are ineffective in preventing a secondary antibody response.[13] HLAs themselves are sufficient to elicit an anamnestic reaction. A similar finding was made in the TRAP trial. It was reported that women with prior pregnancies who were transfused with leukocyte-depleted or leukocyte-inactivated platelets had higher HLA immunization rates (32% to 34%) than those with no prior pregnancies (7% to 15%).[4] Thus, the efficacy of leukocyte-depleted or leukocyte-inactivated blood components in preventing a secondary antibody response is limited. Despite the reduced effectiveness, additional results of the TRAP trial suggest that the use of leukocyte-depleted or leukocyte-inactivated blood components may attenuate or prevent the anamnestic response in some patients with prior HLA alloimmunization.

FUTURE DIRECTIONS

During the 1990s, considerable progress has been made in elucidating the cellular mechanisms of platelet transfusion–induced HLA alloimmunization. Many discoveries have led to the development of effective ways of preventing this immunological complication and have laid the groundwork for further investigation of the immunomodulatory roles of donor leukocytes. According to the current two-signal hypothesis,[135, 136] the expression of the second costimulatory signals such as CD80 and CD86 on the activated APCs (see Fig. 28–2) is essential for mounting effective immune responses, and the absence of such costimulatory signals could render helper T cells unresponsive (anergy) and lead to immunological tolerance.[137–139] Because irradiation of APCs with UVB or UVC inhibits the expression of the costimulatory signals on APCs,[95–97] it will be of interest to learn whether transfusions of donor leukocytes inactivated by UV light can induce immunological tolerance to donor MHC antigens. Initial studies using canine and murine transfusion models showed that immunological tolerance to donor MHC antigens can be induced by transfusions of peripheral mononuclear leukocytes irradiated with UVC or UVB.[95, 96] A more recent study indicated that the use of UVB-irradiated donor leukocytes with little contamination of plasma and platelets is critical for the successful induction of immunological tolerance to donor MHC antigens.[140] The use of highly purified donor leukocytes avoids indirect presentation of plasma and platelet MHC antigens by host APCs, which may interfere with tolerance induction.

As demonstrated by the TRAP trial,[4] transfusion of UVB-irradiated blood components is feasible and safe. The use of UVB-irradiated donor leukocytes for tolerance induction is therefore potentially applicable for the prevention of allograft rejection and for the attenuation of graft-versus-host disease in allogeneic bone marrow transplant patients.[141] Other potential clinical applications of tolerance induction include the establishment of bone marrow mixed chimerism for various hematological diseases, without the significant toxicity associated with myeloablative conditioning, and the induction of tolerance to viral vectors for gene therapy. Before all these applications can be realized, further investigations are needed to understand the cellular basis of tolerance induction by UVB-irradiated leukocytes, to answer questions regarding the appropriate dose schedule for induction and maintenance of tolerance, and to develop new in vitro systems for the assessment of tolerance induction. Further progress in this area should open a new and exciting chapter for blood component therapy in transfusion medicine.

REFERENCES

1. Surgenor DM, Wallace EL, Hao SH, et al. Collection and transfusion of blood components in the United States: 1982–1988. N Engl J Med 1990; 322:1646.
2. Wallace EL, Churchill WH, Surgenor DM, et al. Collection and transfusion of blood and blood components in the United States, 1992. Transfusion 1995; 35:802.
3. Schiffer CA. Prevention of alloimmunization against platelets. Blood 1991; 77:1.
4. TRAP Study Group. Leukocyte reduction and ultraviolet B irradiation of platelets to prevent alloimmunization and refractoriness to platelet transfusions. N Engl J Med 1997; 337:1861.
5. Opelz G, Mickey MR, Terrasaki PI. Unrelated donors for bone marrow transplantation and transfusion support: pool sizes required. Transplant Proc 1974; 6:405.
6. Bolgiano DC, Larson EB, Slichter SJ. A model to determine required pool size for HLA-typed community donor apheresis programs. Transfusion 1989; 29:306.
7. Standard Committee of the AABB. Standards for Blood Banks and Transfusion Services, 17th ed. Bethesda, MD: American Association of Blood Banks, 1996, p 15.
8. Herman JH. Single-donor (apheresis) vs. pooled platelet concentrates. *In* Kurtz SR, Brubaker DB (eds): Clinical Decision in Platelet Therapy. Bethesda, MD: American Association of Blood Banks, 1992, p 19.
9. Lichtiger B, Surgeon J, Rhorer S. Rh-incompatible platelet transfusion therapy in cancer patients: a study of 30 cases. Vox Sang 1983; 45:139.

10. Skinnider L, Wrobel H, McSheffrey B. The nature of the leukocyte "contamination" in platelet concentrates. Vox Sang 1985; 49:309.
11. QC results from the Lifesouth Community Blood Bank, Gainesville, FL.
12. de Villartay JP, Rouger P, Muller JY, et al. HLA antigens on peripheral red blood cells: analysis by flow cytofluorometry using monoclonal antibodies. Tissue Antigens 1985; 26:12.
13. Everett ET, Kao KJ, Scornik JC. Class I HLA molecules on human erythrocytes: quantitation and transfusion effects. Transplantation 1987; 44:123.
14. Everett ET, Scornik JC, Davis G, Kao KJ. Induction of erythrocyte HLA expression during interferon treatment and HIV infection. Hum Immunol 1990; 29:14.
15. Kao KJ. Plasma and platelet HLA in normal individuals: quantitation by competitive enzyme-linked immunoassay. Blood 1987; 70:282.
16. Haga JA, She JX, Kao KJ. Biochemical characterization of 39-kDa class I histocompatibility antigen in plasma: a secretable membrane protein derived from transmembrane domain deletion. J Biol Chem 1991; 266:3695.
17. Allison JP, Ferrone S, Callahan GN, et al. Biologic and chemical characterization of HLA antigens in human serum. J Immunol 1977; 118:1004.
18. Emerson SG, Cone RE. I-K^k and H-$2K^k$ antigens are shed as supramolecular particles in association with membrane lipids. J Immunol 1981; 127:482.
19. Puppo F, Indiveri F, Scudeletti M, et al. Soluble HLA antigens: new roles and uses. Immunol Today 1995; 18:154.
20. Zavazava N, Kronke M. Soluble HLA class I molecules induce apoptosis in alloreactive cytotoxic T lymphocytes. Nat Med 1996; 2:1005.
21. Pellegrino MA, Indiveri F, Fagiolo U, et al. Immunogenicity of serum HLA antigens in allogeneic combination. Transplantation 1982; 33:530.
22. van Rood JJ, van Leeuven A, van Santen MC. Anti HL-A2 inhibitior in normal human serum. Nature 1970; 226:336.
23. Champion AB, Carmen RA. Factors affecting white cell content in platelet concentrates. Transfusion 1985; 25:334.
24. Trucco M, de Petris S, Garotta G, Ceppellini R. Quantitative analysis of cell surface HLA structures by means of monoclonal antibodies. Hum Immunol 1980; 3:233.
25. Aster RH, Miskovich BH, Rodey GE. Histocompatibility antigens of human plasma: localization to the HDL-3 lipoprotein fraction. Transplantation 1973; 16:205.
26. Dunstan RA, Simpson MB. Heterogeneous distribution of antigens on human platelets demonstrated by fluorescence flow cytometry. Br J Haematol 1985; 61:603.
27. Dunstan RA, Simpson MB, Rosse WF. Presence of P blood group antigens on human platelets. Am J Clin Pathol 1985; 83:731.
28. Santoso S, Kiefel V, Mueller-Eckhardt C. Blood group A and B determinants are expressed on platelet glycoproteins IIa, IIIa, and Ib. Thromb Haemost 1991; 65:196.
29. Kelton JG, Hamid C, Aker S, et al. The amount of blood group A substance on platelets is proportional to the amount in plasma. Blood 1982; 59:980.
30. Dunstan RA, Simpson MB, Knowles RW, et al. The origin of ABH antigens on human platelets. Blood 1985; 65:615.
31. Mollicone R, Caillard T, Le Pendu J, et al. Expression of ABH and X (Lex) antigens on platelets and lymphocytes. Blood 1988; 71:1113.
32. Mollison PL, Engelfriet CP, Contreras M. ABO, Lewis, Ii and P groups. *In* Blood Transfusion in Clinical Medicine, 9th ed. Oxford, UK: Blackwell Scientific, 1993, p 149.
33. Lee EJ, Schiffer CA. ABO compatibility can influence the results of platelet transfusion: results of a randomized trial. Transfusion 1989; 29:384.
34. Duquesnoy RJ, Anderson AJ, Tomasulo PA, et al. ABO compatibility and platelet transfusions of alloimmunized thrombocytopenic patients. Blood 1979; 54:59.
35. Heal JM, Blumberg N, Masel D. An evaluation of crossmatching, HLA, and ABO matching for platelet transfusions to refractory patients. Blood 1987; 70:23.
36. Brand A, Sintnicolaas K, Claas FHJ, et al. ABH antibodies causing platelet transfusion refractoriness. Transfusion 1986; 26:463.
37. McFarland JG, Anderson AJ, Slichter SJ. Factors influencing the transfusion response to HLA-selected apheresis donor platelets in patients refractory to random platelet concentrates. Br J Haematol 1989; 73:380.
38. Freireich EJ, Kliman A, Gaydos LA, et al. Response to repeated platelet transfusion from the same donor. Ann Intern Med 1963; 59:277.
39. Tosato G, Appelbaum FR, Deisseroth AB. HLA-matched platelet transfusion therapy of severe aplastic anemia. Blood 1978; 52:846.
40. Shulman NR. Immunological considerations attending platelet transfusion. Transfusion 1966; 6:39.
41. Ogasawara K, Ueki J, Takenaka M, Furihata K. Study on the expression of ABH antigens on platelets. Blood 1993; 82:993.
42. Warkentin TE, Smith JW. The alloimmune thrombocytopenic syndromes. Transfus Med Rev 1997; 11:296.
43. Kunicki TJ, Newman PJ. The molecular immunology of human platelet proteins. Blood 1992; 80:1386.
44. Newman PJ, Valentin N. Human platelet alloantigens: recent findings, new perspectives. Thromb Haemost 1995; 74:234.
45. Kim HO, Jin Y, Kickler TS, et al. Gene frequencies of the five major human platelet antigens in African American, white and Korean population. Transfusion 1995; 35:863.
46. Mcfarland JG. Alloimmunization and platelet transfusion. Semin Hematol 1996; 33:315.
47. Ploegh HL, Orr HT, Strominger JL. Major histocompatibility antigens: the human (HLA-A, B, C) and murine (H-2K, H2-D) class I molecules. Cell 1981; 24:287.
48. Zinkernagel RM, Doherty PC. MHC restricted cytotoxic cells: studies on the biological role of polymorphic major transplantation antigens determine T-cell restriction specificity function and responsiveness. Adv Immunol 1979; 27:51.
49. Zijlstra M, Bix M, Simister NE, et al. β2-microglobulin deficient mice lack CD4−8+ cytolytic T cells. Nature 1990; 344:742.
50. Koller BH, Marrack P, Kappler JW. Normal development of mice deficient in β2M, MHC class I proteins and CD8+ T cells. Science 1990; 248:1227.
51. Kao KJ, Cook DJ, Scornik JC. Quantitative analysis of platelet surface HLA by W6/32 anti-HLA monoclonal antibody. Blood 1986; 68:627.
52. Blumberg N, Masel D, Mayer T, et al. Removal of HLA-A, B antigens from platelets. Blood 1984; 63:448.
53. Kao KJ. Selective elution of HLA antigen and B2-microglobulin from human platelets by chloroquine diphosphate. Transfusion 1988; 28:14.
54. Lalezari P, Driscoll AM. Ability of thrombocytes to acquire HLA specificity from plasma. Blood 1982; 59:167.
55. Santoso S, Mueller-Eckhardt G, Santoso S, et al. HLA antigens on platelet membranes: in vitro and in vivo studies. Vox Sang 1986; 51:327.
56. Santoso S, Kalb R, Kiefel V, et al. The presence of messenger RNA for HLA class I in human platelets and its capability for protein synthesis. Br J Haematol 1993; 84:451.
57. Schiffer CA, Lichtenfeld JL, Wiernik PH, et al. Antibody response in patients with acute non-lymphocytic leukemia. Cancer 1976; 37:2177.
58. Howard JE, Perkins HA. The natural history of alloimmunization to platelets. Transfusion 1978; 18:496.
59. Murphy MF, Metcalfe P, Ord J, et al. Disappearance of HLA and platelet-specific antibodies in acute leukaemia patients alloimmunized by multiple transfusions. Br J Haematol 1987; 67:255.
60. MacPherson BR. HLA antibody formation within the HLA-A1, crossreactive group in multitranfused platelet recipients. Am J Hematol 1989; 30:228.
61. Pamphilon DH, Farrell DH, Donaldson C, et al. Development of lymphocytotoxic and platelet reactive antibodies: a prospective study in patients with acute leukaemia. Vox Sang 1989; 57:177.
62. Godeau B, Fromont P, Seror T, et al. Platelet alloimmunization after multiple transfusions: a perspective study of 50 patients. Br J Haematol 1992; 81:395.
63. Atlas E, Freedman J, Blanchette V, et al. Downregulation of the anti-HLA alloimmune response by variable region reactive (anti-idiotypic antibodies) in leukemic patients transfused with platelet concentrates. Blood 1993; 81:538.
64. Hogge DE, McConnell M, Jacobson C, et al. Platelet refractoriness and alloimmunization in pediatric oncology and bone marrow transplant patients. Transfusion 1995; 35:645.

65. Gleichmann H, Breininger J. Over 95% sensitization against allogeneic leukocytes following single massive blood transfusion. Vox Sang 1975; 28:66.
66. Janeway CA Jr, Travers P. The two classes of MHC molecules are expressed differentially on cells. *In* Immunobiology: The Immune System in Health and Disease, vol 4, 3rd ed. New York: Current Biology Ltd., 1997, p 4:9.
67. Harding CV. Class II antigen processing: analysis of compartments and functions. Crit Rev Immunol 1996; 16:13.
68. Watts C. Capture and processing of exogenous antigens for presentation on MHC molecules. Annu Rev Immunol 1997; 15:821.
69. Natali PG, Bigotti A, Nicotra MR, et al. Distribution of human class I (HLA-A, B, C) histocompatibility antigens in normal and malignant tissues of nonlymphoid origin. Cancer Res 1984; 44:4679.
70. Batchelor JR, Welsh KI, Burgos H. Transplantation antigens per se are poor immunogens within species. Nature 1978; 273:54.
71. Galvao MM, Peixinho ZF, Mendes NF, Sabbaga E. Stored blood—an effective immunosuppressive method for transplantation of kidneys from unrelated donors: an 11 year follow up. Braz J Med Biol Res 1997; 30:727.
72. Claas FHJ, Smeenk RJT, Schmidt AN, et al. Alloimmunization against the MHC antigens after platelet transfusions is due to contaminating leukocytes in the platelet suspension. Exp Hematol 1981; 9:84.
73. Parthenais MA, Soots A, Nemlander A, et al. Immunogenicity of allograft components. II. Relative immunogenicity of rat kidney parenchymal versus passenger cells. Cell Immunol 1981; 57:92.
74. Eernisse JG, Brand A. Prevention of platelet refractoriness due to HLA antibodies by administration of leukocyte-poor blood components. Exp Hematol 1981; 9:77.
75. Schiffer CA, Dutcher JP, Aisner J, et al. A randomized trial of leukocyte-depleted platelet transfusion to modify alloimmunization in patients with leukemia. Blood 1988; 62:815.
76. Fisher M, Chapman JR, Ting A, et al. Alloimmunization to HLA antigens following transfusion with leukocyte poor and purified platelet suspensions. Vox Sang 1985; 49:331.
77. Murphy MF, Metcalfe P, Thomas M, et al. Use of leucocyte poor blood components and HLA-matched platelet donors to prevent HLA alloimmunization. Br J Haematol 1986; 62:529.
78. Sniecinski I, O'Donnell MR, Nowicki B, et al. Prevention of refractoriness and HLA alloimmunization using filtered blood products. Blood 1988; 71:1402.
79. Brand A, Claas FHJ, Voogt PJ, et al. Alloimmunization after leukocyte-depleted multiple random donor platelet transfusions. Vox Sang 1988; 54:160.
80. Andreu G, Dewailly J, Leberre C, et al. Prevention of HLA immunization with leukocyte-poor packed red cells and platelet concentrates obtained by filtration. Blood 1988; 72:964.
81. Panina-Bordignon P, Corradin G, Roosnek E, et al. Recognition by class II alloreactive T cells of processed determinants from human serum proteins. Science 1991; 252:1548.
82. Pawelec G, Adibzadeh M, Bonhak S, et al. The role of endogenous peptides in the direct pathway of alloreactivity to human MHC class II molecules expressed on CHO cells. Immunol Rev 1996; 154:155.
83. Reinsmoen NL. Histocompatibility testing by immunologic methods: cellular assays. *In* Rose NR, de Macario EC, Folds JD (eds): Manual of Clinical Laboratory Immunology, 5th ed. Washington, DC: ASM Press, 1997, p 1080.
84. Kao KJ, del Rosario MLU. Role of class II MHC antigen positive donor leukocytes in transfusion-induced alloimmunization to donor class I MHC antigens. Blood 1998; 92:690.
85. Clark EA, Ledbetter JA. How B and T cells talk to each other. Nature 1994; 367:425.
86. Dubey C, Croft M, Swain SL. Costimulatory requirements of naive CD4+ T cells: ICAM-1 or B7-1 can costimulate naive CD4 T cell activation but both are required for optimal response. J Immunol 1995; 155:45.
87. Bachmann MF, McKall-Faienza K, Schmits R, et al. Distinct roles for LFA-1 and CD28 during activation of naive T cells: adhesion versus costimulation. Immunity 1997; 7:549.
88. Nabavi N, Freeman GJ, Gault A, et al. Signalling through the MHC class II cytoplasmic domain is required for antigen presentation and induces B7 expression. Nature 1992; 360:266.
89. Fleischer J, Soeth E, Reiling N, et al. Differential expression and function of CD80 (B7-1) and CD86 (B7-2) on human peripheral blood monocytes. Immunology 1996; 89:592.
90. Thompson CB. Distinct roles for the costimulatory ligands B7-1 and B7-2 in T helper cell differentiation? Cell 1995; 81:979.
91. Reiser H, Stadecker MJ. Costimulatory B7 molecules in the pathogenesis of infectious and autoimmune diseases. N Engl J Med 1996; 335:1369.
92. Klaus SJ, Pinchuk LM, Ochs HD, et al. Costimulation through CD28 enhances T cell–dependent B cell activation via CD40-CD40L interaction. J Immunol 1994; 152:5643.
93. Yang Y, Wilson JM. CD40 ligand-dependent T cell activation: requirement of B7-CD28 signalling through CD40. Science 1996; 273:1862.
94. Grana NH, Kao KJ. Use of 8-methoxypsoralen and ultraviolet-A pretreated platelet concentrates to prevent alloimmunization against class I major histocompatibility antigens. Blood 1991; 77:2530.
95. Kao KJ. Effects of leukocyte depletion and UVB irradiation on alloantigenicity of major histocompatibility complex antigens in platelet concentrates: a comparative study. Blood 1992; 80:2931.
96. Slichter SJ, Deeg HJ, Kennedy MS. Prevention of platelet alloimmunization in dogs with systemic cyclosporine and by UV-irradiation or cyclosporine-loading of donor platelets. Blood 1987; 69:414.
97. Fujihara M, Takahashi TA, Azuma M, et al. Decreased inducible expression of CD80 and CD86 in human monocytes after ultraviolet-B: its involvement in inactivation of alloantigenicity. Blood 1996; 87:2386.
98. Krutmann J, Khan IU, Wallis RS, et al. Cell membrane is a major locus for ultraviolet B–induced alteration in accessory cells. J Clin Invest 1990; 85:1529.
99. Bang A, Speck ER, Blanchette VS, et al. Recipient humoral immunity against leukoreduced allogeneic platelets is suppressed by aminoguanidine, a selective inhibitor of inducible nitric oxide synthase. Blood 1996; 88:2959.
100. van de Wiel TWM, van de Wiel-Dorfmeyer H, van Loghem JJ. Studies on platelet antibodies in man. Vox Sang 1961; 6:641.
101. Holohan TV, Terasaki PI, Diesseroth AB. Suppression of transfusion-related alloimmunization in intensively treated cancer patients. Blood 1981; 58:122.
102. Pegels JG, Bruynes EC, Engelfriet CP, et al. Serological studies in patients on platelet and granulocyte substitution therapy. Br J Haematol 1982; 52:59.
103. Tejada F, Bias WB, Santos GW, et al. Immunologic response of patients with acute leukemia to platelet transfusions. Blood 1973; 42:405.
104. Dutcher JP, Schiffer CA, Aisner J, et al. Alloimmunization following platelet transfusion: the absence of a dose response relationship. Blood 1981; 57:395.
105. Lee EJ, Schiffer CA. Serial measurement of lymphocytotoxic antibody and response to nonmatched platelet transfusions in alloimmunized patients. Blood 1987; 70:1727.
106. Uhrynowska M, Zupanska B. Platelet-specific antibodies in transfused patients. Eur J Haematol 1996; 56:248.
107. Bishop JF, McGrath K, Wolf M, et al. Clinical factors influencing the efficacy of pooled platelet transfusions. Blood 1988; 71:383.
108. Meenaghan M, Judson P, Yousaf K, et al. Antibodies to platelet glycoprotein V in polytransfused patients with hematological disease. Vox Sang 1993; 64:167.
109. Murata M, Furihata K, Ishida F, et al. Genetic and structural characterization of an amino acid dimorphism in glycoprotein Ib alpha involved in platelet transfusion refractoriness. Blood 1992; 79:3086.
110. Novotny VMJ, van Doorn R, Witvliet MD, et al. Occurrence of allogeneic HLA and non-HLA antibodies after transfusion of prestorage filtered platelets and red blood cells: a prospective study. Blood 1995; 85:1736.
111. Saji H, Maruya E, Fuji H, et al. New platelet antigen, Siba, involved in platelet transfusion refractoriness in a Japanese man. Vox Sang 1989; 56:283.
112. Lagenscheidt F, Kiefel V, Santoso S, et al. Platelet transfusion refractoriness associated with two rare platelet-specific alloantibodies (anti-Bak-a and anti-Pl^{A2}) and multiple HLA antibodies. Transfusion 1988; 28:597.
113. Reznikoff-Etievant MF, Muller JY, Julien F, et al. An immune

response gene linked to MHC in man. Tissue Antigens 1983; 22:312.
114. de Waal LP, Van Dalen CM, Engelfriet CP, et al. Alloimmunization against the platelet specific Zwa antigen resulting in neonatal alloimmune thrombocytopenia or post transfusional purpura is associated with the supertypic DRw52 antigen including DR3 and DRw6. Hum Immunol 1986; 17:45.
115. Valentin N, Vergracht A, Bignon JD, et al. HLA-DRw52a is involved in alloimmunization against PL-A1 antigen. Hum Immunol 1990; 27:73.
116. Mueller-Eckhardt C, Kiefel V, Kroll H, et al. HLA-DRw6, a new immune response marker for immunization against the platelet alloantigen Br[a]. Vox Sang 1989; 57:90.
117. Braud V, Chevrier D, Cesbron A, et al. Susceptibility to alloimmunization to platelet HPA-1a antigen involves TAP1 polymorphism. Hum Immunol 1994; 41:141.
118. Ikeda H, Mitani T, Ohnuma M, et al. A new platelet specific antigen Nak-a, involved in the refractoriness of HLA-matched platelet transfusion. Vox Sang 1989; 57:213.
119. Goldfinger D, McGinniss MH. Rh-incompatible platelet transfusions—risks and consequences of sensitizing immunosuppressed patients. N Engl J Med 1971; 284:942.
120. Baldwin ML, Ness PM, Scott D, et al. Alloimmunization to D antigen and HLA in D-negative immunosuppressed oncology patients. Transfusion 1988; 28:330.
121. Enright H, Gersheimer T, McCullough J, et al. Moderate to severe reactions to platelet transfusion: experience of the TRAP multicenter trial. Blood 1997; 90(suppl 1):267a.
122. Hopkins KA. Basic microlymphocytotoxicity test. *In* Zachary AA, Teresi G (eds): ASHI Laboratory Manual, 2nd ed. Lenexa, KS: ASHI, 1990, p 195.
123. Lou CD, Cunniffe KJ, Garovoy MR. Histocompatibility testing by immunological methods: humoral assays. *In* Rose NR, de Macario EC, Folds JD (eds): Manual of Clinical Laboratory Immunology, 5th ed. Washington, DC: ASM Press, 1997, p 1090.
124. Kao KJ, Scott SJ, Scornik SC. Enzyme linked immunoassay for anti-HLA antibodies: an alternative to panel studies by lymphocytotoxicity. Transplantation 1993; 55:192.
125. Zaer F, Metz S, Scornik JC. Antibody screening by enzyme-linked immunosorbent assay using pooled soluble HLA in renal transplant candidates. Transplantation 1997; 63:48.
126. Mueller-Eckhardt C, Kiefel V. Laboratory methods for the detection of platelet antibodies and identification of antigens. *In* Kunicki TJ, George JN (eds): Platelet Immunobiology: Molecular and Clincial Aspects. Philadelphia: JB Lippincott, 1989, p 436.
127. Kekomaki R. Detection of platelet-bound IgG with ^{125}I-labelled staphylococcal protein A. Med Biol 1977; 55:112.
128. Rachel JM, Sinor LT, Tawfik OW, et al. A solid-phase red cell adherence test for platelet cross-matching. Med Lab Sci 1985; 42:194.
129. Kiefel V, Santoso S, Weisheit M, Mueller-Eckhardt C. Monoclonal antibody-specific immobilization of platelet antigen (MAIPA): a new tool for the identification of platelet reactive antibodies. Blood 1987; 70:1772.
130. Kickler TS, Bell W, Drew H, et al. Depletion of white cells from platelet concentrates with a new adsorption filter. Transfusion 1989; 29:411.
131. Wenz B, Besso N. Quality control and evaluation of leukocyte depleting filters. Transfusion 1989; 29:186.
132. Miyamoto M, Sasakawa S, Ishikawa Y, et al. Leukocyte-poor platelet concentrates at the bed side by filtration through Sepacell-PL. Vox Sang 1989; 57:164.
133. Pamphilon DH, Corbin SA, Saunders J, et al. Application of ultraviolet light in the preparation of platelet concentrates. Transfusion 1989; 29:379.
134. Snyder EL, Beardsley DS, Smith BR, et al. Storage of platelet concentrates after high-dose ultraviolet B irradiation. Transfusion 1991; 31:491.
135. Bretscher P. The two signal model of lymphocyte activation twenty-one years later. Immunol Today 1992; 13:74.
136. Lanzavecchia A. Identifying strategies for immune intervention. Science 1993; 260:937.
137. Schwartz RH. A cell culture model for T lymphocyte clonal anergy. Science 1990; 248:1349.
138. DeSilva DR, Urdahl KB, Jenkins MK. Clonal anergy is induced in vitro by T cell receptor occupancy in the absence of proliferation. J Immunol 1991; 147:3261.
139. Gimmi CD, Freeman GJ, Gribben JG, et al. Human T-cell clonal anergy is induced by antigen presentation in the absence of B7 costimulation. Proc Natl Acad Sci U S A 1993; 90:6586.
140. Kao KJ. Induction of humoral immune tolerance to major histocompatibility complex antigens by transfusions of UVB-irradiated leukocytes. Blood 1996; 88:4375.
141. del Rosario MLU, Zucalis JR, Kao KJ. Prevention of GVHD by induction of immune tolerance with UVB-irradiated leukocytes in H-2 disparate bone marrow donors. Blood 1997; 90(suppl 1):205a.

CHAPTER 29

Transfusion-Associated Graft-Versus-Host Disease

Iain J. Webb
Kenneth C. Anderson

The clinical course of allogeneic bone marrow and peripheral blood stem cell transplant recipients is frequently complicated by graft-versus-host disease (GVHD). This condition results when lymphocytes in the donor hematopoietic stem cell (HSC) component recognize the human leukocyte antigens (HLAs) of the recipient as foreign, generating a characteristic immune response.[1, 2] Fever, diarrhea, liver function test abnormalities, and a characteristic rash are the major clinical manifestations of this condition. However, GVHD may also result from the infusion of viable T lymphocytes within cellular blood components. This condition, which is accompanied by marrow aplasia and pancytopenia, was first described in 1966.[3] Since then, transfusion-associated GVHD (TA-GVHD) has been established as a distinct disease entity. TA-GVHD is resistant to most immunosuppressive therapeutic modalities; thus treatment is rarely successful, and it is essential to recognize patients in whom preventive measures are warranted.

New therapeutic strategies with the potential graft-versus-leukemia (GVL) effect of allogeneic lymphocytes have been developed, which emphasizes the need to further understand the pathogenesis of TA-GVHD. Adoptive immunotherapy, the infusion of allogeneic lymphocytes into patients who have suffered relapse after allogeneic HSC transplantation, has been shown to produce both remissions and a clinical syndrome similar to TA-GVHD.[4–6] Whether the GVL effect is separable from GVHD is the object of ongoing laboratory and clinical studies.

CLINICAL PRESENTATION AND COMPLICATIONS

Symptoms and signs of TA-GVHD typically appear 8 to 10 days after transfusion, and death occurs 3 to 4 weeks after transfusion.[7] As seen in cases of GVHD after HSC transplantation, a characteristic cutaneous eruption appears, in association with watery diarrhea, liver function test abnormalities, and fever. The diarrhea may be profuse, and liver function test elevations may be marked and accompanied by extensive hepatocellular damage. Nonspecific manifestations include anorexia, nausea, and vomiting. The maculopapular exanthem typically develops centrally, then progresses to involve the extremities. In severe cases, generalized erythroderma and bullae may appear.

The development of marrow aplasia distinguishes TA-GVHD from GVHD occurring after allogeneic HSC transplantation. Thrombocytopenia and leukopenia are late features. Complications of pancytopenia such as hemorrhage and infection ensue and lead to death. The course is rapid: death occurs 1 to 3 weeks after the development of clinical symptoms.

DIFFERENTIAL DIAGNOSIS

There are no pathognomonic features that differentiate TA-GVHD from a variety of viral illnesses and drug reactions.[8] Patients who are receiving transfusions typically suffer from comorbid conditions, which may obscure the clinical features of TA-GVHD, particularly if the clinician has a low index of suspicion. Characteristic pathological changes in the skin, liver, and bone marrow may aid in establishing the diagnosis, but only the documentation of donor-derived lymphocytes in the recipient circulation and/or tissues can confirm it. Techniques used to detect donor-derived lymphocytes in the patient are available. Pathological examination of a skin biopsy may reveal degeneration of the epidermal basal cell layer with vacuolization; dermal-epithelial layer separation and bullae formation; mononuclear cell migration into, and infiltration of, the upper dermis; hyperkeratosis; and degenerative dyskeratosis.[9, 10] Liver biopsies reveal degeneration and eosinophilic necrosis of the small bile ducts, with intense periportal inflammation and mononuclear (lymphocytic) infiltration. Bone marrow aspirates reveal lymphocytic infiltration, pancytopenia, and possibly fibrosis.

INCIDENCE

The epidemiological data on TA-GVHD are derived from analysis of reports of single or very small groups of patients. A prospective study on the development of TA-GVHD has never been undertaken and would be difficult to perform. Estimates of the incidence of TA-GVHD and identification of patient groups at risk are therefore subject to the limitations of retrospective data. TA-GVHD is certainly more common than reported, and at least two factors contribute to this underreporting: lack of recognition, and the absence of definitive diagnostic studies. Thus, although over 200 cases of presumed TA-GVHD have been reported or referenced in the Japanese- and English-language literature, definitive diagnostic tests have been performed in only a handful of cases. Lists of published case reports and small series have been compiled in several articles.[11, 12] Rare survivors have been documented, but the overall reported mortality rate is approximately 90%.[7, 13, 14]

PATIENT GROUPS AT RISK

TA-GVHD has been reported in patients with hematological and solid malignancies and congenital immunodeficiency states, as well as in infants and adults with apparently intact immune systems, but not in patients with acquired immunodeficiency syndrome (AIDS). In addition, the disease has been reported rarely in recipients of organ transplants or in patients on immunosuppressive medications (Tables 29–1 and 29–2).

Initially, cases of TA-GVHD were reported in patients with severe combined immunodeficiency and Wiskott-Aldrich syndromes; in newborns with erythroblastosis fetalis; and in patients with Hodgkin's disease and non-Hodgkin's lymphoma, acute myelocytic and lymphoblastic leukemia, and chronic lymphocytic leukemia.[15] Although its true incidence remains unknown, TA-GVHD is estimated to occur in 0.1% to 1% of patients with hematological malignancies or lymphoproliferative diseases, and patients carrying these diagnoses are thought to be at risk for TA-GVHD. Certain subgroups of patients with hematological malignancies, including those suffering from chronic lymphocytic leukemia who are treated with fludarabine, may be at higher risk owing to the prolonged effects of this purine analogue on cell-mediated immune function.[16–18]

Table 29–1. Conditions Predisposing to the Development of Transfusion-Associated Graft-Versus-Host Disease

Congenital Immunodeficiency Syndromes
Severe combined immunodeficiency syndrome
Thymic hypoplasia
Wiskott-Aldrich syndrome
Leiner's disease
5′-nucleotidase deficiency
Nonspecified immunodeficiency
Immunodeficiency States
Hemolytic disease of the fetus or newborn
Prematurity
Neonatal alloimmune thrombocytopenia
Neonatal immunosuppressive medication
Autologous hematopoietic stem cell transplantation for solid tumors
Malignancies
Hematological
Hodgkin's disease
Non-Hodgkin's lymphoma
Acute myelocytic leukemia
Acute lymphocytic leukemia
Chronic lymphocytic leukemia
Aplastic anemia
Solid tumors
Neuroblastoma
Lung carcinoma
Glioblastoma
Rhabdomyosarcoma
Cervical carcinoma
Esophageal carcinoma
Renal adenocarcinoma
Immunocompetence
Pregnancy
Cholecystectomy
Cardiac surgery
Vascular surgery
Gastrointestinal surgery
Abdominal surgery
α-Thalassemia
Liver transplantation
Pancreaticosplenic transplantation

Table 29–2. Patient Groups at Risk for Developing Transfusion-Associated Graft-Versus-Host Disease

Clear Risk
Patients with selected immunodeficiencies:
Congenital immunodeficiencies
Hodgkin's disease
Chronic lymphocytic leukemia treated with fludarabine
Newborns with erythroblastosis fetalis
Recipients of intrauterine transfusions
Recipients of hematopoietic stem cell transplants
Recipients of blood products donated by relatives
Recipients of human leukocyte antigen (HLA)–selected (matched) platelets or platelets known to be homozygous
Probable Risk
Patients with:
Other hematological malignancies
Solid tumors treated with cytotoxic agents
Recipient-donor pairs from genetically homogeneous populations
Premature and possibly term neonates
No Defined Risk
Patients with acquired immunodeficiency syndrome (AIDS)
Patients taking immunosuppressive medications

Cytotoxic drugs and irradiation may be related to the development of TA-GVHD.[19] TA-GVHD was originally recognized in patients with solid tumors who received intensive therapy for neuroblastoma.[20, 21] In one series, 4 of 34 patients with solid tumors (lung and germ cell cancer) who were treated with high doses of chemotherapy and autologous marrow infusions and subsequently received transfusions of nonirradiated blood cells developed TA-GVHD.[22] In addition, case reports documenting TA-GVHD in patients with cervical, renal, esophageal, lung, bladder, and prostate carcinoma who did not receive aggressive chemotherapy indicate that a broader spectrum of patients with solid tumors may be at risk.

TA-GVHD has also been documented in premature infants who received nonirradiated blood products in the setting of hyaline-membrane disease, suspected sepsis, and respiratory distress syndrome, as well as in infants without these complications.[12, 23] Such patients did not have congenital immunodeficiency syndromes or erythroblastosis fetalis.

Finally, TA-GVHD has been reported in apparently immunocompetent adults. Clinical settings in which TA-GVHD has been reported in immunologically normal hosts include pregnancy; cardiac, vascular, and abdominal surgeries; α-thalassemia; rheumatoid arthritis; trauma; and short-course glucocorticoid therapy.[24, 25] The syndrome was initially described in 1986 after blood transfusion to a patient in Japan who had had surgery for an aortic aneurysm and was not recognized to be immunodeficient.[26] A survey of 340 Japanese hospitals documented "postoperative erythroderma," identical to TA-GVHD, in 96 of the 63,257 patients who underwent cardiac surgery, with a mortality rate of 90%.[27]

More recently, fatal GVHD has been reported in a number of HLA-heterozygous transfusion recipients who received transfusions with a "one-way HLA match."[28, 29] These recipients shared a haplotype with related or unrelated HLA-homozygous donors. Directed donations from immediate family members increase the likelihood of TA-GVHD, because such donors share HLAs with recipients; homozygosity for HLA types is likely to be present among not only first-degree relatives but also all related recipient-donor pairs.[30] The frequency of one-way HLA matches has been calculated in different countries.[31] This risk may increase 11- to 21-fold in the setting of directed donations within families.[32] The reported risk varies from 1 in 16,835 in France to 1 in 874 in Japan, where there is less diversity in HLA expression and, consequently, TA-GVHD cases have been reported more frequently.[11, 12, 31]

The transfusion of platelets from donors sharing at least two antigens at the HLA-A and -B loci (HLA-matched platelets) has been demonstrated to result in satisfactory platelet increments in alloimmunized patients refractory to standard platelet therapy.[33] However, the provision of platelets from donors sharing HLAs may also predispose to TA-GVHD.[34, 35]

The risk factors predisposing to TA-GVHD are only partially defined. TA-GVHD does not always occur in immunodeficient patients receiving nonirradiated blood components, and it may affect people with apparently normal immune function, particularly in the setting of a one-way HLA match. Blood transfusion itself may be immunosuppressive.[36] Hence, an argument can be made that almost every patient who requires transfusion of a blood product is potentially immunocompromised in some way that could facilitate the development of TA-GVHD. The low incidence of TA-GVHD in presumably immunocompetent patients may result from underrecognition of the syndrome, but it likely also reflects the effective defense mechanisms in people with truly intact immune functions.

PATHOGENESIS

Both the immune status of the host and the extent of HLA mismatch between donor and recipient determine the extent of any host-versus-graft response. The ability of the transfusion recipient to mount an immune response against donor T lymphocytes is fundamental to the pathogenesis of TA-GVHD. Thus Billingham proposed three requirements for the development of GVHD: (1) differences in histocompatibility antigens (HLAs) between the donor and the recipient, (2) the presence of immunocompetent cells in the graft, and (3) the inability of the host to reject these immunocompetent cells.[37] Usually the larger number of immune cells in an immunocompetent host eliminates the donor-derived T cells via a host-versus-graft reaction. However, if an immunocompetent HLA-heterozygous patient is transfused with even a small number of functional T lymphocytes derived from a donor who is homozygous for one of the recipient's HLA haplotypes, the recipient's immune system does not recognize the major histocompatibility antigens on the donor cells as being foreign and is therefore incapable of eliminating them. Some of the donor-derived T cells recognize the host HLAs that are encoded by the unshared haplotype as being foreign, undergo clonal expansion, and establish TA-GVHD.[28] The TA-GVHD expressed under these circumstances may be expected to occur regardless of the host's immune status, because the failure to eliminate donor-derived T lymphocytes is based on the genetics of the HLA system rather than on variables that contribute to immune competence per se.[38]

Fast and colleagues[39] provided important insights into the pathogenesis of TA-GVHD, implicating recipient $CD4^+$, $CD8^+$, and natural killer cells in the control of TA-GVHD. In a mouse model, varying numbers of parental lymphoid cells were injected into nonirradiated F1 hybrid recipients, providing donor lymphocytes homozygous for an HLA haplotype present in the recipient. The effect of selective depletion of recipient $CD4^+$, $CD8^+$, and natural killer cells on the regulation of TA-GVHD was assessed. Depletion of $CD4^+$ cells increased the number of donor cells necessary to induce TA-GVHD, whereas depletion of recipient $CD8^+$ cells or natural killer cells decreased the number of donor cells required to produce TA-GVHD. Thus $CD4^+$ cells may be involved in the pathogenesis of TA-GVHD, and $CD8^+$ and natural killer cells may be protective. According to this model, patients at high risk for TA-GVHD are those with impaired CD8 and natural killer cell function, especially if they receive blood products with a one-way HLA match.

Other studies have attempted to determine the T cell subsets involved in the pathogenesis of TA-GVHD. The T cell clones expanding in vivo are reportedly limited, based on Vβ gene distribution.[40] In addition, Nishimura and colleagues characterized three types of $CD8^+$ and $CD4^+$ T cell clones derived from the blood of a patient with TA-GVHD, which suggests that both types of cells may be involved in the pathogenesis of TA-GVHD, either through direct cell-mediated cytotoxicity or through cytokine-mediated modulation of the process.[41] This dysregulation of cytokines, with subsequent activation of donor T cells, may be an essential element of the pathogenesis of both TA-GVHD and HSC transplantation–related GVHD.[2, 42, 43]

No reported cases of TA-GVHD have occurred in patients with AIDS, further emphasizing the role of $CD4^+$ and $CD8^+$ lymphocytes in the pathogenesis of TA-GVHD. It is possible that TA-GVHD may account for some of the nonspecific signs and symptoms presently attributed to infections, drug reactions, and other coexistent medical conditions in AIDS patients. Alternatively, it may be that some qualitative aspect of the human immunodeficiency virus (HIV)–related immune deficit may alter the predisposition of AIDS patients to develop TA-GVHD. The murine study reported by Fast and colleagues[39] suggests that the latter explanation may be valid, inasmuch as $CD4^+$ lymphocyte function declines early, whereas CD8+ function is preserved until late in the course of HIV disease. In the mouse model, both these features would be expected to decrease the likelihood of developing TA-GVHD. In contrast, it has been proposed that reactive recipient CD8+ T cells are required for the development of GVHD.[44] Activated HIV-1–infected CD4+ T cells express an HLA class II–derived peptide that is mimicked by the carboxy terminus of the HIV-1 envelope. It is hypothesized that the activation of CD8+ T cells against the HIV-infected CD4+ T cells may preclude the development of GVHD. In addition, HIV infection of the infused CD4+ cells may make them incapable of initiating TA-GVHD.[45] Clarification of the role of both CD4+ and CD8+ cells in AIDS will likely provide further insight into the pathogenesis of GVHD, and vice versa.

In recipients of allogeneic HSC transplants, the spectrum between GVHD and HLA alloimmunization and the extent of mononuclear cell microchimerism depend on the dose of allogeneic cells transfused, the immune competence of the recipient, and the extent of HLA similarity between donor and recipient.[46] For example, in an animal model of GVHD after bone marrow transplantation, reducing the number of cells transplanted resulted in a stepwise increase in the rejection rate of donor cells; conversely, reduction in the size of the marrow inoculum could be compensated by increasing host immunosuppression.[47]

Because transfused cellular blood products are rarely HLA tested or matched, the first of Billingham's three requirements[37]—differences in HLAs between donor and recipient—is almost always present in the setting of blood component transfusion. TA-GVHD is mediated by the viable T lymphocytes that inevitably contaminate nonirradiated transfused cellular blood products. A naturally or iatrogenically immunosuppressed recipient has only a limited capacity to generate an effective host-versus-graft reaction, and greater HLA disparity increases the probability that donor lymphocytes will attack host tissues.

DIAGNOSIS

The differential diagnosis for TA-GVHD is broad; myriad factors such as infections and drug reactions can result in the development of fever, skin rash, and liver function test abnormalities. Histological findings in the skin and gastrointestinal tract may suggest the diagnosis of TA-GVHD but are not pathognomonic. The only definitive approach to the diagnosis of TA-GVHD is the identification of donor-derived lymphocytes in the circulation or tissues of the affected host (Table 29–3). This requires either careful HLA typing or some other technique that reliably distinguishes between host and donor cells.[48–51] Blood samples adequate for HLA typing are frequently not available, because circulating host blood cells are rapidly eliminated. Polymerase chain reaction–based methods for HLA typing may be a useful substitute.[50–53] Otherwise, the patient's HLA type can be deduced from those of surviving first-degree relatives.[28] Cytogenetics have been employed when donor and recipient were different genders or when the disease followed transfusion of granulocytes donated by persons with Philadelphia chromosome–positive chronic myeloid leukemia.[54] Increasingly sophisticated techniques for confirming the diagnosis of TA-GVHD include the detection of polymorphisms of restriction fragment lengths and human microsatellite markers.[29, 51] Even so, this syndrome is still frequently diagnosed only at autopsy.

Table 29–3. Methods Used to Diagnose or Document Transfusion-Associated Graft-Versus-Host Disease

Conventional human leukocyte antigen (HLA) typing
Deduction of patient's HLA type from those of family members
DNA-based HLA typing using polymerase chain reaction
Cytogenetics
Restriction fragment length polymorphisms
Polymorphism of human microsatellite markers
Identification of donor T cells by above techniques in skin biopsies

THERAPY

Treatment of TA-GVHD is only rarely effective. Attempted immunosuppressive therapies have included glucocorticoids, antithymocyte globulin, cyclosporine, cyclophosphamide, and anti–T cell monoclonal antibodies.[10, 25, 27, 55–57] Although some of these agents are usually successful in the treatment of post–HSC transplantation GVHD, they have been ineffective for TA-GVHD. Rare responses to some of the commonly used agents have been reported,[9, 58] contributing to anecdotal experience but making it difficult to extract guidelines for clinical practice. A therapeutic trial of glucocorticoids or other immunosuppressive agents is often attempted but is frequently ineffective in this serious and increasingly common disease. There appears to be no advantage to early diagnosis and treatment, because patients diagnosed early in the course of the disease fare no better than those diagnosed later. Thus prevention is critical.

PREVENTION: GAMMA IRRADIATION

Irradiation of blood components is indicated in patient groups at high risk for the development of TA-GVHD. The relatively low frequency of TA-GVHD in immunocompetent patients receiving blood from unrelated donors has thus far precluded the extension of gamma irradiation to all transfused cellular blood products. Issues relating to cost, reduced lifespan of irradiated red blood cells, logistics of irradiation in emergency and small clinic settings, and the exceedingly low risk of TA-GVHD in most cases have also been raised.[59–61] However, irradiation is indicated within genetically homogeneous populations, because transfusion of nonirradiated products between unrelated donor-recipient pairs may be expected to result in TA-GVHD when a one-way HLA match occurs by chance.

The American Association of Blood Banks (AABB) currently recommends the irradiation of blood components at 25 Gy to the center of the component, with no area receiving less than 15 Gy.[62] Quality control of irradiation procedures is essential to ensure that the correct dose is administered.[63] The 25-Gy irradiation dose is in excess of the 15-Gy level found to abrogate mixed lymphocyte culture reactivity, which is inadequate to prevent TA-GVHD.[64, 65] Instead, the recommended 25-Gy dose is based on limiting dilution assays (LDAs) with visual assessment of T cell proliferation, which demonstrate more than a 5-log reduction in viable T cells. However, levels of host cytotoxic T lymphocyte precursors and interleukin-2–secreting helper T lymphocyte precursors, which are not measured in LDAs, may be more predictive of GVHD development after allogeneic bone marrow transplantation.[66–70]

Significant variability in irradiation practices exists among centers. For example, blood component irradiation practices were examined in a survey of 2250 blood centers, hospital blood banks, or transfusion services that are institutional members of the AABB.[71] Of these institutions, 12.3% had on-site facilities for the irradiation of blood components. Of 9,397,516 components transfused in 1989, 952,516 (10.1%) were irradiated, and 44 cases of TA-GVHD were identified. There was marked variability in blood component irradiation practices, even for those patient groups in whom the risk of TA-GVHD is well defined. For example, 12%, 19%, and 32% of institutions did not provide irradiated components to recipients of allogeneic bone marrow transplants, patients receiving autologous bone marrow transplants, and those with congenital immunodeficiencies, respectively. Irradiated blood components were provided by 51.4%, 34%, 32%, and 20% of institutions to patients with leukemias, Hodgkin's disease, non-Hodgkin's lymphoma, and solid tumors, respectively, and 24.5% provided irradiated blood products to patients with AIDS.

NEW DIRECTIONS

Leukoreduction to Prevent TA-GVHD

In theory, leukodepletion of cellular blood components could be used to decrease the incidence of TA-GVHD. However, because neither the number nor the quality of T cells that mediate GVHD is currently defined, targets for leukodepletion to prevent TA-GVHD cannot be established. Furthermore, TA-GVHD has been reported in both immunocompetent and immunodeficient recipients of transfusions leukodepleted by filtration, which suggests that standard leukodepletion procedures cannot completely prevent TA-GVHD.[72, 73] Newer technologies appear to be capable of decreasing the number of contaminating leukocytes[74]; whether the levels of leukoreduction achieved will be adequate to prevent TA-GVHD remains to be established.[75] Leukodepletion could theoretically deplete sufficient numbers of T helper lymphocyte precursors and cytotoxic T lymphocyte precursors to avoid TA-GVHD. However, the effect of either gamma irradiation or leukodepletion on these cell populations has not yet been determined. Until data demonstrate adequate, highly efficient removal of these precursors by leukodepletion, gamma irradiation of all cellular blood components should be used to prevent TA-GVHD in patient groups judged to be at risk.

Donor Lymphocyte Infusions and TA-GVHD

Patients with leukemia who suffer relapse after allogeneic bone marrow transplantation may respond to infusions of lymphocytes from the original bone marrow donor, without receiving chemotherapy or other treatment. For example, the European Group for Blood and Marrow Transplantation documented complete remissions in 73% of 84 patients with relapsed chronic myelogenous leukemia.[4] Eighty-seven percent of the 73% who achieved complete remissions remained in remission at 3 years. GVHD of grade II or greater developed in 41% of all patients, and myelosuppression occurred in 34% of all patients. The development of these features in association with TA-GVHD was linked to the attainment of remission, which suggests a potential relationship between TA-GVHD and the GVL effect of lymphocyte infusions.

The donor lymphocyte populations responsible for the GVL effect, TA-GVHD, and post–HSC transplantation GVHD have not been determined. $CD4^+$ cells have been implicated in the GVL effect,[76, 77] and it has been observed that depletion of either $CD6^+$ or $CD8^+$ T lymphocytes from donor bone marrow can prevent GVHD at the time of allogeneic transplantation.[6, 78–80] Further experiments to identify the role of both donor and host lymphocyte populations in TA-GVHD and GVL effect are necessary. These studies will be important to determine how best to prevent TA-GVHD and optimize the GVL effect of lymphocytes while minimizing GVHD.

REFERENCES

1. Ferrara JL, Deeg HJ. Graft versus host disease. N Engl J Med 1991; 324:667.
2. Antin JH, Ferrara JLM. Cytokine dysregulation and acute graft-versus-host disease. Blood 1992; 80:2964.
3. Hathaway WE, Brangle RW, Nelson TL, Roeckel IE. Aplastic anemia and alymphocytosis in an infant with hypogammaglobulinemia: graft-versus-host reaction? J Pediatr 1966; 68:713.
4. Kolb HJ, Schattenberg A, Goldman JM, et al. Graft-versus-leukemia effect of donor lymphocyte transfusions in marrow grafted patients. European Group for Blood and Marrow Transplantation Working Party on Chronic Leukemia. Blood 1995; 86:2041.
5. Collins RH Jr, Shpilberg O, Drobyski WR, et al. Donor leukocyte infusions in 140 patients with relapsed malignancy after allogeneic bone marrow transplantation. J Clin Oncol 1997; 15:433.
6. Alyea EP, Soiffer RJ, Canning C, et al. Toxicity and efficacy of defined doses of $CD4^+$ donor lymphocytes for treatment of relapse after allogeneic bone marrow transplant. Blood 1998; 91:3671.
7. Anderson KC. Clinical indications for blood component irradiation. *In* Baldwin ML, Jefferies LC (eds): Irradiation of Blood Components. Bethesda, MD: American Association of Blood Banks, 1992, pp 31–49.
8. Shivdasani RA, Anderson KC. Transfusion-associated graft-versus-host disease: scratching the surface. Transfusion 1993; 33:696.
9. Prince M, Szer J, van der Weyden MB, et al. Transfusion associated graft-versus-host disease after cardiac surgery: response to antithymocyte-globulin and corticosteroid therapy. Aust N Z J Med 1991; 21:43.
10. O'Connor NTJ, Mackintosh P. Transfusion associated graft versus host disease in an immunocompetent patient. J Clin Pathol 1992; 45:621.
11. Ohto H, Anderson KC. Survey of transfusion-associated graft-versus-host disease in immunocompetent recipients. Transfus Med Rev 1996; 10:31.
12. Ohto H, Anderson KC. Posttransfusion graft-versus-host disease in Japanese newborns. Transfusion 1996; 36:117.

13. Andersen CB, Ladefoged SD, Taaning E. Transfusion-associated graft-versus-graft and potential graft-versus-host disease in a renal allotransplanted patient. Hum Pathol 1992; 23:831.
14. Mori S, Matsushita H, Ozaki K, et al. Spontaneous resolution of transfusion-associated graft-versus-host disease. Transfusion 1995; 35:431.
15. von Fliedner V, Higby DJ, Kim U. Graft-versus-host reaction following blood product transfusion. Am J Med 1982; 72:951.
16. Briz M, Cabrera R, Sanjuan I, et al. Diagnosis of transfusion-associated graft-versus-host disease by polymerase chain reaction in fludarabine-treated B-chronic lymphocytic leukaemia. Br J Haematol 1995; 91:409.
17. Briones J, Pereira A, Alcorta I. Transfusion-associated graft-versus-host disease (TA-GVHD) in fludarabine-treated patients: is it time to irradiate blood component? Br J Haematol 1996; 93:739.
18. Williamson LM, Wimperis JZ, Wood ME, Woodcock B. Fludarabine treatment and transfusion-associated graft-versus-host disease. Lancet 1996; 348:472.
19. Kessinger A, Armitage J, Klassen L, et al. Graft versus host disease following transfusion of normal blood products to patients with malignancies. J Surg Oncol 1987; 36:206.
20. Woods WG, Lubin BH. Fatal graft-versus-host disease following a blood transfusion in a child with neuroblastoma. Pediatrics 1981; 67:217.
21. Kennedy J, Ricketts R. Fatal graft versus host disease in a child with neuroblastoma following a blood transfusion. J Pediatr Surg 1986; 21:1108.
22. Postmus PE, Mulder NH, Elema JD. Graft versus host disease after transfusions of non-irradiated blood cells in patients having received autologous bone marrow: a report of 4 cases following ablative chemotherapy for solid tumors. Eur J Cancer Clin Oncol 1988; 24:889.
23. Berger RS, Dixon SL. Fulminant transfusion-associated graft-versus-host disease in a premature infant. J Am Acad Dermatol 1989; 20:945.
24. Sheehan T, McLaren KM, Brettle R, Parker AC. Transfusion-induced graft versus host disease in pregnancy. Clin Lab Haematol 1987; 9:205.
25. Otsuka S, Kunieda K, Kitamura F, et al. The critical role of blood from HLA-homozygous donors in fatal transfusion-associated graft-versus-host disease in immunocompetent patients. Transfusion 1991; 31:260.
26. Hathaway WE, Fulginiti VA, Pierce CW, et al. Graft-vs-host reaction following a single blood transfusion. JAMA 1967; 201:1015.
27. Juji T, Takahashi K, Shibata Y, et al. Post-transfusion graft-versus-host disease in immunocompetent patients after cardiac surgery. N Engl J Med 1989; 321:56.
28. Shivdasani RA, Haluska FG, Dock NL, et al. Graft-versus-host disease associated with transfusion of blood from unrelated HLA-homozygous donors. N Engl J Med 1993; 328:766.
29. Petz LD, Calhoun L, Yam P, et al. Transfusion-associated graft-versus-host disease in immunocompetent patients: report of a fatal case associated with transfusion of blood from a second-degree relative, and a survey of predisposing factors. Transfusion 1993; 33:742.
30. Kanter MH. Transfusion-associated graft-versus-host disease: do transfusions from second-degree relatives pose a greater risk than those from first-degree relatives? Transfusion 1992; 32:323.
31. Ohto H, Yasuda H, Noguchi M, Abe R. Risk of transfusion-associated graft-versus-host disease as a result of directed donations from relatives. Transfusion 1992; 32:691.
32. Wagner FF, Flegel WA. Transfusion-associated graft-versus-host disease: risk due to homozygous HLA haplotypes. Transfusion 1995; 35:284.
33. Yankee RA, Grumet FC, Rogentine GN. Platelet transfusion therapy: the selection of compatible platelet donors for refractory patients by lymphocyte HLA typing. N Engl J Med 1969; 281:1208.
34. Grishaber JE, Birney SM, Strauss RG. Potential for transfusion-associated graft-versus-host disease due to apheresis platelets matched for HLA class I antigens. Transfusion 1993; 33:910.
35. Benson K, Marks AR, Marshall MJ, Goldstein JD. Fatal graft-versus-host disease associated with transfusions of HLA-matched, HLA-homozygous platelets from unrelated donors. Transfusion 1994; 34:432.
36. Perkins HA. Transfusion-induced immunologic unresponsiveness. Transfus Med Rev 1988; 2:196.
37. Billingham RE. The biology of graft-versus-host reactions. Harvey Lect 1966–67; 62:21.
38. Shivdasani RA, Anderson KC. HLA homozygosity and shared HLA haplotypes in the development of transfusion-associated graft-versus-host disease. Leuk Lymphoma 1994; 15:227.
39. Fast LD, Valeri CR, Crowley JP. Immune responses to major histocompatibility complex homozygous lymphoid cells in murine F1 hybrid recipients: implications for transfusion-associated graft-versus-host disease. Blood 1995; 86:3090.
40. Wang L, Tadokoro K, Tokunaga K, et al. Restricted use of T-cell receptor V beta genes in posttransfusion graft-versus-host disease. Transfusion 1997; 37:1184.
41. Nishimura M, Uchida S, Mitsunaga S, et al. Characterization of T-cell clones derived from peripheral blood lymphocytes of a patient with transfusion-associated graft-versus-host disease: Fas-mediated killing by $CD4^+$ and $CD8^+$ cytotoxic T-cell clones and tumor necrosis factor beta production by $CD4^+$ T-cell clones. Blood 1997; 89:1440.
42. Krenger W, Ferrara JL. Dysregulation of cytokines during graft-versus-host disease. J Hematother 1996; 5:3.
43. Ferrara JL, Krenger W. Graft-versus-host disease: the influence of type 1 and type 2 T cell cytokines. Transfus Med Rev 1998; 12:1.
44. Habeshaw JA, Dalgleish AG, Hounsell EF. Absence of GVH in AIDS. J Acquir Immune Defic Syndr 1994; 7:1287.
45. Ammann AJ. Hypothesis: absence of graft-versus-host disease in AIDS is a consequence of HIV-1 infection of $CD4^+$ T cells. J Acquir Immune Defic Syndr 1993; 6:1224.
46. Dzik WH. Mononuclear cell microchimerism and the immunomodulatory effect of transfusion. Transfusion 1994; 34:1007.
47. Uharek L, Gassmann W, Glass B, et al. Influence of cell dose and graft-versus-host disease on rejection rates after allogeneic transplantation. Blood 1992; 79:1612.
48. Kunstmann E, Bocker T, Roewer L, et al. Diagnosis of transfusion-associated graft-versus-host disease by genetic fingerprinting and polymerase chain reaction. Transfusion 1992; 32:766.
49. Suzuki K, Akiyama H, Takamoto S, et al. Transfusion-associated graft-versus-host disease in a presumably immunocompetent patient after transfusion of stored packed red cells. Transfusion 1992; 32:358.
50. Hayakawa S, Chishima F, Sakata H, et al. A rapid molecular diagnosis of posttransfusion graft-versus-host disease by polymerase chain reaction. Transfusion 1993; 33:413.
51. Wang L, Juji T, Tokunaga K, et al. Polymorphic microsatellite markers for the diagnosis of graft-versus-host disease. N Engl J Med 1994; 330:398.
52. Saito M, Takamatsu H, Nakao S, et al. Transfusion-associated graft-versus-host disease after surgery for bladder cancer. Blood 1993; 82:326.
53. Uchida S, Wang L, Yahagi Y, et al. Utility of fingernail DNA for evaluation of chimerism after bone marrow transplantation and for diagnostic testing for transfusion-associated graft-versus-host disease [Letter]. Blood 1996; 87:4015.
54. Matsushita H, Shibata Y, Fuse K, et al. Sex chromatin analysis of lymphocytes invading host organs in transfusion-associated graft-versus-host disease. Virchows Arch B Cell Pathol 1988; 55:237.
55. Arsura EL, Bertelle A, Minkowitz S, et al. Transfusion-associated graft-vs-host disease in a presumed immunocompetent patient. Arch Intern Med 1988; 148:1941.
56. Otsuka S, Kunieda K, Hirose H, et al. Fatal erythroderma (suspected graft-versus-host disease) after cholecystectomy. Transfusion 1989; 29:544.
57. Vogelsang GB. Transfusion-associated graft-versus-host disease in non-immunocompromised hosts. Transfusion 1990; 30:101.
58. Cohen D, Weinstein H, Mihm M, Yankee R. Nonfatal graft-versus-host disease occurring after transfusion with leukocytes and platelets obtained from normal donors. Blood 1979; 53:1053.
59. Lind SE. Has the case for irradiating blood products been made? Am J Med 1985; 78:543.
60. Perkins H. Should all blood from related donors be irradiated? Transfusion 1992; 32:302.
61. Anand AJ, Dzik WH, Imam A, Sadrzadeh SM. Radiation-induced red cell damage: role of reactive oxygen species. Transfusion 1997; 37:160.
62. Klein H. Standards for Blood Banks and Transfusion Services, 17th ed. Bethesda, MD: American Association of Blood Banks, 1996.

63. Moroff G, Leitman SF, Luban NL. Principles of blood irradiation, dose validation, and quality control. Transfusion 1997; 37:1084.
64. Sproul AM, Chalmers EA, Mills KI, et al. Third party mediated graft rejection despite irradiation of blood products. Br J Haematol 1992; 80:251.
65. Lowenthal RM, Challis DR, Griffiths AE, et al. Transfusion-associated graft-versus-host disease: report of an occurrence following the administration of irradiated blood. Transfusion 1993; 33:524.
66. Kaminski E, Hows J, Man S, et al. Prediction of graft versus host disease by frequency analysis of cytotoxic T cells after unrelated donor bone marrow transplantation. Transplantation 1989; 48:608.
67. van Els CA, Bakker A, Zwinderman AH, et al. Effector mechanisms in graft-versus-host disease in response to minor histocompatibility antigens. II. Evidence of a possible involvement of proliferative T cells. Transplantation 1990; 50:67.
68. Irschick EU, Hladik F, Niederwieser D, et al. Studies on the mechanism of tolerance or graft-versus-host disease in allogeneic bone marrow recipients at the level of cytotoxic T-cell precursor frequencies. Blood 1992; 79:1622.
69. Theobald M, Nierle T, Bunjes D, et al. Host-specific interleukin-2–secreting donor T-cell precursors as predictors of acute graft-versus-host disease in bone marrow transplantation between HLA-identical siblings. N Engl J Med 1992; 327:1613.
70. Schwarer AP, Jiang YZ, Brookes PA, et al. Frequency of anti-recipient alloreactive helper T-cell precursors in donor blood and graft-versus-host disease after HLA-identical sibling bone-marrow transplantation. Lancet 1993; 341:203.
71. Anderson KC, Goodnough LT, Sayers M, et al. Variation in blood component irradiation practice: implications for prevention of transfusion-associated graft-versus-host disease. Blood 1991; 77:2096.
72. Akahoshi M, Takanashi M, Masuda M, et al. A case of transfusion-associated graft-versus-host disease not prevented by white cell–reduction filters. Transfusion 1992; 32:169.
73. Hayashi H, Nishiuchi T, Tamura H, Takeda K. Transfusion-associated graft-versus-host disease caused by leukocyte-filtered stored blood. Anesthesiology 1993; 79:1419.
74. Webb IJ, Schott DM, Cook J, et al. Cobe Spectra LRS for preparation of leukoreduced single donor apheresis platelets without laboratory filtration [Abstract 1327]. Blood 1996; 88:335a.
75. Anderson KC. Leukodepleted cellular blood components for prevention of transfusion-associated graft-versus-host disease. Transfus Sci 1995; 16:265.
76. Faber LM, van Luxemburg-Heijs SAP, Veenhof WFJ, et al. Generation of $CD4^+$ cytotoxic T-lymphocyte clones from a patient with severe graft-versus-host disease after allogeneic bone marrow transplantation: implications for graft-versus-leukemia reactivity. Blood 1995; 86:2821.
77. Giralt S, Hester J, Huh Y, et al. CD8-depleted donor lymphocyte infusion as treatment for relapsed chronic myelogenous leukemia after allogeneic bone marrow transplantation. Blood 1995; 86:4337.
78. Champlin R, Ho W, Gajewski J, et al. Selective depletion of $CD8^+$ T lymphocytes for prevention of graft-versus-host disease after allogeneic bone marrow transplantation. Blood 1990; 76:418.
79. Soiffer RJ, Murray C, Mauch P, et al. Prevention of graft-versus-host disease by selective depletion of CD6-positive T lymphocytes from donor bone marrow. J Clin Oncol 1992; 10:1191.
80. Soiffer RJ, Fairclough D, Robertson M, et al. CD6-depleted allogeneic bone marrow transplantation for acute leukemia in first complete remission. Blood 1997; 89:3039.

CHAPTER 30

Transfusion Immunomodulation

Neil Blumberg
Joanna M. Heal

"Phenomena which occur in adult life and which may be cognate with tolerance induced by foetal inoculation include . . . the enchancement of the growth of tumor homografts by treatment . . . with . . . lyophilized tissue preparations."[1]

For the better part of a century, when hematologists and transfusion medicine physicians have considered the immunological effects of blood transfusions, allosensitization has been the primary concern and scientific paradigm. Over the last quarter century, however, a large body of data has accumulated that proves that transfusion's immunomodulatory (or tolerogenic) effects are equally profound. Downregulation of cellular immunity by allogeneic transfusions may be of even greater clinical importance than allosensitization, although controversy exists on this issue. This changing paradigm is ironic, as surgeons have intuitively suspected for some time that transfusions can be deleterious to a patient's well-being under some circumstances. Therefore, it is not surprising that most of the clinical and scientific work on transfusion-induced immunomodulation is in the surgical literature. A number of reviews of various aspects of transfusion as an immunomodulatory influence have appeared over the last decade.[2–11]

This chapter reviews the recent evidence for transfusion as a downregulator of host immune function and then addresses some of the data suggesting that these changes are responsible for significant clinical consequences. Only a few studies have attempted to correlate immunological changes directly with altered clinical outcomes. The immunological basis for these clinical events is imperfectly understood, and it is not ethically or clinically feasible to perform randomized clinical trials in which patients not requiring transfusions are given them, while patients requiring transfusions are treated with alternative modalities. The current state of understanding is (1) that transfusions cause many changes in immune function in animal models and patients, (2) that transfusions are associated with altered clinical outcomes in patients, and (3) that allogeneic leukocytes appear to be the major component of blood mediating these effects. The extent to which a cause-and-effect relationship has been established between transfusion and altered clinical outcome ranges from almost certain (renal allograft enhancement, reduction in spontaneous abortion, increase in postoperative bacterial infection), to likely causal but not definitively proved (increase in cancer recurrence), to largely uncertain because of insufficient data (increase in severity of viral infection, reduction in autoimmune disease activity).

CHANGES IN RECIPIENT IMMUNOLOGICAL FUNCTION ASSOCIATED WITH TRANSFUSION

Transfusion as clinically practiced consists of intravenous administration of relatively large quantities of peripheral blood cells, proteins, lipids, and so forth diluted with preservatives and anticoagulant. Infusion of a gram or more of various antigens is common. From a practical standpoint, the only natural situations in which the immune system confronts such large quantities of intravenous antigen are self-antigens and pregnancy.[12, 13] Teleologically speaking, these two situations require unresponsiveness or tolerance. To provide defense, the immune system has evolved to deal with dangerous foreign antigens.[14] These consist primarily of microorganisms, present in small quantities, at mucosal or skin locations or altered self–tumor cells in small numbers, largely in tissue locations. Therefore, it should not be surprising that large doses of intravenous antigen containing both self- and non–self-determinants often result in tolerance rather than allosensitization. This appears to be especially true when other influences lead to decreased host immune function (e.g., the immaturity of fetal life, surgical stress, radiotherapy, anesthesia, immunosuppressive drugs).

When reading the literature or evaluating the relevance of animal studies, it is well to remember that the cells and substances transfused to patients have changed during the evolution of transfusion therapy and blood storage. Patients now receive red cell concentrates that are partially leukocyte depleted and almost totally plasma depleted, containing a deciliter of anticoagulant and storage solution including adenine, inorganic phosphate, and mannitol. Twenty years ago, transfusions were of whole blood that had no adenine or mannitol and had different amounts of glucose and other metabolic substrates than are currently used. Even the additive solutions may have immunomodulatory properties in vitro.[15] Additionally, blood is almost always stored for days or weeks before transfusion in the clinical setting. The effects of storage have only rarely been studied in the animal model or clinical setting.

Animal Models

In animal studies, blood is often collected into heparin anticoagulant, without the storage conditions and solutions employed clinically. Furthermore, most animal models use heavily inbred subjects that poorly mimic the much more heterogeneous situation in transfused patients. Medawar noted in his Nobel lecture that "perhaps the behaviour of inbred and homozygous mice is not the best theoretical guide to what may be expected of animals so obstinately heterozygous as human beings."[16] If complex immunological differences between donor and recipient are important in transfusion-induced immunomodulation, then most laboratory animals only approximate the clinical setting. Thus one must be cautious in extrapolating animal studies to human patients. Still, animals are the only practical subjects for randomized controlled trials of transfusions versus no transfusions.

Transplantation

The first indication that infusion of allogeneic tissue intravenously could cause immunomodulation or tolerance came from animal models. The classic experiments of Medawar and colleagues demonstrated that exposure during fetal life to foreign tissue could lead to lifelong acceptance of subsequent skin grafts from the tissue donor.[1] It is instructive to remember that some of their animals accepted grafts for only short periods, and that some animals were not rendered tolerant at all. Other early work showed that hyporesponsiveness to a specific antigen could be induced by large intravenous doses of that antigen. Felton found that when pneumococcal antigen was given at high doses, animals were impaired in their subsequent ability to mount a humoral immune response to antigen administered by routes and in doses that invariably cause sensitization ("immune paralysis").[17] These and many other studies gave hope that donor- and organ-specific tolerance could be induced for transplantation in human patients. These hopes have been realized only in small part. Presumably this is because of the greater immunological complexity of transplanting human tissue, especially in adult life, rather than in the fetal or neonatal period, when tolerance may be more readily induced. As for how post-transfusion antigen-specific tolerance occurs, very little is certain. It is now thought that multiple mechanisms of tolerance exist, both to self and non-self. These tolerance mechanisms exist in adult as well as fetal life and include clonal deletion and clonal anergy.

From clinical and animal studies in the late 1960s and early 1970s, it became clear that, contrary to theory, previous blood transfusions facilitated renal allografting.[18] Many animal studies were performed to elucidate the immunological mechanism underlying variations in 1-year graft survival from 40% in never-transfused patients to 70% in those receiving many transfusions (Fig. 30–1).[19] However, these studies were hampered by the almost total lack of basic information concerning the mechanisms of graft rejection. Even today, these mechanisms, largely thought to be cellular rather than humoral and involving primarily T cell and other cytotoxic effector cells, are only partially understood both qualitatively and quantitatively.

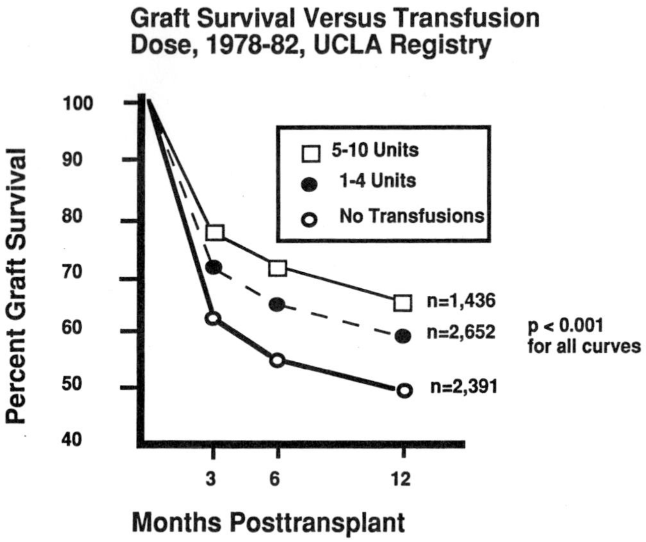

Figure 30–1. The dose-response relationship between pretransplantation transfusions and 1-year renal allograft survival in humans is shown from the UCLA registry for transplantations performed in the late 1970s to early 1980s. (Adapted with permission from Cecka M, Toyotome A. The transfusion effect. *In* Terasaki PI [ed]: Clinical Transplants 1989. Los Angeles: UCLA Tissue Typing Laboratory, 1989, p. 336.)

Nonetheless, a number of candidate effects have been demonstrated with some consistency in at least some animal model systems. Transfusions from genetically disparate animals of the same species lead to impaired mixed lymphocyte culture reactivity, impaired antigen processing by macrophages, increases in both suppressor cells and humoral suppressive substances, reduction in cell killing, and generation of idiotypic antibodies that can be immunomodulatory in vitro.[20] This suggests that downregulation of cellular immunity is a key component to the transfusion effect in renal allografting. Because similar effects have been detected in other solid organ allografts (particularly heart and liver), it seems certain that downregulation is a general property of blood transfusions.

Table 30–1 lists most of the immunological changes that have been demonstrated in studies of animals and human patients who have received blood transfusions.[20]

Table 30–1. Effects of Allogeneic Transfusions on Recipient Immunological Functions

1. Decreased Th1 and increased Th2 cytokine production in vitro
2. Reduced responses in mixed lymphocyte culture
3. Decreased proliferative response to mitogens or soluble antigens in vitro; impaired delayed-type hypersensitivity skin responses
4. Increased CD8 T cell number or suppressor function in vitro
5. Decreased natural killer cell number and activity in vitro
6. Decreased CD4 helper T cell number
7. Decreased monocyte or macrophage function in vitro and in vivo
8. Enhanced production of anti-idiotypic antibodies suppressive of mixed lymphocyte response in vitro
9. Decreased cell-mediated cytotoxicity (LAK) against certain target cells in vitro
10. Humoral alloimmunization to cell-associated and soluble antigens

The degree to which these findings explain the transfusion enhancement effect in organ transplantation is still a matter of active debate. There is general consensus that most components of peripheral blood can mediate this effect but that transfusion of donor white blood cells, especially lymphocytes, is especially effective. There is also evidence that transfusions that are partially matched to the recipient at minor and major histocompatibility loci (i.e., partially "self") are more effective than transfusions that are completely identical or nonidentical at the major histocompatibility loci.[21] Animal data suggest that infusion of viable allogeneic histoincompatible mononuclear cells leads to specific recipient anergy. Cytotoxic T lymphocyte response to the infused cells, but not to unrelated third-party cells, is greatly reduced.[22] Convincing data from other animal models show that allogeneic transfusion decreases the ability of mononuclear cells to secrete interleukin-2 (IL-2) in response to a variety of in vitro stimuli.[23, 24] The transplantation enhancement effect of transfusions almost certainly comprises both antigen-specific and nonspecific tolerogenic effects, but the relative importance of each is not known.

One recent model for post-transfusion immunomodulation that is receiving attention is shown in Figure 30–2.[13, 23–34] Immune deviation toward secretion of T helper type 2 (Th2) cytokines (e.g., IL-10, IL-4) and suppression of Th1 cytokines (e.g., IL-2) is one explanation of why transfusion impairs recipient immune responses to allogeneic organs, tumors, or fetuses. Effective immune responses against tumors and organ allografts have proved to be largely Th1 in nature,[35, 36] as is rejection of the fetus as an allograft.[37, 38] Although this diagram no doubt vastly oversimplifies the detailed biology of such events, it appears from clinical and animal studies that allogeneic transfusions impair cellular immunity by fostering immune responses that involve primarily IL-10, IL-4, and transforming growth factor-β (TGF-β).[13] These cytokines impair natural killer (NK) and T effector cell functions and some phagocytic cell functions and generally act as anti-inflammatory mediators.[39] These functions are critical to maintaining antitumor, antiallograft, and antimicrobial immunity; thus their impairment by allogeneic transfusion provides a reasonable unifying mechanism to explain the altered clinical outcomes that occur.

Tumor Growth

In 1951 Kaliss and Snell showed that infusions of various tissue extracts from allogeneic donors before tumor implantation accelerated tumor growth in the mouse.[40] Even serum infusion before implantation led to death of most of the animals due to tumor growth. The saline-infused control animals easily rejected this tumor and survived. Oddly, among all the tissue extracts infused, only infusions of lyophilized red cells failed to enhance tumor-related mortality. This particular difference has parallels in the clinical setting, in which red cell concentrates appear to be less immunomodulatory than whole blood in renal transplantation, postoperative infection, and cancer recurrence settings.

The notion that transfusion could be immunomodulatory in animal models of cancer was largely forgotten for three decades. However, after that time, a number of investigators reasoned that if transfusion was beneficial and therefore probably immunomodulatory in the renal allograft setting, perhaps it could be immunomodulatory and therefore deleterious in the setting of malignancy. Although occasional studies have demonstrated that transfusion before tumor implantation is beneficial and mediates tumor rejection, almost all recent studies have demonstrated that transfusions either impair host defenses against tumor growth or have no effect.

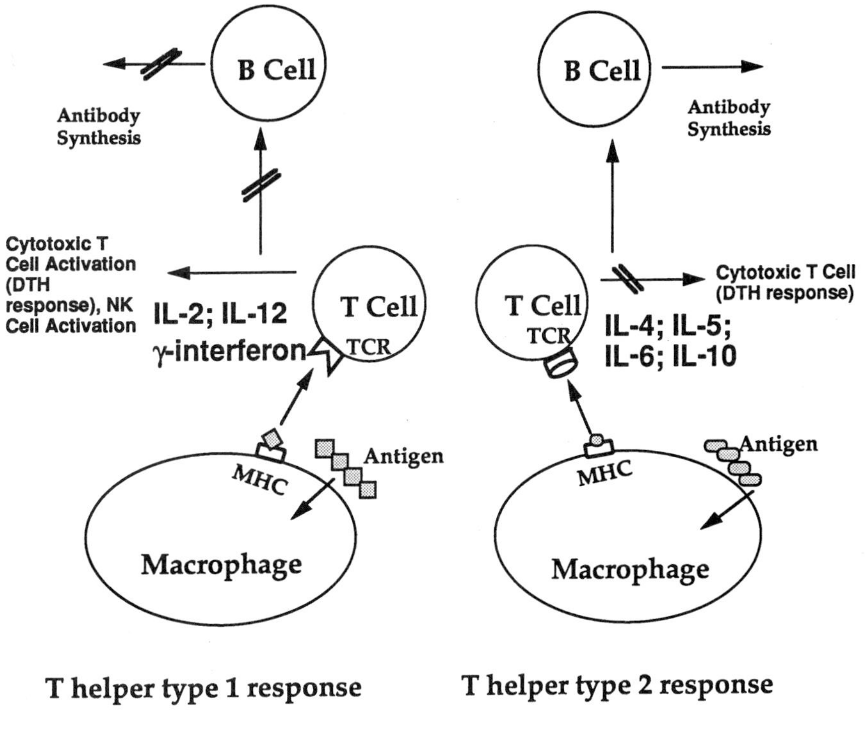

Figure 30–2. A simplified schematic view of how alloantigens are processed by macrophages and presented to T cells, with emphasis on the distinction between responses that primarily involve T helper type 1 or 2 (Th1 or Th2) cytokines. Allogeneic transfusions appear to evoke primarily Th2 cytokine secretion patterns with reciprocal downregulation of Th1 cytokine secretion. Thus many cellular immune functions, including cytotoxic T cell and NK functions, are downregulated.[13, 39] DTH, Delayed-type hypersensitivity; TCR, T cell antigen receptor; MHC, major histocompatibility complex; NK, natural killer; IL, interleukin.

Infection

Surgeons have been interested for many decades in the factors that predispose to postoperative infection, especially in trauma patients or those undergoing major interventions such as cardiac surgery. Although it has been assumed that neutrophils play the predominant role in defenses against bacterial sepsis, it is likely that lymphocytes, NK cells, dendritic cells, and macrophages are critical as well. For example, patients with naturally occurring neutrophil defects such as chronic granulomatous disease are primarily susceptible to gram-positive infections. Patients receiving cytotoxic chemotherapy that impairs both cellular and humoral immunity in addition to granulocytes are susceptible to a much broader range of microbial pathogens.

There are few animal data to suggest that allogeneic transfusion impairs neutrophil chemotaxis or bacterial killing. There is evidence to suggest that macrophage/monocyte phagocytosis, killing, and migration to sites of infection may be impaired in an animal model of peritonitis.[41, 42]

Evidence for Immunological Changes in Transfused Patients

As previously mentioned, patients do not resemble laboratory animals genetically, immunologically, or in terms of the kinds of observations that can be made. Thus, almost all clinical observations are necessarily poorly controlled and involve patients whose treatment aside from transfusion and whose underlying disease vary considerably. For example, prophylactic antibiotics before surgery vary in their specificity, dose, duration, and time of administration, all factors that can greatly affect clinical efficacy in preventing postoperative infections.

Chronically Transfused Patients

A major confounding problem is that patients who have an extensive transfusion history are also potentially subjected to the effects of chronic immunosuppressive viral infection. Even before the discovery of human immunodeficiency virus-1 (HIV-1), viruses such as cytomegalovirus (CMV) and Epstein-Barr virus (EBV) were suspected to cause clinical syndromes involving impairment of immune function. There is no ready way of controlling for this possibility.

Patients Receiving Red Cell Transfusions. Studies of immune function have been performed in hemodialysis patients and individuals with hemoglobinopathies such as thalassemia and sickle cell anemia. Despite the variability of these diseases and their treatment, heavily or recently transfused patients seem to have the same immunological changes described in the animal literature (see Table 30–1).[20]

Patients Receiving Plasma and Plasma Derivatives. Patients with hemophilia receive different sorts of blood components from patients with renal failure or hemoglobinopathy (pooled as opposed to single donor; plasma as opposed to cellular elements). They are much more likely to be infected with HIV-1 and much less likely to be exposed to CMV. Nonetheless, patients with hemophilia treated with unpurified factor concentrates develop the same sort of immunological changes as patients receiving primarily red cell concentrates (see Table 30–1). In some studies of hemophilia A, these effects of factor VIII concentrate are dose related. Monocytes from HIV-1–positive hemophiliacs receiving higher doses of factor VIII concentrate had reduced adherence capability, chemotactic response, and phagocytic indices as compared with monocytes from otherwise similar HIV-1–infected patients receiving lower doses of factor VIII.[43] Studies in vitro have demonstrated inhibition of IL-2 secretion and IL-2 receptor expression by normal human mononuclear cells when they were exposed to factor VIII concentrate.[44, 45] Thus the immunological defects in hemophiliacs are probably not entirely explained by HIV-1 or other viral infections and may relate to direct immunomodulatory effects of the infused plasma and plasma derivatives.

Surgical Patients Who Are Transfused

These patients differ dramatically from chronic transfusion recipients, in that their exposure is episodic, brief, and almost always associated with other immunomodulatory influences such as surgical stress, trauma, and anesthesia. Surgery without transfusion causes immune deviation toward Th2 cytokine secretion, which probably contributes to the reduction in cutaneous delayed-type hypersensitivity responses seen for the first week or two after surgery.[46–48] Whether these effects are due to surgical trauma alone, anesthesia, or other drugs is uncertain. These effects are additive with the effects of transfusion, and there are impairments of cellular immunity that last for days to weeks.[33, 34, 47–50] Immunomodulatory effects are not seen or are seen to a lesser degree in patients receiving only autologous blood or leukocyte-depleted transfusions. Many of the immunological alterations shown in Table 30–1 occur in surgical patients receiving red blood cells or whole blood within hours to days of transfusion, with no evidence of acute illnesses suggestive of viral infection.

CHANGES IN CLINICAL OUTCOME ASSOCIATED WITH TRANSFUSIONS

Organ Transplantation

As mentioned, much of the interest in transfusion-induced immunomodulation, as well as some of the most convincing clinical and laboratory data to date, centers around the role of transfusion in enhancing the success of organ allografting.[51, 52]

Animal Models

Animal models conclusively support the role of blood transfusion in enhancing organ allograft acceptance, whether the organ is the kidney, heart, or other tissue. Most studies suggest that the presence of white cells in the transfused blood is important to the effect, but evidence exists that plasma, red cells alone, and even purified, soluble class I histocompatibility antigens or peptide fragments of class I molecules[53–55] can mediate a similar effect to some degree. That transfusion-induced immunomodulation in the transplant setting is at least in part mediated by a prostaglandin E_2 (PGE_2)–IL-2 pathway is suggested by data that inhibition of PGE_2 by indomethacin or anti-PGE_2 antibody blocks this transfusion allograft enhancement effect.[56] Furthermore, in another model system, administration of exogenous IL-2 reversed the blood transfusion–induced immunomodulatory effect on renal allografting.[57]

Human Patients

Transfusions from the organ donor are particularly effective in mediating renal allograft acceptance, as would be predicted from the early animal work on tolerance. However, transfusions from unrelated third parties also are very effective, although the 1-year graft survival differences between transfused and nontransfused patients have decreased from about 30% to 3% to 8% as graft survival has improved overall (compare Fig. 30–3 with Fig. 30–1).[19] Most of this decreasing difference between transfused and nontransfused patients is due to the dramatically improved results in allografts to nontransfused patients, including improved techniques and immunosuppressive regimens. Some of the decreasing difference may be due to changes in transfusion practice, such as reduced plasma and white cell content of the red cell transfusions given. Recent evidence suggests that for third-party transfusions, sharing of at least one human leukocyte antigen–DR (HLA-DR) phenotype between blood donor and organ recipient leads to better 1-year renal allograft survival than when the recipient is untransfused or shares no HLA-DR antigens with the blood donor.[58] Thus, immunomodulation has been shown to be especially likely in both animal and clinical investigations when self- and non–self-antigens are presented simultaneously.

Cancer Surgery

Unlike with allografts, it is by no means certain that malignant tumors differ antigenically from normal tissue. Many of the "tumor antigens" that have been identified in humans appear to be self-antigens present at incorrect stages of development (e.g., oncofetal antigens), in the wrong cell or tissue, or in dramatically higher quantities than normal. There is also less consensus on the role of immune competence in protecting against the common solid tumors that cause the most morbidity and mortality (e.g., colon, lung, breast). Nonetheless, it seems almost certain that the immune system can play a role in eradicating tumors, usually in the setting of very low tumor cell number. For example, prior or concomitant splenectomy, an immunomodulatory event, adversely affects prognosis in Dukes stage C colon cancer patients.[59] There is a growing body of evidence that tumors actively downregulate local and regional immune responses by secreting or provoking the secretion of cytokines such as IL-10 and TGF-β, which downregulate cellular immunity.[60] Immune deviation toward a Th2 pattern is associated with tumor progression, and Th1 immunity with tumor regression.[61–64]

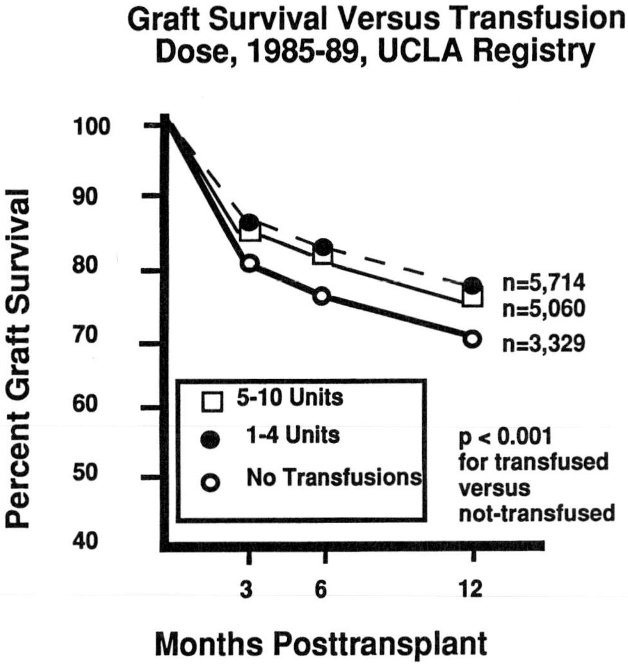

Figure 30–3. The decreasing advantage accruing to transfused patients in terms of 1-year renal allograft survival is shown from the UCLA registry for transplantation performed in the late 1980s. Although all patients, regardless of transfusion status, had improved survival from the early period shown in Figure 30–1, the improvement for the nontransfused patients was most quantitatively impressive (from 49% to 73%). The long-term survival of renal allografts surviving at least 1 year was significantly longer in the patients receiving 5 to 10 units of blood before transplantation (mean, 8.4 years) than in the patients receiving no transfusions (mean, 6.0 years; $p = .001$) (data not shown). (Adapted with permission from Cecka M, Toyotome A. The transfusion effect. *In* Terasaki PI [ed]: Clinical Transplants 1989. Los Angeles: UCLA Tissue Typing Laboratory, 1989, p. 336.)

The use of immunocompetent host cells that have been stimulated to higher levels of activation to treat human tumors is in its infancy but demonstrates the certainty that immune effector cells can kill or control neoplastic cells. IL-2–mediated increases in tumor killing can on rare occasions cause complete regression of widely metastatic disease. Therefore, it is especially interesting that preliminary studies in uremic patients show dramatic increases in PGE_2 secretion accompanied by decreases in IL-2 secretion after transfusion (Figs. 30–4 and 30–5).[30] Furthermore, previously transfused renal cancer patients may have a blunted lymphokine-activated killer (LAK) cell response to exogenous IL-2.[65] High blood and tumor levels of PGE_2 have been associated with an increased likelihood of liver and lung metastases in patients with colorectal carcinoma.[66] Finally, allogeneic transfusion causes immune deviation toward secretion of Th2 cytokines that downregulate cellular immunity (Fig. 30–6).[26, 31, 32, 34] The Th2-promoting effects of allogeneic transfu-

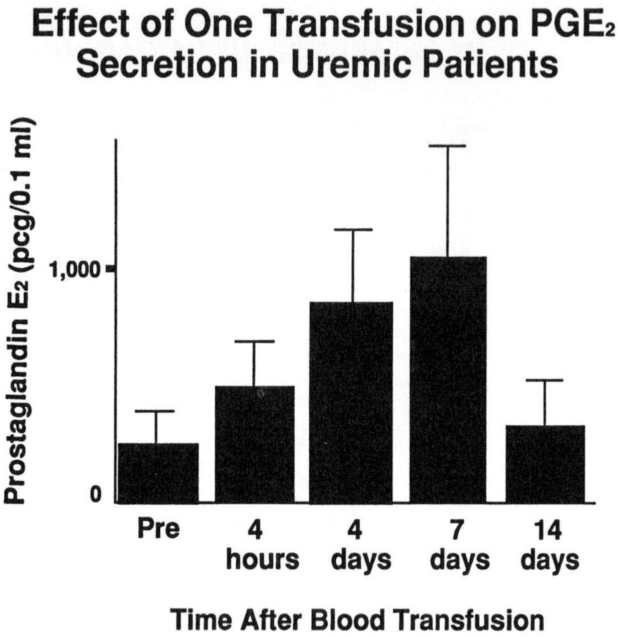

Figure 30–4. Uremic hemodialysis patients who had not recently undergone transfusion received a single unit of red blood cells and the secretion of prostaglandin E_2 (PGE_2) of peripheral blood mononuclear cells after mitogen stimulation was measured in vitro over time. PGE_2 has been shown to impair interleukin-2 (IL-2) secretion (see Figs. 30–2 and 30–5). No control studies were performed with patients who received sham or saline infusion. (Adapted with permission from Kalechman Y, Gafter U, Sobelman D, Sredni B. The effect of a single whole-blood transfusion on cytokine secretion. J Clin Immunol 1990; 10:99.)

sion appear to augment and mimic the "survival strategy" of solid tumors.

Animal Models

Tumors in animal models are, in many instances, rather poor analogs of human cancer. Animal model tumors are often rapidly growing, measurably antigenic, and chemically or virally induced. The degree to which naturally occurring human cancers are similar varies but is much less than ideal. Many (but by no means all) models of tumor implantation after transfusion suggest that transfusion accelerates tumor growth. Waymack and colleagues found that animals receiving allogeneic transfusions had reduced NK cell function and shortened survival owing to tumor metastases, compared with syngeneically transfused animals.[67] Parrott and associates found a dose-response effect between whole blood transfusions and enhanced tumor growth in a rat model.[68] Furthermore, either washed red cells or allogeneic plasma alone could mediate this effect. Sham laparotomy, to mimic the immunomodulatory effect of surgical stress, appeared additive to the transfusion effect in promoting tumor growth. This is consistent with immunological research that demonstrates that surgery alone causes immune deviation toward Th2 cytokine secretion, and this effect is additive with the effects of allogeneic but not autologous transfusion in humans.[26, 33, 34, 47]

Blajchman and colleagues demonstrated in both inbred and outbred animal tumor models that allogeneic transfusions promote tumor metastasis, that this effect is transferable and mediated by soluble factors, and that leukodepletion of the transfused blood abrogates the metastasis-enhancing effect.[69]

Additive or synergistic immunomodulatory effects from surgery, anesthesia, or drugs may determine whether a particular transfusion dose has clinically detectable effects. In this regard, it is worth noting that even drugs thought to be immunologically benign, such as antibiotics, are now being shown to cause immunomodulation.[70]

Human Patients

In contrast with most animal models of cancer recurrence and transfusion, where transfusion precedes tumor implantation, the patient's tumor is always present before transfusion. Given that tumors are often associated with immune deviation toward a Th2 pattern of cytokine secretion, the probability exists that allogeneic transfusion's enhancement of Th2 cytokine secretion can further impair the patient's cellular immune response to the tumor.[36, 61–64]

No Transfusion Versus Transfusion. The first study in humans suggesting that transfusion might lead to increased or earlier cancer recurrence was reported in

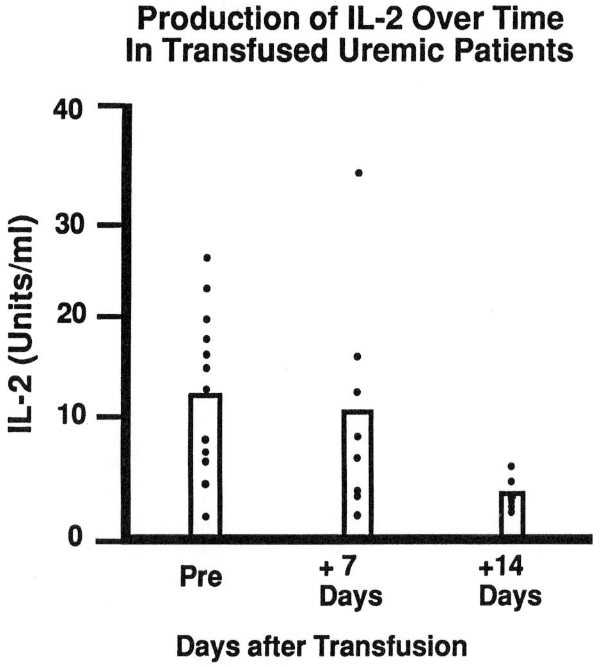

Figure 30–5. The same samples from uremic hemodialysis patients shown in Figure 30–4 were tested for their ability to secrete interleukin-2 (IL-2) in response to in vitro stimulation. A single red cell transfusion led to virtual abrogation of IL-2 synthesis by 2 weeks after transfusion. No control studies were performed with patients who received sham or saline infusion. (Adapted with permission from Kalechman Y, Gafter U, Sobelman D, Sredni B. The effect of a single whole-blood transfusion on cytokine secretion. J Clin Immunol 1990; 10:99.)

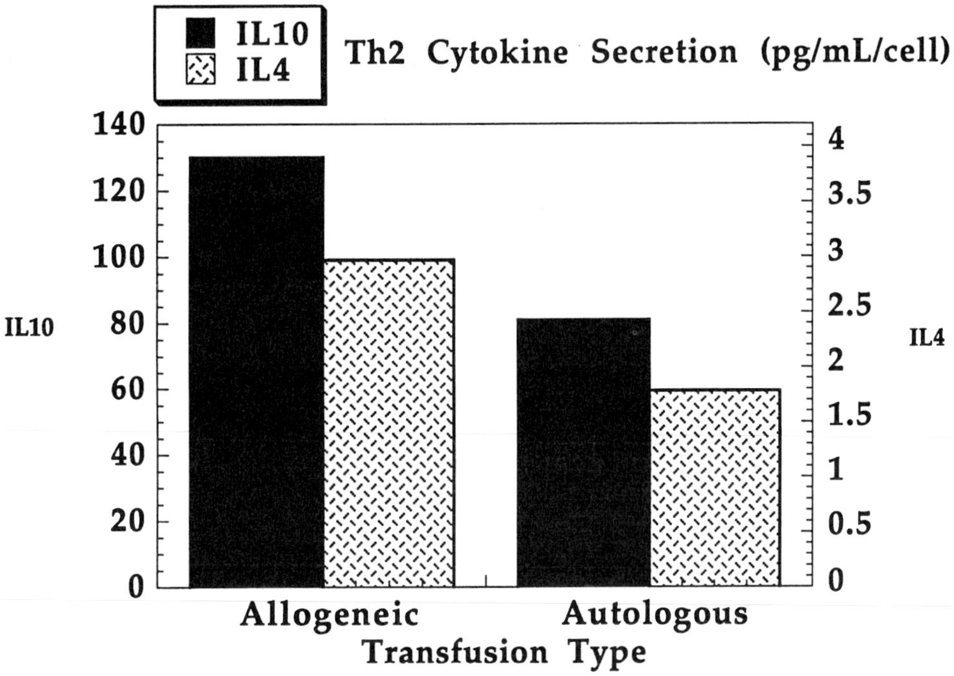

Figure 30–6. In the first such study published, patients undergoing joint replacement surgery with either autologous transfusions or autologous and allogeneic transfusions were compared for in vitro whole blood interleukin-10 and interleukin-4 (IL-10 and IL-4) secretion postoperatively. The IL-10 differences are significant, but the IL-4 differences did not achieve significance in this study.[26] In subsequent studies in both patients and animals, secretion of both IL-10 and IL-4 has been definitively shown to increase after allogeneic transfusions.[30–32, 34]

a letter to *Lancet* by Burrows and Tartter.[71] This and most subsequent data come from retrospective studies. Thus efforts have been made to determine whether tumor recurrence differs in patients with similar amounts of blood loss, stage of tumor spread, and so forth but who have or have not been transfused. About two thirds of the existing studies suggest that after these other factors have been considered, transfusion remains a significant, independent predictor of tumor recurrence; the remainder of the studies conclude that transfusion either is not significant or may be acting as a surrogate marker for other prognostic clinical variables.

However, short of performing a randomized study, which would not be ethically defensible, given the other risks of transfusion, the only likely clinical proof of the correctness or falseness of the hypothesis linking perioperative transfusions with increased tumor recurrence rates will be controlled studies employing modified types of transfusions of lesser immunomodulatory potential (e.g., plasma and leukocyte depleted) or transfusions of autologous blood only. Indeed, two randomized studies of autologous transfusions versus standard allogeneic transfusions have yielded conflicting results, with one showing evidence of benefit[72] and the other no such evidence.[73] Two caveats regarding these studies are that the control arm consisted of buffy coat–depleted red cells, and that many patients in the autologous study arm (about 25% to 30%) also received allogeneic blood. Thus, these are effectively studies of 60% to 80% leukocyte-depleted blood versus autologous transfusion. Given data suggesting the importance of allogeneic white cells in mediating transfusion immunomodulation, these studies had only a small chance of demonstrating efficacy. Nonetheless, Heiss and coworkers found evidence that autologous transfusions can reduce cancer recurrence and postoperative infection, and they have preliminary data that autologous transfusions may foster Th1 cytokine secretion and thus act as a stimulant for cellular immunity.[33, 34, 48, 72]

One multicenter randomized trial in colorectal cancer failed to demonstrate that leukocyte depletion of transfusions is beneficial in reducing cancer recurrence.[74] Two cohort studies in acute leukemia suggested that leukocyte depletion of transfusions yields better outcomes in terms of both morbidity and leukemia recurrence, but these were not randomized trials.[75, 76]

Type of Blood Components Transfused to Cancer Patients. Support for the hypothesis that transfusion actually causes increased recurrence rates of solid tumors comes from the facts that the effect in retrospective studies is often dose dependent and cannot be explained by other known prognostic factors, and that the type of blood component transfused is relevant. Transfusions of plasma- and white cell–rich blood components (e.g., whole blood, fresh frozen plasma, plasma derivatives) have been associated with increased tumor recurrence or death rates, compared with transfusions of similar quantities of red cell concentrates in all four studies that have examined this variable (Fig. 30–7).[77–81] The fact that patients transfused with only a few units of red cells are more likely to have favorable outcomes than those receiving more immunomodulatory components is consonant with theory and with prior observations. In the clinical renal allograft setting, whole blood transfusions are associated with better graft survival than are red cell and washed red cell transfusions.[82] Patients with colorectal cancer receiving whole blood have decreased cell-mediated immunity, as measured by response to skin test antigens, compared with similar patients receiving only red cell concentrates.[46] Neither the clinical nor the laboratory data are likely to be explained by clinical differences among the patients, given that similar amounts of transfusion were received by both groups. The current data

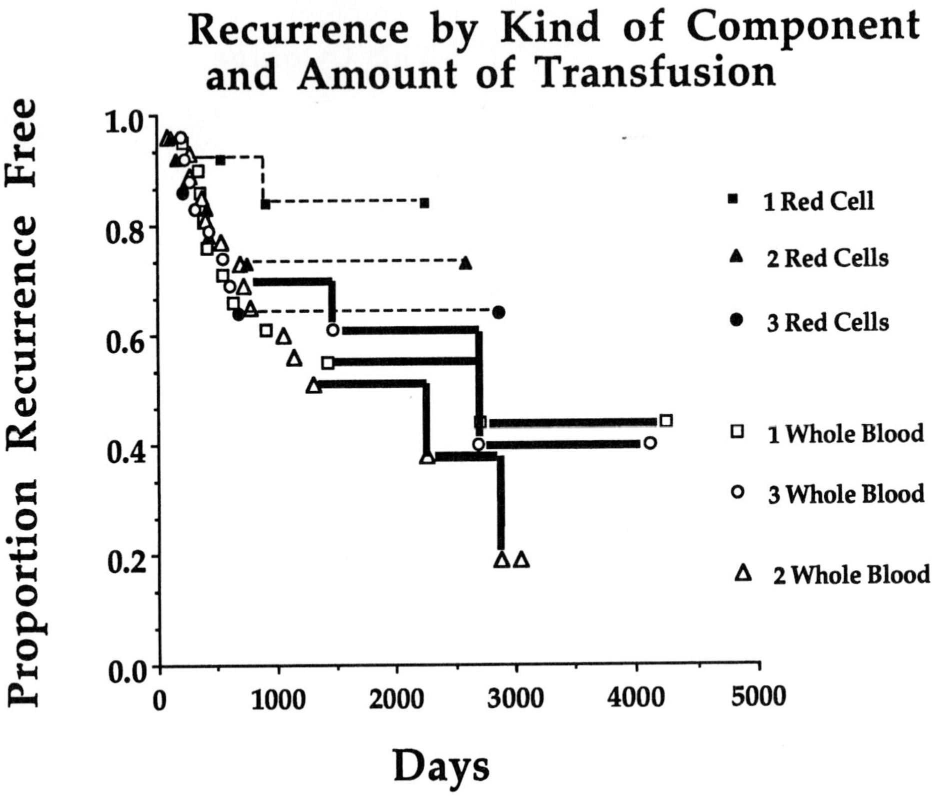

Figure 30–7. Recurrence of cancer in patients with prostate, colorectal, or cervical cancer is shown by type and amount of component transfused. The estimates shown are Kaplan-Meier estimates of patients receiving only red cells and of patients who received any whole blood. The numbers of patients represented by these curves are 17, 16, and 7 for 1, 2, and 3 units of red cells, respectively, and 22, 29, and 24 for 1, 2, and 3 units of whole blood, respectively. The data have been pooled to provide sufficient numbers for statistical analysis, but the trends shown were seen in each tumor group individually. These differences are significant when the 1- and 2-unit red cell curves are compared with the corresponding whole blood curves or when a Cox multivariate regression is performed to compare patients receiving 3 or fewer units of red cells with those receiving the same amount of whole blood. Even when tumor, preoperative anemia, and duration of surgery were considered as prognostic factors, transfusion with whole blood was an independent predictor of earlier tumor recurrence. (Adapted with permission from Blumberg N, Heal JM. Transfusion and host defenses against cancer recurrence and infection. Transfusion 1989; 29: 240.)

and standards of blood component therapy are strong arguments that the use of plasma components and whole blood should be strictly avoided in patients whose anemia and blood loss require only a few units (one to three) of red cells for replacement therapy.

Problems in Interpreting the Literature on Cancer Recurrence and Transfusion. The association between transfusion and cancer recurrence seems plausible on the basis of (1) theoretical immunological considerations, (2) controlled animal models in which a clear effect has been demonstrated, and (3) the difference in outcomes among patients receiving similar amounts of red cells but differing amounts of plasma and white cells. Then why has this effect failed to be detected in about a third of the studies to date? There is no simple answer. The role of cellular immunity probably varies in different tumors. One other possibility is that patients in the negative studies predominantly received small numbers of red cell transfusions, with few transfused patients receiving whole blood or fresh frozen plasma. The failure to distinguish between kinds of blood components transfused or the dose thereof is a potential weakness in many studies. Other medication and surgical technique variables may also impair cellular immunity to a greater or lesser degree and mask the effects of transfusion. The recurrence rates in various studies vary enormously from center to center, giving some support to such a possibility.

Some studies have insufficient numbers of patients or suboptimal statistical methodology. As an example of the latter, the lack of multivariate analyses, such as logistic or Cox regressions, which can analyze the contributions of prognostic variables other than transfusion, could lead to erroneous conclusions about the role of transfusion, positive or negative. When multivariate analyses are performed, missing data for some variables in some patients may represent a problem in retrospective studies. It seems likely from studies that have examined transfusion dose and immunomodulation that transfusions of one or two units of red cells (as opposed to whole blood) may be associated with modest and difficult-to-detect differences in renal allograft survival, colon cancer recurrence, or postoperative bacterial infection. Thus, treating transfusion as a categorical (yes or no) variable, as many earlier studies did, may lead to erroneous negative or positive conclusions about the significance of transfusion.

Other immunomodulatory factors, such as surgical trauma, anesthesia, and drugs, may be necessary to potentiate the transfusion effect, and these factors almost certainly vary among medical centers. Perhaps different types of anesthesia or drugs commonly given perioperatively vary in their ability of potentiate transfusion-induced immunomodulation. For example, laparoscopic cholecystectomy causes less immune deviation toward Th2 cytokine secretion than does open surgery.[47]

Transfusions in the distant past may have long-term immunological significance, and most studies have not investigated this confounding variable. Indeed, transfusion has been linked in preliminary studies to an increased risk of malignancy some years later.[83, 84] Finally, administration of blood components such as albumin and plasma protein fraction may be immunomodulatory if Marsh and colleagues' results are indicative.[81] Few studies have included these components in their analyses of transfusions. Perhaps some of the allegedly nontransfused patients in the literature received plasma protein fraction transfusions, skewing the results reported. Meta-analyses of the epidemiological literature have come to varied conclusions, depending on the biases of the authors,[85–87] but it is clear that transfusion is overall a strong predictor of recurrence and cancer death (Fig. 30–8). Attempts to rationalize that these observations are due to transfusion acting as a surrogate variable for other clinically important factors are hampered mainly by the lack of data to support these theoretical arguments.

In summary, given all the caveats mentioned, the frequent finding that transfusion is a significant unfavorable prognostic variable—even after tumor stage, preoperative anemia, operative blood loss, patient age, and duration of surgery have been accounted for—is highly suggestive but not conclusive evidence that transfusions can increase the risk of cancer recurrence. However, this deleterious effect may not be detectable in all types of tumors or in all clinical settings.

Immunomodulatory Factors in Plasma. When considering which components of plasma might be immunomodulatory, there is no shortage of candidates. As mentioned later in the chapter, intravenous high-dose immunoglobulin G (IgG) infusion is a powerful immunomodulator in many clinical settings.[88, 89] Presentation of high concentrations of either cellular or soluble histocompatibility antigens (both class I and II), or fragments of these antigens, has been shown in animal models to mediate immunomodulation.[90, 91] Clayberger and Krensky and their colleagues have demonstrated both antigen-specific and nonspecific downregulation of T cell function by class I and II fragments.[54, 92] Formation of soluble immune complexes, which almost certainly occurs after plasma transfusions, has been shown to inhibit macrophage cytotoxic functions[93] and inhibit secretion of the important Th1 cytokine IL-12.[94]

As a final point, it remains possible, but remotely so, that the transfusion-associated increase in cancer recurrence is caused by nonimmunological mechanisms. Hoh and colleagues showed that stored blood for transfusion contains greater mitogenic stimulatory activity than fresh blood, and that transfused patients exhibit a 100% increase in plasma mitogenic activity as compared with those not receiving transfusions.[95] They hypothesized that release of tumor-stimulating growth factors during blood storage may contribute to the increased rate of tumor recurrence seen in transfused patients. Another report studying macrophage release of PGE_2 in a rat transfusion model demonstrated that 24-hour storage of blood before transfusion significantly increased PGE_2 synthesis 7 days later for both allogeneic and syngeneic transfusions.[25] Thus blood storage, a variable not heretofore considered in animal or clinical studies, may contribute to both im-

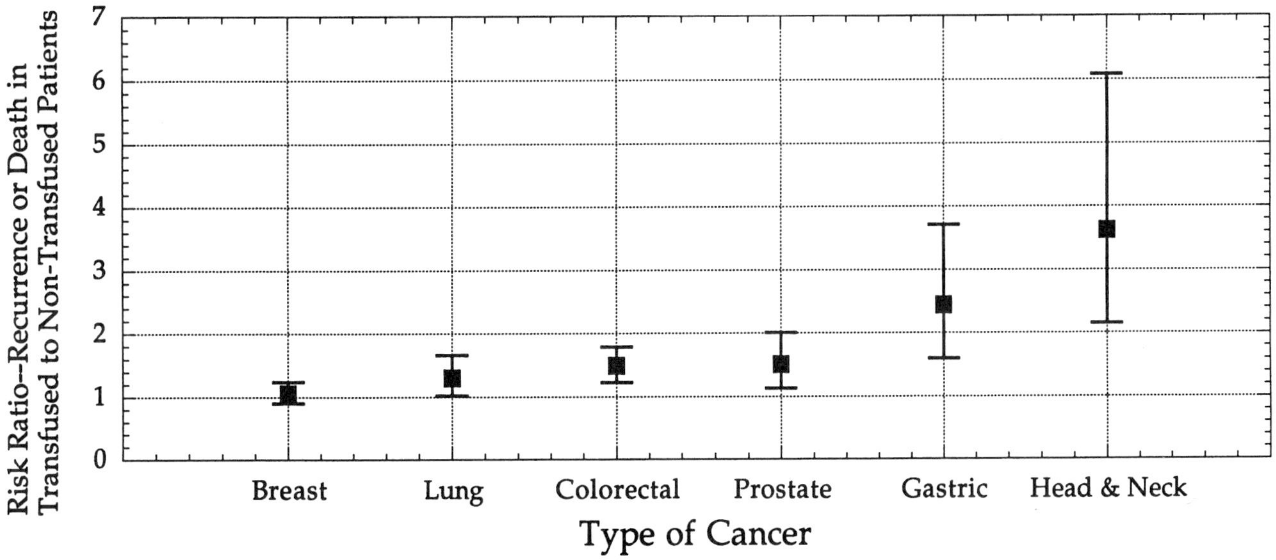

Figure 30–8. The relative risk of cancer recurrence or death in patients receiving allogeneic transfusions in comparison with the risk in those receiving no transfusions is shown for a variety of human cancers, based upon epidemiologic studies; 95% confidence intervals of the estimate are shown. A relative risk of 1.0 indicates no additional risk of recurrence or death beyond that seen in nontransfused patients. For transfused patients, the relative risk is statistically significantly increased for each type of tumor except breast cancer. The relative risk for lung cancer in one-pack-a-day cigarette smokers is about 10 in comparison with nonsmokers, and the relative risk for oral cancer in pipe and cigar smokers is 3.3 in comparison with nonsmokers. (Data plotted are from the meta-analysis results of E. C. Vamvakas.[140])

munological and nonimmunological mechanisms that favor tumor growth.

Perioperative Infection

Some surgeons have long held the opinion that transfusions are associated with more complicated clinical courses in their patients. The difficulty of testing this hypothesis in a controlled fashion has been alluded to previously. Recently, efforts have been made to study the frequency of acute postoperative bacterial infection in animals and patients receiving various amounts of allogeneic (homologous) or syngeneic (autologous) blood, or to compare unmodified and leukocyte-depleted allogeneic transfusions. These last studies have definitively answered the question of causality, because they were randomized and had clear-cut outcomes in three of the four trials.[49, 74, 96, 97]

Animal Models

Most, but not all, data suggest that allogeneic transfusions increase the likelihood of death after experimental bacterial challenge in a dose-dependent fashion. As in the cancer setting, the degree to which animal models can mimic the clinical setting depends on the degree to which conditions such as surgical trauma, anesthesia, and storage of blood are duplicated. Few, if any, studies have attempted to completely replicate the transfusion setting clinically, especially in terms of transfusion variables such as anticoagulant, storage period, use of multiple donors, dosage of transfusion, or administration of other drugs routinely used perioperatively. A series of elegant and thorough animal model experiments demonstrated that allogeneic transfusions impair resistance to experimental infections in a number of animal models and anatomical sites.[41, 42, 98–100] This work supports the notion that transfusion affects systemic resistance to infection rather than local wound factors, and that impaired monocyte or macrophage functions such as chemotaxis, phagocytosis, and bacterial killing are likely to be at least part of the explanation.[100] It is also known that hemorrhage sufficient to cause significant hypotension can depress important host defenses against bacterial infection.[101] Thus transfusion may be an important immunomodulatory influence for perioperative infection, but it is by no means the only one.

Furthermore, Gianotti and coworkers showed that allogeneic white blood cells are the major cause of reduced host defenses against bacteria after transfusion.[102] Babcock and Alexander further showed that allogeneic transfusions in nonoperated animals favor Th2 cytokine secretion.[31] Th2 cytokine secretion may impair some phagocytic cell functions.[103, 104]

Human Patients

The first studies demonstrating an increased rate of perioperative bacterial infection came from Tartter and associates.[105, 106] These and almost all studies to date demonstrate a dose-response relationship between allogeneic transfusion and the likelihood of postoperative infection. In most studies, transfusion is the single best predictor of postoperative infection, superior in many instances to factors such as extent of trauma, anemia, blood loss, hypotension, presence of a contaminated wound, and duration of surgery. The primary concern about these difficult-to-control, nonrandomized observations is that transfusion may be acting as a surrogate marker for other variables that may actually be responsible for the increased risk of infection, such as anemia, degree of tissue destruction, duration of anesthesia and operation, as well as degree of blood loss.[107] But in most studies in which these variables have been studied, the dose of transfusion appears to be an independent predictor of infection that is actually quantitatively more important than the other variables mentioned.[105, 108–111] As an extraordinary example, one prospective study of infection in patients undergoing colorectal surgery found that transfusion was a more significant predictor of postoperative infectious complications than fecal contamination of the abdominal cavity at surgery.[112] Of the 20 patients with fecal contamination, only the 15 transfused patients developed infections. Of those undergoing emergency surgery, the infection rate was 56% in transfused patients versus 0% in those not requiring transfusions.

Recently, susceptibility to fungal infections after liver transplantation has been linked to the dose of transfusion given perioperatively. Other than need for retransplantation, reintubation, and preexisting bacterial infection, transfusion dose was the best predictor of post-transplant fungal infection by discriminant analysis.[113] Transfusion was more important as a predictor of fungal infection than dose of steroids, presence of vascular complications, or types of antibiotics given. Among preoperative or intraoperative variables, transfusion dose was the best predictor of postoperative fungal infection and was more important than emergent versus elective nature of the transplant, level of bilirubin or albumin, length of intensive care stay preoperatively, need for biliary reconstruction, need for intubation, presence of steroid therapy, history of gastrointestinal bleeding, and duration of surgery.

Further support for allogeneic transfusion as a cause of postoperative infection comes from comparisons of outcomes in retrospective cohort studies performed in recipients of autologous versus allogeneic transfusions. When patients with comparable degrees of blood loss and type of surgery are grouped by whether they received autologous or allogeneic blood, it is found that the autologous recipients have a risk of infection comparable to that of patients receiving no transfusions (0% to 5%). The allogeneic recipients have a dose-related increased risk of infection, beginning at approximately two units of transfused blood (Fig. 30–9).[108, 109] The major caveat here is that these observations are not randomized, and the diagnosis of infection is subject to observer bias. Infection is often underreported in the literature on perisurgical patients because of the exclusive reliance on positive bacterial cultures for diagnosis. Most surgical patients currently receive prophylactic antibiotics, which makes culturing much less sensitive. Furthermore, cultures have poor predictive power for diagnosing certain types of infections (e.g., wound, pneumonia, cellulitis). Therefore, broader

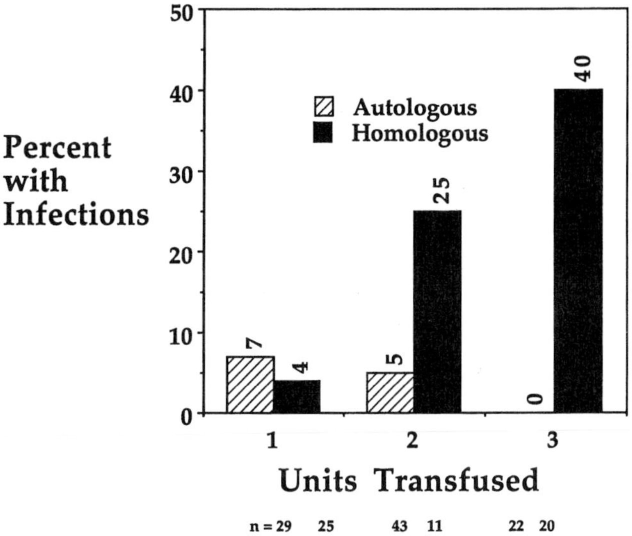

Figure 30–9. Patients undergoing posterior or anterior cervical or lumbar spinal fusion or primary hip replacement surgery, without malignancy, autoimmune diseases, or diabetes, were grouped according to whether they had received only autologous blood or only homologous blood. The proportion with culture-proven or clinically evident infections, grouped according to number of units of blood transfused, is shown. The differences between autologous and homologous recipients are statistically significant at doses of 2 or 3 units but not for 1 unit of blood. This significant dose-response relationship was also evident when days of antibiotics and length of hospital stay were measured. Infections were predominantly away from the wound site: two thirds were cellulitis, urinary tract, or pulmonary infections. (Data are pooled from two studies.[108, 109])

criteria for infection or probable infection are more sensitive tools to use when searching for clinically relevant events that may be due to transfusion-induced immunomodulation.

As an example, in one study in which 17 infections were diagnosed by the broader criteria for postoperative infection, only three were proved by culture.[108] Nonetheless, the mean days of antibiotics in the patients considered "infected" was 7.6, as opposed to 2.3 in those with no infection ($p = .0001$). The mean length of hospital stay was 15.5 days in the infected group versus 12.3 days in the noninfected group ($p = .0001$). Sixteen of these patients had received allogeneic blood, and one had received autologous blood only. Had more traditional and less sensitive criteria for infection been used, this study would have failed to identify most of the clinical events that led to significant morbidity and expense. In patients receiving two or three units of blood, the event rate was 16 of 50 (32%) in recipients of homologous blood and 1 of 34 (3%) in patients receiving only autologous blood ($p = .0029$).

Two randomized trials of autologous versus allogeneic transfusion have yielded divergent results. Heiss and colleagues found significant protection against postoperative infection with autologous transfusions,[48] but Busch and colleagues reported no such benefit.[73] As mentioned previously, these are studies of buffy coat–depleted (60% to 80% leukoreduction) allogeneic red cells versus autologous red cells, which minimizes the opportunity for detecting a benefit if allogeneic white cells are important mediators of the effect. In addition, a critical difference may be that the Munich study[48] was a single-center study and the Rotterdam study[73] was multicenter, with a few dozen patients at each of many centers. So far, all single-center trials of leukocyte depletion (n = 3) or autologous transfusion (n = 1) have been successful in demonstrating reductions in morbidity or mortality in allogeneic transfusion recipients,[48–50, 97] and the two multicenter trials have failed to find such benefits.[73, 74] This suggests that the variability introduced when small numbers of patients are treated by varying clinical protocols may mask any potential benefit. Such procedural variations from center to center have been shown to account for much of the variability in postoperative infection rates in Israel.[114] It is particularly interesting that the multicenter study by investigators in Leiden failed to find a benefit for leukodepletion in colorectal cancer surgery[74] but found a morbidity and mortality benefit to leukodepletion in cardiac surgery when a single-center study was performed.[97]

The findings by Jensen and coworkers in two randomized trials of leukodepletion in colorectal surgery,[49, 96] confirmed by Van der Watering and colleagues in cardiac surgery,[97, 115] provide conclusive evidence that postoperative infection rates can be strikingly reduced by leukodepletion. In Jensen's first study,[49] whole blood was the control arm, and in the second study, buffy coat–depleted red cell transfusion was the control arm.[96] As shown in Figure 30–10, as the amounts of plasma and white cells were reduced, the wound infection rate decreased concomitantly.

Variations in appropriate infection control and surgical techniques, such as time of administration of preoperative prophylactic antibiotics, have an important impact on infection rates, and these variables may compromise studies of transfusion interventions. Nonetheless, it seems clear that allogeneic transfusions, particularly those containing white cells, cause an increased risk of postoperative infection and that this effect can be largely abrogated in some settings by leukocyte depletion.

Public Health and Cost Considerations

Depending on the percentage of the epidemiological association that is causal, the number of transfusion immunomodulation–associated deaths may be tens of thousands per year (Table 30–2), far exceeding those due to other transfusion complications.[13] The opportunity to improve care involves not only lives but also dramatic cost reductions. Investigators in diverse cities such as Rochester, New York, and Aarhus, Denmark, have estimated the additional costs of allogeneic transfusion at $1000 to $2000 per unit given.[116, 117] It has been estimated that the potential savings to the U.S. health care system after the adoption of universal leukocyte reduction of allogeneic transfusions to surgical patients may be as much as $6 billion to $12 billion per year, or 1% to 2% of the national health budget.[13]

Autoimmune Diseases

Patients with diseases such as rheumatoid arthritis or systemic lupus are infrequently transfused. This makes

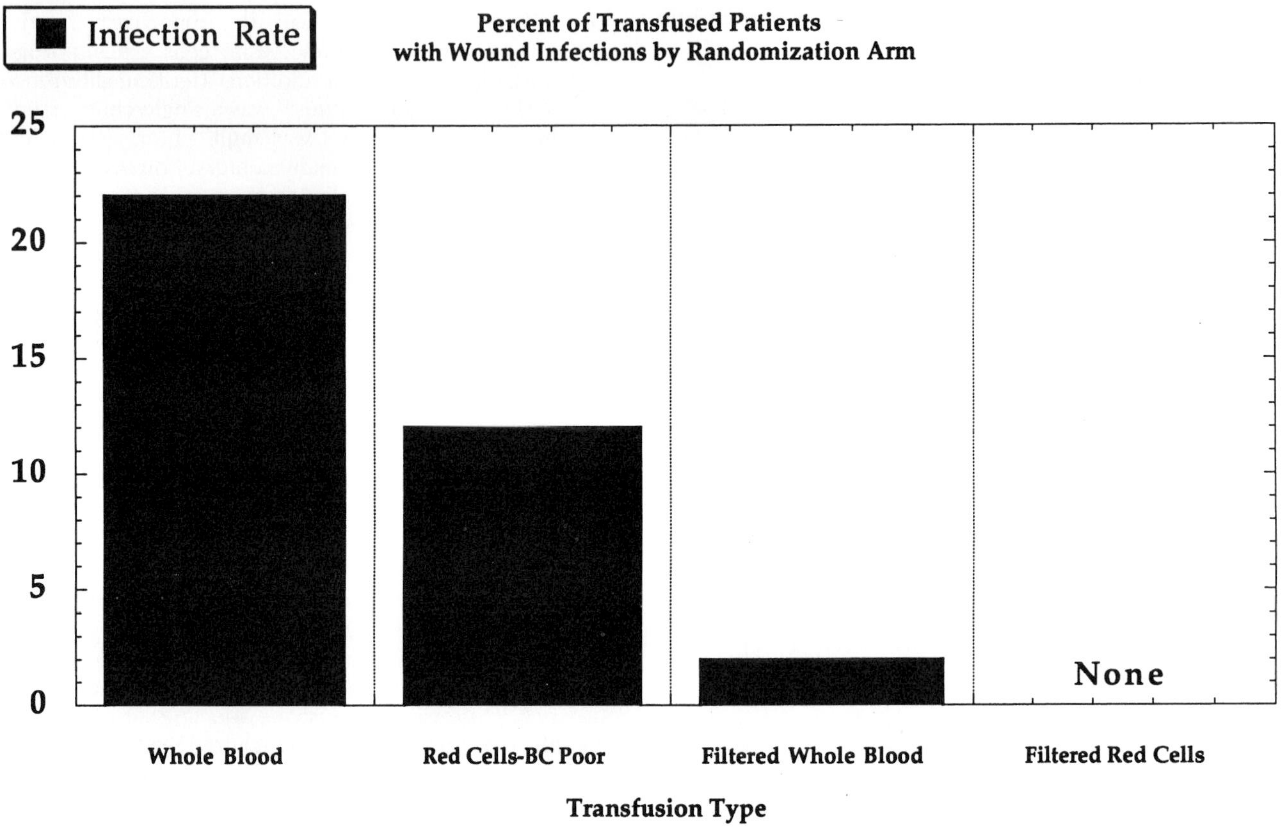

Figure 30–10. The rates of postoperative wound infection are summarized for four randomized groups of patients (from two separate studies) receiving blood components of different degrees of white cell and plasma content.[49, 96] As progressively more white cells (and stored supernatant plasma) are removed, the infection rate decreases; white cell depletion is apparently the major factor. These data from Jensen and coworkers are the most convincing evidence for transfusion immunomodulation's clinical significance.

it difficult to address the hypothesis that transfusion is immunomodulatory, causing Th2 immune deviation, and thus might be beneficial in autoimmune diseases characterized by Th1 responses. There are some modest data to support this concept.

Animal Models

Type I diabetes is an autoimmune disease affecting the pancreas and is apparently due to a Th1-biased cellular immune effector process. It has been shown that transfusion of white blood cell concentrates, particularly T cells, can prevent the spontaneous development of this disease in susceptible animals.[118, 119] Thus the beneficial effects of transfusion may be due to immune deviation toward Th2 immunity and consequent inhibition of Th1 immunity.[120]

Human Patients

Only one study has attempted to use transfusion to alter the course of type I diabetes in humans.[121] This, in large part, failed, perhaps because the transfusions were of

Table 30–2. Estimates of Allogeneic Transfusion Immunomodulation–Related Deaths in the United States Due to Cancer Recurrence and Postoperative Infection

Estimated Proportion of the Effect That Is Causal	Cancer*		Infection†		Total‡	
	Deaths per Year	Death Rate per 10^6 Transfusions	Deaths per Year	Death Rate per 10^6 Transfusions	Deaths per Year	Death Rate per 10^6 Transfusions
100%	20,000	33,000	1500	250	21,500	33,250
50%	10,000	16,667	750	125	10,750	16,892
10%	2000	3300	150	25	2150	3325

*Assumptions: (1) a 10% difference in death rates between transfused and nontransfused patients, (2) mean transfusions per patient = 3, (3) 200,000 transfused cancer patients per year out of approximately 1 million total cancer patients.

†Assumptions: (1) a 15% difference in infection rates between transfused and nontransfused surgical patients, (2) mean transfusions per patient = 3, (3) 6 million transfused surgical patients per year, (4) mortality due to postoperative infection averages 1 in 200 infections.

‡For comparison, Roger Dodd estimates that the number of deaths due to HIV-1 infection from transfusion is currently approximately 2.38 per million units transfused, or about 30 per year total. The corresponding numbers for hepatitis C are a fatality rate of 0.75 to 6.63 per million units, or about 9 to 80 deaths per year total. These data include only red blood cell transfusions.

insufficient dose (one whole blood buffy coat given weekly for 5 weeks), given for too short a period, and given too late in the course of the disease, or because of the inexact analogy between type I diabetes in animals and the same disease in humans. In this randomized study, three remissions (euglycemia without insulin) occurred in two patients, all in the transfusion group, but these remissions were short-lived.

Crohn's disease, an inflammatory bowel disease thought to be primarily Th1 in nature,[122] has been reported to recur less frequently in patients receiving transfusions as part of their surgical treatment (Fig. 30–11).[123] This benefit occurred despite the fact that transfused patients tend to have larger areas of involved bowel to begin with, a factor known to predispose to disease recurrence. Studies in which transfused patients did not have better outcomes of statistical significance, and one negative meta-analysis, have been reported.[124] Nonetheless, the transfused patients in these studies had somewhat lower rates of recurrence despite being at a higher a priori risk for recurrence.[125] The finding of better outcomes in transfused patients with Crohn's disease, despite their poor prognosis, is evidence against the argument that transfused patients with cancer or postoperative infection do poorly merely because of preexisting prognostic factors. If transfusion is merely a surrogate for other prognostic factors, and these factors are the actual predictor of outcomes, transfused patients with Crohn's disease should have significantly worse outcomes, as do cohorts of surgical patients without autoimmune disease, and this is clearly not the case.

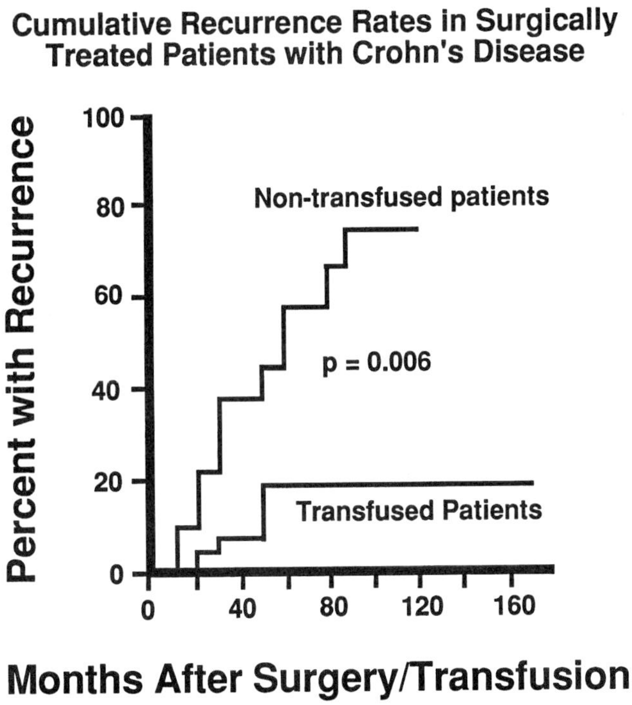

Figure 30–11. Recurrence of Crohn's disease (regional enteritis), a disease with auto-inflammatory characteristics, is shown over the ensuing years for patients who had undergone surgery for their bowel disease. Patients who had received concomitant transfusions perioperatively were significantly less likely to have recurrent disease than were those who did not receive transfusions. This observation suggests a favorable effect of transfusions, hypothetically due to downregulation of the Th1 inflammatory response by transfusion induced immunomodulation. (Adapted with permission from Williams JG, Hughes LE. Effect of perioperative blood transfusion on recurrence of Crohn's disease. Lancet 1989; 2:131.)

Rheumatoid arthritis, a Th1 process in some studies,[126] is also favorably affected by pregnancy and allogeneic white cell transfusions, both of which favor downregulation of Th1 immunity and immune deviation toward a Th2 response.[127, 128]

Miscellaneous Clinical Settings in Which Transfusion Immunomodulation May Play a Role

Recurrent Spontaneous Abortion

Recurrent spontaneous abortion is caused in certain instances by an overly vigorous maternal immune response to paternal antigens present in the fetus. This is at least in part a Th1-mediated process of fetal allograft rejection.[12, 39] Successful pregnancy is associated with Th2 cytokine secretion at the fetal-maternal interface.[38] There are good data, including one controlled randomized trial and a meta-analysis, that suggest that treating recurrent aborters with paternal white cells or blood transfusions improves the likelihood of a successful pregnancy.[129] Thus the immunomodulatory effects of allogeneic transfusion, though clinically modest, can be considered proved in this setting. Mueller-Eckhardt and colleagues reported preliminary evidence that high-dose intravenous IgG infusions may be effective in reducing fetal loss in women with both primary and secondary recurrent spontaneous abortion.[130]

Severity of Viral Infection

Four investigations have suggested that the amount of blood transfused at the time of infection correlates with the rapidity of development of clinically evident HIV-1 disease (acquired immunodeficiency syndrome [AIDS]) in patients infected through transfusion.[131–134] These observations are consonant with the observation that immune deviation toward a Th2 bias favors progression of HIV-1 infection.[135] Likewise, the frequency of seroconversion to CMV appears to be much higher in patients receiving larger amounts of transfused blood.[136] The likelihood of reactivation of previous CMV infection, as indicated by rising antibody titers, appears to be related to the number of units of blood transfused.[137] These observations are compatible with the hypothesis that increased immunomodulation by transfusion can lead to more widespread or severe viral infection after virus transmission or reactivation by transfusion. Given that viral immunity probably requires an intact Th1 immune response, allogeneic transfusion's impairment of such responses, particularly NK and T cell functions, may be an explanation for these observations. A randomized trial of leukocyte-depleted transfusions in HIV-1–infected patients is currently under way.

Effects of Intravenous IgG

There is little doubt that concentrated high-dose intravenous administration of γ globulin (IVIG) is immunomodulatory.[138] The course of many autoimmune diseases, such as autoimmune thrombocytopenia, hemolytic anemia, Kawasaki's disease, and myasthenia gravis, has been reported to be favorably modified by this therapy. It has been shown in a randomized clinical trial that repeated administration of IVIG reduces the incidence of graft-versus-host disease (GVHD) in allogeneic marrow transplant recipients.[88] Consonant with the immunological model of immunomodulation due to IVIG, the same marrow transplant recipients also had a somewhat higher relapse rate for their leukemia. Thus, overall survival was unaffected, with fewer deaths due to acute GVHD in the IVIG group and fewer deaths due to leukemic recurrence in those patients not receiving IVIG.

Whether the immunomodulatory effect of IVIG is mediated by the high levels of monomeric IgG, by smaller contaminating amounts of IgG aggregates, or by copurified biological response modifiers in these infusions is uncertain. The relevance to transfusion-mediated immunomodulation of IgG in stored plasma, whole blood, red cells, or cryoprecipitate is also unknown.

GVHD After Allogeneic Marrow Transplantation

DeGast and colleagues[139] reported that of close to 1000 leukemics receiving HLA-identical sibling transplants, those receiving transfusion within 6 weeks before transplantation had about a 27% lower incidence of chronic GVHD than those with no recent transfusions. This difference remained significant after multivariate analysis of patient age, sex, type of leukemia, stage of disease, and type of GVHD prophylaxis. Because GVHD is probably also a Th1-mediated process, these observations are what would be expected from the immunological effects of allogeneic transfusions.

SUMMARY

Transfusion of allogeneic blood to animals or to human patients is immunomodulatory under many circumstances. Patients with hemophilia, thalassemia, and other disorders requiring multiple transfusions clearly are not immunologically normal, but whether this is owing to viral infection or to transfusion per se is unknown. Whether these changes are of clinical significance is also unknown. There is little evidence to suggest that such patients are at greater risk of infection or malignancy unless they are infected with HIV-1.

Transfused patients are more likely to accept renal allografts. IVIgG recipients are more likely to experience decreased activity of their autoimmune disease. Whole blood recipients have better allograft survival but higher colorectal cancer recurrence rates than similar recipients receiving red cells alone. Allogeneic transfusion recipients are more likely to have postoperative infections than are recipients of identical amounts of autologous transfusion. Recipients of leukocyte-depleted transfusions are less likely to develop postoperative infection than are recipients of buffy coat–poor red cell concentrates. All these observations can be interpreted consistently by the recent finding that many immune processes, including transfusion, can be defined in part by their propensity to foster either Th1- or Th2-predominant responses. Allogeneic transfusions lead to decreased Th1 and increased Th2 cytokine secretion in animal models and in medical and surgical patients. Thus a potential unifying theory of transfusion immunology, including the formation of alloantibodies (primarily a Th2 response), allergic reactions (also Th2 in nature), and downregulation of cellular immunity (a Th2 counterregulated process), can now be proposed for the first time. The single explanation that best fits these clinical and laboratory observations is that allogeneic transfusions cause significant immunomodulation. However, some of these observations have yet to be confirmed in randomized controlled clinical trials, so some caution is still warranted in assuming that all these phenomena are cause and effect. Further study is needed for many of these findings.

REFERENCES

1. Billingham RE, Brent L, Medawar PB. Actively acquired tolerance of foreign cells. Nature 1953; 172:603.
2. Blumberg N, Heal JM. Effects of transfusion on immune function—cancer recurrence and infection. Arch Pathol Lab Med 1994; 118:371.
3. Bordin JO, Heddle NM, Blajchman MA. Biologic effects of leukocytes present in transfused cellular blood products. Blood 1994; 84:1703.
4. Blumberg N, Triulzi DJ, Heal JM. Transfusion-induced immunomodulation and its clinical consequences. Transfus Med Rev 1990; 4:24.
5. Blumberg N, Heal JM. Transfusion and host defenses against cancer recurrence and infection. Transfusion 1989; 29:236.
6. Tartter PI. Immune consequences of blood transfusion in the surgical patient. Surg Immun 1989; 1:13.
7. Tartter PI. Blood transfusion and postoperative infections. Transfusion 1989; 29:456.
8. Tartter PI. Does blood transfusion predispose to cancer recurrence. Am J Clin Oncol 1989; 12:169.
9. Blumberg N, Heal JM. Perioperative blood transfusion and solid tumour recurrence. Blood Rev 1987; 1:219.
10. Triulzi DJ, Blumberg N, Heal JM. Association of transfusion with postoperative bacterial infection. Crit Rev Clin Lab Sci 1990; 28:95.
11. Nielsen HJ. Detrimental effects of perioperative blood transfusion. Br J Surg 1995; 82:582.
12. Wegmann TG, Lin H, Guilbert L, Mosmann TR. Bidirectional cytokine interactions in the maternal-fetal relationship: Is successful pregnancy a T_H2 phenomenon? Immunol Today 1993; 14:353.
13. Blumberg N, Heal JM. The transfusion immunomodulation theory—the Th1/Th2 paradigm and an analogy with pregnancy as a unifying mechanism. Semin Hematol 1996; 33:329.
14. Matzinger P. Tolerance, danger, and the extended family [Review]. Annu Rev Immunol 1994; 12:991.
15. Vliet WC, Dock NL, Davey FR. Factors in the liquid portion of stored blood inhibit the proliferative response in mixed lymphocyte cultures. Transfusion 1989; 29:41.
16. Medawar PB. Immunological tolerance. Nobel lecture, 12 December 1960. Scand J Immunol 1991; 33:337.
17. Felton LD. The significance of antigen in animal tissues. J Immunol 1949; 61:107.
18. Halasz NA, Orloff MJ, Hirose F. Increased survival of renal homografts in dogs after injection of graft donor blood. Transplantation 1964; 2:453.

19. Cecka M, Toyotome A. The transfusion effect. *In* Terasaki PI (ed): Clinical Transplants 1989. Los Angeles: UCLA Tissue Typing Laboratory, 1989, pp 335–341.
20. Blumberg N, Heal JM. Transfusion and recipient immune function. Arch Pathol Lab Med 1989; 113:246.
21. Quigley RL, Wood KJ, Morris PJ. The relative roles of major and minor histocompatibility antigens in the induction of immunologic unresponsiveness by blood transfusion. Transfusion 1989; 29:789.
22. Martin DR, Miller RG. In vivo administration of histoincompatible lymphocytes leads to rapid functional deletion of cytotoxic T lymphocyte precursors. J Exp Med 1989; 170:679.
23. Wood ML, Gottschalk R, Monaco AP. Effect of blood transfusion on IL-2 production. Transplantation 1988; 45:930.
24. Stephan RN, Kisala JM, Dean RE, et al. Effect of blood transfusion on antigen presentation function and on interleukin 2 generation. Arch Surg 1988; 123:235.
25. Ross WB, Leaver HA, Yap PL, et al. Prostaglandin E_2 production by rat peritoneal macrophages: role of cellular and humoral factors in vivo in transfusion-associated immunosuppression. FEMS Microbiol Immunol 1990; 64:321.
26. Kirkley SA, Cowles J, Pellegrini VD Jr, et al. Cytokine secretion after allogeneic or autologous blood transfusion [Letter]. Lancet 1995; 345:527.
27. Blumberg N, Heal JM. Transfusion and the immune system: a paradigm shift in progress? Transfusion 1995; 35:879.
28. Dzik S, Blajchman MA, Blumberg N, et al. Current research on the immunomodulatory effect of allogeneic blood transfusion [Review]. Vox Sang 1996; 70:187.
29. Blumberg N, Heal JM. Immunomodulation by blood transfusion: an evolving scientific and clinical challenge. Am J Med 1996; 101:299.
30. Kalechman Y, Gafter U, Sobelman D, Sredni B. The effect of a single whole-blood transfusion on cytokine secretion. J Clin Immunol 1990; 10:99.
31. Babcock GF, Alexander JW. The effects of blood transfusion on cytokine production by TH1 and TH2 lymphocytes in the mouse. Transplantation 1996; 61:465.
32. Gafter U, Kalechman Y, Sredni B. Blood transfusion enhances production of T-helper-2 cytokines and transforming growth factor b in humans. Clin Sci 1996; 91:519.
33. Heiss MM, Fasolmerten K, Allgayer H, et al. Influence of autologous blood transfusion on natural killer and lymphokine-activated killer cell activities in cancer surgery. Vox Sang 1997; 73:237.
34. Heiss MM, Fraunberger P, Delanoff C, et al. Modulation of immune response by blood transfusion—evidence for a differential effect of allogeneic and autologous blood in colorectal cancer surgery. Shock 1997; 8:402.
35. Dallman MJ. Cytokines and transplantation: Th1/Th2 regulation of the immune response to solid organ transplants in the adult. Curr Opin Immunol 1995; 7:632.
36. Clerici M, Clerici E, Shearer GM. The tumor enhancement phenomenon: reinterpretation from a Th1/Th2 perspective. J Natl Cancer Inst 1996; 88:461.
37. Hill JA, Polgar K, Anderson DJ. T-helper 1–type immunity to trophoblast in women with recurrent spontaneous abortion. JAMA 1995; 273:1933.
38. Piccinni MP, Romagnani S. Regulation of fetal allograft survival by hormone-controlled Th1- and Th2-type cytokines. Immunol Res 1996; 15:141.
39. Mosmann TR, Sad S. The expanding universe of T-cell subsets: Th1, Th2 and more. Immunol Today 1996; 17:138.
40. Kaliss N, Snell GD. The effects of injections of lyophilized normal and neoplastic mouse tissues on the growth of tumor homoisotransplants in mice. Cancer Res 1951; 11:122.
41. Waymack JP, Warden GD, Alexander JW, et al. Effect of blood transfusion and anesthesia on resistance to bacterial peritonitis. J Surg Res 1987; 42:528.
42. Waymack JP, Gallon L, Barcelli U, Alexander JW. Effect of blood transfusions on macrophage function in a burned animal model. Curr Surg 1986; 43:305.
43. Roy G, Pardo A, Leyva-Cobian F. Phenotypic and functional abnormalities in monocytes from patients with haemophilia A treated with factor VIII concentrates. Acta Haematol 1988; 79:26.
44. Thorpe R, Dilger P, Dawson NJ, Barrowcliffe TW. Inhibition of interleukin-2 secretion by factor VIII concentrates: a possible cause of immunosuppression in haemophiliacs. Br J Haematol 1989; 71:387.
45. Hay CRM, McEvoy P, Duggan-Keen M. Inhibition of lymphocyte IL2-receptor expression by factor VIII concentrate: a possible cause of immunosuppression in haemophiliacs. Br J Haematol 1990; 75:278.
46. Nielsen HJ, Hammer JH, Moesgaard F, Kehlet H. Comparison of the effects of SAG-M and whole-blood transfusions on postoperative suppression of delayed hypersensitivity. Can J Surg 1991; 34:146.
47. Decker D, Schöndorf M, Bidlingmaier F, et al. Surgical stress induces a shift in the type-1/type-2 T-helper cell balance, suggesting down-regulation of cell-mediated and up-regulation of antibody-mediated immunity commensurate to the trauma. Surgery 1996; 119:316.
48. Heiss MM, Mempel W, Jauch K-W, et al. Beneficial effect of autologous blood transfusion on infectious complications after colorectal cancer surgery. Lancet 1993; 342:1328.
49. Jensen LS, Andersen AJ, Christiansen PM, et al. Postoperative infection and natural killer cell function following blood transfusion in patients undergoing elective colorectal surgery. Br J Surg 1992; 79:513.
50. Jensen LS, Hokland M, Nielsen HJ. A randomized controlled study of the effect of bedside leucocyte depletion on the immunosuppressive effect of whole blood transfusion in patients undergoing elective colorectal surgery. Br J Surg 1996; 83:973.
51. George CD, Morello PJ. Immunologic effects of blood transfusion upon renal transplantation, tumor operations and bacterial infections. Am J Surg 1986; 152:329.
52. Opelz G. Current relevance of the transfusion effect in renal transplantation. Transplant Proc 1985; 17:1015.
53. Kerman RH, Van Buren CT, Lewis RM, Kahan BD. Blood transfusion experience for cyclosporine/prednisone-treated renal allograft recipients at the University of Texas Medical School at Houston. *In* Terasaki PI (ed): Clinical Kidney Transplants 1988. Los Angeles: UCLA Tissue Typing Laboratory, 1988; pp 167–170.
54. Buelow R, Burlingham WJ, Clayberger C. Immunomodulation by soluble HLA class I. Transplantation 1995; 59:649.
55. Cuturi M-C, Josien R, Douillard P, et al. Prolongation of allogeneic heart graft survival in rats by administration of a peptide (a.a. 75-84) from the a1 helix of the first domain of HLA-B7 01. Transplantation 1995; 59:661.
56. Shelby J, Marushack MM, Nelson EW. Prostaglandin production and suppressor cell induction in transfusion-induced immune suppression. Transplantation 1987; 43:113.
57. Dallman MJ, Wood KJ, Morris PJ. Recombinant interleukin-2 (IL-2) can reverse the blood transfusion effect. Transplant Proc 1989; 21:1165.
58. Lagaaij EL, Hennemann IPH, Ruigrok M, et al. Effect of one-HLA-DR-antigen-matched and completely HLA-DR mismatched blood transfusions on survival of heart and kidney allografts. N Engl J Med 1989; 321:701.
59. Davis CJ, Ilstrup DM, Pemberton JH. Influence of splenectomy on survival rate of patients with colorectal cancer. Am J Surg 1988; 155:173.
60. Maeurer MJ, Martin DM, Castelli C, et al. Host immune response in renal cell cancer: interleukin-4 (IL-4) and IL-10 mRNA are frequently detected in freshly collected tumor-infiltrating lymphocytes. Cancer Immunol Immunother 1995; 41:111.
61. Pellegrini P, Berghella AM, Del Beato T, et al. Disregulation in TH1 and TH2 subsets of CD4+ T cells in peripheral blood of colorectal cancer patients and involvement in cancer establishment and progression. Cancer Immunol Immunother 1996; 42:1.
62. Lowes MA, Bishop GA, Crotty K, Barnetson RS, Halliday GM. T helper 1 cytokine mRNA is increased in spontaneously regressing primary melanomas. J Invest Dermatol 1997; 108:914.
63. Lee PP, Zeng DF, Mccaulay AE, et al. T helper 2–dominant antilymphoma immune response is associated with fatal outcome. Blood 1997; 90:1611.
64. Chouaib S, Asselinpaturel C, Mamichouaib F, et al. The host-tumor immune conflict—from immunosuppression to resistance and destruction. Immunol Today 1997; 18:493.
65. Fujioka T, Kudo T, Ishikura K, et al. Clinical efficacy of recombinant interleukin-2 for renal cell carcinoma and the effect of blood transfusion upon the immune response of these patients. Jpn J Urol 1990; 81:296.

66. Narisawa T, Kusaka H, Yamazaki Y, et al. Relationship between blood plasma prostaglandin E_2 and liver and lung metastases in colorectal cancer. Dis Colon Rectum 1990; 33:840.
67. Waymack JP, Fernandes G, Yurt RW, et al. Effect of blood transfusions on immune function. Part VI. Effect on immunologic response to tumor. Surgery 1990; 108:172.
68. Parrott NR, Lennard TWJ, Proud G, et al. Blood transfusion and surgery: the effect on growth of a syngeneic sarcoma. Ann R Coll Surg Engl 1990; 72:77.
69. Blajchman MA, Bardossy L, Carmen R, et al. Allogeneic blood transfusion–induced enhancement of tumor growth: two animal models showing amelioration by leukodepletion and passive transfer using spleen cells. Blood 1993; 81:1880.
70. Antibiotics as biological response modifiers [Editorial]. Lancet 1991; 337:400.
71. Burrows L, Tartter P. Effect of blood transfusions on colonic malignancy recurrence rate [Letter]. Lancet 1982; 2:662.
72. Heiss MM, Mempel W, Delanoff C, et al. Blood transfusion modulated tumor recurrence: first results of a randomized study of autologous versus allogeneic blood transfusion in colorectal cancer surgery. J Clin Oncol 1994; 12:1859.
73. Busch ORC, Hop WCJ, Hoynck van Papendrecht MAW, et al. Blood transfusions and prognosis in colorectal cancer. N Engl J Med 1993; 328:1372.
74. Houbiers JGA, Brand A, Van de Watering LMG, et al. Randomised controlled trial comparing transfusion of leucocyte-depleted or buffy-coat-depleted blood in surgery for colorectal cancer. Lancet 1994; 344:573.
75. Oksanen K, Elonen E. Impact of leukocyte-depleted blood components on the haematological recovery and prognosis of patients with acute myeloid leukaemia. Br J Haematol 1993; 84:639.
76. Blumberg N, Heal JM, Rowe JM, Kirkley SA. Reduced morbidity and mortality in acute leukemia associated with leukodepleted blood transfusions [Abstract]. Blood 1997; 90(suppl 1):155a.
77. Blumberg N, Heal JM, Murphy P, et al. Association between transfusion of whole blood and recurrence of cancer. BMJ 1986; 293:530.
78. Blumberg N, Heal JM, Chuang C, et al. Further evidence supporting a cause and effect relationship between blood transfusion and cancer recurrence. Ann Surg 1988; 207:410.
79. Hermanek P Jr, Guggenmoos-Holzmann I, Schricker KT, et al. The influence of blood and hemoderivatives on the prognosis of colorectal carcinoma. Langenbecks Arch Chir 1989; 374:118.
80. Wobbes T, Joosen KHG, Kuypers HHC, et al. The effect of packed cells and whole blood transfusions on survival after curative resection for colorectal carcinoma. Dis Colon Rectum 1989; 32:743.
81. Marsh J, Donnan PT, Hamer-Hodges DW. Association between transfusion with plasma and the recurrence of colorectal carcinoma. Br J Surg 1990; 77:623.
82. Horimi T, Terasaki PI, Chia D, Sasaki N. Factors influencing the paradoxical effect of transfusions on kidney transplants. Transplantation 1983; 35:320.
83. Cerhan JR, Wallace RB, Folsom AR, et al. Transfusion history and cancer risk in older women. Ann Intern Med 1993; 119:8.
84. Cerhan JR, Wallace RB, Folsom AR, et al. Medical history risk factors for non-Hodgkins lymphoma in older women. J Natl Cancer Inst 1997; 89:314.
85. Chung M, Steinmetz OK, Gordon PH. Perioperative blood transfusion and outcome after resection for colorectal carcinoma. Br J Surg 1993; 80:427.
86. Vamvakas E, Moore SB. Perioperative blood transfusion and colorectal cancer recurrence: a qualitative statistical overview and meta-analysis. Transfusion 1993; 33:754.
87. Amato A, Pescatori M. Reported noncausal effect of blood transfusions on colorectal cancer recurrence [Letter]. Ann Surg 1997; 225:129.
88. Sullivan KM, Kopecky KJ, Jacom J, et al. Immunomodulatory and antimicrobial efficacy of intravenous immunoglobulin in bone marrow transplantation. N Engl J Med 1990; 323:705.
89. Kaveri S, Vassilev T, Hurez V, et al. Antibodies to a conserved region of HLA class molecules, capable of modulating CD8 T cell–mediated function, are present in pooled normal immunoglobulin for therapeutic use. J Clin Invest 1996; 97:865.
90. Ludwin D, Joseph S, Singal DP. MLC-inhibiting serum in mice after transfusion with 3 M KCI-extracted soluble antigen. J Surg Res 1987; 43:436.
91. Madsen JC, Superina RA, Wood KJ, Morris PJ. Immunological unresponsiveness induced by recipient cells transfected with donor MHC genes. Nature 1988; 332:161.
92. Clayberger C, Krensky AM. Immunosuppressive peptides corresponding to MHC class I sequences. Curr Opin Immunol 1995; 7:644.
93. Virgin HW IV, Kurt-Jones EA, Wittenberg GF, Unanue ER. Immune complex effects on murine macrophages. II. Immune complex effects on activated macrophages cytotoxicity, membrane IL 1, and antigen presentation. J Immunol 1985; 135:3744.
94. Berger S, Chandra R, Ballo H, et al. Immune complexes are potent inhibitors of interleukin-12 secretion by human monocytes. Eur J Immunol 1997; 27:2994.
95. Hoh H, Umpleby H, Cooper A, Taylor I. Recurrence of colorectal cancer and perioperative blood transfusion. Is blood storage time important? Dis Colon Rectum 1990; 33:127.
96. Jensen LS, Kissmeyer-Nielsen P, Wolff B, Qvist N. Randomised comparison of leucocyte-depleted versus buffy-coat-poor blood transfusion and complications after colorectal surgery. Lancet 1996; 348:841.
97. Van der Watering LMG, Hermans J, Houbiers JGA, et al. Beneficial effects of leukocyte depletion of transfused blood on postoperative complications in patients undergoing cardiac surgery. Circulation 1998; 97:562.
98. Waymack JP, Miskell P, Gonce S. Alterations in host defense associated with inhalation anesthesia and blood transfusion. Anesth Analg 1989; 69:163.
99. Waymack JP, Rapien J, Garnett D, et al. Effect of transfusion on immune function in a traumatized animal model. Arch Surg 1986; 121:50.
100. Waymack JP, Yurt RW. The effect of blood transfusions on immune function. V. The effect on the inflammatory response to bacterial infections. J Surg Res 1990; 48:147.
101. Ayala A, Perrin MM, Wagner MA, Chaudry IH. Enhanced susceptibility to sepsis after simple hemorrhage. Arch Surg 1990; 125:70.
102. Gianotti L, Pyles T, Alexander JW, et al. Identification of the blood component responsible for increased susceptibility to gut-derived infection. Transfusion 1993; 33:458.
103. Tascini C, Baldelli F, Monari C, et al. Inhibition of fungicidal activity of polymorphonuclear leukocytes from HIV-infected patients by interleukin (IL)-4 and IL-10. AIDS 1996; 10:477.
104. Roilides E, Kadiltsoglou I, Dimitriadou A, et al. Interleukin-4 suppresses antifungal activity of human mononuclear phagocytes against *Candida albicans* in association with decreased uptake of blastoconidia. FEMS Immunol Med Microbiol 1997; 19:169.
105. Tartter PI. Blood transfusion and infectious complications following colorectal cancer surgery. Br J Surg 1988; 75:789.
106. Tartter PI, Driefuss RM, Malon AM, et al. Relationship of postoperative septic complications and blood transfusions in patients with Crohn's disease. Am J Surg 1988; 155:43.
107. Vamvakas EC, Moore SB. Blood transfusion and postoperative septic complications. Transfusion 1994; 34:714.
108. Murphy P, Heal JM, Blumberg N. Infection or suspected infection after hip replacement surgery with autologous or homologous transfusions. Transfusion 1991; 31:212.
109. Triulzi DJ, Vanek K, Ryan DH, Blumberg N. A clinical and immunologic study of blood transfusion and postoperative bacterial infection in spinal surgery. Transfusion 1992; 32:517.
110. Murphy PJ, Connery C, Hicks GL Jr, Blumberg N. Homologous blood transfusion as a risk factor for postoperative infection after coronary artery bypass graft operations. J Thorac Cardiovasc Surg 1992; 104:1092.
111. Vamvakas EC, Carven JH. Allogeneic blood transfusion, hospital charges, and length of hospitalization—a study of 487 consecutive patients undergoing colorectal cancer resection. Arch Pathol Lab Med 1998; 122:145.
112. Jensen LS, Andersen A, Fristrup SC, et al. Comparison of one dose versus three doses of prophylactic antibiotics, and the influence of blood transfusion, on infectious complications in acute and elective colorectal surgery. Br J Surg 1990; 77:513.
113. Castaldo P, Stratta RJ, Wood RP, et al. Clinical spectrum of fungal infections after orthotopic liver transplantation. Arch Surg 1991; 126:149.

114. Simchen E, Zucker D, Siegman IY, Galai N. Method for separating patient and procedural factors while analyzing interdepartmental differences in rates of surgical infections: the Israeli study of surgical infection in abdominal operations. J Clin Epidemiol 1996; 49:1003.
115. Van der Watering LMG, Houbiers JGA, Hermans J, et al. Leukocyte depletion reduces postoperative mortality in patients undergoing cardiac surgery [Abstract]. Br J Haematol 1996; 93(suppl 2):312.
116. Jensen LS, Grunnet N, Hanberg-Sorensen F, Jorgensen J. Cost-effectiveness of blood transfusion and white cell reduction in elective colorectal surgery. Transfusion 1995; 35:719.
117. Blumberg N, Kirkley SA, Heal JM. A cost analysis of autologous and allogeneic transfusions in hip-replacement surgery. Am J Surg 1996; 171:324.
118. Rossini AA, Mordes JP, Pelletier AM, Like AA. Transfusions of whole blood prevent spontaneous diabetes mellitus in the BB/W rat. Science 1983; 219:975.
119. Mordes JP, Gallina DL, Handler ES, et al. Transfusions enriched for W 3/25$^+$ helper/inducer T lymphocytes prevent spontaneous diabetes in the BB/W rat. Diabetologia 1987; 30:22.
120. Cameron MJ, Arreaza GA, Zucker P, et al. IL-4 prevents insulitis and insulin-dependent diabetes mellitus in nonobese diabetic mice by potentiation of regulatory T helper-2 cell function. J Immunol 1997; 159:4686.
121. Cavanaugh J, Chopek M, Binimelis J. Buffy coat transfusions in early type I diabetes. Diabetes 1987; 36:1089.
122. Plevy SE, Landers CJ, Prehn J, Carramanzana NM, Deem RL, Shealy D. A role for TNF-alpha and mucosal T helper-1 cytokines in the pathogenesis of Crohn's disease. J Immunol 1997; 159:6276.
123. Williams JG, Hughes LE. Effect of perioperative blood transfusion on recurrence of Crohn's disease. Lancet 1989; 2:131.
124. Hollaar GL, Gooszen HG, Post S, et al. Perioperative blood transfusion does not prevent recurrence in Crohn's disease—a pooled analysis. J Clin Gastroenterol 1995; 21:134.
125. Scott ADN, Ritchie JK, Phillips RKS. Blood transfusion and recurrent Crohn's disease. Br J Surg 1991; 78:455.
126. Dolhain RJEM, Vanderheiden AN, Terhaar NT, et al. Shift toward T lymphocytes with a T helper 1 cytokine-secretion profile in the joints of patients with rheumatoid arthritis. Arthritis Rheum 1996; 39:1961.
127. Smith JB, Fort JG. Treatment of rheumatoid arthritis by immunization with mononuclear white blood cells: results of a preliminary trial. J Rheumatol 1996; 23:220.
128. Russell AS, Johnston C, Chew C, Maksymowych WP. Evidence for reduced Th1 function in normal pregnancy—a hypothesis for the remission of rheumatoid arthritis. J Rheumatol 1997; 24:1045.
129. Mowbray JF, Liddell H, Underwood JL, et al. Controlled trial of treatment of recurrent spontaneous abortion by immunisation with paternal cells. Lancet 1985; 1:941.
130. Mueller-Eckhardt G, Heine O, Polten B. IVIG to prevent recurrent spontaneous abortion [Letter]. Lancet 1991; 337:424.
131. Blumberg N, Heal JM. Evidence for plasma-mediated immunomodulation—transfusions of plasma-rich blood components are associated with a greater risk of acquired immunodeficiency syndrome than transfusions of red blood cells alone. Transplant Proc 1988; 20:1138.
132. Ward JW, Bush TJ, Perkins HA, et al. The natural history of transfusion-associated infection with human immunodeficiency virus: factors influencing the rate of progression to disease. N Engl J Med 1989; 321:947.
133. Vamvakas E, Kaplan HS. Early transfusion and length of survival in AIDS: experience with a population receiving medical care at a public hospital. Transfusion 1993; 33:111.
134. Sloand E, Kumar P, Klein HG, et al. Transfusion of blood components to persons infected with human immunodeficiency virus type 1: relationship to opportunistic infection. Transfusion 1994; 34:48.
135. Mosmann TR. Cytokine patterns during the progression of AIDS. Science 1994; 265:193.
136. Preiksaitis JK, Brown L, McKenzie M. The risk of cytomegalovirus infection in seronegative transfusion recipients not receiving exogenous immunosuppression. J Infect Dis 1988; 157:523.
137. Adler SP, McVoy MM. Cytomegalovirus infections in seropositive patients after transfusion: the effect of red cell storage and volume. Transfusion 1989; 29:667.
138. Boshov LK, Kelton JG. Use of intravenous gammaglobulin as an immune replacement and an immune suppressant. Transfus Med Rev 1989; 3:82.
139. deGast GC, Beatty PG, Amos D, et al. Transfusions shortly before HLA-matched marrow transplantation for leukemia are associated with a decrease in chronic graft-versus-host disease. Bone Marrow Transplant 1991; 7:293.
140. Vamvakas EC. Perioperative blood transfusion and cancer recurrence: meta-analysis for explanation. Transfusion 1995; 35:760.

CHAPTER 31

Mechanisms Underlying the Immunomodulatory Effect of Allogeneic Blood Transfusion

Sunny Dzik

It is now widely accepted that some form of immunomodulation may result as a consequence of blood transfusion. The concept of tolerance induction by transfusion has been recognized for nearly half a century. In 1953 Billingham and colleagues demonstrated that the injection of adult allogeneic tissue into fetal mice resulted in the induction of tolerance and the acceptance of skin grafts from the donor strain mice.[1] In the 1970s blood transfusions given before renal allografting were found to improve post-transplant allograft survival. Since then, numerous observations—both clinical and experimental—have gradually increased our understanding of the immune consequences of allogeneic blood transfusion. With the advent of technology for the preparation of leukocyte-depleted blood components in the 1980s, additional research has focused on the role of recipient exposure to allogeneic donor leukocytes as a mediator of transfusion-associated immunomodulation. However, the exact mechanisms by which transfusions may exert a tolerogenic effect have remained elusive. Experimental evidence has been conflicting, often difficult to reproduce, or confined to certain animal models. The scientific literature on the topic is broad, and this chapter reviews only selected publications on the major mechanisms considered responsible for transfusion-associated immunomodulation. Interested readers are directed to additional reviews on this topic.[2–5]

Several specific clinical conditions have been the subject of most investigation into the immunomodulatory effect of transfusion. These include the induction of tolerance before solid organ transplantation, the enhancement of tumor relapse, the development of postoperative bacterial infections, the amelioration of inflammatory bowel disease, and the potential to prevent immune-mediated fetal loss. Clinical studies in these areas have, for the most part, been retrospective analyses, and there are few prospective randomized clinical trials. As a result, it is important to consider the possible effect of clinical confounders that might either obscure or enhance an effect of transfusion.[6, 7] Although the limitations of clinical studies do not allow firm conclusions to be drawn regarding transfusion-associated immunomodulation, there exists a strong experimental literature that has used animal models (especially rodents) to examine the possible mechanisms. These studies have provided key insights into the immune consequences of blood transfusion, although rodent systems also carry some limitations. Transfusions given in animal systems are frequently given as fresh heparinized blood transfusions and may not reflect the character of blood that is given clinically. Donors and recipients in animal models are nearly always inbred strains and may carry restricted major histocompatibility complex (MHC) haplotypes not typical of the human transfusion experience. Other parallels between the rodent and human immune system are not precise. For example, Busch and colleagues observed that transfusion from C57BL6 mice (H-2k) to BALB/c mice (H-2d) resulted in persistence of donor leukocytes for 1 to 3 months after transfusion.[8] In contrast, studies in humans have found that donor leukocytes do not generally persist for more than 1 week.[9] Moreover, conditioning regimens involving blood transfusion that induce tolerance to organ allografts in specific rodent models are often unable to reproduce tolerance in higher primate models. Thus, readers should be cautious about translating the results of preclinical experimental data regarding immune mechanisms of the transfusion effect to humans.

The mechanisms of clonal deletion, anergy, and immune suppression can account for many of the observed experimental findings suggesting that allogeneic transfusions exert an immunomodulatory effect on recipients. Clonal deletion refers to the elimination of alloreactive clones. Removal of reactive clones may occur in the thymus gland (referred to as central clonal deletion) or outside the thymus (referred to as peripheral clonal deletion). In contrast to clonal deletion, in which cells are physically destroyed, anergy refers to immune nonresponsiveness in the presence of stimulators. Immune suppression refers to mechanisms in which the responding cell is prevented from reacting as a result of an external negative stimulus, such as that of a suppressive cytokine.

OVERVIEW OF EXPERIMENTAL VARIABLES IN THE INDUCTION OF TOLERANCE BY TRANSFUSION

Several important variables affect the likelihood and extent of immune effect from pretransplant transfusion protocols. These include the immune conditioning of the recipient, the MHC relationship between donor and recipient, the presentation of antigen, the persistence of antigen, and the immune stability of the recipient. The original experimental induction of tolerance was done in a fetal mouse system, and subsequent experiments have verified that tolerance is more readily established in the immature immune system of a neonatal animal compared with an adult animal. Tolerance induction in the adult always requires some form of immune conditioning before transfusion. Numerous regimens exist and include the use of antithymocyte globulin, anti–T cell monoclonals, chemotherapy agents, or other immunosuppressive treatments. The extent to which a sufficient degree of immune conditioning exists in the setting of routine blood transfusions is speculative.

The MHC relationship between donor and recipient is a key variable in the induction of immune tolerance by transfusion. Rodent tolerance models document that an immunomodulatory effect may be limited to certain strain combinations. Moreover, tolerance induction is frequently donor-specific and thus limited to the MHC type of the donor. Because inbred animals are generally homozygous for MHC antigens, they present a restricted set of haplotypes to the recipient. Although the circumstances in human transfusion are clearly more complex owing to the far greater diversity of outbred MHC combinations, there is evidence from clinical research that the histocompatibility relationship between blood donor and recipient is relevant to the induction of tolerance by transfusion. For example, van Twuyver and colleagues studied 23 untransfused first-time renal transplant candidates who were deliberately transfused with donor-specific transfusions of fresh blood containing donor leukocytes.[10] Cytotoxic T cell precursors (CTL_p) specifically directed against donor-type antigens were studied 1 month following transfusion. Ten of the 23 recipients demonstrated a significant decrease in CTL_p frequency. Among these 10, 9 were found to have a one-haplotype human leukocyte antigen (HLA) match (or HLA-B and HLA-DR match) between the blood donor and recipient. However, subsequent studies from other laboratories could not confirm an effect on CTL_p frequency as a result of HLA-matched transfusions.[11, 12] Other evidence for the role of MHC similarity between donor and recipient comes from Leivestad and Thorsby, who investigated one-haplotype-matched transfusions and showed evidence for donor-specific suppression of in vitro mixed lymphocyte responses following transfusion.[13] One possible clue to the discrepancy in observed experimental findings comes from the work of Breur-Vriesendorp and colleagues, who found that immune responsiveness may depend not only on the degree of HLA matching but also on the particular HLA antigens that are mismatched between the donor and recipient.[14] This finding is akin to the strain specificity observed in animal models. Because of the complexity of the human MHC, clinical studies that seek to observe global changes in immune parameters following transfusion may fail to detect effects that are specific to particular donor-recipient combinations.[12, 15]

The route, dose, timing, and presentation of alloantigen all affect the likelihood of immune suppression following transfusion. The repeated subcutaneous injection of small doses of an antigen in the presence of an immunological adjuvant is an effective way to provoke an alloimmune response in many animals. In contrast, blood transfusion represents the direct intravenous presentation of a high dose of alloantigen—conditions that in some experimental systems result in high-zone tolerance. Because the spleen and the liver are the major organs to receive intravenously administered alloantigen, these organs may be central to immune reactions to transfusion. Studies in mice have induced transplant tolerance by transfusion of allogeneic leukocytes into the portal circulation of the recipient.[16] Numerous studies demonstrate that splenic lymphocytes may be particularly important in the development of immune suppression after blood transfusion. The timing of antigen also affects the likelihood of transfusion-induced immune tolerance. Studies of transplant tolerance in mice have documented that a critical period exists between administration of immunosuppression plus donor-specific blood transfusions and a successful organ transplant.[17] At the cellular level, antigen presentation plays a critical role in the immunological outcome of alloantigen delivered by transfusion. Antigen-presenting cells (APCs) display allopeptides within the structure of the MHC molecule. These cells also display important costimulatory molecules and release cytokines that promote an alloimmune response. As discussed later in this chapter, experimental studies have demonstrated that suppression of the immune response may occur in the absence of costimulation and in the context of down-regulating cytokines.

The persistence of donor antigen is a common experimental requirement for the induction of transplant tolerance. Antigen that is introduced to the immune system once or repeatedly (but intermittently) is more likely to induce an alloimmune response. In contrast, chronic exposure to persistent antigen is more likely to induce tolerance. Thus, most experimental models for the induction of transplant tolerance require persistence of donor antigen. Whether or not donor antigen persists chronically after blood transfusion is an area of active investigation and is discussed later in the section on microchimerism. Finally, stability of the recipient immune system appears to be important for the maintenance of immune tolerance. Experimental models of transplant tolerance demonstrate a breakdown of tolerance during times of immune reactivity or stimulation, as occurs with infection, immune rechallenge, or additional allografting. Such "provocation" of the immune system may result in cytokine patterns that are unfavorable for the maintenance of tolerance.

PERSISTENCE OF DONOR ANTIGEN: THE CONTROVERSIAL ROLE OF MICROCHIMERISM

In the last decade, studies by Starzl and colleagues renewed interest in the potential role of *microchimerism* as a mediator of allograft tolerance.[18] Microchimerism refers to the low-level persistence of donor cells in the tolerant recipient. Studies from several laboratories have confirmed without any doubt that microchimerism occurs following solid organ transplantation. Donor leukocytes migrate out of the allograft and can be found in the spleen, lymph nodes, skin, and other tissue of the recipient. Using either molecular techniques or sensitive immunohistochemical stains, these donor cells can be detected for decades after transplantation. Although no one disputes the presence of microchimerism after solid organ transplantation, there remains controversy over whether the development of microchimerism is a cause of transplantation tolerance or simply evidence of its effect.

It is also controversial whether donor cell microchimerism occurs following blood transfusion. Schechter and associates used a rather insensitive cytogenic assay but were able to document the persistence of donor cells for at least 1 week after transfusion.[19] Adams and colleagues used polymerase chain reaction (PCR) to study the duration of donor-type DNA after routine transfusion and found a positive signal for only 5 to 7 days.[9] However, that study did not examine fresh blood transfusions, and no attempt was made to control for the HLA relationship between donor and recipient. In fact, the development of mononuclear cell microchimerism following transfusion may depend on the number of viable donor cells transfused, the immune status of the recipient, and the HLA relationship between donor and recipient.[20] More recently, Busch and colleagues reported preliminary evidence for extended donor cell microchimerism as a result of transfusion.[21] Using a PCR-based assay that amplified the HLA type of the donor, they found evidence for persistence of donor cells for up to 1.5 years after transfusion. These transfusions, in contrast to those in the study by Adams, occurred in the setting of trauma and consisted of relatively fresh blood that had been stored for less than 1 week. The fresh nature of the transfusions may have increased the number of viable donor cells infused. The blood components were not gamma irradiated. Of note, among those recipients in whom long-term microchimerism was detected, the blood donor and recipient were found to share some HLAs. No obvious immune downregulation or graft-versus-host disease was detected in these recipients. Additional work from the same laboratory highlighted the importance of sample processing to avoid contamination of the PCR amplifications.[22]

Although not the same as a clinical blood transfusion, fetal-maternal hemorrhage may represent a useful model of "fresh transfusion" that occurs under conditions favorable to the development of donor cell microchimerism. By definition, fetal cells transferred to the maternal circulation are HLA haploidentical with the mother, are fresh, and are rich in hematopoietic progenitors. Such cells might be expected to survive in the mother. Bianchi and associates reported long-term microchimerism in women who had given birth to male children.[23] Using PCR to detect the presence of Y-gene DNA, they found positive PCR signals when DNA was extracted from the stem cell fraction of maternal blood. Among eight women tested, six were found to have male-type DNA among the $CD34^+/CD38^+$ fraction of cells, including one subject with persistent male-type DNA more than 27 years after the birth of her male child. The results of studies such as these suggest that recipient exposure to HLA-similar allogeneic stem cells at the time of transfusion may lead to persistence of donor antigen and the opportunity for the induction of tolerance. More research is needed to assess the importance of donor cell microchimerism as a mediator or consequence of transfusion-induced immunomodulation.

CLONAL DELETION AND THE ROLE OF CENTRAL THYMIC TOLERANCE

Protein antigens are broken into small peptide units by APCs. These peptides are deposited in the peptide-binding groove of the MHC structure for presentation to alloreactive T cells. Under normal conditions, individuals are tolerant to self-antigens. The thymus is the major site for development of self-tolerance. T cells directed against self are deleted in the thymus. The process of clonal deletion of autoreactive T cells is depicted in Figure 31–1A. In the cortex of the thymus, developing T cells phenotypically characterized as $CD3^+;CD4^-;CD8^-$ un-

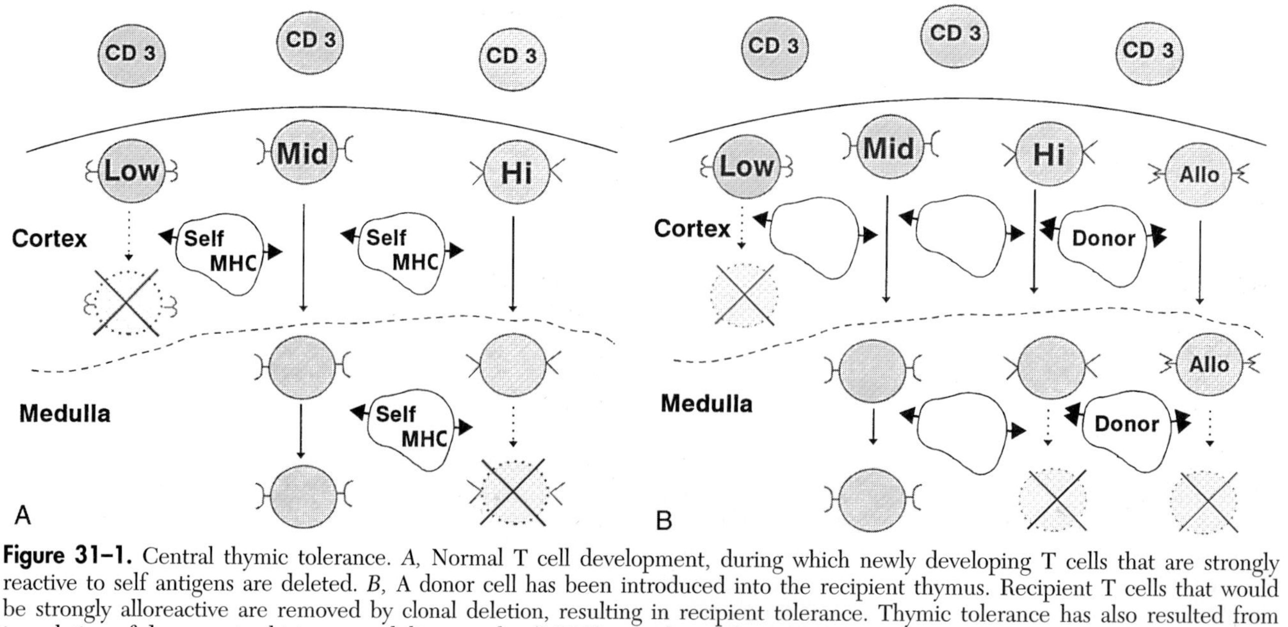

Figure 31–1. Central thymic tolerance. *A*, Normal T cell development, during which newly developing T cells that are strongly reactive to self antigens are deleted. *B*, A donor cell has been introduced into the recipient thymus. Recipient T cells that would be strongly alloreactive are removed by clonal deletion, resulting in recipient tolerance. Thymic tolerance has also resulted from inoculation of donor major histocompatibility complex (MHC) peptides or donor DNA.

dergo combinatory gene rearrangement of their T cell antigen receptor (TCR). The expressed TCR encounters APCs in the cortex that express self-MHC antigens. Positive contact at this stage of T cell development is required to sustain that development and ensures some degree of MHC restriction between T cells and self-MHC. The developing T cells then migrate to the thymic medulla, where they undergo further differentiation into either $CD4^+$ or $CD8^+$ cells. In the medulla, autoreactive T cells are eliminated. High-affinity binding between the TCR and APCs expressing self-MHC results in apoptosis of the T cell.

The powerful role of the thymus as an organ for deletion of autoreactive T cell clones has been used by investigators seeking to induce transplant tolerance.[24, 25] The strategy is to introduce donor antigen in the thymus. A recipient T cell whose TCR binds with high affinity to the donor alloantigen would then be eliminated in the same manner as when T cells encounter self-antigen. Thus, T cells that would otherwise have been strongly alloreactive to donor antigen are clonally deleted (see Fig. 31–1*B*). Several experimental models have documented that this strategy can effectively induce tolerance to foreign MHC antigens. Investigators have achieved transplant tolerance by injecting donor cells or donor MHC peptides into the recipient thymus. For example, Campos and colleagues studied rejection of liver transplants among inbred but MHC-disparate rats.[26] DA rat livers were transplanted into Lewis rat recipients. When only antilymphocyte globulin was used as immunosuppression, the donor livers survived only 29 days. However, if 5×10^7 donor bone marrow cells were injected into the recipient thymus in addition to the antilymphocyte globulin, the donor liver allograft was accepted indefinitely. The tolerance-inducing effect of donor inoculation into the recipient thymus was found to be MHC (strain) specific, and transplants from a third strain were promptly rejected. It was also found that intravenous infusion of donor bone marrow cells rather than intrathymic inoculation was far less effective at inducing tolerance but nevertheless resulted in allograft acceptance that was significantly longer than in control animals who did not receive any transfusion. This study demonstrated principles common to several studies of thymic-induced tolerance, including the need for anti–T cell conditioning therapy, the MHC-specific nature of the induced tolerance, and the better results obtained with thymic injection compared with intravenous injection. Central tolerance to donor antigens has been demonstrated by investigators using injections into the recipient thymus of donor spleen cells, islet cells, kidney cells, and muscle cells.[27–30] Further research has demonstrated that central thymic tolerance can be induced by injecting donor MHC peptide rather than intact cells into the recipient thymus.[31–35] The injected donor peptides, once taken up by resident APCs in the thymus, presumably directed the clonal deletion of alloreactive T cells in a manner similar to that achieved with intact donor cells.

Might central thymic tolerance account for some of the suggested immunomodulatory effect of allogeneic blood transfusion? There is no direct proof in humans that immunomodulation after transfusion results from thymic-based tolerance. However, it is possible that either donor cells or donor plasma proteins could enter the thymic circulation and undergo uptake and processing by APCs within the thymus. Soluble HLA proteins are known to exist in human plasma and could be one source of peptides suitable for recipient thymic processing. This would provide one possible explanation to support those studies that have suggested that transfusion-associated immunomodulation results from recipient exposure to plasma-containing blood components. However, transfusion-induced immunomodulation has been suggested to occur in adult transfusion recipients in whom the thymus gland has largely involuted. Blood transfusions given before thymectomy surgery in patients with myasthenia would provide one clinical model for the detection of donor material in the recipient thymus as a result of transfusion. However, to date, such studies have not been done.

ANERGY: IMMUNOLOGICAL NONRESPONSIVENESS AND TOLERANCE

Activation of T cells is a complex and highly regulated process that involves at least three fundamental processes: binding of the TCR to antigen, binding of costimulatory molecules, and signal activation by local cytokines. The result of effective T cell signaling is the initiation of a second messenger system of intracellular activation and the release of interleukin-2 (IL-2). In recent years, the details of T cell activation have become increasingly clear. Research on the induction of T cell nonresponsiveness (also called T cell anergy) has progressed in parallel with that on T cell activation. An important insight came with the recognition that interruption of costimulatory T cell signals was central to the development of anergy.[36, 37] A number of costimulatory molecules exist for lymphocytes, including CD80/CD28, CD86/CD28, LFA-3(CD58)/CD2, ICAM-1(CD54)/LFA-1, and CD40/CD40L. Interruption of these costimulatory signals was shown to prevent a response in the allogeneic mixed lymphocyte reaction. Three different surface molecules (CD28, CTLA-4, and Fas) are particularly relevant to the induction of immune downregulation (Fig. 31–2).

Research on the induction of T cell anergy has focused on CD28 and CD40. Blockade of the interaction between CD28 on the T cell and CD80 (also called B7-1) on the APC or the interaction between CD28 on the T cell and CD86 (also called B7-2) has proved to be particularly important in the development of T cell nonresponsiveness. For example, fibroblasts transfected with MHC proteins and with CD80 function as APCs and are able to induce T cell proliferation in vitro. However, fibroblasts transfected with MHC but lacking CD80 produce an anergic T cell response that can be overcome only by the addition of exogenous IL-2.[37] A fusion protein (termed CTLA4-Ig) was developed with characteristics of immunoglobulin but with binding characteristics to CD80/CD86. In rodent experiments in which LEW rats received an allogeneic renal allograft from WF rats, a single injection of CTLA4-Ig was able to induce transplant tolerance.[38] Long-term survivors were able to reject

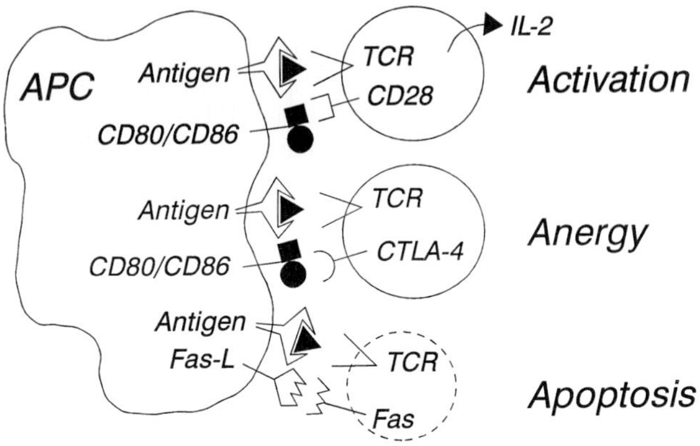

Figure 31–2. Lymphocyte co-stimulatory molecules and the development of T cell activation, anergy, or apoptosis. The antigen presenting cell (APC) is shown at the left. TCR, T cell receptor; IL-2, interleukin 2.

third-party allografts but demonstrated tolerance specific to the original donor strain. Of note, histological examination of the rejecting third-party allografts demonstrated an infiltrate with $CD4^+$ T cells exhibiting T helper type 1 (Th1) cytokine characteristics (releasing IL-2 and interferon-γ), whereas the allografts in tolerant animals exhibited a $CD4^+$ infiltrate with Th2 cytokine characteristics (releasing IL-4 and IL-10). The potential importance of these two different subsets of T cells in the development of tolerance is discussed further later. Additional organ transplant experiments have shown that dual blockade of CD80 and CD40 is sufficiently effective to permit not only allotransplants but also xenotransplants.[39]

Further research on the induction of T cell anergy has highlighted the importance of the CTLA-4 T cell receptor (CD152). CTLA-4 appears to play an essential role in immune downregulation following activation, thereby preventing immune overresponsiveness. Evidence supporting this role comes from CTLA-4 knockout mice that die prematurely of massive T cell overgrowth. CTLA-4 may play an additional role in directing T cell differentiation from a Th1 to a Th2 response. Activation of CTLA-4 can suppress IL-2 production in response to a normal activation signal. Blockade of CTLA-4 exacerbates experimental autoimmune phenomena. One model suggests that CTLA-4 receptor binding by CD80 or CD86 results in T cell downregulation and nonresponsiveness.[40, 41]

Fas protein (also called CD95 or APO-1) is a third cell-surface molecule important in research on immune downregulation. Fas protein is central to the induction of T cell apoptosis. Apoptosis refers to a series of intracellular changes resulting in cell death. These include mitochondrial swelling and nuclear degeneration. Thus, Fas is involved in peripheral clonal deletion of T cells rather than the induction of anergy. Lymphocytes that express Fas and encounter Fas-ligand on APCs receive a signal for apoptosis. Mincheff and Meryman suggested that loss of costimulatory signals and/or apoptosis occurred as a consequence of refrigerated blood storage.[42, 43] Using a rodent transfusion model, they demonstrated that transfusion of apoptotic or necrotic donor leukocytes did not result in the stimulation observed in recipients of viable donor leukocytes.[44] Their results suggest that transfusion of refrigerated stored blood may exert an immune downregulatory effect as a result of the infusion of large numbers of nonviable cells. Indeed, other experimental results have suggested that apoptotic cells are directly immunosuppressive.[45] For example, when cell cultures are stimulated by lipopolysaccharide, the addition of apoptotic cells results in the release of immunosuppressive cytokines such as IL-10 and suppresses the release of stimulatory cytokines such as IL-1 and tumor necrosis factor-α (TNF-α).[45]

Soluble HLA Peptides, Transfusion, and T Cell Anergy

Clinical studies of transfusion and tumor recurrence have suggested that the plasma component of whole blood may be related to transfusion-associated immunomodulation.[46–48] Animal studies have suggested that soluble MHC proteins may play a role. Sumimoto and Kamada studied the timing of rejection of cardiac allografts from DA rats (MHC $RT1^a$) into PVG rats (MHC $RT1^c$) and observed that rejection was slightly delayed if the recipients were transfused for 4 days with serum from donor rats ($RT1^a$). Removal of soluble class I MHC antigens from the transfused serum abolished the beneficial effect of transfusion, suggesting that soluble MHC proteins were responsible.[49] Subsequent research has focused on the infusion of soluble HLA peptides rather than whole serum.

Considerable preclinical research has suggested that infusion of soluble HLA molecules or their peptide fragments may induce recipient immunomodulation.[50–53] Nonpolymorphic peptides derived from HLA class I molecules may induce a general immune downregulation, and polymorphic peptide sequences of HLA class I may have a more antigen-specific immunomodulatory effect. For example, peptides from the polymorphic section of the α_1 or α_2 helix of HLA-A2 inhibited cytotoxic T cells directed against HLA-A2. Peptides from the nonpolymorphic α_3 region inhibited the differentiation of cytotoxic T cells in response to an allogeneic stimulus. Among the different peptides tested, amino acid residues 75–84 from the α_1 helix of HLA-B7 and HLA-B27 have shown the most promise in animal transplant studies and are now undergoing clinical investigation.[53] These peptides, when used in combination with subtherapeutic doses of cyclosporin, inhibited rejection of solid organ allografts in a rodent transplant model. In initial human trials among patients undergoing first-time renal allografts, patients treated with high doses of intravenous class I peptides demonstrated depressed natural killer (NK) cell cytotoxicity.[54] It is interesting that peptides derived from HLA-B7 were found to be among the more effective class I allotypes in studies of soluble HLA proteins. HLA-B7 is also the class I allotype with a high vestigial expression on the surface of human red cells (Bg^a antigen). Thus red cell concentrates from HLA-B7–positive donors may deliver considerable quantities of this peptide to transfusion recipients.

IMMUNE SUPPRESSION AND PERIPHERAL TOLERANCE

The concept of suppressor T cells as a mechanism of immune downregulation is not new, but isolation and characterization of suppressor T cells have been somewhat elusive. Nevertheless, several experimental systems exist to demonstrate functional immune suppression. In vitro co-culture experiments are among the original methods to demonstrate inhibition of cellular immune responses. The use of a diffusion chamber in such experiments can demonstrate that soluble factors released by cells (cytokines) are capable of causing immune downregulation. A more convincing physiological demonstration of immune suppressor cells comes from adoptive transfer experiments in which cells from one animal are either transfused or inserted within a diffusion chamber into a recipient animal.

Th1 and Th2 Cells

Early attempts to characterize suppressor cells solely on the basis of cell surface markers have gradually given way to characterization based on both marker expression and the profile of cytokines released by the cell.[55] T cells have been broadly characterized into two subsets—Th1 and Th2 cells—based on the cytokines released (Fig. 31–3). Th1 cells release IL-2, interferon-γ and TNF-α. Th2 cells release IL-4, IL-5, IL-6, and IL-10. The two subsets are said to be counterregulatory, as expansion of Th1 cells suppresses expansion of Th2, and vice versa.[56] Th1 responses are inflammatory and are seen in allograft rejection, graft-versus-host disease, delayed-type hypersensitivity, and autoimmune tissue destruction. In contrast, Th2 responses are seen in chronic parasitic infection and in the augmentation of humoral immunity. In addition, Th2 responses counter the inflammatory Th1 response and may serve to downregulate an alloaggressive transplantation response.[57] Release of IL-6[58] and IL-10[59] by Th2 cells appears to be particularly relevant for this downregulation. Thus, the development of a Th2 response versus a Th1 response polarizes (or directs) the immune response toward a different functional outcome.

One hypothesis is that blood transfusion promotes the development of a Th2 immune response.[60] Several indirect lines of evidence suggest that transfusion may provoke a Th2 response in the recipient. Babcock and Alexander reported the short-term effects of a single transfusion of fresh blood in mice.[61] Whole blood from BALB/cAnNHsd (H-2d) mice was transfused into AKR/J (H-2k) recipients. Control recipients received either normal saline or blood from syngeneic donors (H-2k). The spleen cells from the recipients were harvested, cultured for 48 hours in concanavalin A, and tested for the pattern of cytokine release. In contrast to the control animals, those transfused with allogeneic blood demonstrated increased in vitro release of IL-4 and IL-10 and decreased secretion of IL-2, consistent with a Th2 response. The cytokine changes were detectable at day 3 post-transfusion and persisted for at least 2 weeks.

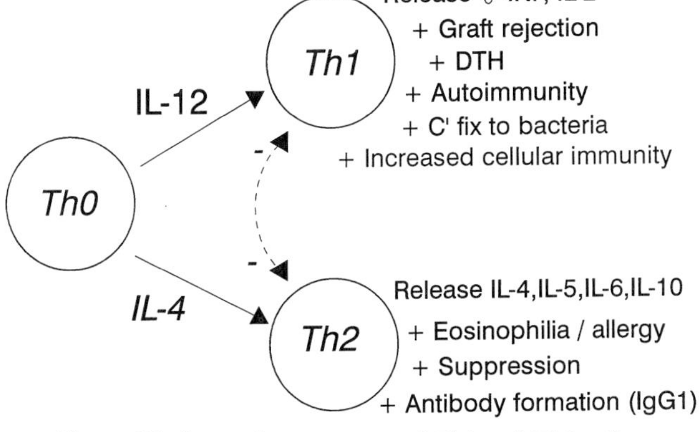

Figure 31–3. Cytokine patterns of Th1 and Th2 cells.

Suppressor Cells and the Role of the Spleen

Just as the thymus has been shown to be the major anatomical site for the production of central tolerance through the mechanism of clonal deletion, recent research has highlighted the importance of the spleen in the development of peripheral tolerance mediated by T cell suppression. Candidate suppressor cells have been identified among the $CD4^+$ subpopulation and particularly among cells exhibiting some Th2 functional characteristics.[55, 62] More recently, Groux and colleagues identified a human $CD4^+$ regulator cell that they designated Tr1.[63] Tr1 cells produce high levels of IL-10 and little IL-2 or IL-4. Tr1 cells were able to suppress the proliferation of other $CD4^+$ T cells in response to antigen. In an animal model of experimental colitis, Tr1 cells were able to suppress the autoimmune response. Experimental work in the field of transplant tolerance has also found evidence for suppressor $CD4^+$ cells. For example, Chen and associates studied heterotopic cardiac allograft rejection in mice and demonstrated that splenic $CD4^+$ cells could prolong allograft acceptance through a mechanism of immune suppression.[63a] BALB/c mice (H-2d) were cardiac donors to MHC-incompatible CBA/Ca (H-2k) recipients. Recipients were conditioned with nonlytic doses of anti-CD4 and anti-CD8. Strain-specific tolerance was then induced by a donor-specific blood transfusion. In the absence of conditioning and transfusion, recipients promptly rejected the donor allografts. Conditioned and transfused animals demonstrated long-term acceptance of the cardiac transplant. These tolerant animals were then sacrificed, and cells from their spleens were used for adoptive transfer to naive CBA/Ca recipients who had received no preparative immunosuppression. The transfusion of splenic lymphocytes from tolerant animals was sufficient to induce tolerance to the cardiac allografts in the new recipients without any other form of immunosuppression. Whereas depletion of $CD8^+$ cells from the spleen cell transfers did not affect the results, depletion of $CD4^+$ cells abrogated the induction of tolerance, suggesting that tolerance was dependent on a subtype of cells bearing the $CD4^+$ marker. Spleen cells removed from the second set of animals could be transferred to a third set of CBA/Ca recipients, with sustained tolerance to the BALB/c cardiac allografts.

Perhaps surprisingly, adoptive transfer of spleen cells was successful through nine passages. Given the loss of cells that occurs with each adoptive transfer, and given the initial number of spleen cells transferred from the original tolerant recipients, Chen and associates estimated that the original cells would not be present in appreciable numbers by the ninth passage, thereby demonstrating either expansion of the adoptively transferred suppressor T cells or polarization of naive cells into CD4+ suppressor cells among the new recipients. Nisco and colleagues also studied tolerance to cardiac allografts but used a rat transplant model.[64] ACI rats were conditioned with cyclosporin. Tolerance was donor strain specific and could be adoptively transferred to naive recipients using spleen cells. Of note, thymectomized animals were still able to develop suppressor cells in the spleen, documenting a purely peripheral-based mechanism of immune tolerance in this model.

Suppression of the immune response has also been suggested as a cause of tumor recurrence. Blajchman and colleagues conducted a series of experiments in animals demonstrating a tumor-promoting effect of allogeneic transfusions that contain donor leukocytes.[65–67] Animals were conditioned with unmodified fresh allogeneic transfusions, leukocyte-depleted allogeneic transfusions, or syngeneic transfusions. Recipients were then challenged with an inoculation of tumor cells, and the number of pulmonary metastases was counted. Although the cells responsible for immune suppression were not characterized, the investigators again found a role for suppressor spleen cells. When spleen cells from animals that had received allogeneic transfusions were transferred to naive recipients, those animals developed greater numbers of pulmonary metastases when challenged with tumor cells than were observed in mice receiving spleen cells from untransfused animals. Of note, the adoptive transfer of cells that supported tumor growth did not occur if the original recipients were transfused with either leukocyte-reduced allogeneic blood or syngeneic blood. The investigators interpreted their results as supporting the hypothesis that recipient exposure to allogeneic donor leukocytes induces an active cell population in the spleens of transfusion recipients that exerts an immunomodulatory effect on tumor growth. Subsequent studies by the same investigators found that the tumor-growth-promoting effect could also be demonstrated by placing in the peritoneum of naive animals a diffusion chamber containing spleen cells obtained from animals transfused with allogeneic blood containing donor leukocytes. This latter observation suggests that the immunoregulatory spleen cells in transfused animals mediate the effect on tumor growth via the release of a soluble factor (cytokine).

Transfusion-associated immunomodulation may suppress humoral as well as cellular immune responses. Kao successfully induced humoral immune tolerance in CBA mice (H-2k) using transfusions from BALB/c donors (H-2d) of leukocytes that were treated with ultraviolet B (UVB) irradiation.[68] When suspensions of donor leukocytes that were depleted of donor platelets or plasma were transfused, the recipients became resistant to alloimmunization. Of interest, the presence of donor platelets or plasma interfered with the effect of UVB irradiation on the donor leukocytes. Animals transfused with UVB-irradiated donor leukocytes became resistant not only to the MHC strain of the donor cells (H-2d) but also to the related MHC types H-2b, H-2r, and H-2n but not to other MHC allotypes. Of particular note, adoptive transfer experiments demonstrated that the spleens of recipient animals contained cells capable of transferring tolerance.

Clinical studies in humans have not been able to address the role of transfusion-associated induction of CD4+ suppressor cells in the spleen. In addition, human studies cannot control for the effects of the illness that necessitates blood transfusion nor account easily for the MHC relationship between donor and recipient. Nevertheless, some preliminary evidence supports the notion that Th2 cells may be activated by transfusion. Kirkley and associates studied in vitro cytokine release on day 7 and day 14 among 43 patients transfused with either allogeneic or autologous blood at the time of hip surgery.[60] They observed that the mean IL-10 release in vitro was slightly higher among recipients of allogeneic blood compared with no allogeneic blood (130 versus 81 pg/mL). Mean IL-4 release was also slightly higher among recipients of allogeneic blood. Jensen and colleagues randomized 60 patients undergoing colorectal surgery to receive either whole blood (unmodified) or leukocyte-reduced whole blood.[69] They observed that recipients of unmodified whole blood demonstrated elevated systemic IL-6 levels (a Th2 cytokine) after transfusion. In contrast, a separate report found increased postoperative IL-6 levels among patients receiving autologous blood at the time of hip replacement surgery,[70] and other studies have found no significant differences in cytokine profiles as a result of transfusion.[71, 72] Thus, data in humans are insufficient to document that transfusions induce either a systemic Th2 response or the development of suppressor T cells.

Transforming Growth Factor-β, Th3 Cells, and the Lung

Transforming growth factor-β (TGF-β) is another cytokine that may play a role in transfusion-associated immunomodulation. TGF-β is not considered to be strictly associated with either a Th1 or a Th2 response and has been assigned by some investigators to a third subset of CD4+ cells, termed Th3 cells.[73] TGF-β is not a single molecule but rather a family of polypeptide growth factors released from several different cell types, including NK cells, macrophages, and lymphocytes.[74] TGF-β is found in high concentrations in gut-associated and lung-associated lymphoid tissue. Because the lung represents the first capillary endothelial circuit exposed to allogeneic transfusion, the potential importance of lung-associated lymphoid tissue and the response to transfusion is of interest and has not yet been adequately explored. When examined in a variety of experimental systems, TGF-β release appears to induce immune downregulation. TGF-β inhibits monocyte hydrogen peroxide production and reduces macrophage cytotoxicity.[75] It can block IL-2 expression by T cells and can suppress T cell expansion in response to an antigen stimulus. It may also play a role in the maternal tolerance to fetal antigens. Whether allogeneic transfusion induces release of pulmonary TGF-β is largely unexplored. However, recent reports have drawn attention to the fact that transfusion may result in the passive transfer of TGF-β from donor to recipient. Studies of factor VIII concentrates prepared from plasma pools were shown to inhibit in vitro T cell proliferation to phytohemagglutinin.[76] The inhibition was considered to result from residual levels of TGF-β in the concentrates.[77] TGF-β concentrations in plasma may increase as a result of platelet storage. Kunz and coworkers demonstrated a transient elevation (1.3 times baseline) of recipient circulating levels of TGF-β following transfusion of platelets.[78] In addition, a recent analysis of commercially available lots of intravenous immunoglobulin preparations found high levels of TGF-β (>10 ng/mL), and there were increased circulating levels of TGF-β in the blood of patients after transfusion with intravenous immunoglobulin.[79] This latter finding raises the possibility that some of the immunomodulatory effects of intravenous immunoglobulin may be mediated by this cytokine.

Veto Cells

Most mechanisms of transplantation tolerance or transfusion-associated immunomodulation are based on recipient immune effector cells. In contrast, the veto cell concept is based on immune suppression mediated by transplanted or transfused *donor* cells. Veto cells act to selectively suppress or clonally delete those recipient immune cells directed against donor alloantigens. The concept of the veto cell is functionally defined, and no cell surface marker or cytokine profile has been identified to specifically characterize veto cells. The location of veto cells is uncertain, but experimental evidence from the literature on solid organ allograft acceptance suggests that veto cells may reside in the bone marrow.[80] This has led to experimental protocols involving the infusion of donor bone marrow as part of conditioning regimens for the induction of tolerance. For example, Thomas and colleagues successfully induced transplant tolerance to renal allografts in a rhesus monkey transplant model.[81] Induction of tolerance in higher primates is much more difficult than in rodent models and lends support to the relevance of this line of research for human investigations. Recipient rhesus monkeys were first conditioned with anti-CD3-immunotoxin plus the transfusion of APC-depleted and T cell–depleted donor bone marrow. After transplantation, all immunosuppression could be stopped, and the recipients demonstrated greatly prolonged allograft acceptance, even though the animals were outbred and donor-recipient pairs were strongly incompatible by in vitro testing. Consistent with the veto cell hypothesis, tolerance persisted as long as the recipient demonstrated PCR evidence of the persistence of donor cells, and tolerance was lost as donor cell signals were lost. Additional studies demonstrated that gamma irradiation of the donor bone marrow abrogated the tolerogenic effect. Recipients treated with donor bone marrow demonstrated in vitro a decrease in cytotoxic T cell activity that was specific to donor targets. Three cell co-culture experiments suggested that veto cells were able to suppress cytotoxicity of donor targets by recipient cells. Sharing of MHC class II antigens between donor and recipient may play a role in the veto phenomenon[82] and would be consistent with the findings of human clinical transplantation.

Studies in humans are under way to identify whether donor bone marrow may represent an important source of immunomodulatory cells. Following a series of initial pilot trials, a prospective clinical study in humans undergoing cadaveric renal transplants was conducted.[83] Patients received infusions of donor marrow harvested from the cadaveric donor at the time of renal harvesting, as well as traditional immunosuppression. Initial allograft survival results at 18 months showed improved survival in the group randomized to receive donor marrow. Further studies using donor peripheral blood hematopoietic cells mobilized by growth factors are under way.

The possibility that donor $CD34^+$ cells mediate transfusion-associated immunomodulation is consistent with numerous experimental findings of tolerance. Donor stem cells are long-lived and would provide for persistence of donor MHC antigen in the recipient circulation. Donor stem cells would be expected to be capable of microchimerism and were identified in studies of persistent fetal cells in the maternal circulation. Donor stem cells express MHC antigens, consistent with studies that have found that tolerance induction depends on the MHC relationship between donor and recipient. Finally, $CD34^+$ cells have cell surface markers involved in the honing of these cells to microenvironments. In the context of routine allogeneic transfusions, it is noteworthy that fresh transfusions contain viable stem cells. A recent study demonstrated that most $CD34^+$ hematopoietic progenitors segregate with packed red cells when whole blood is made into routine components.

GRAFT ENGINEERING AND FUTURE RESEARCH ON TRANSFUSION-ASSOCIATED IMMUNE TOLERANCE

Recent research on the induction of transplant tolerance has taken full advantage of the ability to express foreign genes within viable target cells. Cells harvested from a potential organ recipient can be engineered to express specific donor MHC allotypes. By reintroducing these manipulated autologous transfected cells into a conditioned recipient, transplant tolerance has been demonstrated. For example, Knechtle and coworkers injected into the thymus of recipients muscle cells that had been transfected with donor class I MHC genes.[84] The transfectants induced central thymic tolerance and resulted in a decrease in MHC-specific cytotoxic precursor cells. Wood and colleagues used peripheral transfusion of transfected cells to induce transplant tolerance in mice.[85, 86] Recipient cells from C3H/He mice (H-2k) were transfected with either class I (K,D) or class II (IA) genes from C57BL/10 donor mice (H-2b).[87] The transfected cells were then given as a transfusion to recipients that had been conditioned for transplantation with a nondepleting monoclonal antibody directed against T cells. As a result of the conditioning and the transfusion, recipient animals became fully tolerant to cardiac allografts from donor (H-2b) mice. Tolerance was long-lasting and did not require post-transplant immunosuppression. Similar studies have been reported by other laboratories.[88] Experiments such as these demonstrate a future path for the induction of clinical transplant tolerance and are likely to uncover mechanisms that may help explain the immunomodulatory effect of allogeneic blood transfusions.

Additional strategies for gene-mediated graft engineering are emerging. In a murine heart transplant model, Qin and associates injected allografts with a plasmid carrying the gene for TGF-β1. Transfected hearts survived longer than controls.[89] Other investigators have transfected DNA encoding CLTLA4-Ig into liver cells that were then transplanted.[90] This strategy is designed to block recognition of the allogeneic liver cells by recipient T cells. A third approach investigated eliminating the recipient immune response to an allograft through expression of Fas-ligand on the graft. In a rat renal allograft model, the allograft was transfected with DNA sequences encoding Fas-ligand. The transfectants expressed Fas-ligand for approximately 2 weeks, which was long enough to prolong allograft survival compared with controls.[91] Each of these new methods relies on manipulation of the graft rather than the host, thereby allowing the host to maintain a normal immune system.

SUMMARY OF THE MECHANISMS OF TRANSFUSION-ASSOCIATED IMMUNOMODULATION

Despite decades of laboratory and clinical investigation, the exact mechanisms by which blood transfusion may induce or contribute to an immunosuppressive effect remain incompletely understood. It is likely that no single mechanism applies and that multiple immune responses occur, depending on the dose and timing of antigen, the immune status of the recipient, and the HLA relationship between the donor and recipient. Donor leukocytes (and possibly stem cells) and donor soluble HLA proteins may be critical for the induction of the transfusion effect. Blood cell modifications such as leukocyte reduction, gamma irradiation, or cell washing may have important effects on the likelihood of inducing transfusion-associated immunomodulation. Some form of recipient conditioning appears to be essential for the induction of transplant tolerance induced by transfusion. The extent to which human illnesses, infections, medications, or surgery may serve as surrogate conditioning in the setting of routine blood transfusion remains largely unexplored. The HLA relationship between donor and recipient is likely to be of fundamental importance to the immunomodulatory effect of transfusion. HLA peptide sequences may affect detection and clearance of donor cells by recipient NK cells and other host defenses, may influence the extent of microchimerism resulting from transfusion, and would be expected to influence the range of MHC-peptide responses by recipient T cells. Different immunomodulatory mechanisms may be uniquely localized to different anatomical sites. Substantial experimental evidence supports the hypothesis that central immune tolerance resulting from clonal deletion of alloreactive cells occurs in the thymus gland. Similar evidence supports the development of suppressor T cells in the spleen of conditioned animals. Lung-associated immune tissue may be important in the development of immune suppression mediated by TGF-β. Insight into the balance and interaction among these different immune responses awaits future research.

REFERENCES

1. Billingham RE, Brent I, Medawar PB. Actively acquired tolerance of foreign cells. Nature 1953; 172:603.
2. Blumberg N, Heal JM. Effects of transfusion on immune function, cancer recurrence and infection. Arch Pathol Lab Med 1994; 118:371.
3. Dzik S, Blajchman MA, Blumberg N, et al. Current research on the immunomodulatory effect of allogeneic blood transfusion. Vox Sang 1996; 70:187.
4. Klein HG. Immunomodulation caused by blood transfusion. *In* Petz LD, Swisher SN, Kleinman S, et al. (eds): Clinical Practice of Transfusion Medicine. New York: Churchill Livingstone, 1996, pp 59–69.
5. Bordin JO, Blajchman MA. Transfusion-associated immunosuppression. *In* Rossi E, Simon T, Moss G, Gould SA (eds): Principles of Transfusion Medicine. Baltimore: Williams & Wilkins, 1996, pp 803–812.
6. Vamvakas EC, Carven JH. Transfusion of white-cell-containing allogeneic blood components and postoperative wound infection: effect of confounding factors. Transfus Med 1998; 8:29.
7. Vamvakas EC, Blajchman MA. A proposal for an individual patient data based meta-analysis of randomized controlled trials of allogeneic transfusion and postoperative bacterial infection. Transfus Med Rev 1997; 11:180.
8. Busch MP, Lee TH, Donegan E, Pallavicini M. Use of an inbred model system for studies of allogeneic transfusion-induced immunosuppression. Blood 1993; 82:3509.
9. Adams PT, Davenport RD, Reardon DA, Roth MS. Detection of circulating donor white blood cells in patients receiving multiple blood transfusions. Blood 1992; 80:551.
10. van Twuyver E, Mooijaart RJD, ten Berge IJM, et al. Pretransplantation blood transfusion revisited. N Engl J Med 1991; 325:1210.
11. Baudouin V, de Vitry N, Hiesse C, et al. Cytotoxic T lymphocyte changes after HLA-DR match and HLA-DR mismatch blood transfusions. Transplantation 1997; 63:1155.
12. Young NT, Roelen DL, Iggo N, et al. Effect of one-HLA-haplotype-matched and HLA-mismatched blood transfusions on recipient T lymphocyte allorepertoires. Transplantation 1997; 63:1160.
13. Leivestad T, Thorsby E. Effects of HLA-haploidentical blood transfusion on donor-specific immune responsiveness. Transplantation 1984; 37:175.
14. Breur-Vriesendorp BS, Vingerhoed J, Schaasberg WP, Ivanyi P. Variations in the T-cell repertoire against HLA antigens in humans. Hum Immunol 1990; 27:1.
15. van der Mast BJ, Balk AH. Effect of HLA-DR shared blood transfusion on the clinical outcome of heart transplantation. Transplantation 1997; 63:1514.
16. Sugiura K, Kato K, Hashimoto F, et al. Induction of donor-specific T cell anergy by portal venous injection of allogeneic cells. Immunobiology 1997; 197:460.
17. Saitovitch D, Bushell A, Mabbs DW, et al. Kinetics of induction of transplantation tolerance with a non-depleting anti-CD4 monoclonal antibody and donor-specific transfusion before transplantation: a critical period of time is required for development of immunological unresponsiveness. Transplantation 1996; 61:1642.
18. Starzl T, Demetris A, Murase N, et al. Cell migration, chimerism and graft acceptance. Lancet 1992; 339:1579.
19. Schechter GP, Whang-Peng J, McFarland W. Circulation of donor lymphocytes after blood transfusion in man. Blood 1977; 49:651.
20. Dzik WH. Mononuclear cell microchimerism and the immunomodulatory effect of transfusion. Transfusion 1994; 34:1007.

21. Busch MP, Paglieroni T, Ohto H, et al. Transient and long-term multilineage chimerism of donor leukocytes in transfused patients [Abstract]. Infusionsther Transfusionsmed 1997; 24:295.
22. Reed W, Lee TH, Busch MP, Vichinsky EP. Sample suitability for the detection of minor leukocyte populations by polymerase chain reaction [Abstract]. Transfusion 1997; 37(suppl 1):107S.
23. Bianchi D, Zickwolf GK, Weil GJ, et al. Male fetal progenitor cells persist in maternal blood for as long as 27 years post partum. Proc N Y Acad Sci 1996; 93:705.
24. Naji A. Induction of tolerance by intrathymic inoculation of alloantigen. Curr Opin Immunol 1996; 8:704.
25. Remuzzi G. Cellular basis of long-term organ transplant acceptance: pivotal role of intrathymic clonal deletion and thymic dependence of bone marrow microchimerism-associated tolerance. Am J Kidney Dis 1998; 31:197.
26. Campos L, Alfrey EJ, Posselt AM, et al. Prolonged survival of rat orthotopic liver allografts after intrathymic inoculation of donor-strain cells. Transplantation 1993; 55:866.
27. Ohzato H, Monaco AP. Induction of specific unresponsiveness (tolerance) to skin allografts by intrathymic donor-specific splenocyte injection in antilymphocyte serum-treated mice. Transplantation 1992; 54:1090.
28. Goss JA, Nakafusa Y, Flye MW. MHC class II presenting cells are necessary for the induction of intrathymic tolerance. Ann Surg 1993; 217:492.
29. Remuzzi G, Rossini M, Imberti O, Perico N. Kidney graft survival in rats without immunosuppressants after intrathymic glomerular transplantation. Lancet 1991; 337:750.
30. Posselt AM, Campos L, Mayo GL, et al. Selective modulation of T cell immunity by intrathymic cellular transplantation. Transplant Rev 1993; 7:200.
31. Shirwan H, Mhoyan A, Leamer M, et al. The role of donor class I major histocompatibility complex peptides in the induction of allograft tolerance. Transplant Proc 1997; 2:1134.
32. Chowdhury NC, Murphy B, Sayegh MH, et al. Acquired systemic tolerance to rat cardiac allografts induced by intrathymic inoculation of synthetic polymorphic MHC class I allopeptides. Transplantation 1996; 62:1878.
33. Wang M, Stepkowski SM, Yu J, et al. Localization of cryptic tolerogenic epitopes in the alpha-1 helical region of the RT1.u alloantigen. Transplantation 1997; 63:1373.
34. Oluwole SF, Jin MX, Chowdhury NC, Ohajekwe OA. Effectiveness of intrathymic inoculation of soluble antigens in the induction of specific unresponsiveness to rat islet allografts without transient recipient immunosuppression. Transplantation 1994; 58:1077.
35. Sayegh MH, Perico N, Gallon L, et al. Mechanisms of acquired thymic unresponsiveness to renal allografts: thymic recognition of immunodominant allo-MHC peptides induces peripheral T cell anergy. Transplantation 1994; 58:125.
36. Bashuda H, Takazawa K, Tamatani T, et al. Induction of persistent allograft tolerance in the rat by combined treatment with anti-leukocyte function-associated antigen-1 and anti-intercellular adhesion molecule-1 monoclonal antibodies, donor specific transfusions, and FK506. Transplantation 1996; 62:117.
37. Schultz J, Nadler LM, Gribben JG. B7-mediated costimulation and the immune response. Blood Rev 1996; 10:111.
38. Sayegh MH, Akalin E, Hancock WW, et al. CD28-B7 blockade after alloantigenic challenge in vivo inhibits Th1 cytokines but spares Th2. J Exp Med 1995; 181:1869.
39. Larsen CP, Pearson TC. The CD40 pathway in allograft rejection, acceptance, and tolerance. Curr Opin Immunol 1997; 9:641.
40. Perez VL, Van Parijs L, Biuckians A, et al. Induction of peripheral T cell tolerance in vivo requires CTLA-4 engagement. Immunity 1997; 6:411.
41. Chambers CA, Allison JP. Co-stimulation in T cell responses. Curr Opin Immunol 1997; 9:396.
42. Mincheff MS, Meryman HT, Kapoor V, et al. Blood transfusion and immunomodulation: a possible mechanism. Vox Sang 1993; 65:18.
43. Mincheff MS, Meryman HT. Blood transfusion, blood storage and immunomodulation. Immun Invest 1995; 24:303.
44. Mincheff MS, Getsov SI, Meryman HT. Mechanisms of alloimmunization and immunosuppression by blood transfusion in an inbred rodent model. Transplantation 1995; 60:815.
45. Voll RE, Herrmann M, Roth EA, et al. Immunosuppressive effects of apoptotic cells. Nature 1997; 390:350.
46. Blumberg N, Heal JM. Transfusion and recipient immune function. Arch Pathol Lab Med 1989; 113:246.
47. Wobbes T, Joosen KHG, Kuypers HHC, et al. The effect of packed cells and whole blood on survival after curative resection for colorectal carcinoma. Dis Colon Rectum 1989; 32:743.
48. Marsh J, Donnan PT, Hamer-Hodges DW. Association between transfusion with plasma and the recurrence of colorectal carcinoma. Br J Surg 1990; 77:623.
49. Sumimoto R, Kamada N. Evidence that soluble class I antigen in donor serum induces the suppression of heart allograft rejection in rats. Immunol Lett 1990; 26:81.
50. Krensky AM, Clayberger C. Structure of HLA molecules and immunosuppressive effects of HLA derived peptides. Int Rev Immunol 1996; 13:173.
51. Buelow R, Burlingham WJ, Clayberger C. Immunomodulation by soluble HLA class I. Transplantation 1995; 59:649.
52. Chueh SC, Tian L, Wang M, et al. Induction of tolerance toward rat cardiac allografts by treatment with allochimeric class I MHC antigen and FTY720. Transplantation 1997; 64:1407.
53. Magee CC, Sayegh MH. Peptide-mediated immunosuppression. Curr Opin Immunol 1997; 9:669.
54. Giral M, Cuturi MC, Nguyen JM, et al. Decreased cytotoxic activity of natural killer cells in kidney allograft recipients treated with human HLA-derived peptide. Transplantation 1997; 63:1004.
55. Field EH, Gao Q, Chen NX, Rouse TM. Balancing the immune system for tolerance: a case for regulatory CD4 cells. Transplantation 1997; 64:1.
56. Seder RA, Paul WE. Acquisition of lymphokine-producing phenotype by CD4+ T cells. Annu Rev Immunol 1994; 12:635.
57. Lowry R, Takeuchi T. The Th1, Th2 Paradigm and Transplantation Tolerance. Austin, TX: RG Landes, 1994, pp 1–134.
58. Tomura M, Nakatani I, Murachi M, et al. Suppression of allograft responses induced by interleukin-6, which selectively modulates interferon-gamma but not interleukin-2 production. Transplantation 1997; 64:757.
59. Blancho G, Gianello PR, Lorf T, et al. Molecular and cellular events implicated in local tolerance to kidney allografts in miniature swine. Transplantation 1997; 63:26.
60. Kirkley SA, Cowles J, Pellegrini VD, et al. Cytokine secretion after allogeneic or autologous blood transfusion. Lancet 1995; 345:527.
61. Babcock GF, Alexander JW. The effects of blood transfusion on cytokine production by Th1 and Th2 lymphocytes in the mouse. Transplantation 1996; 61:465.
62. Weigle WO, Romball CG. CD4+ T-cell subsets and cytokines involved in peripheral tolerance. Immunol Today 1997; 18:533.
63. Groux H, O'Garra A, Bigler M, et al. A CD4+ T-cell subset inhibits antigen-specific T-cell responses and prevents colitis. Nature 1997; 389:737.
63a. Chen ZK, Cobbold SP, Woldmann H, Metcalfe S. Amplification of natural regulatory immune mechanisms for transplantation tolerance. Transplantation 1996; 62:1200.
64. Nisco SJ, Hissink RJ, Vriens PW, et al. In vivo studies of the maintenance of peripheral transplant tolerance after cyclosporine: radiosensitive antigen-specific suppressor cells mediate lasting graft protection against primed effector cells. Transplantation 1995; 59:1444.
65. Blajchman MA, Bardossy L, Carmen R, et al. Allogeneic blood transfusion–induced enhancement of tumor growth: two animal models showing amelioration of leukodepletion and passive transfer using spleen cells. Blood 1993; 81:1880.
66. Bordin JO, Bardossy L, Blajchman MA. Growth enhancement of established tumors by allogeneic blood transfusion in experimental animals and its amelioration by leukodepletion: the importance of timing of the leukodepletion. Blood 1994; 84:344.
67. Blajchman MA, Bordin JO. Tumor growth-promoting effect of allogeneic blood transfusion. Immunol Invest 1995; 24:311.
68. Kao KJ. Induction of humoral immune tolerance to major histocompatibility complex antigens by transfusions of UV-B irradiated leukocytes. Blood 1996; 88:4375.
69. Jensen LS, Hokland M, Nielsen HJ. A randomized controlled study of the effect of bedside leucocyte depletion on the immunosuppressive effect of whole blood transfusion in patients undergoing elective colorectal surgery. Br J Surg 1996; 83:973.
70. Avail A, Hyllner M, Bengtson JP, et al. Postoperative inflammatory response after autologous and allogeneic blood transfusion. Anesthesiology 1997; 87:511.

71. Quintiliani L, Iudicone P, DeGirolamo M, et al. Immunoresponsiveness of cancer patients: effect of blood transfusion and immune reactivity of tumor infiltrating lymphocytes. Cancer Detect Prev 1995; 19:518.
72. Tietze M, Kluter H, Troch M, Kirchner H. Immune responsiveness in orthopedic surgery patients after transfusion of autologous or allogeneic blood. Transfusion 1995; 35:378.
73. Chen Y, Kuchroo V, Inobe J, et al. Regulatory T cell clones induced by oral tolerance: suppression of autoimmune encephalomyelitis. Science 1994; 265:1237.
74. Horwitz DA, Gray JD, Ohtsuka K, et al. The immunoregulatory effects of NK cells: the role of TGF-β and implications for autoimmunity. Immunol Today 1997; 18:538.
75. Haak-Frendscho M, Wynn TA, Czuprynski CJ, Paulnock D. Transforming growth factor beta 1 inhibits activation of macrophage cell line RAW 264.7 for cell killing. Clin Exp Immunol 1990; 82:404.
76. Vermont-Desroches C, Rigal D, Blourde C, Bernard J. Immunosuppressive property of a very high purity antihemophilic preparation: a low molecular weight component inhibits an early step of PHA induced cell activation. Br J Haematol 1992; 80:370.
77. Wadha M, Dilger P, Tubbs J, et al. Identification of transforming growth factor-β as a contaminant in factor VIII concentrates: a possible link with immunosuppressive effects in hemophiliacs. Blood 1994; 84:2021.
78. Kunz D, Luley C, Heim MU, Bock M. Transforming growth factor β is increased in plasma of patients with hematologic malignancies after transfusion of platelet concentrates. Transfusion 1998; 38:156.
79. Kekow J, Reinhold D, Pap T, Ansorge S. Intravenous immunoglobulins and transforming growth factor β. Lancet 1998; 351:184.
80. Burlingham WJ, Grailer AP, Fechner JH, et al. Microchimerism linked to cytotoxic T lymphocyte functional unresponsiveness (clonal anergy) in a tolerant renal transplant recipient. Transplantation 1995; 59:1147.
81. Thomas JM, Neville DM, Contreras JL, et al. Preclinical studies of allograft tolerance in rhesus monkeys: a novel anti-CD3-immunotoxin given pretransplant with donor bone marrow induces operational tolerance to kidney allografts. Transplantation 1997; 64:124.
82. Thomas JM, Verbanac KM, Smith JP, et al. The facilitating effect of one-DR antigen sharing in renal allograft tolerance induced by donor bone marrow in rhesus monkeys. Transplantation 1995; 59:245.
83. Barber WH, Mankin JA, Laskow DA, et al. Long-term results of a controlled prospective study with transfusion of donor-specific bone marrow in 57 cadaveric renal allograft recipients. Transplantation 1991; 51:70.
84. Knechtle SJ, Wang J, Jiao S, et al. Induction of specific tolerance by intrathymic injection of recipient muscle cells transfected with donor class I major histocompatibility complex. Transplantation 1994; 57:990.
85. Wood KJ. The induction of tolerance to alloantigens using MHC class I molecules. Curr Opin Immunol 1993; 5:759.
86. Wong W, Morris PJ, Wood KJ. Pretransplant administration of a single donor class I major histocompatibility complex molecule is sufficient for the indefinite survival of fully allogeneic cardiac allografts: evidence for linked epitope suppression. Transplantation 1997; 63:1490.
87. Saitovitch D, Morris PJ, Wood KJ. Recipient cells expressing single donor MHC locus products can substitute for donor-specific transfusion in the induction of transplantation tolerance when retreatment is combined with anti-CD4 monoclonal antibody: evidence for a vital role of CD4+ T cells in induction of tolerance to class I molecules. Transplantation 1996; 61:1532.
88. Schumacher IK, Newberg MH, Jackson JD, et al. Use of gene therapy to suppress the antigen-specific immune responses in mice to an HLA antigen. Transplantation 1996; 62:831.
89. Qin L, Chavin KD, Ding Y, et al. Multiple vectors effectively achieve gene transfer in a murine cardiac transplantation model: immunosuppression with TGF-β1 or vIL-10. Transplantation 1995; 59:809.
90. Olthoff KM, Judge TA, Gelman AE, et al. Adenovirus-mediated gene unresponsiveness following transduction with CTLA4-Ig. Nat Med 1998; 4:194.
91. Swenson KM, Ke B, Wang T, et al. Fas ligand gene transfer to renal allografts in rats: effects on allograft survival. Transplantation 1998; 65:155.

SECTION

X Transfusion-Transmitted Diseases

CHAPTER 32

Epidemiology of Transfusion-Transmitted Diseases

Roger Y. Dodd

HISTORICAL REVIEW

There is little doubt that transmission of infectious agents has been a problem from the time blood transfusion was first attempted. However, recipient infection was not perceived as a major difficulty until the fundamental issues of donor-recipient compatibility and prevention of coagulation and preservation of blood components were resolved. The true magnitude and significance of transfusion-transmitted viruses, particularly hepatitis, then became apparent. Although the first agent to provoke concern and action was *Treponema pallidum,* the etiological agent of syphilis, it is possible that serological tests for syphilis were implemented as a response to perception rather than to demonstrated need—a practice that strangely foreshadowed the events of the late 1980s. However, there is no doubt that acute hepatitis was a serious and frequent outcome of transfusion; at least one author has reported that 1.5% of recipients developed symptomatic, clinical hepatitis.[1] In retrospect, it is alarming to speculate on how many subclinical and chronic infections actually occurred. From the early 1940s to about 1981, hepatitis was the only transfusion-transmitted disease that provoked concern and action.

The recognition of acquired immunodeficiency syndrome (AIDS) in 1981, along with the eventual demonstration that it could be transmitted by transfusion, led to profound changes in both attitude and practice in transfusion medicine. Although rapid actions were taken to reduce the risk of transmitting AIDS by transfusion, it was not easy to select the most appropriate course in the absence of any real knowledge about the etiology of the disease. In fact, from the perspective of current knowledge, many have charged that the response to the AIDS crisis was inadequate, both within and outside transfusion medicine. Largely as a consequence of these perceptions, management of blood safety became focused on the need to prevent recipient infection whenever possible; screening measures, including new tests, were implemented without reference to cost-benefit analyses.

Five additional tests for transfusion-transmitted infections have been implemented since 1985, including three tests to prevent or reduce infection with hepatitis C virus (HCV), plus one directed toward the prevention of transmission of human T cell lymphotropic virus type I (HTLV-I), an uncommon retrovirus that is only rarely associated with clinically apparent disease. Subsequently, tests for HTLV-I have been modified to include the specific ability to detect infection with the very similar HTLV-II. Tests for antibodies to human immunodeficiency virus (HIV), the AIDS virus, have been modified to detect infection with HIV-2 as well as HIV-1. Additional testing to detect the HIV-1 p24 antigen was implemented in 1996. Improved versions of tests for antibody to HCV have also been introduced. Testing of donor blood by genome amplification technology (GAT) was expected to be implemented in 1999. Because technology for testing individual donations will not be available, small to moderate pools of samples will initially be tested for HCV and probably for HIV RNA.

FUNDAMENTAL REQUIREMENTS FOR TRANSMISSION BY TRANSFUSION

Despite the multitude of viruses, bacteria, protozoa, and other parasites that infect humans, only a handful are known to pose problems for blood recipients. The particular characteristics favoring this mode of transmission must therefore be relatively uncommon. First, the infectious agent must, almost by definition, be present in the donor's blood stream. This is hardly a unique characteristic for a pathogen; many bacteria, most viruses, and a fair number of parasites are clearly present in the circulating blood at some stage of an acute or chronic infection. However, for most pathogens, this occurrence is extremely unusual in the absence of symptoms. Thus, simple health screening procedures, such as general questioning and the measurement of body temperature, along with the fact that few people give blood during a bout of malaise, prevent the transmission of many common infections. It is of interest to note that this protection is not complete; there are, for example, infrequent reports of transmission of hepatitis A by transfusion of blood drawn from a donor just before the development of symptoms.[2–4]

A characteristic of most transfusion-transmitted infections is chronicity. Indeed, hepatitis B virus (HBV), HCV, herpesviruses, human retroviruses, and parasites such *Plasmodium malariae* and *Trypanosoma cruzi* may all establish lifelong infection. These infections may be asymptomatic for many years or even for the lifetime of an infected person, and in most instances, there are no significant or recognizable signs of early acute infection. As a consequence, there may be no obvious way to identify an infectious donor on the basis of medical history. However, some infections known to be transmitted from donor to recipient do not appear to be chronic. Hepatitis A virus (HAV) has been mentioned, and the B19 parvovirus and *Yersinia enterocolitica* are other examples of infectious agents that are transmitted as a result of the collection of blood during a brief phase of viremia or bacteremia.

In this context, it is important to note that different agents may be present in different compartments within the blood. Some, such as HBV and HCV, are thought to be found mainly in plasma; others, such as cytomegalovirus (CMV) and HTLV-I, are present only in leukocytes. HIV-1 is present in both plasma and leukocytes; malaria and babesia parasites are found within the red cells. Consequently, not all blood components or fractions are equally capable of transmitting all infectious agents. It is also of interest to note that many transfusion-transmissible agents are characteristically, or incidentally, transmitted by the sexual route.

A final component in the complex of factors leading to infection by transfusion is the susceptibility of the blood recipient. It is well known that the host-parasite response is complex and that there may be both inherent and acquired immunity to infection. Data on the impact of host resistance to blood-transmitted agents are unclear, because the prevalence of preexisting antibodies is generally low. In addition, in most cases, it seems likely that the enormous dose of infectious agents transmitted by a full unit of blood or blood component is sufficient to overwhelm host resistance. Infection occurred among more than 90% of the recipients of blood products that were subsequently found to be positive for anti–HIV-1.[5] Similarly, HBV is transmitted from blood that is positive for hepatitis B surface antigen (HBsAg) in almost all cases, although this is not necessarily true in areas of high endemicity. About 65% of recipients of blood from donors with antibodies to HTLV-I were infected in studies in Japan,[6] and it seems likely that at least 80% to 90% of recipients of blood that tests positive for antibodies to HCV are also infected.[7]

REQUIREMENTS FOR SUCCESSFUL INTERVENTION

How can the transmission of infectious agents during transfusion be prevented? Overall, four activities contribute to the prevention of such transmission. The first is to reduce the number of allogeneic transfusions given, because it is clear that the safest blood unit is the one that remains on the shelf. The second is the selection of safe donors or donor populations; one of the major objectives of epidemiological studies on donors is to improve this process. The third measure is laboratory testing of blood that has already been collected. The last line of defense is to treat blood components to inactivate any residual infectious agents. Until the 1990s, this approach was available only for pooled plasma components. However, solvent-detergent fresh frozen plasma was licensed for use in the United States in 1998; in Europe, virally inactivated plasma had been in use for several years before that time. Virally inactivated cellular components were still in the research phase in mid-1998.

The selection of safe donors or donor populations is the sum of a complex of activities, many of which require the active participation of the donor. The majority of these measures are discussed in relation to the specific agents or diseases involved. However, it is worth summarizing the sequence of donor selection activities at this point.

A relatively unknown but important degree of selection takes place before people enter the donation site. First, it is apparent that the sociodemographic structure of the donor population differs in some important respects from that of the overall population: Donors are often better educated and have higher family incomes than the overall population. This difference is probably a result of both the volitional factors that motivate people to give blood and the way in which donors are recruited.[8] Because the prevalence rates of some infections are inversely related to sociodemographic status, this aspect of donor selection has some impact on safety. In addition, experience showed that certain donor populations were associated with unacceptable frequencies of post-transfusion infections, particularly with hepatitis viruses. As a result, collection from these populations was avoided. The most notable examples were paid donors, prisoners, and certain other institutionalized groups. Finally, it seems clear that at least some potential donors are knowledgeable about factors that would preclude acceptance of their blood and, as a result, do not present for donation. Many are aware that a history of hepatitis excludes a potential donor. Also, the continuing decline in prevalence of anti–HIV-1 antibodies among first-time male donors suggests that many people with risk behaviors for HIV-1 infection are not donating.[9, 10]

The second phase of donor selection is accomplished by direct questioning during the medical history. This process, which depends on the interaction between the medical historian and the donor, is aimed at identifying persons who are considered to be at increased risk of transmitting infectious disease. A part of the medical history is designed to elicit an actual history of the disease in question; for example, donors are routinely asked whether they have had viral hepatitis or symptoms of AIDS. In addition, the donor is asked about the existence of risk factors or behaviors associated with certain infections. Donations from persons reporting a history of any risk behavior for HIV-1 infection are not acceptable and the donor will be permanently or temporarily deferred, depending on the nature of the risk behavior. Similarly, certain geographical exclusions apply, with special reference to residence or travel in areas where malaria is endemic. Interestingly, some questions currently included in the medical history are designed to be indirect indicators of risk. For example, donors are asked whether they have had syphilis or gonorrhea within the past year. Such a history is interpreted as a potential indication of increased risk for HIV-1 infection. It must also be realized that there are real limits to the history-taking process. If a donor is unaware that he or she has been at risk of infection, a history will clearly not be useful. It is also clear from follow-up studies that some donors know that they are at risk but fail to acknowledge this risk at the interview; a study based on a mailed, anonymous questionnaire showed that almost 2% of respondents acknowledged a previously unreported risk that would have resulted in deferral of their donations had it been revealed at the time of donation.[11] This figure greatly exceeds the proportion of people from whom donations are deferred for risk factors revealed at the donation interview. Additional steps in the process of selecting safe donors include record keeping to prevent the collection or issuance of blood from donors previously found unsuitable and the provision of an opportunity for donors to signify that their blood should not be used for transfusion.

Laboratory tests on collected blood currently represent the final line of defense against the transmission of infectious agents. As indicated previously, serological tests for syphilis were the first to be implemented. It was not until the discovery of HBsAg that the modern era of testing began. Subsequently, specific tests for other viruses have depended largely on the identification of virus-specific antibodies. The apparent paradox of testing for antibodies to indicate the presence of active viral infection stems from the persistent nature of infection with these agents. More recently, testing for the transiently expressed HIV p24 antigen has been implemented in the United States, and plans are in place to initiate testing for HCV and HIV genomic materials.

RECIPIENT EPIDEMIOLOGY

Transmission of infections by blood transfusion represents a highly artificial situation. As pointed out previously, host factors have relatively little effect on the outcome of exposure by this route. As a consequence, the epidemiology of transfusion-transmitted infection almost entirely reflects the epidemiology of blood recipients. A clear example is seen in the case of transfusion-associated AIDS, in which the age, sex, and race distribution of patients is closely reflective of the distribution seen in blood recipients and is totally different from that of other AIDS patients.[12] Conversely, a history of transfusion is an independent risk factor for infection with a number of agents. It is important to recognize, however, that only a small minority of infections are a consequence of transfusion. For example, even in the absence of donor testing, only 2% of AIDS cases were transfusion related. Before defining a disease or infection as transfusion transmitted, it is necessary to eliminate other, more common risk factors and, wherever possible, to perform appropriate serological and virological studies on the blood recipient and the implicated donors. The frequency of some transfusion-transmitted infections is now so low that a significant number of apparently transfusion-associated events may represent the coincident occurrence of a natural infection and transfusion.

HEPATITIS B

Epidemiology

During 1996, a total of 10,637 clinical cases of hepatitis B were reported in the United States; the mean number of cases per year for the 8 years 1989 through 1996 was 15,746. The number of cases showed a steady annual decline from 23,419 in 1989.[13] It is likely that hepatitis B is underreported, because active surveillance suggests that only 30% of cases are actually reported. There may be as many as 300,000 new infections annually in the United States. Surveillance studies by Alter and colleagues[14] showed that during the period 1982–1988, the distribution of risk factors for HBV infection changed significantly; fewer cases were associated with homosexual activity (declining from 19.9% to 7.2%), and more cases occurred in the setting of intravenous drug use (increasing from 15.3% to 27.1%). Between 31% and 42% of cases had no identifiable source, and only 0.4% to 4% of cases in this study had a history of transfusion.[14] This and other studies imply that a significant proportion of cases is associated with heterosexual contact (14% to 26%).[14, 15]

Serology

A number of different antigens are expressed by HBV. The outer coat of the virus itself bears HBsAg; this antigen is also shed into the circulation in copious excess as a particulate. There are antigenic variants of HBsAg. The common, or *a,* antigen is expressed in all cases, and two pairs of antigenic specificities, *w/r* and *d/y,* behave like mutually exclusive alleles. Hence, HBV isolates can usually be grouped into one of four antigenic groups: *adw, adr, ayw,* or *ayr.* The antigenic subtypes of HBsAg reflect amino acid substitutions at defined sites. They are of some value in epidemiological tracking. The characteristic antigen of the core, or capsid protein, of HBV is termed hepatitis B core antigen (HBc). There are also other antigenic components or products of HBV; other than the *e* antigen, these are of limited interest in epidemiological terms. The presence of detectable levels of *e* antigen is associated with more aggressive infection and a higher likelihood of infectivity.

The earliest serological sign of infection with HBV is circulating HBsAg. In an acute infection, HBsAg disappears from the circulation as anti-HBs antibody appears, signaling resolution and eventual immunity. In chronic infections, this does not occur, and HBsAg continues to circulate. Antibodies to HBc (anti-HBc) appear shortly after HBsAg is detectable; they may be the only detectable antibody during the early stages of resolution of acute infection. In addition, anti-HBc may occasionally persist after anti-HBs has declined. Overall, the presence of detectable levels of HBsAg defines active infection accompanied by circulating, infectious virions. Anti-HBs reflects a resolved infection. Anti-HBc is an indicator of current or past active infection; in limited circumstances, it may be the sole serological marker of infectivity, particularly when present in the immunoglobulin M (IgM) form. More information may be obtained by the use of

GAT to detect HBV DNA. Detectable DNA may circulate for a few days before, and persist until some time after, detectable HBsAg is present.

Mechanism of Transmission

The underlying mechanism for the transmission of HBV is transfer of body fluids from one person to another. The virus circulates freely in the plasma, and all blood components may transmit infection. HBV nucleic acids have been detected in leukocytes, but it is not clear whether the virus can replicate in these cells. In cases of acute or chronic infection, HBV is frequently present at titers of 10^7 or more virions per milliliter, whether or not the disease is symptomatic. As a consequence, the infection may be transmitted by an extremely small volume of blood, and it is possible that transmission by body fluids other than blood may actually reflect contamination of those fluids by a small amount of blood. It appears that infection requires the virus to enter the blood stream by direct contact via broken skin or mucous membrane. Chimpanzee experiments suggest that infection does not occur as a result of ingestion through the gastrointestinal tract. The virus may, however, enter the body through damaged mucous membranes in the mouth. Similarly, epidemiological data clearly demonstrate that HBV is transmissible by the sexual route, presumably via the mucous membranes.[15] Infection via anal intercourse is particularly efficient. In areas where HBV is endemic, the predominant route of transmission is infection of infants at or around birth. There is no evidence that such infection is strictly vertical or transplacental; rather, it is thought that infants are infected by direct contact with maternal body fluids during birth. Infection at an early age is much more likely to become chronic, contributing to a high prevalence of carriers in the overall population. In the United States, the predominant transmission route is horizontal, between adults.

On the basis of serological studies, it is clear that about 5.7% of the U.S. population has been infected with HBV, suggesting that infection itself is not infrequent. Prevalence rates are higher among African-Americans (13.7%) than among whites (3.2%), and there is an increasing prevalence with age in all populations.[16] A large proportion, if not the majority, of such infected persons appears to have neither risk factors for infection nor a clear history of exposure, suggesting some cryptic route of infection for the virus. Although there is no evidence of a strict aerosol infection route for HBV, it can be transmitted by droplet contamination onto mucous membranes. A variety of theories and concepts have been proposed to account for this "unseen" natural transmission route, but none of them can explain it in full. Transmission most likely occurs via the sexual route in most cases. However, it is important to stress again that only a fraction of a microliter of blood can transmit infection and that the virus may readily enter the body through imperceptible skin lesions. In addition, HBV can survive on surfaces for some time without losing all infectivity. Thus, there are recorded cases of infection from items such as papers and thorns. Other mechanisms have been suggested as occasional routes of transmission, including contact with weeping sores, menstrual fluids, and shared personal grooming equipment.

Of course, transmission of HBV by a variety of non-natural routes, particularly medical procedures, is well known. Perhaps the first outbreak of this nature to be documented and studied was the transmission of HBV through the use of a human-derived smallpox vaccine in Bremen in 1885. Subsequently, hepatitis B outbreaks were associated with multiple use of hypodermic syringes and in a number of situations involving the incorporation of human serum or plasma into biologicals, culminating in 28,585 cases associated with a yellow fever vaccination program in 1942. Hepatitis B infection is a significant risk for health care workers. It has been estimated that 30% of needlesticks involving blood from infected patients result in infection. Laboratory staff were particularly at risk in the past; the risk appeared to be inversely related to experience in handling microbial pathogens. In the United States, regulatory agencies require that any sample of human blood be handled as though it were infectious. It is anticipated that these so-called universal precautions will be effective in reducing the risk of accidental transmission in the workplace.

Risk Factors Among Blood Donors

Risk factors for HBV infection are well known; they have been defined for acute, clinical infection and for serological evidence of infection. There is a high rate of HBV endemicity in some populations; geographical or racial origin can be a risk factor. HBV infection is endemic in many parts of the Far East and Southeast Asia and in many native populations of the Oceanian region, where overall seroprevalence rates may approach 100%. In addition, infection is common in parts of sub-Saharan Africa and among some Native American populations, including those in Alaska. In the United States, the prevalence of infection among Asians, African-Americans, and Hispanics is generally greater than that among whites, although these findings may be confounded by an inverse relationship between socioeconomic status and prevalence of infection.[16]

In the United States, risk factors relating to exposure routes or behavioral factors seem to have the greatest influence on the frequency of infection. Male homosexuals with multiple sex partners have been shown to have seroprevalence rates of 80% to 90% in some studies. A history of current or past intravenous drug abuse involving needle sharing is also associated with greatly increased risk for infection. There is evidence of heterosexual transmission, so a history of multiple sexual partners or of an HBV-infected sexual partner is a risk factor. In addition, a history of household or other types of close contact with HBV-infected persons is associated with infection. People living in institutional settings, particularly prisons and facilities for the mentally retarded, are also in this category. It is not clear in these cases how the infection is transmitted, although there is little reason to suppose that an aerosol or enteric route is involved.

Occupation may also be a significant risk factor for

HBV infection. Health care workers who are exposed to human blood are at highest risk, particularly with needlestick exposure. There are other situations in which people may be infected with HBV as a result of the use of nonsterile skin-piercing implements, such as tattooing. Finally, in the past, people who received multiple blood transfusions or were treated with clotting factor concentrates were at increased risk of infection. Current donor screening and testing and the use of methods to inactivate viruses in plasma products have essentially eliminated this risk.

A number of factors are thought to be associated with higher risk for development of chronic HBV infection. The most important of these is infection at birth or early in life. In addition, persistent infection may be more likely in immunosuppressed patients and among some populations institutionalized for mental retardation.

How does this knowledge about the risk of HBV infection affect the overall safety of the blood supply? The earliest preventive measure to be implemented was the prohibition of donation by those reporting a history of viral hepatitis. This measure was justified to some extent by the finding that prospective donors with such a history clearly had elevated prevalence rates for serological markers of hepatitis B[17]; subsequently, this finding was also shown to extend to hepatitis A and C.[18] The value of this approach is severely compromised by the fact that most cases of HBV infection are subclinical. Deferral of donations from persons with a history of close contact with a case of viral hepatitis or with potential parenteral exposure to blood is also clearly consistent with the known epidemiology of HBV. In contrast, prohibition of donation by prisoners and paid donors was based on observations that such donors were frequently implicated in the transmission of hepatitis.

Interestingly, there was relatively little effort to use the presence of other risk factors to interdict donation, at least until the recognition of transfusion-transmitted AIDS. Developing knowledge about the immunopathology of HBV itself was, however, utilized. For example, the temporary deferral period for donors with parenteral exposure to HBV was increased to 12 months after specific immunoglobulin treatment because clinical studies had suggested that such treatment could extend the incubation period before clinical infection.

Interventions

The frequency of HBV transmission can be reduced by a number of measures designed to prevent exposure to body fluids. Obviously, proper cleansing and sterilization of instruments and fomites and the proper use of gloves are critical in medical practice. The use of condoms would be expected to limit exposure via the sexual route. Effective inactivation procedures have been developed for pooled plasma products. However, the most important intervention is the proper use of HBV vaccine. Highly effective, safe vaccines are available, and they should be used to immunize patients at risk for infection. In some cases, postexposure prophylaxis with specific HBV immunoglobulin plus vaccination is recommended and effective.

Donors and Recipients

The incidence of clinically apparent post-transfusion hepatitis B has declined from 1.5% or more in the 1950s to essentially negligible levels today. The American Red Cross collects about 6 million units of blood annually, and fewer than 150 cases of transfusion-related HBV infection were reported each year from 1987 to 1991; the figure has subsequently declined to fewer than 100. It is highly likely that most of these cases were coincidental and were not causally related to transfusion, because the overall reported rate of hepatitis B in the United States is now about 4 to 5 cases per 100,000 annually. The very low frequency of transfusion-transmitted hepatitis is a result of donor screening and testing measures. Potential donations are deferred if donors report a history of viral hepatitis, of potential parenteral exposure to blood, or of close contact with a known case. In addition, current tests for HBsAg are able to detect the majority of actively infected persons. Finally, although testing for anti-HBc was originally introduced as a surrogate test for non-A, non-B hepatitis (NANBH), it was known that in the later stages of acute HBV infection, virus could be present in the absence of detectable HBsAg; anti-HBc was usually present in such cases. The frequency of post-transfusion hepatitis B declined in association with the introduction of anti-HBc testing, and this measure is now recommended for its value in preventing HBV infection.

The prevalence of detectable HBsAg in the American donor population is around 0.03%, and about 0.75% to 1.25% of donors are reactive in tests for anti-HBc. Schreiber and colleagues reported that the crude incidence rate of HBV infection among repeat voluntary blood donors is 4 per 100,000 person-years. However, recognizing that HBsAg is only transiently detectable, they suggest that the true incidence is more likely on the order of 9.5 per 100,000 person-years. If the infectious window period is 59 days, the residual risk of HBV infection is estimated at 1 per 63,000 donations.[19] However, some of these underlying assumptions may not be accurate, and it seems likely that the actual risk is lower.

At presentation, HBsAg-positive donors do not have any symptoms of hepatitis. However, some of these people appear to be at significantly higher risk of developing severe liver disease, including hepatoma, over their lifetimes, as shown by death record searches.[20, 21] Consequently, appropriate follow-up and counseling may be advisable. In addition, because HBsAg-positive persons can transmit HBV to their sexual partners, and because infected women may transmit HBV to their infants, it is important to provide information about the availability and use of the HBV vaccine.

HEPATITIS C

Before the recognition of HBsAg, viral hepatitis was epidemiologically characterized as either a parenterally transmitted "serum" hepatitis or an epidemic or "infectious" form. It was therefore anticipated that the implementation of blood donor testing for HBsAg around 1971 would eliminate transfusion-transmitted hepatitis. That this did not occur was attributed to the relative insensitivity of the tests then in use. The development of the much more sensitive radioimmunoassay technique offered great promise for the elimination of the remaining cases of post-transfusion hepatitis. This perception was heightened by the fact that the new test actually identified four to five times more reactive samples than did the previous, second-generation methods. However, it soon became apparent that the major part of this increased reactivity was due to nonspecificity of the radioimmunoassay, and confirmatory testing was implemented. Nonetheless, residual post-transfusion hepatitis continued to occur. Once diagnostic reagents for HAV infection became available, it was clear that the major cause of post-transfusion hepatitis was neither HAV nor HBV, and the disease was called NANBH. In 1988, HCV was identified by molecular methods and was subsequently shown to be the cause of almost all cases of post-transfusion NANBH.[22, 23]

Epidemiology

During 1996, 3716 cases (an incidence rate of approximately 1.5 per 100,000) of clinical hepatitis C/NANBH were reported to the Centers for Disease Control and Prevention (CDC).[13] However, this disease is notoriously underreported, and in the past, active surveillance in selected sites revealed that the incidence was closer to 7.1 cases per 100,000.[24] During the period 1982–1988, although the incidence remained relatively constant, there were significant changes in the reported risk factors; the proportion of patients with a history of intravenous drug abuse increased from 21% to 42%. Over the same period, the proportion of cases associated with a history of blood transfusion declined from 17% to 6%. No risk factor was identified among 51% of cases initially, but this declined to 42% by the end of the study. Heterosexual exposure to a contact with hepatitis or to multiple partners accounted for 6% of cases, and household exposure to a case accounted for 3%.[24]

Serology

For many years, NANBH was characterized by a diagnosis of exclusion. It was recognized in the post-transfusion setting as a result of serological tests that showed that cases of hepatitis occurring among recipients of HBsAg-negative blood were not caused by either HAV or HBV. Extensive post-transfusion follow-up studies were initiated to characterize NANBH and to identify the causative agents or their serology. Essentially all these studies involved biweekly evaluation of preselected blood recipients during the 6 months after transfusion. Two successive elevations of serum levels of the enzyme alanine aminotransferase (ALT) were considered to be evidence of hepatitis. In these studies, at least 7% to 10% of the recipient populations evaluated had enzymatic evidence of liver dysfunction, which was classified as NANBH. In 50% of the cases, the dysfunction was chronic, and a majority of patients with chronic NANBH were shown by histological criteria to have serious disease.[25] The infectious etiology of this form of hepatitis was conclusively demonstrated by extensive transmission studies in chimpanzees. However, until the late 1980s, it proved impossible to identify or isolate an etiological principle or any serological markers of infection or infectivity.

Two of the most extensive post-transfusion evaluations, the Transfusion-Transmitted Viruses Study[26, 27] and the National Institutes of Health Study,[28, 29] included extensive investigation of all donors whose blood products were transfused to patients who developed NANBH. Both studies showed that there was a correlation between elevations of ALT levels in the donor and development of NANBH in the recipient. Interestingly, subsequent reevaluation of the study samples showed that there was a similar relationship between the presence of anti-HBc among donors and the development of NANBH in recipients. However, the two markers identified different and largely nonoverlapping populations of donors. Testing for these two markers was implemented in the United States in 1986–1987 as a surrogate for a specific test for NANBH. A small number of blood centers had implemented ALT screening shortly after the original publication of the results of these studies.

Unfortunately, surrogate markers such as ALT elevations and the presence of anti-HBc, along with a nonspecific diagnosis, were blunt tools for the epidemiological dissection of NANBH. The eventual cloning and expression of the genome of HCV, however, and the development of enzyme-linked immunosorbent assays (ELISAs) for antibodies to the viral proteins revolutionized our ability to investigate this disease.[22, 30]

The first tests to be developed were based on the single expressed protein c100, which represents a nonstructural viral component. Subsequent versions of the test included other viral proteins and were much more sensitive.[31] It is now apparent that anti-HCV, as measured by these multiantigen tests, is detectable 80 to 90 days after infection. The appearance of antibody may be immediately preceded by a spike in serum ALT levels. Genome amplification studies suggest that HCV RNA may be detectable some 40 days before there are detectable antibodies.[19] In most cases, circulating RNA is present for many years, although there is some evidence that a minority of infected patients (perhaps 15% to 30%) may eventually clear their infection. In most infected patients, the virus circulates over their lifetimes, and they are at risk for the development of clinical liver disease, including liver failure, cirrhosis, or even primary hepatocellular carcinoma. Nevertheless, such outcomes may take 20 or more years to become apparent and appear to affect less than 20% of those with chronic infection, with an eventual mortality of about 4%.

Mechanism of Transmission

HCV is readily transmitted by a number of parenteral routes. Blood transfusion and the use of clotting factor concentrates without viral inactivation have been associated with frequent transmission of HCV. In addition, populations of intravenous drug users have very high prevalence rates (up to 80%) for HCV antibodies. Some limited data suggest that the virus may be transmitted to health care workers by needlestick.[32] However, these findings do not define the natural routes of transmission of this virus.

Relatively little is known about the mechanism of spread of HCV or its maintenance in the population. The global distribution of HCV infection is strikingly consistent, with seroprevalence rates of 1% in almost every population studied, irrespective of location, genetic makeup of the population, or social practices. This implies that the transmission of HCV occurs by a common mechanism worldwide. The absence of epidemics and of non-iatrogenic, single-source outbreaks of HCV infection shows that the virus is not readily transmitted by casual contact or by the fecal-oral route. It should be noted that some regions, countries, or cohorts do show unusually high prevalence rates for anti-HCV, but these are usually attributed to widespread use of traditional medicine in the past. There is some evidence for transmission from infected mother to child at or around birth; the risk appears to be about 5%. Finally, seroprevalence rates are age dependent; most studies have revealed a peak prevalence between 30 and 35 years, even in cohorts of subjects widely separated chronologically or geographically.[33]

A number of studies indicate modest elevations in prevalence rates for anti-HCV antibodies among sexually active male homosexuals. In addition, case-control studies on HCV-positive patients suggest that a history of multiple sexual partners is significantly associated with infection. Other studies show that family and/or sexual contact with a person with hepatitis is also a risk factor for HCV infection. Again, the literature is inconsistent, but overall, it appears that the risk of sexual transmission of HCV between long-term partners may be 5% or less. Taken together, the data tend to support the concept that HCV may be transmitted, albeit inefficiently, by sexual intercourse or close contact. Whether this is the predominant transmission route for the virus remains to be determined. However, the epidemiological pattern of HCV infection does not appear to be compatible with other major transmission mechanisms.[7, 15]

The implementation of screening tests for HCV antibodies among blood donors has led to a number of epidemiological studies. Conry-Cantilena and colleagues reported that almost all seropositive donors had some kind of risk factor; highly significant findings were that 27% had a history of prior blood transfusion, 42% had a history of intravenous drug use, and 53% had a history of sexual promiscuity. In addition, histories of nasal cocaine use and of ear-piercing among men were highly significant, but both these findings could have been confounded by other behaviors.[34]

Interventions

Relatively few interventions were established specifically to prevent the transmission of NANBH by blood transfusion. In retrospect, those early measures designed to deal with "serum" hepatitis must have had some degree of efficacy. In particular, avoidance of populations traditionally or demonstrably associated with intravenous drug abuse probably had a profound effect on post-transfusion infection rates. Even in the late 1980s, when serological tests for antibodies to HCV-encoded proteins were evaluated, the prevalence of repeatedly reactive test results was 10-fold higher among paid plasma donors than among voluntary donors to community blood centers.[35] In addition, Tegtmeier and colleagues[18] showed that a history of hepatitis among putative donors was associated with an increased prevalence of anti-HCV.

Around the end of 1986, there was widespread introduction of the so-called surrogate screening assays for NANBH. Essentially all donations were tested for elevated levels of ALT and for the presence of anti-HBc. These measures were accompanied by appreciable declines in the rates of post-transfusion hepatitis in the United States.[36] However, it is not entirely clear whether the relationship was causal, because the decline occurred before the impact of testing would have been expected to be detected. Chambers and Popovsky demonstrated that, at least in the Boston area, part of the decline paralleled the overall change in reported rates of viral hepatitis, but that an additional incremental decline in post-transfusion hepatitis was most likely a result of the introduction of surrogate testing.[37] Others hypothesized that changes in donor selection practices implemented in an effort to reduce the risk of transfusion-associated AIDS may have contributed to the reduction in hepatitis.

Once tests for antibodies to HCV proteins became available, it was possible to evaluate the efficacy of surrogate testing, at least with respect to post-transfusion hepatitis due to infection with HCV. In studies performed in the United States, it was clear that anti-HCV antibodies were more common among donors with elevated ALT levels or those with anti-HBc than among donors without these findings.[33] In general, the relationship between elevated ALT levels and HCV antibodies is uniform in a number of studies from around the world. In some studies performed outside the United States, however, there was no significant relationship between anti-HBc and anti-HCV.[38] A Consensus Development Conference found that once anti-HCV testing was in place, these surrogate tests had no demonstrable residual value for the prevention of post-transfusion HCV infection.[38a]

Implementation of a test for antibodies to HCV proteins has clearly had a significant impact on the frequency of recipient infection with this virus, as shown by retrospective analysis of post-transfusion follow-up studies and a limited number of prospective studies. In one such study, Donahue and colleagues[39] showed that the incidence of post-transfusion HCV infection declined significantly after implementation of both surrogate and specific screening measures. Their study of cardiac surgery patients showed that the per-unit risk of HCV infection was 0.45% before any testing, 0.19% after implementation of surrogate testing, and 0.033% after initiation of anti-HCV testing. This last rate approximately doubled when the recipient population was evaluated with the more sensitive second-generation test. It appears that the multi-antigen tests have effected a major improvement in transfusion safety; there have been no reported cases of post-transfusion HCV infection in any U.S. prospective studies undertaken since the implementation of these sensitive tests. It now seems likely that the major risk of infection is due to the donation of blood during the infectious but seronegative window period; that risk has been estimated to be about 1 per 103,000 units.[19] At the same time, concern about post-transfusion infection continues, and new donor questions have been implemented, including one relating to intranasal cocaine use.[34]

OTHER HEPATITIS VIRUSES

After the recognition of HCV, it became apparent that there were still some cases of post-transfusion hepatitis that could not be attributed to known viruses. Two groups identified viruses termed GBV-C[40, 41] and hepatitis G virus (HGV),[42] which now appear to be essentially identical. Although HGV infection is quite frequent among blood donors (approximately 2% are infected, as demonstrated by the presence of HGV RNA) and is transmissible by transfusion, it appears to be detectable in only about 12% of cases of residual post-transfusion hepatitis.[43] Even so, it has not proved possible to attribute any actual disease to this virus, leading to questions about its role as a cause of hepatitis. Even more recently, a Japanese group described another DNA virus termed TTV, which they have tentatively described as a transfusion-transmissible hepatitis virus.[44] It is too early to define the significance of this finding. It should also be realized that post-transfusion liver dysfunction may not necessarily be due to an infectious agent; indeed, post-transfusion hepatitis (as defined by liver function tests) has been observed among recipients of autologous blood.[45]

RETROVIRUSES: HTLV-I AND HTLV-II

HTLV-I was the first human retrovirus to be isolated and characterized.[46] Subsequently, the closely related HTLV-II was isolated. HTLV-I is now known to be the causative agent of adult T cell lymphoma-leukemia (ATL) and is generally accepted as the causative agent in HTLV-associated myelopathy/tropical spastic paraparesis (HAM/TSP). Data are emerging that suggest that some neurological disease states may be associated with HTLV-II infection.[47] In the United States and many other countries, blood donations are routinely tested for the presence of antibodies to HTLV-I, to prevent transmission of this agent by blood transfusion. Because HTLV-II is closely related to HTLV-I at the level of its genetic sequence, it shares many antigenic specificities, and viral lysate-based serological tests for anti–HTLV-I also detect many, if not all, cases of infection with HTLV-II. Even so, combination tests containing specific antigens from both viruses were licensed and mandated for donor screening by early 1998.

Epidemiology

The epidemiology of HTLV-I is characterized by extreme geographical clustering. On a global scale, the infection is endemic in southern Japan, parts of sub-Saharan Africa, and parts of the Caribbean. Even within these areas, there may be considerable clustering of cases. It is probable that this clustering reflects the predominance of transmission from mother to child, along with the characteristic retroviral pattern of lifelong persistence. Interestingly, it appears that the transmission route from mother to child may be via breast milk. Horizontal transmission, primarily from male to female, also occurs via the sexual route. The seroepidemiology of infection is characterized by higher prevalence rates among women and by an age-related increase in antibody prevalence, even among populations in which infection most likely occurred around birth. It is generally accepted that a seropositive person has about a 4% lifetime risk of developing either ATL or HAM/TSP, at least in areas of high endemicity. In countries where HTLV-I infection is not endemic, such as the United States, this relationship is not so clear.

The natural epidemiology of HTLV-II has not been fully characterized. The virus is endemic in certain native populations of the Americas, where it is presumably maintained in the same fashion as HTLV-I. Unfortunately, these populations have not been studied enough to permit an assessment of the natural history of HTLV-II infection. It is also clear that this virus is present among populations of intravenous drug users and presumably is readily transmitted (as is HTLV-I) by shared use of injection equipment.

Serology

Infection with HTLV of either type is accompanied by the development of antibodies to viral components. Such antibodies are detectable weeks to months after exposure to the virus by blood transfusion. However, little is known about the serological response to infection acquired by natural routes. Western blot analyses of the immune response to HTLV-I have shown that a wide range of antibodies may appear in response to infection. The *gag* gene encodes a parent polypeptide, p55, and two derived peptides, p19 and p24. Glycoproteins encoded by the *env* region include gp46, gp68, and even gp61, depending on the cellular source of the virus. There has been some controversy about the significance of antibodies to the p40x peptide, which is the product of the regulatory gene *tax*.[48, 49] Because of the antigenic and structural similarities between HTLV-I and HTLV-II, it is not easy to differentiate infections with these two viruses, other than by the use of virus-specific peptide-based tests or genomic analysis.

Mechanism of Transmission

HTLV establishes persistent and generally nonlytic infection in T lymphocytes. In some cases, the viral genome may be integrated into that of the host cell, but productive infection may also occur. It seems likely, at least for HTLV-I, that transmission of the virus depends on actual transmission of infected lymphocytes, although a role for free virus has not been excluded. There appear to be two major natural infection routes for HTLV-I: from mother to child, mainly via breast milk, and horizontally via sexual intercourse. Transmission from male to female seems to be more efficient than from female to male. Presumably, this accounts for the generally higher seroprevalence levels among women.

The natural infection routes for HTLV-II have not been established, but they are likely similar. Both viruses are transmitted by transfusion of cellular blood components, but apparently not by plasma or plasma derivatives. The efficiency of transfusion-associated transmission does not seem as high as with some other viruses; however, this observation is largely a function of the cell-associated nature of the virus. The efficiency of transmission declines with the length of time the blood component has been stored, presumably reflecting a loss of cell viability.[6, 50] There is evidence that both HTLV-I and HTLV-II are transmitted between intravenous drug users, presumably as a result of needle sharing. There also appears to be an excess prevalence of anti–HTLV-I antibodies among some populations of homosexual males.

Risk Factors Among Blood Donors

In the United States, routine testing for antibodies to HTLV-I probably represents the largest single means of identifying persons infected with HTLV-I or HTLV-II. Before the initiation of such testing, seroepidemiological studies suggested that the prevalence of infection among U.S. blood donors would be on the order of 0.025%.[51] Once large-scale testing was initiated, the actual figure was found to be approximately 0.017%; the prevalence rate has been declining as seropositive repeat donors have been identified and eliminated from the pool and is now on the order of 10 per 100,000 donations.

With a combination of the polymerase chain reaction and ELISA tests based on synthetic antigens, it has proved possible to characterize whether seropositive donors were infected with HTLV-I or HTLV-II in the majority of instances. In one such study, 53% of those that could be typed had been infected with HTLV-II.[50] Interview-based studies on such serotyped donors have defined the distribution of risk factors for infection with the two viruses. Among donors, it is clear that the major risk factors for HTLV-I are birth or sexual contact in endemic areas, whereas for HTLV-II, the predominant risk factor is intravenous drug use or sexual contact with intravenous drug users. Interestingly, studies in the southwestern United States suggest that HTLV-II may be endemic in particular Native American populations.[52] Emerging data support the finding that the predominant risk factors for HTLV-I infection among blood donors in the United States are geographical—that is, a history of birth or residence in an area endemic for HTLV-I, such as Japan or the Caribbean, or of sexual contact with natives of these areas—and that the predominant risk factor for HTLV-II infection is a history of intravenous drug abuse or of contact with intravenous drug users.[53] On the basis of studies on the length of the infectious window period and the incidence of new infections among blood donors, Schreiber and colleagues estimated that the residual risk of infection with HTLV is about 1 per 640,000 blood units.[19]

Interventions

Clearly, measures to prevent HTLV-I infection via sexual contact and breast milk can be defined and implemented. Other than testing for antibodies to HTLVs, there are no specific interventions to prevent the transmission of these viruses by transfusion. Geographical exclusions would be neither specific nor sensitive. Exclusion of donors with risk factors for either HTLV type, such as use of illicit drugs, sex with users of such drugs, and male homosexual behavior, would help prevent infection from donors who circulate the virus but do not have detectable levels of antibodies. Little is known about the frequency or duration of such window periods. It is possible that widespread use of effective methods for leukocyte depletion in blood components will also contribute to reducing any residual risk of transmission.

HIV-1 AND HIV-2

HIV-1 and the closely related HIV-2 are the causative agents of AIDS. HIV-1 is the predominant virus in the United States, most of Europe, Asia, Oceania, and eastern parts of sub-Saharan Africa. HIV-2 appears to be the predominant AIDS virus in parts of sub-Saharan West Africa and its offshore islands. From there, it has apparently spread with population movements, so that it is represented, but by no means predominant, in parts of Europe and possibly South America.

HIV demonstrates three broad patterns of transmission. Pattern I, typically seen in North America, Western Europe, and Australia, involves horizontal transmission of the agent by male homosexual activity and practices associated with intravenous drug abuse. Pattern II, found in much of Africa and parts of South America, is characterized by heterosexual transmission between adults and maternal transmission to infants. In many cases, the transmissibility of the agent appears to be potentiated by concurrent infection with other venereal agents that cause genital ulcers or sores. Finally, pattern III, originally found in parts of East Asia and Eastern Europe, was known as imported AIDS and was typified by small point-source outbreaks, representing viral infection from imported, pooled plasma products or occasional travelers. This pattern has become essentially irrelevant to the understanding of the global AIDS epidemic. The divisions among these patterns are becoming less clear-cut, but pattern II is of the greatest global concern, because it has already resulted in regions where 20% or more of the entire population is infected.[54, 55]

Epidemiology of AIDS and HIV Infection in the United States

By the middle of 1998, 665,357 people had been diagnosed with AIDS in the United States, and of these,

401,028 (60.3%) had died.[56] The epidemic of disease grew exponentially for 12 or more years after it was first observed in 1981. From 1995 to 1996, the occurrence of AIDS-defining illnesses and AIDS deaths declined by 7% and 25%, respectively, largely as a result of the efficacy of combination therapies. Some 14,338 deaths were reported in 1997, compared with a high of almost 50,000 in 1994. It is believed that in the late 1990s there were about 40,000 new HIV infections annually in the United States. It is now clear that, because the disease has such a long incubation period, there must have been extensive transmission of the causative agent many years before the first case was diagnosed.

The demographic structure of the population of AIDS patients differs significantly from that of the population at large: it consists of many more males, nonwhites, and people aged 25 to 44 years. A hierarchical breakdown of risk factors among AIDS patients shows that the majority of adult cases have occurred among homosexual men (49%), followed by intravenous drug users (26%). An increasing proportion of cases, however, is attributed to heterosexual exposure routes (9%). Overall, only about 1% of cases have been attributed to transmission via blood transfusion, and 1% from pooled plasma products prepared before the introduction of viral inactivation procedures. For about 8% of cases, no risk factor can be elicited.[56] Evidence is now emerging that health care workers are at some risk of HIV infection, although only about 0.4% of needlesticks involving HIV-infected blood actually transmit the infection.[57]

Transfusion-associated AIDS is defined as a case of AIDS occurring in a person with no risk factor other than blood transfusion. As of the end of 1997, 8575 cases of transfusion-associated AIDS had been reported. Of these, only 39 were associated with transfusions that had been given since the initiation of testing for antibodies to HIV in April 1985. Only two pediatric cases have occurred as a result of transfusion since that time, despite the somewhat shorter incubation period for HIV in children.[56] The demographics of transfusion-transmitted AIDS patients are similar to those of transfusion recipients in general.

A large number of studies on the epidemiology of HIV infection have been conducted in a variety of population groups. On the basis of such studies, the CDC has estimated that there may have been about 1 million HIV-infected people in the United States in 1989, with approximately 40,000 new infections per year. Incidence rates vary widely, from a low of 1 per 30,000 blood donors per year, to 1 to 3 per 100 male homosexuals in observed cohorts.[58] Seroprevalence studies suggest that the frequency of infection is alarmingly high among minority populations in inner cities. There are indications that the frequency of cases attributable to heterosexual contact is increasing, and it is becoming apparent that some of these cases may be associated with nonintravenous drug abuse involving exchange of sex for drugs.

As of January 1992, 31 cases of infection with HIV-2 had been recorded in the United States. Some of these cases were identified as a result of anonymous surveillance activities, but in all the other cases, it was established that infection had occurred in a person with potential exposure in HIV-2–endemic areas. Widespread surveillance of blood donors was established. Because viral lysate assays for anti–HIV-1 are likely to detect 50% to 96% of HIV-2 infections, large numbers of donor samples that were reactive in the ELISA for HIV-1 were subjected to specific tests for anti–HIV-2. In 1990, it was reported that none of the 24,826 samples tested had been found to be positive for HIV-2[59]; 1 year and about 10,000 samples later, no HIV-2 infections had been identified. Nevertheless, the U.S. Food and Drug Administration (FDA) recommended that, as of June 1, 1992, all donations be specifically screened for antibodies to HIV-2. In the interim, donors with a history of residence in areas endemic for HIV-2 were excluded. Subsequent to the initiation of tests designed to detect HIV-1 and HIV-2 in 1992, only three donors with HIV-2 infection have been identified. Within the Red Cross system, the frequency was 1 in 28 million donations tested.[60] More recently, similar concern has been expressed about HIV-1 group O, a variant that is sufficiently distant from M strains to evade detection by some but not all HIV antibody tests. In the United States, pending modification of screening tests, potential donations by persons from endemic areas of Central Africa (e.g., Gabon, Cameroon) must be deferred. Group O infection seems to be almost totally absent in the United States, and the risk to the blood supply is vanishingly small, at least as of 1998.

Serology

Infection with HIV stimulates the formation of antibodies. In the case of transfusion-associated AIDS, for which the date of infection can be determined, the period between infection and development of detectable antibodies is 8 weeks or less. A variety of estimates suggest that the period is generally similar for infection acquired by other routes. A number of studies have suggested that, in rare instances, the period between infection and the development of antibodies may be much longer—perhaps up to 1 year. Such studies have always been controversial, and some have been retracted by their authors. However, even with these long incubation periods, it seems that the actual evolution of markers takes a similar course—that is, that HIV RNA, HIV p24 antigen, and antibodies to HIV appear in the same sequence and over about the same time frame (in reference to the point at which antibodies are detectable).

Studies based on seroconversion series, usually obtained from commercial plasma donors, show that RNA (as detected by GAT) appears first, followed in about 5 to 6 days by the p24 antigen. Some 6 days later, a Western blot may detect weak antibody bands, usually to the gp120/160 *env* bands and often to the p24 *gag* gene product. Subsequently, antibody is detectable by ELISA, and additional bands are detected by Western blot. Studies on seroconverting voluntary donors through 1990 showed that the infectious window period for HIV was approximately 45 days: that is, a donor was infectious for about 45 days before the appearance of detectable antibodies.[61] Implementation of peptide-based sandwich immunoassays improved detection of anti-HIV, so that infection was detected about 23 days earlier.[62] The p24 antigen test was implemented in 1996 and was expected to reduce the window period by an additional 6 days[19]; this measure has been seen as an interim step on the way to GAT.

The serology of HIV-2 is similar to that of HIV-1. The polypeptides of HIV-2 do differ in molecular weight from those of HIV-1; consequently, the Western blot pattern is somewhat different when the blot is prepared from a lysate of HIV-2. The *gag* encoded peptides are p16, p26, p55, p56, and p68; the *pol* peptide is p34; and the *env* products are gp36 and gp160.[48]

Mechanism of Transmission

HIV is transmitted exclusively by parenteral exposure to body fluids containing the virus. It is presumed that both free and cell-associated virus can be transmitted in this fashion. The predominant route is sexual; it appears that male homosexual receptive intercourse is one of the most efficient transmission routes. Heterosexual transmission is a major route in some parts of the world; the presence of genital ulcers or sores apparently increases the efficiency. Mother-to-child transmission is also an important route, which may be interrupted by appropriate use of antiviral drugs. Intravenous drug use involving shared needles or "works" readily transmits the virus. The major routes of iatrogenic transmission have clearly been via blood components and, in particular, clotting factors prepared from pooled plasma before the introduction of inactivation procedures. There may also have been an extraordinarily small number of transmissions from infected health care providers to patients. Health care workers are themselves at risk of infection from contaminated sharps or from direct splashes to mucous membranes. There does not appear to be any evidence of transmission of HIV by close nonsexual contact or from fomites.

Risk Factors Among Donors

A number of studies have sought to define the characteristics of blood donors found to test positive for anti-HIV. At the initiation of testing, the representation of HIV risk factors among donors was similar to that among the population of people diagnosed with AIDS.[63] Extensive studies published more recently have revealed some changes in this pattern. The predominant risk factor among males is still a history of sex with a man (53%), and among females, it is a history of sex with an intravenous drug user (38%). The proportion of HIV-positive donors without identifiable risk factors is particularly high; 27% of males and 41% of females belong to this category.[64] The major factor accounting for this is probably the efficacy of measures designed to discourage those at risk from giving blood.[10, 65] It should also be recognized, however, that failure to elicit a risk factor does not necessarily mean that there is no risk, but rather that the risk has not been recognized or acknowledged by the person being questioned.

Evaluation of data from such studies on seropositive donors permits some degree of evaluation of indirect measures designed to reduce the risk of HIV transmission. Interestingly, only 5% of 512 HIV-positive donors used the confidential unit exclusion option.[65]

It has become apparent that the interview process itself is quite inefficient in identifying people with a history of behaviors that increase the risk of HIV infection. Indeed, an anonymous, mailed survey showed that approximately 2% of accepted donors acknowledged a risk history that should have led to the deferral of their donations if the history were reported at the initial donor interview. In the absence of linkage, it is not possible to assess whether these donors actually demonstrated an elevated incidence of HIV infection. It is possible that other approaches to the interview process might eliminate more of these people from the donor pool.[11]

Interventions

The recognition that AIDS might be transmissible by blood transfusion initiated extensive and continuing measures to reduce or prevent such infections. In the absence of any knowledge about the actual etiology of the disease, initial efforts were directed at eliciting a history of AIDS symptoms from prospective donors and educating people with AIDS risk factors not to give blood. Such measures have been made increasingly rigorous over the years by redefining exclusion criteria, soliciting direct responses about risk, and providing opportunities for donors to designate that their blood not be used for transfusion. In addition, the recognition and isolation of the causative agent of AIDS led directly to the development of tests for antibodies to the virus. These tests were implemented on all donations as soon as they were licensed for use in early 1985.

At the initiation of testing, the frequency of confirmed positive test results was 38 per 100,000 in the American Red Cross system,[63] and similar frequencies were found in other donor populations. By the end of 1991 and thereafter, the frequency of confirmed positive results was less than 7 per 100,000. Although some part of this decline was obviously a function of the elimination of seropositive repeat donors, it is clear that prevalence rates among first-time donors also declined significantly during this period.[9]

There is continuing pressure to improve the effectiveness of interventions to prevent the transmission of HIV by transfusion. Essentially all avenues for improvement are under evaluation. Demographic and marketing tools may lead to an expansion of the pool of low-risk donors, but such approaches are at an early stage. There is continuing effort to improve the process of interacting with donors during the donor qualification process. Direct questioning, the use of simpler and more precise language, better educational materials, and perhaps the use of a nonhuman interface for donor response all offer some promise of improvement. Clearly, it will not be possible to eliminate collection from people who either are unaware of their risk or will not acknowledge it. It is evident, for example, that some continue to donate in order to learn their HIV infection status.[11, 65] Some attention is also being paid to the use of surrogate markers of

HIV risk, such as a history of sexually transmitted disease. In fact, in late 1991, the FDA required that prospective donations be deferred for 1 year after an episode of syphilis or gonorrhea.

As discussed earlier, testing for the p24 antigen has been implemented; 2-year testing resulted in the detection of only a handful of additional, putatively infectious donations—perhaps fewer than a half or even a quarter of the expected number. On the basis of incidence data and the window period of 16 days, Schreiber and colleagues indicated that the residual risk may be as low as 1 infectious unit per 676,000.[19]

OTHER TRANSFUSION-TRANSMITTED INFECTIONS

Viruses

Cytomegalovirus

CMV is one of the agents most commonly transmitted by blood transfusion. In the majority of cases, immunologically competent recipients do not develop any disease as a result of such infection, but patients with immature or seriously compromised immune systems are at risk of serious or fatal disease. Infants with low birth weights (less than about 1500 g) are specifically defined as being at high risk for CMV disease, and the use of CMV-seronegative blood is recommended for such patients. There is also increasing recognition that transplant (especially bone marrow transplant) recipients, AIDS patients, and oncology patients receiving aggressive therapy are also at risk.

CMV is a herpesvirus, and in common with other viruses of this group, it may establish persistent, lifelong infection. Antibodies to CMV accompany infection; some of these antibodies, such as IgM and those antibodies directed toward the early antigens of the virus, are specific to recent infection.[66, 67] Infection with CMV is widespread. Overall seroprevalence rates of around 50% have been measured among donor populations in the United States, and the figure may be as high as 90% in some parts of the world.[68] Prevalence rates increase with age; correspondingly, incidence rates may be higher among the young adult population. However, the presence of antibody does not necessarily correlate with the ability to transmit infection via the blood. Extensive studies have been undertaken to isolate CMV from the blood or urine of seropositive donors, but remarkably few have been successful. Although seronegativity has not been associated with transmission, there is considerable controversy about the actual prevalence of infectivity among seropositive donors.

It has been suggested that infectivity has wide geographical variation. Although there may be some truth in this suggestion, the variation is more likely related to how blood and blood products are stored and handled.[69] Data strongly suggest that even a relatively modest depletion of leukocytes may prevent CMV transmission by blood products.[70] A randomized study to compare seronegative and leukoreduced products concluded that they were equivalent in terms of reduction of risk, although this issue is still regarded as controversial.[71] It is clear that in the context of transmission by transfusion, the virus is associated with leukocytes, and emerging data suggest that the association may be specific to the granulocyte fraction, but monocytes may also contribute.[72]

Until the late 1990s, the major intervention to prevent transmission of CMV was to use tested, seronegative blood for patients at high risk of developing the disease.[73] Although attempts have been made to identify serological tests with more specificity for infectivity, total antibody tests are the only ones recommended. It is now becoming accepted that leukocyte reduction may supplement or supplant serological testing.[71] In some circumstances, the use of specific CMV globulin preparations may also offer some benefits in the prevention of disease.[74]

Human B19 Parvovirus

The B19 parvovirus is the agent of erythema infectiosum, or fifth disease, an acute infection usually seen in children and characterized by a rash and fever. The disease is usually benign and self-limited, although it may have serious consequences to the fetus if a woman contracts the infection during pregnancy. In addition, the virus may cause aplastic crisis among patients with chronic hemolytic anemias,[75] and there is increasing evidence that it may have similar effects in AIDS patients.[76] The B19 parvovirus is unusual among transfusion-transmitted viruses in a number of respects. First, it does not usually establish persistent infection in immunocompetent patients and is transmitted during the early acute phase. Second, unlike other viruses routinely transmitted by transfusion, it lacks a lipid coat and consequently is not susceptible to inactivation procedures based on organic solvents and detergents. It is, however, inactivated by modern heating protocols for pooled plasma products.

B19 is normally spread by the droplet-inhalation route and has an epidemic pattern with incidence peaking about every 2 years. It is thus difficult to provide a single estimate of the prevalence of viremia. Although some earlier estimates of the prevalence of infectious virus were generally 1 per 20,000 to 40,000 donations, more recent data based on GAT show that virus may be present in 1 or more per 3000 donations.[77] The prevalence of antibodies is much greater as a result of the widespread nature of infection.[75, 78] There have been only a handful of papers clearly linking B19 disease with transfusion of single-donor products, and there are few indications for measures to prevent transfusion transmission of this virus. More recently, some concern has been expressed about the potential increased risk of B19 from solvent-detergent–treated frozen plasma, as it is a pooled product. It is possible, however, that infectivity is neutralized by the natural antibodies present in the pools.

Parasitic Infections

Malaria and Babesiosis

On a worldwide basis, it is estimated that more than 300 to 500 million people are infected with parasites that cause malaria each year. These parasites, as part of their life cycle, establish a long-term, intraerythrocytic infection and are thus readily transmitted by transfusion. In view of the widespread nature of malarial infection, along with extensive population movements and travel, it is surprising that there are so few cases of transfusion-transmitted malaria in the United States. In fact, from 0 to 2.6 such cases per 1 million transfusion recipients have been reported each year during the period 1972–1994. This appears to reflect the efficacy of processes designed to prevent donations by people who have traveled from malarious areas, because there were about 500 to 1000 non–transfusion-related imported cases of malaria each year in the United States over the same period.[79]

Prospective donors are asked whether they have traveled outside the United States; a positive response requires further evaluation to determine whether such travel was to an area where malaria is endemic. Donation is deferred for 1 year after travel in a malarious area or for 3 years after residence in a malarious area or recovery from clinical malaria. In the United States, these measures seem to be sufficient to prevent almost all post-transfusion malaria. In some parts of Europe, a history of travel to malarious areas is quite common, and donors with such a history may be tested for immunological evidence of infection with malaria parasites. In the absence of such evidence, donations may be accepted.

The protozoan parasite *Babesia microti* is widely distributed in the United States; in Europe, the corresponding organism is *Babesia divergens (Babesia bovis).* Both pathogens may be transmitted to humans by the bite of ticks of the genus *Ixodes.* The primary host for the parasite in the United States is the white-footed mouse; the human is an incidental or accidental host. This parasite, like the plasmodia, also establishes an intraerythrocytic phase and may be transmitted by blood transfusion. A number of such cases have been reported in the northeastern United States, where the parasite is considered to be endemic.[80–82] However, data suggest that the range of this parasite is expanding. In some cases, transfusion-transmitted *Babesia* infection results in serious or even fatal disease. Such outcomes seem to be more common among splenectomized patients. There are no clear measures to prevent transmission of *Babesia* by transfusion. Clearly, donations from persons with a history of the disease must be deferred. It is probably not appropriate to elicit a history of tick bites in areas of particularly high endemicity, inasmuch as this measure is neither specific nor sensitive. Finally, studies using immunological tests for *Babesia* infection have suggested that such tests may not be satisfactory, owing to relatively poor specificity and their inability to differentiate populations from areas thought to be endemic and nonendemic.[83] Other piroplasms have been described in the western and midwestern United States; some appear to be more pathogenic than *B. microti*, and at least one has been transmitted by transfusion.[84–86]

Chagas' Disease

Trypanosoma cruzi causes Chagas' disease; it may establish a long-term or lifelong blood-borne infectious state. The parasite is naturally endemic among most mammals and is transmitted to humans by the bite of hematophagous insects of the genera *Triatoma, Panstrongylus,* and *Rhodnius,* which are commonly found in primitive or rural dwellings in South and Central America. In fact, *T. cruzi* is endemic in human populations in almost all parts of South and Central America. Seroprevalence rates up to 62% have been measured among populations in Bolivia, but most seroprevalence rates in South and Central America range from 1% to 20%. In such parts of the world, transfusion-transmitted Chagas' disease is a common and serious problem.[87] Attempts to prevent transmission have included the use of serological tests, although in many cases it was necessary to use multiple procedures. Alternatively, attempts have been made to prevent infection by treating blood with crystal violet, which inactivates the organism. Aggressive vector-control programs are under way in much of Latin America in an attempt to eliminate human infection with this parasite.

In the United States and Canada, there have been four case reports of transfusion-transmitted Chagas' disease, all of which occurred in immunocompromised patients.[88] The infections were traced to donors who had entered North America from South or Central America. It has been estimated that as many as 100,000 infected people had entered the United States legally by 1990.[87] Seroprevalence studies showed that about 1 in every 1000 donors reporting birth or extensive time in Chagas' disease–endemic areas are *T. cruzi* antibody–positive. This translates to a seroprevalence rate of 1 per 8000 to 10,000 donors in Los Angeles and Miami, where there are high proportions of migrants from Latin America. It appears likely that the prevalence rate is about one fifth of this value on a national basis. Case-control studies showed that it is unlikely that donor screening questions could be devised to minimize the risk of *T. cruzi* infection, because risk factors identified in the study were neither sensitive nor specific.[88]

Leishmaniasis

A small number of cases of transmission of leishmanial infection by blood infusion have been reported, but they provoked little attention or action. However, in late 1991, a small number of unusual cases of visceral infection with *Leishmania tropica* were noted among U.S. troops who had returned from active duty in the Persian Gulf. As a result, there was concern that the agent might be transmitted by transfusion, and a temporary policy of deferring donations from people who had visited the area was instituted. Although this is only a footnote in the overall story of the epidemiology of transfusion-transmitted infection, it illustrates the increasingly important concept that population movements also move infectious agents. A continuing area of concern must be the introduction of exotic agents into nonendemic areas. Despite concerns that geographical exclusion of donors appears discriminatory, this option must be retained and used when appropriate.

Bacteria

Very few bacteria are transmissible by blood transfusion, largely because bacteremia is almost always a serious event accompanied by severe disease symptoms. It is rare to have any form of long-term, asymptomatic bacteremia. Syphilis is one of the few infections in which this can occur. Modern blood collection and storage procedures essentially eliminate the chance of transmission, however, because the organism is fragile and does not survive refrigeration. In addition, routine tests for reagins are believed to detect potentially infectious donations. The reader is referred elsewhere for discussion of the issues relating to transfusion-transmitted syphilis.[89]

A real problem that occurs when a unit of blood is contaminated with bacteria is that the contaminating organism multiplies during storage. Consequently, the recipient may be transfused with a product containing 10^7 to 10^9 organisms per milliliter. The consequences are immediate, serious, and dramatic, unlike those of transmission of viral or parasitic agents.

Essentially two circumstances may lead to bacterial contamination of a transfusion product: when blood is drawn from a person who has some level of bacteremia, and when the unit or product becomes contaminated with organisms from outside the blood stream, perhaps from the donor's skin or some other environmental contaminant. Mild, transient bacteremia may occur as a result of a variety of day-to-day activities; only rarely do these events appear to lead to bacterial contamination of donor blood. However, moderate or extensive dental work may result in significant levels of bacteremia. Consequently, recent (within 3 days) dental surgery is a cause for temporary deferral of prospective donation. Nevertheless, a significant proportion of bacteria associated with outgrowth in stored platelet products may reflect donor bacteremia rather than skin or environmental contaminants.[90, 91]

There are relatively few reported cases of bacterial sepsis associated with platelet transfusion. However, Morrow and colleagues[92] evaluated platelet recipients in one hospital and found that bacterial sepsis occurred about once in every 4000 transfusions. Many of these events occurred among recipients of platelets that had been stored for 3 or more days. Prevention of platelet-associated bacterial sepsis does not appear to be simple. In the past, the shelf life of platelets was reduced from 7 to 5 days in an effort to reduce risk. It is not clear whether further reductions could reasonably be achieved at this time. It is possible that the technology of skin preparation before phlebotomy could be improved, and there may be some potential for pretransfusion testing.

It is also apparent that certain enteric pathogens may be the cause of blood product contamination. In particular, *Salmonella* species and *Yersinia enterocolitica* are occasionally implicated in transfusion-associated recipient sepsis. *Yersinia* is of particular interest, because it can grow at refrigerator temperature. Consequently, it is the most common cause of sepsis from red cell concentrates. In 1990, the CDC reported on seven such cases. In all cases, the red cells had been stored for 20 days or more, although there are reports of *Yersinia* sepsis from products that were not stored for such extended periods. It seems likely that the organisms multiplied to levels in excess of 10^7/mL; the major immediate effect on recipients was endotoxin shock.[93] However, this particular complication of transfusion appears to occur with a frequency of less than 1 per 1 million units transfused. Consideration has been given to a number of interventions, including reducing the shelf life of red cells, testing products before transfusion, and asking prospective donors about episodes of enteric disease. None of these measures appears to have a cost-benefit ratio that justifies their being implemented.

Transmissible Spongiform Encephalopathies

Transmissible spongiform encephalopathies (TSEs) are unusual, fatal degenerative neurological diseases thought to be caused by an aberrant conformation of a specific normal protein (prion). The principal human TSE is Creutzfeldt-Jakob disease (CJD), which has an incidence of about 1 per 1 million worldwide. The majority of cases (85%) are spontaneous, but around 15% are familial and are associated with a number of mutations in the prion protein gene sequence. A minority of cases are iatrogenic, illustrating the transmissible nature of the etiological agent. Transmission has been traced to the use of brain-derived human growth hormone, transplantation of dura mater (multiple preparations may have been contaminated as a result of being processed in pools), use of incompletely decontaminated stereotactic electrodes, and, extremely rarely, corneal transplantation. Such events have led to concern that the agent of CJD might be transmissible by blood transfusion, although there was no evidence of any such transmission as of the end of 1999. Nevertheless, a number of precautionary measures have been formalized, including deferral of donations from persons with a history of use of human-derived growth hormones or dura mater transplantation and those with a family history of CJD. In addition, prior donations or plasma products including such donations must be withdrawn if a donor reports CJD risk or is known to have developed CJD after donating blood. Some product shortages have been attributed, at least in part, to these measures, and they may be subject to change.[94]

Perhaps of more concern has been the emergence of new variant CJD (nvCJD) and recognition of its possible linkage to bovine spongiform encephalopathy (BSE). Although BSE originally appeared to be a disease of cattle, spread in epidemic fashion by feeding cattle improperly rendered carcass by-products, it now seems possible that it has been transmitted to humans, presumably as a result of eating meat from affected animals. Currently, almost all cases of BSE and of nvCJD have occurred in the United Kingdom. nvCJD appears to be a completely new TSE in humans, characterized by its onset early in life and by its unusual pathology.[95] A major concern for transfusion medicine is that the characteristics of the disease and of its spread within the body are unknown, so it is not possible to assess whether it may present a greater risk to transfusion recipients than does CJD. As a result, some European countries are proposing additional safety measures to reduce the as-yet theoretical risk. For example, pooled plasma products are no longer manufactured from plasma donations made within the United Kingdom, and it has been suggested that universal leukoreduction of single-donor products should be implemented, because lymphocytes may contribute to the transport of TSE agents within the body, and the BSE agent appears to be more strongly associated with lymphoid tissue than are other TSEs.

SUMMARY AND CONCLUSIONS

The presence of infectious agents in the blood stream, in the absence of disease symptoms or of a specific history of disease, is a clear threat to the safety of the blood supply. That the actual risk of transfusion-transmitted infections is so low in the developed world is a result of the careful application of science over many years. The dissection of the microbiology and immunopathology of infection has been critical to the development of prevention strategies based on testing, but it is perhaps not appreciated that the largest gains in safety have been achieved by the development and exploitation of epidemiological information. Indeed, it might be argued that the limits of sensitivity of both test-based and epidemiological approaches to donor safety are within reach and that, in the absence of inactivation procedures, a zero-risk blood supply may not be achievable in the developed world. This may be true, but it is critical to recognize that the most serious and pervasive threats to the safety of transfusion are found in the developing nations.

REFERENCES

1. Allen JG. The Epidemiology of Posttransfusion Hepatitis: Basic Blood and Plasma Tabulations. Stanford, CA: Commonwealth Fund, 1972.
2. Hollinger FB, Khan NC, Oefinger PE, et al. Posttransfusion hepatitis type A. JAMA 1983; 250:2313.
3. Noble RC, Kane MA, Reeves SA, Roeckel I. Posttransfusion hepatitis A in a neonatal intensive care unit. JAMA 1984; 252:2711.
4. Azimi PH, Roberto RR, Guralnick J, et al. Transfusion-acquired hepatitis A in a premature infant with secondary nosocomial spread in an intensive care nursery. Am J Dis Child 1986; 140:23.
5. Donegan E, Stuart M, Niland JC, et al. Infection with human immunodeficiency virus type 1 (HIV-1) among recipients of antibody-positive blood donations. Ann Intern Med 1990; 113:733.
6. Okochi K, Sato H, Hinuma Y. A retrospective study on transmission of adult T-cell leukemia virus by blood transfusion: seroconversion in recipients. Vox Sang 1984; 46:245.
7. Alter HJ. Descartes before the horse: I clone, therefore I am: the hepatitis C virus in current perspective. Ann Intern Med 1991; 115:644.
8. Piliavin JA. Why do they give the gift of life? A review of research on blood donors since 1977. Transfusion 1990; 30:444.
9. Cumming PD, Wallace EL, Schorr JB, Dodd RY. Exposure of patients to human immunodeficiency virus through the transfusion of blood components that test antibody-negative. N Engl J Med 1989; 321:941.
10. Busch MP, Young MJ, Samson SM, et al. Risk of human immunodeficiency virus (HIV) transmission by blood transfusions before the implementation of HIV-1 antibody screening. Transfusion 1991; 31:4.
11. Williams AE, Thomson RA, Schreiber GB, et al. Estimates of infectious disease risk factors in US blood donors. JAMA 1997; 277:967.
12. Peterman TA, Jaffe HW, Feorino PM, et al. Transfusion-associated acquired immunodeficiency syndrome in the United States. JAMA 1985; 254:2913.
13. CDC. Summary of notifiable diseases, United States, 1996. MMWR 1996; 45(53):1.
14. Alter MJ, Hadler SC, Margolis HS, et al. The changing epidemiology of hepatitis B in the United States: need for alternative vaccination strategies. JAMA 1990; 263:1218.
15. Alter MJ, Coleman PJ, Alexander WJ, et al. Importance of heterosexual activity in the transmission of hepatitis B and non-A, non-B hepatitis. JAMA 1989; 262:1201.
16. McQuillan GM, Townsend TR, Fields HA, et al. Seroepidemiology of hepatitis B virus infection in the United States: 1976 to 1980. Am J Med 1989; 87(suppl 3A):5S.
17. Tabor E, Hoofnagle JH, Barker LF, et al. Antibody to hepatitis B core antigen in blood donors with a history of hepatitis. Transfusion 1981; 21:366.
18. Tegtmeier GE, Parks LH, Blosser JK, et al. Hepatitis markers in blood donors with a history of hepatitis or jaundice [Abstract]. Transfusion 1991; 31(suppl):64.
19. Schreiber GB, Busch MP, Kleinman SH, Korelitz JJ. The risk of transfusion-transmitted viral infections. N Engl J Med 1996; 334:1685.
20. Dodd RY, Nath N. Increased risk for lethal forms of liver disease among HBsAg-positive blood donors in the United States. J Virol Methods 1987; 17:81.
21. Hall AJ, Winter PD, Wright R. Mortality of hepatitis B positive blood donors in England and Wales. Lancet 1985; 1:91.
22. Choo Q, Kuo G, Weiner AJ, et al. Isolation of a cDNA clone derived from a blood borne non-A, non-B viral hepatitis genome. Science 1989; 244:359.
23. Alter HJ, Purcell RH, Shih JW, et al. Detection of antibody to hepatitis C virus in prospectively followed transfusion recipients with acute and chronic non-A, non-B hepatitis. N Engl J Med 1989; 321:1494.
24. Alter MJ, Hadler SC, Judson FN, et al. Risk factors for acute non-A, non-B hepatitis in the United States and association with hepatitis C virus infection. JAMA 1990; 264:2231.
25. Dienstag JL. Non-A, non-B hepatitis. I. Recognition, epidemiology, and clinical features. Gastroenterology 1983; 85:439.
26. Aach RD, Szmuness W, Mosley JW, et al. Serum alanine aminotransferase of donors in relation to the risk of non-A, non-B hepatitis in recipients: the Transfusion-Transmitted Viruses Study. N Engl J Med 1981; 304:989.
27. Stevens CE, Aach RD, Hollinger FB, et al. Hepatitis B virus antibody in blood donors and the occurrence of non-A, non-B hepatitis in transfusion recipients: an analysis of the Transfusion-Transmitted Viruses Study. Ann Intern Med 1984; 101:733.
28. Alter HJ, Purcell RH, Holland PV, et al. Donor transaminase and recipient hepatitis: impact on blood transfusion services. JAMA 1981; 246:630.
29. Koziol DE, Holland PV, Alling DW, et al. Antibody to hepatitis B core antigen as a paradoxical marker for non-A, non-B hepatitis agents in donated blood. Ann Intern Med 1986; 104:488.
30. Kuo G, Choo Q, Alter HJ, et al. An assay for circulating antibodies to a major etiologic virus of human non-A, non-B hepatitis. Science 1989; 244:362.
31. Kleinman S, Alter H, Busch M, et al. Increased detection of hepatitis C virus (HCV)–infected blood donors by a multiple-antigen HCV enzyme immunoassay. Transfusion 1992; 32:805.
32. Kiyosawa K, Sodeyama T, Tanaka E, et al. Hepatitis C in hospital employees with needlestick injuries. Ann Intern Med 1991; 115:367.
33. Stevens CE, Taylor PE, Pindyck J, et al. Epidemiology of hepatitis C virus: a preliminary study in volunteer blood donors. JAMA 1990; 263:49.
34. Conry-Cantilena C, VanRaden M, Gibble J, et al. Routes of infection, viremia, and liver disease in blood donors found to have hepatitis C virus infection. N Engl J Med 1996; 334:1691.
35. Dodd RY. Hepatitis C virus, antibodies, and infectivity: paradox, pragmatism, and policy. Am J Clin Pathol 1992; 97:4.
36. Dodd RY. Screening for hepatitis infectivity among blood donors: a model for blood safety. Arch Pathol Lab Med 1989; 113:227.
37. Chambers LA, Popovsky MA. Decrease in reported posttransfusion hepatitis: contributions of donor screening for alanine aminotransferase and antibodies to hepatitis B core antigen and changes in the general population. Arch Intern Med 1991; 151:2445.
38. Dodd RY, Popovsky MA, Scientific Section Coordinating Committee. Antibodies to hepatitis B core antigen and the infectivity of the blood supply. Transfusion 1991; 31:443.

38a. NIH Consensus Statement. Infectious Disease Testing for Blood Transfusions. January 9–11, 1995, pp 1–29.

39. Donahue JG, Mũnoz A, Ness PM, et al. The declining risk of post-transfusion hepatitis C virus infection. N Engl J Med 1992; 327:369.
40. Simons JN, Pilot-Matias TJ, Leary TP, et al. Identification of two flavivirus-like genomes in the GB hepatitis agent. Proc Natl Acad Sci U S A 1995; 92:3401.
41. Simons JN, Leary TP, Dawson GJ, et al. Isolation of novel virus-like sequences associated with human hepatitis. Nat Med 1995; 1:564.
42. Linnen J, Wages J Jr, Zhang-Keck ZY, et al. Molecular cloning and disease association of hepatitis G virus: a transfusion-transmissible agent. Science 1996; 271:505.
43. Alter HJ, Nakatsuji Y, Melpolder J, et al. The incidence of transfusion-associated hepatitis G virus infection and its relation to liver disease. N Engl J Med 1997; 336:747.
44. Nishizawa T, Okamoto H, Konishi K, et al. A novel DNA virus (TTV) associated with elevated transaminase levels in posttransfusion hepatitis of unknown etiology. Biochem Biophys Res Commun 1997; 241:92.
45. Blajchman MA, Bull SB, Feinman SV. Post-transfusion hepatitis: impact of non-A, non-B hepatitis surrogate tests. Lancet 1995; 345:21.
46. Poiesz BJ, Ruscetti FW, Gazdar AF, et al. Detection and isolation of type C retrovirus particles from fresh and cultured lymphocytes of a patient with cutaneous T-cell lymphoma. Proc Natl Acad Sci U S A 1980; 77:7415.
47. Murphy EL, Fridey J, Smith JW, et al. HTLV-associated myelopathy in a cohort of HTLV-I and HTLV-II–infected blood donors. Neurology 1997; 48:315.
48. Williams AE, Sullivan MT. Other retroviruses transmitted by blood transfusion. *In* Smith DM, Dodd RY (eds): Transfusion-Transmitted Infections. Chicago: American Society of Clinical Pathologists, 1991, pp 81–114.
49. Sandler SG, Fang CT, Williams AE. Human T-cell lymphotropic virus type I and II in transfusion medicine. Transfus Med Rev 1991; 5:93.
50. Sullivan MT, Williams AE, Fang CT, et al. Transmission of human T-lymphotropic virus types I and II by blood transfusion: a retrospective study of recipients of blood components (1983 through 1988). Arch Intern Med 1991; 151:2043.
51. Williams AE, Fang CT, Slamon DJ, et al. Seroprevalence and epidemiological correlates of HTLV-1 infection in U.S. blood donors. Science 1988; 240:643.
52. Hjelle B, Scalf R, Swenson S. High frequency of human T-cell leukemia-lymphoma virus type II infection in New Mexico blood donors: determination by sequence-specific oligonucleotide hybridization. Blood 1990; 76:450.
53. Williams AE, Sullivan MT, Fang CT, et al. Differential characterization of HTLV-I and HTLV-II infection in U.S. blood donors [Abstract]. Transfusion 1991; 31(suppl):40.
54. Mann JM. AIDS—the second decade: a global perspective. J Infect Dis 1992; 165:245.
55. Quinn TC. Global burden of the HIV pandemic. Lancet 1996; 348:99.
56. CDC. HIV/AIDS surveillance report, 1998; 10:1.
57. Marcus R. Surveillance of health care workers exposed to blood from patients infected with the human immunodeficiency virus. N Engl J Med 1988; 319:1118.
58. CDC. HIV prevalence estimates and AIDS case projections for the United States: report based upon a workshop. MMWR Morb Mortal Wkly Rep 1990; 39(RR 16):1.
59. CDC. Surveillance for HIV-2 infection in blood donors—United States, 1987–1989. MMWR 1990; 39:829.
60. Sullivan MT, Guido EA, Metler RP, et al. Identification and characterization of an HIV-2 antibody-positive blood donor in the United States. Transfusion 1998; 38:189.
61. Petersen LR, Satten GA, Dodd R, et al. Duration of time from onset of human immunodeficiency virus type 1 infectiousness to development of detectable antibody. Transfusion 1994; 34:283.
62. Busch MP, Lee LLL, Satten GA, et al. Time course of detection of viral and serologic markers preceding human immunodeficiency virus type 1 seroconversion: implications for screening of blood and tissue donors. Transfusion 1995; 35:91.
63. Schorr JB, Berkowitz A, Cumming PD, et al. Prevalence of HTLV-III antibody in American blood donors. N Engl J Med 1985; 313:384.
64. Petersen LR, Doll LS, HIV Blood Donor Study Group. Human immunodeficiency virus type 1–infected blood donors: epidemiologic, laboratory, and donation characteristics. Transfusion 1991; 31:698.
65. Doll LS, Petersen LR, White CR, Ward JW, HIV Blood Donor Study Group. Human immunodeficiency virus type 1–infected blood donors: behavioral characteristics and reasons for donation. Transfusion 1991; 31:704.
66. Lamberson HV, McMillan JA, Weiner LB, et al. Prevention of transfusion-associated cytomegalovirus (CMV) infection in neonates by screening blood donors for IgM to CMV. J Infect Dis 1988; 157:820.
67. Lentz EB, Dock NL, McMahon CA, et al. Detection of antibody to CMV-induced early antigens and comparison with four serologic assays and presence of viruria in blood donors. J Clin Microbiol 1988; 26:133.
68. Tegtmeier GE. Cytomegalovirus and blood transfusion. *In* Dodd RY, Barker LF (eds): Infection, Immunity and Blood Transfusion. New York: Alan R. Liss, 1985, pp 175–199.
69. Adler SP, McVoy MM. Cytomegalovirus infections in seropositive patients after transfusion: the effect of red cell storage and volume. Transfusion 1989; 29:667.
70. Gilbert GL, Hayes K, Hudson IL, James J, Neonatal Cytomegalovirus Infection Study Group. Prevention of transfusion-acquired cytomegalovirus infection in infants by blood filtration to remove leucocytes. Lancet 1989; 1:1228.
71. Bowden RA, Slichter SJ, Sayers M, et al. A comparison of filtered leukocyte-reduced and cytomegalovirus (CMV) seronegative blood products for the prevention of transfusion-associated CMV infection after marrow transplant. Blood 1995; 86:3598.
72. Taylor-Wiedeman J, Sissons JGP, Borysiewicz LK, Sinclair JH. Monocytes are a major site of persistence of human cytomegalovirus in peripheral blood mononuclear cells. J Gen Virol 1991; 72:2059.
73. Preiksaitis JK. Indications for the use of cytomegalovirus-seronegative blood products. Transfus Med Rev 1991; 5:1.
74. Snydman DR. Prevention of cytomegalovirus disease with intravenous immune globulin. Transplant Proc 1991; 23(suppl 1):20.
75. CDC. Risks associated with human parvovirus B19 infection. MMWR Morb Mortal Wkly Rep 1989; 38:81.
76. Frickhofen N, Abkowitz JL, Safford M, et al. Persistent B19 parvovirus infection in patients infected with human immunodeficiency virus type 1 (HIV-1): a treatable cause of anemia in AIDS. Ann Intern Med 1990; 113:926.
77. McOmish F, Yap PL, Jordan A, et al. Detection of parvovirus B19 in donated blood: a model system for screening by polymerase chain reaction. J Clin Microbiol 1993; 31:323.
78. Cohen BJ, Field AM, Gudnadottir S, et al. Blood donor screening for parvovirus B19. J Virol Methods 1990; 30:233.
79. CDC. Malaria surveillance—United States, 1994. MMWR 1997; 46(suppl):1.
80. Mintz ED, Anderson JF, Cable RG, Hadler JL. Transfusion-transmitted babesiosis: a case report from a new endemic area. Transfusion 1991; 31:365.
81. Popovsky MA. Transfusion-transmitted babesiosis. Transfusion 1991; 31:296.
82. Gerber MA, Shapiro ED, Krause PJ, et al. The risk of acquiring Lyme disease or babesiosis from a blood transfusion. J Infect Dis 1994; 170:231.
83. Popovsky MA, Lindberg LE, Syrek AL, Page PL. Prevalence of *Babesia* antibody in a selected blood donor population. Transfusion 1988; 28:59.
84. Persing DH, Herwaldt BL, Glaser C, et al. Infection with a *Babesia*-like organism in northern California. N Engl J Med 1995; 332:298.
85. Herwaldt BL, Persing DH, Précigout EA, et al. A fatal case of babesiosis in Missouri: identification of another piroplasm that infects humans. Ann Intern Med 1996; 124:643.
86. Herwaldt BL, Kjemtrup AM, Conrad PA, et al. Transfusion-transmitted babesiosis in Washington state: first reported case caused by a WA1-type parasite. J Infect Dis 1997; 175:1259.
87. Schmuñis GA. *Trypanosoma cruzi*, the etiologic agent of Chagas' disease: status in the blood supply in endemic and nonendemic countries. Transfusion 1991; 31:547.
88. Leiby DA, Read EJ, Lenes BA, et al. Seroepidemiology of *Trypanosoma cruzi*, etiologic agent of Chagas' disease, in US blood donors. J Infect Dis 1997; 176:1047.
89. Barnes A. Transfusion-transmitted treponemal infections. *In* Smith

DM, Dodd RY (eds): Transfusion-Transmitted Infections. Chicago: American Society of Clinical Pathologists, 1991, pp 161–166.
90. Goldman M, Blajchman MA. Blood product–associated bacterial sepsis. Transfus Med Rev 1991; 5:73.
91. Wagner SJ, Friedman LI, Dodd RY. Transfusion-associated bacterial sepsis. Clin Microbiol Rev 1994; 7:290.
92. Morrow JF, Braine HG, Kickler TS, et al. Septic reactions to platelet transfusions: a persistent problem. JAMA 1991; 266:555.
93. Tipple MA, Bland LA, Murphy JJ, et al. Sepsis associated with transfusion of red cells contaminated with *Yersinia enterocolitica*. Transfusion 1990; 30:207.
94. Dodd RY, Sullivan MT. Creutzfeldt-Jakob disease and transfusion safety: tilting at icebergs? Transfusion 1998; 38:221.
95. Zeidler M, Stewart GE, Barraclough CR, et al. New variant Creutzfeldt-Jakob disease: neurological features and diagnostic tests. Lancet 1997; 350:903.

CHAPTER 33

Hepatitis

Cathy Conry-Cantilena
Jay E. Menitove

The current risk of non–A-E post-transfusion hepatitis is less than 0.001% per unit infused. This compares favorably with hepatitis rates of 10% or more per patient given transfusions 2 decades ago.

During the 1950s, post-transfusion icterus occurred in 3% of transfused patients; 23% of those older than age 40 died.[1] In the early 1960s, serially performed aspartate aminotransferase (AST) and alanine aminotransferase (ALT) levels were abnormal in 18% of transfusion recipients.[2] Symptomatic hepatitis developed in 2.8% of recipients in the late 1960s, with an associated 0.1% mortality rate.[3] Subsequently, a distinction in post-transfusion hepatitis rates between blood obtained from volunteer and commercial sources led to elimination of paid donors.[4]

Hepatitis B testing was introduced in 1971, but significant strides in decreasing the incidence of post-transfusion hepatitis had already been achieved by shifting the donor base away from renumerated donors. Between 1975 and 1979, hepatitis B antigen–negative blood was associated with a 10% post-transfusion hepatitis rate per patient as defined by elevated ALT levels. By the mid 1980s, surrogate testing (ALT and anti-hepatitis B core testing) was implemented to reduce the risk of post-transfusion hepatitis not attributed to hepatitis A or B (non-A, non-B hepatitis [NANBH]).[5–8]

In 1989, molecular biology techniques led to the discovery of the hepatitis C virus (HCV), the agent responsible for most NANBH cases.[9] Testing with single-antigen hepatitis C assays began in 1990, and testing with multiple-antigen determinants began in 1992. Subsequently, the risk of post-transfusion hepatitis declined to less than 1% of recipients. Hepatitis D and hepatitis E have little impact on transfusion-transmitted hepatitis.

The search for the elusive etiological agent(s) of non–A-E post-transfusion hepatitis implicated the hepatitis G virus (GBV-C) in 1996[10] and the "TT" virus in 1997.[11] Neither virus has been proven to cause clinical hepatitis.[12–15] The pursuit of alternative etiological agents of non–A-G post-transfusion hepatitis is ongoing.

The scientific and clinical factors leading to the reduction in post-transfusion hepatitis rates are discussed in this chapter. Information is presented about the virology, epidemiology, clinical presentation, incubation, transfusion association, and transfusion risk for agents implicated in cases of post-transfusion hepatitis (Table 33–1).

HEPATITIS A

Virology

The hepatitis A virus (HAV) is a small, nonenveloped, RNA-containing virus belonging to the picornavirus family. Mature virions are spherical, are approximately 27 nm in diameter, and have an icosahedral symmetry. The viral genome is a linear, single-stranded RNA of messenger-sense polarity. It has approximately 7500 nucleotides without significant genetic variation.

HAV (enterovirus type 72) is stable and resists heating at 60°C for 1 hour or at 25°C for 3 months. It survives storage in the cold at 5°C or at acidic conditions (pH 3).[16, 17]

Epidemiology

Exact data on the incidence of HAV infection are unavailable because of its frequent asymptomatic nature. Among

Table 33–1. Hepatitis Viruses

Type	Family	Size (nm)	Genome	Length (kb)
A	Picornaviridae	27	Single-stranded RNA	7.8
B	Hepadnaviridae	42	Partially double-stranded DNA	3.2
C	Flaviviridae	30–60	Single-stranded RNA	9.4
D	Defective passenger virus	40	Single stranded RNA	1.7
E	Calicivirus	32–34	Single-stranded RNA	7.2
F		Designation withdrawn		
G (GBV-C)	Flaviviridae	—	Single-stranded RNA	9.4
TT	Parvoviridae	—	Single-stranded DNA	3.7

children and young adults, less than 5% of cases are diagnosed. Most cases occur in the 5- to 30-year age group. It is estimated that more than 100,000 new cases occur in the United States each year.

Spread of HAV is linked to poor hygiene and low socioeconomic status.[17] Americans older than age 50 have a 50% chance of prior exposure, probably related to a high incidence of HAV infection when this cohort of patients was younger and to the declining incidence of hepatitis A during the intervening years.[16, 17]

HAV infections are spread through sporadic or endemic transmission as well as contaminated water supplies and foodstuffs. Most epidemics are traced to a single source in which food or water contamination has occurred, including uncooked food and drinks; steaming of shellfish to open them does not inactivate the virus. Approximately 24% of HAV cases have been traced to person-to-person contact with someone who has had hepatitis; 11% involve homosexual contact; 4% are related to travel to endemic areas; 18% occur among children at day-care centers; and approximately 2% occur in intravenous drug users. In the remaining 40% of cases, no specific risk factor is identified.[16, 17] Most epidemiologists consider fecal-oral transmission the predominant pathway for HAV transfer. Parenteral transmission occurs infrequently, presumably as a result of the limited duration of viremia during HAV infection.

Clinical Presentation

Young children are frequently asymptomatic, whereas up to two thirds of adults are clinically ill and manifest jaundice. Among symptomatic patients, there is a 4- to 10-day prodrome characterized by anorexia, malaise, weight loss, fever, and diarrhea. The first clinical sign is dark urine, followed by jaundice within 1 to 2 days and light-colored stools. Fever resolves, but pruritus, hepatic tenderness, and moderate hepatomegaly may develop. There is controversy concerning HAV recurrence or relapse within 3 months of the initial symptomatology; however, this type of hepatitis does not become chronic.

The case-fatality rate among healthy individuals who develop hepatitis A is 1/1000. Fulminant hepatic failure is rarely associated with HAV in people with no underlying liver disease. However, 41% (7/17) of individuals with chronic hepatitis C and HAV superinfection had their course complicated by fulminant hepatic failure. Death resulted in 6 of these 7 patients.[18] In contrast, most patients with chronic hepatitis B virus (HBV) infection who acquired HAV infection in this study had an uncomplicated course. Thus, these data suggest that vaccination against HAV is appropriate for those patients known to have a high prevalence of chronic HCV infection, such as those who have been multitransfused.

Incubation Period and Viremic Phase

The incubation period is approximately 28 days (range: 15 to 50 days). A brief viremic phase occurs 5 to 28 days before the onset of hepatic disease.[16, 17] The virus appears in the stool shortly after infection, rising to maximal levels during the late incubation period. Stool levels decline 2 weeks after the onset of jaundice.

Immunoglobulin M (IgM) antibody to hepatitis A antigen appears in the serum 5 to 10 days after exposure. The IgM antibodies persist at detectable levels for up to 6 months after infection. Immunity is denoted by IgG antibody that remains indefinitely. Typically, ALT elevations occur 3 to 4 weeks after exposure, peak 7 to 10 days later, and return to baseline within 1 month. Serum bilirubin abnormalities follow a similar pattern but follow ALT abnormalities by 1 week. Anorexia, malaise, fever, headache, and nausea antedate transaminase abnormalities by approximately 1 week. Signs and symptoms usually persist for less than 2 months, but 10% to 15% of patients develop prolonged or relapsing illness that lasts up to 6 months.[17]

Transfusion-Associated Hepatitis A

Transfusion-associated hepatitis A occurs infrequently (1/1 million) because of the short viremic period before symptoms and the lack of an asymptomatic carrier state.[16, 19–27] Several case reports implicate red cell and fresh-frozen plasma transfusions donated 5 to 28 days before onset of illness. The incubation period in the recipient ranges from 22 to 49 days after transfusion. Several outbreaks of hepatitis A in neonatal intensive care units are attributed to blood transfusion. Post-transfusion hepatitis A has been documented despite donor ALT testing.[23]

Although rarely transmitted by single donor blood components, HAV infections have been associated with transfusion of clotting factor concentrates in the United States, Italy, and Ireland despite the solvent detergent treatment of the concentrates that were derived from plasma pools.[24–27]

The solvent detergent treatment of plasma-derived concentrates appears 100% effective for the inactivation of lipid-enveloped viruses such as human immunodeficiency virus (HIV), HBV, and HCV, but it is ineffective for viruses such as HAV and parvovirus B19, which lack an outer lipid envelope.

Donor Screening and Blood Testing to Reduce Post-Transfusion Hepatitis A

Donor questioning is designed to elicit a history of intravenous drug use, hepatitis, jaundice, and foreign travel and treatment with immune globulin prophylaxis within 12 months of donation. Donors providing this information are deferred. In the absence of a chronic carrier state, routine testing for evidence of exposure to this agent is not considered to be warranted.

HAV Vaccination

Although patients who will receive transfusions are not routine targets for pre-exposure prophylaxis with the inactivated HAV vaccine, it might be considered for use in patients who are chronic recipients of pooled plasma products, such as clotting factor concentrates. As noted earlier, vaccination is worthwhile in patients with chronic hepatitis C. Interestingly, postexposure co-administration of immune globulin and HAV vaccine lowers ultimate anti-HAV response levels 50% compared with HAV vaccine alone.[28]

HEPATITIS B

A member of the Hepadaviridae, HBV has a DNA genome that is partially double stranded and has approximately 3200 base pairs. It replicates through an RNA intermediate; viral DNA is formed from an RNA template in a manner similar to RNA retrovirus replication. There are four overlapping open reading frames that encode for surface (S) or envelope, core (C), "X," and polymerase proteins. The S and C genes have pre-S and pre-C regions that are located upstream. More than one half of the nucleotides are involved in more than one open reading frame (Fig. 33–1).

The infective virion, known as the Dane particle, has a 42-nm diameter and contains surface and core, or nucleocapsid, components. The core HBV contains the circular DNA and DNA polymerase. The surface antigen, or HBsAg, is present on the virion coat or is found in serum as small spheres or rods 20 to 22 nm in diameter. The viral envelope contains large, middle, and major proteins transcribed by the pre-S1, pre-S2, or S genes. The pre-S1 messenger RNA (mRNA), 2.4 kilobases, encodes for the larger surface protein, Pre-S1 + Pre-S2 + S. The middle surface protein, Pre-S2 + S, and the small surface protein, S, arise from codons present in the Pre-S2/S mRNA.[29–31]

The HBV viral genome becomes circular after entering the hepatocyte nucleus. Messenger RNAs, transcribed by a cellular DNA-dependent RNA polymerase, derive from the covalently closed circular DNA. The C mRNA initiates within the pre-C gene and serves as the template for the hepatitis B core antigen (HBcAg) and polymerase proteins. The pre-C mRNA initiates upstream of the pre-C start codon and transcribes only the HBe antigen.[30]

The hepatitis B e antigen (HBeAg), a nonstructural protein, shares approximately 90% of the amino acids contained in HBcAg. The two proteins differ conformationally. In animal models, linear HBeAg stimulates humoral immune reactions mediated by T-helper 2 lymphocytes. In contrast, HBcAg stimulates cellular immune reactions through a T-helper 1 response.[30] In general, seroconversion from HBeAg to anti-HBe signals a reduc-

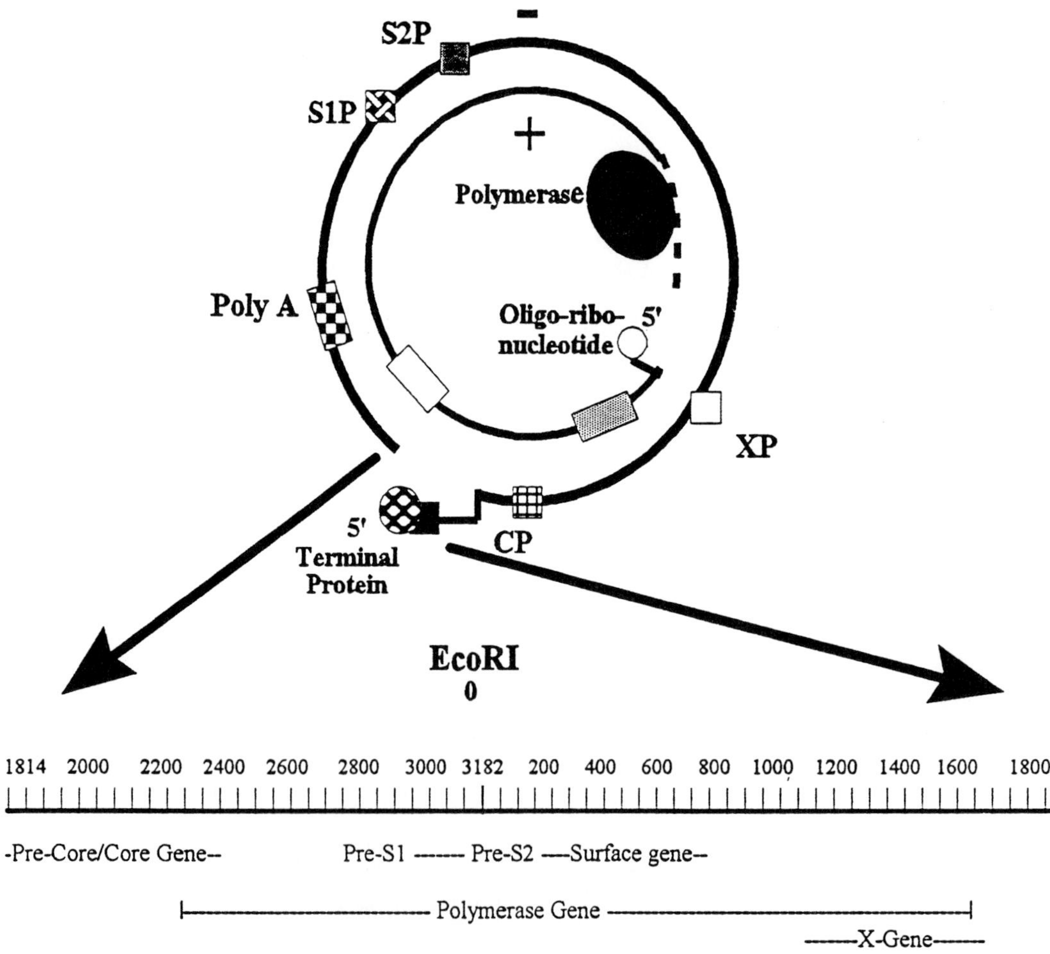

Figure 33–1. Schematic representation of the hepatitis B virus genome. CP, core promoter; S1P, Pre-S1 promoter; S2P, Pre-S2 promoter; XP, X gene promoter; EcoRI, restriction site for EcoRI enzyme used as starting point for numbering. (From Torre F, Naoumov NV. Clinical implications of mutations in the hepatitis B virus genome. Eur J Clin Invest 1998; 28:604.)

tion in viral replication. However, HBsAg-positive/anti-HBe positive patients with circulating HBV-DNA have been described with blocked HBcAg translation or abated transcription of pre-C mRNA. The HBe-negative HBV strains retain the ability to replicate and infect.

HBe-negative mutants have been associated with excessive production of HBcAg, enhanced viral replication, and fulminant hepatitis. Mutant, surface gene proteins have been reported in conjunction with prolonged administration of hepatitis B immune globulin (HBIG) to HBV-infected patients undergoing orthotopic liver transplantation. Apparently, the mutant strains "escaped" as a result of changes in the surface antigen "a" determinant region.[31]

The P gene encodes the DNA polymerase. The polymerase also has a reverse-transcriptase function because HBV replication requires RNA intermediates. The X gene encodes two transcriptional transactivators that aid viral replication.

HBV particles are assembled in the hepatocyte cytoplasm. The polymerase proteins mediate the circular shape of the double-stranded DNA. The assembled nucleocapsid is enveloped by a lipoprotein membrane from cell-derived lipid bilayer and virus surface proteins. The virus is exported through a secretory pathway. Part of the nucleocapsid particles reenter the nucleus and maintain the pool of covalently closed circular DNA.[29, 30]

A serological based system is used to classify the HBV for epidemiological purposes. There is one constant epitopic region, the "a" determinant (amino acids 124–147), which is flanked by mutually exclusive d/y determinants and w/r determinants.[29–31] A genome-based classification system allows for up to 8% divergence in the HBV genomic sequence. Genotype A through F designations are given when the level of divergence exceeds this threshold.[30] The immune response induced by recombinant vaccines targets the "a" determinant of the surface envelope and confers protective immunity. Antibody to the surface or envelope antigen is also found in patients who have recovered from an acute HBV infection. It becomes undetectable in some patients with fully recovered HBV infection.[29]

Hepatitis B surface antigen (HBsAg) is produced by the envelope or surface gene and is detected at serum levels of approximately 200 pg/mL. Its presence in serum indicates ongoing infection. However, the level of HBsAg does not correlate with amount of active virus because HBsAg is found on the surface of virions as well as subviral particles. Absence of HBsAg, in contrast, does not confirm uniform protection from HBV transmission. Recipients of liver transplants from HBsAg-negative but anti-HBc–positive donors have developed de novo HBV infections.[32] The virus may persist in hepatocytes despite serological evidence of resolution. Alternatively, serological resolution may be insensitive despite HBsAg assays that detect 200 pg/mL or 10^7 particles/mL. Hybridization techniques detect 1 pg of DNA or 10^5 HBV genomes/mL, and polymerase chain reaction (PCR) assays detect approximately 20 HBV copies/mL.[33]

Epidemiology

During the past decade, 140,000 to 320,000 acute cases of hepatitis B occurred in the United States each year. One half of these patients had jaundice or other symptoms; an average of 350 died of fulminant disease and approximately 5000 from cirrhosis and hepatoma that is associated with chronic HBV infection. There are an estimated 1.0 to 1.25 million people chronically infected with hepatitis B in the United States. One fourth of these patients are at risk for chronic active hepatitis, which may lead to cirrhosis. HBV carriers have a 12 to 300 times greater risk of hepatocellular carcinoma.[34, 35]

HBV is transmitted through percutaneous or mucous membrane exposures, including sexual contact and intravenous drug use. In 1994, heterosexual activity accounted for 33% of reported cases; intravenous drug users, 19%; homosexual men, 12%; household contacts of persons with hepatitis, 2%; and occupational exposures such as needle stick injuries, 1%. No known risk factors were identified in 8% of those with HBV infection. Twenty-five percent had other high-risk factors, such as a history of other sexually transmitted diseases, imprisonment, or noninjection illicit drug use.[34] More than 98% of infants born of HBsAg-positive mothers in the United States receive HBIG vaccination and are protected from HBV.

Clinical Presentation

The initial symptoms of hepatitis B are nonspecific, consisting of malaise, fatigue, anorexia, nausea, vomiting, and arthralgia. Some patients describe a loss of taste for coffee or cigarettes. Arthritis may occur in 10% to 15%. Urticaria and other rashes and, less commonly, glomerulonephritis and vasculitis, occur.[29]

Fifty to 70 percent of infected adults are asymptomatic. Some have a mild flu-like illness without jaundice; and others develop jaundice, dark urine, fatigue, anorexia, and abdominal pain. Most new cases occur in persons aged 20 to 39. Thirty to 90 percent of infants and children younger than age 5 years become infected chronically, whereas only 2% to 10% of adults develop chronic infections.[34] Hepatomegaly with abdominal tenderness is present frequently; approximately 20% of patients have associated splenomegaly.

Laboratory abnormalities are variable; however, ALT usually is elevated to a greater extent than AST. Serum bilirubin levels may reach 15 to 20 mg/dL. The alkaline phosphatase level is moderately increased, and diffuse hypergammaglobulinemia is observed frequently. Jaundice usually persists for several weeks. Laboratory parameters return to normal within 4 months in patients resolving their infection. The acute-phase fatality rate is 0.5% to 1.0%. Among those chronically infected, 15% to 25% die prematurely as a result of infection.[34, 35] The progression rate to cirrhosis and hepatocellular carcinoma is 8.0% and 2.1% at 5 years, 21.2% and 4.9% at 10 years, and 37.0% and 18.8% 15 years after infection, respectively, in a report involving Japanese patients with chronic hepatitis.[36]

HBV per se is not cytopathic. Hepatic damage results from the immune response against viral antigens on the surface of the hepatocyte, particularly HBcAg. A limited array of HBV peptide fragments processed within the hepatocyte are displayed on the hepatocyte surface, in conjunction with HLA class I molecules. Host CD8 + cytotoxic T lymphocytes subsequently initiate cell killing by means of apoptosis mediated by the Fas ligand, cytokines, and perforin. HBV antigens present in plasma may be processed by macrophages with subsequent HLA class II–restricted presentation to CD4-positive helper T lymphocytes. This results in increased synthesis of cytokines, augmentation of T-cell proliferation, increased display of HLA class I molecules on hepatocytes, and decreased viral replication. CD4-positive cells may, in certain circumstances, become cytolytic.[29]

Incubation and Viremic Phase

The period between infection and development of clinical symptoms ranges from 45 to 180 days, with an average of 60 to 90 days. HBsAg, HBV DNA, and HBeAg are present approximately 6 weeks after infection, 2 to 4 weeks before increase in ALT, and 3 to 5 weeks before the development of symptoms and jaundice. Anti-HBc appears at the onset of symptoms or liver function test abnormalities and persists indefinitely. IgM anti-HBc is detected at the onset of acute hepatitis and persists for only 3 to 12 months, if the disease resolves. Anti-HBe is detected when HBeAg is lost. Anti-HBs indicates resolution of the acute infection[29, 34, 35] (Fig. 33–2).

An alternative description of the HBV life cycle in humans divides the acute illness into four stages: the initial two involve the replicative phase and other two involve the integrative phase.[29] The first or incubation stage lasts 2 to 4 weeks and is characterized by immune tolerance. Active viral replication manifested by high-titer HBV DNA and presence of HBeAg, HBsAg, and antibody to HBc is not associated with symptoms or aminotransferase elevations. Stage 2, symptomatic hepatitis, lasts 3 to 4 weeks in acute infections and for many years in those infected chronically. An immunological response with cytokine stimulation, direct cell lysis, and an inflammatory reaction is associated with a decline in HBV DNA defected by hybridization and PCR methods. In the third stage, the infection is cleared. By 12 weeks after infection, HBeAg gives rise to anti-HBe and HBV DNA levels are detectable by PCR only. Serum HBsAg remains detectable because of integration of the S gene into hepatocytes. The final, or immune stage, occurs approximately 5 months after infection and is associated with anti-HBs instead of HBsAg and lack of HBV DNA. Anti-HBc persists.

In approximately 5% of those infected the acute infection does not resolve and, instead, becomes chronic (Fig. 33–3).

Transfusion-Associated Hepatitis B

Estimates of the residual risk of hepatitis B transmission by blood transfusion are obscured by underreporting associated with absence of symptoms and lack of consensus about mathematical modeling methods. Using one approach involving persons making repetitive blood donations, investigators assumed only 42% of donors previously infected with HBV would be identified by HBsAg testing.[37] This proportion derived from an estimate that 70% of HBV-infected donors have transient antigenemia, 25% have a primary antibody response without HBsAg, and 5% became chronic carriers. HBsAg testing would detect the carriers and those with circulating viremia during the transient, average 63-day, antigenemic phase. These investigators did not include anti-HBc testing in their model because of the nonspecificity associated with this test. The derived risk of a donor giving blood when infectious but serologically negative (window period donation) was 1 in 63,000 (range: 1 in 31,000 to 1 in 147,000).

Taking an alternative approach that includes the use of anti-HBc testing, the risk is approximately 1 in 233,000.[38] This analysis assumes HBV is found in 0.03% of blood donors, HBsAg testing is 99.9% sensitive, and anti-HBc testing is 99% sensitive.

In addition to the analyses just provided, there is a small risk of transfusion-associated hepatitis B by HBV mutants, especially those with mutations affecting HBsAg "a" determinants.[39] Nonetheless, donors with most of these HBV mutants have anti-HBc or HBV DNA. The latter would be detected by PCR test methodology.

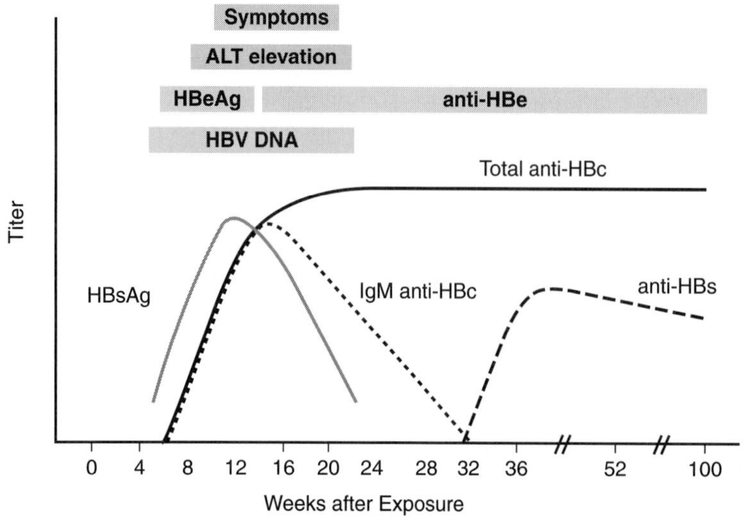

Figure 33–2. Acute hepatitis B virus infection with recovery: typical serological course. ALT, alanine aminotransferase; HBsAg, hepatitis B surface antigen; anti-HBc, antibody to hepatitis B core antigen; HBV DNA, hepatitis B virus deoxyribonucleic acid; HBe, hepatitis B e antigen. (Modified from Centers for Disease Control and Prevention home page: http://www.cdc.gov/ncidod/diseases/hepatitis/hepatitis.htm)

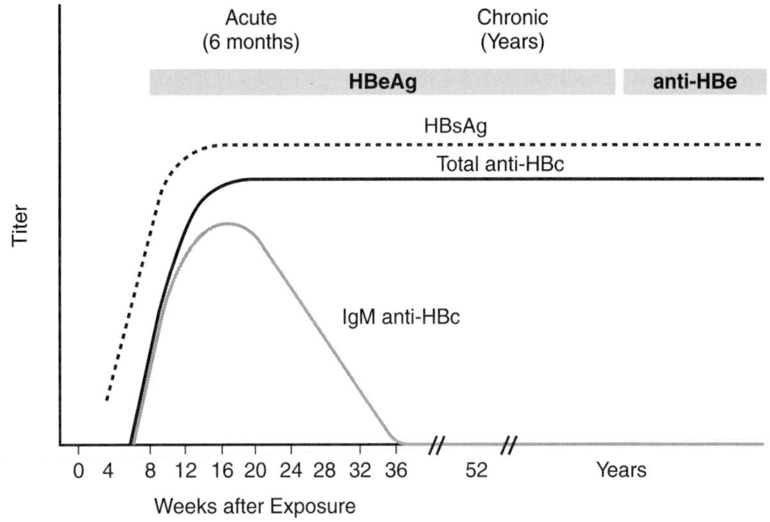

Figure 33–3. Progression to chronic hepatitis B virus infection: typical serological course. HBsAg, hepatitis B surface antigen; anti-HBc, antibody to hepatitis B core antigen; HBe, hepatitis B e antigen; anti-HBe, antibody to hepatitis B e antigen. (Modified from Centers for Disease Control and Prevention home page: http://www.cdc.gov/ncidod/diseases/hepatitis/hepatitis.htm)

Donor Screening and Testing for Hepatitis B

The multilayer approach to donor screening and testing involves questioning and subsequent deferral of donors giving a history of behaviors or exposures that place them at risk for hepatitis B (e.g., injecting drug use, needle stick exposures, body piercing, tattoos).

Laboratory testing includes determination of HBsAg, anti-HBc, and HBV DNA by PCR or nucleic acid amplification testing (NAT). The nonspecificity (a high rate of false-positive results associated with anti-HBc testing) leads to unnecessary deferral of donors and discarding of collected blood. Nonetheless, anti-HBc testing closes serological windows in the setting of acute, resolving infections when HBsAg titers decrease before appearance of anti-HBs; low-level HBV infections with undetectable HBsAg; and some infections with HBV variants.[40]

Routine donor testing for HBV DNA by PCR or NAT methodology, theoretically, should reduce the window between infection and HBV detection by 25 days.[41] This estimate and the continued need for anti-HBc testing in conjunction with NAT will be assessed after evaluation of data derived during NAT clinical trials initiated in 1999. Preliminary results with pooled donor samples do not suggest any major advantage with NAT methods for HBV.

HEPATITIS C

Virology

The etiological agent of NANBH was identified as a result of molecular biology techniques by scientists at Chiron Corporation in collaboration with Daniel W. Bradley of the Centers for Disease Control and Prevention (CDC).[9, 42–45] A novel strategy was devised using pooled plasma samples from chimpanzees infected with NANBH by factor VIII concentrates as the source material for virus isolation. The plasma underwent intensive ultracentrifugation, and nucleic acids were extracted from the sedimented material. After denaturation, both RNA and DNA were transcribed using random primers. The resultant complementary DNA was inserted into a lambda gt11 bacteriophage cloning vector and expressed in *Escherichia coli.* Subsequently, the bacteria were lysed, adhered to an overlying filter, and screened with serum presumably containing antibody against the putative virus derived from patients with chronic NANBH.

A single clone (5-1-1), from more than 1 million in the screening library, was identified only when there was an NANBH infection. With the use of clone 5-1-1 as a hybridization probe, overlapping clones were identified that coded for a 363-amino acid polypeptide. This larger clone (c100-3), which contained 5-1-1 and two adjacent clones, was fused with a human superoxide dismutase gene to facilitate efficient expression of foreign proteins in recombinant yeast. The c100 antigen subsequently became the basis for solid-phase assays for detecting antibodies in patients with NANBH. The excellent correlation between NANBH and anti-c100 confirmed the discovery of HCV.[9]

The nucleotide sequence of HCV is composed of approximately 9400 single-stranded RNA nucleotides that encode a polyprotein precursor of either 3010 or 3011 amino acids. A 19-kD nucleocapsid protein (C) is encoded at the 5′ end of the genome, followed by the putative envelope glycoproteins E1 (33 kD) and E2/NS1 (72 kD).[44, 45] The remainder of the HCV polyprotein codes for a variety of nonstructural proteins, including a membrane-bound protein in the nonstructural two (NS2) region (23 kD) and a soluble protein (60 kD) presumably corresponding to a viral helicase in the NS3 region. The function of NS4 is unknown, although it probably contains polypeptides with membrane-binding functions. An RNA polymerase is contained within the NS5 region.

An analysis of the genetic structure of HCV indicates a similarity to flaviviruses and pestiviruses. Of interest, flaviviruses, such as those that cause yellow fever and dengue fever, are transmitted by arthropods. In comparison, pestiviruses, such as those that cause hog cholera and the bovine viral diarrhea virus, have natural reservoirs in swine, cattle, and sheep. The age distribution, seasonal appearance, and geographic location of HCV does not suggest arthropod spread. These findings are consistent with earlier studies showing cytoplasmic tubular structures in hepatic cells of experimentally infected chimpanzees. The "tubule-forming" agent is sensitive to organic solvents, passes through 80-nm pore-size filters, and has other features suggesting that it is an enveloped virus related to togaviruses or flaviviruses.[46]

In a classification proposed by Simmonds and colleagues, there are six major HCV genotypes with a series of subtypes (designated by a lower case letter following the Arabic numeral) used to characterize HCV infection.[47] Although infection can result from any of these genotypes, the most common genotypes in Western nations are 1a and 1b.[48, 49] Considerable sequence variation between HCV genotypes, its subtypes, and a high spontaneous mutation rate contribute to the complicated picture of HCV diagnostics and therapeutics. Hypervariability probably contributes to the inability of most persons to develop a protective humoral antibody response. Infection with multiple HCV genotypes is not common, but HCV has been shown to circulate as a heterogeneous population in the form of "quasi-species" in patients years after initial infection.[50] This is a result of sequence divergence, an inherent feature of RNA viral replication. From a virological standpoint, HCV, like HIV, may exist as a number of variants even within the same patient. Identification of antibodies that neutralize HCV remains elusive.

Epidemiology

Hepatitis C virus is the most common chronic bloodborne infection in the United States, and it is estimated that 3.9 million Americans are infected. From 1989 to 1996, there was a decline in the incidence of acute HCV infection by more than 80% to 36,000 cases/year.[49, 51] The reasons for this decline are unclear, but it correlates with a decrease in cases among injection drug users. The proportion of cases that are associated with the two most common exposures, transfusions and injection drug use, has changed with time. In fact, since 1994, the CDC viral hepatitis surveillance system has detected no cases of transfusion-associated acute HCV infection.

HCV is transmitted primarily through direct percutaneous exposure to blood. Intensive surveillance for acute NANBH was conducted by CDC investigators in four sentinel counties in various parts of the United States between 1981 and 1988 to determine NANBH risk factors.[52] All of the enrolled patients had elevated ALT levels, and 77% were icteric. In 1988, 42% reported a history of parenteral drug use, 6% gave a history of blood transfusion, 6% had heterosexual exposure to a contact with hepatitis or to multiple sexual partners, 3% had household exposure to a contact with hepatitis, 2% reported health care employment with frequent blood contact, and 0.6% were undergoing hemodialysis. No identifiable risk factor other than low socioeconomic status was identified in 40% of cases.

Sexual activity and other types of nonpercutaneous contact are relatively inefficient modes of HCV transmission. In the CDC sentinel county study, 12% of NANBH patients reported heterosexual contact with more than two partners during the previous 6 months, compared with only 1% of control subjects.[52] However, no homosexual men with NANBH were identified. Because homosexual activity is usually associated with sexually transmitted viruses, this observation argues against sexual transmission of NANBH. In a study conducted in Spain, only 8% of homosexual men infected with HIV were anti-HCV positive.[53] In another Spanish study, 16% of homosexual men had antibodies against hepatitis C, but 84% were HIV antibody positive and 81% had evidence of prior hepatitis B.[54] In a cohort study of homosexual men conducted in Denmark, 1.6% were reactive for anti-HCV in 1981, compared with 4.1% in 1989.[55] During that interval, the rate of hepatitis B increased from 44% to 59% and the prevalence of anti-HIV increased from 8.8% to 30.1%.

None of 37 sexual partners of patients with chronic NANBH followed at the National Institutes of Health (NIH) Clinic Center was found to have anti-HCV.[56] Another NIH study found no HCV cases among sexual partners of HCV-infected blood donors that could not be accounted for by another established risk factor.[57] In a Spanish study in which spouses of patients with HCV were followed, additional risk factors for HCV were also present among the 2.3% who were found to be anti-HCV positive.[58] Likewise, a study of a cohort of women who were infected with HCV through contaminated Rh immune globulin in the late 1970s demonstrated that none of their sexual partners had acquired HCV without having additional risk factors.[59] In contrast, a report from Japan indicated that spousal HCV infection increased with the duration of marriage. However, it is possible that this reflects inapparent, nonsterile percutaneous exposures occurring as a result of traditional folk medicine practices in Japan.[60] A single case of sexual transmission of HCV infection to a blood donor was reported by Capelli and colleagues and confirmed by a molecular analysis of the HCV genotype.[61] Taken altogether, data indicate that HCV is generally not associated with sexual transmission. The efficiency of sexual spread is low and estimated at most to be 5%,[62] much lower than either HIV or HBV.

Another potential mode of transmission is from mothers to their newborns. It appears the average rate of HCV infection among infants born to HCV-positive HIV-negative mothers is 5% to 6%, whereas it is higher (14%–17%) in mothers who are coinfected with HIV.[63, 64] In one report of 17 infants of mothers infected with HCV, only one was anti-HCV positive.[63] In a Japanese study, Ohto and colleagues reported a rate of mother to child transmission of 5.6% as measured by HCV RNA.[64] In a study of former blood donors deferred for HCV infection, none of 6 children born to five mothers were HCV RNA positive at birth even though antibodies to HCV were present.[57] Results of further studies are needed to place conflicting observations in proper perspective and to clarify the risk of perinatal HCV transmission.

Clinical Presentation

In general, the symptoms and signs of acute hepatitis C are less severe than those associated with either hepatitis

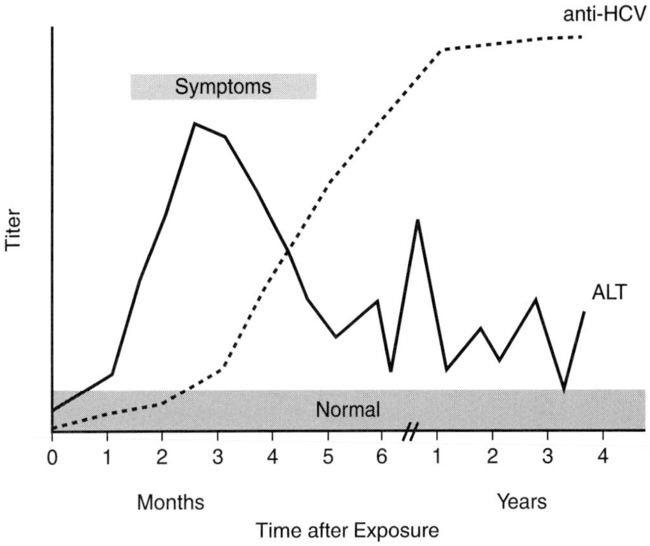

Figure 33–4. Hepatitis C virus infection: typical serological course. Anti-HCV, antibody to HCV; ALT, alanine aminotransferase. (Modified from Centers for Disease Control and Prevention home page: http://www.cdc.gov/ncidod/diseases/hepatitis/hepatitis.htm)

A or hepatitis B. Nonspecific symptoms such as fatigue, anorexia, nausea and vomiting, abdominal pain, and weight loss are reported in 10% to 20% of infected patients. Sixty to 70 percent of infected persons have no discernible symptoms. The average period between exposure and symptoms is 6 to 7 weeks. The average time between exposure and seroconversion is 8 to 9 weeks[49] (Fig. 33–4).

Twenty to 30 percent of patients with acute NANBH become jaundiced. ALT levels increase to approximately 20 times the upper limit of normal, ranging from 2-fold to 82-fold. Fewer than one third of patients have ALT levels higher than 800 IU/L, and the bilirubin level is usually lower than 10 mg/dL. The acute illness may persist for up to 10 weeks. Hepatitis C infections rarely result in fulminant clinical hepatitis. However, in the CDC sentinel county study that included predominantly symptomatic patients, the case-fatality rate was 1.6%.[52] Fulminant hepatic failure is rare after acute hepatitis C. However, chronic liver disease related to chronic hepatitis C results in 8,000 to 10,000 deaths per year in the United States.[49]

At least half the patients infected through transfusion develop chronic hepatitis. Of 32 patients with chronic post-transfusion NANBH who underwent liver biopsy at the NIH Clinical Center, 69% had chronic active hepatitis, 9% had cirrhosis, 3% had nonspecific lesions, and 19% had chronic persistent hepatitis. Repeat liver biopsy, performed 1 to 3 years after the first biopsy, showed evidence of histological improvement in 46%, with evidence of deterioration in 39% cases. One patient developed more severe chronic active hepatitis, and 4 had cirrhosis.[65] In a study involving anti-HCV–positive blood donors in Barcelona, Spain, 60% had chronic active hepatitis and 9% had cirrhosis. Among those with normal ALT levels, 47% had chronic persistent hepatitis and 35% had chronic active hepatitis, suggesting that histological changes may be present in patients without liver function abnormalities.[58] However, histological changes are more likely to be mild in patients who have normal or near-normal ALT levels.[66]

Whether reinfection or recurrent episodes of NANBH occur after a subsequent exposure is uncertain. In rechallenge experiments in chimpanzees, 75% of reexposed animals developed signs of reinfection regardless of whether the same or a different HCV strain was used. Thus, postinfection immunity to HCV appears to be weak.[67]

An association between NANBH and hepatocellular carcinoma (HCC) has been suspected for some time. Antibodies to hepatitis C are found in 29% of patients with HCC in South Africa and the United States and in 39% to 76% of patients in Europe.[68, 69] In a long-term follow-up study of post-transfusion NANBH patients in Japan, there was a 10-year interval between transfusion and chronic hepatitis. Cirrhosis was present 21 years after transfusion, and HCC developed 29 years after transfusion. Anti-HCV was detected in each of the patients with HCC for intervals as long as 14 years before carcinoma was detected.[69] Apparently, cirrhosis occurs in 10% to 20% of persons with chronic hepatitis C over a 20- to 30-year interval, and HCC occurs in 1% to 5%. Alcohol intake of 10 g/day or more accelerates progression of liver injury.[49, 66] When cirrhosis is established, the rate of HCC onset is 1% to 4% per year.[49] Although an epidemiological link between hepatitis C and HCC is apparent, a causative relationship has not been established. One hypothesis is that hepatitis C induces cirrhosis, which in turn increases the risk of HCC.[68]

Patients with hepatitis-associated aplastic anemia usually lack markers of HAV or HBV infection. Hence, NANBH was implicated by exclusion. A study reported in 1992 described 28 patients who had aplastic anemia within 90 days of acute hepatitis and 3 patients who had aplastic anemia after liver transplantation, indicating that HCV is rarely present in the serum or marrow of patients with hepatitis-associated aplastic anemia.[70] However, anti-HCV is commonly present as a result of blood transfusion. Acute hepatitis apparently causes an autoreactive immune response, which in turns leads to aplasia. Because hepatitis viruses A through G have not been implicated and HCV RNA has not been found in these patients, the existence of a novel non–A-G hepatitis virus has been postulated.[71–72]

Incubation and Viremic Phase

Precise estimates of the incubation and viremic phase of HCV infections depend on the sensitivity and specificity of available test systems. Enzyme immunoassays (EIAs) for c100 antibodies were supplanted by multiple-antigen tests that included recombinant polypeptides derived from the NS3 region (c33c) and the core region (c22-3), in addition to c100. A composite antigen (c200) was constructed by combining c100 with c33c. The most recent "third-generation" assays use three recombinant antigens (c22-3, c200, and NS5) derived from four different regions of the HCV genome. Nonspecificity inherent in tests using this format is addressed by the use of supplemental assays, either the recombinant immunoblot assay (RIBA) or a neutralization assay. Detection of HCV RNA is attained by PCR using pairs of nested primers that anneal to conserved regions of the HCV genome, such as in the third and fourth nonstructural regions. One hundred to 1000 viral genome copies per milliliter are detected by this methodology. HCV RNA is detectable in serum within 1 to 2 weeks of exposure and weeks before ALT elevations occur.[49] Patients with chronic hepatitis C have 10^5 to 10^7 HCV genome copies/mL[49] (Fig. 33–5).

Serology

Supplemental assays are used to clarify reactive EIA results, although they are not considered confirmatory tests because they employ the same antigens present in the screening test. Supplemental tests identify a significant number of donors implicated as the cause of post-transfusion hepatitis. For example, only 7% to 25% of anti-c100 EIA positive blood components transmitted HCV, compared with 88% of units reactive by RIBA.[73] Blood components from donors who were c100 EIA positive but RIBA negative were either not implicated or were found to be negative in PCR assays for HCV RNA.

Third-generation anti-HCV assays were available in Europe in 1993, but only one manufacturer obtained licensure for the third version of the anti-HCV EIA in the United States. Both types of third-generation assays for anti-HCV (EIA 3.0 and RIBA 3.0) were designed to further improve sensitivity and specificity by adding more antigens to favor specific over nonspecific reactivity. As noted earlier, EIA 3.0 uses three recombinant antigens (c22-3, c200, and NS5) derived from four different regions of the HCV genome. RIBA 3.0 employs modified c33c and recombinant NS5 antigens. In addition, two synthetic peptides (c100p and c22p) replace these two recombinant proteins used in RIBA 2.0, to reduce the number of false-positive reactive sera.

EIA 3.0 is slightly more sensitive and specific than earlier tests. In the United States, it is estimated that the residual risks of HCV transmission, after the implementation of anti-HCV testing using EIA 2.0 and EIA 3.0, are 1/92,000 and 1/103,000 units of blood, respectively.[37] Both EIA 2.0 and 3.0 are highly specific (>99.8%) in blood donors, but the latter has its advantage in blood screening because of its ability to detect anti-HCV several days earlier than the second-generation assays.

Although the use of NS5 in third-generation antibody assays allows for broader detection of HCV-encoded epitopes, and HCV infected individuals occasionally seroconvert first to NS5, these are not the basis for this assay's increased sensitivity.[74, 75] Rather, it appears that the differences in sensitivity between the second- and third-generation EIA tests are due to the conformational changes in the NS3-derived antigen (c33c).

Similar to EIA 3.0, the configuration of RIBA 3.0 offers increased sensitivity and specificity compared with RIBA 2.0. In a study of American blood donors, HCV RNA was demonstrated in 86%, 3%, and 0% of RIBA 2.0–positive, RIBA 2.0–indeterminate, and RIBA 2.0–negative donors, respectively.[76] RIBA 3.0 reduces the number of sera considered anti-HCV "indeterminate" in HCV RNA–positive persons.[77] However, isolated reactivity of either the modified c33 antigen or NS5-encoded antigen produced a small new population of RIBA 3.0 indeterminate, HCV RNA–negative individuals. In blood donor specimens with no detectable HCV RNA, RIBA 3.0 was useful in eliminating many of the c22-3, RIBA 2.0–indeterminate reactions.[78] The use of new antigens such as the E2 protein in future generations of anti-HCV tests might offer higher sensitivity and specificity.[79] The ideal immunoblot might require representation of all the antigenic domains. In summary, although serological diagnostic accuracy has greatly improved, anti-HCV assays are still not absolutely dependable in correctly identifying and confirming all cases of infection in all patients. Molecular testing therefore plays an integral role in the evaluation of possible HCV infection.

Molecular Testing

HCV RNA is the marker detected earliest after infection. Subsequently, ALT levels become elevated and then sero-

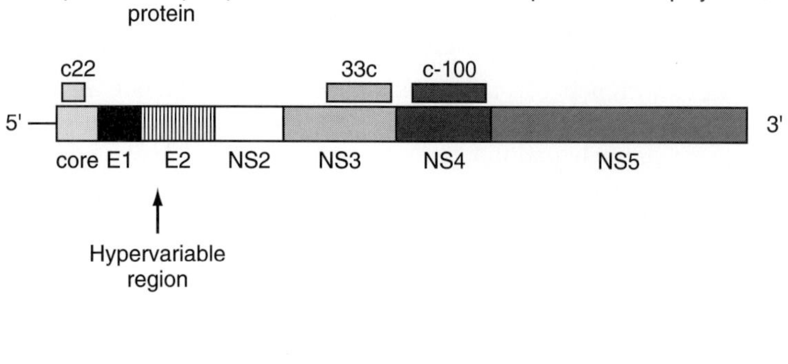

Figure 33–5. Hepatitis C virus genomic structure. E1 and E2 refer to envelope regions. NS2 to NS5 refer to nonstructured regions 2 through 5. The c22, 33c, and c-100 refer to expressed viral epitopes. Not pictured: c200 = composite antigen combining 33c and c-100; 5-1-1 = the initial HCV epitope used in first-generation HCV tests contained within c-100. (Modified from Centers for Disease Control and Prevention home page: http://www.cdc.gov/ncidod/diseases/hepatitis/hepatitis.htm)

conversion occurs. Hepatitis C viremia is transient in acute self-limited hepatitis but persists for decades in the majority of people with chronic hepatitis. HCV antibody may not be detectable in patients with transient acute hepatitis, in part because the level of HCV is not sufficient to stimulate a response. In patients with chronic hepatitis, anti-HCV usually persists. PCR assays for detecting HCV RNA are becoming more available routinely, and results of this test appear to correlate most closely with transaminase abnormalities and the clinical aspects of the disease. Persistent viremia is found in more than 85% patients with chronic hepatitis C.[57, 80–83]

PCR is the most sensitive tool for identifying HCV-infected patients. HCV RNA was detected within 1 to 3 weeks of infection in five patients with post-transfusion hepatitis. Chimpanzees inoculated with aliquots of serum obtained during this period became infected with HCV, as determined by seroconversion and HCV RNA detection.[80] In attempting to close the window period of infectivity of blood for HCV, genomic amplification technology was applied on a large scale for the screening of pooled blood components in 1999.

Transfusion-Associated Hepatitis C

Prospective monitoring of transfusion recipients for extended intervals is required to determine the incidence of post-transfusion hepatitis. Two studies, the Transfusion Transmitted Virus (TTV) Study and the NIH series of open heart surgery cases, were conducted during the late 1970s. Approximately 10% of transfused patients developed post-transfusion hepatitis, but 3% of nontransfused patients in the control groups had similar evidence of hepatitis. More than 90% of the post-transfusion hepatitis cases were considered to be NANBH.[84]

In the TTV study, 39% of the hepatitis cases occurred in recipients of blood from donors with elevated ALT levels.[85] In the NIH series, 42% of hepatitis cases occurred in similar recipients.[86] Anti-HBc was also investigated as a surrogate test for reducing the incidence of post-transfusion NANBH. Approximately 35% and 66% of hepatitis cases occurred in recipients of anti-HBc positive blood in the TTV and NIH studies, respectively.[87, 88] Only 8% to 9% of anti-HBC positive donors had elevated ALT levels. On the basis of sophisticated mathematical models, the predicted efficacy for either ALT or anti-HBc testing was approximately 30%. If both tests were performed, a 40% to 58% reduction in the incidence of post-transfusion hepatitis was predicted. These estimates were corroborated partially by a study conducted in Tübingen, Germany, between 1980 and 1982 involving recipients of blood with normal ALT levels from donors who were either anti-HBc negative or not screened. The rate of post-transfusion NANBH was 42% lower among those receiving anti-HBc negative blood.[85]

Prospective, randomized, controlled studies were not conducted when the surrogate tests ALT and anti-HBc were introduced in the United States in the mid 1980s. The lack of a large, multicenter, prospective study to determine the incidence of post-transfusion hepatitis precluded an opportunity to evaluate the effectiveness of these tests and to assess the risk of post-transfusion hepatitis from blood collected after the donor pool changed in response to an acquired immunodeficiency syndrome prevention measure. This is unfortunate, because there was preliminary evidence that the rate of post-transfusion NANBH was declining in the United States before implementation of surrogate testing.[51] Similar observations were seen in Italy, where the incidence of post-transfusion NANBH has decreased over time: 11% in 1986; 6.6% in 1987; 5.6% in 1988; and 4.3% in 1989.[86]

In Canada between 1988 and 1992, allogeneic transfusion recipients were randomly assigned to two study groups in a prospective, intervention study. One group received blood that included some donations with positive NANBH surrogate markers, and the others received blood from which donations with surrogate markers were withheld.[87] Not infusing blood with NANBH surrogate markers reduced the overall post-transfusion hepatitis rate by 40% and the hepatitis C rate by 70%. Additional information is provided by a study performed at hospitals in Baltimore and Houston.[88] Through retrospective testing of post-transfusion blood samples for anti-HCV, seroconversion was found in 3.3% of persons transfused before surrogate testing was introduced. This was significantly different from the 1.2% seroconversion rate in recipients of ALT-screened and anti-HBc–negative blood.

Surrogate tests were implemented when a specific test for NANBH was considered distant, but evidence linking HCV and post-transfusion NANBH was reported within months of surrogate test implementation.[9] Kuo and associates[42] reported that approximately 80% of chronic post-transfusion NANBH patients from Italy and Japan had circulating HCV antibody. Alter and colleagues[43] selected 15 patients with unequivocal chronic post-transfusion NANBH documented by liver biopsy. All showed seroconversion to anti-HCV. Among five patients with acute resolving post-transfusion NANBH, only three (60%) had seroconversion.

Samples from 1,247 patients who underwent transfusion and 1,235 matched control subjects who did not receive transfusion as part of the TTV study were evaluated for anti-HCV.[89] Of the 111 patients who developed post-transfusion NANBH, 46% had positive first-generation anti-HCV tests, and an additional 14% had positive second-generation assays. Interestingly, control patients believed to have NANBH as a result of ALT elevations after transfusion had negative anti-HCV results. If this rate of nonspecificity is factored into the rate of post-transfusion hepatitis in transfusion recipients, only 74 of the 111 cases of hepatitis could be attributed to transfusion. Of these, 91% were reactive in multiple-antigen or second-generation anti-HCV tests.[89]

In hemophiliac patients who received large quantities of unheated or dry heat–treated factor VIII or IX concentrates, up to 90% are anti-HCV positive. Effective procedures for inactivating HCV were introduced for factor VIII concentrates in 1985 and for factor IX concentrates in 1987.[49]

Renal dialysis patients represent another group of heavily transfused patients. In one report from a southeastern U.S. renal transplant center, 30% of patients were anti-HCV positive at the time of renal allograft surgery.[90] Interestingly, the survival of patients who were seropositive and seronegative for anti-HCV was similar 10 years after transplant.

Donor Screening and Testing to Decrease Post-Transfusion Hepatitis C

Testing for anti-HCV with the c100-based EIA was introduced in the United States in May 1990. Since then, the seroprevalence of HCV in the blood donors population decreased continuously owing to the exclusion of donors who were repeatedly anti-HCV positive. Initially, approximately 1.4% of donors were repeatedly reactive,[91, 92] but this has declined over the ensuing years to about 0.16%.[49] Early on, reports indicated that only 19% to 26% were confirmed positive, 20% to 24% had indeterminate status in supplemental assays, and the remainder apparently had false-positive reactions.[91, 92] Nowadays, the majority of anti-HCV–positive donors are confirmed positive by supplemental assays.

Although the first generation of testing for HCV had poor specificity in a population with a low incidence of hepatitis C, its efficacy was demonstrated in Japan, where the incidence of post-transfusion NANBH declined from 4.9% in patients who received 1 to 10 units of blood before screening to 1.9% after implementation of c100-based tests.[93] Among those patients receiving 11 to 20 units, hepatitis decreased from 16.3% before testing to 3.3% after testing. Preliminary observations in Baltimore and Houston reveal that none of 256 recipients of HCV antibody–negative blood had seroconversion after transfusion.[88] These observations are consistent with a retrospective analysis in which 88% of recipients of anti-HCV–positive blood had transfusion-associated hepatitis and anti-HCV.[94] In the TTV study, 73% of recipients of anti-HCV positive blood became anti-HCV positive.[89]

In March 1992, the multiple-antigen or second-generation EIA was introduced in the United States. Using sera stored in the TTV study repository, these assays detected 31% more HCV seroconversions than the first-generation assay.[89] In the NIH series, 89% of the patients were anti-HCV positive according to the second-generation assay, versus 78% in the c100-based test.[94] Only 62% of cases were anti-c100 positive by 20 weeks after transfusion, but all were positive in the multiple-antigen assay.

In prelicensure clinical trials, multiple-antigen HCV tests detected anti-HCV seroconversion earlier in 73% of 15 transfusion-associated NANBH patients. This anti-HCV test detected a positive reaction 21 to 77 days before c100-based assays. Among patients with sporadic NANBH, the multiple-antigen tests detected anti-HCV earlier in 72% of 57 cases. Antibodies were detected 1 to 100 days earlier in 32 cases, 101 to 200 days earlier in 6 cases, and more than 200 days earlier in 3 cases.[95] In patients with post-transfusion hepatitis, antibodies to the HCV core region were detected at 13.7 weeks after transfusion, and antibodies against c33c at 17.1 weeks after transfusion, compared with anti-c100 reactivity, which was observed at 20.6 weeks.[96] In clinical trials for second-generation test license approval involving 14,068 blood donors, the c100-based assay identified 11 EIA-positive and supplemental test positive donors but the multiple-antigen assay found an additional 16 (59%) cases.[94] For these reasons, the significantly improved second-generation test immediately replaced the earlier version.

By 1995, it was shown that EIA 3.0 had slightly increased sensitivity over EIA 2.0, detecting seroconversion earlier in 24% (5/21) of post-transfusion HCV cases.[97] Subsequently, EIA 3.0 was licensed for use in the United States.

Since anti-HCV testing of the blood supply began, the utility of surrogate testing (ALT and anti-HBc) has been questioned. In fact, ALT testing is no longer mandated in the United States, although it is still performed by most blood collection centers. Before the introduction of anti-HCV testing, surrogate markers including ALT may have reduced the overall post-transfusion hepatitis rate by 30% to 40% on a per-unit basis. Improved donor recruitment and selection also contributed to this reduction. However, since anti-HCV testing began, it appears that ALT testing of blood donors has little additional value. With specific anti-HCV testing, the risk of post-transfusion hepatitis was equivalent in groups receiving blood screened with or without surrogate markers, suggesting redundancy of ALT testing. Theoretically, ALT might pick up donors during the anti-HCV seronegative "window period," since ALT rises approximately 4 weeks before anti-HCV appears. However, there are no clinical studies to prove that ALT screening now improves the safety of blood transfusion.[98] With nucleic acid amplification testing for HCV, the window period will be reduced even further. In addition, although the direct cost of ALT testing is low, it incurs high indirect costs to the blood supply through discarded units and donor deferrals. ALT testing continues to be a requirement in some European countries that import U.S. plasma.

Like ALT screening, it appears that anti-HBc testing does not identify donors capable of transmitting HCV. However, it is retained as a screening tool to prevent post-transfusion HBV and some cases of transfusion-transmitted HIV from donors who test negative for anti-HIV and HIV p24 antigen. Its ability to serve as a surrogate marker for HIV stems from the overlapping epidemiology of HIV and HBV, owing to common parenteral and sexual transmission risk factors.[40, 98]

The persistent risk of transfusion-transmitted HCV infection is due to those individuals who donate during the seronegative window period of acute HCV infection. Viral inactivation using solvent detergent treatment of clotting factor concentrates and plasma can eliminate lipid-enveloped HCV and other lipid-enveloped viruses from these products. There are other promising methods that may soon be available to apply on a universal basis to both cellular and acellular blood products for the purpose of sterilizing blood. In the interim, NAT testing will be used by blood centers in the United States. It has been postulated that such testing will reduce the risk of post-transfusion HCV infection by an additional 72%.[41]

HEPATITIS D

Virology

The delta agent is a "defective" RNA-containing passenger virus that requires HBV to act as a "helper" for assembling envelope proteins.[29, 99] The hepatitis D virus (HDV) particles contain a ribonucleoprotein core containing the circular 1.7-kilobase single-stranded RNA genome and multiple copies of the delta antigen, the sole HDV encoded protein. HDV resembles plant viruses; it cannot replicate by itself. HDV requires HBV envelope protein domains, in addition to HDV antigen proteins, for genome replication and packaging.[29, 100, 101]

Epidemiology

Delta hepatitis occurs only in patients who are HBsAg positive. Persons at risk therefore include those at risk for hepatitis B, especially injection drug users. Sexual transmission is less compared with HBV, and perinatal HDV transmission occurs infrequently. In Italy, the HDV incidence rate declined from 3.1 per million population in 1987 to 1.2 million in 1992.[102] Approximately one half were HBV/HDV coinfections and one half were superinfections in chronic HBsAg carriers. Blood transfusion was not found to be an independent risk factor.

Clinical Features

HDV infection occurs either as an acute coinfection with patients acquiring HBV and HDV simultaneously or as a superinfection in a previous HBV carrier. The acute coinfection is usually self-limited because of HBV clearance but has a higher incidence of fulminant hepatitis than that occurring with HBV alone. Superinfection should be suspected when a chronic HBsAg carrier has evidence of additional liver damage or when active disease persists in a patient with a negative HBeAg test.[29, 99] Among HBsAg carriers with HDV superinfection, 70% to 80% develop chronic liver disease and cirrhosis compared with 15% to 20% of patients with HBV infection alone. The mortality rate is 2% to 20% in patients with coinfection and up to 30% in cases with superinfection.

Incubation and Viremic Phase

The incubation period ranges from 21 to 90 days.

In HBV/HDV coinfection, IgM and IgG antibodies against HDV appear. In approximately 15% of patients, the only serological evidence of HDV infection is IgM anti-HDV during the early acute phase or IgG anti-HDV during convalescence. Anti-HDV declines after resolution of the infection; no long-term markers persist. HDAg is found in one fourth of patients with HDV coinfection and becomes undetectable in conjunction with HBsAg clearance.

In HBV/HDV superinfection, the titer of HBsAg declines when HDAg appears. HDAg and HDV RNA persist, because most patients develop chronic HDV infection. High titers of IgM and IgG anti-HBV remain. The diagnosis may be confirmed by finding HDAg in hepatocytes.[29, 99]

Transfusion-Associated Hepatitis D

Among recipients of blood, blood components, or plasma derivatives, hemophilic patients are considered at highest risk for hepatitis D.

Donor Screening and Testing to Decrease Transmission of Delta Hepatitis

Screening for hepatitis B should be effective in preventing transmission of HDV by transfusion. No specific tests are used to detect HDV: HBsAg and anti-HBc appear to be adequate for this purpose.[103]

HEPATITIS E

The hepatitis E virus (HEV), a calicivirus, is a single-stranded RNA virus of approximately 7.2 kilobases without an envelope. The virus contains at least three open reading frames encoding proteins to which antibodies are made. HEV affects young adults predominantly and is associated with symptoms similar to those occurring in patients with hepatitis A. Transmission occurs through the fecal-oral route and usually involves contaminated water. Epidemics have been reported in Mexico, Africa, and Asia. Preliminary reports suggest transmission by blood transfusion, but other reports refute this conclusion.[104]

HEV is shed into feces approximately 1 week before symptoms occur; the incubation period is approximately 45 days (range: 2 to 9 weeks). The virus has been detected in serum before and during clinical disease.[105, 106] Studies using various anti-HEV tests in United States blood donors show significant inter-test variability, suggesting that further investigation is needed to permit interpretation of anti-HEV test results in non-HEV endemic areas.[107]

HEPATITIS G VIRUS

Virology and Immunology

Although HBV and HCV explain the majority of cases of viral hepatitis, studies investigating causes of hepatitis suggest that up to 20% of acute cases and 5% of chronic hepatitis remain unexplained. Thus, a relentless search to define their etiologies using sophisticated molecular biological techniques continues. A novel single-stranded (ss) RNA virus of the Flaviviridae discovered recently was designated hepatitis G virus (HGV)[10] by one and hepatitis GBV-C virus by another group.[108, 109] Sequence analysis has shown that they are different isolates of the same virus. HGV is approximately 25% homologous with HCV over the entire polyprotein sequence, depending on the genotype of HCV strain used for comparison. Unlike HCV, whose envelope proteins can vary significantly, HGV is 90% to 100% conserved at the amino acid level and there is no evidence that a hypervariable region exists. Sequences of HGV do not seem to evolve over

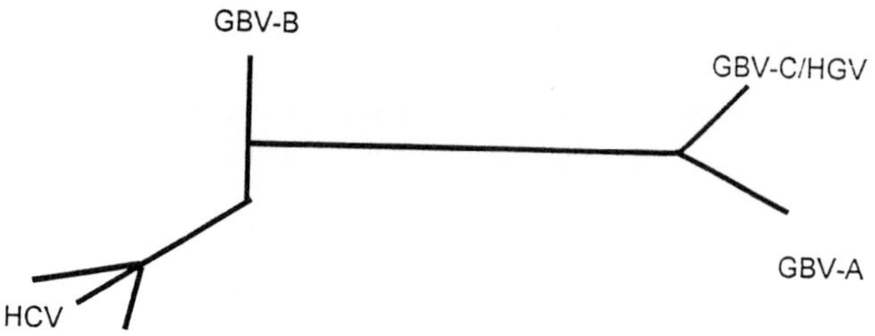

Figure 33–6. Hepatitis G virus/GBV-C. GB viruses A and C (HGV) are related closely, but GBV-B and HCV share less homology. (From Leary TP, Muerhoff AS, Simon JHM, et al. Sequence and genomic organization of GBV-C: a novel member of the flaviviridae associated with human non–A-E hepatitis. J Med Virol 1996; 48:60.)

time as do those from chronically infected HCV patients. Likewise, there is little variation of HGV at the nucleotide level (Fig. 33–6).

An antibody response to HCV proteins makes a sero-diagnosis of HCV infection very reliable. HCV viremia and antibodies generally coexist. However, the humoral immune response to HGV is more akin to HBV infection in which clearance of HBV surface antigen takes place when antibodies to HBV surface antigen appear. In serial plasma samples from patients with post-transfusion HGV infection, antibodies to the envelope (E2) protein coincide with the disappearance of serum HGV RNA. Likewise, the presence of anti-E2 and HGV RNA is nearly mutually exclusive in blood donors and injection drug users, suggesting that anti-E2 in HGV infection is neutralizing antibody.[110, 111] Currently, anti-E2 is the only link to resolution of HGV infection and there is no information on its false-positive rate or a cellular immune response to HGV.

Epidemiology: Prevalence and Transmission

HGV prevalence in volunteer eligible donors is 1% to 2% in the United States[112] and in most areas of Europe and Japan, although rates as high as 4% have been reported in France. These rates are HGV RNA PCR rates of viremia and not simply the detection of antibody. Such viremia rates are 5-fold to 10-fold higher than the estimated prevalence of HCV viremia (0.3%) when HCV testing of the blood supply was first introduced. HGV viremia and anti-E2 are useful to define the active infection rate and exposure or recovery rate, respectively. It appears that the viremia rate may be as high as 15% to 20% in persons at risk for parenteral exposures, such as hemophiliacs and intravenous drug users, whereas the exposure rate (presence of anti-E2) is 80% to 90%. In contrast to HCV infection, which is most often chronic, these data suggest that most HGV carriers eventually clear the virus. Although anti-E2 is useful for defining the epidemiology of HGV infection, it has little use as a donor screening measure. When prevalence is measured by the presence of anti-E2, the rate is usually three to five times that for HGV RNA. Anti-E2 was found in 3% to 9% of blood donations and in 8.1% of units with abnormal ALT.[111, 112] In data summarized from various countries, the prevalence of HGV RNA is high in "at-risk" populations such as hemophiliacs (13.7%–37.7%), intravenous drug users (15.8%–43.3%), and hemodialysis patients (3.1%–26.0%).[113] Among HCV-infected individuals, 10% to 20% are coinfected with HGV, presumably related to common routes of exposure.[111] HGV RNA is present in 10% to 20% of patients with non–A-E hepatitis, accounting for the minority of such cases. It is no more common in non–A-E hepatitis than in patients with hepatitis B or C or than in patients with nonviral liver disease.[114]

HGV is efficiently transmitted by blood transfusion. It is possible that 8% to 12% of blood transfusion recipients may acquire HGV infection from transfusion.[13] Almost 50% of HCV-infected blood units transmitted infection in one study.[115] In the NIH prospective post-transfusion study, HGV infection accounted for only 4% of transfusion-associated non-A, non-B, non-C hepatitis cases. Although HGV RNA is present in up to 50% of patients with fulminant hepatic failure, these patients may have acquired it from their multiple transfusions. High rates of serum HGV RNA have been reported in liver transplant patients (10%–30% in cases of cryptogenic cirrhosis and up to 70% of patients after liver transplant); however, these results do not prove that liver damage was due to HGV.[116] HGV appears reliably inactivated by virucidal methods such as vapor heating, pasteurization, and treatment with solvent detergent mixtures.[117]

Modes of transmission other than parenteral exposures are poorly defined. Mother-to-child transmission of HGV infection has been reported and appears to occur at higher rates (30%–62%) than the vertically acquired HCV infection.[118, 119] Confounding the rates of transmission in these studies is that most mothers were coinfected with other viruses such as HCV and HIV. Likewise, sexual transmission is difficult to assess since a high rate of HGV RNA (11%) was found among female prostitutes who also have high rates of HBV surface antigen and anti-HCV.[120]

Clinical Importance

Although HGV is common among blood donors, there does not appear to be an association of biochemical liver disease and HGV RNA.[112] In fact, there is poor correlation between ALT levels and the presence of HGV RNA in all populations tested including blood recipients, dialysis patients, hemophiliacs, and intravenous drug users. Because evidence for biochemical liver disease is uncommon, few HGV-infected patients have undergone liver biopsy. However, one report suggested that biochemical and histological changes in HGV infection are very mild and quite different from those of HCV infection.[121] HGV has not yet been shown to reside in hepatocytes or replicate in the liver.

HGV accounted for only 4% of the transfusion-associated non-A, non-B, non-C hepatitis cases in the NIH prospective transfusion study.[112] Even in this small number, causality was *not* established because there was dissociation of HGV RNA and ALT levels. Importantly, a non–A-G agent appeared three times more prevalent than HGV. In the community, a CDC study showed that HGV infection was identified in only 9% of patients presenting with acute hepatitis. Furthermore, acute hepatitis resolved while HGV RNA persisted in the few cases that were HGV positive, suggesting a superimposed acute hepatitis of undefined cause.[121] HGV was originally suspected to play a role in hepatitis-associated aplastic anemia, but the finding of HGV in such patients is related to transfusion after the onset of aplasia.[122]

Despite inadvertent transfusion of HGV in 1% to 2% of blood transfusion recipients in the United States, there is no apparent hepatitis burden associated with transmission, and the rate of post-transfusion hepatitis is now near zero and not rising. Therefore, it seems that the term *hepatitis G virus* may be a premature misnomer. At present, the issue of screening the blood supply for HGV is hypothetical, because the appropriate technology is lacking. Because significant hepatic or extrahepatic disease due to HGV infection is not yet proven, it is questionable whether donor screening for HGV should be routinely implemented once a test is developed.

"TT" VIRUS

A transfusion-transmissible virus discovered by means of molecular methods was reported in 1997.[11] Unfortunately, it was named the "TT" virus after the patient from which it was first reported. This should not be confused with the acronym TTV, which is used widely in transfusion medicine to refer to any transfusion-transmitted virus. Molecular characterization is proceeding quickly. It appears to be a nonenveloped ssDNA virus of the Parvoviridae with a worldwide distribution and high prevalence. Serum "TT" virus DNA appears widespread in blood donors but may not be associated with ALT elevations in this population. It appears to be present at greater rates in multitransfused populations.[12, 123, 124] In hemophiliacs, a greater "TT" virus DNA prevalence was associated with disease severity and having had a greater number of transfusions. Like HGV, preliminary data have not established a definitive disease association for "TT" virus, and further work is necessary (Table 33–2).

CONCLUSION AND FUTURE DIRECTIONS

Molecular biology techniques provide significant insight into an understanding of the various hepatitis viruses and post-transfusion hepatitis. Currently, the risk of transfusion-associated hepatitis from known hepatitis viruses primarily relates to serological testing failures. This problem should diminish after widespread implementation of NAT or PCR testing for hepatitis B and C.[125]

Active research involving viral inactivation procedures is intended to prevent transmission of unknown or emerging agents. Benefits associated with some of these processes may be offset by risks associated with pooling multiple donations required by manufacturing and cost efficiencies. For example, up to 2500 plasma donations are pooled in the production of solvent/detergent treated frozen plasma products.[126] Inactivation processes intended for red cells and platelets using psoralen and phthalocyanine compounds are under development for treatment of individual rather than pooled components.[127] Factor VIII and factor IX concentrates prepared by recombinant technology eliminate exposures to human plasma. These technologies should continue to reduce the risk of post-transfusion hepatitis.

Table 33–2. Epidemiology of TT virus

Country	Number Tested	% TT Positive
Japan		
Blood donors	320	12
Hemophiliac patients	28	68
Chronic liver disease patients	90	46
Fulminant hepatic failure	19	47
United Kingdom		
Healthy controls	30	10
Non-B, non-C chronic liver disease	13	38
Chronic HCV	33	21
Non–A–G liver transplant	16	25
Scotland		
Blood donors	1000	1.9

Data from references 11, 123, and 124.

REFERENCES

1. Allen JG, Sayman WA. Serum hepatitis from transfusions of blood. JAMA 1962; 180:1079.
2. Hampers CL, Prager D, Senior JR. Post-transfusion anicteric hepatitis. N Engl J Med 1964; 271:747.
3. Grady GF, Bennett AJE. Risk of posttransfusion hepatitis in the United States. JAMA 1972; 220:692.
4. Gocke DJ. A prospective study of posttransfusion hepatitis. JAMA 1972; 219:1165.
5. Aach RD, Szmuness W, Mosley JW, et al. Serum alanine aminotransferase of donors in relation to the risk of non-A, non-B hepatitis in recipients: the Transfusion Transmitted Viruses Study. N Engl J Med 1981; 204:989.
6. Alter HJ, Purcell RH, Holland PV, et al. Donor transaminase and recipient hepatitis: impact on blood transfusion services. JAMA 1981; 246:630.
7. Stevens CE, Aach RD, Hollinger FB, et al. Hepatitis B virus antibody in blood donors and the occurrence of non-A, non-B hepatitis in transfusion recipients: an analysis of the Transfusion Transmitted Viruses Study. Ann Intern Med 1984; 101:733.
8. Koziol DE, Holland PV, Alling DW, et al. Antibody to hepatitis B core antigen as a paradoxical marker for non-A, non-B hepatitis agents in donated blood. Ann Intern Med 1986; 104:488.
9. Choo Q-L, Kuo G, Weiner AJ, et al. Isolation of a cDNA clone derived from blood-borne non-A, non-B viral hepatitis genome. Science 1989; 244:359.
10. Linnen J, Wages J, Zhang-Keck ZY, et al. Molecular cloning and disease association of hepatitis G virus: a transfusion-transmissible agent. Science 1996; 271:505.
11. Nishizawa T, Okomoto H, Konishi K, et al. A novel DNA viruses (TTV) associated with elevated transminase levels in post transfusion hepatitis of unknown etiology. Biochem Biophys Res Comm 1997; 241:92.
12. Cosart Y. TTV a common virus, but pathogenic? Lancet 1998; 352:164.
13. Alter HJ. G-pers creepers, where'd you get those papers? A reassessment of the literature on the hepatitis G virus. Transfusion 1997; 37:569.
14. Alter MJ, Gallagher M, Morris TT, et al. Acute non–A-E hepatitis in the United States and the role of hepatitis G virus infection. N Engl J Med 1997; 336:741.
15. Alter HJ, Nakatsuji Y, Melpolder J, et al. The incidence of transfusion-associated hepatitis C virus infection and its relation to liver disease. N Engl J Med 1997; 336:747.
16. Lemon SM: The natural history of hepatitis A: The potential for transmission by transfusion of blood or blood products. Vox Sang 1994; 67(suppl 4):19.

17. Centers for Disease Control and Prevention. Prevention of hepatitis A through active or passive immunization: recommendations of the Advisory Committee on Immunization Practices. MMWR 1996; 45(RR-15):1.
18. Vento S, Garfano T, Renzini C, et al. Fulminant hepatitis associated with hepatitis A virus superinfection in patients with chronic hepatitis C. N Engl J Med 1998; 338:286.
19. Hollinger FB, Khan NC, Olfinger PE, et al. Posttransfusion hepatitis type A. JAMA 1983; 250:2313.
20. Sherertz RJ, Russell BA, Reuman PD. Transmission of hepatitis A by transfusion of blood products. Arch Intern Med 1984; 144:1579.
21. Noble RC, Kane MA, Reeves SA, Roeckel I. Posttransfusion hepatitis A in a neonatal intensive care unit. JAMA 1984; 252:2711.
22. Azimi PH, Roberto RR, Guralnik J, et al. Transfusion-acquired hepatitis A in a premature infant with secondary nosocomial spread in an intensive care nursery. Am J Dis Child 1986; 140:23.
23. Giacoia GP, Kasprisin DO. Transfusion-acquired hepatitis A. South Med J 1989; 82:1357.
24. Soucie JM, Robertson BH, Bell BP, et al. Hepatitis A virus infections associated with clotting factor concentrates in the United States. Transfusion 1998; 38:573.
25. Mannucci PM, Gdovin S, Gringeri A, et al. Transmission of hepatitis A to patients with hemophilia by factor VIII concentrates treated with organic solvent and detergent to inactivate viruses. Ann Intern Med 1994; 120:1.
26. Lawlor E, Graham S, Davidson E, et al. Hepatitis A transmission by factor IX concentrates. Vox Sang 1996; 71:126.
27. Lawlor E, Johnson Z, Thornton L, et al. Investigation of an outbreak of hepatitis A in Irish hemophilia patients. Vox Sang 1994; 675:18.
28. Bader TF. Hepatitis A vaccine. Am J Gastroenterol 1996; 91:217.
29. Lee WM. Hepatitis B virus infection. N Engl J Med 1997; 337:1733.
30. Torre F, Naoumov NV. Clinical implications of mutations in the hepatitis B virus genome. Eur J Clin Invest 1998; 28:604.
31. Locarnini SA. Hepatitis B virus surface antigen and polymerase gene variants: potential virological and clinical significance. Hepatology 1998; 27:294.
32. Dickson RC, Everhart JE, Lake JR, et al. Transmission of hepatitis B by transplantation of livers from donors positive for antibody to hepatitis B core antigen. Gastroenterology 1997; 113:1668.
33. Nagaraju K, Misra S, Saraswat S, et al. High prevalence of HBV infectivity in blood donors detected by the dot blot hybridisation assay. Vox Sang 1994; 67:183.
34. Alter M. Epidemiology and disease burden of hepatitis B and C. Antiviral Ther 1996; 1:9.
35. Centers for Disease Control. Public Health Service inter-agency guidelines for screening donors of blood, plasma, organs, tissues, and semen for evidence of hepatitis B and hepatitis C. MMWR 1991; 40(RR-4):1.
36. Ikeda K, Saitoh S, Suzuki Y, et al. Disease progression and hepatocellular carcinogenesis in patients with chronic viral hepatitis: a prospective observation of 2215 patients. J Hepatol 1998; 28:930.
37. Schreiber GB, Busch MP, Kleinman SH, et al. The risk of transfusion-transmitted viral infections: the Retrovirus Epidemiology Donor Study. N Engl J Med 1996; 334:1685.
38. United States General Accounting Office. Report to the Ranking Minority Member, Committee on Commerce, House of Representatives. Blood Supply, Transfusion-Associated Risks. GAO/PEMD 97-2, 1997.
39. Jongerius JM, Wester M, Cuypers HTM, et al. New hepatitis B virus mutant form in a blood donor that is undetectable in several hepatitis B surface antigen screening assays. Transfusion 1998; 38:56.
40. Busch MP. Prevention of transmission of hepatitis B, hepatitis C and human immunodeficiency virus infections through blood transfusion by anti-HBc testing. Vox Sang 1998; 74(suppl 2):147.
41. Lee HH, Allain JP. Genomic screening for blood-borne viruses in transfusion settings. Vox Sang 1998; 74:119.
42. Kuo G, Choo Q-L, Alter HJ, et al. An assay for circulating antibodies to a major etiologic virus of human non-A, non-B hepatitis. Science 1989; 244:362.
43. Alter HJ, Purcell RH, Shih JW, et al. Detection of antibody to hepatitis C virus in prospectively followed transfusion recipients with acute and chronic non-A, non-B hepatitis. N Engl J Med 1989; 321:1494.
44. Alter HJ. Descartes before the horse: I clone, therefore I am: the hepatitis C virus in current perspective. Ann Intern Med 1991; 115:644.
45. Houghton M, Weiner A, Han J, et al. Molecular biology of the hepatitis C viruses: implication for the diagnosis, development and control of viral disease. Hepatology 1991; 14:381.
46. Bradley DW, Maynard JE, Popper H, et al. Post-transfusion non-A, non-B hepatitis: physicochemical properties of two distinct agents. J Infect Dis 1983; 148:254.
47. Simmonds P, Alberti A, Alter HJ, et al. A proposed system for the nomenclature of hepatitis C viral genotypes. Hepatology 1994; 19:1321.
48. Lau JY, Davis GL, Prescott LE, et al. Distribution of hepatitis C virus determined by line probe assay in patients with chronic hepatitis C seen at tertiary referral centers in the United States: Hepatitis Interventional Therapy Group. Ann Intern Med 1996; 124:868.
49. Centers for Disease Control and Prevention. Recommendations for prevention and control of HCV infection and HCV-related chronic disease. MMWR 1998; 47:1.
50. Genetic diversity of hepatitis C virus: implications for pathogenesis, treatment and prevention. Lancet 1995; 345:562.
51. Alter MJ, Hadler SC, Judson FN. Risk factors for acute non-A, non-B hepatitis in the United States and association with hepatitis C virus infection. JAMA 1990; 264:2231.
52. Alter MJ, Coleman PJ, Alexander WJ: Importance of heterosexual activity in the transmission of hepatitis B and non-A, non-B hepatitis. JAMA 1989; 262:1201.
53. Esteban JI, Viladomiu L, Gonzalez A, et al. Hepatitis C virus antibodies among risk groups in Spain. Lancet 1989; 2:294.
54. Tor J, Libre JM, Carbonell M, et al. Sexual transmission of hepatitis C virus and its relation with hepatitis B virus and HIV. BMJ 1990; 301:1130.
55. Melbye M, Biggar RJ, Wantzin P, et al. Sexual transmission of hepatitis C virus: cohort study (1981–9) among European homosexual men. BMJ 1990; 301:210.
56. Everhart JE, Di Bisceglie AM, Murray LM, et al. Ann Intern Med 1990; 112:544.
57. Conry-Cantilena C, VanRaden M, Gibble J, et al. Routes of infection, viremia and liver disease in blood donors found to have hepatitis C virus. N Engl J Med 1996; 334:1691.
58. Esteban JI, Lopez-Talavera JC, Genesca J, et al. High rate of infectivity and liver disease in blood donors with antibodies to hepatitis C virus. Ann Intern Med 1991; 115:443.
59. Power J, Lawlor E, Davidson F, et al. Hepatitis infection from anti-D immunoglobulin. Lancet 1995; 346:372.
60. Akahane Y, Kojima M, Sugai Y, et al. Hepatitis C virus infection in spouses of patients with type C chronic liver disease. Ann Intern Med 1994; 120:748.
61. Capelli C, Prati D, Bosoni P, et al. Sexual transmission of hepatitis C virus to a repeat blood donor. Transfusion 1997; 37:436.
62. Dienstag J. Sexual and perinatal transmission of hepatitis C virus. Hepatology 1997; 26(3 suppl 1):66S.
63. Reesink HW, Wong VCW, Ip HMH, et al. Mother-to-infant transmission and hepatitis C virus. Lancet 1990; 335:1216.
64. Ohto H, Terazawa S, Sasaki N, et al. Transmission of hepatitis C from mothers to infants. N Engl J Med 1994; 330:744.
65. Dienstag JL, Alter HJ. Non-A, non-B hepatitis: evolving epidemiologic and clinical perspective. Semin Liver Dis 1986; 6:67.
66. Shakil AO, Conry-Cantilena C, Alter HJ, et al. Volunteer blood donors with antibody to hepatitis C virus: clinical, biochemical, virologic and histologic features. Ann Intern Med 1995; 123:330.
67. Prince AM, Brotman B, Huima T, et al. Immunity in hepatitis C infection. J Infect Dis 1992; 165:438.
68. Simonetti RG, Camma C, Fiorello F, et al. Hepatitis C virus infection as a risk factor for hepatocellular carcinoma in patients with cirrhosis: a case control study. Ann Intern Med 1992; 116:97.
69. Kiyosawa K, Sodeyama T, Tanaka E, et al. Interrelationship of blood transfusion, non-A, non-B hepatitis and hepatocellular carcinoma: analysis by detection of antibody to hepatitis C virus. Hepatology 1990; 12:671.
70. Hibbs JR, Frickhofen N, Rosenfelt SJ, et al. Aplastic anemia and viral hepatitis: non-A, non-B, non-C? JAMA 1992; 267:2051.
71. Pol S, Driss F, Devergie A, et al. Is hepatitis C virus involved in hepatitis-associated aplastic anemia? Ann Intern Med 1990; 113:435.

72. Brown KE, Wong S, Young N. Prevalence of hepatitis G, a novel hepatitis virus in patients with aplastic anemia. Br J Hematol 1997; 97:492.
73. Van Der Poel CL, Cuypers HTM, Reesink HW, et al. Confirmation of hepatitis C virus infection by new four-antigen recombinant immunoblot assay. Lancet 1991; 337:317.
74. Barrerra JM, Francis B, Ercilla G, et al. Improved detection of post-transfusion hepatitis by a third generation ELISA. Vox Sang 1995; 68:15.
75. Courouce AM, Lemerraac N, Girault A, et al. Anti-HCV seroconversion in patients undergoing hemodialyis: comparison of 2nd and 3rd generation anti-HCV. Transfusion 1994; 34:790.
76. Damen M, Zaaiger HL, Cuypers HT, et al. Reliability of the third generation recombinant immunoblot assay for hepatitis C virus. Transfusion 1995; 35:745.
77. Tobler LH, Busch M, Francis BS. Evaluation of indeterminate CZZ-3 reactivity in volunteer blood donors. Transplantation 1994; 34:130.
78. Zaaijer HL, Vallaris DS, Cunningham M, et al. E2 and NS5: new antigens for detection of hepatitis C virus antibodies. J Med Virol 1994; 44:395.
79. Allain J-P, Coghlan PJ, Kenrick KG, et al. Prediction of hepatitis C virus infectivity in seropositive Australian blood donors by supplemental immunoassays and detection of viral RNA. Blood 1991;78:2462.
80. Farci P, Alter HJ, Wong D, et al. A long-term study of hepatitis C virus replication in non-A, non-B hepatitis. N Engl J Med 1991; 325:98.
81. Tremolada F, Casarin C, Tagger A, et al. Antibody to hepatitis C virus in post-transfusion hepatitis. Ann Intern Med 1991; 114:277.
82. Shibata M, Morishima T, Kudo T, et al. Serum hepatitis C virus sequences in post-transfusion non-A, non-B hepatitis. Blood 1991; 77:1157.
83. McHutchison JG, Kuo G, Houghton M, et al. Hepatitis C virus antibodies in acute icteric and chronic non-A, non-B hepatitis. Gastroenterology 1991; 101:1117.
84. Menitove JE. Rationale for surrogate testing to detect non-A, non-B hepatitis. Trans Med Rev 1988; 2:65.
85. Zuck TJ, Sherwood WC, Bove JR. A review of recent events related to surrogate testing of blood to prevent non-A, non-B post-transfusion hepatitis. Transfusion 1987; 27:203.
86. Sirchia G, Giovanetti AM, Parravicini A, et al: Prospective evaluation of post-transfusion hepatitis. Transfusion 1991; 31:299.
87. Blajchman MA, Bull SB, Feinman SV, et al. Post-transfusion hepatitis: impact of non-A, non-B hepatitis surrogate tests. Lancet 1995; 345:21.
88. Donahue J, Nelson K, Munoz A, et al. Risk of hepatitis C virus (HCV) infection in cardiac surgery patients, and effectiveness of screening. Transfusion 1991; 31S:55S.
89. Aach RD, Stevens CE, Hollinger FB, et al. Hepatitis C virus infection in post-transfusion hepatitis. N Engl J Med 1991; 325:1325.
90. Roth D, Fernandez JA, Burke GW, et al. Detection of antibody to hepatitis C virus in renal transplant recipients. Transplantation 1991; 51:396.
91. Menitove JE, Richards WA, Destree M. Early US experience with anti-HCV kit in blood donors. Lancet 1990; 336:244.
92. Zuck TF, Rose GA, Dumaswala UJ, Geer NJ. Experience with a transfusion recipient education program about hepatitis C. Transfusion 1990; 30:759.
93. Japanese Red Cross Non-A, Non-B Hepatitis Research Group. Effect of screening for hepatitis C virus antibody and hepatitis B virus core antibody on incidence of post-transfusion hepatitis. Lancet 1991; 338:1040.
94. Alter HJ. New kit on the block: evaluation of second-generation assays for detection of antibody to the hepatitis C virus. Hepatology 1992; 15:350.
95. Hepatitis C virus encode antigen (recombinant c100-3, c200 and c22-3) HCV 2.0 ELISA Test System (package insert). Raritan, NJ: Ortho Diagnostic Systems, 1992.
96. Clemens JM, Taskar S, Chau K, et al. IgM antibody response in acute hepatitis C viral infection. Blood 1992; 79:169.
97. Lee SR. Improved detection of anti-HCV in post-transfusion hepatitis by a third-generation ELISA. Vox Sang 1995; 68:15.
98. NIH Consensus Conference: Infectious disease testing for blood transfusions. 1995; 13:1.
99. Polish LB, Gallagher M, Fields HA, Hadler SC. Delta hepatitis: molecular biology and clinical and epidemiological features. Clin Microbiol Rev 1993; 6:211.
100. Hourioux C, Sureau C, Poisson F, et al. Interaction between hepatitis delta virus-encoded proteins and hepatitis B virus envelope protein domains. J Gen Virol 1998;79:1115.
101. Dingle K, Bichko V, Zuccola H, et al. Initiation of hepatitis delta virus genome replication. J Virol 1998; 72:4783.
102. Stroffolini T, Ferrigno L, Cialdea L, et al. Incidence and risk factors of acute delta hepatitis in Italy: results from a national surveillance system: SEIEVA Collaborating Group. J Hepatol 1994; 21:1123.
103. Holland PV. Post-transfusion hepatitis: current risks and causes. Vox Sang 1998; 74:135.
104. Mateos ML, Lasa E, Camarero C, et al. Is hepatitis E virus transfusion-transmitted to children? Transfus Med 1997; 7:319.
105. Chauhan A, Jameel S, Gilawari JB. Hepatitis E transmission to a volunteer. Lancet 1993; 341:149.
106. de Groen PC. Hepatitis E in the United States: a case of "hog fever." Mayo Clin Proc 1997; 72:1197.
107. Mast EE, Alter MJ, Holland PV. Evaluation of assays for antibody to hepatitis E virus by serum panel. Hepatology 1998; 27:857.
108. Simon JN, Leary TP, Dawson GJ, et al. Isolation of novel virus-like sequences associated with human hepatitis. Nat Med 1995; 1:564.
109. Leary TP, Muerhoff AS, Simon JM, et al. Sequence and genomic organization of GBV-C: A novel member of the flaviviridae associated with human non-A-E hepatitis. J Med Virol 1996; 48:60.
110. Tacke M, Kiyosawa K, Stark K, et al. Detection of antibodies to a putative hepatitis G virus envelope protein. Lancet 1997; 349:318.
111. Dille BJ, Surowy TK, Gutierrez RA, et al. An ELISA for detection of antibodies to the E2 protein of GB virus C. J Infect Dis 1997; 175:458.
112. Alter HJ, Nakatsuji Y, Melpolder J, et al. The incidence of transfusion-associated hepatitis G virus infection and its relation to liver disease. N Engl J Med 1997; 336:747.
113. Hadlock KG, Foung SK. GBV-C/HGV: a new virus within the Flaviviridae and its clinical implications. Trans Med Rev 1998; 94.
114. Haddziyannis SJ, Daws GJ, Vrettou E, et al. Infection with novel GB-C virus in multiply transfused patients and in various forms of chronic liver disease. Hepatology 1996; 22:218A.
115. Roth WK, Waschk D, Marx S, et al. Prevalence of hepatitis G virus and its strain variant, the GB agent, in blood donations and their transmission to recipients. Transfusion 1997; 37:651.
116. Berenguer M, Teerault NA, Piatak M, et al. Hepatitis G virus infection in patients with hepatitis C virus infection undergoing liver transplantation. Gastroenteroloy 1996; 111:1569.
117. Uhle C, Zimmerman R, Goeser T, et al. Virus inactivation and prevalence of GBV-C in hemophiliacs. Br J Hematol 1997; 99:837.
118. Lin HH, Kao JH, Yeh KY, et al. Mother to infant transmission of GB virus C/hepatitis G virus: the role of high titered maternal viremia and mode of delivery. J Infect Dis 1998; 177:1202.
119. Zannetti AR, Tanzi E, Ramano L, et al. Multicenter trial on mother-to-infant transmission of GBV-C virus. J Med Virol 1998; 54:107.
120. Kao JH, Chen W, Chen PJ, et al. GB virus C/hepatitis G virus infection in prostitutes: possible role of sexual transmission. J Med Virol 1997; 52:381.
121. Alter MJ, Gallagher M, Morris TT, et al. Acute non–A-E hepatitis in the US and the role of hepatitis G virus infection. N Engl J Med 1997; 336:741.
122. Brown KE, Wong S, Young NS. Prevalence of GBV-C/HGV, a novel hepatitis virus in patients with aplastic anemia. Br J Hematol 1997; 97:492.
123. Naoumov NV, Petrova EP, Thomas MG, et al. Presence of a newly described human DNA virus (TTV) in patients with liver disease. Lancet 1998; 352:195.
124. Charleston M, Adjei P, Poterucha J, et al. TT-virus infection in North American blood donors, patients with fulminant hepatic failure and cryogenic cirrhosis. Hepatology 1998; 28:839.
125. Cardoso MS, Koerner K, Kubanek B. Mini-pool screening by nucleic acid testing for hepatitis B virus, hepatitis C virus, and HIV: preliminary results. Transfusion 1998; 38:905.
126. Mohr H. Inactivation of fresh plasma. Vox Sang 1994; 74:171.
127. Corash L. Inactivation of viruses, bacteria, protozoa, and leukocytes in platelet concentrates. Vox Sang 1994; 74:173.

CHAPTER 34

Cytomegalovirus

Naomi L. C. Luban
Jeanne A. Lumadue

Cytomegalovirus (CMV) is a herpesvirus belonging to the family Herpetoviridiae. Other viruses in this family include herpes simplex virus (HSV) types 1 and 2, Epstein-Barr virus (EBV), and varicella zoster virus. In the immunocompetent host, CMV, like EBV and varicella, produces self-limited disease states. In the immunocompromised host, all three of these viruses can produce significant morbidity and mortality. They share a unique characteristic: the ability to remain latent in tissues following an acute infection. Unlike herpes simplex and varicella viruses, which have restricted tissue expression, CMV can be isolated from many different organs, excretions, and secretions, as well as from both fresh and anticoagulated stored blood components. As organ transplantation has expanded and treatment modalities for malignancies have become more immunosuppressive, CMV has become a major problem whose epidemiology is just now being elucidated.

MOLECULAR STRUCTURE OF CMV

The CMV genome is a linear, double-stranded DNA molecule, approximately 229 kb in length. The genome is helically associated with protein, forming a viral core particle that is encapsulated in an envelope composed of both viral envelope proteins and portions of the phospholipid bilayer (derived from the internal nuclear membrane and the endoplasmic reticulum of the infected cell). The total virion is 180 nm in size.[1]

The CMV genome is divided into two regions. The unique short (U_S) region is 35 kb in length and is bounded by two 2.5-kb repeats that are designated IR_S and TR_S. The unique long (U_L) region is approximately 170 kb in length and is flanked by two 11-kb repeats (the IR_L and TR_L regions). The U_S and U_L segments can be oriented in either direction with respect to each other, resulting in four distinct isomeric forms of the virion DNA, which are generally present in equimolar amounts in CMV-infected cells. Studies utilizing restriction fragment length polymorphisms (RFLPs) have shown that clinical isolates of CMV are distinct in that they contain different sized fragments when digested with restriction endonucleases. Most of this genetic heterogeneity is located in the U_S and U_L segments. The entire CMV genome is rich in guanine and cytosine residues (G-C rich), accounting for the cross-hybridization seen with human genomic DNA, even under stringent hybridization conditions.[1a]

Between the U_L and U_S sequence is an area called the L-S junction. The hypervariability in the repeat elements within this junction represents strain differences. This area, also termed *seq* (or alpha sequence), has homology to HSV types 1 and 2. In HSV, the *seq* directs viral DNA packaging in single-genome length. This region was examined by Zaia and colleagues[4] in analyses of clinical viral isolates from bone marrow transplant patients and day-care center personnel. Using polymerase chain reaction (PCR) and RFLP analysis, they compared the *seq* of the clinical isolates with that of laboratory strains. Although matching was successful in most cases, several clinical isolates failed to amplify, probably because of primer site mismatches resulting in poor or absent amplification. Thus there is notable genetic heterogeneity in *seq* between isolates.

When CMV infects its host cell, the viral genome is released from the capsid and immediately circularizes. After infection, the genes of CMV are expressed in three distinct phases, designated immediate early (IE), early (E), and late (L), or α, β, and γ, respectively.[1a] For purposes of clinical diagnosis, the most important antibodies are made to these antigens. Immediate early antigens (IEAs) are produced independent of DNA synthesis, within 1 to 4 hours following infection.[1, 1a] The IE region contains four major transcription units—IE1, IE2, IE3, and IE4—that function as transactivators for the promoters of both viral and cellular genes and hence are necessary for progression of the viral infection.[1a, 2]

The expression of the E genes is dependent on the IE gene products. Early antigens (EAs) are produced after IEAs and have been mapped to all regions of the CMV genome. These gene products include the viral encoded DNA polymerase that allows for viral replication, as well as other DNA binding proteins.[1b] The L genes encode the late structural antigens (LAs), which are required for production of an infective viral particle and include matrix and tegument proteins as well as the envelope glycoproteins.[1, 1b]

There are an estimated 35 to 40 structural proteins in the infectious CMV viral particle,[1b] which can be categorized as structural (that is, found in the virion) or nonstructural (which include enzymes present in the infected cell).[1a] Using restriction endonuclease mapping, some of these proteins have been assigned to particular regions of the genome. Four of nine known phosphoproteins (pp150, pp71, pp65, and pp28) are located in the matrix region of the viral particle and are among the most consistently recognized proteins by antibodies in human sera.[1b]

The viral envelope consists of at least three glycoprotein complexes. Glycoprotein B (gB; gp 58 or gcI) is the carboxy terminus of a 160-kD glycosylated protein precursor that is proteolytically cleaved to a 58-kD mature product. It shows considerable homology to the major membrane glycoproteins of the other herpesviruses. In both human and murine systems, the gB region is critical to host humoral and cellular immune responses and, therefore, to the development of vaccines that can induce both classes of immune response.[3] Glycoprotein H (gH; gp 86 or gcII) is expressed on the viral envelope and the plasma membrane of CMV-infected cells and shows less homology between species than gB. Both gB and gH have been localized to the U_L55 region. Glycoprotein gcII is a complex of two envelope glycoproteins, gp 47-52.[1a, 2]

Many other proteins have been mapped genetically to particular regions of the genome, but their functions are unclear. Many of these regions of DNA are conserved, which indicates their importance in the viral life cycle. Characterization of the CMV genome may help explain many of the paradoxes of CMV infection: antibody neutralization of laboratory but not clinical strains, variability of cellular and humoral immune response using in vitro systems versus in vivo protective immunity in some clinical settings but not others, and degree of infectivity.

PATTERNS OF INFECTION

Three patterns can develop after infection with CMV. Primary infection occurs in a seronegative recipient of blood or of an organ from a donor who is actively or latently infected. Viremia, viruria, and immunoglobulin M (IgM)–specific antibody response, and later an immunoglobulin G (IgG)–specific antibody response occur. Secondary infection may occur as either reactivation or coinfection. Reactivation of latent virus occurs in a previously CMV-seropositive recipient of either seropositive or seronegative donor blood or organ. The pathogenesis of this response is described later. Reactivation infections are accompanied by a fourfold or greater titer rise in CMV IgG and shedding of the virus. Occasionally, an IgM response may be elicited; alternatively, viral shedding may occur without a rise in IgG or IgM antibody response. Reinfection, which is better defined as coinfection, occurs in a seropositive patient who is exposed to a strain of CMV different from the one that caused the original infection. In this case, an IgM antibody response, viral shedding, and an IgG CMV antibody response will be seen.

The frequency of reactivation and coinfection has not been determined in different patient groups because of the difficulty in distinguishing these two types of infection using antibody quantification or immunoblotting assays. Molecular epidemiological techniques, however, permit identification of strain differences. Tolpin and coworkers[5] were the first to identify two different strains of CMV by restriction endonuclease DNA patterns in a neonate who received blood from a seropositive donor. Since that report, similar molecular epidemiological studies have been performed in transfused infant-donor pairs,[6] in transplant recipients,[7, 8] and in the setting of day-care centers.[9] Such techniques have not been applied to large enough populations of immunoincompetent individuals to permit calculation of frequency of reactivation or coinfection. However, the rate of seroconversion alone can be used to calculate the risk of primary infection from seropositive donor units. The incidence varies widely according to patient group and year of study. The incidence of primary post-transfusion CMV in one study ranged from 10% to 50%,[10] although figures of 1.2%[11] and 0.9%[12] were reported in large populations of hospitalized patients admitted for burns, major surgery, pregnancy and delivery, neonatal complications, and oncological treatment. In both these studies, no morbidity or mortality was attributed to primary CMV infection acquired through transfusion.

In primary infection, an immunoblot assay demonstrates that the IgM and IgG responses are directed toward a polypeptide of 66 kD; in reactivation infection (e.g., in renal transplant patients), the IgG response is more intense and is directed toward glycoproteins 150, 66, and 61, whereas the IgM reactivity is toward gp 38 and gp 66 polypeptides.[13, 14] In both primary infection and reactivation, the IgG response to gp 150, the most immunogenic of the polypeptides, appears later in infection but lasts longer than the antibody to the other epitopes.[13] Despite this dissection of antibody response on a molecular level, total IgG and IgM are most often measured; commercial tests utilizing epitope patterns to distinguish patterns of infection have not yet been developed.

The distinction between CMV infection identified by seroconversion or viral isolation and CMV disease is important when interpreting the vast literature on post-transfusion CMV. CMV disease is defined as laboratory evidence of infection coupled with specific symptoms attributable to the virus in the absence of other culpable pathogens or the patient's primary disease. The clinical manifestations of post-transfusion CMV range from a heterophile-negative mononucleosis syndrome to disseminated disease. Lymphadenopathy, lymphocytosis, fever, and pharyngitis with hepatitis constitute the mononucleosis-like syndrome. Interstitial pneumonitis, thrombocytopenia, hemolytic anemia, meningoencephalitis, and polyneuropathy are other associated findings. In the immunocompromised host, there is a wide range of associated symptoms and signs. These include all the aforementioned findings as well as retinitis, colitis, gastritis, nephritis, and rash. Renal allograft rejection[15] and atherosclerosis of transplanted hearts[16] have also been associated with primary CMV infection.

DONOR AND RECIPIENT FACTORS PREDISPOSING TO INFECTION

CMV and the White Blood Cell

Not all seropositive donor units are capable of causing infection. Both recipient and donor factors predispose certain recipients to acquire post-transfusion CMV and certain donors to transmit this cell-associated virus. In seroepidemiological studies, post-transfusion CMV has been attributed to the transfusion of all cellular blood components but has not been associated with the transfusion of plasma products. Leukocytes, as either buffy coats or granulocytopheresis products, transmit CMV, often with fatal results.[17, 18] Fresh frozen plasma (FFP) does not transmit CMV.[19, 20] High-titer antibody to CMV, in the form of either CMV hyperimmune globulin[21] or intravenous (IV) IgG,[22] protects against CMV and has been used prophylactically in transplant recipients, with variable results. It is unknown whether platelets transmit CMV more readily than red blood cells. Leukodepletion through washing of blood[23] reduces and deglycerolization eliminates the potential[24–26] for CMV transmission, even when the red blood cell units are seropositive for CMV. Third-generation white blood cell removal filters also appear to be effective.[27–29]

The seroepidemiology of the virus, coupled with attenuation or prevention of post-transfusion CMV by leukoreduction, implies that CMV is harbored in the white blood cell. Several studies have attempted to grow CMV from both blood donor units and asymptomatic healthy individuals, using standard culture techniques, and have been unsuccessful.[30] In 1985, Schrier and colleagues[31] were able to detect CMV RNA in circulating mononuclear cells using a hybridization probe unique to the IE proteins. These probes were selected because they were likely to be heavily transcribed in early infection. Furthermore, this group established through flow cytometry that 24% of CMV-hybridizing cells have CD4 marker, whereas 0.8% have CD8 marker, suggesting that the lymphocyte was the major source of CMV.[31] In another study using dot blot of mononuclear and neutrophil DNA samples from 458 healthy blood donors, there was no difference in signal intensity among donors who were seronegative, IgG and IgM seropositive, or IgG seropositive only.[32] Only samples from patients with CMV disease were positive in this study. It is likely that the sensitivity limit of this assay was not met and that the infected donor cells contained less than one CMV genome per 20 cells. When the same group used RNA transcripts, they were able to detect CMV DNA in 0.03% to 2% of peripheral blood mononuclear cells in eight seropositive asymptomatic individuals,[32] but the exact cell type was not specified.

The transplantation literature provides further information on the cell type responsible for CMV transmission. Direct detection of CMV antigens in the nuclei of polymorphonuclear leukocytes by immunoperoxidase staining and indirect fluorescent antibody (IFA) techniques has provided some of this additional information. One of the more commonly used techniques is detection of early antigen fluorescent foci (DEAFF). Heparinized buffy coat samples are inoculated onto cellular monolayers for up to 72 hours, with refreshment of culture media in 5% CO_2. Monolayers are fixed in acetone, stained indirectly through immunofluorescence with mouse anti-CMV monoclonal antibody and fluorescein isothiocyanate (FITC)–conjugated anti-immunoglobulin, and scored on a fluorescent microscope. Urine, saliva, or blood can be analyzed with this method.

PCR techniques have been optimized for peripheral blood leukocytes by several groups. PCR positivity appears to be a better marker of acute CMV infection than is DEAFF. In one study, PCR failed to detect CMV in asymptomatic seropositive and seronegative controls and became negative following acute viremia in patient samples. In serial samples obtained from 13 kidney or bone marrow transplant patients, PCR was more sensitive than DEAFF in 8 patients because it permitted isolation of CMV DNA for a longer time than DEAFF (at $p < .05$), with an estimate of greater than 69 genomes per sample of 10^5 leukocytes.[7] Latent infection with CMV could not be identified, implying that healthy seropositive individuals have fewer CMV genome-bearing cells. Another study used different primers and compared two different assays—a modified immunofixation assay with IEA to determine antigenemia, and a standard shell vial assay to quantify viremia.[33] Fourteen patients in this study who underwent cardiac transplantation were categorized as having primary infection on the basis of IgG seroconversion. IgM seroconversion was seen in 3 of 10 patients with recurrent CMV infection and all 3 patients with primary CMV infection. Clinical symptoms appeared to be correlated with the level of antigenemia. PCR detected CMV DNA in 48 samples that were consistently negative for both viremia and antigenemia, usually obtained early or late in infection after ganciclovir therapy was initiated. PCR was consistently positive 1 week before the appearance of positivity in other assays and remained positive longer following negative tests for antigenemia and viremia.[33]

A similar dissociation between antigenemia and presence of CMV DNA was reported by Saltzman and associates.[34] In this study, DNA dot blot hybridization was used in place of PCR, and DNA was quantitated in mononuclear and polymorphonuclear populations of blood and saliva from transplant patients by means of an optical scanning system. Viral genome equivalents were calculated using a formula. CMV DNA was recovered from 16 of 17 (94%) polymorphonuclear cell specimens and from 7 of 15 (47%) mononuclear cell specimens obtained from EDTA specimens of viremic patients. The number of cells required for detection was 1.6×10^5 (range, 5.5×10^3 to 1.3×10^6) for polymorphonuclear cells and 2.3×10^5 (range, 8.6×10^3 to 1×10^6) for mononuclear cells. More viral DNA was present in polymorphonuclear cells (13.1 viral genome equivalents per 100 cells) than in mononuclear cells (9.1 viral genome equivalents per 100 cells). In patients without positive viral cultures, less viral DNA was obtained (4 viral genome equivalents per 100 cells), with no difference in cell type. No CMV DNA was detected in the leukocytes of 25 IgG CMV-seropositive blood donors.

The disparity between culture and the molecular hybridization techniques for identifying virus in mononuclear cells is not easily explained. One can speculate that CMV exists within the granulocyte in a mature infectious form. In the mononuclear fraction, the infection may be primarily abortive or may require cell-cell interaction to induce transcription. Understanding the cellular harbinger of infectious or latent viruses has implications for the screening of infectious donors and for the processing of donor blood to make it noninfectious.

IMMUNOLOGY OF CMV INFECTION

The interaction of CMV with both the humoral and cellular immune systems is complex. CMV can both suppress and enhance host response to specific viral and nonviral antigens. Antibody response to CMV may develop but does not result in protective immunity. Further, therapeutic immunosuppression activates viral expression and replication. Patients with congenital immunodeficiency who lack the ability to mount antibody responses are at risk for fulminant CMV disease.

Humoral Immune Response

Humoral immune response, initially with IgM and later with IgG anti-CMV antibody production, provides a means of classifying the type of CMV infection. In the presence of preexisting antibody, there may be moderation of pathogenicity but not prevention of disease. Specifically, in prenatal CMV, mothers with preexisting antibody are less likely to develop CMV disease, as are their fetuses.[35] In renal transplantation, CMV antibody–positive recipients of CMV-seropositive renal allografts have less morbidity from CMV than do CMV-seronegative recipients of CMV-seropositive, living related donor allografts.[36] Discordant heart, heart-lung, liver, and bone marrow donor-recipient pairs have been reported with similar results. In solid organs and allografts, it is either the allograft itself or blood remaining in the allograft after processing that is implicated as the source of CMV. CMV is latent in a number of tissues of CMV-seropositive adults, including those of the kidneys, lungs, liver, and brain.[37] CMV-seropositive premature infants receiving seropositive blood have been reported to suffer severe morbidity.[38, 39] Although not mentioned or specifically investigated in these studies, other sexually transmitted diseases in the mother, particularly gonorrhea,[40] might have compounded the clinical course of the infants. Alternatively, loss of protective immunity from the mother over time may have resulted in viral activation and CMV disease.

Probably the most supportive evidence of humoral attenuation of CMV infection and disease comes from the bone marrow transplantation literature. Studies have evaluated the efficacy of CMV hyperimmune plasma,[41] IV IgG,[22] and intramuscular[42] and IV CMV-specific immunoglobulin.[21, 41, 43, 44] Results have been conflicting, with some studies demonstrating a decrease in the incidence of CMV pneumonia[22, 41–43] and others not.[21, 42] Reasons for the discrepancies include variability in the titers of antibody to CMV in the product, total dose and dosage schedule, and discordance in kind of blood product used or in serostatus of donor-recipient pairs. Bowden and associates[45] used a CMV IgG product, prepared from donors selected for high concentrations of "naturally" occurring CMV antibody, in a randomized placebo-controlled study of 123 seronegative recipients of seropositive bone marrow. The product was administered at 200 mg/kg on days 8 and 6 before transplantation, on the day of marrow infusion, and weekly for 7 weeks, for a total of 10 doses. There was less CMV infection and viremia in the treated group. However, similar numbers of patients (14 in the treatment group, 17 in the control group) developed a CMV syndrome with CMV disease documented by tissue invasion. There was also no difference in the median days after transplantation until onset of infection, viremia, or tissue-invasive CMV disease. The results of this study differ from those of others[22, 41, 43] and may be due in part to the failure of CMV IV IgG to affect the incidence of acute graft-versus-host disease (GVHD). The authors speculate that the reduction in incidence of CMV disease in previous studies may have been due to reduction in incidence of GVHD by IV IgG; the mechanism by which IV IgG attenuates GVHD is still not understood.[46]

Neutralizing antibodies are responsible for inactivating extracellular virions by binding to the virus. Purified gB envelope protein induces neutralizing antibodies in both human and murine models. In one study, 40% to 70% of neutralizing antibodies were directed toward gB[47]; in recombinant vaccinia-gB vaccine studies, 50% to 88% of total virus-neutralizing activity was directed toward gB protein.[48] Evaluation of 20 immunocompetent CMV-seropositive individuals for neutralizing antibody to gB protein, with the use of a radioimmunoprecipitation assay and specific absorption experiments, demonstrated that 48% of specimens had neutralizing activity to gB.[49] Intracellular viral proliferation and reactivation are under the control of helper and cytotoxic T cells. Cytotoxic T cells respond to gB protein by increasing cytolysis,[50] and in one study, the gB-specific cytotoxic response was isolated to the N-terminal 513 amino acids of gB.[51] Exposing helper T cell clones derived from CMV-seropositive and CMV-seronegative donors to whole virus and immunoaffinity-purified segments of the gB glycoprotein complex demonstrated variability in the response of different clones to the different epitopes. This study implies that helper T cell precursors recognize a variety of immunodominant epitopes on gB.[3]

Another possible explanation for the conflicting clinical trials using different IV IgG and plasma preparations is that the products have varying levels of neutralizing antibody. In an effort to avoid such variability, two human monoclonal antibodies with neutralizing characteristics have been used in a phase I clinical trial in bone marrow transplant recipients. The target antibodies are of IgG isotope: SOZ 109 neutralizes by binding to an 82-kD complex characterized as gpB (gp59), and SDZ 104 binds to a disulfide-bonded complex that includes 58-kD, 107-kD, and 163-kD proteins.[52] These antibodies were chosen because of identification of the neutralizing epitope on glycoprotein gp58 of human CMV.[53] Because this was a phase I study, only half-life data and kinetics were measured, and no data on efficacy were provided.

Data from a study by Chou and Dennison[54] support future development of monoclonal antibodies of high purity and specificity. They showed peptide homology ranging from 91% to 98% in the gB gene of more than 28 clinical strains and suggested that the number of gB variants among clinical strains is limited. They also speculated that sequence differences may determine tissue tropism, as occurs in HSV, in which gB sequence differences correlate with neurovirulence.[53] However, the role of strain-specific neutralizing antibody in attenuating CMV remains incompletely understood.

Vaccination is yet another mechanism that can be used to study humoral response. In a study evaluating the efficacy of the Towne vaccine, 237 renal transplant recipients were entered into a double-blind, randomized, placebo-controlled trial. The vaccine was ineffective in protecting against CMV disease in seropositive recipients. In seronegative recipients of seropositive kidneys, there was less severe CMV disease and improved graft survival, although the infection rate was the same in both the placebo and vaccination groups. RFLP analysis showed that the virus excreted after transplantation differed from the live vaccine virus, confirming that Towne virus does not become latent in vaccine recipients. Antibody response did not correlate with outcome. The authors of this study speculate that the cellular immune response to the vaccine might provide more information on protection against CMV.[55]

Cell-Mediated Immunity

The importance of cell-mediated immunity in CMV infection is probably best defined by CMV's variable expression in individuals with defects in cellular immunity. The more cellular immunosuppression an individual has, the more likely he or she is to develop CMV disease when exposed to the virus, or to reactivate latent virus. For example, renal allograft recipients are less adversely affected than heart, heart-lung, or liver transplant recipients. Bone marrow recipients with the potential for CMV pneumonitis rank next, followed by reactivation of CMV in patients with acquired immunodeficiency syndrome (AIDS), in whom CMV becomes disseminated to different sites than in immunosuppressed transplant recipients.

Several early studies evaluated cell-mediated immunity through measurements of lymphocyte transformation and blastogenesis to different mitogens and antigens. CMV-immune individuals were found to have proliferative responses to both mitogens and viral antigens, the latter occurring within 1 to 2 months after primary infection. In contrast, congenitally infected infants and their mothers were found to have decreased proliferative response to CMV antigens as well as mitogen-specific responses. Cardiac, renal, and bone marrow transplant recipients were found to have similar laboratory test results.[56, 57] Possible explanations for these findings include (1) a direct effect of the virus on T cell proliferation; (2) release of soluble factors that suppress T cell function; and (3) maximal stimulation of effector cells by virus, rendering them incapable of further stimulation.

Using murine CMV (MCMV) as an animal model of human CMV, researchers have evaluated many different cellular immune responses. During acute MCMV infection, humoral immune response to other antigens is suppressed, as well as specific T cell response to mitogens; monocyte excretion of interleukin-1 is also decreased. Cytotoxic T lymphocyte (CTL) response to MCMV has been extensively investigated and appears to be restricted by the major histocompatibility locus, H-2. The process in mice might be due to recognition of an H-2 complex modified by viral antigens or to simultaneous recognition of independent viral and histocompatibility antigens. In the mouse, CTLs respond to the immunogenic protein encoded by the IEA or the structural gB protein. In several studies, $CD8^+$ T cells were found to confer resistance to MCMV; in the presence of selective deficiency of $CD8^+$ cells, $CD4^+$ T cells facilitate the production of CMV-specific antibodies that neutralize virus.[58] Alternatively, selective deficiency of $CD4^+$ cells in immunocompetent mice resulted in persistent viral latency; remaining $CD8^+$ T cells functioned independently of $CD4^+$ T cells to restrict virus to acinar glandular epithelial cells of the salivary gland.[59] In adoptive transfer experiments, immune $CD8^+$ T cells protected immunosuppressed mice from primary MCMV and attenuated disease in mice with established MCMV infection. Other investigators have evaluated antibody-dependent cell-mediated cytotoxicity (ADCC) and natural killer (NK) cell function in MCMV. There is a lack of H-2 restriction for NK cells that appear early in infection, whereas ADCC is more likely to be found in chronic and latent phases of murine infection and is likely to be H-2 restricted.[1]

Viral-specific CTLs are also responsible for at least some of the cytopathic effects of CMV. Murine lymphocytic choriomeningitis virus, for example, when injected into immunocompromised mice, produces neither encephalitis nor hepatitis; when immune spleen cells are coinjected, an encephalitis develops, and if $CD8^+$ T cells ($Ly2^+$) are adoptively transferred, hepatic necrosis and periportal infiltrates form. This and other models indicate that CTLs may well be protective in early infection through lysis of small numbers of infected cells and provocation of the cytokine response, whereas in late infection, cytolysis of infected tissues and the subsequent inflammatory response produce pathology. Pasternack and coworkers[60] reviewed some of the parameters that might be involved in the balance between protective immunity and cytopathology in the mouse model. The size and route of the inoculum, temporal relationship between infection and development of T cell–mediated immunity or adoptive transfer, strain of virus, characteristics of host, and nature of immunosuppressive regimen used[60] may all be critical to the development of CMV-mediated disease. Many parallels can be drawn to human CMV infection in the immunocompromised host.

ANALYZING CELLULAR IMMUNE RESPONSE WITH FLOW CYTOMETRY

Early studies in lymphocyte transformation and mitogen- and antigen-induced blastogenesis[56, 57] have been further extended by flow-cytometric analysis. Patients with CMV mononucleosis have elevated suppresser-cytotoxic $CD8^+$ T cells, activation marker (I^a), and an inverted $CD4^+/CD8^+$ ratio. Peripheral blood mononuclear cells from healthy CMV-seropositive donors undergo B cell activation with production of IgG, IgM, and IgA antibody, which is likely dependent on $CD4^+$ lymphocytes.[61] Organ transplant recipients have been shown to have total T cell depletion, $CD4^+/CD8^+$ ratio inversion, polyclonal B cell activation, and a wide variety of immune perturbations that might be due in part to the use of pretransplantation immunosuppression and degree of rejection.

In a study by Gratama and colleagues[62] of 112 normal volunteer blood donors stratified according to their CMV IgG and IgM antibody status, flow-cytometric analysis, including human natural killer (HNK) fluorescent intensity, and morphology were evaluated. CMV-seropositive individuals had larger numbers of $HNK1^+$ (Leu 7^+) lymphocytes than CMV-seronegative individuals. In addition, lymphocytes with strong HNK1 fluorescence showed greater granularity, suggesting that these cells with HNK1 epitopes may serve as adhesion or interaction sites between cytotoxic lymphocytes and their targets.[62] This study was an outgrowth of a previous smaller study in which CMV carrier status was found to be associated with increases both in $CD3^+$, $CD4^+$, $HNK1^+$, $CD16^-$ and in $CD3^+$, $CD8^+$, $HNK1^+$, $CD16^-$ lymphocyte subsets in peripheral blood.[63] CMV-seronegative individuals lacked $HNK1^+$ phenotype. That study evaluated ADCC as a function of seropositivity, as well as $HNK1^+$ function. A second study by Gratama and colleagues[63] found that $HNK1^+$ cells of CMV-seropositive individuals were more efficient in assays of ADCC and NK function than were those of CMV-negative individuals with the same markers. The authors further speculated that a subpopulation of lymphocytes with strong HNK expression, present in 1:18 lymphocytes in CMV-seropositive individuals, may be the CMV-specific cytotoxic cells that function to keep CMV replication under control.

Additional work from the same laboratory has attempted to characterize subpopulations of lymphocytes responsible for regulating pokeweed mitogen (PWM)–induced B cell differentiation.[64] Identification of a subpopulation that regulates CMV-specific antibody production would be of obvious importance. The researchers used three-color fluorescent activated cell sorter (FACS) analysis and functional co-culture assays in 17 IgG-seropositive and 42 IgG-seronegative individuals. Specifically, they evaluated expression of CD11b, which is the third receptor for complement and belongs to a group of cell surface molecules called integrins that facilitate intercellular contacts between target and effector cells or trigger cell lysis. Gratama and colleagues[64] could not demonstrate CD11b preferentially on the lymphocytes of seropositive individuals. In addition, both $CD8^+$, $HNK1^+$ and $CD8^+$, $HNK1^-$ lymphocytes suppressed PWM-driven B cell differentiation. The authors theorized that following CMV activation, both $CD4^+$ and $CD8^+$ lymphocytes acquire both HNK1 and CD11b epitopes, permitting interaction with virally infected target cells. When the lymphocytes return to a resting state, they retain HNK1 and downregulate CD11b. The $CD8^+$, $HNK1^+$ population does not appear to be solely responsible for the inhibition of PWM B cell antibody production.[64]

In humans, $CD8^+$ CTLs are likely to be restricted by the major histocompatibility complex (MHC).[57] The $CD8^+$ CTLs usually recognize endogenously synthesized viral proteins processed in the infected cell and presented with class I MHC molecules. In MCMV, the IEA or gB is the target antigen. In human CMV infection, $CD8^+$ CTLs are also critical to controlling infection, but the specific viral proteins that serve as target antigens are still under investigation. In one study using autologous CMV-infected fibroblasts and limiting dilution analysis of peripheral blood lymphocytes, IEA was reported as a major and gB as a minor target antigen.[50] Using CTL clone methods, Riddell and associates[65] demonstrated that the CMV-specific, class I–restricted response in latently infected individuals was due to structural virion proteins introduced into the cell following viral penetration, in the absence of specific cell surface gene expression.

In a prospective study of 20 human leukocyte antigen (HLA)–matched bone marrow transplant recipients, 16 of whom were seropositive and received seropositive allogeneic bone marrow, CMV-specific CTL reactivity was evaluated with a short-term in vitro culture system at 1, 2, and 3 months after transplantation, and results were compared with the incidence of CMV disease. All 20 donors had CMV-specific $CD8^+$ CTL activity (estimated at between 1 in 5000 and 1 in 20,000 peripheral blood T cells), whereas 10 marrow recipients developed a detectable class I MHC-restricted, CMV-specific CTL response within the first 3 months after transplantation. Moderate to severe (grades II to IV) acute GVHD developed in all 10 patients who failed to develop CTLs. Six of 10 patients who did not develop CTLs developed CMV pneumonia, in contrast to none of the 10 patients with CTLs.[66] The authors hypothesized that the correlation between GVHD and lack of detectable CTL response might be due to the direct effect of GVHD or might be secondary to the immunosuppression used to treat GVHD.

The same group has developed methods to produce CTL clones that can specifically lyse CMV-infected target cells, home appropriately, and enter a resting phase after a single lytic cycle. Ultimately, such clones could be used in adoptive immunotherapy of selected patients at risk for CMV disease.[67] Further work to unravel MHC restriction through clinical trials of cloned CTLs from HLA-matched donors is under way.[67] The possible cross-reactivity between CMV structural proteins of either the IE or L nuclear antigen and T cell receptor molecules may contribute to controlling the regulatory network involved in CMV and transplantation.[68]

As in the mouse system, at least some of the failure of human CTLs is due to HLA restriction and to the production of soluble mediators. Using short-term in vivo culture of human fibroblasts from 16 normal volunteers, 13 seropositive and 3 seronegative, Laubscher and colleagues[69] were able to demonstrate that CMV-specific killing was caused by a CTL of CD8 phenotype. The killing was inhibited by HLA class I monoclonal antibodies, but not by class II, and was modified by pretreatment of target fibroblasts with interferon-γ, which increased expression of HLA class I antigens.[69] These authors did not evaluate HNK phenotype but did suggest that the experimental system was not optimized for evaluation of class II–restricted CTL identification. Furthermore, they theorized that a CTL subpopulation other than CD8 or CD4, possibly an NK cell, was responsible for at least some of the CMV-specific killing.

Using the same cytotoxicity assay with CMV-infected and uninfected HLA-mismatched fibroblasts and more complex FACS analysis than in the previous investigation, Bowden and associates[70] evaluated 45 CMV-seropositive bone marrow transplant recipients. Thirty-five of these patients became culture positive, and 10 remained uninfected. These researchers found reduction of cytotoxic activity as measured by percentage of lysis in infected patients; when stratified according to invasive or noninvasive disease, cytotoxic responses were lower in those patients who developed pneumonia than in those who recovered or had CMV enteritis. Acute GVHD occurred in 17 patients, all of whom were CMV culture–positive. When studied 20 to 40 days after transplantation, the period coinciding with the peak incidence of GVHD, the patients had significantly lower cytotoxic responses against both CMV-infected and uninfected target cells than did CMV-infected patients without acute GVHD. Bowden and associates[70] characterized the cytotoxic cells phenotypically as NK cells.

Soluble mediators of T cell activation or of monocytes may be involved in the immunopathogenesis of CMV. In the mouse, tumor necrosis factor (TNF), interferon-α, and interleukin-2 (IL-2) are all thought to induce resistance to viral infection in different cell lines. Peripheral blood monocytes secrete interferon-α with an antiviral capability that is thought to be important in the control of HSV infection,[71] but monocyte and monokine production has been studied infrequently.[72] TNF secreted from monocytes has been better investigated; it provides antiviral protection against several different RNA and DNA viruses and induces cytotoxicity in viral-infected cells of several different cell lines in vitro. Different mouse strains have different susceptibility for bacterial lipopolysaccharides, based on ability to transcribe TNF mRNA.[73] Mouse strains with different susceptibilities to CMV were exposed to lipopolysaccharides and studied for viral recovery in different organs; the strains that were known to have blocks in TNF transcription and translation were more likely to succumb to CMV, which implies that TNF may well modulate CMV cytopathology.

The correlation between these findings in mice and their potential importance in humans is again best defined in the setting of bone marrow transplantation. TNF-α has many functions in the protection of early human bone marrow progenitors against 4-hydroperoxycyclophosphamide, may be selectively tumoricidal for certain acute myelocytic leukemia cells,[74] and may be important in progenitor homing. In the early post-transplantation period, a subpopulation of cells secretes TNF and interferon-α. In some transplantation centers, TNF-α is monitored to predict transplant-related conditions before they became clinically apparent.[75] CMV delays bone marrow engraftment, inhibits myelopoiesis, and destroys bone marrow stroma.[76, 77] A logical connection between TNF production and CMV infection should therefore exist.

Duncombe and colleagues[78] explored this relationship in 13 bone marrow transplant recipients, 12 of whom were CMV seropositive. These researchers demonstrated that both interferon-γ and TNF were constitutively produced in the recipient by recipient $CD3^+$ and $CD16^+$ lymphocytes, but not by their marrow fibroblasts. These authors demonstrated that after bone marrow transplantation, CMV regulates both interferon-γ and TNF production, which blocks viral replication, whereas the decline in cytokine production correlates with the time of highest risk from CMV.[78] Co-culture of MHC-matched marrow fibroblasts with peripheral blood mononuclear cells in the presence or absence of CMV demonstrates that interferon-γ and TNF are able to protect against CMV infection of bone marrow fibroblasts. Duncombe and colleagues[78] further speculated that unrestricted production of TNF and interferon-γ might be responsible for suppression of hematopoietic recovery, as has been previously suggested.[79, 80]

Other cytokines and interleukins are likely also involved in support of bone marrow growth, which may or may not be influenced by concomitant CMV infection. IL-2 is another putative inhibitor of fibroblast growth,[81] which is probably less important in CMV-induced pathogenicity but is critical in the development of GVHD (i.e., IL-2–positive alloreactive T cells are increased in GVHD).

In an attempt to correlate interferon-γ, CMV, and the incidence of rejection in heart and heart-lung recipients, 37 adult patients were followed serially by means of viral cultures, assays of cell-mediated immunity with passive hemagglutination (PHA) stimulation, assessment of the supernatant for interferon-γ, and lymphocyte proliferation assays. Morbidity due to CMV was 62% in CMV-seropositive individuals; mortality was 6% in CMV-seronegative cases, compared with 19% in CMV-seropositive cases. CMV-induced interferon-γ production in vitro was lower than in normal adult controls, although only for up to 3 months after transplantation. No clear-cut association with graft rejection was made. The lower interferon-γ concentrations were thought to be secondary to the functional T cell impairment associated with immunosuppression, not specifically to CMV infection.[82]

BLOOD PRODUCT VARIABLES INFLUENCING INFECTIVITY

Several variables are important in the transmissibility of CMV in a blood product: the number of white blood cells containing CMV virions capable of proliferating in the recipient; the cellular and humoral immune status of the recipient; the presence of immune or neutralizing antibody in the product, the recipient, or both; and, at least for some patients, particularly those who are seropositive, the development of subclinical GVHD that can reactivate latent virus.

Blood products vary widely in the quantity of leukocytes present, owing at least in part to the method of collection (Table 34–1). Those products with the greatest number of leukocytes would be expected to transmit CMV infection most efficiently, as has been borne out by studies of individuals receiving granulocyte transfusions.[17, 18] With increase in storage time, fewer lymphocytes can be isolated from either red blood cell concentrates[83] or random platelet concentrates.[84] Platelets express only class I MHC antigens, whereas white blood cells express both class I and class II MHC antigens.

Table 34–1. White Blood Cell (WBC) Content of Different Blood Components

Component	Volume (mL)	Average WBC Content
Whole blood	450	1–2 × 10^9
Red blood cells	250	2–5 × 10^9
Washed red blood cells	Variable	<5 × 10^8
Deglycerolized red blood cells	250	~10^7
Platelet concentrate	50–75	4 × 10^7
Plateletpheresis unit	200–500	3 × 10^8*
Cryoprecipitate	25	0
Fresh frozen plasma	125	0
Pediatric frozen plasma	Variable	0
Liquid plasma	125	1.5 × 10^5
Single-donor plasma	125	0
Granulocyte concentrate	200–500	1 × 10^{10}

Adapted from Luban NLC. Basics of transfusion medicine. *In* Fuhrman BP, Zimmerman JJ (eds): Pediatric Critical Care. St. Louis: Mosby–Year Book, 1992, pp 829–840.

*Less with new modified chambers.

The white cell contamination of platelet concentrates, specifically through expression of both class I and class II MHC antigens, is thought to be necessary to evoke primary sensitization and platelet refractoriness.

Using FACS analysis and mixed lymphocyte culture, Sherman and Dzik[84] determined that there was progressive decline in HLA class II antigen expression over time in platelets stored at room temperature, whereas HLA class I antigens were consistently expressed throughout storage in 95% of the platelet concentrates analyzed. These findings may well have implications for CMV transmission. As the total white cell count decreased, presumably by cytolysis, the percentage of cells remaining as lymphocytes increased.[84] If polymorphonuclear cells or mononuclear cells harbor CMV, then the incidence of infection in "aged," leukocyte-reduced products would be less.

Data from four studies constitute conflicting information in this regard, at least in part because of differences in study design. Two papers report higher rates of seroconversion to CMV in recipients of fresh red blood cells,[11, 85] and two papers correlate the higher seroconversion rate with greater transfusion number and volume.[12, 86] Red blood cell storage of 3 to 8 days versus 20 to 42 days was specifically assessed in a group of 84 seropositive patients undergoing surgery; there was no statistically significant increase in antibody titer as a determinant of reactivation between the two groups.[86] Despite variable rates of seroconversion in different studies,[11, 12, 85, 86] and viral excretion noted in one study,[85] no mortality or morbidity was attributable to CMV. It appears that at least for patients who are not severely immunocompromised, reactivation of latent CMV remains subclinical.

Although the study by Sherman and Dzik[84] confirmed that platelets stored at 22°C have less class II antigenicity than fresh platelets, similar data are not available for lymphocytes in red blood cell units. At least one study in renal transplant recipients showed that those receiving stored refrigerated red blood had less HLA sensitization than those receiving fresh red blood cells.[87] T lymphocytes (as measured by E rosetting) in red blood cell units collected in citrate-phosphate-dextrose (CPD) and stored for up to 14 days lose their ability to respond to antigens and mitogens by day 6 of storage.[88] Diminished class II–dependent allogeneic stimulation from older red blood products may contribute to the lower rate of reactivation of CMV in recipients of both CMV-seropositive and CMV-seronegative aged blood units. Furthermore, human CMV-specific CTLs expressing class I antigenicity have been identified in the lymphocytes of symptomatic, persistently CMV-infected individuals. These cells may be the T cells responsible for establishing latent infection in nonimmune hosts and for further immune perturbations in the immune host, and they may be selectively depleted under certain storage conditions.

GVHD develops when there are histocompatibility differences between an immunocompetent donor and an immunoincompetent recipient. When histocompatibility is minimal (i.e., when there is heterozygosity for a specific allele), engraftment occurs. This is followed in time by recognition by the transfused donor lymphocytes of the "foreign" nature of the histocompatibility antigens of the host. Proliferation of cytotoxic T cells ensues, with organ dysfunction that may result in mortality or significant morbidity. GVHD can be abrogated by gamma irradiation of blood products, which inhibits the proliferation of T lymphocytes to both mitogen and antigen in standard lymphocyte cultures as well as in limiting dilution analysis.[89] Irradiation will not prevent post-transfusion CMV as either primary infection or reactivation, as evidenced by the fact that gamma irradiation is standard for all blood products given to bone marrow transplant recipients, many of whom develop reactivation CMV.

Despite the use of irradiated blood products, there is a strong association between the development of GVHD and CMV, particularly in the setting of bone marrow transplantation; CMV interstitial pneumonia is the primary cause of morbidity and mortality. In the setting of autologous transplantation, in which there is less GVHD and less post-transplantation immunosuppressive therapy, there is less CMV disease. In one study of 159 autologous transplant recipients, 31% developed CMV infection, as opposed to 51% of 545 allograft recipients from the same institution.[90] Positive pretransplantation serology was the only identifiable risk for CMV infection, and 9 of 11 cases of pneumonia were fatal. The probability of CMV interstitial pneumonia was 7% in seronegative and 11.3% in seropositive autologous marrow recipients in this study, compared with 10% and 50%, respectively, in allograft recipients. The exact nature of the defective T cell function in GVHD that results in a higher rate of CMV interstitial pneumonitis has yet to be established.

Two animal studies may help in understanding the CMV and GVHD connection. In murine systems, when there is class I MHC disparity between donor and host, the introduction of CMV with donor cells results in both cellular and humoral dysfunction. This includes failure to produce IgG antiviral antibody as well as increases in NK activity and in CTLs. In an effort to determine whether attenuated virus or T cell–dependent antigens are responsible for exacerbation of GVHD, mice were injected with lethal doses (400 LD_{50}) of MCMV, ultraviolet (UV)–light inactivated MCMV, or DNP-BSA, a T cell–dependent antigen. Mice were sacrificed and analyzed for CTL, NK cells, and phenotypic changes through FACS analysis. There was no GVHD with either UV-inactivated MCMV or DNP-BSA. However, the introduction of MCMV plus donor cells plus DNP-BSA was associated with antiviral IgM and IgG response, implying that a generic serological response occurred but did not exacerbate GVHD.[91] Although an increase in NK activity was not seen in experiments done with DNP-BSA plus donor cell inoculum or UV-inactivated MCMV plus inoculum alone, other studies have shown that polyclonally activated alloreactive T cells contribute to GVHD, and that this can occur with MCMV and other herpesviruses.[92]

Bean and coworkers[93] have used heat and gamma irradiation to prevent transfusion-induced sensitization to minor histoincompatibility antigens in DLA (MHC)–identical canine marrow grafts. This study was prompted by looking at mechanisms to prevent transfusion-induced sensitization from dendritic or mononuclear cells in transfused blood products that prohibit marrow engraftment in DLA-identical littermates. Unexpectedly, treatment of blood before transplantation with gamma radiation at 2000 cGy alone prevented the transfusion-induced sensitization, presumably by inhibiting dendritic cell presentation of minor histocompatibility antigens.[93] The mechanisms that result in CMV activation in marrow transplant are multifactorial. If activation of latent CMV is due in part to this mechanism, then irradiation of blood products might well serve as at least one method to attenuate transfusion-transmitted CMV.

RECIPIENT GROUPS AT RISK FOR TRANSFUSION-TRANSMITTED CMV

Risk for CMV infection through transfusion varies among different groups of immunosuppressed recipients according to their native CMV immune status and the extent and nature of their T cell dysfunction. On the basis of a review of the English language literature on transfusion-transmitted CMV, Sayers and colleagues[94] formulated a classification of risk (Table 34–2). This review and others[10, 30, 95, 96] have attempted to classify patients in order to streamline provision of blood products that may be difficult to obtain. One should note that recipients may switch between classification groups as chemotherapy, adoptive immunotherapy, and treatment protocols increase in immunosuppressive intensity.

METHODS OF PREVENTION

Blood obtained from seronegative donors is considered by many authorities to be the standard of care for individuals requiring CMV-negative blood products. Seronegativity may be defined using one of several methods. The commercial assays measure either IgG-specific or total anti-CMV antibody and use indirect hemagglutination, latex agglutination, enzyme-linked immunosorbent assay (ELISA), or solid-phase immunofluorescence techniques. A review of those methods commonly available in clinical laboratories has shown differences in sensitivity and specificity, which may account for the few anecdotal cases of post-transfusion CMV in seronegative recipients of seronegative blood and blood products.

IgM testing of donors is another serological technique that has not been used widely, predominantly because assay systems for IgM CMV are not well established. Theoretically, IgM-seropositive donors would be most likely to be harboring infectious virus that could produce fulminant disease. In one study, 7 of 22 seronegative infants who had seroconversion and shed virus had received at least one IgM-seropositive donor transfusion. In the second phase of this study, 1 of 141 seronegative infants receiving IgM-seronegative blood showed seroconversion; the donor was later found to be seropositive using another assay system.[97] IgM seroprevalence in donor populations ranges from less than 1% to 6%,[23, 94, 97] far lower than the reported 70% seroprevalence for IgG. Owing to the paucity of clinical trials with IgM-seronegative, IgG-seropositive blood, other methods of prevention have received more attention.

Because CMV is probably harbored in the white blood cell, leukocyte depletion of blood products has been advocated as a method to abrogate CMV transmission. This is supported by clinical studies demonstrating no or reduced seroconversion with either untested or seropositive frozen deglycerolized and washed red blood

Table 34–2. Patients at Risk for Transfusion-Transmitted Cytomegalovirus (CMV) Infection

Patients for whom the risk is well established	CMV-seronegative pregnant women Premature infants (<1200 g) born to CMV-seronegative mothers CMV-seronegative recipients of allogeneic bone marrow transplants from CMV-seronegative donors CMV-seronegative patients with acquired immunodeficiency syndrome
Patients for whom the risk is less well established but sufficient to merit consideration	CMV-seronegative patients receiving tissue transplants (renal, heart, liver, lung) from CMV-seronegative donors CMV-seronegative patients who are potential candidates for bone marrow transplantation (allogeneic, autologous, or both) CMV-seronegative autologous bone marrow transplant recipients CMV-seronegative patients with evidence of infection with human immunodeficiency virus type 1 CMV-seronegative patients undergoing splenectomy
Patients for whom the risk is not established	CMV-seronegative recipients of bone marrow from CMV-seropositive donors CMV-seropositive recipients of bone marrow transplants Premature infants (<1200 g), regardless of the mother's CMV antibody status CMV-seropositive recipients of solid organ allografts (e.g., heart, kidney)

Adapted from Sayers MH, Anderson KC, Goodnough LT, et al. Reducing the risk for transfusion-transmitted cytomegalovirus. Ann Intern Med 1992; 116:55.

cells and FFP. Filtration, particularly with the recently developed leukodepletion filters capable of several-log removal of white blood cells, has become a method used to avoid CMV transmission.

Although the minimum number of infected white blood cells and the specific subtype of white cell (monocyte, granulocyte, lymphocyte) harboring sufficient virus to cause CMV disease remain unknown, early clinical studies using filtration or double spinning of platelet concentrate pools or pheresis platelets were promising in leukemic patients,[98] bone marrow transplant recipients,[99] and neonates.[27] Each of these studies used filters not available in the United States. Bowden and colleagues[100] used CMV-seronegative red blood cells and double-spun platelets versus unscreened blood and blood products in a randomized study of 77 seronegative bone marrow transplant recipients of either autologous or CMV-seronegative marrow allografts. They found no CMV infections in 35 evaluable patients who were studied until day 100 after transplantation, compared with 7 infections in the 30 control patients. They estimated a 1.5- to 2-log reduction of white blood cells in the platelets used. Donor exposures were significant, with a mean of 164 platelet concentrates and 25 units of red blood cells in the leukodepletion group and 165 platelet concentrates and 20 units of red blood cells in the control group.[100]

The investigators subsequently undertook a prospective randomized trial in CMV-seronegative marrow recipients to determine whether filtered, 3-log leukocyte-reduced red cells and platelets were as effective as CMV-seronegative blood products for the prevention of transfusion-transmitted CMV infections after marrow transplantation.[101] Five hundred two patients were randomized to receive either type of product and were monitored for the development of CMV infection or disease between days 21 and 100 after transplantation. CMV infection was defined as the identification of CMV (antigen-based or culture-positive) from weekly urine, throat, or blood cultures, and CMV disease was defined as the presence of CMV in tissue specimens or bronchoalveolar lavage with associated clinical symptoms. There was no significant difference between the randomized groups as far as the number of products received. In a primary analysis of the data (end point at day 100 after transplantation), the group documented a total of five CMV infections in the two population groups: two in the 249 recipients receiving seronegative products, and three in the 247 recipients receiving filtered blood products. This difference was not statistically significant. In a secondary analysis, five additional patients were documented who developed early CMV infection between the time of randomization and day 21 post-transplant: two in the seronegative arm and three in the leukoreduced arm. Their conclusion was that the rate of infection from leukoreduced and seronegative products was comparable (2.4% versus 1.4%), but the probability of developing CMV disease was higher in persons receiving the leukodepleted products (2.4% versus 0%, $p = .03$). This incidence was within a prestudy clinically defined rate of less than 5%, and the group concluded that filtration was an effective alternative to seronegative blood products.[101]

Another prospective study comparing the rate of CMV infection in 60 seronegative bone marrow transplant recipients originated in Europe. In this study, 23 allogeneic and 37 autologous bone marrow transplant recipients were given filtered (leukodepleted) blood products, and none developed positive CMV serology.[102]

A subsequent study in the pediatric population examined the practice of using "CMV-safe" (seronegative or leukoreduced) blood products in patients with newly diagnosed malignancies that might ultimately be treated by transplantation.[103] This study attempted to determine the rate of CMV infectivity in persons receiving seronegative and untested products. Seventy-six CMV-seronegative children with hematopoietic or solid malignancies were randomized to receive CMV-untested or CMV-seronegative red cells and platelets. The patients were followed monthly for 1 year after diagnosis or 6 months after their last transfusion. Serological tests for CMV-specific IgG and IgM were performed, as were throat swabs and urine collection for culture. Additional specimens were obtained from various sources when there was a clinical suspicion of CMV disease. There were no significant differences in the number or type of blood products received by the two groups. Children in the CMV-seronegative group and the untested group were followed for a median of 19 and 24 months, respectively. No case of transfusion-acquired CMV was documented. One factor that may have contributed to this observation was the relatively low number of donor exposures (a median of 7 and 9 red blood cell products and a median of 11 and 14 platelet products for the untested and seronegative groups, respectively). Moreover, donor characteristics may have been important in determining the infectivity of the blood product. In this population, there was a relatively low frequency of CMV IgM in the donors (0.9%), indicating a low incidence of acute or subacute infection in these persons.[103]

An additional study of note examined CMV-seropositive products for the presence of free infectious viral particles in the plasma. This study found that the plasma of seropositive blood and platelets contained CMV DNA by PCR, but it also contained viral particles that were able to infect tissue culture cells in vitro. The presence of these infective viral particles was associated with an increased length of storage and was attributed to the release of infective agents with the progressive breakdown of the white blood cells.[104]

Recent recommendations from the American Association of Blood Banks summarize the indications for using CMV-safe (seronegative or leukodepleted) blood. The use of CMV-safe products is not indicated for general hospital patients, persons receiving non–neutropenia-promoting chemotherapy, persons receiving corticosteroids, and full-term infants, regardless of CMV status. Those persons who are CMV seropositive and who are receiving chemotherapy that may promote neutropenia, who are pregnant, or who are infected with human immunodeficiency virus (HIV) do not warrant CMV-seronegative products, and the use of leukodepleted products is currently being evaluated. Persons of similar demographics who are CMV seronegative should receive CMV-safe products.[105]

Persons who are solid organ allograft recipients and who are CMV seronegative receiving CMV-seronegative allografts should receive CMV-safe products. CMV-seropositive transplant recipients or persons receiving allografts from CMV-positive individuals do not warrant CMV-safe products. In persons undergoing bone marrow transplantation, the CMV status of the donor is not considered, and CMV-safe blood is indicated except when the allograft recipient is CMV seropositive. Some institutions may opt to give CMV-seropositive recipients undergoing bone marrow transplantation leukoreduced products, and formal evaluation of this practice is under way. All low-birth-weight or premature infants (<1200 g) require CMV-safe blood products.[105]

Certain seronegative patient populations may require a compromise between acquisition of CMV and induction of tolerance. In renal transplantation, for example, transfusion of cells with a common HLA haplotype or shared HLA-B and HLA-DR antigens induces tolerance to donor antigens. In one study of 23 renal allograft recipients who received buffy coat–depleted red blood cells up to 36 hours after donation, CTLs were quantitated over time. The disappearance of T cell response against donor alloantigens occurred 4 to 16 weeks after transfusion and was long lasting.[106] The authors of this study theorize that under certain conditions, donor lymphocytes may home in on certain sites and induce low-grade mixed chimerism, resulting in T cell inactivation and improvement in graft survival. Another theory is that peripheral blood stem cells present in blood units might produce permanent chimerism, but this is probably less likely in the case of buffy coat–poor transfusion. If either transient or permanent chimerism is the cause of transplant tolerance, viable leukocytes with adequate HLA antigen presentation would be needed. Filtration of blood units would be disadvantageous in this setting.

Filtration is of particular interest, as it may provide the opportunity to remove dendritic antigen-presenting cells, monocytes, and activated T cells that might contribute to the immune perturbations accompanying transfusion. In particular, the removal of certain T cell subsets might prevent reactivation of CMV; at present, no data are available on this added potential benefit of filtration.

REFERENCES

1. Landini MP, Michelson S. Human cytomegalovirus proteins. Prac Med Virol 1988; 35:152.
1a. Emery VC, Griffiths PD. Molecular biology of cytomegalovirus. Int J Exp Pathol 1990; 71:905.
1b. Mach M, Stamminger R, Jahn G. Human cytomegalovirus: recent aspects from molecular biology. J Gen Virol 1989; 70:3117.
2. Lehner R, Stamminger J, Mach M. Comparative sequence analysis of human cytomegalovirus strains. J Clin Microbiol 1991; 29:2494.
3. Gerna G, Revello MC, Percivalle E, et al. Quantification of human cytomegalovirus viremia by using monoclonal antibodies to viral different proteins. J Clin Microbiol 1990; 28:2681.
4. Zaia J, Gallez-Hawkins G, Churchill MA. Comparative analysis of human cytomegalovirus sequence in multiple clinical isolates by using polymerase chain reaction and restriction length polymorphism assays. J Clin Microbiol 1990; 28:2602.
5. Tolpin MD, Stewart JA, Warren D, et al. Transfusion transmission of cytomegalovirus confirmed by restriction endonuclease analysis. J Pediatr 1985; 107:953.
6. Adler SP, Baggett J, Wilson M, et al. Molecular epidemiology of cytomegalovirus in a nursery: lack of evidence for nosocomial transmission. J Pediatr 1986; 108:117.
7. Jiwa NM, Van Gemert GW, Raap AK, Van de Rijke FM. Rapid detection of human cytomegalovirus DNA in peripheral blood leukocytes of viremic transplant patients by the polymerase chain reaction. Transplantation 1989; 48:72.
8. Chou S. Differentiation of cytomegalovirus strains by restriction analysis of DNA sequences amplified from clinical specimens. J Infect Dis 1990; 162:738.
9. Adler SP. Cytomegalovirus and child day care. N Engl J Med 1989; 321:1290.
10. Tegtmeier GE. Cytomegalovirus infection as a complication of blood transfusion. Semin Liver Dis 1986; 6:82.
11. Wilhelm JA, Matter L, Schopfer K. The risk of transmitting cytomegalovirus to patients receiving blood transfusion. J Infect Dis 1986; 154:169.
12. Preiksaitis JK, Brown L, McKenzie M. The risk of cytomegalovirus infection in seronegative transfusion recipients not receiving exogenous immunosuppression. J Infect Dis 1988; 157:523.
13. Landini MP, Rossier E, Schmitz H. Antibodies to human cytomegalovirus structural polypeptides during primary infection. J Virol Methods 1988; 22:309.
14. Landini MP, Mirolo G, Coppolecchia P, et al. Serum antibodies to individual cytomegaloviral structural polypeptides in renal transplant recipient during viral infection. Microbiol Immunol 1986; 30:693.
15. Rubin RH, Tolkoff-Rubin NE, Oliver D, et al. Multicenter seroepidemiologic study of the impact of cytomegalovirus infection on renal transplantation. Transplantation 1985; 40:243.
16. Grattan MT, Moreno-Cabral E, Starnes VA, et al. Cytomegalovirus infection is associated with cardiac allograft rejection and atherosclerosis. JAMA 1989; 261:3561.
17. Luban NLC, Williams AE, MacDonald MG, et al. Low incidence of acquired cytomegalovirus infections transfused with washed red blood cells. Am J Dis Child 1987; 141:416.
18. Hersman J, Meyers JD, Thomas ED, et al. The effect of granulocyte transfusions on the incidence of cytomegalovirus infection after allogeneic marrow transplantation. Ann Intern Med 1982; 96:149.
19. Adler SP. Data that suggests that FFP does not transmit CMV [Letter]. Transfusion 1988; 28:604.
20. Bowden RA, Sayers M. The risk of transmitting cytomegalovirus by fresh frozen plasma. Transfusion 1990; 30:762.
21. Bowden RA, Sayers M, Flounoy N, et al. Cytomegalovirus immune globulin and seronegative blood products to prevent primary cytomegalovirus infection after marrow transplantation. N Engl J Med 1986; 314:1006.
22. Winston DJ, Ho WG, Lin C, et al. Intravenous immune globulin for prevention of cytomegalovirus infection and interstitial pneumonia after bone marrow transplantation. Ann Intern Med 1987; 106:12.
23. Luban NLC, Williams AE, MacDonald MG, et al. Low incidence of acquired cytomegalovirus infections transfused with washed red blood cells. Am J Dis Child 1987; 141:416.
24. Brady MT, Milam JD, Anderson DC, et al. Use of deglycerolized red blood cells to prevent posttransfusion infection with cytomegalovirus in neonates. J Infect Dis 1984; 150:334.
25. Taylor BJ, Jacobs RF, Baker RL, et al. Frozen deglycerolized blood prevents transfusion acquired cytomegalovirus infection in neonates. Pediatr Infect Dis J 1986; 5:188.
26. Simon T, Johnson J, Koffler H, et al. Impact of previously frozen deglycerolized red blood cells in cytomegalovirus transmission to newborn infants. Plasma Ther Transfus Technol 1987; 8:51.
27. Gilbert GL, Hayes K, Hudson IL, James J. Prevention of transfusion-acquired cytomegalovirus infection in infants by blood filtration to remove leukocytes. Lancet 1989; 2:1228.
28. De Graan-Hentzen YCE, Gratama JW, Mudde GC, et al. Prevention of primary cytomegalovirus infection in patients with hematologic malignancy by intensive white cell depletion of blood products. Transfusion 1989; 29:757.
29. Dewitte T, Schattenberg A, Van Dijk BA, et al. Prevention of primary cytomegalovirus infection after allogeneic bone marrow transplantation by using leukocyte-poor random blood products from cytomegalovirus-unscreened blood bank donors. Transplantation 1990; 50:964.
30. Preiksaitis JK. Indications for the use of cytomegalovirus-seronegative blood products. Transfus Med Rev 1991; 5:1.

31. Schrier RD, Nelson JA, Oldstone MBA. Detection of human cytomegalovirus in peripheral blood lymphocytes in a natural infection. Science 1985; 230:1048.
32. Jackson JB, Orr HJ, McCullough JJ, Jordan MC. Failure to detect human cytomegalovirus DNA in IgM-seropositive blood donors by spot hybridization. J Infect Dis 1987; 56:1013.
33. Gerna G, Zipeto D, Parea M, et al. Monitoring of human cytomegalovirus infections and gancyclovir treatment in heart transplant recipients by determination of viremia, antigenemia and DNAemia. J Infect Dis 1991; 164:488.
34. Saltzman RL, Quirk MR, Jordan MC. Disseminated cytomegalovirus infection: molecular analysis of virus and leukocyte interaction in viremia. J Clin Invest 1988; 81:75.
35. Stagno S, Cloud GA. Changes in the epidemiology of cytomegalovirus. Adv Exp Med Biol 1990; 278:93.
36. Weir MR, Henry ML, Blackman M, et al. Incidence and morbidity of cytomegalovirus disease associated with a seronegative recipient receiving seropositive donor-specific transfusion and living-related donor transplantation. Transplantation 1988; 45:111.
37. Toorkey CB, Carrigan DR. Immunohistochemical detection of immediate early antigens of human cytomegalovirus in normal tissue. J Infect Dis 1989; 160:741.
38. deCates CR, Roberton NRC, Walker JR. Fatal acquired cytomegalovirus infection in a neonate with maternal antibody. J Infect 1988; 17:235.
39. Griffin MP, O'Shea M, Brazy JE, et al. Cytomegalovirus infection in a neonatal intensive care unit: subsequent morbidity and mortality of seropositive infants. J Perinatol 1990; 10:43.
40. Fowler KB, Pass RF. Sexually transmitted diseases in mothers of neonates with congenital cytomegalovirus infection. J Infect Dis 1991; 164:259.
41. Winston DJ, Pollard RB, Hu WG, et al. Cytomegalovirus immune plasma in bone marrow transplant recipients. Ann Intern Med 1982; 97:11.
42. Meyers JD, Leszczynski J, Zaia JA, et al. Prevention of cytomegalovirus infection by cytomegalovirus immune globulin after marrow transplantation. Ann Intern Med 1983; 98:442.
43. Condie RM, O'Reilly RJ. Prevention of cytomegalovirus infection by prophylaxis with an intravenous, hyperimmune mature, unmodified cytomegalovirus globulin. Am J Med 1984; 76(suppl 3A):134.
44. Kubanek B, Ernest P, Ostendorf P, et al. Preliminary data of a controlled trial of intravenous hyperimmune globulin in the prevention of cytomegalovirus in bone marrow transplant recipients. Transplant Proc 1985; 17:468.
45. Bowden RA, Fisher LD, Rogers K, et al. Cytomegalovirus (CMV)-specific intravenous immunoglobulin for the prevention of primary CMV infection and disease after marrow transplantation. J Infect Dis 1991; 164:483.
46. Sullivan KM, Kopecky KJ, Jocorn J, et al. Immunomodulatory and antimicrobial efficacy of intravenous immunoglobulin in bone marrow transplantation. N Engl J Med 1990; 323:705.
47. Britt WJ, Vugler L, Butfiloshi EJ, Stephens EB. Cell surface expression of human cytomegalovirus (HCMV) gp 55-116 (gB): use of HCMV recombinant vaccinia virus–infected cells in analysis of the human neutralizing antibody response. J Virol 1990; 64:1079.
48. Gönczöl E, de Taisne C, Hirka G, et al. High expression of human cytomegalovirus (HCMV) gB protein in cells infected with a vaccinia gB recombinant: the importance of the gB protein in HCMV immunity. Vaccine 1991; 9:631.
49. Marshall GS, Rabalais GP, Stout GG, Waldeyer SL. Antibodies to recombinant-derived glycoprotein B after natural human cytomegalovirus infection correlate with neutralizing activity. J Infect Dis 1992; 165:381.
50. Borysiewicz LK, Hickling JK, Graham S, et al. Human cytomegalovirus–specific cytotoxic T cells. J Exp Med 1988; 168:919.
51. Liu Y-N, Klaus A, Kari B, et al. The N-terminal 513 amino acids of the envelope glycoprotein gB of human cytomegalovirus stimulates both B and T cell immune responses in humans. J Virol 1991; 65:1644.
52. Aulitsky WE, Schulz TF, Tilg H. Human monoclonal antibodies neutralizing cytomegalovirus (CMV) for prophylaxis of CMV disease: report of a phase I trial in bone marrow transplant recipients. J Infect Dis 1991; 163:1344.
53. Utz V, Britt W, Vugler L, Mach M. Identification of a neutralizing epitope or the glycoprotein gp58 of human cytomegalovirus. J Virol 1989; 63:1995.
54. Chou S, Dennison KM. Analysis of interstrain variation in cytomegalovirus glycoprotein B sequences encoding neutralization-related epitopes. J Infect Dis 1991; 163:1229.
55. Plotkin SA, Starr SE, Friedman HM, et al. Effect of Towne live virus vaccine on cytomegalovirus disease after renal transplant. Ann Intern Med 1991; 114:525.
56. Quinnan GV, Ennis FA. Cell-mediated immunity in cytomegalovirus: a review. Comp Immunol Microbiol Infect Dis 1980; 3:283.
57. Quinnan GV, Kirmani N, Rook AN, et al. HLA-restricted T-lymphocyte cytotoxic responses correlate with recovery from cytomegalovirus infection in bone marrow transplant recipients. N Engl J Med 1982; 307:7.
58. Koszinowski UH. Molecular aspects of immune recognition of cytomegalovirus. Transplant Proc 1991; 23:70.
59. Jonjic S, Mutter W, Weiland F, et al. Site-restricted persistent cytomegalovirus infection after selective long-term depletion of $CD4^+$ T lymphocytes. J Exp Med 1989; 169:1199.
60. Pasternack MS, Medearis DN, Rubin RH. Cell-mediated immunity in experimental cytomegalovirus infections: a perspective. Rev Infect Dis 1990; 12:3720.
61. Yachie A, Tosato G, Straus SE, Blaese RM. Immunostimulation by cytomegalovirus (CMV): helper T cell–dependent activation of immunoglobulin production in vitro by lymphocytes from CMV immune donors. J Immunol 1985; 135:1395.
62. Gratama JW, Kluin-Nelemans HC, Langelaar RA, et al. Flow cytometric and morphologic studies of $HNK1^+$ (Leu 7^+) lymphocytes in relation to cytomegalovirus carrier status. Clin Exp Immunol 1988; 74:190.
63. Gratama JW, Kardol M, Naipal AMIH, et al. The influence of cytomegalovirus carrier status on lymphocyte subsets and natural immunity. Clin Exp Immunol 1987; 68:16.
64. Gratama JW, Langelaar RA, Oosterveer MAP, et al. Phenotypic study of $CD4^+$ and $CD8^+$ lymphocyte subsets in relation to cytomegalovirus carrier status and its correlation with pokeweed mitogen–induced B lymphocyte differentiation. Clin Exp Immunol 1989; 77:245.
65. Riddell SR, Rabin M, Geballe AP, et al. Class I MHC–restricted cytotoxic T lymphocyte recognition of cells infected with human cytomegalovirus does not require endogenous viral gene expression. J Immunol 1991; 146:2795.
66. Reussner P, Riddell SR, Meyers JD, Greenberg DD. Cytotoxic T-lymphocyte response to cytomegalovirus after human allogeneic bone marrow transplantation: pattern of recovery and correlation with cytomegalovirus infection and disease. Blood 1991; 78:1373.
67. Greenberg P, Goodrich J, Riddell S. Adoptive immunotherapy to human cytomegalovirus infection: potential role in protection from disease progression. Transplant Proc 1991; 23:97.
68. Yang WC, Carreno M, Esquenazi V, et al. Evidence that antibodies to cytomegalovirus and T cell receptor (TCR)/CD3 complex may have common ligands. Transplantation 1991; 51:490.
69. Laubscher A, Bluestein HG, Spector SA, Zvaifler NJ. Generation of human cytomegalovirus–specific cytotoxic T lymphocytes in short term culture. J Immunol Methods 1988; 110:69.
70. Bowden RA, Dobbs S, Amos D, Meyer JD. Comparison of interleukin 2 and gamma interferon production by peripheral blood mononuclear cells in response to cytomegalovirus after marrow transplantation. Transplantation 1990; 50:38.
71. Morse SS, Morahan PS. Activated macrophages mediate interferon-independent inhibition of herpes simplex virus. Cell Immunol 1981; 58:72.
72. Manor E, Sarov I. Inhibition of CMV replication in human fibroblasts by human monocyte–derived macrophages: implication for CMV persistent infection. Microb Pathog 1988; 5:97.
73. Beutler B, Krochen N, Milsark LW, et al. Control of cachectin (tumor necrosis factor) synthesis: mechanism of endotoxin resistance. Science 1986; 232:977.
74. Moreb J, Zucali JR, Rueth S. The effects of tumor necrosis factor on early human hematopoietic progenitor cells treated with 4-hydroperoxycyclophosphamide. Blood 1990; 76:681.
75. Holler E, Kolb HJ, Möller A, et al. Increased serum levels of tumor necrosis factor 2 precedes major complications of bone marrow transplantation. Blood 1990; 75:1011.
76. Preksaitis JK, Janowski-Wieczorek A. Cytomegalovirus (CMV) rep-

lication in human long term marrow cultures (LT MC): effect on myeloid (CFU-GM) and erythroid (BFU-E) progenitor cells. 2nd International Cytomegalovirus Workshop, USCD Abstract 107, 1989.
77. Apperly JF, Dowding C, Hibbin J, et al. The effect of cytomegalovirus on hemopoiesis: in vitro evidence for selective infection of marrow stromal cells. Exp Hematol 1989; 17:38.
78. Duncombe AS, Meager A, Prentice HG, et al. γ-Interferon and tumor necrosis factor production after bone marrow transplantation is augmented by exposure to marrow fibroblasts infected with cytomegalovirus. Blood 1990; 76:1046.
79. Broxmeyer HE, Williams DE, Lu L, et al. The suppressive influence of human tumor necrosis factors on bone marrow hematopoietic progenitor cells from normal donors and patients with leukemia: synergism of tumor necrosis factor and interferon gamma. J Immunol 1986; 136:4487.
80. Murase T, Hotta T, Saito H, Ohno R. Effect of recombinant human tumor necrosis factor on colony growth of human leukemia progenitor cells and normal hematopoietic progenitor cells. Blood 1987; 69:467.
81. MacDonald D, Adams JA, McCarthy D, Barrett AJ. Interleukin 2 inhibits growth of fibroblasts derived from human bone marrow. Acta Haematol 1990; 83:26.
82. Van Tiel FH, Rasmussen L, Merigan TC. Cytomegalovirus-specific cell-mediated immune responses in heart and heart-lung transplant recipients are not predictive for the occurrence of symptomatic CMV disease or tissue rejection. J Interferon Res 1991; 11:221.
83. McCullough J, Yunis EJ, Benson SJ, Quie PG. Effect of blood bank storage on leucocyte function. Lancet 1969; 1:1333.
84. Sherman ME, Dzik WH. Stability of antigens in leukocytes in banked platelet concentrates: decline in HLA-DR antigen expression and mixed lymphocyte culture stimulating capacity following storage. Blood 1988; 72:867.
85. Paloheimo JA, von Essen R, Klemola JE, et al. Subclinical cytomegalovirus infections and cytomegalovirus mononucleosis after open heart surgery. Am J Cardiol 1968; 22:624.
86. Adler SP, McVoy MM. Cytomegalovirus infections in seropositive patients after transfusion. Transfusion 1989; 29:667.
87. Light JA, Metz S, Oddenino K, et al. Donor-specific transfusion with diminished sensitization. Transplantation 1982; 34:322.
88. Khan A, Wakasugi K, Hill N, et al. Changes in the immunocompetence and surface markers of lymphocytes in stored blood. Exp Hematol 1977; 5:8.
89. Dobryski W, Thibodeau S, Truitt RL, et al. Third-party–mediated graft rejection and graft-versus-host disease after T-cell depleted bone marrow transplantation, as demonstrated by hypervariable probes and HLA-DR polymorphism. Blood 1989; 74:2285.
90. Reusser P, Fisher LD, Buckner CD, et al. Cytomegalovirus infection after autologous bone marrow transplantation: occurrence of cytomegalovirus disease and effect on engraftment. Blood 1990; 75:1888.
91. Cray C, Levy BB. The presence of infectious virus but not conventional antigen can exacerbate graft versus host reactions. Scand J Immunol 1990; 32:177.
92. Yang H, Welsh RA. Induction of alloreactive cytotoxic T cells by acute virus infection of mice. J Immunol 1986; 136:1186.
93. Bean MA, Storb R, Graham T, et al. Prevention of transfusion induced sensitization to minor histocompatibility antigens in DLA-identical canine marrow grafts by gamma irradiation of marrow donor blood. Transplantation 1991; 52:956.
94. Sayers MH, Anderson KC, Goodnough LT, et al. Reducing the risk for transfusion-transmitted cytomegalovirus. Ann Intern Med 1992; 116:55.
95. Hillyer CD, Snydman DR, Berkman EM. Risk of cytomegalovirus infection in solid organ and bone marrow transplant recipients: transfusion of blood products. Transfusion 1990; 30:659.
96. Luban NLC, Sacher RA. Transfusion-transmitted cytomegalovirus and Epstein-Barr diseases. *In* Rossi E, Simon TL, Moss GW (eds): Principles of Transfusion Medicine. Baltimore: Williams & Wilkins, 1991, pp 573–583.
97. Lamberson HV, McMillan JA, Weiner LB, et al. Prevention of transfusion-associated cytomegalovirus (CMV) infection in neonates by screening donors for IgM to CMV. J Infect Dis 1988; 157:820.
98. De Graan-Hentzen YCE, Gratama JW, Mudde GL, et al. Prevention of primary cytomegalovirus infection during induction treatment of acute leukemia using at random leukocyte poor blood products. Br J Haematol 1987; 66:421.
99. Verdonck LF, De Graan-Hentzen YC, Dekker AW, et al. Cytomegalovirus seronegative platelets and leukocyte poor red blood cells can prevent primary cytomegalovirus infection after bone marrow transplantation. Bone Marrow Transplant 1987; 2:73.
100. Bowden RA, Slichter SJ, Sayers MH, et al. Use of leukocyte-depleted platelets and cytomegalovirus seronegative red blood cells for prevention of primary cytomegalovirus infection after marrow transplant. Blood 1991; 78:246.
101. Bowden RA, Slichter SJ, Sayers MH, et al: A comparison of filtered leukocyte reduced and cytomegalovirus (CMV) seronegative blood products for the prevention of transfusion-associated CMV infection after marrow transplant. Blood 1995; 86:3598.
102. van Prooijen HC, Visser JJ, van Oostendorp WR, et al. Prevention of primary transfusion-associated cytomegalovirus infection in bone marrow transplant recipients by the removal of white cells from blood components with high-affinity filters. Br J Haematol 1994; 87:144.
103. Preiksaitis JK, Sesai S, Vaudry W, et al. Transfusion and community-acquired cytomegalovirus infection in children with malignant disease: a prospective study. Transfusion 1997; 37:941.
104. James DJ, Sikotra S, Sivakumaran M, et al. The presence of free infectious cytomegalovirus (CMV) in the plasma of donated CMV-seropositive blood and platelets. Transfus Med 1997; 7:123.
105. American Association of Blood Banks Association Bulletin #97-2: leukocyte reduction for the prevention of transfusion-transmitted cytomegalovirus (TT-CMV). AABB Press 1997; 2:1.
106. van Twuyver E, Mooijaart RJD, ten Berge IJM, et al. Pretransplantation blood transfusion revisited. N Engl J Med 1991; 325:1210.

CHAPTER 35

Human Immunodeficiency Viruses

Ricardo S. Diaz
Michael P. Busch

The human immunodeficiency virus (HIV) has influenced virtually every aspect of clinical medicine and biomedical research. Few fields have been affected more than transfusion medicine. It is estimated that during late 1982 and early 1983, more than 1% of all transfusions in some metropolitan regions in the United States were contaminated with HIV type 1 (HIV-1).[1] During this same period, more than 50% of hemophiliacs acquired HIV infections.[2] Even though the blood supply in developed countries is now extremely safe, public concern over HIV and transfusion continues.

Although the tragedy of the transfusion-associated acquired immunodeficiency syndrome (AIDS) epidemic has left a cloud over the field, the response of transfusion medicine physicians and scientists, with the collaboration of basic science colleagues, has been impressive and relentless. Early studies of hemophiliacs and of linked blood donors and recipients involved in transfusion-associated AIDS cases were instrumental in pointing to the infectious etiology of the syndrome,[3] as well as in the subsequent validation of HIV as the primary etiological agent and the development of serological screening and confirmatory assays.[4, 5] These widely recognized accomplishments actually represent only a small element in a continually evolving series of contributions to HIV research by investigators focused on the transfusion setting.

In this chapter, we review those areas in which the combined efforts of blood bankers and their colleagues in basic science, epidemiology, and public health have contributed to progress in understanding HIV virology and pathogenesis and combating HIV infection and disease. We first establish a framework for this discussion by presenting an overview of the virology of HIV infection, emphasizing the dynamic interplay of viral, cellular, and immunological factors in determining the course of infection and disease. We then discuss several aspects of HIV transmission and pathogenesis in which studies of HIV infection in the context of linked donor-recipient clusters have yielded powerful insight into the infectious process.

STRUCTURE AND LIFE CYCLE OF HIV

HIV is a member of the lentivirus subfamily of retroviruses,[6] of which visna virus (which causes demyelinating encephalomyelitis and interstitial pneumonia in sheep) is the prototype. Other, more recently discovered members of this group, such as simian immunodeficiency virus (SIV) and feline immunodeficiency virus (FIV), cause AIDS-like illnesses in specific animal hosts and provide useful animal models for the in vivo study of AIDS.[7, 8] Lentiviruses differ from other retroviruses in that, in addition to carrying genes for the enzyme reverse transcriptase *(pol)* and the structural core *(gag)* and envelope proteins *(env)*, they carry genes for at least six other proteins *(tat, rev, nef, vpu, vif,* and *vpr)*. Some of these genes are thought to contribute to the regulation of HIV infection.

Two copies of the 9-kb, single-stranded RNA genome are contained in each icosahedral virion (Fig. 35–1).[9] The RNA molecules in the virions are associated with the *pol* gene–encoded enzymes reverse transcriptase, integrase, and protease. The viral core structure, consisting of p24, p17, p9, and p7 proteins, surrounds the nucleic acid molecules and is in turn encapsulated by a lipid-containing envelope containing the viral glycoproteins gp120 (external) and gp41 (transmembrane). The viral envelope is derived from the host cell membrane and contains many host proteins, including class I and class II major histocompatibility molecules.

Many of the details of the intracellular life cycle of HIV (see Fig. 35–1) have been elucidated by the study of infection of activated peripheral blood mononuclear cells (PBMCs) and various immortalized T cell lines in tissue culture.[6, 9–11] Adsorption of the virus to a cell occurs through a specific interaction between the viral gp120 envelope protein and the CD4 protein present on the cell surface of helper T cells. Several critical co-receptors (CCR5, CCR2, CXCR4) have been identified that are important determinants of virus susceptibility and disease progression. A viral gp41-mediated fusion process probably introduces the viral core into the cell's cytoplasm. Reverse transcription of the RNA viral genome into a double-stranded DNA molecule occurs in the cytoplasm and is accomplished by virion-associated reverse transcriptase. Short terminal repeats (STRs) in the RNA molecule are critical for this process and are converted into long terminal repeats (LTRs) in the DNA product. It is this reverse transcriptase step that is inhibited by the antiviral drug zidovudine (AZT). Viral DNA is transported into the nucleus of the host cell, where it is integrated into cellular DNA by means of virion-associated integrase activity. Early viral messenger RNAs (mRNAs) are doubly spliced 2-kb transcripts encoding regulatory genes *tat,*

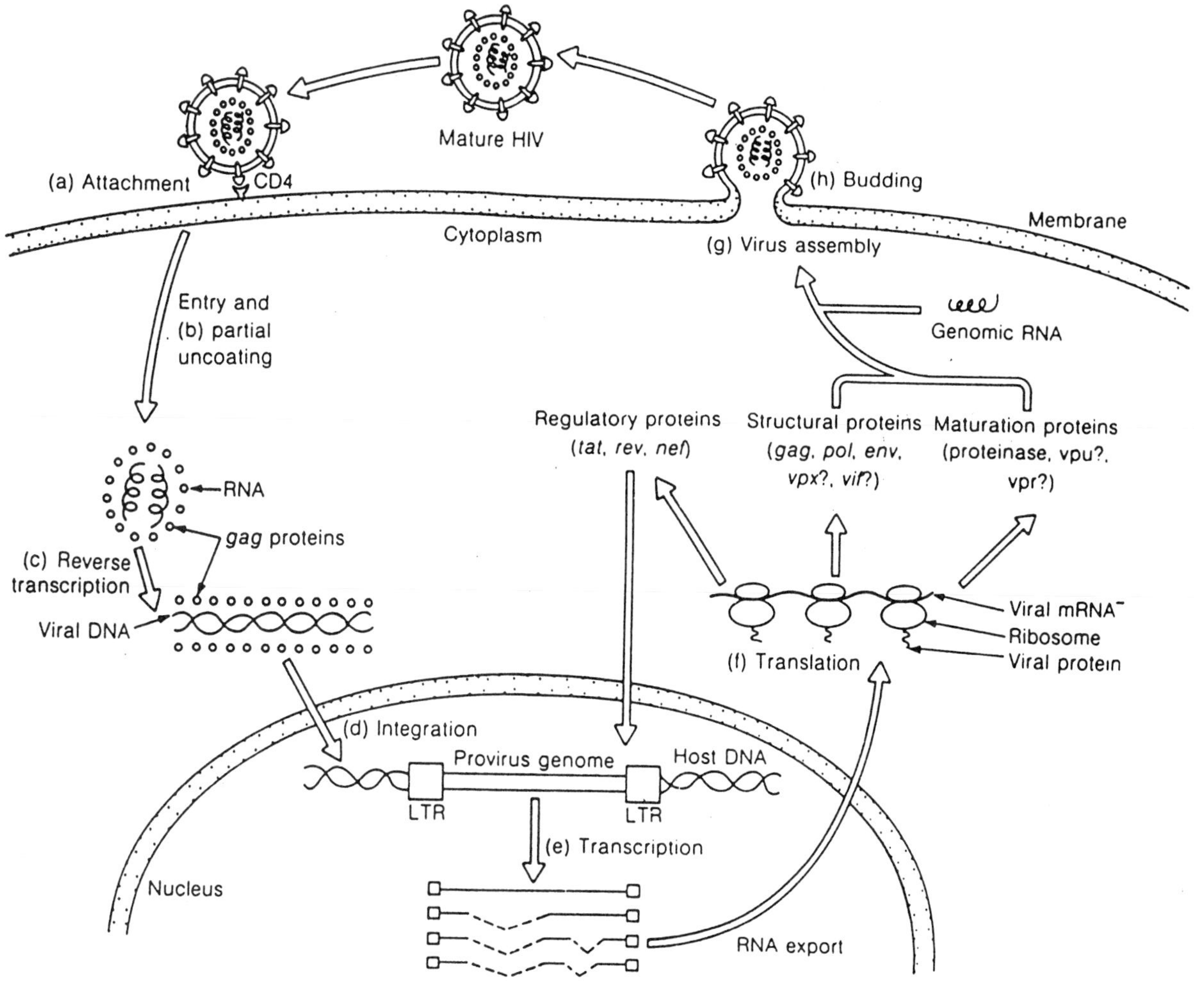

Figure 35–1. Replication cycle of human immunodeficiency virus type 1 (HIV-1). After attachment of virus particles to the CD4 and secondary receptor molecules, virus enters the cell by a pH-dependent mechanism and/or endocytosis (a). The outer lipid envelope of the virus is removed when the particle undergoes fusion with cytoplasmic vacuoles (b). The core particle that remains is the site for reverse transcription of the virion RNA into DNA (c). After translocation into the nucleus, integration into the DNA of the cell occurs (d). The integrated provirus genome is transcribed by cellular RNA polymerase II (e). Translation of viral messenger RNA (mRNA) produces regulatory proteins, which stimulate synthesis of maturation proteins and the structural proteins of the virion (f). Accumulation of structural proteins in the cell membrane permits the assembly of virus particles (g). Maturation, and release from the cell by budding (h). LTR, long terminal repeat. (From Cann AJ, Karn J. Molecular biology of HIV: new insights into the virus life-cycle. AIDS 1989; 3[suppl 1]:S19.)

nef, and *rev*. The *tat* gene product transactivates (enhances) viral transcription by binding to a specific regulatory site in the LTR. The resulting increase in *rev* gene transcription plays a key role in translation of virion proteins. *Rev* promotes the cytoplasmic accumulation of singly spliced *env* mRNA and full-length unspliced *gag/pol* mRNA, which also serves as genomic RNA for progeny virions. The polyprotein products of these mRNAs are cleaved into virion structural proteins (core and envelope) by both cellular and HIV proteases and associate with viral RNA genomes. Progeny virions are released from infected cells by a budding process from the cell surface in which they acquire their lipid envelopes.

TIME COURSE OF PRIMARY HIV INFECTION

An understanding of the time course of viremia and antibody seroconversion after initial HIV infection is extremely important for ensuring the use of optimal assays to guard the blood supply, as well as for developing testing recommendations for recently exposed or infected persons. Since the mid-1980s, studies from the blood bank setting have yielded important insights into the viral dynamics and the so-called window periods from exposure to antibody seroconversion.[12] One of the major contributions came from "lookback" investigations of recipients of blood from seroconverting donors.[13] Because of the enormous scope of blood donor screening (>14 million whole blood donations are tested each year in the United States), a large number of cases have been identified in which a donor who previously tested negative subsequently seroconverted. Determining the HIV status of the recipients of pre-seroconversion transfusions from these donors gives the most accurate understanding of the duration of the infectious or viremic pre-seroconversion window period. Useful data have also been generated from extensive studies of seroconverting plasma donor panels. These panels consist of series of plasmapheresis components (each 200 to 500 mL in volume) collected approximately twice weekly from paid plasma donors who were subsequently found to have seroconverted to anti-HIV. When a seroconverting donor is detected, his or her prior donations that had been held in frozen quarantine are retrieved and aliquoted into seroconversion panels. Characterizing these panels by using HIV RNA, p24 antigen, and various antibody assays has demonstrated the pattern of evolution of virological and immunological markers and the sensitivity of improved screening assays.

The data coming from these investigations, plus data generated from studies of patients with primary HIV infection and of SIV animal models, suggest the following sequence of events during primary HIV infection (Fig. 35–2).[12] After a person is first infected with HIV, there is a variable period (usually 1 to 2 weeks, but occasionally up to 6 months) of viral replication in mucosal and regional lymphoid tissue. During this early tissue phase of replication, the peripheral blood tests negative for virus, and a blood donation is unlikely to be infectious. This is followed by massive hematogenous dissemination of the virus, evidenced by a subsequent rapid increase in plasma viremia first detected by HIV RNA analysis in plasma, followed about 5 days later by detectable levels of p24 antigen. RNA and p24 antigen levels peak, on average, 20 to 30 days after exposure as the immune response matures. Infected PBMCs are detectable by DNA polymerase chain reaction (PCR) approximately 5 days later than free virus and remain present at stable low levels through complete seroconversion. Anti-HIV appears between days 20 and 30 post viremia, with an early immunoglobulin M (IgM) spike followed by progressive development of immunoglobulin G (IgG) over several months.

VIRAL REPLICATION DYNAMICS

Quantitative analysis of viral RNA dynamics from plasma donor seroconversion panels indicates a median viral doubling time before antibody seroconversion of 0.9 day

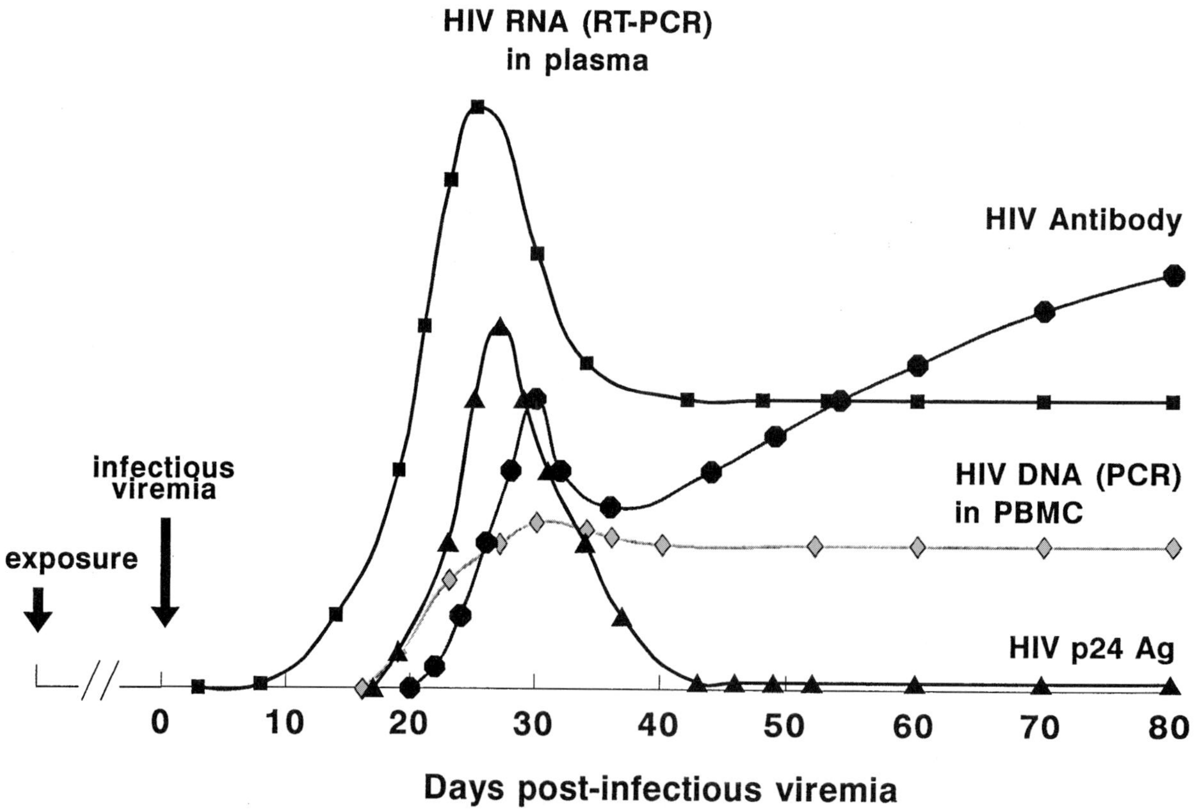

Figure 35–2. Approximate sequence and time course of virological and serological events during primary human immunodeficiency virus (HIV) infection. Following exposure, there is a variable period (usually 1 to 2 weeks, but occasionally up to 6 months) of viral replication in mucosal and lymphoid tissue draining the inoculation site, followed by hematogenous dissemination consistent with an infectious blood donation (day 0 in figure). The subsequent rapid increase in plasma viremia is first detectable by reverse transcriptase polymerase chain reaction (RT-PCR) for HIV RNA in plasma *(squares)* on approximately day 10 and by p24 antigen (Ag) assays *(triangles)* on day 15, with RNA and p24 Ag levels peaking between days 20 and 30. Infected (DNA PCR-positive) peripheral blood mononuclear cells (PBMCs) *(diamonds)* are detected later than free virus at approximately day 15 and remain present at stable, low levels through complete seroconversion. HIV antibody *(circles)* appears between days 20 and 30 post viremia, with an early immunoglobulin M spike followed by progressive development of immunoglobulin G over several months. Seroconversion is associated with clearance of viremia to set-points that correlate with long-term outcome of disease, as well as with probability of secondary transmission of virus. (From Busch MP, Satten GA. Time course of viremia and antibody seroconversion following human immunodeficiency virus exposure. Am J Med 1997; 102[suppl 5B]:117.)

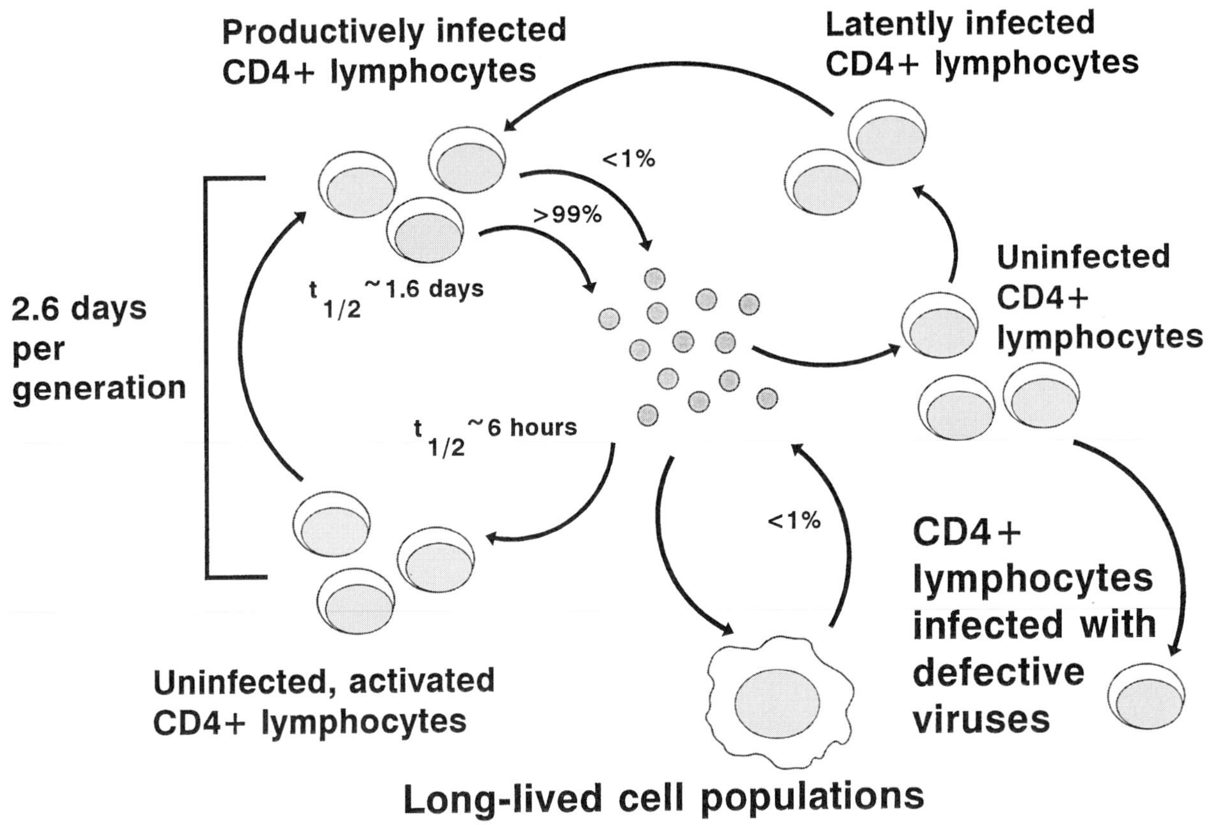

Figure 35–3. Schematic summary of the dynamics of human immunodeficiency virus type 1 infection in vivo. Shown in the center is the cell-free virion population that is sampled when viral load in plasma is measured. $t_{1/2}$, half-life. (From Perelson AS, Neumann AU, Markowitz M, et al. HIV-1 dynamics in vivo: virion clearance rate, infected cell lifespan, and viral generation time. Science 1996; 271:1582. Copyright 1996 by the American Association for the Advancement of Science.)

(range 0.53 to 4 days). This finding indicates that once virus appears in the blood stream, the rate of replication and dissemination is rapid. Viral RNA levels fall 2 to 3 log units during seroconversion and reach steady-state levels by approximately 30 to 50 days.

Studies have shown that during the seemingly quiescent period after the primary infection with HIV, which often lasts 8 to 12 years, the body is producing and eliminating almost 10 billion virions a day. At the same time, about 100 million CD4 T cells are being destroyed daily.[14, 15] The half-life ($t_{1/2}$) of the virus is approximately 6 hours[16] (Fig. 35–3). The $t_{1/2}$ of productively infected CD4 cells is estimated at 1.6 days. There are also long-lived infected mononuclear cells ($t_{1/2}$ of 1 to 4 weeks) and latently infected lymphocytes that are minor sources of cell-free virus but important reservoirs for viral recurrence after antiviral treatment.

Data also indicate that the virion (but not the provirus) is highly associated with platelets during all stages of infection.[17] The high capacity of platelets to adsorb virus may have important implications. On the one hand, platelet binding of HIV could mediate viral clearance by the reticuloendothelial (RE) system. On the other hand, platelets may facilitate viral dissemination and persistence, possibly sheltering the virus from neutralizing antibody or expanding viral tropism by infecting RE cells in spleen, liver, brain, and elsewhere.

The replication rate, as reflected in steady-state viral load levels, is correlated with disease progression, as well as with probability of secondary transmission of the virus. Viral load can be measured in clinical practice with highly sensitive quantitative assays based on the PCR, branched DNA, nucleic acid sequence-based amplification, or transcription-mediated amplification assays. These assays have also been of great value in predicting progression to AIDS and determining the relative effectiveness of antiretroviral therapies, and for the short-term evaluation of viral dynamics in both research and clinical practice. The level of viremia is also an important determinant of viral transmission. Studies of infected transfusion recipients suggest that there is a threshold level of viral load below which heterosexual transmission is unlikely to occur.[18–20] The level of viremia in a donor at the time of donation—or, more precisely, in a component at the time of transfusion—is the primary factor influencing the probability of infection.[21] A similar relationship between virus titer and HIV-1 transmission has been proposed for perinatal[22] and needlestick exposures.[23, 24] Low virus burden has also been posited as an explanation for the lower transmission rate of HIV-2 compared with HIV-1.[25, 26]

VIRAL DIVERSITY

HIV is extraordinary in its genetic mutability, which ranges from within-individual (quasi-species) diversity to population-level diversity (subtypes and groups). The mechanisms thought to contribute to HIV genetic diversity include point mutations, hypermutation, insertions and deletions, and intergenic recombination. Mutations during reverse transcription have been demonstrated to occur in vitro[27] and in vivo,[28, 29] with an error rate estimated at 5 to 10 misincorporations per HIV genome per replication cycle.[27, 30, 31] This high rate is the consequence of the negligible proofreading exonuclease activity of the reverse transcriptase. Hypermutation is defined as the process by which individual proviruses acquire several mutations in a single replication cycle. Hypermutation may underlie the preponderance of G to A substitutions commonly observed in HIV and SIV. Moreover, G to A substitutions account for 90% of all substitutions in the HIV genome (dislocation mutagenesis).[32] Insertions and deletions, usually involving multiples of three nucleotides, have been observed in virtually every study of HIV quasi-species. They predominate in the envelope V5 region. HIV-1 intergenic recombination has been documented in cell culture, where experimental manipulation can achieve dual infection by two defined parental strains differing at linked genetic loci.[32–34]

Recombination between different HIV-1 strains has also been demonstrated to occur in vivo by analysis of an unusual case of an infant concurrently transfused with two HIV-1–seropositive units from two different donors. Through extensive sequence analysis of viruses from the donors and the recipient, the first unequivocal evidence of dual infection was documented, as well as recombination between the two infecting HIV-1 strains.[35] Although this transfusion case was unusual, dual infection may be occurring relatively often among people engaging in frequent high-risk activities. Indeed, a case of alleged multiple infection as a result of homosexual activity[36] and reports of recombinants between different subtypes of HIV-1[37] and HIV-2[38] provide additional evidence that dual infection and recombination may be relatively frequent. Several instances of recombination between members of the same quasi-species have also been reported.[39–42] Therefore, it is likely that recombination within and between strains may constitute a significant factor in the generation of HIV-1 diversity.

QUASI-SPECIES DIVERSITY

As noted earlier, the genetic diversification of HIV-1 is occurring over time within each infected person. Of course, because the current pandemic constitutes the sum of infected persons, HIV-1 has been diversifying over time and space at the level of the entire viral species as well. First we focus on the characteristics and ramifications of diversity at the individual level, and then move to the pandemic level.

Virological studies of primary infections indicate that HIV-1 in acute seroconverters is relatively homogeneous in both sequence and phenotype (typically macrophage-tropic and non–syncytium-inducing [NSI]). Of note, studies of linked epidemiological clusters indicate that the transmitted strain is homogeneous, even though the corresponding source of infection (transmitter) harbors a quasi-species mixture of genotypes and/or phenotypes.[36, 43] Analyses of HIV-1 sequences in seroconverters show a stronger pressure to conserve the *env* gene than other viral core genes, such as *gag*.[36, 43] Although it is not yet clear what accounts for this sequence "bottleneck" during transmission, several hypotheses have been proposed. First, the homogeneity found in the recipient of the infection might reflect the restricted sequence diversity present in the inoculum (e.g., semen, vaginal fluid) of the transmitter. The fact that the transmitted virus sometimes represents only a minor variant in the blood of the transmitter argues against this explanation, however.[36] Another model, termed selective transmission, proposes that some HIV-1 variants have an advantage in penetrating the mucosal barrier of the new host. This would explain not only the sequence homogeneity but also the finding that HIV-1 isolated during the primary infection is predominantly macrophage-tropic and NSI; that is, macrophages or related antigen-processing cells in the submucosal space may allow NSI viruses that are most efficient at replicating in these cells to penetrate. (Some new insights related to the interaction between the virus and cell co-receptors are described later.) Third, it is proposed that multiple HIV-1 variants penetrate the new host, but one outcompetes other variants to become the dominant population because of its biological growth characteristics (selective amplification). This explanation is supported by the homogeneity found in seroconverting hemophiliacs who were presumably inoculated parenterally with multiple HIV-1 variants.[43] A fourth possible explanation for bottlenecking is that multiple variants are transmitted but only one strain predominates early after seroconversion. Other transmitted strains, present at low copy numbers at the time of contagion, eventually emerge at detectable levels later when immune pressures suppress the abundant early replicating strains.[44] This model would explain why a health care worker who was accidentally infected with a clone of HIV-1 showed an unusual homogeneity in the genotypes found up to 5 years after the primary infection.[45]

The bottleneck at transmission happens irrespective of the route of transmission (sexual, maternal-fetal, or parenteral).[46, 47] We described a case in which a person was exposed to two different HIV-1 quasi-species by transfusion from two different blood donors and yet was infected by the quasi-species of only one of the donors.[48] This case exemplifies a previously unreported instance of a transmission bottleneck selecting for specific genomes from different inoculated HIV quasi-species.

In general, more virulent strains (i.e., those with cytopathic properties and high replication rates) tend to appear late in the asymptomatic period (see the review by Nowak and colleagues[49]). Thus, HIV-1 isolates from asymptomatic carriers tend to grow slowly in vitro and yield low titers of p24 antigen and reverse transcriptase activity, whereas isolates from patients with clinical AIDS grow rapidly, induce multinucleated cell syncytia more frequently, and show rapid kinetics of p24 antigen expression and reverse transcriptase activity.[49] There is substantial evidence, particularly from studies of symptomatic patients, that the virus changes to "escape" immune antiviral responses in the host. In general, serum from an individual is not able to neutralize the replicating strain present in the person at that time as effectively as it neutralizes previous autologous strains or strains from other people.[50–52] The generation of viruses that have "escaped" neutralization by serum antibodies has been demonstrated by in vitro studies in which HIV-1 strains cultured in the presence of neutralizing monoclonal antibodies mutate to become resistant to neutralization.[53–55] A few nucleotide substitutions in the HIV-1 genome are enough to confer resistance to neutralization by antibodies[56, 57] or resistance to antiretroviral drugs.[58] In vivo studies show that after the decline of V3-specific antibodies, there is a simultaneous increase in genomic RNA levels in plasma, with the emergence of a new variant with major genomic changes, forming a new homogeneous population of sequences.[57] We described an extensive analysis of a cluster of infected donors and recipients that shows that when mixed populations of virus are present in an infected person, viral motifs can be fixed on escape recombinant viruses, depending on the selective advantage due to their ability to elicit host selective (immune) pressure.[59] Thus, recombination and natural selection acting together can greatly expand the adaptive potential of HIV-1.

Analyses of the rates of diversity within the *env* genes of HIV-1 between infected persons within a point-source cluster suggest that they may be diverging at rates up to 1% per year.[60–62] This intrapatient evolution contributes to the existence at the population level of many closely related but distinguishable "swarms" of HIV variants.[63] The average intrapatient *env* gene distance from randomly selected HIV-1–positive patients in the United States between 1983 and 1985 was 1% to 4%, while the interpatient distance ranged from 4% to 10%. The average intrapatient *env* distance for U.S. samples reached 6.5% between 1990 and 1993, while the interpatient variation remained between 4% and 10%. The rates of intracluster genetic variation are always between the intra- and interpatient variation rates.[64] Furthermore, insights on viral evolution coming from donor-recipient sets show that the evolution of the same viral strain in different hosts is individual-specific, presumably reflecting distinct immune pressures in the different hosts.[64] As HIV-1 evolves in a person, there is a preponderance and accumulation of nonsynonymous (resulting in a changed amino acid) rather than synonymous (no change in amino acid) substitutions in immunodominant regions such as *env* over time.[62] This strongly argues in favor of a dominant role for positive immune selection for amino acid change in governing the pattern and process of HIV-1 evolution in vivo, and argues against hypotheses of neutral or mutation-driven evolution or completely chance events.

SUBTYPE DIVERSITY

At a level beyond this intraindividual genetic variation, HIV continues to evolve over time and space in the human population. HIV-1 and HIV-2 are at the extremes of this diversity. Within the HIV-1 family, analyses of *gag* and *env* genes from genomes sampled at different times in the epidemic and from different regions of the world reveal that HIV-1 has evolved into two major groups termed M and O.[65, 66] At least nine distinct subtypes, or clades, that belong to group M are now circulating in the centers of the AIDS pandemic. It is conceivable that these distinct forms (in both *gag* and *env* sequences) diverged from a single common ancestor as recently as the 1950s. In 1998, viral sequences from a 1959 African plasma sample were characterized.[67] This is probably the oldest known HIV infection, and a phylogenetic analysis indicates that this viral sequence is probably the ancestor of subtypes B and D, suggesting that all the M group viruses may have evolved from a single introduction into the African population not long before 1959. The HIV-2 family is similarly subdivided into at least six subtypes.[38] The amino acid composition of each HIV-1 clade differs from that of the others by at least 20% in the *env* region and 15% in the *gag* region.[65] Their interrelationship has been portrayed by star-shaped phylogenetic trees, which are indicative of exponentially growing viral populations, further indicating the explosive nature of the AIDS pandemic (Fig. 35–4).

The HIV-1 clades are widely distributed geographi-

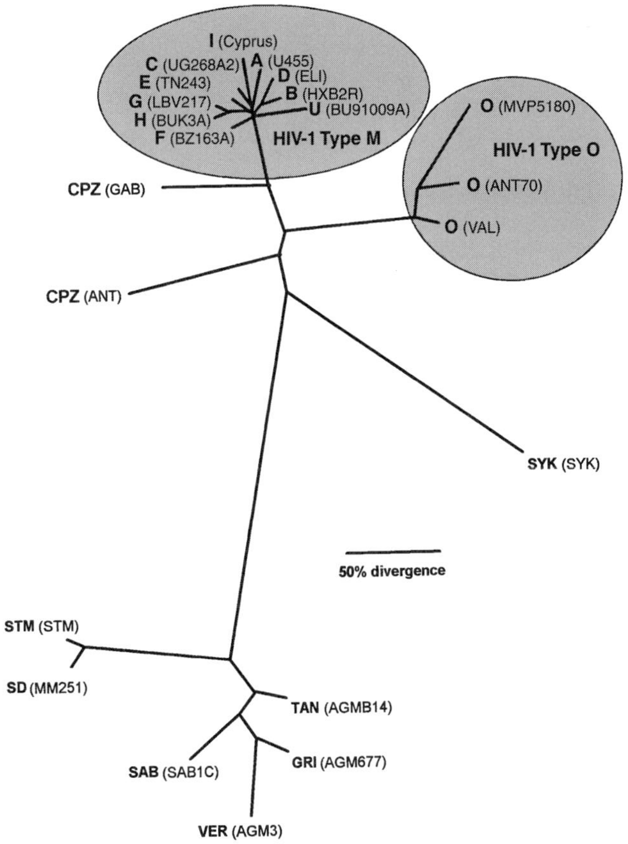

Figure 35–4. A neighbor-joining tree, based on C2-V3 sequences, showing the interrelations between the major subtypes of human immunodeficiency virus type 1 group M (main; clades A–I) and the O (outlier) group. The two groups are separated by the simian immunodeficiency virus sequence CPZ, which suggests that the M and O groups could be the result of two separate cross-species transmissions (founder effect). The star-shaped phylogenetic tree makes clear the evolutionary equidistance within the sequences from different subtypes. U, unclassified to date. (Courtesy of Paolo Zanotto.)

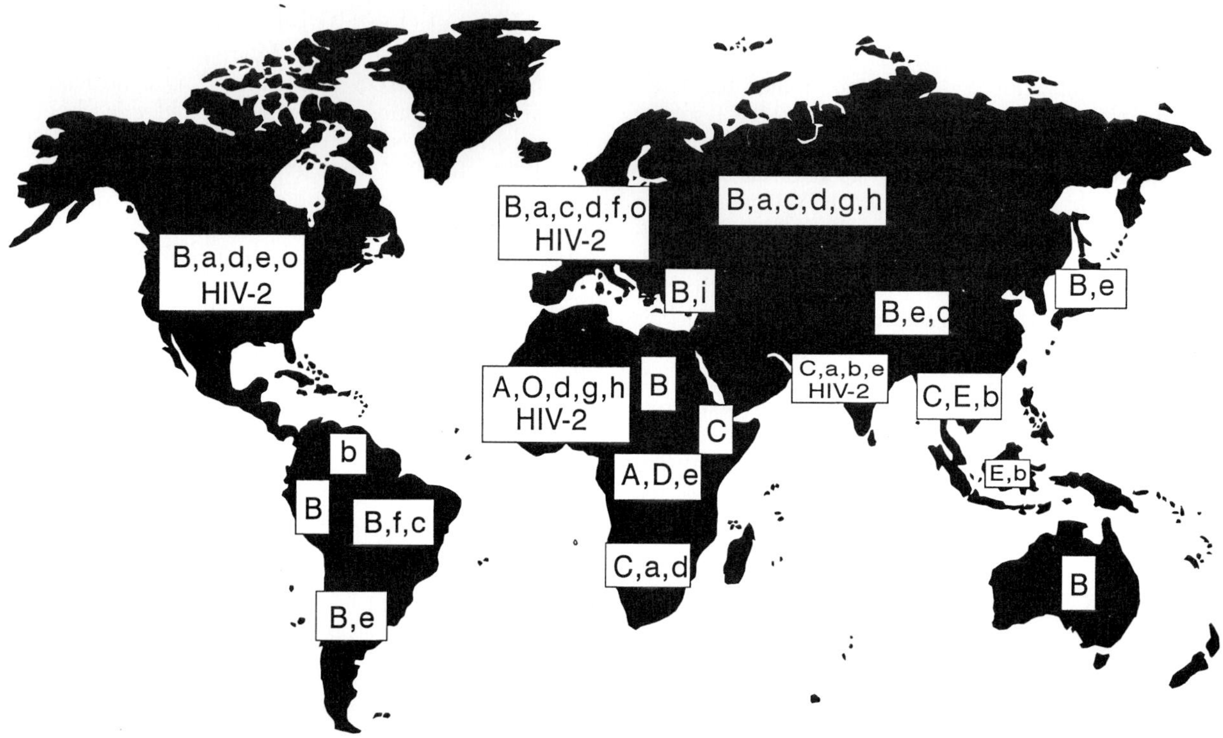

Figure 35–5. Distribution of human immunodeficiency virus (HIV) throughout the world according to the prevalence of its types and subtypes (clades). The distribution of HIV-1 clades is indicated by letters A to I (more prevalent in capital letters). Clades of HIV-2 are not shown separated.

cally and show changing distributions in different parts of the world, probably due to distinct "founder viruses" initiating localized epidemics in different regions (Fig. 35–5).[38, 68] Subtype A is found primarily in Central Africa, subtype B in North and South America and Europe, subtype D in Central Africa, subtype E in Thailand, and subtype F in Romania[69] and among intravenous drug users in Brazil.[70] Other potential sequence subtypes, described as G, H, and I, include viruses from Africa, Russia, and Taiwan.[65, 71, 72] All the clades identified so far can be found in Africa. It is remarkable that whereas increasing clade diversity is well established in Europe, South America, and Asia, clade B is virtually the exclusive epidemic subtype in North America. It is also of note that subtype B has evolved in a specific fashion in parts of the world such as South America. A second lineage of HIV-1 group B, which harbors an unusual amino acid motif (GWGR) at the crown of the V3 loop, has been present since the early epidemic in Brazil, whereas North American–European strains present only the GPGR motif.[73] This previously rare strain now accounts for nearly half the detected B strains in Brazil.[74] This strain has unique genetic and antigenic properties and is probably a result of a founder effect rather than mere evolution.[73]

HIV-2 was discovered in 1985 in several countries in West Africa and was initially called human T cell leukemia/lymphoma virus (HTLV)–IV and lymphadenopathy-associated virus (LAV)–2. More recently, HIV-2 has spread at low rates into Western Europe, where a number of infected blood donors have been detected and cases of transfusion transmission have been documented.[75] HIV-2 is transmitted in the same manner as HIV-1—by sexual contact, by intravenous drug use, and, at a lower rate than for HIV-1, from mother to child. HIV-2 causes progressive immunodeficiency, with susceptibility to a similar array of opportunistic infections as seen with HIV-1. Studies indicate that rates of disease progression and secondary viral transmission are lower in persons infected with HIV-2 compared with HIV-1, possibly owing to lower viral burden in HIV-2 infection.[76] Although only a small number of HIV-2–infected persons have been identified in the United States, screening of blood donors through combination HIV-1/HIV-2 antibody assays was mandated in 1991. Since then, only two HIV-2–infected donors have been identified.[77]

In 1990, a divergent strain of HIV-1, now characterized as group O,[65] was first reported in patients from west-central Africa.[78, 79] This subtype is now endemic in Cameroon and Gabon and has been detected in Europe. However, these variants do not represent a single subtype and may be as different from each other as are the variants that make up subtypes A through I. The worldwide distribution of these divergent HIV-1 strains is not yet known, but they have been reported in Cameroon,[78, 80] Gabon,[80] and France.[81] Despite being rare in many parts of the world, the prevalence of HIV-1 group O among HIV-1–infected people was 3% in Gabon[80] and between 5% and 8% in Cameroon.[80, 82, 83]

In mid-1994, French investigators first reported that a significant proportion of persons infected with HIV-1 subtype O tested negative on a number of HIV-1 and HIV-1/HIV-2 combination assays,[81, 84] an observation later confirmed by investigators at the Centers for Disease Control and Prevention.[85] Antibody assays employing synthetic peptides or recombinant antigens on the solid phase, and those using the so-called third-generation antigen-sandwich format, were particularly prone to false-negative results. Two HIV group O infections were identified in the United States in the late 1990s, precipitating the Food and Drug Administration to require incorporation of HIV-1 group O antigens into screening enzyme immunoassays over the next several years.

As summarized earlier, there is a phenomenal breadth of HIV diversity in central Africa,[38, 66] with increasing evidence of an accelerating "trafficking" of subtypes around the world. Co-circulating lineages of HIV-1 are being tracked in Thailand,[86] Brazil,[74, 87] Russia,[72] and Central Africa.[80] In Cameroon, besides group O, five additional HIV-1 subtypes (A, B, E, F, and H) were identified.[66] In view of the rampant spread of HIV variants and the fast rate of evolution of the virus, sustained vigilance and careful assessment of the implications of the growing genetic diversity are clearly warranted. A thorough understanding of the extent of genetic diversity is critical for implementing effective control measures, including vaccination programs and antiviral drug therapies, and good-quality diagnostic tests.

We have been monitoring the prevalence of HIV subtypes in the U.S. blood donor base by using the heteroduplex mobility assay, a technique based on the mobility of DNA heteroduplex in polyacrylamide gels.[88] We analyzed 100 samples from HIV-positive blood donors from 1984 and over 300 from 1993 to 1997. All but four samples typed as clade B. The exceptions were two clade A and two clade C infections. Two of these infections (one clade A and one clade C) were from African immigrants, but two donors who had never traveled outside the United States were identified as harboring subtype A and C infections.[89] This suggests that migration of diverse forms of HIV-1 will play a major role in the molecular epidemiology of HIV in North America in the near future.

CO-RECEPTORS FOR HIV-1 AND VIRUS-CELL INTERACTION

Attachment of HIV-1 to cells is mediated between specific sequences of the gp120 envelope glycoprotein and the CD4 receptor, which usually functions as a receptor for the major histocompatibility complex class II (MHC-II) molecules. Although the CD4 receptor is the principal binding protein, it is not sufficient for HIV-1 entry into cells. Evidence suggesting additional receptors first came from the fact that HIV-1 could not efficiently replicate in other animal cells engineered to express human CD4.[90–92] The co-receptors (or secondary receptors) such as CCR5, CCR2, CCR3, and CXCR4 (formerly fusin) have provided insights into this phenomenon (reviewed by D'Souza and Harden[93]). In fact, different HIV-1 strains have distinct cell tropism: viruses with T cell tropism use the CXCR4 co-receptor, whereas those with selective macrophage-monocyte tropism use the CCR5 or CCR2 co-receptor. The strain involved in the primary infection (the macrophage-tropic isolates) is the strain that uses the CCR5 or CCR2 co-receptor expressed on mucosal dendritic cells—the strain that leads to central nervous system complications. The more cytopathic (syncytium-inducing [SI]) T cell–tropic strains, which evolve during the course of infection and precipitate accelerated T cell depletion and progression to AIDS, use the CXCR4 receptor. The identification of dual tropic HIV-1 strains over the course of infection suggests that such strains may represent an intermediate form between macrophage- and T cell–tropic populations.[94, 95] This transition in cell tropism indicates that viral adaptation enabling broader co-receptor use may be a key step in progression to AIDS.[96]

Another insight that came from the discovery of co-receptors relates to the observation that some people lack evidence of infection with HIV-1 despite multiple sexual contacts with HIV-1–infected partners.[97, 98] The leukocytes from these exposed, uninfected subjects were found to be highly resistant to infection with multiple primary HIV-1 isolates. This relative resistance to HIV-1 infection did not extend to T cell line–adapted strains. Shortly after that observation, a 32–base pair deletion (CCR5Δ32) in the CCR5 gene, which encodes a membrane cytokine receptor, was identified in some white persons.[99, 100] This mutated allele causes truncation of the CCR5 co-receptor on lymphoid cell surfaces. In the homozygous state, the truncated allele is epidemiologically related to HIV-1–seronegative persons with multiple exposure. The allele frequency coding CCR5Δ32 has been estimated among different ethnic groups. Among whites, approximately 15% are heterozygous and 1% are homozygous (reviewed in Bradbury[101]). In contrast, the diluted allele is rare among persons from Africa, Japan, and Venezuela. In an analysis focused on Brazil, the prevalence of heterozygosity was similar to that found in North America and Western Europe.[102]

Although several HIV-positive CCR5Δ32-homozygous patients have been identified,[103–105] numerous epidemiological studies have confirmed that the absence of full-length CCR5 confers a high degree of resistance to HIV infection. Studies of transfusion recipients and hemophiliacs indicate that this resistance is seen even when the parenteral route is considered.[106]

More recently, a second mutation in CCR5 that is 1% prevalent in the European population was described.[107] A single base-pair mutation, m303, introduces a stop codon that prevents the formation of the CCR5 receptor. Thus, m303 homozygosity or its association with the CCR5Δ32 allele could account for unexplained cases of HIV-1 resistance in people who carry an apparent wild-type CCR5 or are heterozygous. Polymorphism of other genes coding for other co-receptors related to MT strain infection, such as CCR2, apparently exerts no influence on HIV-1 infection incidence.

FACTORS INFLUENCING DISEASE PROGRESSION

It is now known that active replication of HIV is the cause of progressive immune system damage in infected persons.[14, 15] In the absence of effective inhibition of HIV replication, nearly all infected patients suffer progressive deterioration of immune function, which results in their susceptibility to opportunistic infections, malignancies, and neurological diseases and in wasting, ultimately leading to death. The rate of disease progression is predicted by the magnitude of active HIV replication taking place in an infected person, reflected by the RNA viral load in plasma.[108, 109] These viral load assays reflect the immediate status of ongoing viral replication and clearance within an infected person and are of great value in determining the relative risk of clinical progression. The extent of immune system damage that has already occurred in an infected person is indicated by the CD4 cell count, which permits assessment of the risk of developing specific opportunistic infections and other complications. When used with viral load assays, CD4 cell counts enhance the accuracy with which the risk of disease progression and death can be predicted.[109]

The genetic diversity of the virus may be related to pathogenicity and disease progression as well. For example, there is a trend toward isolation of viruses that do not readily form syncytia in cell culture (NSI viruses) from asymptomatic patients.[110] These isolates frequently demonstrate relatively slow, low-level replication in vitro and are generally monocyte-tropic. In contrast, approximately 50% of patients who have rapid progression to AIDS have a shift in phenotype to the more lymphocyte-tropic, SI viral isolates that replicate rapidly and to higher levels in culture.[111, 112] The emergence of SI variants increases the risk for accelerated CD4 cell decline and subsequent onset of AIDS.[113, 114] In the era before highly effective antiretroviral therapy, opportunistic infections generally occurred within 6 to 8 months of this transition to SI virus.[115] There is also evidence that rapid disease progression occurs in rare cases in which SI viruses are transmitted and predominate in primary infection.[116, 117] In the minority of patients in whom disease progression occurs in spite of low viral load levels, more cytopathic strains (i.e., with a higher capacity for cell destruction) such as SI viruses may be the cause of progression.

The increasing genetic diversity during the course of infection may also be related to disease progression for reasons other than SI strain appearance. The increase in the number of virus variants may be an important factor leading to the breakdown of the immune system. Theoretically, the control of HIV-1 replication is lost when the antigenic diversity of HIV-1 within an infected host exceeds the capacity of that person's immune system to respond effectively. When this diversity threshold is crossed, viremia increases, CD4 cells decline, and disease progresses.[49]

A study from Australia of a group of seven long-term asymptomatic transfusion recipients who were infected from 1982 to 1984 with blood from a single donor emphasized the potential importance of the infecting viral strain and its diversity.[118] HIV-1 sequencing revealed deletions in the *nef* LTR region in this group and in a few other long-term survivors.[119–121] However, other researchers failed to identify mutations in *nef* or other critical viral genes influencing replication in similar subjects.[122, 123] To investigate the relative effects of viral and host characteristics on disease course, we compared patients infected by the same and different subtype B strains. Forty-three infection chain clusters were identified, each defined by an infected blood donor, that donor's recipients, and the recipients' sexual partners, representing second and third generations of infection. Analysis of levels and rates of change in CD4 lymphocyte counts and viral load showed that there was more similarity in rates of change in $CD4^+$ lymphocyte counts or viral RNA levels among members within a cluster than among clusters. Differences in entry viral RNA levels by cluster were marginal and markedly smaller than interindividual differences. These results argue that, in general, host factors outweigh differences in viral strain in determining HIV-1 disease progression.[124]

There is also a relationship between genetic polymorphisms in host cell co-receptors and disease progression. The onset of AIDS seems to be postponed 2 to 4 years in persons heterozygous for the CCR5Δ32 and CCR5+ alleles.[125–128] However, identification of the heterozygous state for CCR5 can account for only a small proportion of the long-term nonprogressors who remain AIDS-free 10 to 20 years after HIV-1 infection. For example, more than 60% of long-term nonprogressors are homozygous for the common allele CCR5+/+.[125–128] Another chemokine receptor gene implicated as an HIV-1 co-receptor, the CCR2 gene, also presents polymorphisms that might be related to disease progression. A point mutation described as CCR2-*64I* occurs at an allele frequency of 10% to 15% among whites and African-Americans.[129] Data from one large cohort indicate that HIV-1–infected persons carrying this allele progressed to AIDS 2 to 4 years later than did people homozygous for the common allele,[129] whereas another study failed to detect this association.[127] Further studies are needed to define the role of CCR2-*64I* and other chemokine polymorphisms in HIV-1 pathogenesis.

Although CD4 depletion is the most important finding in AIDS as a mechanism of immunosuppression, diverse qualitative and quantitative effects of HIV-1 can be found in the humoral and cellular immune responses (reviewed by Levy[6]). Many HIV-1–infected patients with relatively high CD4 cell counts are anergic to skin testing, suggesting that cellular immune defects are more complex than a simple decrease in T helper cell numbers. Antibody responses to vaccinations, for example, are frequently suboptimal even before AIDS develops in patients infected with HIV-1. Surprisingly, the pathogenic pathway that leads to CD4 depletion during HIV-1 infection remains unclear and controversial. As mentioned earlier, the dynamic inverse relation between viral load and CD4 cell count suggests that direct cell killing is more likely than indirect mechanisms, such as autoimmune phenomena or cytokine-mediated pathways. However, apoptosis, or programmed cell death, can be triggered by the binding of a primed T cell to gp120, and this mechanism is a potential explanation for the rapid loss of CD4 cells when virus load increases in plasma.[130, 131]

CONCLUSION

The transfusion-transmitted AIDS epidemic has been a tragedy beyond anyone's imagination. As conscientious physicians and scientists involved in transfusion medicine, we have borne and continue to bear the responsibility to learn from the epidemic and to contribute to the battle to control the spread of HIV and its consequent morbidity and mortality. If there is a silver lining to the black cloud of this epidemic, it is that the blood banking community has gained a number of insights that have enabled us to further safeguard the blood supply from both known and unknown infectious agents.[132, 133] The blood supply today is safer than it has ever been. In addition, studies of HIV infection and disease in the transfusion setting have contributed important findings that have furthered HIV research efforts on virtually every front.

REFERENCES

1. Busch MP, Young MO, Samson SS, et al. Risk of human immunodeficiency virus transmission by blood transfusions prior to the implementation of HIV antibody screening in the San Francisco Bay area. Transfusion 1991; 31:4.
2. Ragni MV, Winkelstein A, Kingsley L, et al. 1986 update of HIV seroprevalence, seroconversion, AIDS incidence, and immunologic correlates of HIV infection in patients with hemophilia A and B. Blood 1987; 70:786.
3. Curran JW, Lawrence DN, Jaffe H, et al. Acquired immunodeficiency syndrome (AIDS) associated with transfusions. N Engl J Med 1984; 310:69.
4. Feorino PM, Jaffe HW, Palmer E, et al. Transfusion-associated acquired immunodeficiency syndrome: evidence for persistent infection in blood donors. N Engl J Med 1985; 312:1293.
5. Jaffe HW, Sarngadharan MG, DeVico AL, et al. Infection with HTLV-III/LAV and transfusion-associated acquired immunodeficiency syndrome: serologic evidence of an association. JAMA 1985; 254:770.
6. Levy JA. HIV and the Pathogenesis of AIDS, 2nd ed. Washington, DC: American Society for Microbiology/ASM Press, 1998.
7. Schneider J, Hunsmann G. Simian lentiviruses: the SIV group [Editorial review]. AIDS 1988; 2:1.
8. Jarrett O, Yamamoto JK, Neil JC. Feline immunodeficiency virus as a model for AIDS vaccination. AIDS 1990; 4(suppl 1):S163.
9. Cann AJ, Karn J. Molecular biology of HIV: new insights into the virus life-cycle. AIDS 1989; 3(suppl 1):S19.
10. Greene WC. The molecular biology of human immunodeficiency virus type 1 infection. N Engl J Med 1991; 324:308.
11. Coffin JM. The virology of AIDS: 1990. AIDS 1990; 4(suppl 1):S1.
12. Busch MP, Satten GA. Time course of viremia and antibody seroconversion following human immunodeficiency virus exposure. Am J Med 1997; 102(suppl 5B):117 (discussion, pp 125–126).
13. Petersen LR, Lackritz E, Lewis WF, et al. The effectiveness of the confidential unit exclusion option. Transfusion 1994; 34:865.
14. Ho DD, Neumann AU, Perelson AS, et al. Rapid turnover of plasma virions and CD4 lymphocytes in HIV-1 infection. Nature 1995; 373:123.
15. Wci X, Ghosh SK, Taylor ME, et al. Viral dynamics in human immunodeficiency virus type 1 infection. Nature 1995; 373:117.
16. Perelson AS, Essunger P, Cao Y, et al. Decay characteristics of HIV-1–infected compartments during combination therapy. Nature 1997; 387:188.
17. Lee T-H, Stromberg RR, Heitman JW, et al. Distribution of HIV type 1 (HIV-1) in blood components: detection and significance of high levels of HIV-1 associated with platelets. Transfusion 1998; 38:580–588.
18. Operskalski EA, Stram DO, Busch MP, et al. Role of viral load in heterosexual transmission of human immunodeficiency virus type 1 by blood transfusion recipients. Am J Epidemiol 1997; 146:655.
19. O'Brien TR, Busch MP, Donegan E, et al. Heterosexual transmission of human immunodeficiency virus type 1 from transfusion recipients to their sex partners. J AIDS 1994; 7:705.
20. Lee T-H, Sheppard W, Reis M, et al. Circulating HIV-1–infected cell burden from seroconversion to AIDS: importance of post seroconversion viral load on disease course. J AIDS 1994; 7:381.
21. Busch MP, Operskalski EA, Mosley JW, et al. for the Transfusion Safety Study Group. Factors influencing HIV-1 transmission by blood transfusion. J Infect Dis 1996; 174:26.
22. Wilfert CM, Wilson C, Luzuriaga K, et al. Pathogenesis of pediatric human immunodeficiency virus type 1 infection. J Infect Dis 1994; 170:286.
23. Gerberding JL. Incidence and prevalence of human immunodeficiency virus, hepatitis B virus, hepatitis C virus, and cytomegalovirus among health care personnel at risk for blood exposure: final report from a longitudinal study. J Infect Dis 1994; 170:1410.
24. Cardo DM, Culver DH, Ciesielski CA, et al. A case-control study of HIV seroconversion in health care workers after percutaneous exposure. Centers for Disease Control and Prevention Needlestick Surveillance Group. N Engl J Med 1997; 337:1485.
25. De Cock KM, Adjorlolo G, Ekpini E, et al. Epidemiology and transmission of HIV-2: why there is no HIV-2 pandemic. JAMA 1993; 270:2083.
26. Simon F, Matheron S, Tamalet C, et al. Cellular and plasma viral load in patients infected with HIV-2. AIDS 1993; 7:1411.
27. Roberts JD, Bebenek K, Kunkel TA. The accuracy of reverse transcriptase from HIV-1. Science 1998; 242:1171.
28. Boucher CAB, O'Sullivan E, Mulder JW, et al. Ordered appearance of zidovudine resistance mutations during treatment of 18 human immunodeficiency virus–positive subjects. J Infect Dis 1992; 165:105.
29. Larder BA, Darby G, Richman DD. HIV with reduced sensitivity to zidovudine (AZT) isolated during prolonged therapy. Science 1989; 243:1731.
30. Preston BD, Poiesz BJ, Loeb LA. Fidelity of HIV-1 reverse transcriptase. Science 1988; 242:1168.
31. Bebenek K, Abbots J, Roberts JD, et al. Specificity and mechanism of error-prone replication by human immunodeficiency virus-1 reverse transcriptase. J Biol Chem 1989; 264:16948.
32. Vartanian J-P, Meyerhans A, Asjo B, et al. Selection, recombination and G-A hypermutation of HIV-1 genomes. J Virol 1991; 65:1779.
33. Clavel F, Hoggan MD, Willey RL, et al. Genetic recombination of human immunodeficiency virus. J Virol 1989; 63:1455.
34. Tan W, Fredriksson R, Bjorndal A, et al. Cotransfection of HIV-1 molecular clones with restricted cell tropism may yield progeny virus with altered phenotype. AIDS Res Hum Retroviruses 1993; 9:321.
35. Diaz RS, Sabino EC, Mayer A, et al. Dual human immunodeficiency virus type 1 infection and recombination in a dually exposed transfusion recipient. The Transfusion Safety Study Group. J Virol 1995; 69:3273.
36. Zhu T, Mo H, Wang N, et al. Genotypic and phenotypic characterization of HIV-1 in patients with primary infection. Science 1993; 261:1179.
37. Sabino EC, Shapaer EG, Morgado MG, et al. Identification of human immunodeficiency virus type 1 envelope genes recombinant between subtypes B and F in two epidemiologically linked individuals from Brazil. J Virol 1994; 68:6340.
38. Gao F, Yue L, Robertson DL, et al. Genetic diversity of human immunodeficiency virus type 2: evidence for distinct sequence subtypes with differences in virus biology. J Virol 1994; 68:7433.
39. Zhu T, Wang N, Carr A, et al. Evidence for coinfection by multiple strains of human immunodeficiency virus type 1 subtype B in an acute seroconvertor. J Virol 1995; 69:1324.
40. Delassus S, Cheynier R, Wain-Hobson S. Evolution of human immunodeficiency virus type 1 *nef* and long terminal repeat sequences over 4 years in vivo and in vitro. J Virol 1991; 65:225.
41. Groenink M, Andeweg AC, Fouchier RAM, et al. Phenotype-associated *env* gene variation among eight related human immunodeficiency virus type 1 clones: evidence for in vivo recombination and determinants of cytotropism outside the V3 domain. J Virol 1992; 66:6175.
42. Howell RM, Fitzgibbon JE, Noe M, et al. In vivo sequence variation of the human immunodeficiency virus type 1 *env* gene: evidence for recombination among variants found in a single individual. AIDS Res Hum Retroviruses 1991; 7:869.
43. Zhang LQ, MacKenzie P, Cleland A, et al. Selection for specific sequences in the external envelope protein of human immunodeficiency virus type 1 upon primary infection. J Virol 1993; 67:3345.
44. Delwart EL, Busch MP, Kalish ML, et al. Rapid molecular epidemiology of human immunodeficiency virus transmission. AIDS Res Hum Retroviruses 1995; 11:1081.
45. Reitz MS, Hall L, Robert-Guroff M, et al. Viral variability and serum antibodies response in a laboratory worker infected with

HIV type I (HTLV type IIIB). AIDS Res Hum Retroviruses 1994; 10:1143.
46. Wolinsky SM, Wilke CM, Korber BT, et al. Selective transmission of human immunodeficiency virus type-1 variants from mothers to infants. Science 1992; 255:1134.
47. Wolfs TF, Zwart G, Bakker M, et al. HIV-1 genomic RNA diversification following sexual and parenteral virus transmission. Virology 1992; 189:103.
48. Diaz RS, Sabino EC, Mayer A, et al. Lack of dual HIV infection in a transfusion recipient exposed to two seropositive blood components. AIDS Res Hum Retroviruses 1996; 12:1291.
49. Nowak MA, Anderson RM, McLean AR, et al. Antigenic diversity thresholds and the development of AIDS. Science 1991; 254:963.
50. Homsy J, Meyer M, Levy JA. Serum enhancement of human immunodeficiency virus (HIV) correlates with disease in HIV infected individuals. J Virol 1990; 64:1437.
51. Gegerfelt AV, Albert J, Morfeldt-Manson L, et al. Isolate-specific neutralizing antibodies in patients with progressive HIV-1 related disease. Virology 1991; 185:162.
52. Wrin T, Crawford L, Sawyer L, et al. Neutralizing antibody responses to autologous and heterologous isolates of human immunodeficiency virus. J AIDS 1994; 7:211.
53. McKeating JA, Griffiths PD, Goudsmit J, et al. Characterization of HIV-1 neutralization escape mutants. AIDS 1989; 3:777.
54. Reitz MS Jr, Wilson C, Naugle C, et al. Generation of a neutralization-resistant variant of HIV-1 is due to selection of a point mutation in the envelope gene. Cell 1988; 54:57.
55. Robert-Guroff M, Reitz MS, Robey WG, et al. In vitro generation of an HTLV-III variant by neutralizing antibodies. J Immunol 1986; 137:3306.
56. Thali M, Charles M, Furman C, et al. Resistance to neutralization by broadly reactive antibodies to the human immunodeficiency virus type 1 gp120 glycoprotein conferred by a gp41 amino acid change. J Virol 1994; 68:674.
57. Wolfs TFW, Zwart G, Bakker M, et al. Naturally occurring mutations within HIV-1 V3 genomic RNA lead to antigenic variation dependent on a single amino acid substitution. Virology 1991; 185:195.
58. Richman DD. New strategies to combat HIV drug resistance. Hosp Pract 1996; (August 15):47.
59. Diaz RS, Zanotto PMA, Mayer A, et al. Escape recombinants of HIV-1 in a dual infected transfusion recipient. Submitted for publication.
60. Kuiken CL, Zwart G, Baab E, et al. Increasing antigenic and genetic diversity of the HIV-1 V3 domain in the course of AIDS epidemic. Proc Natl Acad Sci U S A 1993; 90:9061.
61. Chang SYP, Bowman B, Weiss JB, et al. The origin of HIV-1 isolate HTLV-IIIB. Nature 1993; 363:466.
62. Zhang L, Diaz RS, Ho DD, et al. Host-specific driving force in human immunodeficiency virus type 1 evolution in vivo. J Virol 1997; 71:2555.
63. Eigen M, Gardiner W, Schuster P, et al. The origin of genetic information. Sci Am 1981; 244:88.
64. Diaz RS, Zhang L, Busch MP, et al. Divergence of HIV-1 quasispecies in an epidemiologic cluster. AIDS 1997; 11:415.
65. Myers G, Korber B, Wain-Hobson S, et al. (eds). Human Retroviruses and AIDS 1993, I–IV. A Compilation and Analysis of Nucleic Acid and Amino Acid Sequences. Los Alamos, NM: Los Alamos National Laboratory, 1993 (and subsequent years).
66. Nkengasong JN, Janssens W, Heyndrickx L, et al. Genotypic subtypes of HIV-1 in Cameroon. AIDS 1994; 8:1405.
67. Zhu T, Korber BT, Nahmias AJ, et al. An African HIV-1 sequence from 1959 and implications for the origin of the epidemic. Nature 1998; 391:594.
68. Korber BTM, MacInnes K, Smith RF, et al. Mutational trends in V3 loop protein sequences observed in different genetic lineages of human immunodeficiency virus type 1. J Virol 1994; 68:6730.
69. Dumitresco O, Kalish M, Kliks SC, et al. Characterization of HIV-1 strains isolated from children in Rumania: identification of a new envelope subtype. J Infect Dis 1994; 169:281.
70. Sabino E, Diaz RS, Brigido L, et al. Prevalence of HIV-1 subtypes in Sao Paulo City, Brazil. AIDS 1996; 10:1579.
71. Janssens W, Heyndrickx L, Fransen K, et al. Genetic and phylogenetic analysis of *env* subtypes G and H in central Africa. Aids Res Hum Retroviruses 1994; 10:877.
72. Bobkov A, Cheigsong-Popov R, Garaev M, et al. Identification of an *env* G subtype and heterogeneity of HIV-1 strains in the Russian Federation and Belarus. AIDS 1994; 8:1649.
73. Diaz RS, Hendry M, Sabino E, et al. Genetic and antigenic heterogeneity of V3 region of HIV-1 from Brazilian homosexual males from 1983 [Abstract I25]. 35th Interscience Conference on Antimicrobial Agents and Chemotherapy, San Francisco, 1995, p 209.
74. Morgado MG, Sabino EC, Shpaer EG, et al. V3 region polymorphisms in HIV-1 from Brazil: prevalence of subtype B strains divergent from the North American/European prototype and detection of subtype F. AIDS Res Hum Retroviruses 1994; 10:569.
75. O'Brien TR, George JR, Holmberg SD. Human immunodeficiency virus type 2 infection in the United States: epidemiology, diagnosis, and public health implications. JAMA 1992; 267:2775.
76. Marlink R, Kanki P, Thior I, et al. Reduced rate of disease development after HIV-2 infections as compared to HIV-1. Science 1994; 265:1587.
77. Sullivan MT, Guido EA, Metler RP, et al. Identification and characterization of an HIV-2 antibody-positive blood donor in the United States. Transfusion 1998; 38:189.
78. DeLeys R, Vanderborght B, van den Haesevelde M, et al. Isolation and partial characterization of an unusual human immunodeficiency retrovirus from two persons of west-central African origin. J Virol 1990; 64:1207.
79. van den Haesevelde M, Decourt JL, deLeys RJ. Genomic cloning and complete sequence analysis of a highly divergent African human immunodeficiency virus isolate. J Virol 1994; 68:1586.
80. Nkengasong J, Peters M, van der Haesevelde M, et al. Antigenic evidence of the presence of the aberrant HIV-1 ANT70 virus in Cameroon and Gabon. AIDS 1993; 7:1536.
81. Loussert-Ajaka I, Ly TD, Chaix ML, et al. HIV-1/HIV-2 seronegativity in HIV subtype O infected patients. Lancet 1994; 343:1393.
82. Gurtler L, Hauser PH, Eberle J, et al. A new subtype of human immunodeficiency virus type 1 (MVP-5180) from Cameroon. J Virol 1994; 68:1581.
83. Zekeng L, Gurtler L, Afane ZE, et al. Prevalence of HIV-1 subtype O infection in Cameroon: preliminary results [Letter]. AIDS 1994; 8:1626.
84. Simon F, Ly TD, Baillou-Beaufils A, et al. Sensitivity of screening kits for anti–HIV-1 subtype O antibodies. AIDS 1994; 8:1628.
85. Schable C, Zekeng L, Pau C-P, et al. Sensitivity of United States HIV antibody tests for detection of HIV-1 group O infections. Lancet 1994; 344:1333.
86. Ou C, Takebe Y, Weniger B, et al. Independent introduction of two major HIV-1 genotypes into distinct high-risk populations in Thailand. Lancet 1993; 341:1171.
87. Louwagie J, Delwart EL, Mullins JI, et al. Genetic analysis of HIV-1 isolates from Brazil reveals presence of two distinct genetic subtypes. AIDS Res Hum Retroviruses 1994; 10:561.
88. Delwart EL, Shpaer EG, Louwagie J, et al. Genetic relationships determined by a DNA heteroduplex mobility assay: analysis of HIV-1 *env* genes. Science 1993; 262:1257.
89. de Oliveira CF, Diaz RS, Sullivan M, et al. Surveillance of HIV-1 subtypes in US blood donors: 1994–1996. Transfusion 1997; 37(suppl 9):97S.
90. Clapham PR, Blanc D, Weiss RA. Specific cell surface requirements for the infection of CD4-positive cells by human immunodeficiency virus types 1 and 2 and by simian immunodeficiency virus. Virology 1991; 181:703.
91. Ashorn PA, Berger EA, Moss B. Human immunodeficiency virus envelope glycoprotein/CD4-mediated fusion of nonprimate cells with human cells. J Virol 1990; 64:2149.
92. Simon JH, James W. Heterokaryons formed between a rat myeloma and a mouse fibroblast are permissive for entry of HIV type 1. AIDS Res Hum Retroviruses 1994; 10:1609.
93. D'Souza MP, Harden VA. Chemokines and HIV-1 second receptors: confluence of two fields generates optimism in AIDS research. Nat Med 1996; 2:1293.
94. Zhang L, Huang Y, He T, et al. HIV-1 subtype and second-receptor use. Nature 1996; 383:768.
95. Koot M, van't Wout AB, Kootstra NA, et al. Relation between changes in cellular load, evolution of viral phenotype, and the clonal composition of virus populations in the course of human immunodeficiency virus type 1 infection. J Infect Dis 1996; 173:349.

96. Shibata R, Hoggan MD, Broscius C, et al. Isolation and characterization of a syncytium-inducing, macrophage/T cell line–tropic human immunodeficiency virus type 1 isolate that readily infects chimpanzee cells in vitro and in vivo. J Virol 1995; 69:4453.
97. Detels R, Liu Z, Hennessey K, et al. Resistance to HIV-1 infection. Multicenter AIDS Cohort Study. J AIDS 1994; 7:1263.
98. Paxton WA, Martin SR, Tse D, et al. Relative resistance to HIV-1 infection of CD4 lymphocytes from persons who remain uninfected despite multiple high-risk sexual exposure. Nat Med 1996; 2:412.
99. Liu R, Paxton WA, Choe S, et al. Homozygous defect in HIV-1 coreceptor accounts for resistance of some multiply-exposed individuals to HIV-1 infection. Cell 1996; 86:367.
100. Samson M, Libert F, Doranz BJ, et al. Resistance to HIV-1 infection in Caucasian individuals bearing mutant alleles of the CCR-5 chemokine receptor gene. Nature 1996; 382:722.
101. Bradbury J. HIV-1–resistant individuals may lack HIV-1 coreceptor. Lancet 1996; 348:463.
102. Acceturi CA, Pardini R, Turcato G, et al. Indinavir (IDV) in combination with zidovudine (ZDV) and lamivudine (3TC) in a Brazilian population, and the role of CCR5-32bp heterozygosity in antiretroviral response [Abstract 375]. Presented at the Fifth National Conference on Human Retroviruses and Related Infections, Chicago, 1998, p 149.
103. Biti R, Ffrench R, Young J, et al. HIV-1 infection in an individual homozygous for the CCR5 deletion allele. Nat Med 1997; 3:252.
104. O'Brien TR, Winkler C, Dean M, et al. HIV-1 infection in a man homozygous for CCR5 delta 32. Lancet 1997; 349:1219.
105. Theodorou I, Meyer L, Magierowska M, et al. HIV-1 infection in an individual homozygous for CCR5 delta 32. Seroco Study Group. Lancet 1997; 349:1219–1220.
106. Wilkinson DA, Operskalski EA, Busch MP, et al. A 32 bp deletion within the CCR5 locus protects against transmission of parenterally-acquired human immnodeficiency virus but does not affect disease progression. J Infect Dis 1998; 178:1163.
107. Quillent C, Oberlin E, Braun J, et al. HIV-1-resistance phenotype conferred by combination of two separate inherited mutations of CCR5 gene. Lancet 1998; 351:14.
108. Mellors JW, Rinaldo CR Jr, Gupta P, et al. Prognosis in HIV-1 infection predicted by the quantity of virus in plasma. Science 1996; 272:1167.
109. Mellors JW, Munoz A, Giorgi JV, et al. Plasma viral load and $CD4^+$ lymphocytes as prognostic markers of HIV-1 infection. Ann Intern Med 1997; 126:946.
110. Sheppard HW, Lang W, Ascher MS, et al. The characterization of non-progressors: long-term HIV-1 infection with stable $CD4^+$ T-cell levels. AIDS 1993; 7:1159.
111. Tersmette M, Miedema F. Interactions between HIV and the host immune system in the pathogenesis of AIDS. AIDS 1990; 4(suppl 1):S57.
112. Koot M, Vos AH, Keet RP, et al. HIV-1 biological phenotype in long-term infected individuals evaluated with an MT-2 cocultivation assay. AIDS 1992; 6:49.
113. Koot M, Keet IP, Vos AH, et al. Prognostic value of HIV-1 syncytium-inducing phenotype for rate of $CD4^+$ cell depletion and progression to AIDS. Ann Intern Med 1993; 118:681.
114. Connor RI, Mohri H, Cao Y, et al. Increased viral burden and cytopathicity correlate temporally with $CD4^+$ T-lymphocyte decline and clinical progression in human immunodeficiency virus type 1–infected individuals. J Virol 1993; 67:1772.
115. Tersmette M, Lange JM, de Goede RE, et al. Association between biological properties of human immunodeficiency virus variants and risk for AIDS and AIDS mortality. Lancet 1989; 1:983.
116. Nielsen C, Pederson C, Lundgren D, et al. Biological properties of HIV isolates in primary HIV infection: consequences for the subsequent course of infection. AIDS 1993; 7:1035.
117. Roos MTL, Lange JMA, Goed REY, et al. Viral phenotype and immune response in primary human immunodeficiency virus type 1 infection. J Infect Dis 1992; 165:427.
118. Learmont J, Tidall B, Evans L, et al. Long-term symptomless HIV-1 infection in recipients of blood products from a single donor. Lancet 1992; 340:863.
119. Deacon NJ, Tsykin A, Solomon A, et al. Genomic structure of an attenuated quasi species of HIV-1 from a blood transfusion donor and recipients. Science 1995; 270:988.
120. Kirchoff F, Greenough TC, Brettler DN, et al. Absence of intact *nef* sequences in a long-term survivor with nonprogressive HIV-1 infection. N Engl J Med 1995; 332:228.
121. Iversen AKN, Shpaer EG, Rodrigo AG, et al. Persistence of attenuated *rev* genes in a human immunodeficiency virus type 1–infected asymptomatic individual. J Virol 1995; 69:5743.
122. Huang Y, Zhang L, Ho DD. Biological characterization of *nef* in long-term survivors of human immunodeficiency virus type 1 infection. J Virol 1995; 69:8142.
123. Michael NL, Chang G, D'Arcy LA, et al. Function characterization of human immunodeficiency virus type 1 *nef* genes in patients with divergent rates of disease progression. J Virol 1995; 69:6758.
124. Operskalski EA, Busch MP, Mosley JW, et al. Comparative rates of disease progression among persons infected with the same or different HIV-1 strains. J AIDS Hum Retrovirol 1997; 15:145.
125. Dean M, Carrington M, Winkler C, et al. Genetic restriction of HIV-1 infection and progression to AIDS by a deletion allele of the CKR5 structural gene. Hemophilia Growth and Development Study, Multicenter AIDS Cohort Study, Multicenter Hemophilia Cohort Study, San Francisco City Cohort, ALIVE Study. Science 1996; 273:1856.
126. Huang Y, Paxton WA, Wolinsky SM, et al. The role of a mutant CCR5 allele in HIV-1 transmission and disease progression. Nat Med 1996; 2:1240.
127. Michael NL, Chang G, Louie LG, et al. The role of viral phenotype and CCR-5 gene defects in HIV-1 transmission and disease progression. Nat Med 1997; 3:338.
128. Zimmerman PA, Buckler-White A, Alkhatib G, et al. Inherited resistance to HIV-1 conferred by an inactivating mutation in CC chemokine receptor 5: studies in populations with contrasting clinical phenotypes, defined racial background, and quantified risk. Mol Med 1997; 3:23.
129. Smith MW, Dean M, Carrington M, et al. Contrasting genetic influence of CCR2 and CCR5 variants on HIV-1 infection and disease progression. Hemophilia Growth and Development Study (HGDS). Science 1997; 277:959.
130. Newell MK, Haughn LJ, Maroun CR, et al. Death of mature T cells by separate ligation of CD4 and the T-cell receptor for antigen. Nature 1990; 347:286.
131. Meyaard L, Otto SA, Jonker RR, et al. Programmed death of T cells in HIV-1 infection. Science 1992; 257:217.
132. Dodd RY. Will blood products be free of infectious agents? *In* Nance SJ (ed): Transfusion Medicine in the 1990's. Arlington, VA: American Assocoiation of Blood Banks, 1990, pp 223–251.
133. AuBuchon JP, Birkmeyer JD, Busch MP. Cost-effectiveness of expanded HIV test protocols for donated blood. Transfusion 1997; 37:45.

SECTION

XI Emerging Technologies Applied to Transfusion

CHAPTER 36

Principles of Immunoassay

Fred V. Plapp
Jane M. Rachel

Antigens and antibodies are defined by their ability to interact with one another. During the past hundred years, a variety of methods for detecting and quantitating antigen-antibody reactions have been developed. This chapter describes general principles of past, current, and future immunoassays that have applications in the field of transfusion medicine.

EARLY IMMUNOASSAYS

In 1889, Charrin and Roger[1] mixed bacteria with serum from a previously infected animal and observed distinct clumps, or agglutinates. Kraus[2] demonstrated in 1897 that serum from an animal previously inoculated with bacterial culture filtrate formed a cloudy precipitate when mixed with the filtrate. These early discoveries illustrate the fundamental difference between agglutination and precipitation. Agglutination assays detect antibodies that react with particulate antigens, including those expressed on bacteria and blood cells. Precipitation assays detect antibodies to soluble antigens, which encompasses a much wider range of analytes.

The molecular mechanisms of agglutination and precipitation were elucidated in 1934 when Marrack[3] proposed the lattice theory of immune reactions. The central component of this theory is that antibody molecules are bivalent and antigens are multivalent. Formation of visible antigen-antibody complexes, whether agglutinates or precipitates, occurs in two stages. During the initial sensitization stage, antibody molecules bind univalently to antigens. The second stage, lattice formation, occurs when antibodies react bivalently with adjacent antigens to form a network of linked reactants. As lattice size increases, agglutinates or precipitates become visible. Lattice formation is critically influenced by relative concentrations of antigen and antibody in solution (Fig. 36–1). Excessive amounts of antibody or antigen prevent lattice formation by inhibiting bivalent antibody binding to separate antigen molecules. Although sensitization occurs under these conditions, a lattice is not formed and the end product is not visually detectable.

Antibody-induced clumping of erythrocytes was first reported in 1869 by Creite,[4] who observed that irregular aggregates formed when rabbit blood was mixed with blood from other animals. In 1888, Stillmark[5] described agglutination of erythrocytes by seed extracts of *Ricinus communis*. Ehrlich and Morgenroth[6] reported in 1900 that erythrocytes could be agglutinated by antibodies. Shortly thereafter, Landsteiner[7] discovered ABO blood groups using hemagglutination. In spite of what now seems the obvious importance of this discovery, blood groups were not considered relevant to transfusion until 1908, when Ottenberg[8] performed the first pretransfusion compatibility tests.

The hemagglutination reactions described by Landsteiner and Ottenberg were produced by mixing serum

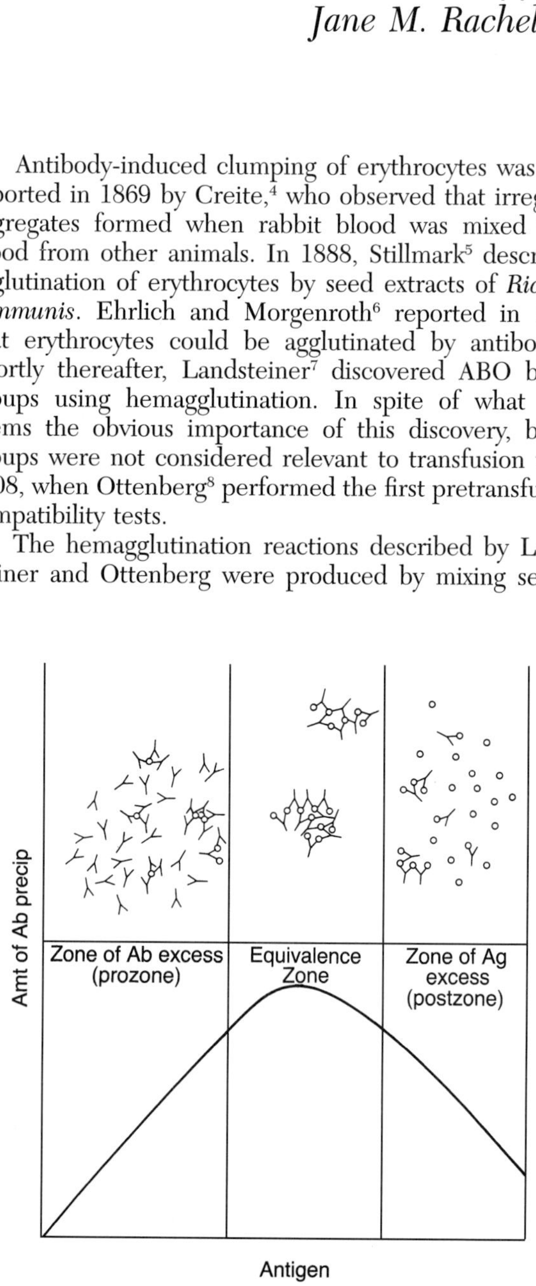

Figure 36–1. Lattice theory of immune reactions. (From Clark WR. The Experimental Foundations of Modern Immunology, 2nd ed. New York: John Wiley & Sons, 1983, p 115.)

with red blood cells (RBCs) on slides or in test tubes and observing for agglutination. At that time, all immunological reactions were believed to produce visible agglutinates. In 1944, Race[9] and Wiener[10] separately described antibodies to Rh blood group antigens that were capable of sensitizing but not agglutinating Rh-positive RBCs. The presence of nonagglutinating antibodies was proved indirectly, by their ability to inhibit hemagglutination with known Rh antisera.

In 1945, Coombs and associates[11] rediscovered the antiglobulin reaction, which was first described in 1908 by Moreschi.[12] RBCs were mixed with serum and incubated to allow sensitization and then washed to remove unbound antibodies. Sensitization was detected by adding serum from a rabbit immunized against human immunoglobulins. The rabbit antiglobulin serum bound bivalently to adjacent sensitized cells to produce agglutination.

The success of the antiglobulin technique provided conclusive support for Marrack's hypothesis that agglutination is a two-stage phenomenon. Sensitization that occurs during the initial reaction is detected by using a second antibody to facilitate lattice formation. Although the antiglobulin test greatly expanded the scope and usefulness of pretransfusion testing, its true significance was far greater. The antiglobulin test was the first instance in which a primary immunological reaction was detected by deliberate production of a secondary immunological reaction. It was a milestone in immunoassay development, because virtually all current assays are based on this concept.

HEMAGGLUTINATION

Hemagglutination methods are still widely used for pretransfusion testing. The sensitivity, simplicity, and economy of hemagglutination account for its persistence in clinical laboratories that bear little resemblance to those of a century ago. The most traditional formats for hemagglutination testing are test tube methods, although slides, cards, capillary tubes, microplate wells, and plastic microtubes have also been used.

Test Tube Methods

For the past half century, most pretransfusion hemagglutination tests have used glass or plastic test tubes. Serum and cells are added to tubes and mixed gently. Tubes are then incubated if necessary to allow sensitization, the first stage of hemagglutination, to occur. The volumes and concentrations of serum and cells are optimized to promote both sensitization and lattice formation.[13]

Antibody binding to RBCs can be enhanced by manipulation of environmental conditions. In general, physiological temperature and pH promote RBC antigen-antibody reactions. Enzyme modification of RBCs reduces net surface charge and distance between cells. Lowering the ionic strength of the reaction medium increases the speed and quantity of antibody binding.

The second stage of hemagglutination is affected primarily by RBC antigen density and physical properties of antibody molecules. Because immunoglobulin M (IgM) molecules are large and multivalent, they are capable of sensitizing and directly agglutinating RBCs (Fig. 36–2). Smaller, bivalent immunoglobulin G (IgG) molecules sensitize RBCs very efficiently but usually require antiglobulin to produce agglutination (Fig. 36–3). For this procedure, sensitized RBCs are washed with physiological saline to remove unbound immunoglobulins. If washing is inadequate, antiglobulin reagent may bind to serum immunoglobulins rather than sensitized RBCs. Addition of antiglobulin reagent facilitates lattice formation and produces hemagglutination (Fig. 36–4). Commercially available antiglobulin reagents may have multiple specificities but typically include reactivity against human IgG and the C3d component of human complement. Tubes are centrifuged briefly to pellet RBCs; then pellets are gently resuspended and examined for agglutinates. The strength of tube hemagglutination reactions is graded as shown in Table 36–1.

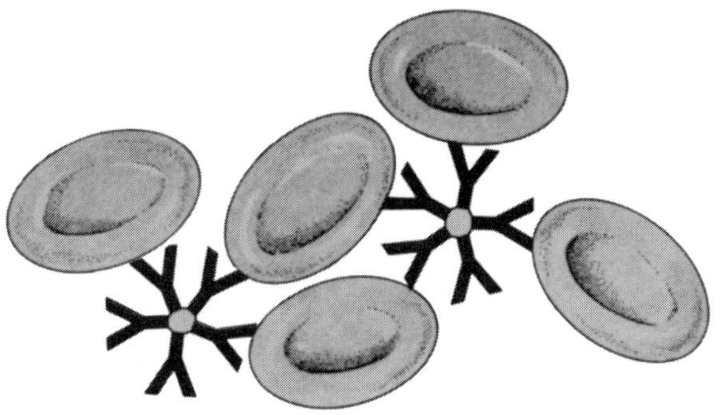

Figure 36–2. Direct agglutination of red blood cells by immunoglobulin M (IgM) antibodies. (From Stroup M, Treacy M. Blood Group Antigens and Antibodies. Raritan, NJ: Ortho Diagnostic Systems, Inc., 1982.)

Slide and Card Methods

Although tube hemagglutination methods were initially used by Ottenberg, they were largely supplanted by slide methods until the 1940s, when antiglobulin techniques were incorporated into pretransfusion compatibility tests. Slide and card methods are now most commonly used in extralaboratory settings for rapid ABO grouping. Slide and card methods are convenient and inexpensive, and

Table 36–1. Grading the Strength of Agglutination

Description	Grade
Button of cells in one clump; background is clear	4+
Button breaks into many large clumps; background is clear	3+
Button breaks into many small clumps; background is cloudy	2+
Button breaks into numerous tiny clumps; background is very cloudy	1+
Very fine agglutinates in a sea of free red cells	+/−
No visible agglutinates	Negative

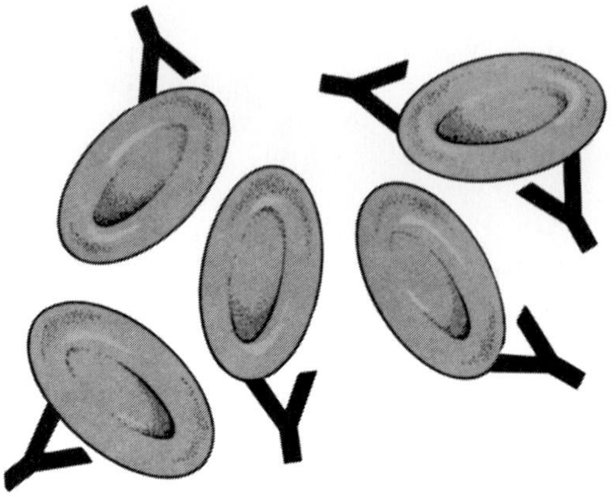

Figure 36–3. Sensitization of red blood cells by immunoglobulin G (IgG) antibodies. (From Stroup M, Treacy M. Blood Group Antigens and Antibodies. Raritan, NJ: Ortho Diagnostic Systems, Inc., 1982.)

they can be read and interpreted accurately with minimal training.

In 1955, a procedure for pretransfusion bedside confirmation of ABO group and Rh type was described by Eldon.[14] The method used cardboard cards with ABO and Rh antisera dried onto defined areas. Antisera were reconstituted with a drop of water and then mixed on the card with a measured amount of fresh whole blood. After 1 minute of incubation and 3 minutes of rotation, agglutination results were read and interpreted. Similar cards for bedside ABO grouping and Rh typing are currently marketed.

Slide hemagglutination procedures are commonly used for ABO grouping of potential blood donors. Liquid ABO reagents are dispensed onto separate areas of a glass microscope slide and mixed with fresh whole blood obtained by fingerstick. The slide is gently rotated for 2 minutes, then observed for agglutination.

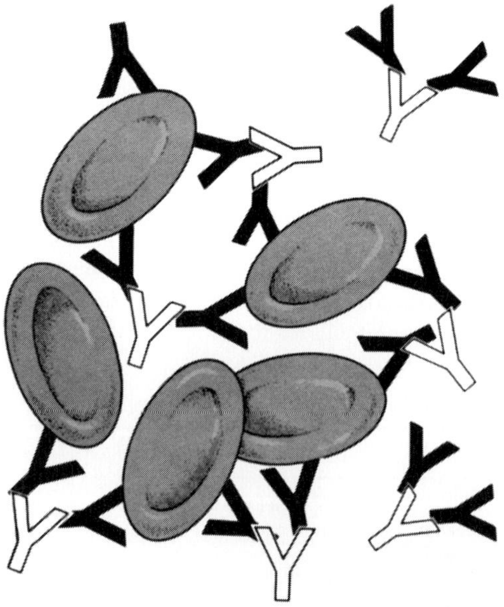

Figure 36–4. Antiglobulin reaction: IgG-sensitized red blood cells are agglutinated by antihuman serum. (From Stroup M, Treacy M. Blood Group Antigens and Antibodies. Raritan, NJ: Ortho Diagnostic Systems, Inc., 1982.)

Capillary Methods

In the 1940s, Chown and Lewis began using 0.4-mm glass capillary tubes to perform hemagglutination tests.[15] The main advantage of capillary testing is economy of RBCs and serum. The conservation of reagents was an important consideration at the time, because available quantities of rare cells and antisera were limited, and those that were commercially available were expensive. Capillary tests are performed by loading the tube with minute quantities of serum and RBCs and then inverting the tube and sealing the lower end by placing it in clay at a 45-degree angle. Agglutinates form as RBCs descend through the serum layer. A negative result is characterized by a smooth line of cells throughout the length of the tube, whereas a positive result appears as clumps, beads, or spirals of agglutinated cells. Reactions can be enhanced by flipping the capillary tubes to allow multiple passes, or trips. Capillary techniques have been described for virtually all pretransfusion compatibility tests.[16]

Microplate Methods

In 1962, Sever reported the use of 96-well conical and radial plastic microplates for virological hemagglutination procedures.[17] Between 1966 and 1968, Wegmann and Smithies[18, 19] and McCloskey and Zmijewski[20] used microplates for pretransfusion hemagglutination testing. Because microplate wells are analogous to small test tubes, the procedures are similar but require only microliter volumes of serum and RBCs. Reactants are mixed in the wells; then RBCs are pelleted by centrifugation or allowed to settle into discrete buttons. Agglutination is detected by tilting the microplates at a 75-degree angle for several minutes. Agglutinated cells remain clumped in the bottom of the wells, whereas nonagglutinated cells stream down the sides of the wells. Microplate methods have been described for ABO grouping, RBC phenotyping, and antibody screening, identification, and titration. The major advantage of microplate testing is economy of reagents and ease of handling when used for large-volume testing. Microplate systems may also be more amenable to automation than tube hemagglutination methods.

In 1986, Olympus Corporation introduced a novel terraced-well microplate design that featured wells with concentric rings engraved into the sides.[21] Upon standing, agglutinated RBCs settle evenly onto the terraces across the surface of the wells. Unagglutinated RBCs fall down the terraces, forming small buttons that are not easily dislodged during handling. Terraced wells eliminate the need for centrifugation, and results can be interpreted without tilting the plate. These unique features facilitated development of a fully automated microplate analyzer for ABO grouping and Rh typing. This instrument has also been adapted to perform pretransfusion infectious disease testing.

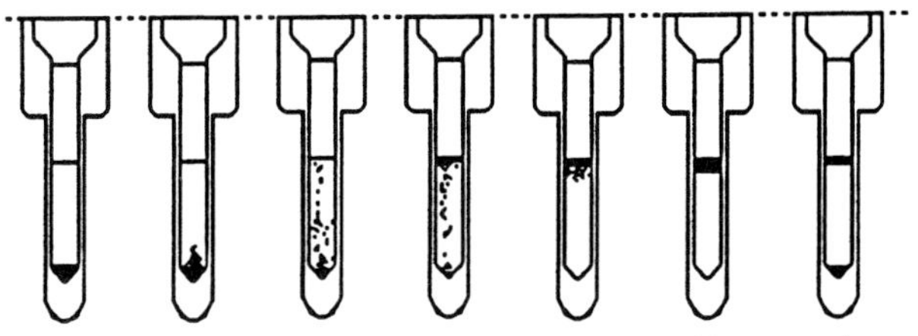

Figure 36–5. Gel test reaction patterns: negative reaction (0), positive reactions of increasing strength (1 to 5), and mixed field agglutination (+/−). (From LaPierre Y, Rigal D, Adam J, et al. The gel test: a new way to detect red cell antigen-antibody reactions. Transfusion 1990; 30:109.)

Gel Methods

A significant modification to standard hemagglutination techniques was described by LaPierre and coworkers in 1990.[22] Gel methods use specially designed microtubes that are wider at the top and form a narrow test tube at the bottom. The wider upper portion of the tube serves as an incubation chamber for serum and RBCs. The narrower lower part contains dextran acrylamide gel suspended in isotonic or low-ionic-strength solution (neutral gel), specific antisera (specific gel), or antiglobulin reagent (antiglobulin gel). Neutral gels are used solely for gradient separation of agglutinates by size exclusion. Upon centrifugation, strongly agglutinated RBCs are trapped in the upper part of the gel, and unagglutinated RBCs pass through the gel to pellet in the conical bottom of the tube. Weak agglutinates are dispersed throughout the gel. Mixed cell suspensions demonstrate a biphasic reaction. Reaction strength is graded as shown in Figure 36–5.

Specific gels are microtubes in which the gel is suspended in antisera, such as ABO grouping or Rh typing sera. RBCs are added to the reaction chamber; then microtubes are centrifuged to propel RBCs into contact with sera. As agglutinates form, they are trapped in the gel as previously described.

Antiglobulin gels contain gel suspended in antiglobulin solution. Serum and RBCs are added to the upper reaction chamber, and microtubes are incubated to allow sensitization. Alternatively, sensitized RBCs may be applied to the chamber. During centrifugation, sensitized RBCs are agglutinated by antiglobulin solution and become trapped in the gel. Unagglutinated cells pellet in the bottom of the tube. Antiglobulin gels differ from tube hemagglutination procedures, which require several wash steps after sensitization to remove unbound serum components before antiglobulin reagent is added. Because the gel is capable of separating RBCs from serum, no washing is required. Elimination of wash steps is a clear advantage in terms of labor and expense. In addition, gel antiglobulin tests do not require large quantities of saline for washing, and less biohazardous waste is generated. Tube antiglobulin procedures that produce negative results are validated by addition of IgG-sensitized RBCs, which ensures adequate washing and addition of antiglobulin reagent. This quality control procedure is unnecessary for gel tests. Additional advantages of gel tests are economy of sera and of RBCs and increased room temperature stability of reagents.

Centrifugation is a critical and comparatively lengthy step in gel procedures; the angle of rotation, speed, and duration must be strictly controlled by using specially designed centrifuges. For ease of handling, several microtubes are attached to rigid cards. Each card may contain a mixture of neutral, specific, or antiglobulin gels, depending on the intended use.

Gel methods have been developed for all aspects of pretransfusion compatibility testing, including ABO grouping; Rh typing; RBC phenotyping; antibody detection, identification, and titration; crossmatching; and fetomaternal hemorrhage.[23]

Column Agglutination Methods

In 1993, Reis and coworkers described column agglutination technology (CAT), a modification of the gel method that uses glass bead microparticles in place of dextran acrylamide gels.[24] CAT was originally described for antiglobulin testing only, but the system has been expanded to include ABO grouping, Rh typing, RBC phenotyping, antibody screening, and crossmatching.

Affinity Column Methods

Affinity column technology uses a similar microtube format to perform antiglobulin testing. Commercially prepared microtubes are attached to a plastic card for ease of handling. Serum and RBCs are added to an upper reaction chamber, which is separated from the microtube by a viscous barrier. After incubation, cards are centrifuged to propel RBCs through the barrier, which traps serum components. The microtube contains a protein G–agarose matrix that binds IgG-sensitized RBCs. Unsensitized RBCs pellet in the bottom of the microtube. This technology differs from other microtube formats in that the agarose matrix is immunologically active and acts as a solid-phase antiglobulin reactant.

SOLID-PHASE IMMUNOASSAYS

The immunoassays described thus far in this chapter are liquid-phase assays, in which antigen and antibody are present in liquid form and reactions take place in solution. During the first half of this century, liquid-phase reactions were the predominant format for immunological assays. Solid-phase immunoassays, in which either antigen or antibody is immobilized on a solid support, had not yet been developed. A solid phase is any solid surface capable of supporting an immunological reaction. Many solid phases have been used, including latex and paramagnetic particles, gels, all types of plastic tubes, microplates and beads, and paper membranes.

Solid-Phase Particle Assays

The first batch of uniform latex particles was inadvertently produced in 1947 by a scientist at Dow Chemical Company, a major manufacturer of polystyrene. Electron microscopy of a polystyrene latex suspension revealed that the particles were perfect spheres of identical diameter. This unexpected uniformity was unique to that particular lot of latex. Attempts to develop a second lot of uniform particles were unsuccessful until 1952, when the critical parameters were rediscovered.

In 1956, Singer and Plotz[25] introduced solid-phase serologic testing when they reported that latex particles passively adsorbed γ globulin and could be substituted for sheep erythrocytes in an agglutination test for rheumatoid arthritis. The particles were more stable and exhibited fewer nonspecific reactions than sheep erythrocytes. Several variables were investigated, including particle composition and size, buffer effects, temperature, quantity of γ globulin, order of reagent addition, and effect of centrifugation. A subsequent paper described the adaptation of latex particle agglutination to a more rapid slide method that used whole blood samples obtained by fingerstick.[26] In addition to direct agglutination assays, latex agglutination inhibition tests, analogous to hemagglutination inhibition, were developed.

Individual latex particles consist of polymers of polystyrene or other derivatives. Particles contain functional surface groups that serve as chemical side chains for protein coupling. They can be passively or covalently coated with proteins or other substances without altering their appearance or basic properties. Latex particle suspensions contain large numbers of uniform spheres with identical size, shape, and behavior. They are manufactured in sizes ranging from 0.018 to 1000 μm in diameter. A variety of colors and intensities are available, from pastels to dark shades to black. Paramagnetic particles are polystyrene particles with incorporated iron particles. They are also available in a wide range of sizes with a variety of functional surface groups. Paramagnetic particles are attractive solid-phase supports for automated systems because they can be removed from solution by a magnet, thus eliminating the requirement for centrifugation.

Latex agglutination methods are currently used in more than 100 immunoassays marketed by nearly as many manufacturers. In the field of transfusion medicine, latex tests are available for hepatitis B surface antigen (HBsAg), cytomegalovirus (CMV), and human immunodeficiency virus type 1 (HIV-1) antibody detection.

Solid-Phase Red Cell Adherence Assays

In 1959, Högman performed the first solid-phase red cell adherence (SPRCA) assay when he added ABO antisera to the surface of human embryonic kidney tissue cells grown as monolayers in glass test tubes.[27, 28] A and B antigens were detected on tissues that had corresponding RBC antigen expression.

In 1961, Fagraeus and Espmark described the technique of mixed hemadsorption, which introduced sheep RBCs coated with antiglobulin reagent as a solid-phase reagent.[29, 30] This novel indicator system combined the intense color of RBCs with the versatility of antiglobulin reagent. In 1972, Juji and coworkers used mixed hemadsorption to detect antigens on platelets and platelet antibodies in human sera.[31] For testing in their solid-phase RBC antiglobulin indicator system, platelets were immobilized on glass tubes or slides. The use of antiglobulin-coated indicator RBCs was also advocated by Coombs, who used chromium chloride to directly couple specific antiglobulin reagents or other proteins to RBCs.[32]

Rosenfield and colleagues were the first investigators to describe solid-phase techniques for routine pretransfusion compatibility tests.[33] Their system used RBC monolayers bound to plastic test tubes. The RBC monolayer was used to adsorb specific antibody from solution. The antigenic composition of the RBC monolayer and the antibody specificity varied for each test.

In the 1980s, SPRCA immunoassays were developed as an alternative to liquid-phase hemagglutination for pretransfusion testing.[35] These methods use U-bottom polystyrene microplate wells as the solid phase and RBCs as the indicator system. For each assay, addition of test or indicator RBCs followed by centrifugation produces a pattern of RBC effacement over the surface of the well (positive reaction) or a discrete pellet in the bottom of the well (negative reaction). Assays for ABO grouping, Rh typing, RBC and platelet antibody screening and crossmatching, IgA-deficiency screening, HIV-1 antibody, CMV antibody, HBsAg, and syphilis serologic testing have been described. Table 36–2 summarizes the solid-phase reactant and indicator RBCs for each SPRCA assay.

To prepare solid phases for antigen testing, antibodies are passively adsorbed onto microplate wells (Fig. 36–6). ABO cell grouping and Rh typing require only centrifugation after addition of test RBCs to antibody-coated wells. For antibody detection assays, RBCs, platelets, or microbial antigens are bound to wells (Fig. 36–7). Test serum is added and incubated to allow antibody to bind to the solid phase. Unbound serum components are removed by washing. Bound antibody is detected by addition of indicator RBCs, followed by centrifugation.

Screening for HBsAg uses specific antibody bound to the wells. Antigen contained in test serum binds to solid-phase antibody and then subsequently binds anti-HBsAg–coated RBCs to produce a positive reaction.

Syphilis serologic testing uses a modified Venereal

Table 36–2. Solid-Phase Reactants and Indicator RBCs for Solid-Phase Red Cell Adherence Assays

Test	Solid-Phase Reactant	Indicator RBCs
ABO cell grouping	Anti-A or anti-B	Patient/donor
Rh typing	Anti-D	Patient/donor
ABO serum grouping	A or B membranes	A and B
Red cell antibody	O membranes	Anti-IgG–coated
Platelet antibody	Platelets	Anti-IgG–coated
HBsAg	Anti-HBsAg	Anti-HBsAg–coated
HIV-1 antibody	Viral antigens	Anti-IgG–coated
CMV antibody	Viral antigens	Anti-IgG + M–coated
IgA	Anti-IgA	IgA-coated
Syphilis	VDRL antigen	Anti-IgG + M–coated

CMV, cytomegalovirus; HBsAg, hepatitis B surface antigen; HIV, human immunodeficiency virus; Ig, immunoglobulin; RBC, red blood cell; VDRL, Venereal Disease Research Laboratory.

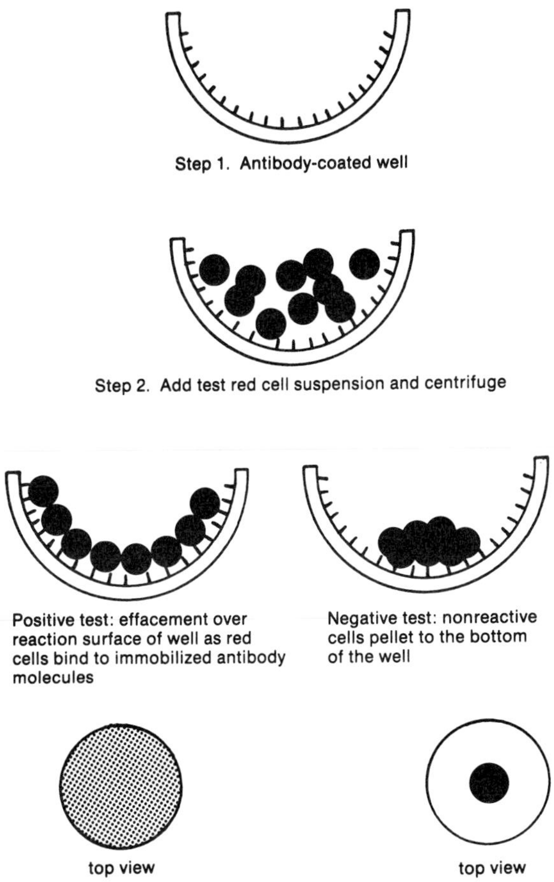

Figure 36–6. Solid-phase red-cell adherence (SPRCA) assays for antigen detection. (From Rolih SD. New frontiers in serologic testing. *In* Wallace CH, McCarthy LJ [eds]: New Frontiers in Blood Banking. Arlington, VA: American Association of Blood Banks, 1986, p 138.)

Disease Research Laboratory (VDRL) antigen bound to the solid phase, which detects reagin antibodies. Serum or plasma is added to wells and incubated to allow binding to solid-phase antigen. Bound antibody is detected by addition of anti-IgG– and anti-IgM–coated RBCs.[35]

For IgA-deficiency screening, microplate wells are coated with anti-IgA, which binds IgA in the test serum.[36] Reactions are detected by adding IgA-coated RBCs. Sera that lack sufficient IgA to neutralize the solid-phase antibody demonstrate a positive reaction.

These SPRCA immunoassays are commercially available for platelet and RBC antibody screening. An automated system for pretransfusion testing uses SPRCA technology. In another SPRCA method for pretransfusion antibody screening and identification, sensitization takes place in uncoated microplate wells. RBCs are then washed, resuspended in polyspecific antiglobulin reagent, and transferred into microplate wells pretreated to bind IgG. Sensitized RBCs adhere to the wells upon centrifugation, and unsensitized RBCs pellet in the bottom of the wells.

IMMUNOFLUORESCENCE

Fluorescence occurs when a molecule absorbs light at one wavelength and emits it at a longer wavelength. In the early 1940s, methods were developed for conjugating fluorescent dyes to antibody molecules. The dyes most commonly used are fluorescein isothiocyanate (fluorescein or FITC), which emits green light, and tetramethylrhodamine isothiocyanate (rhodamine or TRITC), which emits red light. An ultraviolet light is used to excite the conjugates, and emitted light is observed microscopically.

Fluorescence immunoassays detect antigens or antibodies, either directly or indirectly. Direct immunofluorescence is most commonly used for antigen detection. Labeled antibody is added to immobilized cell or tissue samples. After incubation, binding of labeled antibody to antigen in the test sample is detected directly by fluorescence microscopy. Indirect immunofluorescence is generally used for antibody detection. Test sample is added to cells or tissues that express the antigen, and antibody binding is detected indirectly by addition of labeled anti-immunoglobulin.

Fluorescence immunoassays were a significant improvement over agglutination and precipitation methods. The development of labeled antibody conjugates provided a direct means of visualizing primary antigen-antibody reactions that did not require lattice formation. The indirect immunofluorescence method was an extension of the

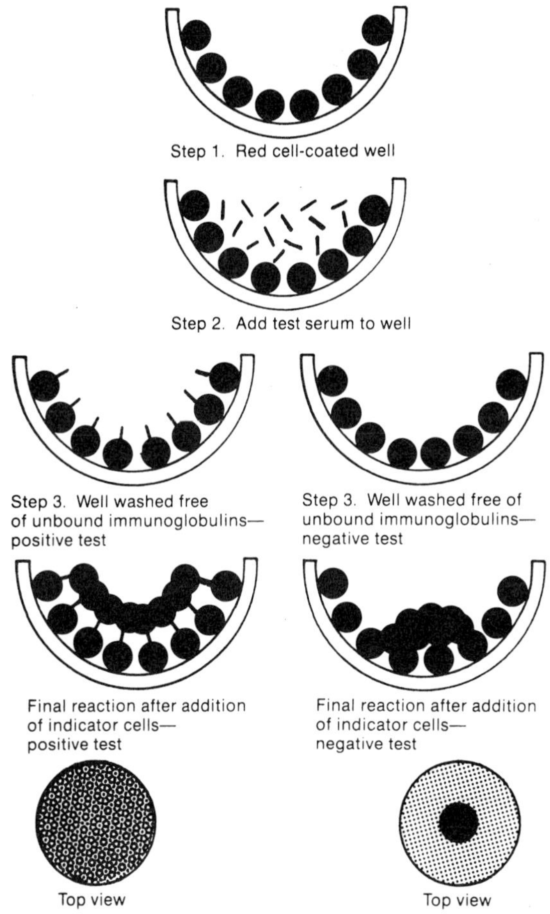

Figure 36–7. SPRCA assays for red blood cell (RBC) antibody detection. (From Rolih SD. New frontiers in serologic testing. *In* Wallace CH, McCarthy LJ [eds]: New Frontiers in Blood Banking. Arlington, VA: American Association of Blood Banks, 1986, p 140.)

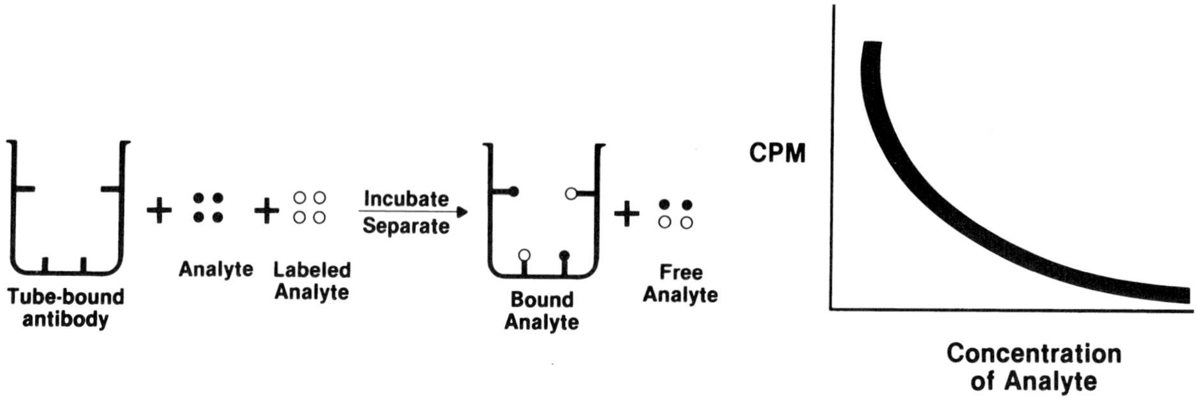

Figure 36–8. Radioimmunoassay (RIA) by competitive inhibition. CPM, counts per minute. (From Shamel LB. The immunoradiometric assay. Am Clin Prod Rev 1983; 2[6]:44. Copyright 1983 by International Scientific Communications, Inc.)

antiglobulin technique and was an important step because it introduced the concept of labeling immune reactants for use in immunoassay procedures.

Most immunofluorescence assays involve solid-phase attachment of cells to glass slides for microscopic analysis and interpretation. One advantage of these methods is their ability to correlate cell morphology with antibody-induced fluorescence. A significant disadvantage is the requirement for visual examination and interpretation of results, which is time-consuming, tedious, and difficult to standardize. In addition, a relatively small number of cells is analyzed.

Flow Cytometry

Flow cytometry is one of the most sophisticated adaptations of liquid-phase technology. The basic principle of flow cytometry is direct immunofluorescence. However, instead of observing fluorescence of single cells under a microscope, fluorescence is detected using a flow cytometer. The instrument arranges cells in a fluid stream so that they pass rapidly through a laser beam in single file. Flow rates can approach several thousand cells per second. Light scattered and emitted by white blood cells (WBCs) is evaluated by a series of filters, mirrors, and detectors and then converted into a digital signal and displayed as frequency distribution data. Thousands of individual cells can be analyzed for cell size, granularity, and fluorescence.

WBC phenotyping is accomplished by mixing whole blood with fluorescence-labeled WBC monoclonal antibodies, usually specific for cell surface molecules termed CD (cluster designation) antigens.[37] After an incubation period, RBCs are lysed to eliminate interference, and sensitized WBC suspensions are analyzed by flow cytometry. In addition to WBC phenotyping, flow cytometry has been used to phenotype platelets, detect WBC and platelet antibodies, and quantitate stem cells in peripheral blood stem cell collections. It has also been used for direct antiglobulin testing and investigating minor RBC populations, including fetomaternal hemorrhage.[38]

RADIOIMMUNOASSAYS

Radioimmunoassay (RIA) was developed in 1959 by Berson and Yalow[39] as a means of measuring small quantities of biological molecules. RIA is based on the principle of competitive inhibition (Fig. 36–8). Antigen in a test sample competes with radioactively labeled antigen for a limited number of antibody-binding sites. Labeled and unlabeled antigens bind equally, so unlabeled antigen in the sample inhibits binding of labeled antigen. After incubation, bound and free labeled antigen moieties are separated, and bound radioactivity is measured in a scintillation or gamma counter. Antigen concentration in the sample is inversely proportional to the amount of bound radioactive antigen, as indicated in Figure 36–8. Results are quantitated by plotting radioactivity on a dose-response curve constructed from standards with known antigen concentrations.

The original RIA technique had two major limitations. The first was that the reaction was carried out in liquid phase and antigen-antibody complexes had to be separated from free labeled antigen before measurement of bound antigen. Separation of small unbound molecules was achieved by charcoal adsorption. In assays for high-molecular-weight proteins or glycoproteins, labeled complexes were precipitated with a second xenogeneic anti-immunoglobulin antibody. In either case, separation required multiple centrifugation and wash steps that were labor-intensive and time-consuming and often resulted in loss of immune complexes.

A major improvement in RIA procedures came in 1967, when Catt and Tregear[40] discovered that plastic test tubes passively adsorb antigens and antibodies. They described a solid-phase RIA technique that uses antibody bound to the inner surface of polypropylene or polystyrene test tubes. Centrifugation steps are eliminated because antigen-antibody complexes immobilized on the plastic surface are easily separated from unbound antigen by simply filling tubes with wash solution and decanting. The use of antibody-coated test tubes is simple, rapid, inexpensive, and amenable to automation. Later solid-phase techniques used large plastic beads rather than tubes as the solid phase. Beads provide more surface area for the solid-phase reaction, thereby accelerating antigen-antibody binding and decreasing incubation times.

The second limitation of classical RIA techniques is the need for radioactive labeling of relatively large quantities of highly purified antigen. The labeling process sometimes alters the antigen's structure, so that antibody binds to labeled antigen and unlabeled antigen with different affinities. Detection limits of RIA procedures are ultimately determined by antibody affinity, so structural changes that influence binding markedly affect sensitivity.

IMMUNORADIOMETRIC ASSAYS

In 1968, Miles and Hales[41] reported an immunoradiometric assay (IRMA) in which antibody, rather than antigen, is radioactively labeled. IRMAs are also called double-antibody or two-site "sandwich" assays, because they employ a combination of solid-phase antibody and labeled antibody (Fig. 36–9). The solid-phase antibody is coated onto plastic tubes in high enough concentrations to bind all antigen in test samples. The addition of sample and an excess of radioactively labeled second antibody results in a "sandwich" that contains antigen bound between labeled and solid-phase antibodies. Unbound labeled antibody is removed by washing. Radioactivity bound to the solid phase is directly proportional to antigen concentration in the sample. This construct is the opposite of classical RIA, which demonstrates an inverse relationship between bound radioactivity and antigen concentration.

Several IRMA variants have been described. The simplest but least sensitive is the simultaneous assay just described, in which all reactants are incubated together. This procedure is not suitable for steroids, most drugs, and small peptides. Alternatively, a two-step protocol can be used in which antigen is incubated with either solid-phase or radiolabeled antibody before the addition of second antibody.

IRMAs offer several advantages over RIAs. Labeled antibodies are more stable than labeled antigens, so antibody affinity and test performance are less variable. The use of labeled antibody is more economical, because antibodies are usually available in much larger quantities than are antigens. Also, the common properties of immunoglobulins permit use of a single reagent or labeling procedure for different assays. IRMA reactions proceed more quickly to completion and have better sensitivity, because antibody is present in excess and traps all antigen in the reaction. Specificity is also improved by the combined selectivity of two antibodies, either monoclonal or polyclonal, that recognize different epitopes on the same molecule. First-generation immunoassays for HBsAg were based on IRMA.

RIA and IRMA techniques are sensitive, specific, precise, and versatile. However, techniques that use radioactive isotopes have serious disadvantages. Reagents are costly and have short shelf lives. Instruments that measure radioactivity are expensive. Potential health hazards are associated with handling and disposal of radioactive waste. Because of these limitations, considerable effort has been expended to develop nonisotopic labels for antigens and antibodies.

ENZYME IMMUNOASSAYS

The first nonisotopic alternative, enzyme immunoassay (EIA), was introduced in the early 1970s by Engvall and Perlmann.[42] The novel feature of EIAs is the detection system, which consists of enzymes covalently conjugated to antigens or antibodies in such a way that the conjugate retains both immunological and enzymatic activity. EIAs have been given many names, including *enzyme-linked immunoassay, immunoenzymatic assay,* and *enzyme-linked immunosorbent assay.* Three major types of EIA were originally described (Table 36–3),[43] but many different variations exist. They differ largely in the choice of solid-phase support and end point detection system. Solid-phase supports can be tubes, large or small latex beads, microplates, membranes, paramagnetic particles, or single-use devices. Detection systems include visible color, fluorescence, and chemiluminescence.

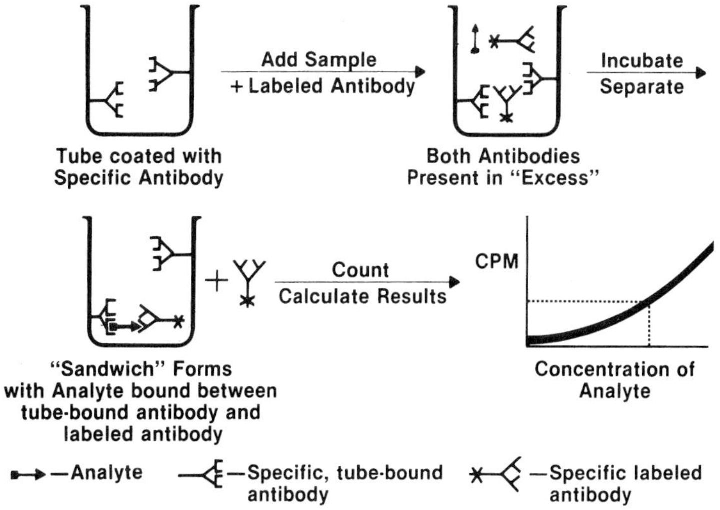

Figure 36–9. Immunoradiometric assay (IRMA). CPM, counts per minute. (From Shamel LB. The immunoradiometric assay. Am Clin Prod Rev 1983; 2[6]:44. Copyright 1983 by International Scientific Communications, Inc.)

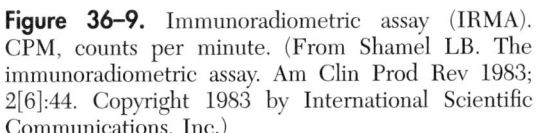

Table 36–3. Enzyme Immunoassay Formats

Assay Type	Substance Being Assayed	Solid-Phase Component	Labeled Component
Competitive	Antigen	Antibody	Antigen
Immunometric	Antigen	Antibody	Antibody
Indirect	Antibody	Antigen	Anti-immunoglobulin

EIA Formats

The first major type of EIA is the competitive EIA, which measures antigen and is analogous to classical RIA. Antibody bound to a solid phase is incubated with test sample and enzyme-labeled antigen, which compete for a limited number of antibody-binding sites. After incubation, unbound antigen is removed by washing. Labeled antigen bound to the solid phase is detected by adding substrate and measuring color development. The presence of unlabeled antigen in the test sample decreases the binding of labeled antigen to the solid phase. Therefore, antigen concentration in the sample is inversely proportional to the intensity of color development. The primary disadvantage of this procedure, as with RIA, is the need to purify and label large quantities of antigen. Also, competitive immunoassays are relatively slow and require long incubation times to reach equilibrium. This problem has been partially solved by the use of kinetic measurements that assess the initial rate of reaction. Competitive EIA is most effective for measuring small-sample analytes such as drugs or hormones. One of the original screening tests for HIV-1 antibody in Europe was a competitive EIA.

An alternative EIA for antigen detection is the immunometric or double-antibody "sandwich" method, which is analogous to IRMA. An excess of capture monoclonal or polyclonal antibody, specific to the antigen of interest, is adsorbed to a solid-phase support. Test sample and excess enzyme-labeled signal antibody are added, either simultaneously or sequentially. If antigen is present in the sample, it is captured by the solid-phase antibody at a unique epitope. The signal antibody binds antigen at a different epitope, forming a sandwich. After washing to remove unbound reactants, substrate is added and color development is measured. Color intensity is directly proportional to antigen concentration in the test sample. The advantages of this method are similar to those cited for IRMA. Current screening tests for HBsAg use this format.

A variation of the immunometric EIA is the capture assay. An example of this format is the syphilis IgG enzyme immunoassay for qualitative detection of IgG antibodies to *Treponema pallidum*. Anti–human IgG is attached to microplate wells to capture IgG in donor serum. Purified *T. pallidum* antigen is added, which reacts with bound IgG antibodies directed toward *T. pallidum*. An enzyme-labeled monoclonal antibody to *T. pallidum* and substrate are then added to detect anti–*T. pallidum* IgG–antigen complexes.

Indirect EIA measures antibody that reacts with antigen bound to a solid phase. Reactions are detected by enzyme-labeled anti-immunoglobulin and substrate. Color intensity is proportional to antibody concentration in the sample. Current tests for antibodies to HIV-1 and -2, human T cell lymphotropic virus (HTLV)-I and -II antibody, and hepatitis C virus and hepatitis B core antigen use this format.

Another example of indirect EIA that is used to detect platelet-specific antibodies is the monoclonal antibody-specific immobilization of platelet antigens (MAIPA) assay.[44] In this procedure, washed platelets are first incubated with monoclonal antibody specific for a platelet glycoprotein antigen. The targeted glycoprotein is then released from the membrane by solubilization with nonionic detergent. The solubilized fraction is added to microplate wells coated with goat anti–mouse IgG, which captures the glycoprotein antigen–monoclonal antibody complexes. In this way, specific platelet antigens are immobilized on a solid-phase support. Patient serum is then added to the well. If platelet antibody is present, it binds to immobilized platelet glycoprotein. Bound antibody is detected by adding enzyme-labeled goat anti–human IgG and substrate. A color change indicates a positive reaction. By using a set of monoclonal antibodies recognizing different platelet membrane antigens, the specificity of human platelet antibodies can be determined in a single procedure.

A solid-phase EIA based on MAIPA is commercially available for detection of human leukocyte antigen (HLA) class I and platelet-specific antibodies. Microplate wells are precoated with purified glycoprotein and HLAs. Test serum or platelet eluate is added to each well, followed by labeled anti–human IgG and substrate.

Enzyme Conjugates and Substrates

The most suitable enzymes for labeling antibodies are those that conjugate easily without loss of activity, convert substrate rapidly to stable products, lack interference from biological fluids, and produce products that are read spectrophotometrically at common wavelengths. Horseradish peroxidase (HRP) and alkaline phosphatase (ALP) are most commonly used. HRP is inexpensive, readily available, and simple to conjugate, and it metabolizes substrate rapidly (300 molecules per second). ALP shares many of these properties but converts substrate at a more rapid rate (1450 molecules per second).

Characteristics of the most common substrates for ALP and HRP are listed in Table 36–4. Insoluble or partially soluble end products are acceptable for qualitative EIA procedures that are read and interpreted visually. Quantitative EIAs require soluble end products and spectrophotometric readout. Ortho-phenylenediamine (OPD) may be the best substrate for HRP because it is readily soluble and has high absorptivity, which is a measure of

Table 36–4. Enzyme Substrates

Enzyme	Substrate	Product Solubility	Color	Wavelength (nm)
Horseradish peroxidase	ABTS	Soluble	Blue-green	415
	OPD	Soluble	Orange	492
	TMB	Soluble	Yellow with acid	450
			Blue without acid	655
	Iodophane	Soluble	Violet	540
	5AS	Partially soluble	Brown	449
	4CN	Insoluble	Purple	
	DAB	Insoluble	Brown	
	AEC	Insoluble	Red	
	Pyronin	Insoluble	Red	
Alkaline phosphatase	PNPP	Soluble	Yellow	405
	BCIP	Insoluble	Purple	
	NBT	Insoluble	Purple	
	Fast red	Insoluble	Rose	
	NP-ADPDS	Insoluble	Brown	
	NASMXP red	Insoluble	Red	
	NASMXP blue	Insoluble	Blue	

ABTS, 2,2′-azinobis-(3-ethylbenzthiazolone-6-sulfonic acid); AEC, 3-amino-9-ethyl carbazole; 5AS, 5-aminosalicylic acid; BCIP, 5-bromo-4-chloro-3-indolyl phosphate; 4CN, 4-chloro-1-naphthol; DAB, 3,3′-diaminobenzidine; NASMXP red or blue, naphthol-AS-MX phosphate with fast red TR or blue; NBT, nitroblue tetrazolium; NP-ADPDS, alpha-naphthyl phosphate and 4-aminodiphenylamine diszonium sulfate; OPD, ortho-phenylenediamine; PNPP, para-nitrophenyl phosphate; TMB, tetramethylbenzidine.

the amount of light energy absorbed by a solution. Although less sensitive, 2,2′-azinobis-(3-ethylbenzthiazolone-6-sulfonic acid) (ABTS) is more stable in light. The most commonly used ALP substrate is para-nitrophenyl phosphate (PNPP), which is readily available and sensitive enough for most immunoassays.

Measurement of enzyme activity by fluorometry and luminometry can increase EIA sensitivity, but these methods require more sophisticated instrumentation than spectrophotometry. The relative sensitivity of these detection systems is as follows: chemiluminescence>fluorescence>colorimetry. The most common fluorogenic substrate for ALP is 4-methylumbelliferyl phosphate, which increases sensitivity 3 to 100 times over that with use of standard colorimetric substrates (Table 36–5). This fluorogenic substrate is employed in many immunoassay analyzers.

Luminescent substrates have also been used to increase EIA sensitivity and dynamic range.[45] Luminescence is simply the conversion of energy into light. It occurs when a molecule is excited to a higher energy level by an oxidative reaction and then emits light upon returning to the resting state. The intensity of emitted light is measured by a luminometer, which consists of a photomultiplier detector, a microplate or tube holder, and a microprocessor. For every photon of light striking the surface of the photomultiplier, there is a millionfold electronic amplification of the signal.

Table 36–5. Relative Sensitivities of Different Enzyme Labeling Systems

	Detection Limit (mol/L)	
Detection System	**Horseradish Peroxidase**	**Alkaline Phosphatase**
Colorimetry	2×10^{-15}	5×10^{-17}
Fluorimetry	6×10^{-15}	5×10^{-19}
Bioluminescence	4×10^{-19}	1×10^{-20}
Chemiluminescence	2×10^{-17}	1×10^{-21}

Bioluminescence and chemiluminescence refer to biological and chemical reactions, respectively, that result in emission of light. Bioluminescent EIAs use a natural substrate, firefly D-luciferin-*O*-phosphate. ALP cleaves the phosphate group to produce D-luciferin, which reacts with firefly luciferase and adenosine triphosphate (ATP) to produce light. The detection limit for ALP with this substrate is in the range of 10^{-20} M (see Table 36–5).

The traditional chemiluminescent HRP substrate is luminol. In the presence of hydrogen peroxide, HRP catalyzes oxidation of luminol to produce radicals, which decay to ground state and emit light (Fig. 36–10). Enhancers such as benzothiazoles, phenols, or naphthols significantly improve the "signal-to-noise" ratio by increasing the intensity of emitted light and decreasing background emission. Emitted light is extremely stable, allowing measurement up to 30 minutes after initiation of the reaction. Sensitivity is in the range of 10^{-17} M (see Table 36–5).

A very popular chemiluminescent substrate for ALP is adamantyl 1,2-dioxetane phosphate (AMPPD).[45] ALP cleaves the phosphate group from dioxetane, destabilizing the molecule and causing it to decompose (see Fig. 36–10). Energy stored in the dioxetane ring is released as a long-lived light emission rather than a quick flash. This chemiluminescent assay for ALP is very sensitive, with a detection limit of 10^{-21} M (see Table 36–5). AMPPD is used in another immunoassay system that is used to test for antibody to CMV in the United States and for HBsAg and core antigen in other countries.

By studying bioluminescence, investigators were eventually able to synthesize molecules, such as acridinium esters, that emit light in vitro without an enzyme catalyst.[46] This molecule decomposes in the presence of hydrogen peroxide and sodium hydroxide to give a flash of light that lasts for less than 5 seconds (see Fig. 36–10).

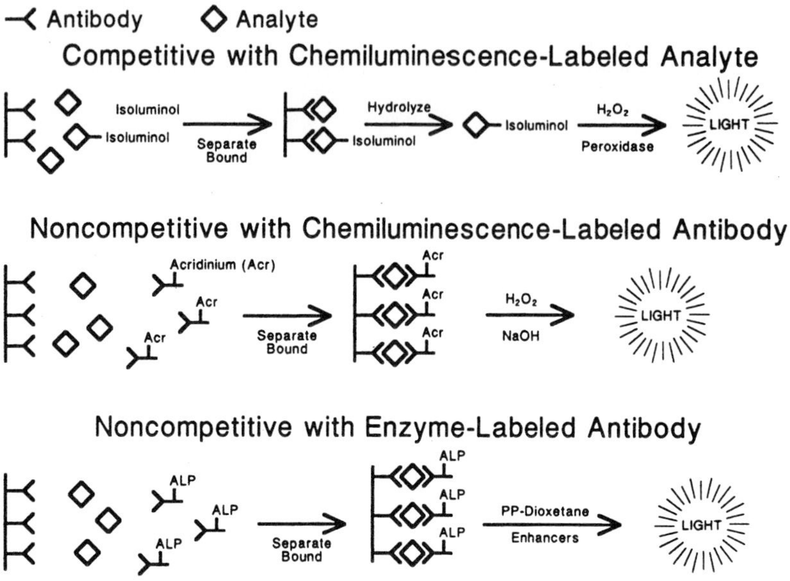

Figure 36–10. Examples of chemiluminescent reactions with isoluminol and HRP (*top*), acridinium ester (*middle*), and dioxetane and alkaline phosphatase (*bottom*). (From Stabler TV. Chemiluminescence. Clin Chem News 1991; 17[October]:12.)

Acridinium esters offer several advantages over luminol, including greater sensitivity (10^{-21} M) and less protein interference.

Microparticle Enzyme Immunoassay

Microparticle enzyme immunoassay (MEIA) incorporates many features of classical enzyme immunoassays: a double-antibody sandwich format, an enzyme label, and a colorimetry or fluorometry detection system. Its distinguishing characteristic is the use of submicron microparticles that provide increased surface area for antigen-antibody reactions. Incubation times are shorter because of increased reaction kinetics.

For MEIA assays, microparticles are coated with antibody directed toward the antigen of interest. Test sample is added to a suspension of microparticles and incubated to allow binding of antigen to solid-phase antibody. Following incubation, the reaction mixture is transferred to a glass fiber membrane. Microparticles bind irreversibly to the membrane, whereas other constituents pass through unimpeded. Following a wash step to remove unbound proteins, enzyme-labeled second antibody is added. If antigen is present in the sample, enzyme-labeled antibody binds to immobilized antigen, forming a sandwich. Substrate is then added, and the product of the enzymatic reaction is detected either fluorometrically or colorimetrically. Signal intensity is directly proportional to the amount of antigen in the test sample. An automated immnunoassay analyzer is available that uses microparticles and chemiluminescence detection to screen donor sera for infectious diseases.[47] Serum samples are tested simultaneously for the following infectious disease markers: HTLV-I and -II antibody, hepatitis C virus antibody, HIV-1 and -2 antibody, HIV-1 group O antibody, HBsAg, and hepatitis B core antibody. Microparticles are coated with monoclonal antibody for the HBsAg assay and recombinant antigens for antibody assays. Donor serum and microparticles are incubated in an incubation well and then transferred to a detection well, where a porous matrix captures the microparticles. After washing, acridinium-labeled second antibody is added, the acridinium label is activated, and emitted light photons are counted. This instrument has been used by blood centers outside the United States for donor screening since February 1996.

MEMBRANE ENZYME IMMUNOASSAYS

The assays previously discussed use polystyrene tubes, large polystyrene beads, microparticles, or microplate wells as solid-phase components in EIA. These materials are widely used because of their optical clarity, which is ideal for quantitative spectrophotometric analysis. They are also ideal for handling large numbers of test samples. However, immobilization of immune reactants on these relatively large surface areas requires proportionately large amounts of antigen or antibody. When only qualitative analysis is needed or the supply of immune reactants is limited, other solid-phase matrices are preferable. Membranes have become a popular alternative.

Membrane EIA procedures offer several advantages over classical EIA methods. They are simple, reliable, and optimally designed for low-volume tests that require only a qualitative visual readout. The amount of antigen or antibody required for immobilization is minimal. A wide variety of macromolecules bind with high affinity and no loss of immune activity, even after drying and storage. Labile proteins often stabilize when bound to membranes. Precision and sensitivity are increased because protein loss during washing steps is minimized. Weak positive reactions are easily interpreted because the final color reaction is viewed against a white background rather than translucent plastic.

Dot Immunobinding

In 1982, Hawkes and colleagues[48] and Herbrink and associates[49] independently reported dot immunobinding assays for antibody detection. Dot immunobinding is commonly referred to as dot blotting, but the terms *spot immunodetection* and *antigen spot detection* are synonymous. This technique involves direct spot application of minute quantities of antigen (1 μL) to a small area of membrane (Fig. 36–11). Unoccupied membrane sites are blocked to reduce nonspecific binding, and test sample is applied to the prepared area. The binding of antibody to immobilized antigen is detected by EIA with an insoluble chromogenic substrate. Positive reactions appear as colored dots at the site of antigen application, and negative reactions remain colorless.

Antigens that bind to membranes include proteins, glycoproteins, glycolipids, polysaccharides, intact cells, cell membranes, nucleic acids, bacteria, viruses, and yeasts.[50] Dot immunobinding assays can also detect antigens using a double-antibody sandwich format.[51]

Different types of membranes can be used as the solid phase. Positively charged nylon has the highest protein-binding capacity (500 μg/cm^2), but nonspecific binding is also high. Nitrocellulose membranes, which bind proteins almost irreversibly through hydrophobic interactions, are most commonly used for dot blotting. Their binding capacity is 90 μg/cm^2.

A variety of procedures are used to detect antigens or antibodies bound immunologically to membranes. The enzyme-conjugated reagent may be primary antibody, secondary antibody, or streptavidin. The amount of conjugate that binds to immune complexes on the membrane determines signal intensity. Primary-antibody conjugate systems exhibit the least nonspecific staining but are also the least sensitive. Secondary-antibody conjugates react with multiple sites on each primary antibody, as do streptavidin conjugates, thereby amplifying the signal and increasing sensitivity. Labeling of secondary antibody or streptavidin also eliminates the need for single-specificity primary-antibody conjugates, but this advantage must be weighed against the higher number of steps and longer assay times.

Solubility of the end product is an important determinant of dot blot sensitivity. Because completely soluble products migrate away from the reaction site, color intensity and resolution are decreased. When the end product is completely insoluble, enzyme activity is smothered by product deposition at the reaction site. The preferred substrate for HRP is 4-chloro-1-naphthol (4CN), because of its high sensitivity and low background staining. ALP conjugates with 5-bromo-4-chloro-3-indolyl phosphate–nitroblue tetrazolium (BCIP-NBT) substrate achieve similar sensitivity without excessive background staining.

Immunoblotting (Western Blotting)

Although dot immunobinding is a simple and efficient technique for detecting antigens or antibodies, it cannot identify specific antigens within a complex mixture. Prior separation of protein or glycoprotein antigens by electrophoresis allows individual reactions with specific antibodies to be detected.

The development of immunoblotting (Western blot-

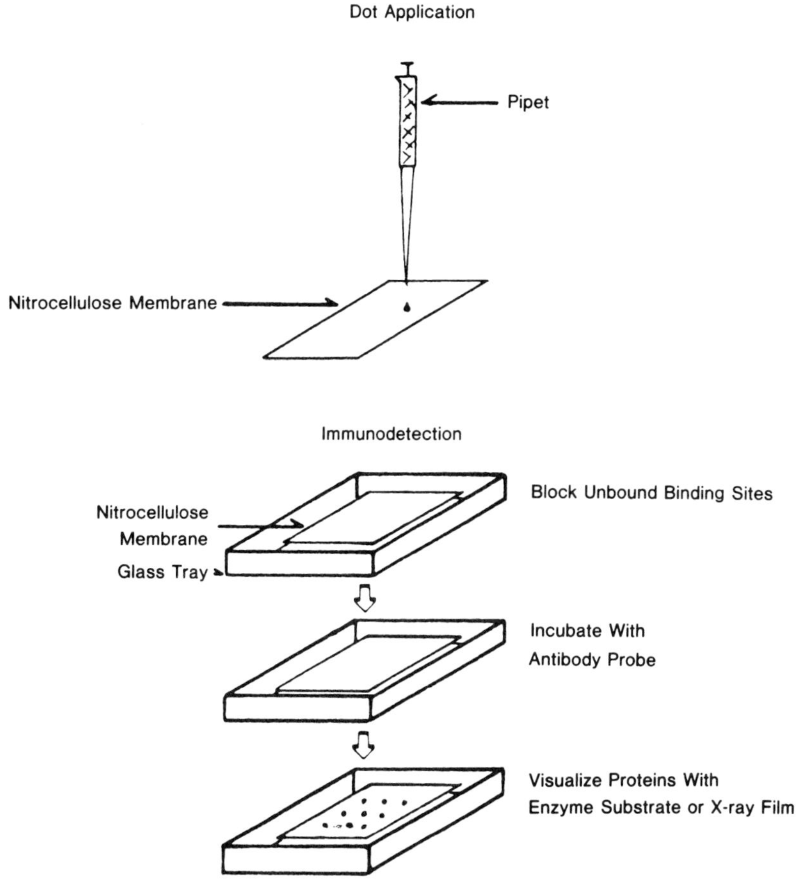

Figure 36–11. Dot immunobinding assay. (From Renner SW. Immunoblotting and dot immunobinding. Arch Pathol Lab Med 1988; 112:780–786. Copyright 1988, American Medical Association.)

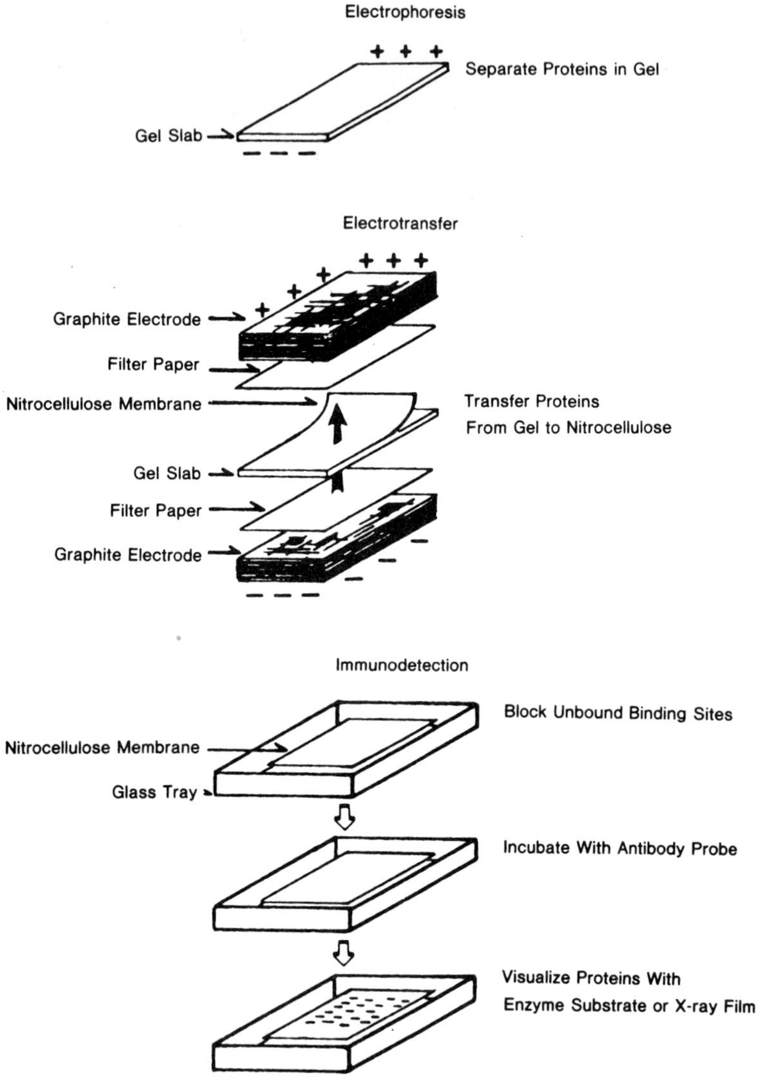

Figure 36–12. Immunoblotting (Western blotting) technique with electrophoretic transfer. (From Renner SW. Immunoblotting and dot immunobinding. Arch Pathol Lab Med 1988; 112:780–786. Copyright 1988, American Medical Association.)

ting) by Renart and colleagues[52] and Towbin and associates[53] in 1979 revolutionized immunological detection of separated proteins. With this technique, proteins are first separated in a gel by electrophoresis and then transferred onto a membrane. The transfer step concentrates and immobilizes separated proteins on a flat surface (membrane) that is easier to handle, more durable, and more accessible to antibody than a gel. The term *blotting* is used because the transfer method produces an exact membrane replica of the separated antigen bands in the gel.

The simplest technique for blotting proteins from gels to membranes is diffusion.[50] Membranes are laid on both sides of a gel and immersed in buffer for 36 to 48 hours. Proteins diffuse outward in both directions to produce replicate blots. The disadvantage to this approach is that transfer is not quantitative and band resolution is lost during the lengthy time required for diffusion. This problem can be partially overcome by inducing solvent flow, with or without a vacuum pump, to accelerate and focus protein transfer in one direction toward a single membrane. This modification works well for agarose gels, but transfer from polyacrylamide gels is less satisfactory.

Electrophoretic transfer, as illustrated in Figure 36–12, is the most rapid and quantitative method for blotting proteins from polyacrylamide gels. A gel and wet membrane are laid together between buffer-saturated filter paper and sponge pads. This "sandwich" is clamped together and inserted into an electrotransfer apparatus. Electric current flowing through aqueous buffer causes charged protein molecules to migrate from the gel onto the membrane. Electrophoretic blotting onto nitrocellulose is usually performed in buffers containing 20% methanol, which prevents gel swelling and increases protein binding to membranes. Nitrocellulose membranes with a pore size of 0.45 μm are most commonly used, but low-molecular-weight proteins may require a pore size of 0.1 or 0.2 μm. After protein transfer, unoccupied membrane binding sites must be blocked with an inert protein solution to prevent nonspecific binding of antibody.

When clinical samples are being assayed for specific antibody, the primary antibody source is patient sera. If blotted antigens are being characterized, the primary antibody is polyclonal or monoclonal antisera of known specificity, either labeled or unlabeled. Primary antibodies are usually diluted in blocking solution to decrease nonspecific binding. Following primary-antibody incubation, the membrane is washed with buffer. If the primary

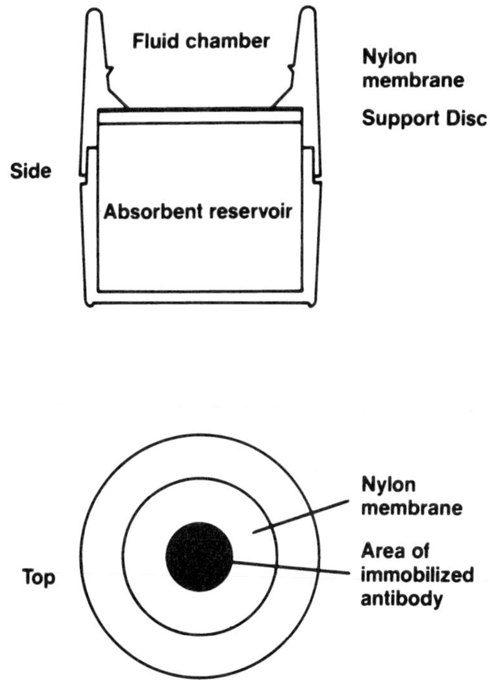

Figure 36–13. Flow-through immunoassay device. (From Morris DL, Ledden DJ, Boguslaski RC. Dry-phase technology for immunoassays. J Clin Lab Anal 1987; 1:243. Copyright 1987, Alan R. Liss, Inc.)

antibody is unlabeled, a second, labeled antibody with specificity for the primary antibody is applied. Enzyme labels with insoluble chromogenic substrates, which detect 100 pg of protein per band, are sensitive enough for most diagnostic applications. Iodine 125 is the most sensitive label, but development of images on radiographic film requires several days. Sensitivity comparable to that of iodine 125 can be achieved with HRP-labeled antibodies and chemiluminescent substrates and enhancers.

Commercially available Western blots are available as supplemental tests for antibodies to HIV-1 and -2 and HTLV-I. In these tests, viral antigens are separated into discrete bands by electrophoresis of viral lysates and then are transferred to membrane strips. These membranes are commercially available. Patient or control serum is added to these prepared strips and analyzed using the steps outlined earlier to detect antibody to individual viral antigens.

A commercially available modification of dot blot and Western blot techniques is a strip immunoblot assay for detection of antibodies to hepatitis C virus. This qualitative enzyme immunoblot assay detects antibodies to four recombinant hepatitis C virus antigens that are precoated as individual bands onto nitrocellulose strips.[54] Because the assay uses recombinant proteins, it is commonly referred to as RIBA, or recombinant immunoblot assay. To perform this assay, test serum is diluted and incubated with the strip to allow antibodies to bind to antigens on the strip. HRP-labeled anti–human IgG conjugate is then added and binds to immobilized human IgG–hepatitis C virus (HCV) antigen complexes. After washing, hydrogen peroxide and 4CN substrate are added. Wherever conjugate is bound to the strip, the enzymatic reaction produces an insoluble blue-black band. Color intensity of each band is proportional to the amount of specific antibody bound and is reported semiquantitatively.

RAPID IMMUNOASSAYS

The availability of blotting membranes, latex particles, and enzyme-labeled antibodies eventually led to the development of rapid immunoassays. These disposable single-use devices are ideal for low-volume testing and usually have self-contained negative and positive test controls. Rapid immunoassays fall into two broad categories: flow-through and lateral flow immunoassays.

Flow-Through Devices

Flow-through devices generally consist of a plastic container with upper and lower chambers separated by a blotting membrane (Fig. 36–13).[55, 56] An antigen or antibody, specific for the analyte of interest, is immobilized onto the blotting membrane. In some cases, antigen or antibody is actually coated onto latex particles, which are then trapped within the membrane. The use of particles increases sensitivity because they have larger surface areas for protein binding than do membranes (Table 36–6). Particles can also be arranged more easily in shapes such as positive and negative symbols to facilitate interpretation. Following immobilization, remaining protein-binding sites on the membrane are blocked to minimize nonspecific interactions. The prepared membrane is placed on top of an absorbent cellulose acetate pad that fills the lower chamber. The absorbent pad enhances capillary flow of liquid through the membrane and serves as a reservoir for waste liquids. Sample flow through the area of membrane containing immobilized antibody speeds up antigen-antibody reaction kinetics and shortens assay time.

To use a flow-through device, test sample is added to the upper chamber and allowed to flow through the membrane into the absorbent pad (Fig. 36–14). Immune complexes form rapidly when analyte in the sample contacts antigen or antibody on the membrane. A wash solution is then added to remove unbound antibody, followed by enzyme-labeled antibody and insoluble chromogenic substrate. If antigen is present in the sample, a color change occurs on the membrane.

A more recent modification of the vertical flow principle is the particle agglutination filtration assay, which uses dyed latex particles for detection (Fig. 36–15).[57] In

Table 36–6. Particle Sizes Commonly Used for Particle Immunoassays

Assay Type	Particle Diameter (μ)
Slide agglutination	0.2–0.9
Latex IRMA, EIA	0.01–0.3
Vertical flow—particle capture	0.3–0.9
Vertical flow—particle agglutination	0.1–0.4
Lateral flow—immunochromatography	0.1–0.4

EIA, enzyme immunoassay; IRMA, immunoradiometric assay.

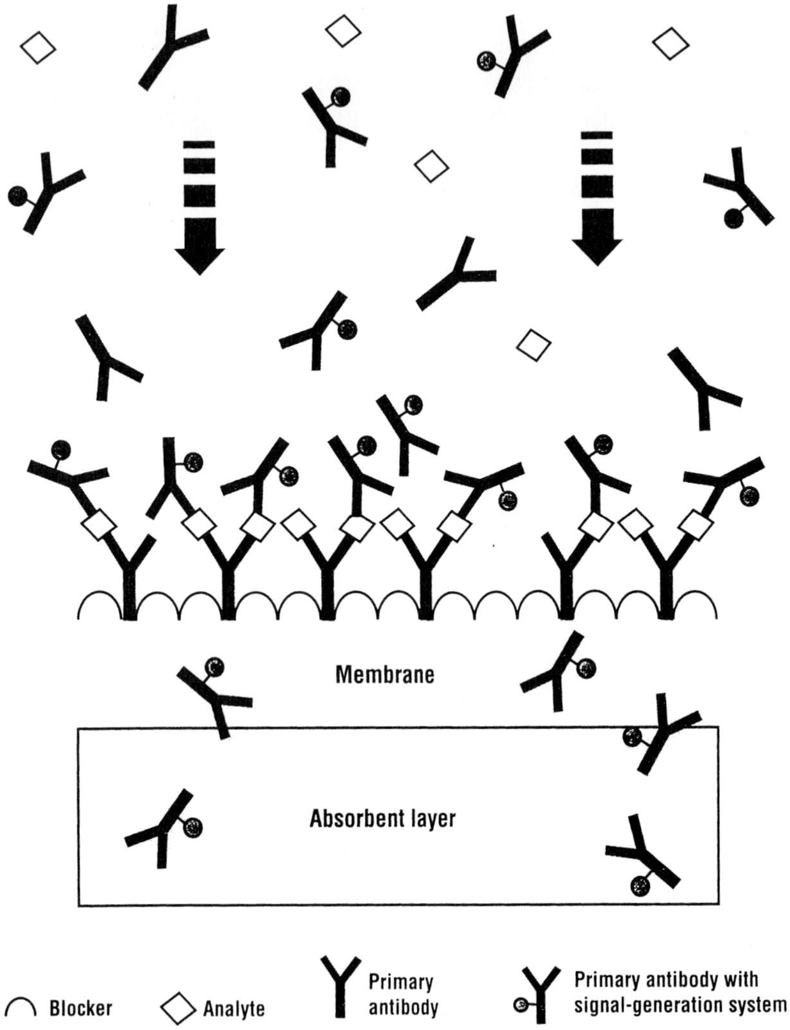

Figure 36–14. Flow-through immunoassay reaction scheme. (From Harvey MA, Audette CA, McDonogh R. The use of microporous polymer membranes in immunoassays. IVD Technology 1996; 2[May/June]:34.)

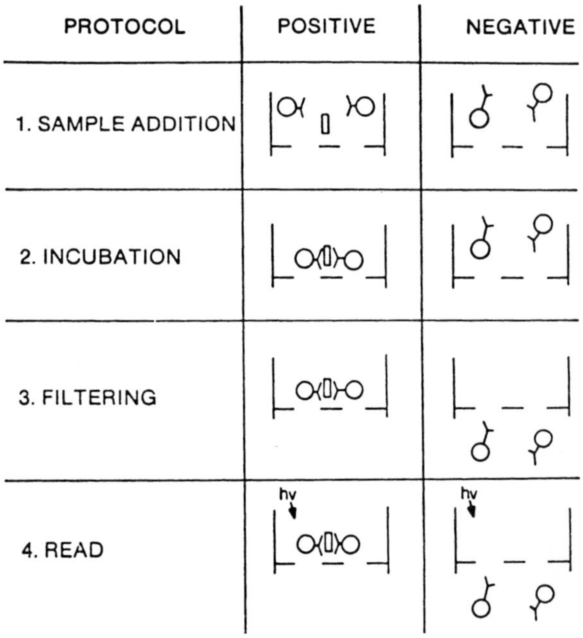

Figure 36–15. Particle agglutination filtration assay. (From Bangs LB. New developments in particle-based tests and immunoassays. J Int Fed Clin Chem 1990; 2:188.)

the first step of this assay, test sample is added to a suspension of particles coated with antibody. During a brief incubation, antigen in the sample agglutinates the particles. The suspension is poured through a cellulose acetate membrane, which traps agglutinated particles while allowing smaller individual particles to pass through. A positive reaction is detected as an intensely colored dot on the white membrane.

The principles of particle agglutination filtration have been used to develop a platelet filtration assay for the detection of HLA or platelet-specific antibodies.[58] Platelet filtration assays are rapid, are technically simple, and require no specialized equipment. The single-use filtration module is well suited for individual testing, and reagents are stable at room temperature for at least 1 year. Patient serum or plasma is incubated with one drop of a pooled platelet suspension. After incubation, platelets are washed briefly and applied to a vertical flow device, which traps them on the surface of a membrane. Platelet-bound antibodies are detected by addition of enzyme-conjugated anti–human IgG and insoluble chromogenic substrate. Positive reactions produce a distinct blue color, and negative reactions remain white. The platelet filtration assay has also been used to detect in vivo platelet-associated IgG.

A particle agglutination assay for HIV-1 uses an enzyme-labeled antibody to enhance sensitivity. White latex particles are coated with a mixture of affinity-purified *gag* p24 antigen and synthetic *env* peptide antigen. Patient serum is mixed with diluent and coated latex particles in a sample cup, incubated, and poured into the vertical flow device. If HIV-1 antibody is present, latex particles are agglutinated and trapped by the membrane. Trapped particles are washed, and bound antibody is detected by adding enzyme-labeled anti–human immunoglobulin conjugate and an insoluble chromogenic substrate. A reactive sample produces a blue dot on the membrane.

Lateral Flow Devices

More recently, lateral flow immunoassay devices have been developed that are single-step assays, requiring only the addition of sample.[57, 59] Most commercial lateral flow devices include self-contained positive, negative, and procedural controls to indicate that the test was performed properly. Intensely dyed latex particles or gold or selenium colloidal particles coated with specific antibody are embedded on a blotting membrane at the sample application zone of the device (Fig. 36–16). The particles must be large enough to provide a strong visual signal, yet small enough to diffuse freely along the membrane. A detection zone is created by immobilizing a second antibody with the same specificity at the opposite end of the membrane. Absorbent material is attached at the distal end of the device to help draw sample through the membrane.

The test is performed by adding patient sample to the application zone and waiting a sufficient time to allow it to flow laterally across the membrane. As the sample

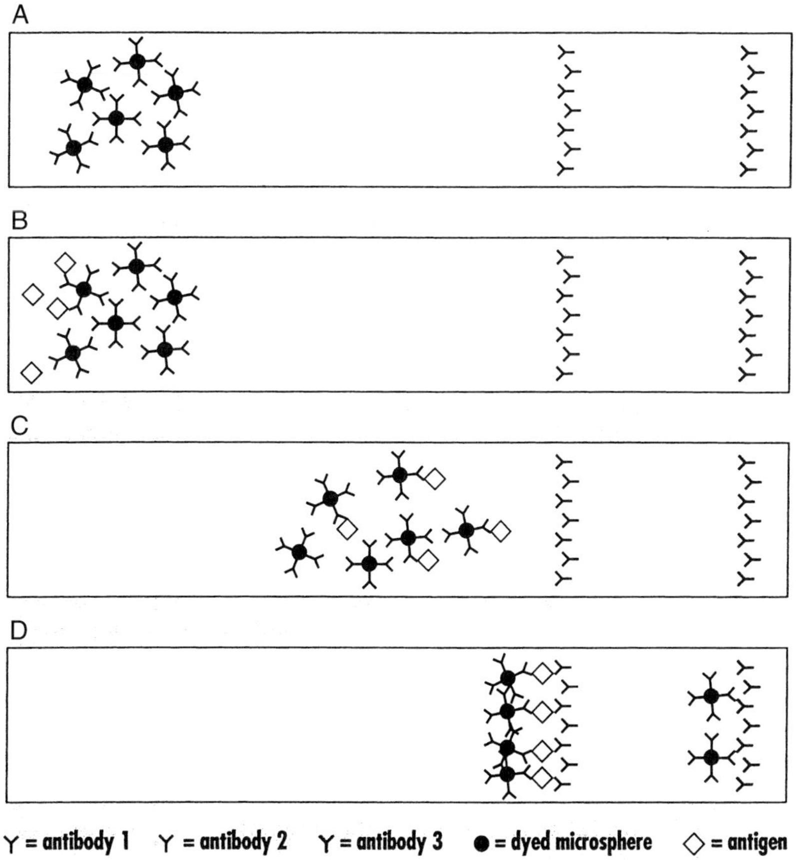

Figure 36–16. Lateral flow immunoassay (immunochromatography). *A*, Dry membrane strip with immobilized latex particles and antibodies. *B*, Addition of sample containing antigen. *C*, Sample flow solubilizes particles, which bind to antigen. *D*, Latex particle–antigen complex is immobilized by a solid-phase second antibody, and a colored line is formed for positive test results and controls. (From Bangs LB, Meza MB. Microspheres, part 2: ligand attachment and test formulation. IVD Technology 1995; 1[April]:20.)

flows through the membrane, it solubilizes the antibody-coated particles. If antigen is present in the sample, it complexes with antibody-coated particles and is captured by immobilized antibody in the detection zone (see Fig. 36–16). The formation of a colored dot in the detection zone is interpreted as a positive reaction. Unreacted antibody-coated particles flow past the detection zone to an end-of-assay indicator zone.

SUMMARY

Early immunoassays were based on agglutination and precipitation. The recognition that not all antigen-antibody reactions produced visible end points led to the development of the antiglobulin test and immunofluorescence methods, which solved the problem of detecting immune reactions that did not result in lattice formation. The modern era of quantitative immunoassays began with the introduction of RIA.

Several key technological developments in the last three decades have had a major impact on the evolution of immunoassays and their applicability to laboratory medicine. The first was the concept of binding antigens and antibodies to a solid phase, which greatly simplified separation steps in RIA procedures and led to the development of other immunoassay formats such as IRMA. The subsequent introduction of plastic beads and microplates as solid phases further enhanced convenience and facilitated semiautomated sample handling. The use of membranes ushered in dot blotting and immunoblotting techniques.

The second major development was the conjugation of enzymes to antigens and antibodies, which led to EIAs. These assays eliminated potential biohazards associated with radioactivity and increased the flexibility of immunoassay design. The combination of enzyme-labeled antibodies with membrane solid phases spurred the development of numerous innovative diagnostic tests that are ideally suited for emergency and decentralized testing. Attempts to further simplify these assays resulted in the use of particles as labels. The need to improve the sensitivity of EIAs led to fluorogenic and chemiluminescent substrates. These investigations enabled the discovery of alternative fluorescent and chemiluminescent labels, such as dioxetane and acridinium esters.

The third major development was the introduction of hybridoma technology, which engendered a proliferation of monoclonal antibodies with unique specificities. Their availability refined the specificity of double-antibody "sandwich" immunoassays.

Developments in the last few years have focused on increasing automation. Centralized laboratories are demanding fully automated, random-access analyzers to provide higher throughput and faster turnaround times. Increasing computerization and more precise engineering are meeting this demand. Paramagnetic particles and vertical flow technology are making it possible to fully automate immunoassays for an increasing number of analytes. Hybridoma and recombinant DNA techniques allow molecular engineering of purified high-affinity antibodies and antigens. Chemiluminescent labels are sensitive enough to permit rapid detection of analytes in the attomole range.

Rapid advances are also occurring in molecular diagnostics. Eventually, these immunoassay principles will be adopted to automate amplified DNA and RNA testing. The greater sensitivity and specificity afforded by these advances will eventually allow detection and monitoring of heretofore undetectable substances.

REFERENCES

1. Humphrey JH, White RG. Immunology for Students of Medicine. Oxford, UK: Blackwell Scientific, 1971, p 6.
2. Kraus R. Uber spezifische reaktionen in keimfreien filtraten aus cholera, typhus and pestbouillonculturen, erzeugt durch homologes serum. Wien Klin Wochenschr 1897; 10:736.
3. Marrack JR. The chemistry of antigens and antibodies. London: MRC Special Report Series, No. 194, 1934.
4. Creite A. Versuche uber die wirkung des serumeiweisses nach injection in das blut. Rat Med 1869; 26:90.
5. Stillmark H. Uber ricin ein giftiges ferment aus den samen von *Ricinus communis* L und einigen anderen Euphorbiaceen. Dorpat, Germany, 1888 thesis.
6. Ehrlich P, Morgenroth J. Uber haemolysine dritte mitteilung. Berl Klin Wochenschr 1900; 37:681.
7. Landsteiner K. Uber agglutinationserscheinungen normalen menschlichen blutes. Wien Klin Wochenschr 1901; 14:1132.
8. Ottenberg R. Transfusion and arterial anastomosis. Ann Surg 1908; 47:486.
9. Race RR. An "incomplete" antibody in human serum. Nature 1944; 153:771.
10. Wiener AS. A new test (blocking test) for Rh sensitization. Proc Soc Exp Biol Med 1944; 56:173.
11. Coombs RRA, Mourant AE, Race RR. A new test for the detection of weak and "incomplete" Rh agglutinins. Br J Exp Pathol 1945; 26:255.
12. Moreschi C. Neue tatsachen uber die blutkorperchenagglutination. Zentralbl Bakt 1908; 46:49.
13. Beattie KM. Control of the antigen-antibody ratio in antibody detection/compatibility tests. Transfusion 1980; 20:277.
14. Eldon K. Simultaneous ABO and Rh groupings on cards, in the laboratory or at the bedside. Dan Med Bull 1955; 2:33.
15. Chown B, Lewis M. Further experience with the slanted capillary method for Rh typing of red blood cells. Can Med Assoc J 1946; 55:66.
16. Weiland DL. Capillary tube techniques. *In* Myers M, Reynolds A (eds): Micromethods in Blood Group Serology. Arlington, VA: American Association of Blood Banks, 1984.
17. Sever JL. Application of microtechnique to viral serological investigations. J Immunol 1962; 88:320.
18. Wegmann TG, Smithies O. A simple hemagglutination system requiring small amounts of red cells and antibodies. Transfusion 1966; 6:67.
19. Wegmann TG, Smithies O. Improvement of the microtiter hemagglutination method. Transfusion 1968; 8:47.
20. McCloskey RV, Zmijewski CM. A semi-microtechnic for the detection of human blood group isohemagglutinins. Am J Clin Pathol 1967; 48:240.
21. Gibbons DS, Kano T, Edelmann M. A terraced microplate system for automated ABO and Rh grouping. Am Clin Prod Rev 1986; 5:42.
22. LaPierre Y, Rigal D, Adam J, et al. The gel test: a new way to detect red cell antigen-antibody reactions. Transfusion 1990; 30:109.
23. Malyska H, Weiland D. The gel test. Lab Med 1994; 25:81.
24. Reis KJ, Chachowski R, Cupido A, et al. Column agglutination technology: the antiglobulin test. Transfusion 1993; 33:639.
25. Singer JM, Plotz CM. The latex fixation test. I. Application to the serologic diagnosis of rheumatoid arthritis. Am J Med 1956; 21:888.
26. Singer JM, Plotz CM. Slide latex fixation test: a simple screening method for the diagnosis of rheumatoid arthritis. JAMA 1958; 168:180.
27. Högman C. The principle of mixed agglutination applied to tissue

culture systems: a method for the study of cell-bound blood group antigens. Vox Sang 1959; 4:12.
28. Högman C. Blood group antigens A and B determined by means of mixed agglutination on cultured cells of human fetal kidney, liver, spleen, lung, heart, and skin. Vox Sang 1959; 4:319.
29. Fagraeus A, Espmark A. Use of a mixed haemadsorption method in virus-infected tissue cultures. Nature 1961; 190:370.
30. Fagraeus A, Espmark JA, Jonsson J. Mixed haemadsorption: a mixed antiglobulin reaction applied to antigens on a glass surface. Immunology 1965; 9:161.
31. Juji T, Kano K, Milgrom F. Mixed agglutination with platelets. Int Arch Allergy 1972; 42:474.
32. Coombs RRA. Assays utilizing red cells as markers. *In* Voller A (ed): Immunoassays for the 80's. Lancaster, England: MTP Press, 1981, pp 17–34.
33. Rosenfield RE, Kochwa S, Kaczera Z. Solid-phase serology for the study of human erythrocytic antigen-antibody reactions. *In* Program and Abstracts of the Proceedings of the 15th Congress of the International Society for Blood Transfusion, Paris, 1976.
34. Plapp FV, Sinor LT, Rachel JM. The evolution of pretransfusion testing: from agglutination to solid-phase red cell adherence tests. Crit Rev Clin Lab Sci 1989; 27:179.
35. Stone DL, Moheng MC, Rolih S, et al. Capture-S, a nontreponemal solid-phase erythrocyte adherence assay for serological detection of syphilis. J Clin Microbiol 1997; 35:217.
36. Schulenburg BJ, Plapp FV, Rachel JM. A rapid screening test for detection of IgA deficiency. Transfusion 1991; 31:633.
37. Kipps TJ, Meisenholder G, Robbins BA. New developments in flow cytometric analyses of lymphocyte markers. Clin Lab Med 1992; 12:237.
38. Garratty G, Arndt P. Applications of flow cytofluorometry to transfusion science. Transfusion 1995; 35:157.
39. Berson SA, Yalow RS. Quantitative aspects of the reaction between insulin and insulin-binding antibody. J Clin Invest 1959; 38:1996.
40. Catt K, Tregear GW. Solid phase radioimmunoassay in antibody-coated tubes. Science 1967; 158:1570.
41. Miles LEM, Hales CN. Labeled antibodies and immunological-assay systems. Nature 1968; 219:186.
42. Engvall E, Perlmann P. Enzyme-linked immunosorbent assay (ELISA): quantitative assay of immunoglobulin G. Immunochemistry 1971; 8:871.
43. Voller A, Bartlett A, Bidwell DE. Enzyme immunoassays with special reference to ELISA techniques. J Clin Pathol 1978; 31:507.
44. Kiefel V, Santoso S, Weisheit M, Mueller-Eckhardt C. Monoclonal antibody-specific immobilization of platelet antigens (MAIPA): a new tool for the identification of platelet-reactive antibodies. Blood 1987; 70:1722.
45. Bronstein I, Kricka LJ. Clinical applications of luminescent assays for enzymes and enzyme labels. J Clin Lab Anal 1989; 3:316.
46. Kricka LJ. Luminescent immunoassays. J Int Fed Clin Chem 1989; 1:24.
47. Khalil OS, Zurek TF, Tryba J, et al. Abbott prism: a multichannel heterogeneous chemiluminescence immunoassay analyzer. Clin Chem 1991; 37:1540.
48. Hawkes R, Niday E, Gordon J. A dot-immunobinding assay for monoclonal and other antibodies. Anal Biochem 1982; 119:142.
49. Herbrink P, van Bussel FJ, Warnaar SO. The antigen spot test: a highly sensitive assay for the detection of antibodies. J Immunol Methods 1982; 48:293.
50. Stott DI. Immunoblotting and dot blotting. J Immunol Methods 1989; 119:153.
51. Towbin H, Gordon J. Immunoblotting and dot-immunobinding—current status and outlook. J Immunol Methods 1984; 72:313.
52. Renart J, Reiser J. Stark GR. Transfer of proteins from gels to diazobenzyloxymethyl paper and detection with antisera: a method for studying antibody specificity and antigen structure. Proc Natl Acad Sci U S A 1979; 76:3116.
53. Towbin H, Staehelin T, Gordon J. Electrophoretic transfer of proteins from polyacrylamide gels to nitrocellulose sheets: procedure and some applications. Proc Natl Acad Sci U S A 1979; 76:4350.
54. Wilber J. Development and use of laboratory tests for hepatitis C infection: a review. J Clin Immunoassay 1993; 16:204.
55. Valkirs GE, Barton R. Immunoconcentration—a new format for solid-phase immunoassays. Clin Chem 1985; 31:1427.
56. Anderson RR, Lee TT, Saewert DC, et al. Internally referenced immunoconcentration assays. Clin Chem 1986; 32:1692.
57. Bangs LB. New developments in particle based tests and immunoassays. J Int Fed Clin Chem 1990; 2:188.
58. Rachel JM, Plapp FV, Hawk SE, Thompson KS. A rapid qualitative assay for platelet associated IgG. Transfusion 1992; 32:13S.
59. Harvey MA, Audette CA, McDonogh R. The use of microporous polymer membranes in immunoassays. IVD Technology 1996; 2:34.

CHAPTER 37

Principles of Cell Survival, Kinetics, and Imaging

Richard J. Davey

RADIONUCLIDES IN TRANSFUSION MEDICINE

Gray and Sterling[1] described the first clinically useful red cell radiolabel, chromium-51, in 1950. Fisher and colleagues[2] introduced technetium-99m as a cell label in 1967, and the importance of indium-111 was recognized after an evaluation of leukocyte radiolabels by McAfee and Thakur[3] in 1976. Other cell radiolabels have been evaluated and used, with varying degrees of success. However, the three radionuclides named here are used for the vast majority of cell survival and imaging studies.

An ideal radiolabel for red cells, platelets, or leukocytes does not exist, however. Each of the three commonly used radionuclides has advantages and disadvantages that must be fully appreciated by the investigator or clinician who uses it. The desirable characteristics of a cell radiolabel are as follows:

Minimal radiation dose to the recipient
Nontoxic to the recipient
Nontoxic to the cell
Specific for the cell
No metabolism of the label by the cell
Radioactive half-life appropriate for the study
Radioactive emissions suitable for detection or imaging
Minimal manipulation of the cell required
No elution of the label
No relabeling of other cells in vivo

The radioactive half-life, elution characteristics, and gamma-photon energy are the primary determinants of the clinical utility of chromium-51, technetium-99m, and indium-111. These features are listed in Table 37–1. The optimal range for detection of photoelectric events in a standard gamma counting instrument (gamma counter) is 100 to 300 keV. The "yield" of gamma-photon emissions is the number of photons emitted per 100 radioactive decays. A high yield means that a lower radiation dose can be used to achieve adequate detection levels.

Chromium-51

Chromium-51 is produced in a reactor by neutron activation. It decays by electron capture, with a radioactive half-life of 27.7 days. The principal gamma-photon emission occurs by electron capture at 320 keV, slightly above the optimum detection range of standard gamma counters. The yield of gamma-photon emissions is quite low (9.8%). The high energy and low yield mean that higher doses of this radionuclide must be given for adequate detection in a gamma counter. The dose of chromium-51 required for imaging studies, which require a high yield of gamma-photon emissions, is unacceptably high for most applications in transfusion medicine. The radioactive half-life of chromium-51 is quite long for most cell recovery studies.

Chromium-51 is supplied as sodium radiochromate ($Na_2{}^{51}CrO_4$) for cell labeling purposes. Hexavalent chromate labels red cells by first binding rapidly and reversibly to the red cell membrane. After reduction to the trivalent state, the chromic ion binds more slowly and firmly to the β-globin chain of intracellular hemoglobin, and probably to other intracellular ligands as well. Labeling efficiency is about 90%. Younger red cells take up slightly more label than do older cells. Trivalent chromium that elutes from the labeled cells is rapidly excreted in the urine and does not relabel other cells in vivo.

Chromium elutes from red cells in two phases. There is an early loss of 1% to 4% of the label within 24 hours, which may represent elution of a loosely bound fraction of the label.[4] Garby and Mollison[5] found that subsequent elution varies from 0.56% to 2.04% per day, similar to the 0.70% to 1.55% reported by Bentley and associates.[6] An estimated elution rate of 1% per day is satisfactory for most investigational and clinical purposes.[7]

Moroff and colleagues[8] have described the technical steps for labeling red cells with chromium-51 to evaluate blood storage and preservation systems. The International

Table 37–1. Major Features of Radionuclides Used for Cell Labeling

	Chromium-51	Technetium-99m	Indium-111
Radioactive half-life	27.7 days	6.0 hours	2.8 days
Major-photon emissions (yield)	320 keV (9.8%)	140 keV (90%)	173/247 keV (90%/94%)
Elution (red cell)	1%/day	1–7%/hour	4–8%/day
Target organ	Spleen	Total body	Spleen
Suitable for imaging	No	Yes	Yes

Committee for Standardization in Hematology[9] has described the slightly different technique necessary for labeling red cells for the determination of transfusion compatibility. The technical simplicity of the labeling process, excellent red cell uptake, low toxicity, and relatively low and stable rate of elution are the major advantages of chromium-51 as a red cell label.

Baldini and colleagues[10] first described the use of chromium-51 as a platelet radiolabel. The platelet-labeling efficiency of chromium-51 is low (9%) compared with its red cell–labeling efficiency (90%). Therefore, it is important that platelet preparations be free of red cells before being labeled.[11] The procedure for labeling platelets with chromium-51, which is more difficult than that for red cells, has been described by Snyder and colleagues.[12]

Technetium-99m

Technetium-99m is widely used as an imaging agent in nuclear medicine and has a useful role as a red cell label. This metastable radionuclide is produced in a molybdenum generator and is a product of molybdenum-99 decay. Technetium-99m decays, in turn, to technetium-99 with a half-life of 6.02 hours. Technetium-99m emits a gamma-photon at 140 keV with a yield of 90%. This photon energy falls within the optimal range of gamma counters. The high yield is useful for external imaging.

Technetium-99m, as pertechnetate, diffuses across the red cell membrane into the cell, where it binds to hemoglobin and other intracellular ligands with a labeling efficiency of about 90%. The short half-life of technetium-99m precludes its use for long-term red cell survival studies. Groups of samples must be counted rapidly, or a correction must be made for radioactive decay that occurs during the counting procedure.

The nuclide also has a high and variable rate of elution. The use of stannous compounds as intracellular reducing agents in the labeling process has permitted firmer binding of technetium-99m, but elution rates of 4% per hour with considerable variation may be expected.[13, 14] Heaton and colleagues[15] have described the technical steps necessary to minimize variability in labeling and elution with this nuclide. Because of its short half-life, technetium-99m is useful as a red cell label when a series of survival studies must be performed for transfusion compatibility. This radionuclide is also useful for the accurate determination of red cell volume as part of longer-term red cell recovery studies.

Indium-111

Indium-111 can be used as a label for red cells, platelets, and leukocytes. It is prepared in a cyclotron by proton bombardment of a cadmium target. It has two major gamma-photon emissions, 173 keV (90.5% yield) and 247 keV (94% yield), which are excellent for counting in a gamma counter and for external imaging. The radioactive half-life of the nuclide is 2.83 days, making it appropriate for leukocyte imaging studies that extend over several days. Indium-111 is also used for red cell mass determinations, for short-term red cell survival studies, and for platelet recovery studies.

Indium-111 must be complexed with a lipophilic chelating agent if it is to traverse cell membranes and label intracellular proteins. Although several lipophilic chelates have been studied, 8-hydroxyquinoline (oxine) is the only agent currently licensed for this purpose in the United States. Technical procedures have been published for labeling red cells,[16] platelets,[12] and leukocytes[17] with indium-111.

Indium-111 is a nonselective label, with preferential uptake as follows: platelets > leukocytes > red cells.[18] Cell preparations therefore must be free of extraneous elements before being labeled. Like technetium-99m, indium-111 has a high and variable rate of elution from red cells. AuBuchon and Brightman[16] have shown that 8% to 10% of the label elutes within 24 to 48 hours, with a 4% per day loss after that time. This problem with elution renders indium-111 unsuitable for long-term red cell survival studies. It is useful for determining red cell volume and for short-term recovery studies when precision is not critical.

BLOOD CELL LIFE SPAN AND SURVIVAL STUDIES

Red Cells

The normal red cell life span (110 to 120 days) was first approximated by differential absorption techniques[19] and subsequently confirmed by radioisotopic labeling studies using cohort (marrow) labels[20] and random (peripheral blood) labels.[5] When chromium-51 is used as the label, the time at which the recovered counts are 50% of the originally injected counts is the $T_{50}Cr$, normally 31 ± 6 days. Correction for elution will yield the true red cell life span. The $T_{50}Cr$ is useful for evaluating the extent of hemolysis in a chronic hemolytic anemia. Modest reductions in the $T_{50}Cr$ can correlate with a substantial increase in the rate of red cell destruction.[21]

Red cell life span studies have been conducted to assess the therapeutic benefit of red cell units that are enriched in young red cells ("neocytes"). The transfusion of such units has the theoretical benefit of reducing the iron burden in the patient who undergoes frequent transfusions by increasing the number of long-lived red cells in the circulation.[22] Chromium-51 life span studies have demonstrated that neocytes survive 30% to 60% longer in the circulation than do red cells derived from standard red cell units.[23, 24] However, neocyte units contain only about half of the hemoglobin of standard units and are costly to prepare. Studies have shown that transfusion of neocyte units results in only a modest reduction in transfusion requirements.[25, 26] The transfusion of neocytes, therefore, has not achieved wide clinical acceptance.

In contrast to long-term life span studies, short-term red cell survival studies are useful in identifying patterns of immune red cell destruction. These studies are clinically important when standard pretransfusion serological testing cannot clearly identify or characterize red cell alloantibodies or autoantibodies in a transfusion recipient.

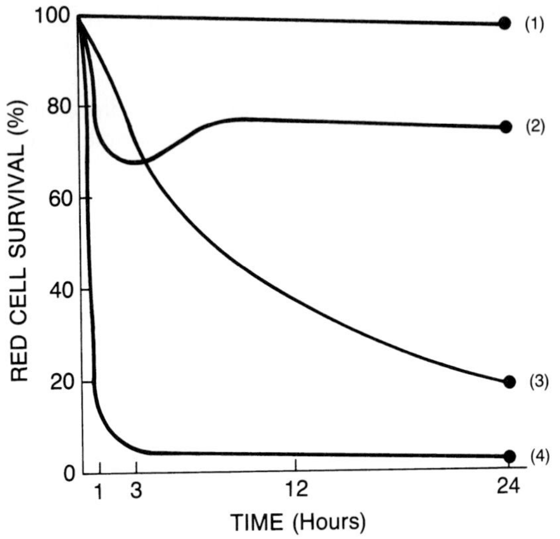

Figure 37–1. Red cell survival patterns representing different mechanisms of immune red cell destruction. (1), Normal survival; (2), two-component curve with partial complement activation to C3b→C3d,g; (3), single exponential curve characteristic of IgG non–complement-activating antibodies; (4), complete complement activation to C5b-C9 complex with intravascular hemolysis.

The various factors that contribute to immune red cell destruction have been discussed in detail elsewhere.[27–29] Of primary importance are the immunoglobulin class and subclass of the recipient red cell alloantibody,[30] and the extent to which that antibody activates complement.[31, 32]

Four characteristic survival patterns can be recognized in a 24-hour red cell survival study conducted to determine transfusion compatibility (Fig. 37–1). They are (1) normal survival, (2) extravascular destruction characterized by a "two-component" survival curve, (3) extravascular destruction characterized by a "single exponential" survival curve, and (4) intravascular destruction.

Normal Survival

The normal range for recovery of transfused red cells is 97% to 102% at 60 minutes and 95% to 100% at 24 hours.

Extravascular Destruction Characterized by a "Two-Component" Survival Curve

Most immunoglobulin M (IgM) red cell alloantibodies and some IgG alloantibodies (e.g., anti-Jk[a]) activate complement. IgM antibodies directly activate complement, with 20 to 40 IgM molecules per red cell being required to initiate red cell clearance. IgG antibodies can activate complement if two or more molecules are physically adjacent on the red cell membrane[33]; thus, many more IgG molecules are required for complement activation to occur. In most cases, the kinetics of complement activation result in generation of the membrane-bound C3b fragment but not the final C5b-C9 "membrane attack" complex. Plasma factor I, with plasma factor H as a cofactor, cleaves C3b to C3bi. Red cell–bound C3b and C3bi adhere to the complement receptors CR1 and CR3 on reticuloendothelial system (RES) macrophages in the liver and spleen. These red cells may be removed from the circulation by either antibody-dependent cell-mediated cytotoxicity or complete phagocytosis, or they may sustain membrane damage through partial phagocytosis. Alternatively, C3bi may be degraded before red cell damage occurs.[34, 35] Plasma factors I and H further cleave C3bi to C3c, which detaches from the cell, and C3d,g, which remains attached to the cell membrane (Fig. 37–2).

Because C3d,g binds weakly to CR3 receptors, most red cells coated with C3d,g detach from RES macrophages and survive relatively normally.[36] The inactive C3d,g fragments may protect the red cell from further complement-mediated damage by occupying complement-binding sites. A "two-component" recovery curve, therefore, represents the early loss of C3b-coated red cells and more normal survival of those cells on whose membranes C3b has degraded to C3d,g. A "two-component" survival curve with more than 70% recovery at 24 hours indicates that the patient can safely receive larger quantities of similar red cells with little risk of rapid immune hemolysis.

Extravascular Destruction Characterized by a "Single Exponential" Survival Curve

Many IgG red cell alloantibodies (e.g., Rh antibodies) do not activate complement. Instead, there is progressive removal of sensitized red cells with a survival curve described by a single exponential. Factors such as the con-

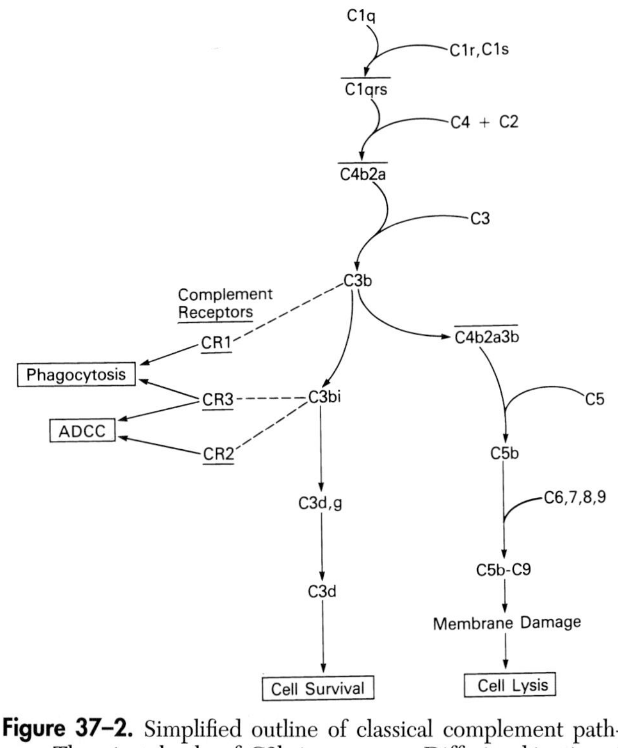

Figure 37–2. Simplified outline of classical complement pathway. The pivotal role of C3b is apparent. Differing kinetics of complement activation can result in red cell lysis, opsonization with reticuloendothelial system phagocytosis or antibody-dependent cell-mediated cytotoxicity (ADCC), or generation of inactive complement fragments with cell survival.

centration and IgG subclass of the antibody determine the rate of removal of the cells. The efficiency of the four IgG subclasses in binding with Fc receptors on RES macrophages is IgG3 > IgG1 > IgG4 > IgG2. IgG1 is present in higher titer than the other subclasses and is most often involved in IgG-mediated red cell destruction.[30] Red cell survival studies that demonstrate an IgG-mediated "single exponential" pattern of cell destruction indicate that the transfusion of similar cells may result in a delayed hemolytic transfusion reaction.

Intravascular Destruction

IgM antibodies that are efficient activators of complement, such as anti-A and anti-B, can drive the kinetics of the reaction to the formation of the terminal C5b-C9 "membrane attack" complex. Insertion of this complex into the red cell membrane results in loss of membrane integrity and osmotic lysis of the cell. Transfused cells that generate complement activation of this magnitude are usually hemolyzed within minutes.

Synergistic Effect of Complement and IgG

Complement and IgG appear to act synergistically in promoting red cell opsonization. Studies have demonstrated that the addition of complement to red cells sensitized with IgG alone will enhance phagocytosis.[37, 38] A hybrid red cell survival curve may occur when both IgM and IgG antibodies are active. There is a rapid loss of a minor population of the cells from IgM-mediated complement activation, and a slower phase of cell destruction mediated primarily by the IgG antibody.

Platelets

Most studies of platelet life span and kinetics have been performed with chromium-51 using labeling procedures defined by the ICSH.[39] However, the drawbacks of this radionuclide (low labeling efficiency, long half-life, poor imaging characteristics) have led to its replacement by indium-111 as the platelet radiolabel of choice.[40] Standard technical methods for preparation of indium-111-oxine–labeled platelets have been published by the ICSH and others.[12, 41] The major drawback of indium-111-oxine is its high affinity for red cells, leukocytes, and plasma proteins, primarily transferrin. The washing and centrifugation steps that are therefore necessary to prepare a "clean" platelet preparation cause a substantial loss of platelets (~ 40%) and a "collection injury" that can distort test results. Other compounds that form lipophilic complexes with indium-111, notably acetylacetone,[42] tropolone,[43] and 2-mercaptopyridine-N-oxide (merc),[44] have been extensively studied as possible agents to overcome these problems. Tropolone is widely used in Europe, but oxine remains the only licensed agent in the United States.

There are four methods for the calculation of platelet lifespan—linear, exponential, weighted mean, and γ-function (multiple hit)—each of which yields slightly different results. The γ-function analysis is the recommended method for the determination of platelet lifespan,[12, 39] but investigators often report their results using one or more additional statistical methods.

Because no radioactive tracer selectively labels newly formed platelets, cohort studies have not been practical to measure platelet production in humans. Instead, the kinetics of normal platelet production have been measured indirectly by determining the turnover rate of circulating platelets (platelet count divided by platelet survival corrected for recovery). Estimates of daily platelet production in the steady state using this method have ranged from 35,000 to 66,000/µL of blood.[45] The lifespan of platelets in the human ranges between 8 and 12 days; Harker and Finch[46] found it to be 9.5 ± 0.6 days. Senescent platelets are removed from the circulation by RES macrophages in the liver and spleen and, to a lesser extent, by bone marrow and lungs.[47, 48]

There is also evidence of a fixed platelet requirement necessary to maintain vascular integrity. Hanson and Slichter[49] have proposed that 82% of platelet turnover in normal persons is due to senescence, and 18% (~ 7100 platelets/µL/day) is due to the fixed requirement. The fixed requirement becomes an increasingly large component of platelet removal as thrombocytopenia from bone marrow hypoplasia worsens. Thus, platelet lifespan correlates directly with the platelet count; an increasing reduction in lifespan is noted as platelet counts decrease below 50,000/µL. The shortened platelet lifespan observed in thrombocytopenic patients, therefore, does not necessarily indicate increased platelet destruction.

Patients with increased peripheral platelet destruction, such as those with idiopathic thrombocytopenic purpura,[50] have platelet lifespans that are shorter than predicted by Hanson and Slichter's model.[49] Thus, platelet life span studies using indium-111 are useful in discriminating between thrombocytopenia caused by decreased platelet production and that caused by increased platelet destruction (Fig. 37–3). Platelet lifespan studies are not generally useful in the alloimmunized patient, however. Post-transfusion platelet counts usually provide the clinician with the necessary information for the management of these patients.

Leukocytes

Although granulocytes, lymphocytes, and monocytes derive from a common pluripotent stem cell, they have widely variant functions and kinetics. Radionuclides have permitted the study of the normal kinetics of these various leukocyte classes.[51] Indium-111-oxine is now the nuclide of choice for leukocyte radiolabeling. Because labeling with indium-111-oxine is nonselective, the leukocytes must be separated from other cells and plasma before being labeled.[52]

Granulocytes

Studies done with granulocytes labeled with diisopropylflurophosphate demonstrated that the circulating cells had a half-life of 3.8 to 6.7 hours. About half of the injected cells were recoverable in the circulation, with

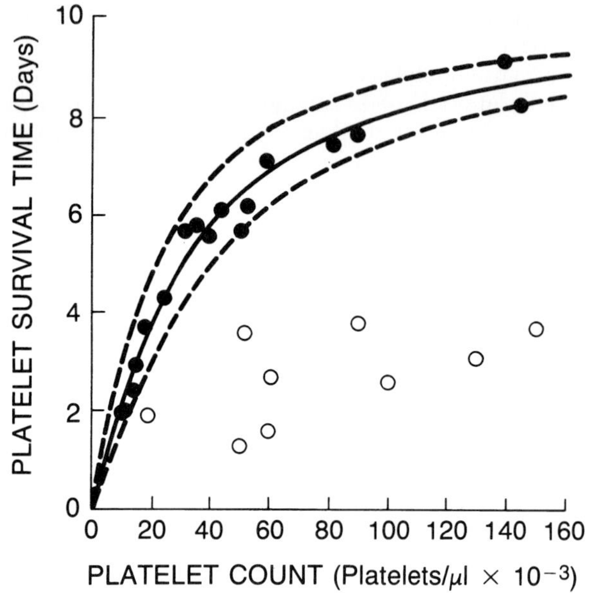

Figure 37–3. The relationship between the survival of indium-111–labeled autologous platelets and the circulating platelet count. *Solid circles* identify patients with impaired platelet production (hypoplasia, n = 17). *Open circles* identify patients with increased peripheral platelet destruction (ITP, n = 9). *Solid line* is best fit to data from the hypoplastic patient group. Platelet survival could be predicted by platelet count in the hypoplastic patient. The "fixed requirement" is increasingly apparent in this group at platelet counts below 50,000/μL. (Adapted from Tomer A, Harker LA. Megakaryocytopoiesis and platelet kinetics. *In* Rossi EC, Simon TL, Moss GS [eds]: Principles of Transfusion Medicine. Baltimore: Williams & Wilkins, 1991, p 175.)

the remainder constituting a "marginating pool" of cells.[53, 54] More recent studies done with indium-111–labeled granulocytes have shown a mean recovery of 30% of the labeled cells and a mean circulating half-life of 5.0 hours.[55] Imaging studies have shown that labeled and transfused granulocytes transiently sequester in the lungs. The extent and duration of the pulmonary sequestration appear to be more severe when the labeled cells are suspended in saline rather than plasma.[56] Alloimmunized patients demonstrate a more prolonged and intense pulmonary sequestration phase than normal subjects.[57] In addition, human leukocyte antigen and granulocyte-specific antibodies appear to reduce the intravascular half-life of transfused granulocytes[58] and to impair their ability to migrate to a site of active infection.[59]

Lymphocytes

The extreme radiosensitivity of lymphocytes has hampered the conduct of kinetic and imaging studies. Autologous lymphocytes labeled with a low dose of indium-111 (<20 μCi/10^8 cells) move rapidly from the circulation and sequester in the lung, liver, and spleen. A more gradual accumulation of radiolabel in the lymph nodes follows.[60] These findings are consistent with studies indicating that most lymphocytes are part of a large recirculating pool consisting of long-lived, nondividing small cells.[61, 62] Lymphocytes in this pool migrate from the circulation to the various lymphoid tissues, where they have opportunity to interact with foreign antigen. The migration patterns are not random but are modified by the lymphocyte class and immunological history of the cell. T cells preferentially migrate to lymph nodes, whereas B cells tend to migrate to mucosal lymphoid tissue.[62] Lymphocytes collected from a specific type of lymphoid tissue (e.g., gut mucosa) move to that tissue because of "homing receptors" expressed on the cell after specific antigenic stimulation.[63]

Activated Mononuclear Cells

Kinetic studies of human monocytes have been limited because of the difficulty of obtaining a homogeneous collection of cells, and because of technical problems with cell activation and clumping during preparation. However, monocytes prepared by leukopheresis, density gradient separation, and countercurrent elutriation have been activated with interferon-γ and infused intraperitoneally in patients with peritoneal spread of colorectal cancer.[64] In two patients, indium-111–labeled cells remained in the peritoneal cavity for up to 5 days after infusion, supporting the observation of clinical improvement in a larger group of patients treated with nonlabeled, activated monocytes.

A subpopulation of peripheral blood lymphocytes activated with the cytokine interleukin-2 has been found to exhibit antitumor activity. These lymphokine-activated killer cells presumably migrate to tumor sites, but cell trafficking and imaging studies have been inconclusive.[65] Lymphocytes directly harvested from tumor sites (tumor-infiltrating lymphocytes), however, have been shown to localize at tumor sites and persist in the circulation after activation.[66]

CELL RECOVERY STUDIES TO EVALUATE BLOOD STORAGE AND PRESERVATION

The two critical advances that led to modern blood preservation techniques were the introduction of acid-citrate-dextrose in 1943[67] and the development of plastic blood containers in the early 1950s. Now, blood components are stored in various anticoagulant-preservative solutions, in plastic containers with differing characteristics, and at nonphysiological temperatures for extended periods. The safety and efficacy of new or modified storage conditions must be determined by both in vitro and in vivo evaluation of cell function and viability.

Red Cells

The 24-hour post-transfusion recovery of red cells stored under experimental conditions is the standard measure of acceptability of the new conditions. The U.S. Food and Drug Administration (FDA) now requires that a mean of 75% or more of the transfused red cells be recovered 24

Table 37–2. Features of Red Cell Survival Studies to Evaluate Transfusion Compatibility and Red Cell Storage Systems

Purpose of Evaluation	Features of Study
Transfusion compatibility	Allogeneic cells; chosen by specific phenotype
	Fresh cells (<5 days old); avoids storage lesion
	Small volume infused (1 to 3 mL); reduces risk of transfusion reaction
	Zero-time (100% recovery) point determined after mixing is complete (3–5 minutes)
	Interpretation: shape of 24-hour survival curve predictive of clinical significance of recipient antibody
Red cell storage	Autologous cells; avoids risks of allogeneic transfusion
	Larger volume infused (15 mL); easy to manipulate and smaller radiation dose per cell
	Zero-time (100% recovery) point determined by independent red cell mass study (double-label method) or back-extrapolation (single-label method)
	Interpretation: precise determination of recovery at 24 hours (>75% mean recovery required)

hours after infusion. Other measures, such as post-storage adenosine triphosphate and supernatant hemoglobin levels, contribute to the assessment of storage condition acceptability. Red cell recovery data have been important in studies evaluating the effect of gamma-irradiation,[68] blood bag plasticizing agents,[69] and prestorage leukocyte depletion[70] on stored red cells.

The technique for performing post-transfusion recovery studies to assess new storage conditions differs in important ways from red cell recovery studies to assess transfusion compatibility. As noted in Table 37–2, autologous red cells are chosen for storage studies, thus avoiding the risks of transmissible disease and transfusion reactions inherent in allogeneic transfusion compatibility studies. The shape of the recovery curve is most important, however, in transfusion compatibility studies. The recovery percentage at 24 hours is of prime importance for studies evaluating storage systems.

Because a precise determination of 24-hour recovery is necessary, the method of establishing the zero-time, or 100% recovery, point is of critical importance. A direct measurement of the zero-time recovery value is not possible, however, because an infused blood sample is not completely mixed until approximately 3 minutes in a normal person.[71] Senescent infused cells, and cells damaged during storage, are removed from the circulation by the spleen, with loss of these cells beginning immediately after infusion. By 3 minutes, a significant loss of the infused cells may have occurred that is not detected if the 3-minute sample is regarded as representing 100% survival. The radioactive counts in the 3-minute sample are falsely low, and the 24-hour recovery value is falsely elevated. Two methods for calculating the zero-time recovery value are useful in red cell storage evaluation studies: the single-label and the double-label techniques.

Single-Label Technique With Back-Extrapolation

The in vivo destruction of damage, stored red cells begins immediately and can be assumed to continue at a first-order rate. If so, the extrapolation of the logarithm of the post-transfusion counts to the y-intercept should yield an accurate determination of the zero-time counts, or the 100% recovery point. Beutler and West[72] compared the red cell mass calculated by the extrapolation method with the red cell mass determined independently using red cells labeled with technetium-99m.[72] They found that extrapolation using fresh red cells yielded red cell mass values that were almost identical to those determined independently. When red cells had been stored for 35 to 49 days, however, there was a consistent overestimation of red cell mass (0.6% to 3.6%) by the extrapolation method, suggesting that the kinetics of the early removal of stored red cells is not described solely by a first-order rate (Fig. 37–4).

The removal of damaged and senescent red cells occurs within 15 to 20 minutes of transfusion. Moroff and colleagues[8] have shown that there is a break in the recov-

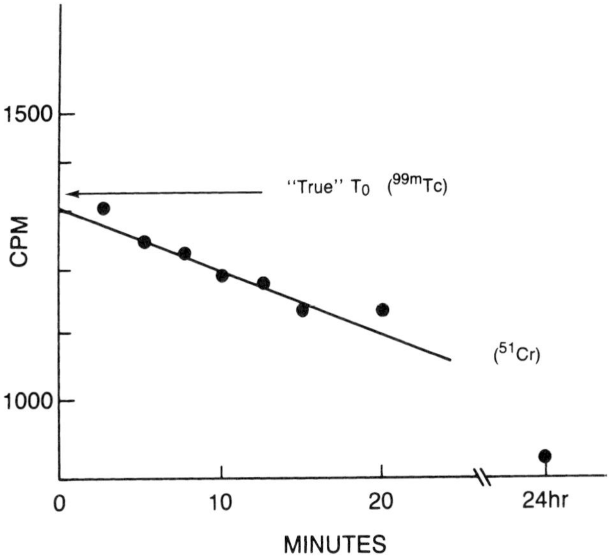

Figure 37–4. Two methods to calculate the counts per minute (CPM) at zero-time (T_0) for determination of red cell mass. With the single-label technique *(solid dots),* the chromium-51–labeled test cells are infused and samples are obtained at 5, 7.5, 10, 12.5, and 15 minutes after infusion. A regression line is plotted, and the y-intercept (T_0) is determined. In the double-label technique, an independent, or "true," measure of T_0 is determined *(arrow)* with fresh autologous red cells labeled with ^{99m}Tc. The single-label regression technique underestimates CPM at T_0 and, therefore, overestimates 24-hour red cell recovery, with the error increasing as red cell storage time increases. (Adapted from Beutler E, West C. Measurement of the viability of stored red cells by the single-isotope technique using ^{51}Cr. Transfusion 1984; 24:100.)

ery curve at 15 minutes, with red cells persisting after that time having more normal survival. The recovery points used for extrapolation to the *y*-intercept, therefore, should be those obtained after 5 minutes, to ensure complete mixing, and before 15 minutes, to avoid the break in the recovery curve. Moroff and colleagues[8] and others[28, 73] have described the technique and interpretation of red cell recoveries using the single-label method.

Double-Label Technique With Direct Measurement of the Red Cell Mass

A precise determination of the recipient's red cell mass provides an accurate volume of dilution for the experimental red cell sample. Simultaneous infusion of fresh, autologous red cells labeled with technetium-99m and stored, experimental red cells labeled with chromium-51 permits this determination. The fresh, autologous red cells labeled with technetium-99m are not removed by the spleen. Early samples, obtained after complete mixing, can be used to determine a precise red cell mass. Subsequent samples counted for the chromium-51–labeled experimental cells can be compared with a zero-time chromium determination calculated from the counts of chromium-51 injected and the volume of dilution, or red cell mass. The major gamma-photon emissions of chromium-51 and technetium-99m permit simultaneous counting of these radionuclides. Alternatively, the red cell mass can be determined and the technetium-99m be allowed to decay before the samples are counted for chromium-51.

The double-label method is very accurate when properly performed. It is technically more difficult than the single-label method, especially in the preparation of the technetium-99m–labeled cells. Heaton and colleagues,[15] who have described the double-label technique in detail, have stressed the importance of keeping the technetium-99m–labeled sample at 4°C to retard elution of the label before infusion.[15]

Platelets

The evaluation of platelet storage and preservation has been complex and challenging. Investigators generally conduct studies using normal volunteer subjects, with each subject serving as his or her own control. Data are usually reported as platelet recovery at 1 hour and as platelet survival or half-life over several days. Both chromium-51 and indium-111 are suitable radiolabels for platelet storage studies,[74–76] and Keegan and associates[77] have reported a combined technique using indium-111–labeled fresh platelets and chromium-51–labeled stored platelets. Platelet recovery and survival studies have been critical to the development of plastics that permit 5-day platelet storage,[78, 79] to the identification of the optimal temperature for platelet storage,[80, 81] to the determination of proper agitation of the platelet concentrates,[82] and to the comparison of manual platelet preparation with automated plateletpheresis techniques.[83]

Granulocytes

Granulocytes labeled with indium-111 and prepared by either centrifugation and hydroxyethyl starch (HES) sedimentation, filtration leukopheresis, or continuous-flow centrifugal leukopheresis migrate equally well to sites of infection. They demonstrate a similar kinetic pattern in the lung, liver, and spleen.[84, 85] McCullough and colleagues[86] demonstrated that post-transfusion granulocyte migration to skin window chambers was impaired when the cells were stored for 8 hours at 1°C to 6°C or for 24 hours at 22°C. Granulocytes stored for 8 hours at 22°C, however, migrated as well as unstored controls.

DISEASE LOCALIZATION AND IMAGING

Blood cells labeled with appropriately chosen radionuclides migrate to sites of disease where they can be detected by collimated scintillation cameras. These devices consist of a sodium iodide crystal that interacts with collimated gamma-photons emitted from the source. Visible light is produced, which is recorded by photomultiplier tubes and converted into an image by means of a dedicated computer interfaced with the camera. The imaging of radiolabeled granulocytes is especially useful in clinical medicine, and the imaging of platelets and red cells can also be important in selected situations.

Red Cells

The diagnostic uses of imaged, radiolabeled red cells have included the localization and sizing of the spleen or accessory spleen, blood pool scanning, and the detection of gastrointestinal bleeding and vascular anomalies such as hemangiomas. Colloids such as rhenium sulfur labeled with technetium-99m are often used to determine spleen size and location. Radiolabeled colloids also image the liver. On occasion, it is desirable to image the spleen alone, especially when an enlarged liver interferes with splenic images or when an accessory spleen is suspected. Red cells damaged by heat and labeled with technetium-99m localize in the spleen without significant hepatic uptake.[87]

The blood pool can be imaged, and related red cell kinetics determined, with red cells labeled with indium-111. Quantitative sequential counting and imaging are possible, focusing on a selected target organ such as the spleen. This procedure can determine the rate of splenic sequestration when increased peripheral destruction of red cells is suggested (Fig. 37–5).

Platelets

Platelets labeled with indium-111 can be detected and imaged at the sites of their deposition, such as in intravascular thrombi. Applications for the use of radiolabeled platelets include detection of venous, arterial, and intraventricular thrombi, pulmonary emboli, and aneu-

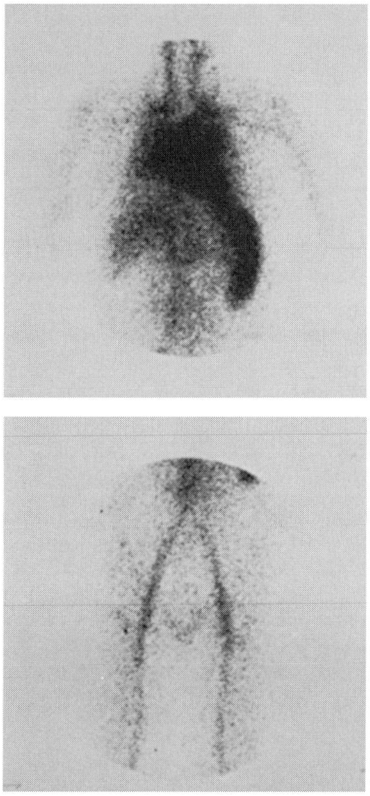

Figure 37–5. Indium-111–labeled red cell blood pool scan. The heart, great vessels, liver, and enlarged spleen are clearly imaged. Differential counting over selected organs can identify sites of red cell sequestration.

rysms.[88, 89] In addition, this technique can aid in the evaluation of the status of renal transplants[90] and arterial grafts.[91]

An actively forming clot incorporates platelets. Therefore, radiolabeled platelets are useful in identifying areas of new thrombus formation but do not label older thrombi. A venogram is often used to confirm a positive platelet scan. However, platelet scanning is reliable as a single diagnostic test and is especially useful in patients who are allergic to intravenous contrast material. If a suspicious area is identified on the early scans, the situation is followed for several days to note whether the area persists or increases in activity as blood pool activity decreases. In a prospective study of high-risk gynecological patients, 29% demonstrated increased platelet deposition in the major veins or lungs that were presumptive sites of thrombus formation.[92]

Granulocytes

Indium-111–labeled granulocytes are used to identify areas of infection and inflammation, such as suspected abscesses[93] or osteomyelitis,[94] or to evaluate a fever of unknown origin.[95] Indium-111–labeled granulocytes are usually preferred over gallium-67 citrate, an agent that is incorporated into phagocytic cells in vivo, because of the former's superior image quality and the absence of accumulation of the tracer in the gastrointestinal and urinary systems.[96] The technique for preparing granulocytes for imaging studies has been described by Loken and colleagues.[17] For most imaging studies in adults, 1 to 3 $\times$ 10^8 granulocytes are labeled with 400 to 500 of μCi of indium-111. Autologous cells are used whenever possible, but allogeneic granulocytes must be used for patients with granulocytopenia or functional granulocyte defects.

FUTURE DIRECTIONS AND NEW APPLICATIONS

The necessity to identify and label formed hematopoietic blood elements, and to follow their in vivo kinetic and localization patterns, will continue. Modified cells specifically designed for targeted clinical applications will need to be labeled and evaluated. Modified mononuclear cells for adoptive immunotherapy of cancer and cells modified by genetic transfer procedures are two exciting areas in which knowledge of in vivo cell behavior is incomplete.

Direct in vivo labeling of cells avoids damage to cells that may occur during in vitro labeling procedures. Coller[97] has described a monoclonal antiplatelet antibody that binds to platelet glycoprotein IIb–IIIa in vivo. This monoclonal antibody can be radiolabeled for localization of thrombi and other vascular lesions.

Improvements in the currently used radionuclides will enhance their clinical utility. Specifically, new chelates of indium-111 and modifications in labeling procedure using technetium-99m can reduce the high rates of elution that complicate their use. Stannous glucoheptonate, for example, results in a more stable technetium-99m red cell label than can be achieved with the standard method using stannous citrate.

Nonradioactive isotopes avoid the delivery of an absorbed radiation dose to the recipient. Chromium-50 binds easily to red cells but is cumbersome to produce and detect. Heaton and colleagues[98, 99] have demonstrated, however, that chromium-52 can be detected using advanced atomic absorption spectrophotometric techniques and is comparable to chromium-51 in red cell volume and post-transfusion survival studies. Flow cytometry can be useful in detecting small populations of heterologous red cells, thus avoiding chromium-51 labeling studies for transfusion compatibility.[100]

The necessity to perform and accurately interpret cell survival, kinetic, and imaging studies will increase as new cell storage and preservation systems are introduced and new clinical applications for standard and modified blood cells are developed. Close collaboration between specialists in transfusion medicine and other disciplines, especially nuclear medicine, will permit the opportunities in this exciting area to be fully explored.

REFERENCES

1. Gray SJ, Sterling K. The tagging of red cells and plasma proteins with radioactive chromium. J Clin Invest 1950; 29:1604.
2. Fisher J, Wolfe R, Leon A. Technetium-99m as a label for erythrocytes. J Nucl Med 1967; 8:229.

3. McAfee JG, Thakur ML. Survey of radioactive agents for in vitro labeling of phagocytic leukocytes: I. Soluble agents. J Nucl Med 1976; 17:480.
4. Mollison PL, Veall N. The use of the isotope ^{51}Cr as a label for red cells. Br J Haematol 1955; 1:62.
5. Garby L, Mollison PL. Deduction of mean red cell life-span from ^{51}Cr survival curves. Br J Haematol 1971; 20:527.
6. Bentley SA, Glass HI, Lewis SM, Szeur L. Elution correction in ^{51}Cr red cell survival studies. Br J Haematol 1974; 26:179.
7. Mollison PL, Engelfriet CP, Contreras M. Blood Transfusion in Clinical Medicine, 8th ed. Oxford: Blackwell Scientific Publications, 1987, p 104.
8. Moroff G, Sohmer PR, Button LN. Proposed standardization of methods for determining the 24-hour survival of stored red cells. Transfusion 1984; 24:109.
9. International Committee for Standardization in Hematology. Recommended method for radioisotope red-cell survival studies. Br J Haematol 1980; 45:659.
10. Baldini M, Costea N, Dameshek W. The viability of stored human platelets. Blood 1960; 16:1669.
11. Eyre HJ, Rosen PJ, Perry S. Relative labeling of leukocytes, erythrocytes and platelets in human blood by ^{51}Cr. Blood 1970; 36:250.
12. Snyder EL, Moroff G, Simon T, Heaton A. Recommended methods for conducting radiolabeled platelet survival studies. Transfusion 1986; 26:37.
13. Jones J, Mollison PL. A simple and efficient method of labeling red cells with ^{99m}Tc for determination of red cell volume. Br J Haematol 1978; 38:141.
14. Holt JT, Spitalnik SL, McMican AE, et al. A technetium-99m red cell survival technique for in vivo compatibility testing. Transfusion 1983; 23:148.
15. Heaton WAL, Keegan T, Holme S, Momoda G. Evaluation of ^{99m}technetium/^{51}chromium posttransfusion recovery of red cells stored in saline, adenine, glucose, and mannitol for 42 days. Vox Sang 1989; 57:37.
16. AuBuchon JP, Brightman A. Use of indium-111 as a red cell label. Transfusion 1989; 29:143.
17. Loken MK, Clay ME, Carpenter RT, et al. Clinical use of indium-111 labeled blood products. Clin Nucl Med 1985; 10:902.
18. Mountford PJ, Allsopp MJ, Hall FM, et al. Leucocyte and contaminant cell-bound activities resulting from the labeling of leucocytes with indium-111 oxine. Eur J Nucl Med 1985; 10:304.
19. Callender STE, Powell EO, Witts LJ. The life-span of the red cell in man. J Pathol Bacteriol 1945; 57:129.
20. Berlin NI. Determination of red cell life span. JAMA 1964; 188:375.
21. Mollison PL. Determination of red cell survival using ^{51}Cr. *In* Bell CA (ed): A Seminar on Immune-Mediated Cell Destruction. Washington, DC: American Association of Blood Banks, 1981, pp 45–69.
22. Propper RD, Button LN, Nathan DG. New approaches to the transfusion management of thalassemia. Blood 1980; 55:55.
23. Corash L, Klein H, Deisseroth A, et al. Selective isolation of young erythrocytes for transfusion support of thalassemia major patients. Blood 1981; 57:599.
24. Simon TL, Sohmer P, Nelson EJ. Extended survival of neocytes produced in a new system. Transfusion 1989; 29:221.
25. Cohen AR, Schmidt JM, Martin MB, et al. Clinical trial of young red cell transfusions. J Pediatr 1984; 104:865.
26. Marcus RE, Wonke B, Bantok HM, et al. A prospective trial of young red cells in 48 patients with transfusion-dependent thalassemia. Br J Haematol 1985; 60:153.
27. Engelfriet CP, von dem Borne AEG, Beckers D, et al. Immune destruction of red cells. *In* Bell CA (ed): A Seminar on Immune-Mediated Cell Destruction. Washington, DC: American Association of Blood Banks, 1981, pp 93–130.
28. Davey RJ. Mechanisms of premature red cell destruction. *In* Judd WJ, Barnes A (eds): Clinical and Serological Aspects of Transfusion Reactions. Arlington, VA: American Association of Blood Banks, 1982, pp 1–35.
29. Mollison PL. Survival curves of incompatible red cells. Transfusion 1986; 26:43.
30. Garratty G. Factors affecting the pathogenicity of red cell allo- and autoantibodies. *In* Nance ST (ed): Immune Destruction of Red Blood Cells. Arlington, VA: American Association of Blood Banks, 1987, pp 114–22.
31. Garratty G. The significance of complement in immunohematology. CRC Crit Rev Clin Lab Sci 1984; 20:25.
32. Freedman J. The significance of complement on the red cell membrane. Transfus Med Rev 1987; 1:58.
33. Jaffe CJ, Atkinson JP, Frank MM. The role of complement in the clearance of cold agglutinin–sensitized erythrocytes in man. J Clin Invest 1976; 58:942.
34. Lachmann PJ, Pangburn MK, Oldroyd RG. Breakdown of C3 after complement activation. J Exp Med 1982; 156:205.
35. Lachmann PJ, Voak D, Oldroyd RG, et al. Use of monoclonal anti-C3 antibodies to characterize the fragments of C3 that are found on erythrocytes. Vox Sang 1983; 45:367.
36. Atkinson JP, Frank MM. Studies on the in vivo effects of antibody: interaction of IgM antibody and complement in the immune clearance and destruction of erythrocytes in man. J Clin Invest 1974; 54:339.
37. Gaither TA, Vargas I, Inada S, Frank MM. The complement fragment C3d facilitates phagocytosis by monocytes. Immunology 1987; 62:405.
38. Ehlenberger AG, Nussenzweig V. The role of membrane receptors for C3b and C3d in phagocytosis. J Exp Med 1977; 145:357.
39. International Committee for Standardization in Hematology. Recommended methods for radioisotope platelet survival studies. Blood 1977; 50:1137.
40. Thakur ML, Walch MJ, Malek HL, Gottschalk A. Indium-111–labeled human platelets: improved method, efficacy, and evaluation. J Nucl Med 1981; 22:381.
41. International Committee for Standardization in Hematology. Recommended method for indium-111 platelet survival studies. J Nucl Med 1988; 29:564.
42. Mathias CJ, Heaton WA, Welch MJ, et al. Comparison of ^{111}In-oxine and ^{111}In-acetyl acetone for the labeling of cells: in vivo and vitro biological testing. Int J Appl Radiat Isot 1981; 32:651.
43. Dewanjee MK, Rao SA, Rosemark JA, et al. Indium-111 tropolone, a new tracer for platelet labeling. Radiology 1982; 145:149.
44. Thakur ML, McKenney SL, Park CH. Simplified and efficient labeling of human platelets in plasma using indium-111-2-mercaptopyridine-N-oxide: preparation and evaluation. J Nucl Med 1985; 26:510.
45. Paulus JM, Aster RH. Platelet kinetics: production distribution, lifespan, and fate of platelets. *In* Williams W, Beutler E, Erslev A, Lichtman M (eds): Hematology, 3rd ed. New York: McGraw-Hill, 1983, pp 1185–1196.
46. Harker LA, Finch CA. Thrombokinetics in man. J Clin Invest 1969; 48:963.
47. Heyns A du P, Lotter MG, Badenhorst PN, et al. Kinetics, distribution and sites of destruction of indium-111–labelled human platelets. Br J Haematol 1980; 44:269.
48. Klonizakis I, Peters AM, Fitzpatrick ML, et al. Radionuclide distribution following injection of In-111–labelled platelets. Br J Haematol 1980; 46:595.
49. Hanson SR, Slichter SJ. Platelet kinetics in patients with bone marrow hypoplasia: evidence for a fixed platelet requirement. Blood 1985; 66:1105.
50. Tomer A, Harker LA. Megakaryocytopoiesis and platelet kinetics. *In* Rossi EC, Simon TL, Moss GS (eds): Principles of Transfusion Medicine. Baltimore: Williams & Wilkins, 1991, p 175.
51. Read EJ. Leukocyte radiolabeling. *In* Davey RJ, Wallace ME (eds): Diagnostic and Investigational Uses of Radiolabeled Blood Elements. Arlington, VA: American Association of Blood Banks, 1987, pp 93–114.
52. McAfee JG, Subramanian G, Gagne G. Technique of leukocyte harvesting and labeling: problems and perspectives. Semin Nucl Med 1984; 12:83.
53. Athens JW, Haab OP, Raab SO, et al. Leukokinetic studies: IV. The total blood, circulating and marginal granulocyte pools and granulocyte turnover rate in normal subjects. J Clin Invest 1961; 40:989.
54. Alexanian R, Donahue DM. Neutrophilic granulocyte kinetics in normal man. J Appl Physiol 1965; 20:803.
55. Weiblen BJ, Forstrom L, McCullough J. Studies of the kinetics of indium-111–labeled granulocytes. J Lab Clin Med 1979; 94:246.
56. Savermuttu SH, Peters AM, Danpure HJ, et al. Lung transit of ^{111}indium-labelled granulocytes: relationship to labelling techniques. Scand J Haematol 1983; 30:151.

57. Dutcher JP, Fox JJ, Riggs C, et al. Pulmonary retention of indium-111–labeled granulocytes in alloimmunized patients. Blood 1982; 58:177a.
58. McCullough J, Clay M, Hurd D, et al. Effect of leukocyte antibodies and HLA matching on the intravascular recovery, survival, and tissue localization of ^{111}In granulocytes. Blood 1986; 67:522.
59. Dutcher JP, Schiffer CA, Johnston CS, et al. Alloimmunization prevents the migration of transfused indium-111–labeled granulocytes to sites of infection. Blood 1983; 62:354.
60. Read EJ, Keenan AM, Carter CS, et al. In vivo traffic of indium-111-oxine labeled human lymphocytes collected by automated apheresis. J Nucl Med 1990; 31:999.
61. Ford WL, Gowans JL. The traffic of lymphocytes. Semin Hematol 1969; 6:67.
62. Butcher EC. The regulation of lymphocyte traffic. Curr Top Microbiol Immunol 1986; 128:85.
63. Gallatin M, St. John TP, Siegelman M, et al. Lymphocyte homing receptors. Cell 1986; 44:673.
64. Stevenson HC, Keenan AM, Woodhouse C, et al. Fate of interferon-activated killer blood monocytes adoptively transferred into the peritoneal cavity of patients with peritoneal carcinomatosis. Cancer Res 1987; 47:6100.
65. Mazumder A, Eberlein TJ, Grimm EA, et al. Phase I study of the adoptive immunotherapy of human cancer with lectin activated autologous mononuclear cells. Cancer 1984; 53:896.
66. Fisher B, Packard BS, Read EJ, et al. Tumor localization of adoptively transferred indium-111 labeled tumor infiltrating lymphocytes in patients with metastatic melanoma. J Clin Oncol 1989; 7:250.
67. Loutit JF, Mollison PL. Advantages of a disodium-citrate-glucose mixture as a blood preservative. BMJ 1943; 2:744.
68. Davey RJ, McCoy NC, Yu M, et al. The effect of pre-storage irradiation on posttransfusion red cell survival. Transfusion 1992; 32:525.
69. AuBuchon JP, Estep TN, Davey RJ. The effect of the plasticizer di-2-ethylhexylphthalate on the survival of stored red cells. Blood 1988; 71:448.
70. Brecher ME, Pineda AA, Torloni AS, et al. Prestorage leukocyte depletion: effect on leukocyte and platelet metabolites, erythrocyte lysis, metabolism, and in vivo survival. Semin Hematol 1991; 28 (suppl 5):3.
71. Mollison PL, Engelfriet CP, Contreras M. Blood Transfusion in Clinical Medicine, 8th ed. Oxford: Blackwell Scientific Publications, 1987, pp 71–73.
72. Beutler E, West C. Measurement of the viability of stored red cells by the single-isotope technique using ^{51}Cr. Transfusion 1984; 24:100.
73. Garratty G. Predicting the clinical significance of alloantibodies and determining the in vivo survival of transfused red cells. *In* Judd JW, Barnes A (eds): Clinical and Serological Aspects of Transfusion Reactions. Arlington, VA: American Association of Blood Banks, 1982, pp 91–120.
74. Heaton WAL. Indium-111 (^{111}In) and chromium-51 (^{51}Cr) labeling of platelets. Are they comparable? Transfusion 1986; 26:16.
75. Snyder EL. Effect of storage conditions on radiolabeling of stored platelet concentrates. Transfusion 1986; 26:6.
76. Moroff G, Simon TL. Use of radioisotopically-labeled platelets to determine the survival characteristics of stored platelets. Transfusion 1986; 26:1.
77. Keegan T, Heaton A, Holme S, et al. Paired comparison of platelet concentrates prepared from platelet-rich plasma and buffy coats using a new technique with ^{111}In and ^{51}Cr. Transfusion 1992; 32:113.
78. Murphy S, Kahn RA, Holme S, et al. Improved storage of platelets for transfusion in a new container. Blood 1982; 60:194.
79. Simon TL, Nelson EJ, Carmen R, Murphy S. Extension of platelet concentrate storage. Transfusion 1983; 23:207.
80. Murphy S, Sayar SN, Gardner FH. Storage of platelet concentrates at 22°C. Blood 1970; 35:549.
81. Filip DJ, Aster RH. Relative hemostatic effectiveness of human platelets stored at 4° and 22°C. J Lab Clin Med 1978; 91:618.
82. Snyder EL, Pope C, Ferri PM, et al. The effect of mode of agitation and type of plastic bag on storage characteristics and in vivo kinetics of platelet concentrates. Transfusion 1986; 26:125.
83. Buchholz DH, Porten JH, Menitove JE, et al. Description and use of the CS-3000 blood cell separator for single-donor platelet collection. Transfusion 1983; 23:190.
84. Alavi JB, Alavi A, Staum MM. Evaluation of infection in neutropenic patients with indium-111–labeled donor granulocytes. Clin Nucl Med 1980; 5:397.
85. Anstall HB, Coleman RE. Donor leukocyte imaging in granulocytopenic patients with suspected abscesses. J Nucl Med 1982; 23:319.
86. McCullough J, Weiblen BJ, Fire D. Effect of storage on granulocytes and their fate in vivo. Transfusion 1983; 23:20.
87. Sty JR, Conway JJ. The spleen: development and functional evaluation. Semin Nucl Med 1985; 15:299.
88. Powers WJ, Siegel BA. Thrombus imaging with indium-111 platelets. Semin Thromb Hemost 1983; 9:115.
89. Smith EO, Snyder EL. Radiolabeled platelets. *In* Davey RJ, Wallace ME (eds): Diagnostic and Investigational Uses of Radiolabeled Blood Elements. Arlington, VA: American Association of Blood Banks, 1987, pp 79–84.
90. Sinzinger HF, Leithner CW. The use of indium-111–labeled platelets in the management of renal transplant patients. *In* Thakur ML, Ezekowitz MD, Hardeman MR (eds): Radiolabeled Cellular Blood Elements. New York: Plenum Press, 1985, pp 201–228.
91. Hanson SR, Kotz HF, Pieters H, Heyns AD. Analysis of indium-111 platelet kinetics and imaging in patients with aortic grafts and abdominal aortic aneurysms. Arteriosclerosis 1990; 10:1037.
92. Clark-Pearson DL, Coleman RE, Siegel R, et al. Indium-111 platelet imaging for the detection of deep venous thrombosis and pulmonary embolism in patients without symptoms after surgery. Surgery 1985; 98:98.
93. Segal AW, Arnot RN, Thakur ML, Lavender JP. Indium-111–labeled leukocytes for localization of abscesses. Lancet 1976; 2:1056.
94. King AD, Peters AM, Stuttle AW, Lavender JP. Imaging of bone infection with labelled white blood cells: role of contemporaneous bone marrow imaging. Eur J Nucl Med 1990; 17:148.
95. Davies SG, Garvie NW. The role of indium-labelled leukocyte imaging in pyrexia of unknown origin. Br J Radiol 1990; 63:850.
96. Froelich JW, Swanson D. Imaging of inflammatory processes with labeled cells. Semin Nucl Med 1984; 14:128.
97. Coller B. Theoretical considerations in designing monoclonal antibodies for imaging thrombi with platelet directed antibodies. Presented at Colloquium on Coronary Thrombosis, the Future of Imaging Techniques. Oklahoma City, Oklahoma Cardiovascular Institute, 1984.
98. Heaton WAL, Hanbury CM, Keegan TE, et al. Studies with nonradioisotopic sodium chromate: I. Development of a technique for measuring red cell volume. Transfusion 1989; 29:696.
99. Heaton WAL, Keegan T, Hanbury CM, et al. Studies with nonradioisotopic sodium chromate: II. Single-and double-label ^{52}Cr/^{51}Cr posttransfusion recovery estimations. Transfusion 1989; 29:703.
100. Nance SJ, Garratty G. Application of flow cytometry to immunohematology. J Immunol Methods 1987; 101:127.

CHAPTER 38

Polymerase Chain Reaction and Transfusion-Related Infections

Kevin P. Whitby
Jeremy A. Garson
John A. J. Barbara

The prevention of transfusion transmission of microbial infection is largely dependent on careful donor selection and reliable screening assays. However, there remains a small but significant transfusion risk for each of the major viral agents.[1, 2] This risk typically occurs for one of four reasons: (1) a failure of current serological screening methods to detect infection during the pre-seroconversion "window" period; (2) the presence of antigenically variant viruses that do not share epitopes detected by current assays; (3) the absence of a detectable immune response because of immunosuppression; and (4) a failure in the testing procedure itself.

The usually small residual risk caused by each of these types of screening failures could be significantly reduced by the introduction of sensitive assays designed to detect the genome of transfusion-transmissible microbial agents. A wide variety of nucleic acid detection methods are now commercially available (e.g., polymerase chain reaction [PCR], nucleic acid sequence–based amplification [NASBA], ligase chain reaction [LCR], Quantiplex assay [bDNA]), but PCR remains the most sensitive and versatile of these methods.

PCR is an exquisitely sensitive tool for the detection and analysis of specific nucleic acid sequences. As such, it represents a very significant advance, and its potential applications impinge on a wide range of biological sciences. One important application relates to the study of microbial infection.[3] This chapter considers the potential impact of PCR on the diagnosis of transfusion-transmitted infections in particular.

THE BASIC PRINCIPLES OF PCR

The PCR was devised and developed by Kary Mullis.[4] Its first practical application was to amplify the human β-globin gene to detect the mutation leading to sickle-cell anemia.[5] The purification of a thermostable polymerase from the eubacterium *Thermus aquaticus* (*Taq* polymerase) has allowed the practical application of this process to large areas of molecular biology.

PCR is an in vitro reaction involving the thermal separation of the two strands of DNA, the annealing of short oligonucleotide primers complementary to each of the DNA strands, and the extension of these primers by a DNA-dependent DNA polymerase. The consequence of this process is a doubling of the original number of DNA copies. If this doubling is repeated a number of times, the resulting twofold geometric increase in DNA copy number leads to a huge amplification of the number of DNA copies identical to the original target sequence.

The basic steps involved in a PCR are as follows (Fig. 38–1):

Strand separation: Incubating DNA at temperatures exceeding 90°C results in the breakage of the hydrogen bonds that hold the two strands together, which leads to their separation.

Priming: Once the strands of DNA are separated, the reaction mix is allowed to cool, thus allowing two synthetic oligonucleotides, usually 15 to 40 bases in length, to bind to the complementary target sequence. One oligonucleotide binds to the sense strand and one to the antisense strand at a predetermined distance apart. The distance between the 5′ ends of the two oligonucleotides, typically 50 to 10,000 bases, determines the size of the PCR product. The exact location where the oligonucleotides bind is dictated by their sequence. Optimized conditions for PCR allow only one binding location for each primer, dictated by the annealing temperature of the reaction and the laws of thermodynamics.

Strand extension: The annealed primers are extended to complete the second strand by heating the reaction to a temperature optimal for the incorporation of deoxyribonucleotide triphosphates (dNTPs) by the thermostable polymerase, usually 68°C to 75°C. During the first cycle of replication, the strand extension proceeds beyond the binding site of the second primer, but on subsequent cycles, the number of molecules with their 3′ end determined by the binding site of the second primer increases logarithmically. The final size of PCR product after many cycles of replication is predominantly that determined by the distance between the binding sites of the two primers. The number of product molecules generated from a single target molecule, assuming a theoretical twofold increase at each cycle and a more realistic 1.7-fold total increase, is shown in Figure 38–2.

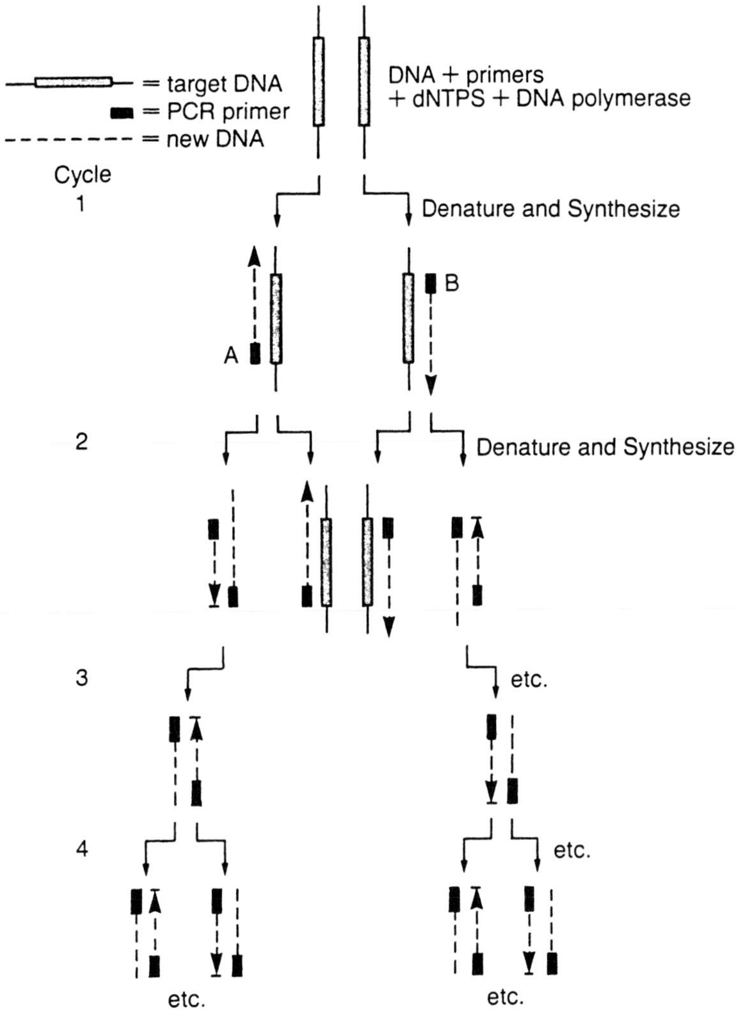

Figure 38–1. Polymerase chain reaction (PCR). DNA is denatured at more than 90°C, oligonucleotides A and B are annealed, and extension from primers of a complementary DNA strand occurs in the presence of a thermostable DNA polymerase and the four deoxyribonucleotide triphosphates (dNTPs). Subsequent cycles of denaturation of the template, annealing of the primers to their complementary sequences, and extension of the annealed primers with a DNA polymerase result in the amplification of the segment, defined by the 5′ ends of the PCR primers. (From White TJ, Arnheim N, Erlich HA. The polymerase chain reaction. Trends Genet 1989; 5(6):185.)

In reality, it is unlikely that the efficiency of PCR is constant from cycle to cycle, because the enzyme loses activity, as a result of either of its thermal inactivation or its incorporation into the PCR product. In addition, depletion of reaction substrates such as nucleotides or primers become limiting as the reaction progresses. As is clearly illustrated in Figure 38–2, small differences in reaction efficiency produce dramatic differences in the rate of accumulation of PCR products. Careful optimization of the factors influencing reaction efficiency is therefore important in the amplification of the target sequence.

In practice, PCR requires the optimization not only of the parameters just described but also of several methods peripheral to the reaction itself. In general, the practical application of PCR to transfusion microbiology can be divided into five stages:

1. *Sample handling:* The stage from phlebotomy to nucleic acid extraction is often a major source of variation. Blood samples stored or transported at or above room temperature may exhibit a rapid loss of viral RNA.[6]

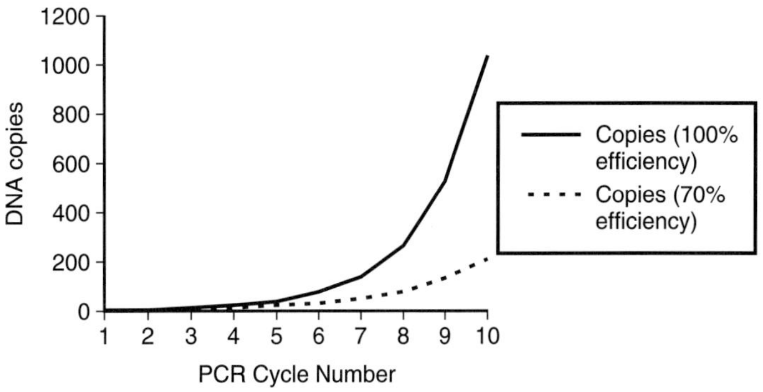

Figure 38–2. The exponential relationship between product numbers and polymerase chain reaction (PCR) cycles. Small differences in reaction efficiency can result in large differences in the final product concentration. It is therefore important to ensure that reaction conditions are carefully optimized and are reproduced faithfully between reaction vessels.

2. *Nucleic acid preparation:* The efficiency and reproducibility of stages 3 to 5 (to be described) are dependent on the yield and purity of the nucleic acid isolated. RNA is inherently less stable than DNA in that it is more thermolabile and readily digested by enzymes. The following processes are essential to the efficiency of extraction:
   - *Inactivation of nucleases present in all living tissues.* This is achieved either by proteinase digestion of the enzymes or by the chemical denaturation with chaotropic agents. Unlike deoxyribonucleases, ribonucleases, by virtue of their small size and highly crosslinked secondary structure, readily reform after heat or chemical denaturation. Meticulous preparation of reaction vessels and buffers to remove contaminating nucleases is necessary to ensure a high yield.
   - *Lysis of cells and viral particles.* This is usually achieved with detergents such as *N*-lauryl sarcosine, Triton X-100, or NP40.
   - *Physical separation of nucleic acids from potential inhibitors.* PCR is particularly susceptible to inhibition by proteins containing porphyrin rings, such as hemoglobin,[7] and by the anticoagulant heparin. Avoidance of these inhibitors is achieved by limiting analysis to that of fresh or fresh frozen serum or heparin-free plasma. The nucleic acids can be separated from small amounts of contaminating hemoglobin and other proteins during phase separation by means of organic solvents[8] or by selective binding to either silica[9] or oligonucleotides.[10]
   - *Concentration.* This is achieved either by precipitation with alcohol or during the selective binding described earlier, followed by elution or resuspension in a small volume of water or appropriate buffer.
3. *Complementary DNA synthesis by reverse transcription of viral RNA:* PCR is a method for the amplification of DNA; therefore, amplification of RNA targets such as the hepatitis C virus (HCV) or human immunodeficiency virus (HIV) genomes first requires that the RNA be reverse-transcribed into DNA.
4. *Amplification by PCR:* Practical considerations for PCR optimization include the following:
   - *The concentrations of reaction components.* Concentrations of the following must be optimized: oligonucleotide primers, dNTPs, and thermostable DNA polymerase (e.g., *Taq, Tth, Tfl, Pfu*). Thermostable polymerases are now supplied with preoptimized reaction buffers containing divalent cations (magnesium ions [Mg^{2+}] or manganese ions [Mn^{2+}], which can be buffered with bicine), hydrogen ions (pH buffer), potassium or sodium ions (which serve to alter the stringency), and a variety of detergents, carriers, and reducing agents that improve reaction efficiency but are not essential components.
   - *Primer design.* Oligonucleotide primers used in PCR are chemically synthesized. Their design is based primarily on the known sequence of the target nucleic acid. Ideally, their sequence should be 100% homologous to the target sequence; however, because of the inherent variability of the genomes of RNA viruses such as HCV and HIV, this is not always possible.
   - *Cycling parameters.* PCR is now invariably performed with an automated programmable heating block (Fig. 38–3). Reaction vessels (5 to 100 μL) are placed in the PCR machine, and the three stages of PCR each occur during predetermined incubation periods and at predetermined temperatures. Denaturation occurs at temperatures above 90°C; too low a temperature or too short an incubation time leads to a loss of sensitivity as a result of incomplete denaturation; too high a temperature or too long an incubation time leads to a loss of sensitivity as a result of thermal inactivation of the polymerase. Annealing temperature is the most variable component between primer sets. If the temperature is not allowed to drop sufficiently, little or no primer will hybridize to its target, but if the annealing temperature is too low, sequences other than the target may be amplified. The optimal annealing temperature is dependent on the nucleotide composition of the primer (GC:AT ratio and length), the variability of the target sequence, and the monovalent cation concentration of the reaction buffer. Primer extension occurs at a temperature near the optimum for the polymerase

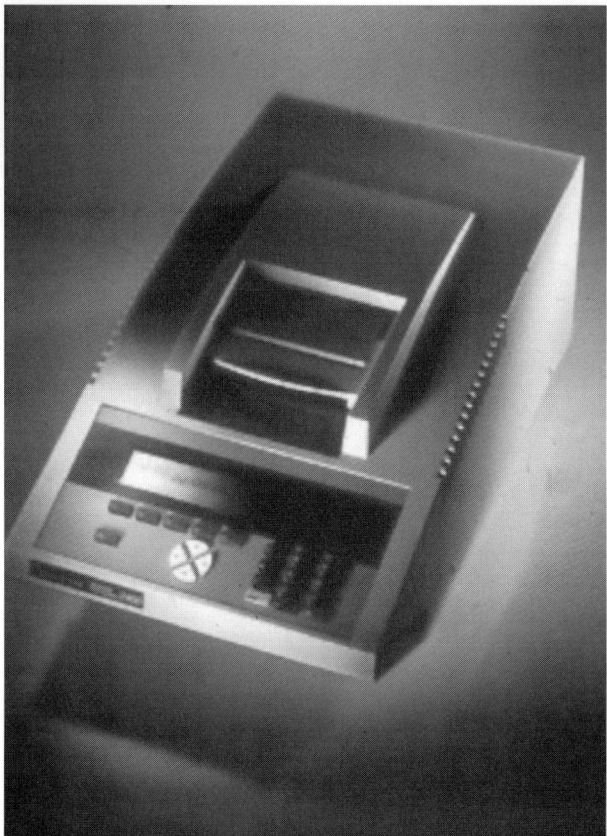

Figure 38–3. Photograph of an automated, electronically controlled "thermal cycler." Thermal cyclers are now available in an increasing variety of formats. The machine featured here amplifies tubes in an 8 × 12 "microtiter" format allowing easier downstream processing of PCR products. (Photograph kindly provided by Perkin Elmer Ltd.)

used. For *Taq* polymerase, the optimum is 72°C, but for other polymerases, this may be different (e.g., *Pfu* polymerase extends optimally at 75°C). The optimal extension time is dependent on the length of the PCR product generated. For short products (<100 base pairs), extension times need be only a few seconds. The number of cycles performed is limited by the amount and stability of polymerase added, but it usually does not exceed 35 to 40.

- *Number of rounds of cycling (nested PCR).* For the reasons outlined earlier, the number of PCR product molecules that can be accumulated in a single reaction is finite.[11] The sensitivity and specificity of PCR can be greatly increased by the use of "nested," or double, reactions.[12] In this method, the products of a PCR are used as the input sample in a second PCR with primers internal to the primer pair that was used in the first PCR. The use of four PCR primers in this way allows the specific detection of even a single initial target molecule.[13, 14]
- *Contamination avoidance.* Because of the extreme sensitivity of PCR, false-negative results are much less likely to occur than they are with other nucleic acid detection techniques. However, as outlined previously, PCR results in the production of large numbers of PCR products, typically more than 10^9, in a small reaction volume, usually less than 100 μL; thus, contaminating volumes of less than 1 pL from a previous reaction with the same primers results in a false-positive result. PCR contamination is therefore a major potential problem that can be avoided only by adherence to stringent precautions, such as those previously outlined by Kwok and Higuchi.[15]

5. *Analysis of the PCR product:* The nature of the analysis performed on PCR products depends primarily on the initial purpose of the PCR. PCR has been applied to a bewildering array of different uses within molecular biology. In brief, the analysis of PCR products falls into three broad categories:
   - *The qualitative detection of PCR products* (i.e., whether a specific product of the expected size has been generated). This is most commonly achieved either by electrophoresis with ethidium bromide–stained agarose gels or with microtiter format product detection assays.[15a]
   - *Quantitative PCR.* Quantification with PCR is dependent on the optimization of the reaction conditions to produce a range of product concentrations that can be related to the amount of virus in the starting material.[15b]
   - *Sequence analysis.* PCR is a convenient method of generating large quantities of DNA for sequence analysis. This analysis may be performed by direct sequence determination of the PCR product or after cloning of the products. The sequence can be determined directly through chain termination methods or indirectly inferred from hybridization or restriction fragment analysis.[15c]

THE POTENTIAL VALUE OF PCR IN TRANSFUSION MEDICINE

The potential advantages of PCR in the context of transfusion microbiology are as follows:

- Sensitivity (detects approximately 10^{-18} g nucleic acid).
- Identification of viral contamination in products made from large pools of plasma.
- Marker for *infectivity* (but may detect nucleic acid in inactivated blood products).
- Reduction of the "window" period (although the timing of sampling may be critical); that is, diagnosis of acute infections is possible.
- Detection of "latent" infections.
- Differentiation of passive antibody from active infection (e.g., HIV in newborns).
- Strain differentiation.
- Detection of novel viral infections.
- Supplement to "confirmation" of traditional blood screening assays.

INTERPRETATION OF A NEGATIVE PCR RESULT

Much attention has been focused on "confirmation" (this term is enclosed in quotation marks because an antibody test cannot strictly be *confirmed* by a test for nucleic acid) of anti-HCV screen test reactivity by PCR. HCV therefore serves as an example to illustrate several possibilities that must be considered in interpreting a negative PCR result.

1. If complete viral clearance occurs, as it probably does in a minority of HCV infections, the PCR assay for serum HCV RNA would not be positive, despite what might be a genuine antibody response.
2. Because the volume of sample being tested (0.1 to 1 mL) is much smaller than the volume of blood or blood component transfused, low-level viremia in potentially infectious blood may go undetected by PCR.
3. Unless highly conserved viral sequences common to all strains are chosen for PCR, strain variation could lead to false-negative results. This problem can be avoided by using PCR primers that are based on highly conserved regions of the viral genome: for example, the 5′ noncoding region (5′NCR) of HCV.
4. If samples containing viruses are not stored frozen under optimal conditions or are subjected to numerous freeze/thaw cycles, degradation of the genome may occur, leading to a false-negative PCR result.[6]

LIMITATIONS OF PCR

No assay system is perfect, and despite the benefits of PCR, several caveats and disadvantages, especially in a transfusion context, must be considered. First, the extreme sensitivity of PCR exacerbates the problem of false positivity that results from contamination of the test sample. Carryover during sampling is a particular problem in transfusion laboratories,[16] in which automated sampling for serological screening, often with washable sample probes, is becoming increasingly common.[17] Where such devices are in use, specially taken PCR samples will be required in order to avoid even minimal carryover. Great care must be taken to avoid contamination of samples by amplified PCR products from previous reactions, which will contain enormous numbers of copies of the DNA sequences under test. Sample preparation and amplification procedures should be carried out in different laboratories or, ideally, in different buildings. Facilities for changing gowns, gloves, and overshoes should be available, and only pipettes dedicated to PCR should be used, and disposable tips are required for mass sampling automation. Kwok and Higuchi[15] and Erlich and colleagues[18] summarized the essential precautions for avoiding contamination in PCR laboratories. Significant progress has been made in developing strategies to prevent amplification of rogue PCR products. These typically involve chemical alteration or destruction of PCR products after amplification and/or enzymatic cleavage immediately before amplification.[19] However, it is extremely important to remember that no strategy has been developed by which to identify false-positive results caused by sample cross-contamination, and special vigilance is required in this area.

False positivity in PCR may also occur if primers are not carefully chosen to avoid similarity with related human endogenous sequences. This caution applies particularly when retroviral *pol* genes are being amplified, because the human genome contains many thousands of endogenous retroviral *pol*-related sequences. Choice of sample may be important, because some viruses, such as human T cell leukemia/lymphoma virus (HTLV), are strongly cell-associated, and peripheral blood mononuclear cells rather than serum are required for nucleic acid extraction before PCR.

The application of PCR to the large-scale routine screening of blood donations has been limited largely by the labor-intensive and time-consuming nature of the technique. In 1990 Jackson[20] estimated that 20 samples would take one person approximately 3 days to complete, although this number could be reduced considerably if a 1-hour DNA extraction protocol is used. However, at that time, PCR was a relatively novel technique, and much progress has been made in streamlining each stage of the procedure. Commercially available PCR assays that allow results to be generated within a single working day are now available.[20a] RNA extraction can be performed robotically, reverse transcription and PCR can be performed in a single tube in less than half an hour, and PCR products can be quantified as they are being produced.[20b] Nevertheless, PCR has remained a technique with a primary application in research,[16] and its main contribution to transfusion microbiology is currently in reference and confirmatory work. However, with increasing automation and allied economies of scale, it seems likely that the use of nucleic acid–based detection in transfusion microbiology will increase rapidly in the near future. Although it seems unlikely that PCR detection will replace serological assays for screening blood donations, PCR does offer the significant advantage of being able to directly detect virus before the development of a detectable immune response. This approach theoretically has the potential to reduce the "window" period by 11 days for HIV (from 22 days to 11 days), by 26 days for HBV infection (from 56 days to 30), and by 59 days for HCV infection (from 82 days to 21 days) if individual donations are tested.[2] More recent data based on retrospective analysis of seroconverting blood donors suggest that these estimates may be a little optimistic (R. Dodd and S. Stramer, American Red Cross, personal communications).

It is also worth noting that detection of viral nucleic acid does not necessarily prove infectivity. First, free nucleic acid may not necessarily be infectious; second, defective or inactivated viral particles will give rise to PCR signals even if they are unable to establish an infection. Nevertheless, it seems prudent to assume infectivity in most situations when genomic sequences can be detected.

ALTERNATIVES TO PCR FOR NUCLEIC ACID DETECTION

Ligase Chain Reaction

The LCR is composed of three steps analogous to those of PCR.[21] The DNA is converted into the single-stranded form by heating (90°C to 100°C), the reaction temperature is reduced to allow the annealing of four primers, and two pairs of primers are annealed to adjacent primer binding sites on each DNA strand. Unlike DNA polymerase, DNA ligase is unable to incorporate nucleotides, and in the ligation phase of LCR, both primer pairs are joined by a thermostable DNA ligase to form two molecules of double-stranded DNA. Repeated doubling reactions can occur, allowing the amplification of target DNA in a similar way to that seen in PCR.

Nucleic Acid Sequence–Based Amplification

NASBA is able to amplify either RNA or DNA through a combination of three enzymes.[22] Amplification begins with the extension of an oligonucleotide primer that incorporates the T7 promoter by AMV reverse transcriptase on a single-stranded DNA or RNA template. If the initial template strand was RNA, this strand is degraded by the ribonuclease RNase H, and a second DNA strand is synthesized by extension from a second primer. Finally, a new RNA template is synthesized by T7 RNA polymerase, allowing the cycle to begin again. For all three enzymes, the optimal temperature for activity is approximately 37°C, thus allowing the whole process to occur at a constant temperature (Fig. 38–4). This system has also been referred to as self-sustained sequence replication (3SR) and is identical in all but minor detail to an assay called transcription-mediated amplification (TMA).

Strand Displacement Amplification (SDA)

Strand displacement amplification (SDA) is an isothermal, in vitro nucleic acid amplification technique based on the

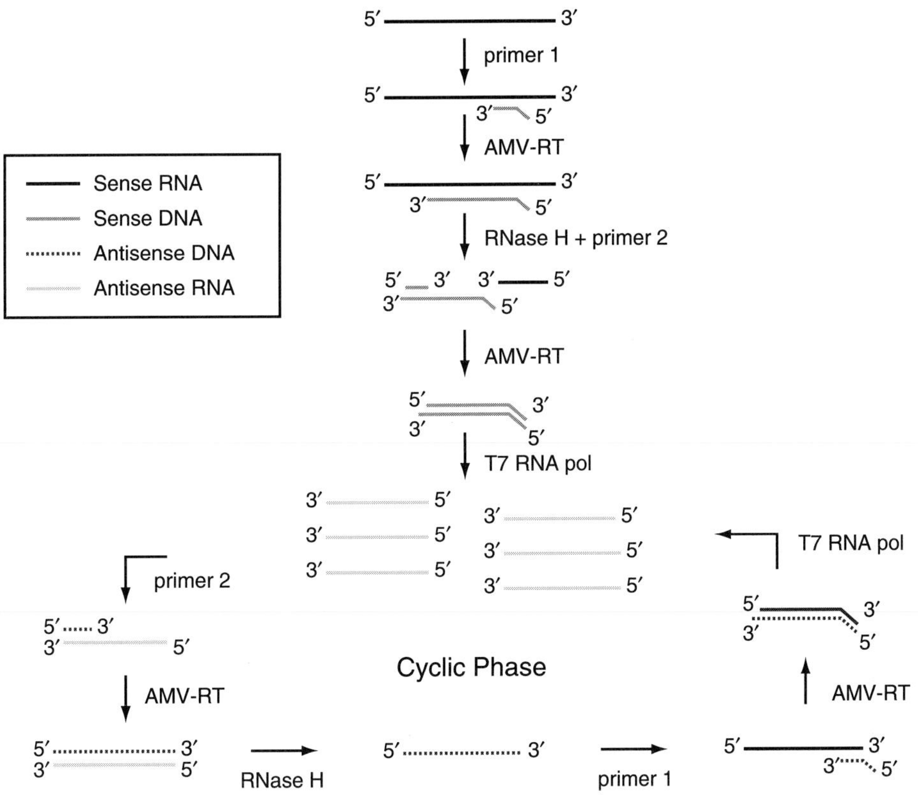

Figure 38–4. Nucleic acid sequence–based amplification (NASBA). NASBA involves the use of a combination of three enzymes, each with an optimal temperature of approximately 37°C for amplification, to amplify either DNA or RNA in an isothermal reaction.

ability of the restriction enzyme *Hinc* II to nick the unmodified strand of a hemiphosphorothioate form of its recognition site and on the ability of the Klenow fragment of DNA polymerase to extend the 3′ end at the nick and displace the downstream DNA strand. Exponential amplification results from coupling sense and antisense reactions, in which strands displaced from a sense reaction serve as targets for an antisense reaction and vice versa.[23]

*Q*β Replicase Amplified Assay

This assay system differs from the target amplification systems in that its strategy is based on probe amplification. *Q*β replicase is a tetrameric enzyme complex capable of inducing the amplification of single-stranded RNA molecules containing a specific recognition sequence and a terminal nucleotide sequence required for polymerase recognition. One of the four subunits of the enzyme complex is derived from the *Q*β bacteriophage; the other three are produced by its host, *Escherichia coli*. Probes for *Q*β replicase–based assays are generated by modifying the single-stranded RNA genome of the *Q*β bacteriophage MDV-1. The target-specific sequence is inserted into the phage genome to generate a hybridization probe, which can then be used to bind target sequences. Once the unbound probe is removed (by careful washing), the enzyme complex is added, which leads to the exponential amplification of the probe.[24] Although this system has largely been applied to the detection of bacterial and *Chlamydia* targets, its adaptation to the detection of viral nucleic acid should be possible. The sensitivity of this assay is limited largely by the level of the background signal generated as a result of nonspecific hybridization. This can be overcome at least in part by dividing the sequence-specific probe into two parts, each half containing only one of the sequence elements required for amplification. A ligase-dependent step would proceed only if both sections of the probe were perfectly aligned.[25]

Chiron Quantiplex Assay and the Ampliprobe System

The Chiron Quantiplex assay involves the use of oligonucleotide probes with complementary sequences to the target nucleic acid.[26] Modification of some of the nucleotide bases allows the construction of DNA probes with a branched, treelike structure. Alkaline phosphatase–labeled oligonucleotides are bound to the branches of the treelike DNA probes, thereby allowing amplification of the signal produced on addition of a dioxetane substrate. The detection limit of this assay is 2×10^5 genomes/mL for HCV RNA, a sensitivity significantly lower than that of comparable nucleic acid amplification methods. This method is illustrated in Figure 38–5.

This assay, although less sensitive than nucleic acid amplification methods, is both rapid and reproducible. The technique is considerably less prone to contamination than PCR is, and it does not require modification to yield quantitative results. The method has been widely used

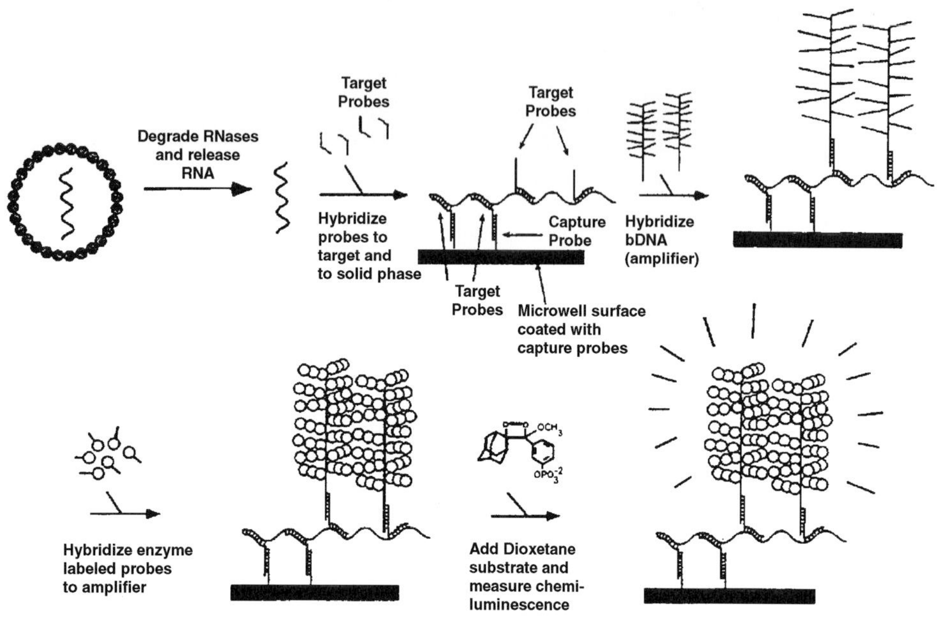

Figure 38–5. Quantiplex assay (bDNA). Chiron's Quantiplex assay differs from nucleic acid amplification techniques such as PCR in that the signal produced, rather than the target nucleic acid, is amplified. This is achieved by virtue of the branched oligonucleotide probes that bind multiple copies of an alkaline phosphatase–labeled probe. (Courtesy of M. Houghton, Chiron Corporation.)

for the quantification of HCV RNA during trials of antiviral therapy.

The principle of signal amplification is also used by the AmpliProbe system (ImClone Systems); however, the chemical methods used to construct probes are considerably less complicated. The single-stranded RNA genome of the bacteriophage M13 is modified to include a region complementary to the target sequence (e.g., viral RNA) fixed to a solid support. Secondary probes bind to multiple sites in the M13 genome, and these secondary probes either directly or indirectly incorporate alkaline phosphatase.[26a]

IMPLICATIONS OF NUCLEOTIDE SEQUENCE VARIATION

Once bloodborne infectious agents have been identified, there is great pressure to develop methods for serological screening. The first assays produced are inevitably biased toward the detection of prototype strains. There are examples of immunologically divergent strains, which have presented problems for these first-generation assays, for each of the major transfusion-transmissible viruses.

For HBV, mutant strains have been reported in which the "*a*" determinant of hepatitis B surface antigen (HBsAg), the target antigen in the HBsAg assay, is undetectable by standard screening tests. Although these mutant strains are rare in the United Kingdom and as yet unreported in the United States, their frequency appears to be increasing in areas where large-scale vaccination programs have been instigated. These mutant strains have been shown to be detectable by PCR testing.[27]

HIV is classified as either HIV-1 or HIV-2; HIV-1 is also divided into main (M) and outlier (O) groups.[28] Group M is further subdivided into at least 10 subtypes, or clades, designated by a letter code from A to J. Group O is also subdivided into a set of divergent clades. HIV-1 group M clade B was by far the predominant subtype in the United States at the outset of the acquired immunodeficiency syndrome (AIDS) epidemic. Consequently, the antibody assays that were initially developed used HIV-1 clade B viral lysate as antigen. Subsequent assays were based on immunodominant regions of the *gag*- and *env*-encoded antigens expressed through recombinant DNA techniques. The DNA sequences expressed were also derived from HIV-1 group M clade B prototypes. Fortunately, these assays have demonstrated a high level of sensitivity to infections by HIV-1 group M clades A to H.[28] However, they fail to detect a proportion of samples from persons with more diverse variants, such as HIV-2 and HIV-1 group O.[29, 30]

HIV-1 and HIV-2 genomes are flanked by two noncoding regions: the long terminal repeats (LTRs). This region is characterized by a high level of sequence homology between clade B and non–clade B sequences of HIV-1 and non–clade A sequences of HIV-2.[30a] The LTR is thus a suitable target for diagnostic PCR. An alternative approach involves using a combination of PCR tests targeted at multiple points within the viral genome. This strategy has been used successfully for the detection of both HIV-1 groups M and O viruses.

HCV is as genetically complex as HIV, with a diverse phylogeny. The major genotypes have been designated a number from 1 to 6; five more have been proposed (7 to 11).[31, 32] Subtypes have been allocated a letter (1a, 1b, etc.). Subtypes 7a, 7b, 8a, 8b, 9a, and 11a are similar to genotype 6, whereas subtype 10a is considered to be a variant of genotype 3.[32] The first-generation screening assays were based on the c100 antigen derived from HCV type 1a, again the predominant strain in the United States at the time the virus was first cloned. Although these first-generation assays missed only an estimated 0.1% of infected donations in the United States,[33] the majority of which were genotype 2 and 3,[34] genotype 1 viruses are not the predominant genotype in large parts of Africa and South East Asia (where genotypes 4, 5, and 6 predominate). Serological assays now contain an expanded representation of antigens in second- and third-generation screening and confirmatory assays. These changes appear to have eliminated the problem of inadequate sensitivity for genotypes 1 to 3.[35]

It is clear that in order to avoid similar problems, the nucleotide sequences targeted by PCR assays must be highly conserved across divergent strains. This is especially true when a single region of the genome is specifically targeted. The most highly conserved regions of both HIV and HCV are those that interact with cellular factors in a sequence-dependent manner. The HCV genome is flanked by two regions of RNA that do not code for protein. The 5′ noncoding region is highly structured and contains an internal ribosome entry site, the sequence of which varies little across all the genotypes. PCR primers directed against this region of the genome have clearly been shown to have an advantage over other areas of the viral genome.[36]

STREAMLINING PCR FOR HIGH THROUGHPUT APPLICATIONS

The number of samples that can reliably be assayed by PCR in a given space of time has significant increased since the early 1990s. This increase has been achieved largely by simplification of the methods: first, by reducing the number of rounds of amplification from two to one and, second, by using protocols that allow reverse transcription and amplification in a single reaction tube.[36a] Both of these time-saving modifications have been achieved without a loss in the sensitivity of the technique. Further improvements will undoubtedly be achieved by the increasing use of automated techniques. It seems likely that liquid-handling robots, such as those currently available for RNA extraction, will be developed in parallel with methodological improvements to allow the automation of the entire process. Increased automation is attractive for several reasons, not least of which is the removal of the operator and therefore operator error from many of the stages of the procedure. When automation has been applied to large-scale DNA-based applications, such as those used for the Human Genome Mapping Project, a clear reduction in the number of processing errors has been observed.[37, 38] Routine serological screening for microbial agents in blood transfusion has advanced to a high degree of process control and information tracking after the introduction of automation, computer tracking of samples, quality control panels, and a national system for surveillance and collation of data. These sorts of requirements must be fulfilled before any routine form of PCR testing of blood donations can be performed with confidence.

The advantages of automation are, however, potentially negated if the handling of large numbers of samples in close proximity increases the risk of cross-contamination. Data generated by international collaborative studies for quality control have shown that a large number of laboratories performing PCR to detect HCV RNA on a routine basis fail to achieve acceptable levels of sensitivity or contamination avoidance.[39] There has undoubtedly been improvement, as evidenced by more recent studies,[40] and it has been suggested[41] that improvements in PCR technology have made it a more reliable technique; however, not all laboratories are able to perform PCR without contamination problems. The introduction of contamination-prevention strategies such as the use of uracil-*N*-glycosylase (UNG),[42] which destroys any contaminating amplified product (based on the incorporation of uracil in place of thymidine), may prevent the reamplification of contaminating PCR products but cannot prevent false-positive results caused by sample cross-contamination. It is therefore difficult to approve the use of any new protocol for performing PCR without assessing the ability of the individual laboratory to produce accurate results. This may best be assessed by using panels of coded standards and by participation in externally organized quality control schemes.

THE APPLICATION OF PCR TO POOLED PLASMA SCREENING

The most striking characteristic of PCR is its exquisite sensitivity, which if ideally optimized can enable detection of a single copy of a DNA sequence. The ability to detect very small numbers of viral genomes in a sample can be exploited to provide an assay for contaminating virus in large pools of plasma.

Serological screening of blood donations has dramatically reduced the number of units containing HCV entering the blood supply. However, occasional incidents of blood product–related viral infection still occur.[43] These incidents frequently result from the transfusion of blood products from donors in the "window period" between infection and the development of a specific antibody response. The risk of infection increases with the number of units transfused, and so a higher risk of infection is associated with the use of products generated from pooled plasma.

Since August 1996, all pooled plasma products not treated with viral inactivation procedures, such as intramuscular immunoglobulin preparations, have been tested for HCV RNA by genome amplification methods. European directives dictate that this policy be extended to include all pooled plasma products by mid-1999. Viremia levels encountered in HCV-infected patients generally range from 10^3 to 10^8 HCV genomes/mL, with a modal value of approximately 10^6 HCV genomes/mL.[44] Plasma pools may contain samples from up to 20,000 donations, so that the final concentration of HCV RNA in a pool containing a single HCV-contaminated donation would be approximately 10^2 HCV genomes/mL, assuming a "typical" concentration of 10^6 HCV genomes/mL in the infected donor. The lower limit of detection of most genome detection methods is approximately 10^3 HCV genomes/mL, and so a significant proportion of HCV-contaminated pools may be missed. The disposal of such large pools as a result of viral contamination would clearly result in the wastage of large quantities of plasma. Currently strategies to detect viral contamination at an earlier stage are being developed. This may involve applying PCR testing to smaller pools (composed of 48 to 480 blood donor samples) or to individual donations. The various alternative approaches, such as the use of two- and three-dimensional intersecting pools, which could be applied to such large-scale testing, have been reviewed.[44a, 44b, 44c]

A quantitative PCR assay with a detection limit of 40 HCV genomes/mL has been described.[45] The increase in sensitivity gained by using this or similar systems should increase the proportion of infected plasma pools detected. The World Health Organization has now produced a calibration standard for HCV RNA to improve the regulation of laboratory screening of plasma pools. The policy of PCR testing of plasma pools may well eventually be extended to include assays for the detection of HIV, HBV, and possibly hepatitis A virus and parvovirus B19.

IDENTIFICATION OF NEW TRANSFUSION-TRANSMISSIBLE AGENTS

Sequences present in the serum after transfusion but absent before transfusion can be selectively amplified with a technique called representational difference analysis (RDA). RDA is performed by preparing two "pools" of nucleic acid from the same patient: one infected and one uninfected. The infected pool is ligated to a priming sequence and hybridized with an excess of nucleic acid from the unligated, uninfected pool. Sequences contained in both pools and hybridized to each other produce double-stranded DNA that is unamplifiable by PCR because it contains only one amplification primer binding site. Sequences unique to the infected material are able to hybridize only to other sequences from the same pool. The double-stranded DNA thus produced is able to bind a primer to both strands and is therefore amplification competent.[45a] The RDA technique is particularly applicable to transfusion-transmissible infectious agents because pretransfusion and post-transfusion samples can readily be used to prepare the uninfected and infected nucleic acid pools.

Two viruses have been isolated from patients with post-transfusion hepatitis, through RDA. The first of these to be isolated was GB virus C (GBV-C; also known as hepatitis G virus [HGV] or human orphan flavivirus [hofv]).[46–49] This virus is a member of the Flaviviridae and is closely related to HCV. Although there is an increased prevalence of GBV-C RNA among groups with frequent exposure to blood or blood products,[49] other modes of transmission, including vertical[50] and sexual,[51] have also been reported. This may in part explain the relatively high prevalence of GBV-C RNA even among healthy blood donors. Coinfection with HBV, HCV, or both is common,[51a] presumably because of similar modes of transmission. It remains unclear what disease state, if any, GBV-C infection causes acutely or in the long term. Although caution and vigilance must be maintained, there is a growing consensus that GBV-C is "a virus looking for a disease" and may in fact prove not to be a cause of viral hepatitis.[52]

The second virus identified through RDA in the serum of a patient with post-transfusion hepatitis was TT virus (TTV).[53] This virus has a DNA genome similar in structure to those of the parvoviruses. TTV DNA has been found in 1% to 4% of blood donors[54] and in 27% of hemophiliacs.[55] The high prevalence of viremia even among healthy blood donors suggests that this virus is not a significant cause of hepatitis. This high prevalence is in part explained by the observation that the virus can be transmitted vertically (70% of children born to infected mothers become infected[55]) and by feco-oral transmission.[54]

A significant amount of hepatitis still occurs without an obvious cause, and virologists continue to search for infectious etiologies. This is especially the case when the hepatitis appears to be triggered by a particular event such as blood transfusion. PCR-based techniques, such as RDA and amplification with degenerate oligonucleotides, are extremely powerful tools for the identification of new viruses. It is plausible that many of the viruses discovered in this way will be found not to be involved in the etiopathogenesis of the disease state from which they are isolated. Special care needs to be taken to establish clear criteria that establish a minimal level of evidence required to define causality.[45a] Many such schemes have already been proposed since Koch's postulates were published,[56, 57] and refinement of these ideas will undoubtedly be required as new technological developments further stretch these definitions.

CONCLUSIONS

Nucleic acid detection techniques, such as PCR, are becoming increasingly important weapons in the armory of the transfusion microbiologist. The progress in this field since the early 1990s has been dramatic. Improvements in the speed and ease with which PCR can be performed have caused the technique to move from highly specialized research laboratories to diagnostic laboratories, thus allowing its use to expand from reference and confirmation work to include plasma screening before the production of blood products. It seems likely that PCR will remain an adjunct to, rather than a replacement of, current serological screening methods for the immediate future, largely because of its relatively low cost, reliability, and proven track record.

Increasing automation of PCR based assays and improvements in contamination prevention strategies may allow PCR to be used to screen blood components as well as pooled blood products. If the target genome has regions of sufficient genetic stability and care is taken with primer design and other technical aspects, PCR screening of blood donations should reduce the albeit small number of samples undetectable by current screening techniques. However, before PCR screening becomes the accepted practice, several hurdles must be overcome, not least of which is the development and validation of techniques for full process control of the systems. Special care must be taken to ensure that both the techniques and the technologists are sufficient to achieve acceptable levels of sensitivity, specificity, and reproducibility. Quality control trials suggest that although progress has been made, not all laboratories are able to produce reliable results. It would therefore be prudent to suggest that all laboratories used for PCR-based screening undergo a rigorous process of accreditation and maintain those high standards through regular internal and external quality control exercises.

REFERENCES

1. Holland PV. Viral infections and the blood supply [Editorial]. N. Eng. J. Med. 1996; 334(26):1734.
2. Schreiber GB, Busch MP, Kleinman SH, et al. The risk of transfusion-transmitted viral infections. N Engl J Med 1996; 334(26):1685.
3. Kwok S, Sninsky JJ. Application of PCR to the detection of human infectious diseases. *In* Erlich HA (ed): PCR Technology. New York: Stockton Press, 1989.
4. Mullis K, Faloona F, Scharf S, et al. Specific enzymatic amplification of DNA in vitro: the polymerase chain reaction. Cold Spring Harbour Symp Quant Biol 1986; 51(part 1):263–273.
5. Saiki RK, Scharf S, Falloona F, et al. Enzymatic amplification of β-globin genomic sequences and restriction site analysis for the diagnosis of sickle cell anemia. Science 1985; 230:1350.
6. Busch MP, Wilber JC, Johnson P, et al. Impact of specimen handling and storage on detection of hepatitis C virus RNA. Transfusion 1992; 32(5):420.
7. Higuchi R. Simple and rapid preparation of samples for PCR. *In* Erlich HA (ed): PCR Technology. New York: Stockton Press, 1989.
8. Chomczynski P, Sacchi N. Single-step method of RNA isolation by acid guanidinium thiocyanate-phenol-chloroform extraction. Anal Biochem 1987; 162(1):156.
9. Boom R, Sol CJ, Salimans MM, et al. Rapid and simple method for purification of nucleic acids. J Clin Microbiol 1990; 28(3):495.
10. Van Doorn LJ, van Belkum A, Maertens G, et al. Hepatitis C virus antibody detection by a line immunoassay and (near) full length genomic RNA detection by a new RNA-capture polymerase chain reaction. J Med Virol 1992; 38:298.
11. Mullis KB. The polymerase chain reaction in anaemic mode: how to avoid cold oligodeoxyribonuclear fusion. PCR Methods Appl 1991; 1:1.
12. Mullis KB, Faloona FA. Specific synthesis of DNA in vitro via a polymerase-catalyzed chain reaction. Methods Enzymol 1987; 155:335.
13. Simmonds P, Balfe P, Peutherer JF, et al. Human immunodeficiency virus–infected individuals contain provirus in small numbers of peripheral mononuclear cells and at low copy numbers. J Virol 1990; 64:864.
14. Garson JA, Tedder RS, Briggs M, et al. Detection of hepatitis C viral sequences in blood donations by "nested" polymerase chain reaction and prediction of infectivity. Lancet 1990; 335:1022.
15. Kwok S, Higuchi R. Avoiding false positives with PCR. Nature 1989; 339:237.
15a. Kemp DJ, Smith DB, Foote SJ, et al. Colorimetric detection of specific DNA segments amplified by polymerase chain reaction. Proc Natl Acad Sci U S A 1989; 86:2423.
15b. Whitby K, Garson JA. Optimisation and evaluation of a quantitative chemiluminescent polymerase chain reaction assay for hepatitis C virus RNA. J Virol Methods 1995; 51:75.
15c. Tuke P, Luton P, Garson JA. Differential diagnosis of HTLV-I and HTLV-II infections by restriction enzyme analysis of "nested" PCR products. J Virol Methods 1992; 40:163.
16. Bevan IS, Daw RA, Day PJR, et al. Polymerase chain reaction for detection of human cytomegalovirus infection in a blood donor population. Br J Haematol 1991; 78:94.
17. Barbara JAJ, Contreras M. Microbiological screening of blood donations. *In* Contreras M (ed): Blood Transfusion: The Impact of New Technologies. Ballière's Clinical Haematology, vol 3. London: Baillière Tindall, 1990, pp 339–354.
18. Erlich HA, Gelfand D, Sninsky JJ. Recent advances in the polymerase chain reaction. Science 1991; 252:1643.
19. Abravaya K, Hu HY, Khalil O. Strategies to avoid amplicon contamination. *In* Lee H, Morse S, Olsvik Ø (eds): Nucleic Acid Amplification Technologies: Application to Disease Diagnosis. Natick, MA: BioTechniques Books, Eaton Publishing, 1997, pp 125–134.
20. Jackson JB. The polymerase chain reaction in transfusion medicine. Transfusion 1990; 30:51.
20a. Lina B, Pozzetto B, Andreoletti L, et al. Multicenter evaluation of a commercially available PCR assay for diagnosing enterovirus infection in a panel of cerebrospinal fluid specimens. J Clin Microbiol 1996; 34(12):3002.
20b. Wittwer CT, Ririe KM, Andrew RV, et al. The LightCycler: a microvolume multisample fluorimeter with rapid temperature control. Biotechniques 1997; 22(1):176.
21. Zebala JA, Barany F. Implications for the ligase chain reaction in gastroenterology. J Clin Gastroenterol 1993; 17(2):171.
22. Kievits T, van Gemen B, van Strijp D, et al. NASBA™ isothermal enzymatic in vitro nucleic acid amplification optimized for the diagnosis of HIV-1 infection. J Virol Methods 1991; 35:273.
23. Walker GT, Little MC, Nadeau JG, et al. Isothermal in vitro amplification of DNA by a restriction enzyme/DNA polymerase system. Proc Natl Acad Sci U S A 1992; 89:392.
24. Olive DM. Qβ replicase assays for the clinical detection of infectious agents. *In* Lee H, Morse S, Olsvik Ø (eds): Nucleic Acid Amplification Technologies: Application to Disease Diagnosis. Natick, MA: BioTechniques Books, Eaton Publishing, 1997, pp 101–113.
25. Carrino JJ, Chan C, Canavaggio M, et al. Ligation-based nucleic acid probe methods. *In* Lee H, Morse S, Olsvik Ø (eds): Nucleic Acid Amplification Technologies: Application to Disease Diagnosis. Natick, MA: BioTechniques Books, Eaton Publishing, 1997, pp 61–79.
26. Urdea MS, Warner BD, Running JA, et al. A comparison of non radioisotopic hybridisation assay methods using fluorescent, chemiluminescent and enzyme labeled synthetic oligodeoxyribonucleotide probes. Nucleic Acids Res 1988; 16:937.
26a. Yang JQ, Tata PV, Park-Turkel HS, et al. The application of AmpliProbe in diagnostics. Biotechniques 1991; 11(3):392.
27. Karthigesu VD, Allison LM, Fortuin M, et al. A novel hepatitis B virus variant in the sera of immunized children. J Gen Virol 1994; 75(part 2):443.
28. Hu DJ, Dondero TJ, Rayfield MA, et al. The emerging genetic diversity of HIV. The importance of global surveillance for diagnostics, research, and prevention. JAMA 1996; 275(3):210.
29. O'Brien TR, George JR, Holmberg SD. Human immunodeficiency virus type 2 infection in the United States: epidemiology, diagnosis and public health implications. JAMA 1992; 267:2775.
30. Loussert-Ajaka I, Ly TD, Chaix ML, et al. HIV-1/HIV-2 seronegativity in HIV-1 subtype O infected patients. Lancet 1994: 343(8910):1393.
30a. Berry N, Ariyoshi K, Jaffar S, et al. Low peripheral blood viral HIV-2 RNA in individuals with high CD4% differentiates HIV-2 from HIV-1 infections. J Human Virol 1998; 1:457–468.
31. Tokita H, Okamoto H, Tsuda F, et al. Hepatitis C virus variants from Vietnam are classifiable into the seventh, eighth, and ninth major genetic groups. Proc Natl Acad Sci U S A 1994; 91(23):11022.
32. Tokita H, Okamoto H, Iizuka H, et al. Hepatitis C virus variants from Jakarta, Indonesia classifiable into novel genotypes in the second (2e and 2f), tenth (10a) and eleventh (11a) genetic groups. J Gen Virol 1996; 77(part 2):293.
33. Kleinman S, Alter H, Busch MP, et al. Increased detection of hepatitis C virus (HCV)–infected blood donors using a multiple antigen HCV enzyme immunoassay. Transfusion 1992; 32:805.
34. McOmish F, Chan S-W, Dow BC, et al. Detection of three types of hepatitis C virus in blood donors: investigation of type specific differences in serological reactivity and rate of alanine aminotransferase abnormalities. Transfusion 1993; 33(1):7.
35. Dow BC, Buchanan I, Munro H, et al. Relevance of RIBA-3 supplementary test to HCV PCR positivity and genotypes for HCV confirmation of blood donors. J Med Virol 1996; 49:132.
36. Garson JA, Ring C, Tuke P, et al. Enhanced detection by PCR of hepatitis C virus RNA. Lancet 1990; 336(8719):878.
36a. Young KKY, Resnick RM, Myers TW. Detection of hepatitis C virus RNA by a combined reverse transcription polymerase chain reaction assay. J Clin Microbiol 1993; 31(4):882.
37. Jones P, Watson A, Davies M, et al. Integration of image analysis and robotics into a fully automated colony picking and plate handling system. Nucleic Acids Res 1992; 20:4599.
38. Landegren U, Kaiser R, Caskey C, et al. Large scale and automated DNA sequence determination. Science 1991; 254:59.
39. Zaaijer HL, Cuypers HT, Reesink HW, et al. Reliability of polymerase chain reaction for detection of hepatitis C virus. Lancet 1993; 341(8847):722.

40. Damen M, Cuypers HT, Zaaijer HL, et al. International collaborative study on the second EUROHEP HCV RNA reference panel. J Virol Methods 1996; 58(12):175.
41. Dore GJ, Kaldor JM, McCaughan GW. Systematic review of role of polymerase chain reaction in defining infectiousness among people infected with hepatitis C virus. BMJ 1997; 315(7104):333.
42. Longo MC, Berninger MS, Hartley JL. Use of uracil DNA glycosylase to control carry-over contamination in polymerase chain reactions. Gene 1990; 93:125.
43. Gomperts ED. HCV and Gammagard in France. Lancet 1994; 344:201.
44. Brillanti S, Garson JA, Tuke PW, et al. Effect of alpha interferon therapy on hepatitis C viremia in community acquired non-A, non-B hepatitis: a quantitative polymerase chain reaction study. J Med Virol 1991; 34:136.
44a. Busch MP, Stramer SL, Kleinman SH. Evolving applications of nucleic acid amplification assays for prevention of virus transmission by blood components and derivatives. *In* Garratty G (ed): Applications of Molecular Biology to Blood Transfusion Medicine. Bethesda, MD: American Association of Blood Banks, 1997, pp 123–176.
44b. Allain JP. Screening blood for viral genomes: which way to go? Transfus Med 1998; 8:5.
44c. Flanagan P, Snape T. Nucleic acid technology (NAT) testing and the transfusion service: a rationale for the implementation of minipool testing. Transfus Med 1998; 8:9.
45. Whitby K, Garson JA. A single tube two compartment reverse transcription polymerase chain reaction system for ultrasensitive quantitative detection of hepatitis C virus RNA. J Virol Methods 1997; 66:15.
45a. Lisitsyn N, Lisitsyn N, Wigler M. Cloning the differences between two complex genomes. Science 1993; 259:946.
46. Simons JN, Leary TP, Dawson GJ, et al. Isolation of novel virus-like sequences associated with human hepatitis. Nat Med 1995; 1(6):564.
47. Muerhoff AS, Leary TP, Simons JN, et al. Genomic organization of GB viruses A and B: two new members of the Flaviviridae associated with GB agent hepatitis. J Virol 1995; 69(9):5621.
48. Leary TP, Muerhoff AS, Simons JN et al. Consensus oligonucleotide primers for the detection of GB virus C in human cryptogenic hepatitis. J Virol Methods 1996; 56(1):119.
49. Linnen J, Wages J Jr, Zhang-Keck ZY, et al. Molecular cloning and disease association of hepatitis G virus: a transfusion-transmissible agent. Science 1996; 271(5248):505.
50. Viazov S, Riffelman M, Sarr S, et al. Transmission of GBV-C/HGV from drug-addicted mothers to their babies. J Hepatol 1997; 27(1):85.
51. Scallan MF, Clutterbuck D, Jarvis LM, et al. Sexual transmission of GB virus C/hepatitis G virus. J Med Virol 1998; 55(3):203.
51a. Jarvis LM, Davidson F, Hanley JP, et al. Infection with hepatitis G virus among recipients of plasma products. Lancet 1996; 348(9038):1352.
52. Alter HJ, Nakatsuji Y, Melpolder J, et al. The incidence of transfusion-associated hepatitis G virus infection and its relation to liver disease. N Engl J Med 1997; 336(11):747.
53. Nishizawa T, Okamoto H, Konishi K, et al. A novel DNA virus (TTV) associated with elevated transaminase levels in posttransfusion hepatitis of unknown etiology. Biochem Biophys Res Commun 1997; 241(1):92.
54. Mizakawa Y. Epidemiology of viral hepatitis, new trends. Presented at the 41st Berzalius Symposium: Viral Hepatitis—Toward Effective Treatment and Prevention. Lund, Sweden: University Hospital, May 11–12, 1998.
55. Simmonds P. WHO international working group on the standardization of genomic amplification techniques for the virological safety testing of blood and blood products. Presented at SoGAT VIII. Amsterdam, Netherlands, June 4, 1998.
56. Hill AB. The environment and disease: association or causation? Proc R Soc Med 1965; 58:295.
57. Fredricks DN, Relman DA. Sequence based identification of microbial pathogens: a reconsideration of Koch's postulates. Clin Microbiol Rev 1996; 9(1):18.

CHAPTER 39

Principles of Apheresis

Harvey G. Klein

HISTORICAL DEVELOPMENT

Bloodletting was a cornerstone of the ancient art of healing. Therapeutic hemapheresis is a distant relative of this ancient practice, but unlike phlebotomy, apheresis has its origins in the research laboratory and relies heavily on science and technology. In 1914, John Jacob Abel coined the term *plasmapheresis*, from a Greek verb meaning to take away or withdraw, to describe removal of plasma and return of the remaining blood components to the donor. Abel and colleagues[1] described the technique of plasma removal as an investigational treatment for toxemia in nephrectomized dogs but foresaw a variety of additional potential applications. Their studies, like those of contemporaries in Germany and Russia, relied on cumbersome phlebotomy, centrifugation, and resuspension techniques, as well as anticoagulation with the leech-derived protein hirudin. Their results were clouded by the technique-related deaths of several experimental animals.

The first manual plasmapheresis procedures in humans were likewise conducted for experimental purposes, to determine the normal rate of protein regeneration in six volunteer donors.[2] The procedure proved safe, although one volunteer experienced a pyrogenic reaction, most likely related to the reusable glass bottle system employed for blood donation in the 1940s. A similar manual technique was put into practice by Grifols-Lucas[3] in 1952, the first use of an apheresis procedure to provide components for transfusion. Whole blood was removed from the donor, and red cells were either allowed to sediment by gravity or packed by centrifugation, removed, and returned to the donor, often as long as a week after the initial phlebotomy. In the same report, Grifols-Lucas described the use of manual plasmapheresis to treat a few patients with hypertension and recorded what is probably the first placebo effect with therapeutic apheresis, noting a "striking subjective improvement, which, however, is not matched by a corresponding betterment of the objective symptoms."[3] A further refinement of manual plasmapheresis relied on a closed-system vacuum bottle technique to remove plasma from a patient with macroglobulinemia.[4]

Although the early manual methods demonstrated the feasibility of plasmapheresis for collecting components and for therapy, glass bottles proved awkward, and reusable equipment raised concern about contamination with bacteria and pyrogens. With the introduction of sterile, disposable, interconnected plastic blood bags, plasmapheresis became relatively safe and easy (Fig. 39–1).[5] The integral-bag procedure required only minor modifications in centrifuge technique for single-donor platelet collections.[6] However, manual apheresis proved too slow, inefficient, and labor intensive for large component volumes and engendered concerns that the separated units of red cells might accidentally be returned to the wrong donor or patient, with potentially fatal consequences. The introduction of automated on-line blood cell separators solved these problems.

Automated on-line blood processing arose from the seminal studies of Cohn and collaborators,[7] who developed an ex vivo refrigerated, sealed-bowl system for centrifugal separation of blood components. This system evolved into a single-arm instrument capable of separating plasma or cellular blood elements in a disposable plastic bowl and returning the unwanted components to the donor in a batch-processing fashion.[8] Almost concurrently, a scientific team from the IBM Corporation and the National Cancer Institute developed a continuous-flow instrument, modeled after the first mechanical heart-lung oxygenator, for collecting granulocytes and platelets from blood donors.[9, 10] These early instruments had reusable parts, rotating seals on the centrifuge bowls, and numerous rings and external connections. A system that eliminates seals for continuous-flow centrifuges has been designed and is now used by several manufacturers.[11]

Although centrifugal cell separation was the earliest and most widely used apheresis technique, automated equipment was also designed to collect granulocytes by filtration or, more accurately, by granulocyte adhesion to nylon filters.[12] Problems with hemocompatibility and donor reactions led to the abandonment of this technique. However, the success of hemodialysis and the desire to effect more selective separation of plasma proteins spurred further development of filtration technology. A wide variety of blood-compatible filters and columns are now either available or under investigation.[13]

PRINCIPLES OF APHERESIS

The primary objective of apheresis is efficient removal of a circulating blood component, either cells (cytapheresis) or a plasma solute (plasmapheresis, plasma exchange). For most disorders, the treatment goal is to remove the circulating cell or substance directly responsible for the disease process. Apheresis can also mobilize cells and plasma components from tissue depots. Depletion of peripheral lymphocytes reportedly reduces the size of the

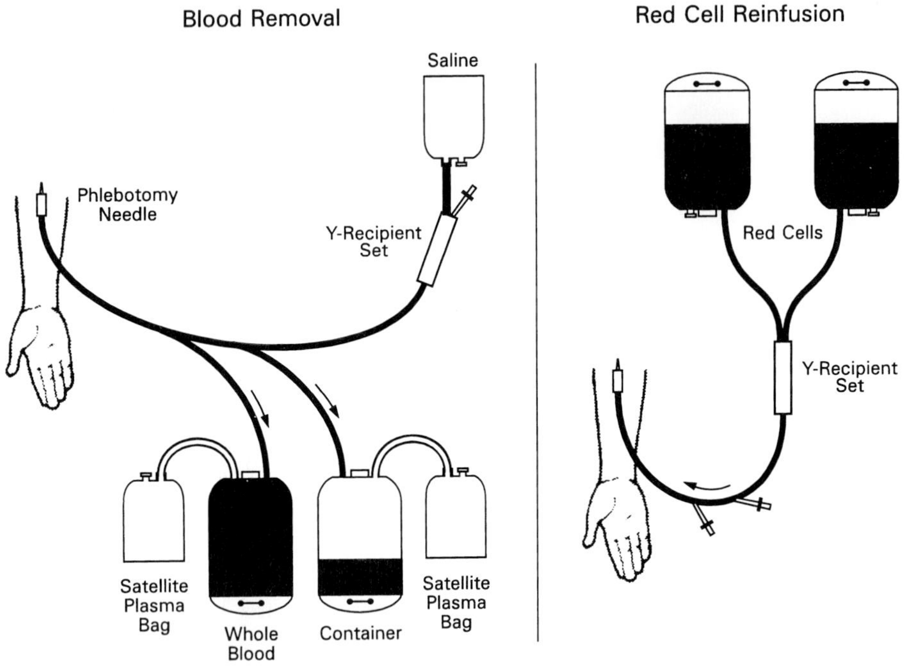

Figure 39–1. Manual apheresis. *Left*, Whole blood is drawn into a system of four to eight sterile, disposable, interconnected plastic bags. Whole blood and a satellite bag are disconnected and then are centrifuged to separate the desired component. *Right*, The packed red cells are returned to the donor through the original infusion set, and the process is repeated.

spleen and lymph nodes in some patients with chronic lymphocytic leukemia. Removal of low-density lipoproteins (LDLs) in serum can result in mobilization of LDLs from tissue stores in patients with familial hypercholesterolemia. Apheresis may also have other, less obvious effects. Lymphocyte depletion appears to modify immune responsiveness in some disease states, possibly by disturbing the control mechanisms of cellular immune regulation.[14] Plasmapheresis enhances splenic clearance of immune complexes in certain autoimmune disorders.[15, 16] Plasmapheresis with plasma exchange is the primary form of treatment for only one disease: thrombotic thrombocytopenic purpura (TTP). However, removal of plasma and cellular components is helpful adjunctive therapy in a variety of clinical situations.

Current automated apheresis instruments use microprocessor technology to administer an anticoagulant, collect the treated blood, separate components either by centrifugation or by filtration, isolate the desired component, and recombine the remaining components for return to the patient or donor. Controlling algorithms have automated the most commonly performed procedures. The equipment has disposable plastic software in the blood path and uses anticoagulants containing citrate or combinations of citrate and heparin, which do not result in clinical anticoagulation. Most instruments function well at blood flow rates of 30 to 80 mL/minute and can operate from peripheral venous access or from a variety of multilumen central venous catheters.[17]

CENTRIFUGAL TECHNIQUES

Centrifugal instruments are capable of collecting both cells and plasma. Separation is effected by manipulating centrifugal force and blood flow rate. These instruments use optical sensors to detect the desired interface and can be programmed to achieve optimal efficiency for the desired procedure.[18] Centrifugal cell separators are generally categorized as either intermittent flow (batch processing) or continuous flow. With intermittent-flow equipment, blood is drawn through a single venipuncture into a processing chamber, where the components separate in the centrifugal field. As the chamber fills, the lighter elements exit sequentially from the chamber into collection containers (Fig. 39–2). Once the desired component is collected, the centrifuge is halted, and the remaining components are returned through the same venipuncture. The process is then repeated. Continuous-flow instruments generally require both a draw line and a return line. Blood is drawn into a centrifugal field, where a continuous interface is established for the duration of the procedure. The individual components are removed continuously through separate ports that lead either to a collection container or to the patient (Fig. 39–3). The intermittent-flow instruments are small and require only a single venipuncture, but they have a relatively large extracorporeal blood volume and return anticoagulant in a bolus fashion. Continuous-flow instruments are less portable and generally require two venipunctures or a multilumen catheter, but the procedure time is shorter. Single-venipuncture procedures have now been described for continuous-flow instruments, but these techniques decrease collection efficiency and prolong collection time.

Several mathematical models formulated for different clinical conditions describe the kinetics of apheresis.[19–21] Most blood components are removed logarithmically, as described by the following equation:

$$C/C_0 = e^{-x},$$

where C_0 is the initial concentration of the component, C is the concentration at some point in time after the procedure has begun, and x is the number of blood or

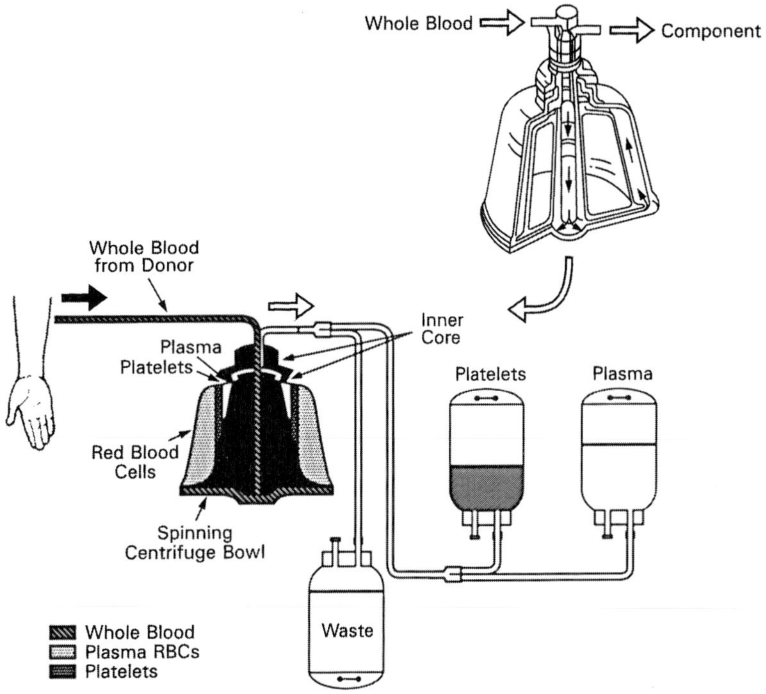

Figure 39–2. Intermittent-flow apheresis. Whole blood enters the separation chamber through a center channel. Cells are separated with continuous centrifugation, and components exit sequentially as the chamber fills. Different fractions are directed into separate disposable containers. When the chamber is filled, the flow is reversed to return unwanted components, and the process is repeated. RBCs, red blood cells.

plasma volumes exchanged up to that point. This model assumes that the component removed is neither synthesized nor degraded substantially during the procedure and that it remains within the intravascular compartment. A further assumption for therapeutic plasmapheresis is that the solute mixes instantaneously and completely with the plasma replacement solution. This model has been validated for removal of immunoglobulins G and M (IgG and IgM) in patients without paraproteinemia. Less efficient removal of paraproteins in patients with multiple myeloma may reflect an underestimate of the expanded plasma volume in patients with this disorder.

A more complex model of solute kinetics in plasma exchange requires a solute diffusion coefficient, transmembrane sieving coefficient, and lymphatic return flow rate between the extravascular and intravascular space.[22] This model has been validated with both a high-molecular-weight, primarily intravascular solute (LDL) and a

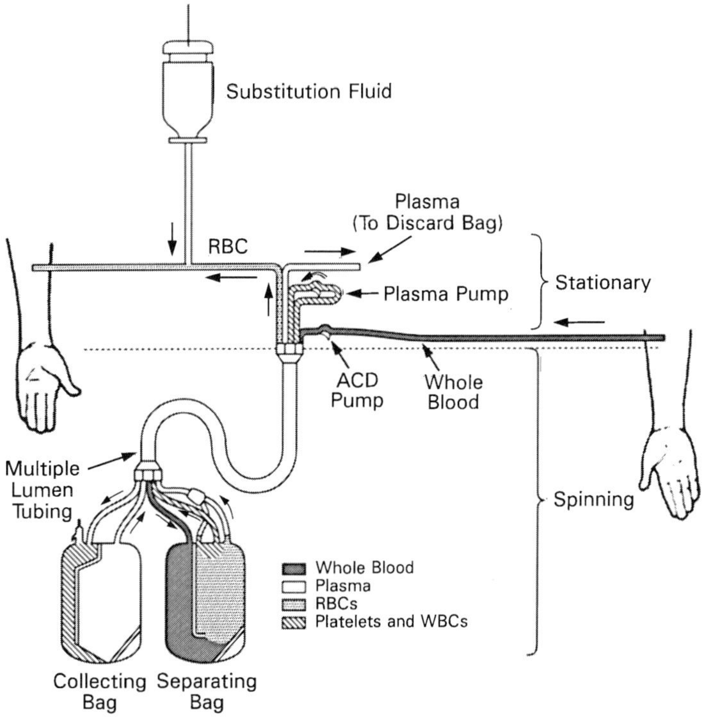

Figure 39–3. Continuous-flow separation. Whole blood is drawn into a separation chamber, where an interface is established in a centrifugal field. Different components are removed simultaneously by separate pumps and ports. Unwanted components are combined (with a replacement solution, in this example of therapeutic plasmapheresis) and returned to the patient. ACD, acid citrate dextrose anticoagulant; RBCs, red blood cells; WBCs, white blood cells.

readily diffusible solute (bilirubin). The results confirm the relatively slow reequilibration of large molecules between the extravascular and intravascular space and the impracticality of using plasma exchange as a means of removing diffusible small molecules.

Different mathematical expressions have been derived for continuous-flow procedures, in which withdrawal and reinfusion are simultaneous, and for intermittent exchange, in which equal volumes are withdrawn and infused sequentially. In practice, there is little difference in efficiency between the two methods (Fig. 39–4). When the goal of apheresis is to supply some deficient cell or solute, e.g., red cells during exchange for sickle cell disease or plasma factors for the treatment of TTP, replacement will follow logarithmic kinetics similar to those developed for solute removal. From Figure 39–4, it is evident that removal of 1.5 to 2 volumes will reduce an intravascular substance by about 60% and that processing larger volumes in a single session will remove little additional solute.

Specific cell removal with centrifugal automated cell separators depends on the number of cells available, the volume of blood processed, the efficiency of the particular instrument, and the separation characteristics of the different cells. Most commercially available instruments remove platelets and lymphocytes extremely efficiently and with little loss of unwanted cells. Granulocytes and monocytes cannot be cleanly separated from other cells by standard centrifugal apheresis equipment (Fig. 39–5). Optimal harvesting of granulocytes requires special techniques, such as stimulating the donor with corticosteroids or growth factors and adding sedimenting agents to enhance cell separation.[23] Peripheral collections can also mobilize a variety of cell types from extravascular sites.[24, 25]

A modification of centrifugal separation, countercurrent elutriation, separates particles on the basis of their size, density, and flow characteristics.[26] The principle of

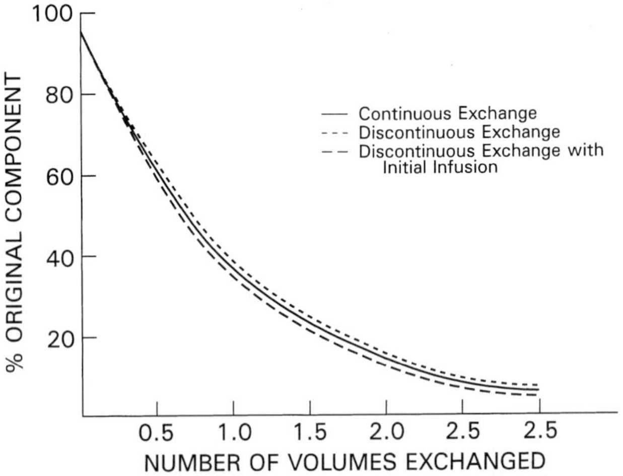

Figure 39–4. Relationship between volumes removed by apheresis and percentage of the target component remaining. The relationship is valid for blood volumes during red cell exchange and for plasma volumes during plasmapheresis, if the target solute remains primarily within the intravascular compartment. (Modified from McCullough J, Chopek M. Therapeutic plasma exchange. Lab Med 1981; 12:745.)

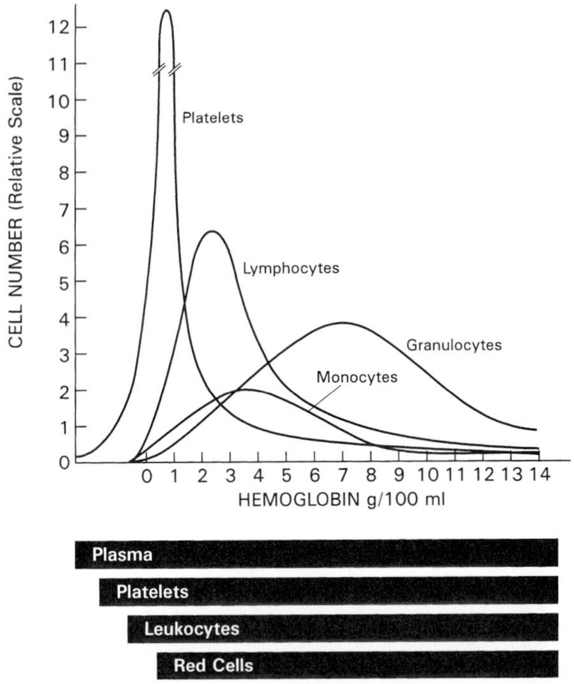

Figure 39–5. Schematic distribution of cells at the interface of a centrifugal cell separator collection chamber. The number and percentage of each cell type collected can be varied by adjusting the site of collection along the interface or by changing centrifugal force, blood flow rate, or rate of cell removal. (From Klein HG. Apheresis. *In* Hoffman R [ed]: Hematology. New York: Churchill Livingstone, 1991, pp 1638–1644.)

elutriation—placing a cell suspension in a centrifugal force field in which fluid flow and centrifugal forces oppose each other—effects precise separation of cells such as monocytes and granulocytes, which are otherwise extremely difficult to separate. Depending on the nature of the fluid and the rate of flow, as well as the centrifugal force, cells either exit the chamber with the fluid or remain behind on the basis of cell size and density. Although the currently available research instrument is an "open" system, has a reusable chamber, and is not useful as an on-line separation device, several commercial companies have applied the elutriation principle to their separation devices.[27]

FILTRATION TECHNIQUES

Filtration instruments used both for therapeutic plasmapheresis and for source plasma collection depend on the sieving properties of a wide variety of membranes to selectively separate plasma solutes. The advantages of filtration technology over centrifugal systems are the smaller size of the instruments, the lower extracorporeal volume, and the potential for obtaining plasma that is free of cells and cell fragments. A further technical refinement involves specific removal of a plasma component, which can be achieved by adding a secondary separation step, e.g., an adsorption column, to the separated plasma.

The ideal method for treating disorders mediated

by abnormal plasma components is to remove only the offending substance, thus avoiding loss of essential plasma components and eliminating the need for a plasma replacement solution. Because many of the proposed target solutes have a molecular weight greater than 100 kD and are therefore larger than albumin, physical separation by various filtration techniques (ultrafiltration) or by phase separation (cryoprecipitation, dextran sulfate precipitation, heparin acidification) followed by ultrafiltration is both effective and practical. These techniques may not achieve as selective a removal as is possible with adsorption and immunoadsorption methods, but they have proved useful for removing LDLs from patients with hypercholesterolemia and IgM from patients with symptomatic paraproteinemia.[28, 29]

Cascade filtration uses two or more filters in serial fashion, first to separate plasma from cells (primary filter) and then to pass or reject plasma solutes on the basis of their molecular weight (Fig. 39–6).[30] The principle of this technique is differential filtration based on membranes of different pore size. In practice, however, several combinations of centrifugal devices, depth filters, and molecular sieves have been used in cascade fashion. Most cascade systems align filters in tandem. Although the concept of cascade filtration is simple, the filtration kinetics are complex.[31] Because of poor filter selectivity, clogging of the filters, and excessive extracorporeal volume, cascade filtration systems have not gained clinical acceptance.

Cryofiltration has been studied since the 1980s as a method of treating patients with rheumatoid arthritis.[32] This procedure involves cooling the plasma to a selected

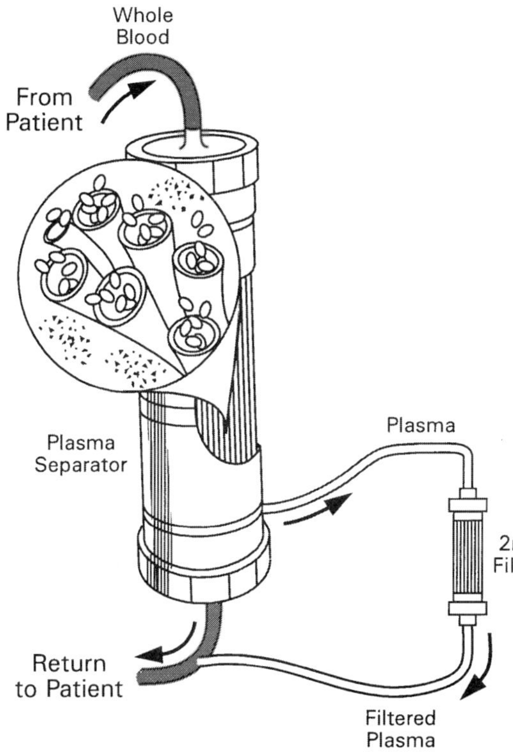

Figure 39–6. Cascade filtration. The filter separates cells from plasma. A second-stage filter is designed to retain plasma solutes according to specific molecular weight.

temperature, usually between 4°C and 10°C, but not below the freezing point of plasma. The material that precipitates in the cold is then filtered from the plasma. Cryofiltration is more selective than ultrafiltration but not as specific as adsorption. Different cryoproteins circulate in a variety of apparently unrelated disorders, including certain malignancies and several autoimmune and connective tissue diseases associated with circulating immune complexes. The relation of these cryoproteins to the disease processes, as well as the effects of removing them, is unknown. Instruments designed to perform this function on-line have been licensed but are no longer commercially available in the United States.

Other on-line methods of phase separation followed by filtration have been used, primarily in the treatment of hypercholesterolemia. One novel system uses paired dialyzers to alter plasma monovalent cation concentration, elevate calcium, and precipitate LDL and very-low-density lipoprotein (VLDL) with dextran sulfate. Advantages of this system include selective removal of LDL and VLDL, with conservation of high-density lipoprotein (HDL) and other macromolecules. An alternative scheme prepares heparinized plasma at a final pH of 5.12 to precipitate LDL and fibrinogen. This system has been widely used in experimental settings.[33] The importance of these techniques lies in the recognition that different well-studied physiochemical separation methods can be adapted to remove specific pathogenic substances during plasmapheresis.

ADSORPTION TECHNIQUES

Removal by adsorption, potentially the most selective apheresis technique, is based on the principle of affinity chromatography. A ligand is bound tightly to an insoluble matrix, over which plasma is passed. The ligand may be a relatively nonspecific chemical binder, such as charcoal or heparin, or an exquisitely specific monoclonal antibody or recombinant protein antigen.

Although adsorption and immunoadsorption systems have been used since the early 1990s, most of the published studies have been performed in vitro or in animal models. Of the general adsorptive materials, charcoal columns, dextran sulfate columns, and staphylococcal protein A columns have been most widely used. Charcoal has a strong affinity for bile acids and is available with a purity that meets United States Pharmacopeia standards. Some patients with cholestasis have noted improvement of previously intractable pruritus after plasma perfusion over columns constructed with charcoal-coated glass beads.[34] Studies of these patients have all lacked appropriate controls, leaving the relationship between bile acid adsorption and clinical efficacy in question. Proposed applications for charcoal columns include management of poisoning and manipulation of chemotherapy during cancer treatment.[35–38] None of these has been effectively applied in practice.

A more specific adsorbent than charcoal, staphylococcal protein A, has long been used as a laboratory reagent because of its high affinity for the Fc portion of IgG1, IgG2, and IgG4 and for immune complexes containing these IgG subtypes. The protein A cell wall constituent of the Cowen I strain of *Staphylococcus aureus* carries five regions at its N-terminus that bind IgG. Binding to other plasma proteins, and to IgG3, IgM, and IgA, is insignificant. Plasma adsorption with "homemade" protein A columns enjoyed short-lived enthusiasm when early reports suggested a tumoricidal effect in plasma passed over these columns.[39, 40] The early success proved difficult to reproduce, and the columns were associated with significant treatment-related side effects.[41] The mode of action was never adequately elucidated.

Current commercial protein A columns have stimulated new interest in this area. A protein A–silica column has been licensed in the United States as treatment for patients with refractory immune thrombocytopenic purpura (ITP).[42] Forty-six percent of patients refractory to steroids and splenectomy responded to treatment with an elevation of platelet count; in the majority, the effect lasted 8 months or more. Because the reported effect seems to be mediated by as little as 250 mL of treated plasma or a calculated removal of as little as 1 g of IgG and 100 mg of circulating immune complex (CIC), these investigators postulated a mechanism by which the removal of a small amount of CIC may result in altered lymphocyte and macrophage immune function and even stimulate production of protective antibody. However, protein A complexed with immunoglobulin activates both the classical and the alternative complement pathways and may therefore have a variety of nonspecific effects.[43] Complement activation, bradykinin activation, and cytokine release may account for the frequent and severe reactions that may be seen with this treatment.[44]

Several other applications of protein A columns have been reported. Six of 10 alloimmunized patients with thrombocytopenia refractory to random donor platelet transfusions responded to treatment with the protein A–silica column.[45] Forty-five percent of patients with chemotherapy-associated TTP responded to therapy with improvement in pretreatment defined laboratory values that was maintained for at least 30 days.[46] Favorable results have been reported with a protein A–agarose column used to remove alloantibody from patients awaiting renal transplantation, patients with rapidly progressing glomerulonephritis, and patients with inhibitors to factor VIII or IX.[47–49] Numerous case reports and small series attest to the ability of these columns to remove IgG and immune complexes in a variety of disease states. Clinical response is more variable. In none of these instances has the use of immunoadsorption achieved the status of routine therapy.

The most specific immunoadsorption techniques involve binding of antigens or antibodies to the inert column matrix. Several examples are promising. Sheep anti-LDL (anti-apolipoprotein B) antibodies have been linked to sepharose to prepare reusable columns that have already been tested in more than 3000 procedures.[50] Specific antigen columns have also long been used clinically. DNA bound to collodion charcoal and synthetic sugar chains analogous to A and B blood group substances linked to crystalline silica have been packed into columns to remove specific antibody from patients' plasma.[51, 52]

Although the technology is available to remove these and other specific immune reactants, the inability to identify the immune pathogen in many disease states limits application of this technology.

CLINICAL APPLICATIONS

Therapeutic Cytapheresis

Erythrocytapheresis

Common indications for therapeutic cell removal are listed in Table 39–1. Red cell exchange (erythrocytapheresis) is used most often to manage complications of sickle cell disease. When such exchanges are indicated, mechanical cell separators offer the advantages of speed and ease of use over earlier manual techniques. Automated procedures can be performed with all centrifugal instruments, which contain integral software programs that permit the operator to tailor the procedure to the requirements of the particular patient.

The original rationale behind exchange transfusion involved improving tissue oxygenation and preventing microvascular sickling by diluting the patient's abnormal red cells, thus simultaneously correcting anemia and favorably altering whole blood viscosity and rheology.[53] However, the pathophysiology of sickle cell disease appears to be far more complex than was originally appreciated.[54] Changes in vascular endothelium and in platelet function may play important roles in the disease process, and an inflammatory response to chronic hemolysis may further contribute to endothelial changes. There is evidence that red cell adhesion, especially to the endothelial layer of small venules, plays a significant role in the sickling process. Sickle cells may interfere with the normal control of vascular smooth muscle relaxation and may induce receptors for von Willebrand factor.[55, 56] Occult viral infection may initiate or contribute to the process.[57] It is not clear whether or how the evolving understanding of the pathophysiology of clinical sickling will affect the role of transfusion therapy.

No clinical data support a single optimal level of hemoglobin A; however, mixtures with as few as 30% transfused cells markedly decrease blood viscosity, whereas mixtures with 50% or more transfused cells normalize resistance to membrane filterability.[58, 59] In nonemergent situations, such levels can easily be achieved

Table 39–1. Common Indications for Therapeutic Cytapheresis

Procedure	Indications
Red cell exchange	Sickle cell disease
	Acute complications (e.g., acute chest syndrome, priapism)
	Prophylaxis for stroke
	Frequent, severe pain crises
	Malaria or babesiosis with hyperparasitemia
Leukapheresis	Hyperleukocytic leukemias
	Rheumatoid arthritis (selected cases)
Photopheresis	Cutaneous T cell lymphoma
	Solid organ allograft rejection
	Graft-versus-host disease
Plateletpheresis	Symptomatic thrombocythemia

with a simple transfusion regimen. Whereas 50% hemoglobin A is a frequently quoted target level for exchange transfusion, some patients remain symptomatic when their hemoglobin A is maintained at levels of 80% and above. Such failures may be due in part to preexisting, irreversible ischemic organ damage. In a randomized study of sickle cell disease patients undergoing surgery, a conservative, simple transfusion regimen was as effective as an aggressive regimen with respect to perioperative non–transfusion-related complications.[60] The group undergoing the aggressive regimen received twice as many units of blood, had a proportionally increased alloimmunization rate, and experienced more hemolytic transfusion reactions. Prophylactic exchange transfusion in the perioperative setting should be limited to those patients undergoing high-risk surgical procedures in whom simple transfusion cannot raise the hemoglobin A level to the 70% range.

Although there is little doubt that exchange transfusion improves some patients with acute sickling crises, clinical indications remain controversial. Simple transfusion has improved renal concentrating ability and splenic function in young sickle cell patients, whereas exchange transfusion has improved exercise tolerance and has reversed the periodic oscillations in cutaneous blood flow noted in this disease.[61–64] These observations have encouraged the use of exchange transfusion for such complications of sickle cell disease as acute chest syndrome, priapism, retinal artery occlusion, pain crisis, and intrahepatic cholestasis.[65–68] A multicenter, randomized trial of transfusion during pregnancy demonstrated that transfusion sufficient to reduce the incidence of painful crises did not reduce the rate of other maternal morbidity or perinatal mortality.[69]

Transfusion prophylaxis, well documented as effective in preventing recurrent stroke in children with sickle cell disease, is now clearly indicated for children designated "high risk" by transcranial Doppler ultrasonography.[70, 71] A randomized, controlled study[71] demonstrated a risk reduction of 92% in patients who received transfusions to reduce the hemoglobin S concentration to less than 30% of total hemoglobin concentration. This result confirms earlier anecdotal experience and indicates that in this group of children, transfusion therapy should begin before the first event and continue indefinitely. Long-term erythrocytapheresis may be preferable for patients at high risk for stroke who have developed iron overload levels that are associated with organ damage.[72]

Exchange transfusion, although relatively safe and convenient, carries all the complications of red cell transfusion. Patients are exposed to a large number of donors, placing them at substantial risk for contracting parvovirus infection and other blood-borne diseases. As many as a third of all patients develop red cell alloantibodies, and life-threatening delayed hemolytic transfusion reactions have been reported.[73, 74] Despite the removal of cells during exchange, patients remain in positive iron balance. Iron accumulation is slow, and chelation is rarely required to prevent transfusional hemosiderosis.

Other indications for red cell exchange are rare. The procedure has been used for overwhelming red cell parasitic infections, such as severe and complicated malaria and babesiosis.[75, 76] In these situations, red cell exchange decreases the circulating parasite load and may help sustain life until conventional therapy and natural immunity take effect. The rate of disease progression and the circulating parasitic load are probably the best guides for therapy. A review of published cases suggests that erythrocytapheresis be considered for patients with parasitemia in the 10% to 15% range or higher or an absolute count of 500,000/μL. Automated red cell removal with volume replacement (isovolemic hemodilution) can be performed rapidly and safely in polycythemic subjects.[77] This maneuver should be reserved for polycythemic patients in whom there is an urgent clinical need to lower hematocrit (e.g., evolving thrombotic stroke) for which standard, single-unit, manual phlebotomy might be inadvisably slow.

Leukapheresis

Therapeutic leukapheresis has been used most successfully to help manage acute or chronic leukemia in patients with extremely high white blood cell numbers, so-called hyperleukocytic leukemias.[78–80] When the fractional volume of leukocytes (leukocrit) exceeds 20%, blood viscosity increases, and leukocytes can interfere with pulmonary and cerebral blood flow and compete with tissue for oxygen in the microcirculation.[81] A single 8- to 10-L leukapheresis procedure generally reduces the white blood cell count by 20% to 50%. However, the results often fall short of predictions concerning cell removal. Circulating cell counts at the end of the procedure likely depend on both the nature of the cells and the degree of mobilization of cells into the circulation from large extramedullary reservoirs, such as the spleen. When the cells of concern are blast cells, neutrophils, eosinophils, or metamyelocytes, use of a red cell sedimenting agent, usually 6% hydroxyethyl starch, improves the separation of leukocytes from erythrocytes and increases collection efficiency substantially.

Ordinarily, leukapheresis is indicated when the peripheral count exceeds 100,000 μL or when blast counts exceed 50,000 μL (leukocrit greater than 10%), especially when central nervous system or pulmonary symptoms appear.[82] In acute leukemia, rapidly rising counts in these ranges, especially in the presence of neurological or pulmonary symptoms, represent an oncological emergency. Leukapheresis can effect rapid clinical improvement.[83] Cell type seems to be as important as cell number, and symptomatic leukostasis occurs more often with acute nonlymphocytic leukemias than with lymphocytic leukemias, and more frequently with cells of M4,M5 morphology than with those of M1,M2 type.[84] A review of 16 patients with chronic lymphocytic leukemia and peripheral counts of 500,000 to 1,700,000 leukocytes/μL found only three patients with signs or symptoms of leukostasis. Circulating leukocyte count does not appear to be a reliable measure for initiating leukapheresis in this disease.[85] The ability to maintain an individual patient with a normal white blood cell count by leukapheresis alone depends on the kinetics of the disease.

Therapeutic leukapheresis plays a smaller role in chronic granulocytic leukemia. Some patients with markedly elevated white cell counts (>300,000/μL) develop symptomatic leukostasis and show dramatic response to cytoreduction.[86, 87] Repeated procedures are generally required. The response is temporary and by no means curative. Repeated leukapheresis adequately reduced the white cell count in a series of 15 patients with chronic myelocytic leukemia treated with more than 900 procedures. However, median patient survival was not significantly different from that in similar patients treated with conventional chemotherapy.[88]

The commonly observed continued decline in peripheral cell counts after a course of leukapheresis probably represents the effects of removing committed progenitor cells.[89] Repeated leukapheresis can provide acceptable control of the peripheral white cell count in clinical situations such as pregnancy, when cytotoxic agents are best avoided. Cytoreduction by leukapheresis does not appear to alter the course of the granulocytic leukemias.

Cytoreduction for managing other leukemic processes has limited usefulness. Some studies of patients with chronic lymphocytic leukemia suggested short-term clinical benefit, but long-term support of cases refractory to chemotherapy does not appear to prolong life.[90, 91] Transient responses to leukapheresis used alone or in combination with low-dose chemotherapy have been reported in a variety of lymphoproliferative disorders, but most cases relapse quickly and become unresponsive to further leukapheresis therapy.[92–95]

Lymphocyte depletion has been used therapeutically to modify patient immune responsiveness. Removal of large numbers of lymphocytes over a few weeks can suppress peripheral lymphocyte counts in rheumatoid arthritis patients for as long as a year and can alter skin test reactivity and lymphocyte mitogen responsiveness to a variety of stimulants.[96] Selected patients experience a modest but significant reduction in disease activity, but the subset of patients who may derive substantial benefit from this therapy is difficult to identify.[97, 98] Lymphocyte removal has also been used to treat patients with multiple sclerosis, to enhance allograft survival, and to reverse graft rejection; objective evidence of clinical efficacy is scarce.

Photopheresis, a novel modification of leukapheresis, was introduced as a treatment for cutaneous T cell lymphoma and subsequently applied to autoimmune disorders, solid organ graft rejection, graft-versus-host disease, and human immunodeficiency virus type 1 (HIV-1) infection.[99–101] With photopheresis, the photosensitizing agent 8-methoxypsoralen is either ingested by the patient before cell separation or added to the collection bag. The patient's collected leukocytes are subsequently exposed to ultraviolet A radiation in a closed extracorporeal chamber before being reinfused. The mechanism of action involves the well-recognized photoconjugation reaction between psoralens and the thymidine base pairs of DNA in the presence of ultraviolet light. Although DNA crosslinking clearly alters leukocyte function and interferes with cell proliferation, it seems unlikely that destruction of a small number of leukocytes alone could account for the broad immunological effects attributed to this therapy. One proposed mechanism postulates that photodamaged alloreactive T cells might elicit a limited cytolytic response directed against the pathological clone; however, the precise mechanism of action that initiates a beneficial immune response remains unexplained.

Photopheresis was categorized as a therapy of choice for the erythrodermic stage of cutaneous T cell lymphoma at an international consensus conference.[102] Its role in other clinical situations is best described as encouraging but unconfirmed. Promising results have emerged from studies in systemic sclerosis,[103] rheumatoid arthritis,[104] systemic lupus erythematosus,[105] and pemphigus vulgaris.[106] Small studies support a role for photopheresis in the treatment of cardiac transplant rejection episodes[107] and in rejection prophylaxis; treated patients had fewer rejection episodes, fewer infections, and improved survival compared with a control group.[108]

One of the more interesting applications of this technology is to the difficult problem of chronic graft-versus-host disease after bone marrow transplantation. Early reports suggest that photopheresis may play a role, particularly in the dermatological complications.[109]

Plateletpheresis

Therapeutic plateletpheresis is generally reserved for patients with myeloproliferative disorders and hemorrhage or thrombosis associated with the increased numbers of circulating platelets. Because thrombocytosis from other causes such as iron deficiency and splenectomy, so-called reactive thrombocytosis, is usually asymptomatic, a clone of functionally abnormal cells probably accounts for the symptoms attributed to elevated platelets in patients with myeloproliferative disorders. Although most centers consider plateletpheresis for any symptomatic patient whose peripheral platelet count exceeds $10^6/\mu L$, there is no consistent relationship between the extent of platelet elevation and the occurrence of symptoms.[110, 111] Unfortunately, neither is there a generally accepted assay of platelet dysfunction to indicate which patients are at risk.[112]

When therapeutic plateletpheresis is indicated, a single procedure can lower the count by 30% to 50%. Attempts to maintain thrombocythemic patients at normal platelet counts by cytapheresis alone have not been successful; chemotherapy should be instituted along with a cytapheresis program.[113] Symptomatic patients generally respond promptly to plateletpheresis.[114] Most patients with thrombocytosis, however, even those with myeloproliferative disorders and strikingly elevated platelet counts, do not have symptoms.[115, 116] Prophylactic plateletpheresis, except for possibly the rare pregnant patient with thrombocythemia in whom placental infarction and fetal death present a reasonable concern, seems unwarranted regardless of the platelet count.[117, 118]

Nontraditional Component Collections

Apheresis has also been used to collect cellular blood components that can be described as nontraditional. One of the earliest applications of the blood cell separator involved lymphocyte collection for the adoptive transfer of immunity from immune donors to nonimmune recipients.[119] In this regard, the wheel has come full circle. Lymphocytes are now collected or prepared from leukocyte collections for numerous forms of immunotherapy.[120]

Independent studies confirm a durable graft-versus-leukemia effect of donor-derived lymphocytes transfused to patients in relapsed chronic-phase chronic myelocytic leukemia and a potent effect against the Epstein-Barr virus–associated lymphoproliferative disease that complicates lymphocyte-depleted bone marrow transplants. Collection and ex vivo expansion of lymphocytes are done for the immunotherapy of infectious diseases and to generate vehicles for cellular gene therapy.[121, 122] Although these applications are not strictly therapeutic, they represent the widening therapeutic potential of cytapheresis. Harvesting hematopoietic progenitor cells from cytokine-stimulated patients and donors for reconstituting bone marrow is now a standard practice.

Therapeutic Plasmapheresis

Dramatic growth of therapeutic plasmapheresis since the early 1970s reflects the development of new technology more than new insight into the pathophysiology of the diseases under treatment. Most of the initial applications of the technology were designed to remove some toxic metabolite, protein, poison, or immune mediator, often in rare disorders not amenable to critical evaluation by controlled trials. Therapeutic indications increasingly derive from carefully designed studies or at least from small series of uncontrolled cases in which there is some objective measurement of clinical or laboratory improvement. However, technical developments continue to outpace scientifically demonstrated clinical applications. Common clinical indications for plasmapheresis are listed in Table 39–2, and postulated mechanisms of action are discussed later. A detailed listing of diseases for which successful plasmapheresis therapy has been reported has been published.[123]

The earliest and most firmly established application of plasmapheresis involves treating the neurological, cardiovascular, and hemorrhagic complications of the hyperviscosity syndrome. Plasma hyperviscosity complicates about 20% of cases of Waldenström's macroglobulinemia and a smaller proportion of cases of other paraproteinemias.[4, 5, 124] Symptoms of hyperviscosity, including headache, nausea, blurred vision, confusion, congestive heart failure, and coma, are rarely subtle, correlate well with measurements of viscosity, and respond promptly to plasmapheresis.[125, 126] The relationship between plasma viscosity and paraprotein concentration is exponential. Therefore, removal of relatively small volumes of plasma may have dramatic clinical effects. Serial measurements of the paraprotein level may underestimate the extent of removal, as predicted by the kinetics shown in Figure 39–4. Patients with hyperviscosity syndrome generally develop a markedly increased plasma volume, which fluctuates during the course of therapy. Hyperviscosity can be managed for years with repeated plasmapheresis procedures, but plasmapheresis does not alter the course of the underlying disease. Occasionally, symptoms suggestive of hyperviscosity syndrome are present in the absence of an elevated plasma viscosity. Such cases merit a trial of plasmapheresis. Syndromes other than hyperviscosity that result from paraproteins, such as cryoglobulinemia and cold agglutinin disease, may also respond to a course of plasmapheresis.[127–129]

Table 39–2. Common Indications for Therapeutic Plasmapheresis

Paraprotein-Related Disorders
- Hyperviscosity syndrome
- Cryoglobulinemia
- Cold agglutinin disease

Diseases Caused by Toxic Metabolites
- Refsum's disease
- Fabry's disease
- Familial hypercholesterolemia

Immunologically Mediated Disorders
- Goodpasture's syndrome
- Myasthenia gravis
- Eaton-Lambert syndrome
- Guillain-Barré syndrome
- Chronic inflammatory demyelinating polyneuropathy
- Pemphigus
- Immune thrombocytopenic purpura
- Post-transfusion purpura
- Coagulation factor inhibitors

Vasculitides
- Systemic lupus erythematosus (selected cases)
- Mesangiocapillary glomerulonephritis
- Wegener's granulomatosis

Plasma Factor Deficiencies
- Thrombotic thrombocytopenic purpura

Removal of Poisons or Drugs
- Protein-bound drugs and toxins

Another early use of therapeutic plasmapheresis involved mobilization of tissue stores of toxic metabolites in relatively rare inherited disorders such as Refsum's disease and Fabry's disease.[130, 131] Although plasma solute reduction and tissue mobilization are readily measured in these disorders, clinical efficacy has been more difficult to demonstrate. The best example of the therapeutic value of this application involves removal of LDL as treatment or prophylaxis for coronary artery disease. Nonselective reduction of LDL by plasmapheresis reduces xanthomas, decreases symptoms, results in regression of coronary atherosclerosis as measured by serial angiography, and appears to prolong survival in patients with homozygous familial hypercholesterolemia.[132–135] Treatment is now also given to heterozygous patients with demonstrated disease and LDL levels that are poorly controlled by optimal diet and drug therapy.

A variety of procedures for increasingly selective removal of LDL have now been introduced. These methods have the advantages of preserving plasma proteins unrelated to the diseases and sparing HDL, which may have a protective effect in atherosclerosis.[13, 28, 33, 136, 137] Although the ideal plasma LDL level is controversial, frequency of apheresis necessary to achieve a target value can be predicted by using a reference chart constructed for the specific apheresis procedure (Fig. 39–7). Individual variations in cholesterol synthesis, degradation, and tissue mobilization will alter predictions slightly.

Plasmapheresis has been used to treat a number of diverse immunologically mediated diseases. Success was

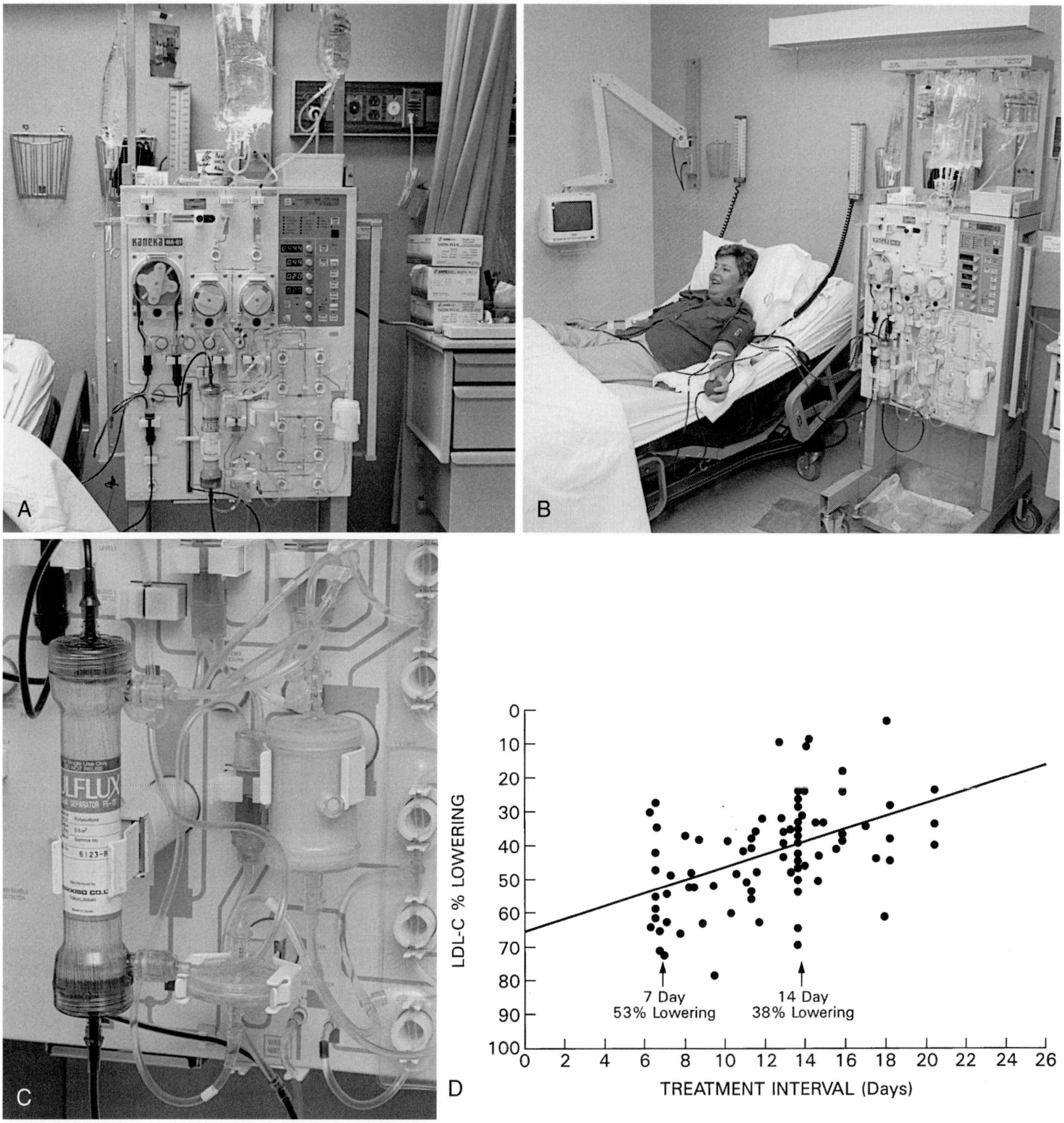

Figure 39–7. *A*, Two-stage therapeutic plasmapheresis. *B*, Plasma is separated from cells by filtration and passed through parallel adsorption columns to remove low-density lipoproteins (LDLs) from a patient with homozygous familial hyperlipoproteinemia. *C*, Hollow-fiber filter. *D*, Frequency at which LDL apheresis achieves a target serum cholesterol level, calculated by using a dextran sulfate cellulose precipitation column. (*D* reprinted courtesy of the Liposorber Study Group.)

first reported in patients with Goodpasture's syndrome, a disorder associated with a specific pathogenic autoantibody, anti–glomerular basement membrane (anti-GBM), directed at the renal glomerular and pulmonary alveolar basement membrane.[138, 139] The treatment rationale proposed that circulating immune complexes were responsible for tissue injury and that removal of both antibody and immune complexes should prove beneficial. Because immune deposits may form in situ, the mechanism of action of plasmapheresis is probably more complex than simple removal. Retrospective analysis of serial samples from these patients suggests that anti-GBM titer correlates with disease progression and that a declining titer during therapy predicts improving renal function.[140] Similar success has been reported with plasmapheresis in other disorders associated with specific autoantibodies, such as myasthenia gravis (anti–acetylcholine receptor), Eaton-Lambert syndrome, Guillain-Barré syndrome (anti–peripheral nerve myelin), pemphigus, ITP, and antibody-mediated hemorrhagic diathesis.[141–146]

Controversy surrounds the practice of combining cytotoxic drug therapy with plasmapheresis to prevent rapid resynthesis of antibody, so-called antibody rebound. The rebound phenomenon after blood exchange is well established in animal models and is further supported by the observed increase in 19S antibody-forming cells in the guinea pig spleen.[147–149] Conversely, investigational studies involving a healthy volunteer, seven patients with nonimmune disorders, and seven patients with immune-mediated disease suggest that rebound is not a common phenomenon.[150] Although post-treatment increases in immunoglobulin levels, especially IgG, and in specific antibody titers accompany anecdotal reports of therapeutic plasma exchange, there is no general agreement on this finding or on its relevance to the course of immune-mediated disease. Because many treatment protocols introduced the simultaneous use of immunosuppressive drugs and plasmapheresis, it is not possible to determine whether favorable outcomes are the result of the independent effects of either treatment or of some synergistic effect.[151–153]

Immune complexes are associated with and may play a pathogenic role in a number of vasculitic disorders for which plasmapheresis had been recommended as adjunctive therapy. Systemic lupus erythematosus (with immune complexes containing complement components and antibodies to DNA and nucleoprotein antigens), mesangiocapillary glomerulonephritis (with complexes containing IgA and anti–mesangial cell antibodies), and Wegener's granulomatosis (with antineutrophil cytoplasmic antibodies) are a few such examples.[154–156] Little convincing evidence indicates that removing circulating complexes by plasmapheresis either mobilizes immune complexes fixed to tissue sites or prevents end-organ damage. Therapeutic plasmapheresis is employed in these disorders, however, often with an immunosuppressive drug regimen, in life-threatening or organ-threatening circumstances.

Treatment of neurological disorders accounts for a majority of plasmapheresis procedures. Guillain-Barré syndrome, an ascending areflexic paralysis, occurs with an annual incidence of 1 to 2 cases per 100,000 population in the United States. Acute demyelination characterizes the pathological process, and an autoimmune basis, possibly as a result of cross-reacting antibodies directed originally against an antigen from infection or vaccination, is postulated.[143, 157] Randomized, controlled trials indicated that plasmapheresis effects a shorter and milder course of disease, possibly as a result of antibody removal or, alternatively, of an immunomodulatory effect of apheresis on the disease process.[158, 159] The observation that intravenous immunoglobulin is as effective as plasma exchange suggests that antibody removal alone is insufficient to explain the clinical response.[160] Immunoglobulin does not appear to have an additive or synergistic effect when used as an adjunct to plasmapheresis.[161] Plasmapheresis can also effect remissions in patients with chronic inflammatory demyelinating polyneuropathies, disorders long recognized as responding to immunotherapy with corticosteroids.[162]

As a general rule, the hematological disorders responsive to plasmapheresis therapy are those mediated by immune complexes or by autoantibodies. These same disorders usually respond to high-dose corticosteroids or a course of intravenous immunoglobulin. One of the first such examples was post-transfusion purpura, a disorder in which patients with platelet-specific alloantibodies destroy transfused platelets as well as their own circulating platelets.[163, 164] Autoimmune thrombocytopenia and hemolytic anemia respond less predictably to plasmapheresis and often do not respond at all in the absence of other modes of therapy. Immune disorders mediated by alloantibodies, such as alloimmune platelet refractoriness, maternal alloimmunization, and alloimmune hemolysis, respond poorly if at all to plasmapheresis. Plasmapheresis to treat these conditions is reserved for desperate clinical circumstances.

Therapeutic plasmapheresis may be used to restore plasma factors as well as to remove noxious agents. The prototypical disorder in which plasma replacement seems to effect remission is TTP. Early empirical treatment with fresh blood exchanges and plasma infusion indicated that serial plasmapheresis was beneficial in the spectrum of syndromes now referred to as thrombotic microangiopathies.[165, 166] Subsequent studies confirmed that 70% to 90% of patients survive an acute episode of TTP when plasmapheresis is part of the therapeutic regimen.[167, 168] How plasma or plasmapheresis mediates the acute episode is not clear. Evidence supports both the removal of platelet-aggregating agents, possibly an antibody to von Willebrand factor–cleaving protease, and the replacement of some factor, such as this protease contained in plasma that dissociates large von Willebrand multimers.[169, 170] There is evidence suggesting a key role for von Willebrand factor–cleaving protein, absent in familial TTP and inhibited in acquired TTP. This protease appears to be unaffected in hemolytic-uremic syndrome (HUS), which may explain the poor response of this disorder to plasma exchange.[171, 172]

In some cases of TTP in which plasmapheresis has failed, replacement of plasma with the supernatant of cryoprecipitated plasma has proved effective.[173] Cryosupernatant seems particularly rich in some factor that reduces the size of the ultralarge von Willebrand multimers that interact with platelet glycoprotein Ib and glycoprotein IIb/IIIa molecules to induce platelet aggregation. TTP is one of the few conditions in which composition of the plasmapheresis replacement fluid seems important. With most disorders, the primary function of the replacement solution is to maintain intravascular volume, but additional desirable features include restoration of specific plasma proteins, maintenance of colloid osmotic pressure, maintenance of electrolyte balance, and preservation of trace elements lost during a prolonged course of plasmapheresis procedures. In moderately well-nourished subjects, normal homeostatic mechanisms usually obviate precise composition and plasma replacement. "Brittle" patients should receive solutions prepared specifically to meet their individual requirements.

COMPLICATIONS OF APHERESIS

In experienced hands, apheresis procedures have proved remarkably safe. Although 59 deaths associated with therapeutic apheresis had been reported through 1984, the majority occurred in patients who were critically ill before treatment. The estimated mortality rate of 3 in 10,000 procedures may more accurately reflect the condition of patients selected for treatment than the true risk of the procedure.[174] National incidence figures for Canada in 1985 indicated that 12% of 5235 therapeutic plasmapheresis procedures (40% of the 627 patients) were associated with side effects; most of these adverse effects were of little clinical significance. No procedure-related deaths occurred.[175] A survey of 3429 therapeutic procedures performed at 18 selected centers reported clinically significant adverse events in 6.9% of first-time and 4.3% of repeat procedures.[176] The great majority were mild, reversible adverse events. Only 11 of 664 (1.6%) autologous peripheral blood progenitor cell collections were associated with adverse effects, a rate substantially lower than that for blood component exchanges. Three deaths reported in this study were all attributed to the primary disease. Only one death attributed to the procedure has ever been reported in a volunteer donating blood components by apheresis.

Apheresis complications are associated with vascular access, hemodynamic changes, mechanical problems related to instrumentation, depletion of cellular and plasma components, reactions to replacement fluids (including anticoagulants), allergic reactions, and infection. Hemodynamic changes are readily prevented, even in patients with underlying cardiovascular disorders, by careful attention to fluid replacement calculations and familiarity with the extracorporeal volume requirements of the different blood cell separators. Vascular access problems occur primarily when catheters are used for long-term access. The most common problems are catheter occlusion, infection, vessel thrombosis, and vascular perforation.[177, 178] Their frequency and severity are determined by the nature and location of the catheter. A variety of soft, flexible multilumen catheters are now available for therapeutic apheresis, with procedures to maintain catheter patency and decrease local thrombosis.[179]

Depletion of plasma electrolytes, plasma proteins, platelets, and lymphocytes has concerned practitioners since the advent of apheresis procedures. Electrolytes and small molecules are not removed efficiently by plasmapheresis. Although small fluctuations in calcium and potassium levels can result in important clinical consequences, changes during apheresis are minimal and transient. In certain clinical situations, e.g., when citrated plasma is used as replacement in patients with hepatic and renal dysfunction, symptomatic hypocalcemia may require intravenous calcium replacement. Signs of severe hypocalcemia may range from involuntary carpopedal spasm to frank tetany and life-threatening laryngospasm.[180] An analysis of therapeutic plasma exchange procedures performed with and without 10% calcium gluconate infusion demonstrated that continuous calcium infusion prevents mild to moderate citrate toxicity.[181] However, careful monitoring is necessary to prevent accidental overdose, and most procedures require no electrolyte supplementation.[182, 183]

Many plasma proteins are removed efficiently by apheresis, but clinical problems such as bleeding and immunosuppression related to specific protein depletion are rare.[184] Acute decrease in platelets has not been accompanied by bleeding, probably because platelet removal becomes increasingly less efficient as the platelet count falls. Clinical problems related to frequent protein, platelet, and leukocyte removal have been sought for years, but there is little evidence that serial apheresis has these deleterious effects.[185, 186]

Adverse reactions related to replacement solutions other than plasma are unusual. However, albumin solutions readily support microbial growth. Glass containers should be examined for evidence of contamination, and once opened, albumin solutions should not be stored for use during subsequent procedures. A 5% solution may be prepared from the 25% solution by dilution with 0.9% sodium chloride injection; sterile water must not be used as a diluent, because the reduction in tonicity increases the risk of hemolysis during plasmapheresis. When plasma is used as a replacement fluid, allergic reactions are distressingly common.[187] Although most of these reactions are mild and transient, fatal anaphylaxis has occurred. Hypotension and flushing have been observed in patients medicated with angiotensin-converting enzyme (ACE) inhibitors, presumably related to their effect on metabolism of eicosanoids and endogenous bradykinin activated by blood contact with plastic surfaces.[188] ACE inhibitors are best discontinued for at least 24 hours before apheresis. Because plasma carries most of the infectious risks of whole blood, including hepatitis and HIV, 5% albumin in saline is the commonly used replacement solution. Concern that removal of circulating immunoglubulins during plasmapheresis with albumin replacement somehow predisposes patients with glomerulonephritis to a higher risk of bacterial infection appears to be unfounded.[189]

Anaphylactoid reactions to ethylene oxide, an agent used in the sterilization of plastic disposables, are well documented.[190] About 1% of subjects who undergo repeated apheresis procedures develop IgE antibodies detected in a radioallergosorbent assay. These reactions may include a variety of signs and symptoms, including pruritic eruption, conjunctivitis, sneezing, coughing, wheezing, abdominal cramping, and diarrhea. Although clinical severity has not been associated with other evidence of atopy or with the titer of the IgE antibody, the only reported death occurred in a normal apheresis donor who had a history of asthma.

The current generation of blood cell separators is extremely reliable and equipped with sensitive detection and alarm systems. Procedures for operator training and competency assessment have become more standardized and rigorous. Experience since the late 1970s confirm the safety of apheresis procedures when they are carried out for appropriate indications by experienced operators and under close medical supervision.[175, 176]

REFERENCES

1. Abel JJ, Rowntree LG, Turner BB. Plasma removal with return of corpuscles (plasmaphaeresis). J Pharmacol Exp Ther 1914; 5:625.
2. Tui B, Barrter FC, Wright AM, et al. Red cell reinfusion and the frequency of plasma donations: preliminary report of multiple donations in eight weeks by each of six donors. JAMA 1944; 124:331.
3. Grifols-Lucas J. Use of plasmapheresis in blood donors. BMJ 1952; 1:854.
4. Adams WS, Blahd WH, Bassott SH. A method of human plasmapheresis. Proc Soc Exp Biol Med 1952; 80:377.
5. Skoog WA, Adams WS. Plasmapheresis in a case of Waldenstrom's macroglobulinemia. Clin Res 1959; 7:96.
6. Kliman A, Gaydos LA, Schroeder LR, et al. Repeated plasmapheresis of blood donors as a source of platelets. Blood 1961; 18:303.
7. Tullis JL, Surgenor DM, Tinch RJ, et al. New principle of closed system centrifugation. Science 1956; 124:792.
8. Freireich EJ, Judson G, Levin RH. Separation and collection of leukocytes. Cancer Res 1965; 25:1516.
9. Latham A. Early developments in blood cell separation technology. Vox Sang 1986; 51:249.
10. Jones AL. The IBM blood cell separator and blood cell processor: a personal perspective. J Clin Apheresis 1988; 4:171.
11. Ito Y, Suaudfau J, Bowman RL. New flow-through centrifuge without rotating seals applied to plasmapheresis. Science 1975; 189:999.
12. Djerassi I, Kim JS, Mitrakul C, et al. Filtration leukapheresis for separation and concentration of transfusable amounts of normal human granulocytes. J Med (Basel) 1970; 1:358.
13. Sawada K, Malchesky PS, Nose Y. Available removal systems. *In* Nydegger UE (ed): Therapeutic hemapheresis in the 1990's. Curr Stud Hematol Blood Transfus 1990; 57:51.
14. Wright DG, Karsh J, Fauci AS, et al. Lymphocyte depletion and immunosuppression with repeated leukapheresis by continuous flow centrifugation. Blood 1981; 58:451.
15. Lockwood SM, Worlledge S, Nicholas A, et al. Reversal of impaired splenic function in patients with nephritis or vasculitis by plasma exchange. N Engl J Med 1979; 300:524.
16. Walport MJ, Peters M, Elkon KB, et al. The splenic extraction ratio of antibody-coated erythrocytes and its response to plasma exchange and pulse methylprednisolone. Clin Exp Immunol 1985; 60:465.
17. Hodgson WJB, Mercan S. Hemapheresis listening post: optimal venous access. Transfus Sci 1991; 12:274.
18. Hester JP, Kellogg RM, Mulzet AP, et al. Principles of blood separation and component extraction in a disposable continuous-flow single-stage channel. Blood 1978; 54:254.
19. Weiner AS, Wexler IB. The use of heparin when performing exchange blood transfusions in newborn infants. J Lab Clin Med 1946; 31:1016.
20. Collins JA. Problems associated with the massive transfusion of stored blood. Surgery 1974; 75:274.
21. McCullough J, Chopek M. Therapeutic plasma exchange. Lab Med 1981; 12:745.
22. Caspar CB, Reinhard AS, Burger J, et al. Effective stimulation of donors for granulocyte transfusions with recombinant methionyl granulocyte colony-stimulating factor. Blood 1993; 81:2866.
23. Lee JH, Leitman SF, Klein HG. A controlled comparison of the efficacy of hetastarch and pentastarch in granulocyte collections by centrifugal leukapheresis. Blood 1995; 86:4662.
24. Hillyer CD, Tiegerman KO, Berkman EM. Increase in circulating colony-forming units–granulocyte-macrophage during large-volume leukapheresis: evaluation of a new cell separator. Transfusion 1991; 31:327.
25. Lee EJ, Schiffer CA. Evidence for rapid mobilization from the spleen during intensive plateletpheresis. Am J Hematol 1985; 19:161.
26. Jemionek JF, Monroy R. Special techniques for the separation of hemopoietic cells: elutriation. Bibl Haematol 1984; 48:12.
27. Schouten HC, Kessinger A, Smith DM, et al. Counterflow centrifugation apheresis for the collection of autologous peripheral blood stem cells from patients with malignancies: a comparison with a standard centrifugation apheresis procedure. J Clin Apheresis 1990; 5:140.
28. Leitman SF, Smith JW, Gregg RE. Homozygous hypercholesterolemia: selective removal of low density lipoproteins by secondary membrane filtration. Transfusion 1989; 29:341.
29. Valbonesi M. Cascade filtration in the management of paraproteinemic and immune complex disease. *In* Lysaght MJ, Gurland H (eds): Plasma Separation and Plasma Fractionation: Current Status and Future Directions. Basel: Karger, 1983, p 245.
30. Agishi T, Kaneko I, Hasuo Y, et al. Double filtration for selective removal or retrieval of plasma fractions. Am Soc Artif Intern Organs 1979; 8:70.
31. Lysaght MJ, Samtleben W, Schmidt B, et al. Closed-loop plasmapheresis. *In* MacPherson JL, Kasprisin DO (eds): Therapeutic Hemapheresis, vol 1. Boca Raton, FL: CRC Press, 1985, p 149.
32. Malchesky PS, Asanuma Y, Zawicki I, et al. On line separation of macromolecules by membrane filtration with cryofiltration. Artif Organs 1980; 4:205.
33. Seidel D, Armstrong VW, Schuff-Werner P, et al. Removal of low density lipoproteins (LDL) and fibrinogen by precipitation with heparin at low pH: clinical application and experience. J Clin Apheresis 1988; 4:78.
34. Lauterburg BH, Pineda AA, Burgstaler EA, et al. Treatment of pruritus of cholestasis by plasma perfusion through USP-charcoal-coated glass beads. Lancet 1980; 1:53.
35. Marks DH, Medina F, Lee S, et al. Removal of bacteria from blood by charcoal hemoperfusion. Biomater Artif Cells Artif Organs 1988; 16:135.
36. Kuhnen E, Schaal KP, Keller F, et al. Clinical evaluation of diagnostic hemoperfusion for in vivo enrichment of bacteria and fungi in comparison with a conventional blood culture system. J Clin Microbiol 1988; 26:1609.
37. Lynn KL, Buttimore AL, Begg EJ, et al. Treatment of theophylline poisoning with haemoperfusion. N Z Med J 1988; 101:4.
38. Relling MV, Stapleton FB, Ochs J, et al. Removal of methotrexate, leukovorin, and their metabolites by combined hemodialysis and hemoperfusion. Cancer 1988; 62:884.
39. Terman DS, Young JB, Shearer WT, et al. Preliminary observations of the effects on breast adenocarcinoma of plasma perfused over immobilized protein A. N Engl J Med 1981; 305:1195.
40. Messerschmidt GL, Henry DH, Snyder HW Jr, et al. Protein A immunoadsorption in the treatment of malignant disease. J Clin Oncol 1988; 6:203.
41. Ainsworth SK, Pilia PA, Pepkowitz SH, et al. Toxicity following protein A treatment of metastatic breast adenocarcinoma. Cancer 1988; 61:1495.
42. Snyder HW Jr, Cochran SK, Balint JP, et al. Experience with protein A–immunoadsorption in treatment-resistant adult immune thrombocytopenic purpura. Blood 1992; 79:2237.
43. Sato H, Yamagata Y, Kidoka T. Studies on quantitative levels of complement activation induced by mobilized and soluble forms of protein A and IgG. Transfus Sci 1991; 12:299.
44. Huestis DW, Morrison FS. Adverse effects of immune adsorption with staphylococcal protein A columns. Transfus Med Rev 1996; 10:62.
45. Christie DJ, Howe RB, Lennon SS, et al. Treatment of refractoriness to platelet transfusion by protein A column therapy. Transfusion 1993; 33:234.

46. Snyder HW, Mittelman A, Oral A, et al. Treatment of cancer chemotherapy-associated thrombotic thrombocytopenic purpura/hemolytic-uremic syndrome by protein A immunoadsorption of plasma. Cancer 1993; 71:1882.
47. Ross CN, Gaskin G, Gregor-MacGregor S, et al. Renal transplantation in highly sensitized patients. Transplantation 1993; 55:785.
48. Palmer A, Cairns T, Gluck G, et al. Treatment of rapidly progressive glomerulonephritis by extracorporeal immunoadsorption, prednisolone, and cyclophosphamide. Nephrol Dial Transplant 1991; 6:536.
49. Nilsson IM. The management of hemophilia patients with inhibitors. Transfus Med Rev 1992; 6:285.
50. Borberg H, Gaczkowski A, Hombach V, et al. Treatment of familial hypercholesterolemia by means of specific immunoadsorption. J Clin Apheresis 1988; 4:59.
51. Terman DS, Buffaloe G, Mattioli C, et al. Extracorporeal immunoadsorption: initial experience in human systemic lupus erythematosus. Lancet 1979; 2:824.
52. Bensinger WI, Baker DA, Buckner CD, et al. Immunoadsorption for removal of A and B blood group antibodies. N Engl J Med 1981; 304:160.
53. Piomelli S, Seaman C, Ackerman K, et al. Planning an exchange transfusion in patients with sickle cell syndromes. Am J Pediatr Hematol Oncol 1990; 12:268.
54. Bunn HF. Pathogenesis of sickle cell disease. N Engl J Med 1997; 337:762.
55. Kaul DK, Fabry ME, Nagel RL. Microvascular sites and characteristics of sickle cell adhesion to vascular endothelium in shear flow conditions: pathophysiological implications. Proc Natl Acad Sci U S A 1989; 86:3356.
56. Kaul DK, Nagel RL, Chen D, et al. Sickle erythrocyte-endothelial interactions in the microcirculation: the role of von Willebrand factor and implications for vaso-occlusion. Blood 1993; 81:2429.
57. Smolinski PA, Offermann MK, Eckman JR, et al. Double-stranded RNA induces sickle erythrocyte adherence to endothelium: a potential role for viral infection in vaso-occlusive episodes in sickle cell anemia. Blood 1995; 85:2945.
58. Anderson R, Cassell M, Mullinax GL, et al. Effect of normal cells on viscosity of sickle-cell blood: in vitro studies and report of six years experience with a prophylactic program of "partial exchange transfusion." Arch Intern Med 1963; 111:286.
59. Lessin LS, Kurantsin-Mills J, Klug PP, et al. Determination of rheologically optimal mixtures of AA and SS erythrocytes for transfusion. Prog Clin Biol Res 1978; 20:123.
60. Vichinsky EP, Haberkern CM, Neumayr L, et al. A comparison of conservative and aggressive transfusion regimens in the perioperative management of sickle cell disease. N Engl J Med 1995; 333:206.
61. Keitel HG, Thompson D, Itano HA. Hyposthenuria in sickle cell anemia: a reversible renal defect. J Clin Invest 1956; 35:998.
62. Pearson HA, Cornelius EA, Schwartz AD, et al. Transfusion-reversible functional asplenia in young children with sickle-cell anemia. N Engl J Med 1970; 283:334.
63. Miller DM, Winslow RM, Klein HG, et al. Improved exercise performance after exchange transfusion in subjects with sickle cell anemia. Blood 1980; 56:1127.
64. Rodgers GP, Schechter AN, Noguchi CT, et al. Periodic microcirculatory flow in patients with sickle cell disease. N Engl J Med 1984; 311:1534.
65. Vichinsky EP, Styles LA, Colangelo LH, et al. Acute chest syndrome in sickle cell disease: clinical presentation and course. Blood 1997; 89:1787.
66. Powell RW, Levine GL, Yang YM, et al. Acute splenic sequestration crisis in sickle cell disease: early detection and treatment. J Pediatr Surg 1992; 27:215.
67. Hassell KL, Eckman JR, Lane PA. Acute multiorgan failure syndrome: a potentially catastrophic complication of severe sickle cell pain episodes. Am J Med 1994; 96:155.
68. Fowler JE, Koshy M, Strub M, et al. Priapism associated with the sickle hemoglobinopathies: prevalence, natural history, and sequelae. J Urol 1991; 145:65.
69. Koshy M, Burd L, Wallace D, et al. Prophylactic red-cell transfusions in pregnant patients with sickle cell disease. N Engl J Med 1988; 319:1447.
70. Cohen AR, Martin MB, Silber JH, et al. A modified transfusion program for prevention of stroke in sickle cell disease. Blood 1992; 79:1657.
71. Adams RJ, McKie VC, Files B, et al. Prevention of first stroke by transfusions in children with sickle cell anemia and abnormal results on transcranial ultrasonography. N Engl J Med 1998; 339:5.
72. Kim HC, Dugan NP, Silber JH, et al. Erythrocytapheresis therapy to reduce iron overload in chronically transfused patients with sickle cell disease. Blood 1994; 83:1136.
73. Coles SM, Klein HG, Holland PV. Alloimmunization in two multitransfused patient populations. Transfusion 1981; 21:462.
74. Diamond WJ, Brown FL, Bitterman P, et al. Delayed hemolytic transfusion reactions presenting as sickle cell crisis. Ann Intern Med 1980; 93:231.
75. Miller KD, Greenberg AE, Campbell CC. Treatment of severe malaria in the United States with a continuous infusion of quinidine gluconate and exchange transfusion. N Engl J Med 1989; 321:65.
76. Jacoby JA, Hunt JV, Kosinski KS, et al. Treatment of transfusion-transmitted babesiosis by exchange transfusion. N Engl J Med 1980; 303:1098.
77. Winslow RM, Monge CC, Brown EG, et al. The effect of hemodilution on O_2 transport in high altitude polycythemia. J Appl Physiol 1985; 59:1495.
78. Freireich EJ, Thomas LB, Frei E III, et al. A distinctive type of intracerebral hemorrhage associated with "blastic crisis" in patients with leukemia. Cancer 1960; 13:146.
79. McKee LC, Collins RD. Intravascular leukocyte thrombi and aggregates as a cause of morbidity and mortality in leukemias. Medicine 1974; 53:463.
80. Lester TJ, Johnson JW, Cuttner J. Pulmonary leukostasis as the single worst prognostic factor in patients with acute myelocytic leukemia and hyperleukocytosis. Am J Med 1985; 79:43.
81. Lichtman MA, Rowe JM. Hyperleukocytic leukemias: rheological, clinical, and therapeutic considerations. Blood 1982; 60:279.
82. Cuttner J, Holland JF, Norton L, et al. Therapeutic leukapheresis in acute myelocytic leukemia. Med Pediatr Oncol 1983; 11:76.
83. Lane TA. Continuous-flow leukapheresis for rapid cytoreduction in leukemia. Transfusion 1980; 20:455.
84. Biggs JC. Cytapheresis in the treatment of leukemia. *In* Valbonesi M, Pineda AA, Biggs JC (eds): Therapeutic Hemapheresis. Bonn: Wichtig Editore Milano, 1986, pp 155–162.
85. Baer M, Stein R, Dessypres E. Chronic lymphocytic leukemia with hyperleukocytosis: the hyperviscosity syndrome. Cancer 1985; 56:2865.
86. Bloom R, Taveira Da Silva AM, Bracey A. Reversible respiratory failure due to intravascular leukostasis in chronic myelogenous leukemia. Am J Med 1979; 67:679.
87. Kar DD, Beck JR, Cornell CJ. Chronic granulocytic leukemia with respiratory distress. Arch Intern Med 1981; 141:1353.
88. Hester JP, McCredie KB, Freireich EJ. Response to chronic leukapheresis procedures and survival of chronic myelogenous leukemia patients. Transfusion 1982; 22:305.
89. Lowenthal RM, Buskard NA, Goldman JM, et al. Intensive leukapheresis as an initial therapy for chronic granulocytic leukemia. Blood 1975; 46:835.
90. Curtis JE, Hersh EM, Freireich EJ. Leukapheresis therapy of chronic lymphocytic leukemia. Blood 1972; 39:163.
91. Goldfinger D, Capostagno V, Lowe C, et al. Use of longterm leukapheresis in the treatment of chronic lymphocytic leukemia. Transfusion 1980; 20:450.
92. Cooper IA, Ding JC, Adams PB. Intensive leukapheresis in the management of cytopenias in patients with chronic lymphocytic leukemia (CLL) and lymphocytic lymphoma. Am J Hematol 1979; 6:387.
93. Fay JW, Moore JO, Logue GL, et al. Leukapheresis therapy of leukemic reticuloendotheliosis (hairy cell leukemia). Blood 1979; 54:747.
94. Edelson R, Facktor M, Andrews A, et al. Successful management of the Sézary syndrome: mobilization and removal of extravascular neoplastic T cells by leukapheresis. N Engl J Med 1974; 291:293.
95. Golomb HM, Kraut EH, Oviatt DL, et al. Absence of prolonged benefit of initial leukapheresis therapy for hairy cell leukemia. Am J Hematol 1983; 14:49.
96. Wilder RL, Yarboro CH, Decker JL. The effects of repeated leukapheresis in patients with severe refractory rheumatoid arthri-

tis. *In* Tindall RSA (ed): Therapeutic Apheresis and Plasma Perfusion. New York: Alan R. Liss, 1982, pp 49–59.
97. Karsh J, Klippel JH, Plotz PH, et al. Lymphapheresis in rheumatoid arthritis: a randomized trial. Arthritis Rheum 1981; 24:867.
98. Wallace DJ, Goldfinger D, Lowe C, et al. A double-blind controlled study of lymphoplasmapheresis versus sham apheresis in rheumatoid arthritis. N Engl J Med 1982; 306:1406.
99. Edelson R, Berger C, Gasparro F, et al. Treatment of cutaneous T-cell lymphoma by extracorporeal photochemotherapy: preliminary results. N Engl J Med 1987; 316:297.
100. Edelson R, Perez M, Heald P, et al. Extracorporeal photochemotherapy. Biol Ther Cancer Updates 1994; 4:1.
101. Bisaccia E, Berger C, Klainer AS. Extracorporeal photopheresis in the treatment of AIDS-related complex: a pilot study. Ann Intern Med 1990; 113:270.
102. Lim HW, Edelson RL. Photopheresis for the treatment of cutaneous T-cell lymphoma. Hematol Oncol Clin North Am 1995; 9:1117.
103. Rook AH, Freundlich B, Jegasothy BV, et al. Treatment of systemic sclerosis with extracorporeal photochemotherapy—results of a multicenter trial. Arch Dermatol 1992; 128:337.
104. Malawista S, Trock D, Edelson R. Treatment of rheumatoid arthritis by extracorporeal photochemotherapy: a pilot study. Arthritis Rheum 1991; 34:646.
105. Knobler RM. Extracorporeal photochemotherapy for the treatment of systemic lupus erythematosus: preliminary observations. Semin Immunopathol 1994; 16:323.
106. Gollnick H, Owsianowski M, Taube K, et al. Unresponsive severe pemphigus vulgaris successfully controlled by extracorporeal photopheresis. J Am Acad Dermatol 1993; 28:122.
107. Constanzo-Nordin MR, Hubbell EA, O'Sullivan EJ, et al. Photopheresis versus corticosteroids in the therapy of heart transplant rejection. Circulation 1992; 86:242.
108. Barr ML, McLaughlin SN, Murphy SP, et al. Prophylactic photopheresis and effect on graft atherosclerosis in cardiac transplantation. Transplant Proc 1995; 27:1993.
109. Owsianowski M, Gollnick H, Siegert W, et al. Successful treatment of chronic graft-versus-host disease with extracorporeal photopheresis. Bone Marrow Transplant 1994; 59:149.
110. Chievitz E, Thiede T. Complications and causes of death in polycythemia vera. Acta Med Scand 1962; 172:51.
111. Dawson AA, Ogston D. The influence of the platelet count on the incidence of thrombotic and hemorrhagic complications in polycythemia vera. Postgrad Med J 1970; 46:76.
112. Schafer AI. Bleeding and thrombosis in the myeloproliferative disorders. Blood 1984; 64:1.
113. Goldfinger D, Thompson R, Lowe C, et al. Long-term plateletpheresis in the management of primary thrombocytosis. Transfusion 1979; 19:336.
114. Orlin JB, Berkman EM. Improvement of platelet function following plateletpheresis in patients with myeloproliferative diseases. Transfusion 1980; 20:540.
115. Buss DH, Stuart JJ, Lipscomb GE. The incidence of thrombotic and hemorrhagic disorders in association with extreme thrombocytosis: an analysis of 129 cases. Am J Hematol 1985; 20:365.
116. Kessler CM, Klein HG, Havlik RJ. Uncontrolled thrombocythemia in myeloproliferative disorders. Br J Haematol 1982; 50:157.
117. Falconer J, Pineo G, Blahey W, et al. Essential thrombocythemia associated with recurrent abortion and fetal growth retardation. Am J Hematol 1987; 25:345.
118. Mercer B, Drouin J, Jolly E, et al. Primary thrombocythemia in pregnancy: a report of two cases. Am J Obstet Gynecol 1988; 159:127.
119. Curtis JE, Hersh EM, Freireich EJ. Antigen specific immunity in recipients with leukocyte transfusions from immune donors. Cancer Res 1970; 30:2921.
120. Lee JH, Klein HG. Mononuclear cell transfusion: immunotherapy using allogeneic donor-derived lymphocytes. *In* Mintz PD (ed): Transfusion Therapy: Clinical Principles and Practice. Bethesda, MD: AABB Press, 1999, pp 251–265.
121. Lane HC, Zunich KM, Wilson W, et al. Syngeneic bone marrow transplantation and adoptive transfer of peripheral blood lymphocytes combined with zidovudine in human immunodeficiency virus infection. Ann Intern Med 1990; 113:512.
122. Blaese RM, Culver KW, Miller AD, et al. T lymphocyte–directed gene therapy for ADA deficiency (SCID): initial trial results over four years. Science 1995; 270:475.
123. American Association of Blood Banks Hemapheresis Committee. Guidelines for Therapeutic Hemapheresis. Bethesda, MD: American Association of Blood Banks, 1995.
124. Powles R, Smith C, Kohn J, et al. Method of removing abnormal protein rapidly from patients with malignant paraproteinemias. BMJ 1971; 3:664.
125. McGrath MA, Penny R. Paraproteinemia: blood hyperviscosity and clinical manifestations. J Clin Invest 1976; 58:1155.
126. Beck JR, Quinn BM, Meier FA, et al. Hyperviscosity syndrome in paraproteinemia: managed by plasma exchange; monitored by serum tests. Transfusion 1982; 22:51.
127. Berkman EM, Orlin JB. Use of plasmapheresis and partial plasma exchange in the management of patients with cryoglobulinemia. Transfusion 1980; 20:171.
128. Geltner DF, Kohn RW, Gorevic PD, et al. The effect of combination chemotherapy (steroids, immunosuppressives and plasmapheresis) on 5 mixed cryoglobulinemia patients with renal, neurologic and vascular involvement. Arthritis Rheum 1981; 24:1121.
129. Taft EG, Propp RP, Sullivan SA. Plasma exchange for cold agglutinin hemolytic anemia. Transfusion 1977; 17:173.
130. Gibberd FB, Billimoria JD, Page NGR, et al. Heredopathia atactica polyneuritiformis (Refsum's disease) treated by diet and plasma exchange. Lancet 1979; 1:575.
131. Moser HW, Braine H, Pyeritz RE, et al. Therapeutic trial of plasmapheresis in Refsum disease and Fabry disease. Birth Defects 1980; 16:491.
132. Thompson GR, Lowenthal R, Myant NB. Plasma exchange in the management of homozygous familial hypercholesterolemia. Lancet 1975; 1:1208.
133. Thompson GR. Plasma exchange for hypercholesterolemia. Lancet 1981; 1:246.
134. Thompson GR, Miller JP, Breslow JL. Improved survival of patients with homozygous familial hypercholesterolemia treated with plasma exchange. BMJ 1985; 201:1671.
135. Stein EA, Adolph R, Rice V, et al. Nonprogression of coronary artery atherosclerosis after 31 months of repetitive plasma exchange. Clin Cardiol 1986; 9:115.
136. Yokoyama S, Hayashi R, Satani M, et al. Selective removal of low density lipoprotein by plasmapheresis in familial hypercholesterolemia. Arteriosclerosis 1987; 6:613.
137. Borberg H, Gaczkowski A, Hombach V, et al. Treatment of familial hypercholesterolemia by means of specific immunoadsorption. J Clin Apheresis 1988; 4:59.
138. Lockwood CM, Boulton-Jones JM, Lowenthal RM, et al. Recovery from Goodpasture's syndrome after immunosuppressive treatment and plasmapheresis. BMJ 1975; 2:252.
139. Pusey CD, Lockwood CM, Peters DK. Plasma exchange and immunosuppressive drugs in the treatment of glomerulonephritis due to antibodies to the glomerular basement membrane. Int J Artif Organs 1983; 6:15.
140. Savage COS, Pusey CD, Bowman C, et al. Antiglomerular basement membrane antibody mediated disease in the British Isles 1980–84. BMJ 1986; 1:301.
141. Newsom-Davis J, Willcox N, Schluep M, et al. Immunologic heterogeneity and cellular mechanism in myasthenia gravis: biology and treatment. Ann N Y Acad Sci 1987; 505:12.
142. Dau PC, Denys EH. Plasmapheresis and immunosuppressive drug therapy in the Eaton-Lambert syndrome. Ann Neurol 1982; 11:570.
143. Koski CL, Gratz E, Sutherland J, et al. Clinical correlation with anti-peripheral myelin antibodies in Guillain-Barré syndrome. Ann Neurol 1986; 19:573.
144. Roujeau JC, Kalis B, Lauret P, et al. Plasma exchange in corticosteroid resistant pemphigus. Br J Dermatol 1982; 106:103.
145. Blanchette V, Hogan A, McCombie N, et al. Intensive plasma exchange therapy in 10 patients with idiopathic thrombocytopenic purpura. Transfusion 1984; 24:388.
146. Wensley R, Stevens R, Burn A, et al. Plasma exchange and human factor VIII concentrate in managing hemophilia A with factor VIII inhibitors. BMJ 1980; 381:1388.
147. Bystryn JC, Schenkein I, Uhr JW. A model for the regulation of antibody synthesis by serum antibody. Prog Immunol 1971; 1:627.
148. Terman DS, Garcia-Rinaldi R, Dannemann B, et al. Specific suppression of antibody rebound after extracorporeal immunoadsorption. Clin Exp Immunol 1978; 34:32.

149. Sturgill BC, Wozniak MJ. Stimulation of proliferation of 19S antibody-forming cells in the spleens of immunized guinea pigs after exchange transfusion. Nature 1970; 228:1304.
150. Derksen RHWM, Schuurman HJ, Gmelig Meyling FHJ, et al. Rebound and overshoot after plasma exchange in humans. J Lab Clin Med 1984; 104:35.
151. Wilson CB, Dixon FJ. Antiglomerular basement membrane antibody–induced glomerular nephritis. Kidney Int 1973; 3:74.
152. Auerbach R, Bystryn JC. Plasmapheresis and immunosuppressive therapy: effect on levels of intracellular antibody in pemphigus vulgaris. Arch Dermatol 1979; 115:728.
153. Huston DP, White MJ, Mattioli C, et al. A controlled trial of plasmapheresis and cyclophosphamide therapy of lupus nephritis. Arthritis Rheum 1983; 26:S33.
154. Mannik M. Pathophysiology of circulating immune complexes. Arthritis Rheum 1982; 27:783.
155. Nicholls K, Walker RG, Kincaid-Smith P, et al. Malignant IgA nephropathy. Am J Kidney Dis 1984; 5:42.
156. Van der Woude FJ, Lobatto S, Permin H, et al. Autoantibodies against neutrophils and monocytes: tool for diagnosis and marker of disease activity in Wegener's granulomatosis. Lancet 1985; 1:425.
157. Rees JH, Soudain SE, Gregson NA, et al. *Campylobacter jejuni* infection and Guillain-Barré syndrome. N Engl J Med 1995; 333:1374.
158. Guillain-Barré Study Group. Plasmapheresis and acute Guillain-Barré syndrome. Neurology 1985; 35:1096.
159. French Cooperative Study Group on Plasma Exchange in Guillain-Barré Syndrome. Plasma exchange in Guillain-Barré syndrome: one-year follow-up. Ann Neurol 1992; 32:94.
160. van der Meche FGA, Schmitz PIM, Dutch Guillain-Barré Study Group. A randomized trial comparing intravenous immune globulin and plasma exchange in Guillain-Barré syndrome. N Engl J Med 1992; 326:1123.
161. Plasma Exchange/Sandoglobulin Guillain-Barré Syndrome Trial Group. Randomised trial of plasma exchange, intravenous immunoglobulin, and combined treatments in Guillain-Barré syndrome. Lancet 1997; 349:225.
162. Dyck PJ, Daube J, O'Brien P, et al. Plasma exchange in chronic inflammatory demyelinating polyneuropathy. N Engl J Med 1986; 314:461.
163. Shulman NR, Aster RH, Leitner A, et al. Immunoreactions involving platelets. V. Post-transfusion purpura due to a complement-fixing antibody against a genetically controlled platelet antigen. A proposed mechanism for thrombocytopenia and its relevance in "autoimmunity." J Clin Invest 1961; 40:1597.
164. Shulman NR. Posttransfusion purpura: clinical features and the mechanism of platelet destruction. *In* Nance SJ (ed): Clinical and Basic Aspects of Immunohematology. Arlington, VA: American Association of Blood Banks, 1991, p 137.
165. Rubinstein MA, Kagan BM, MacGillviray MH, et al. Unusual remission in a case of thrombotic thrombocytopenic purpura syndrome following fresh blood exchange transfusions. Ann Intern Med 1959; 51:1409.
166. Byrnes JJ, Khurana M. Treatment of thrombotic thrombocytopenic purpura with plasma. N Engl J Med 1977; 287:1386.
167. Rock GA, Shumak KH, Buskard NA, et al. Comparison of plasma exchange and plasma infusion in the treatment of thrombotic thrombocytopenic purpura. N Engl J Med 1991; 325:393.
168. Bell WR, Braine HG, Ness PM, et al. Improved survival in thrombotic thrombocytopenic purpura–hemolytic uremic syndrome. N Engl J Med 1991; 325:398.
169. Moake JL, McPherson PD. Abnormalities of von Willebrand factor multimers in thrombotic thrombocytopenic purpura and the hemolytic uremic syndrome. Am J Med 1989; 87(suppl 3N):1N.
170. Moore JC, Murphy WG, Kelton JG. Calpain proteolysis of von Willebrand factor enhances its binding to platelet membrane glycoprotein IIb/IIIa: an explanation for platelet aggregation in thrombotic thrombocytopenic purpura. Br J Haematol 1990; 74:457.
171. Tsai H-M, Lian EC-Y. Antibodies to von Willebrand factor–cleaving protein in acute thrombotic thrombocytopenic purpura. N Engl J Med 1998; 339:1585.
172. Furlan M, Robles R, Galbusera M, et al. Von Willebrand factor–cleaving protease in thrombotic thrombocytopenic purpura and the hemolytic uremic syndrome. N Engl J Med 1998; 313:1578.
173. Byrnes JJ, Moake JL, Klug P, et al. Effectiveness of the cryosupernatant fraction of plasma in the treatment of refractory thrombotic thrombocytopenic purpura. Am J Hematol 1990; 34:169.
174. Huestis DW. Complications of therapeutic apheresis. *In* Valbonesi M, Pineda AA, Biggs JC (eds): Therapeutic Hemapheresis. Milan: Wichtig Editore, Milano, 1986, pp 179–186.
175. Sutton DMC, Nair RC, Rock G, et al. Complications of plasma exchange. Transfusion 1989; 29:124.
176. McLeod BC, Sniecinski I, Ciavarella D, et al. Frequency of immediate adverse effects associated with therapeutic apheresis. Transfusion (in press).
177. Cassidy FP, Jajko AB, Bron KM, et al. Noninfectious complications of long-term central venous catheters: radiologic evaluation and management. AJR Am J Roentgenol 1987; 149:671.
178. Jacobs MB, Yeager M. Thrombotic and infectious complications of Hickman-Broviac catheters. Ann Intern Med 1984; 144:1597.
179. Haire WD, Edney JA, Landmark JD, et al. Thrombotic complications of subclavian apheresis catheters in cancer patients: prevention with heparin infusion. J Clin Apheresis 1990; 5:188.
180. Strauss RG. Mechanisms of adverse effects during hemapheresis. J Clin Apheresis 1996; 11:160.
181. Weinstein R. Prevention of citrate reactions during therapeutic plasma exchange by constant infusion of calcium gluconate with the return fluid. J Clin Apheresis 1996; 11:204.
182. Orlin JB, Berkman EM. Partial plasma exchange using albumin replacement: removal and recovery of normal plasma constituents. Blood 1980; 56:1055.
183. Chopek M, McCullough J. Protein and biochemical changes during plasma exchange. *In* Therapeutic Hemapheresis, a Technical Workshop. Washington, DC: American Association of Blood Banks, 1980, p 13.
184. Klein HG. Effect of plasma exchange on plasma constituents: choice of replacement solutions and kinetics of exchange. *In* McPherson JL, Kasprisin DO (eds): Therapeutic Hemapheresis, vol 2. Boca Raton, FL: CRC Press, 1985, pp 3–14.
185. Wasi S, Santowski T, Murray SA, et al. The Canadian Red Cross Plasmapheresis Donor Safety Program: changes in plasma proteins after long-term plasmapheresis. Vox Sang 1991; 60:82.
186. Sniecenski IJ. Safety of apheresis donation. Infusionstherapie 1987; 14(suppl):52.
187. Heal JM, Horan PK, Schmitt TC, et al. Long-term follow-up of donors cytapheresed more than 50 times. Vox Sang 1983; 45:14.
188. Owen HG, Brecher ME. Atypical reactions associated with use of angiotensin-converting enzyme inhibitors and apheresis. Transfusion 1994; 34:891.
189. Pohl MA, Lan S-P, Berl T, et al. Plasmapheresis does not increase the risk of infection in immunosuppressed patients with severe lupus nephritis. Ann Intern Med 1991; 114:924.
190. Leitman SF, Boltansky H, Alter HJ, et al. Allergic reactions in healthy plateletpheresis donors caused by sensitization to ethylene oxide gas. N Engl J Med 1986; 315:1192.

CHAPTER 40

Alternatives to Allogeneic Blood Transfusion

Lawrence T. Goodnough
George Despotis

The 1990s was a period of explosive growth in the use of alternatives to allogeneic blood; this growth resulted largely from concern over the risk of transfusion-transmitted diseases.[1] Numerous professional organizations and federal agencies have endorsed autologous blood transfusion; the use of agents to reduce perioperative bleeding in patients undergoing cardiac bypass surgery has become common; and recombinant human erythropoietin (EPO) therapy has been approved worldwide for use in patients with medical anemias (associated with renal insufficiency, human immunodeficiency virus [HIV] infection, and cancer) and in the perisurgical setting. However, advances in blood safety and the increased costs associated with blood conservation have prompted reevaluation of alternatives to blood transfusion. This chapter summarizes these developments and provides perspective on the evolving role of blood conservation strategies.

AUTOLOGOUS BLOOD PROCUREMENT

Preoperative Autologous Blood Donation

Some advantages and disadvantages of preoperative autologous blood donation (PAD) are summarized in Table 40–1. Preoperative collection of autologous blood can, in selected patient subgroups, significantly reduce exposure to allogeneic blood. Patients are considered candidates for receiving autologous blood when scheduled for surgical procedures for which a blood transfusion is considered likely. For procedures that are unlikely to necessitate transfusion (i.e., a maximal surgical blood-ordering schedule does not suggest that blood be prepared for crossmatch),[2] preoperative blood collection has not been recommended. This technique has undergone reevaluation of its safety, efficacy, and cost effectiveness.[3]

Selection of Patients

Several recent guidelines that identify patients who are not suitable for PAD have been published.[4–7] Table 40–2 details guidelines published by the British Committee for Standards in Hematology.[7] The American Association of Blood Banks recommends that patients with evidence of systemic infection or unstable angina be excluded. If the units are to be shipped, the first unit collected from a given patient during a 30-day period must have the same testing for infectious disease markers as allogeneic units[8]; however, subsequent units need not be tested, unless they are to be transferred from the collection facility.[8, 9] Supplemental iron is prescribed ideally before the first blood collection, because iron-restricted erythropoiesis is a limiting factor to the collection of multiple units of blood over a short interval.[10, 11]

Autologous blood collection can be performed for patients who would not, under normal circumstances, be considered for allogeneic donation. With suitable volume modification and parental cooperation, pediatric patients can participate in preoperative collection programs.[12] Significant cardiac disease is generally considered a poor risk factor for autologous collection. Despite reports of safety in small numbers of patients scheduled for coronary artery bypass grafting who undergo autologous blood donation,[13] mortality risks associated with autologous blood donation[14] in these patients are probably higher than current estimated mortality risks of allogeneic transfusion.[15] Collecting blood from pregnant women is rarely indicated.[16] In routine pregnancy and delivery or in uncomplicated cesarean section, blood is needed so seldom that autologous collection is considered inappropriate. Potential candidates for autologous blood collection include women with alloantibodies to multiple or high-incidence antigens, with placental previa, or with other conditions that place them at high risk for antepartum or intrapartum hemorrhage.[17]

Preoperative autologous collection is most beneficial for patients undergoing procedures with substantial blood loss, such as orthopedic joint replacement, vascular surgery, cardiac or thoracic surgery, and radical prostatectomy.[3] Autologous blood should not be collected for procedures that seldom (for fewer than 10% of patients) necessitate transfusion, such as transurethral resection of the prostate, cholecystectomy, herniorrhaphy, vaginal hysterectomy, and uncomplicated obstetric delivery.[18]

It is important to establish guidelines for the appropriate number of units to be collected. A sufficient number of units should be drawn, whenever possible, so that the patient can avoid exposure to allogeneic blood. Collection of units should be scheduled as far in advance of surgery as possible for liquid blood storage, in order to allow compensatory erythropoiesis to prevent anemia.[19] Studies have shown that the endogenous erythropoietin response at the level of mild blood-loss anemia from PAD

Table 40–1. Autologous Blood Donation

Advantages
1. Prevents transfusion-transmitted disease
2. Prevents red cell alloimmunization
3. Supplements the blood supply
4. Provides compatible blood for patients with alloantibodies
5. Prevents some adverse transfusion reactions

Disadvantages
1. Does not affect risk of bacterial contamination
2. Does not affect risk of ABO incompatibility
3. More costly than allogeneic blood
4. Blood not transfused is wasted
5. Causes preoperative anemia and increases likelihood of perioperative transfusion

Table 40–2. Scenarios in Which Autologous Blood Donation Should Be Deferred

1. Evidence of infection and risk of bacteremia
2. Scheduled for surgery to correct aortic stenosis
3. Unstable angina
4. Active seizure disorder
5. Myocardial infarction or cerebrovascular accident within 6 months of donation
6. Patients with significant cardiac or pulmonary disease who have not yet been cleared for surgery by their treating physician
7. High-grade left main coronary artery disease
8. Cyanotic heart disease
9. Uncontrolled hypertension

Data from British Committee for Standards in Hematology, Blood Transfusion Task Force: Guidelines for autologous transfusion. Transfus Med 1993; 3:307.

is suboptimal.[20–23] As detailed in Table 40–3, between 25% and 75% of blood that is donated is replaced through compensatory erythropoiesis, so that the hematocrit is not maintained during the donation interval. A mathematical model has predicted that the predeposit of autologous blood may therefore be harmful,[24] which was confirmed in a study of patients undergoing hysterectomy[25] in which PAD resulted in an increased likelihood of blood transfusion.

Efficacy

The relationship between autologous blood ordering and collection and subsequent allogeneic blood transfusion in orthopedic surgical patients has been examined.[26] Donation success is dependent primarily on whether donors are anemic (hematocrit ≤ 39%) at first donation. Of the patients for whom the number of units requested is successfully donated, only 10% subsequently receive allogeneic blood. In contrast, of the patients who are unable to store the number of autologous blood units requested, 27% subsequently receive allogeneic blood.

Although the most important indicator for autologous blood procurement is the reduction in allogeneic transfusions, the "wastage" rate of autologous units is an index of its efficiency and costs. Even for procedures such as joint replacement or radical prostatectomy, a well-designed program may result in discard rates of up to 50% of collected units.[17] Of the autologous blood that is collected for procedures that seldom necessitate transfusion, such as vaginal hysterectomies and normal vaginal deliveries, up to 90% of units collected are wasted.[17, 18, 25] The additional costs associated with the collection of autologous units and the inherent "wastage" rate of these units, along with advances in the safety of allogeneic blood, decrease the cost effectiveness of autologous blood predonation.[27–30] Suggestions to make autologous blood programs less costly include abbreviation of the donor interview for autologous collection; utilization of only whole blood without component production; limiting the use of frozen autologous blood; applying the same transfusion guidelines for autologous and allogeneic blood; and testing only the first donated autologous blood unit for infectious disease markers.

A mathematical model was developed to help identify patients who might benefit from PAD versus those patients who do not need PAD.[3] Figure 40–1 illustrates an algorithm using anticipated surgical blood losses and level of hematocrit to be maintained perioperatively, to determine the indication for autologous blood donation for individual patients, as follows:

1. Measure the patient's initial hematocrit.
2. Set the minimum tolerable hematocrit (transfusion trigger). This value should take into account individual patient characteristics such as age and medical status.
3. Apply these values to the graph shown in Figure 40–1 to derive the estimated blood loss (EBL) necessary to reach this transfusion trigger.
4. Compare this EBL to the predicted EBL for the particular surgical procedure.

Table 40–3. Compensatory RBC Production During Autologous Blood Donation

Reference	Units		Interval (weeks)	RBC (mL) Production		% RBC "Replaced"
	Requested	Donated		Mean	Range	
20	2	2	2	100		25%
21	3	2.7	3	351	9–719	60%
22	6*	4.1*	3	Female: 549	499–599	60%
				Male: 602	564–640	75%
23						
Oral iron	6	2.6	3	328	250–406	60%
IV iron	6	3.3	3	432	353–511	66%

*Total for both male and female.
Modified from Goodnough LT, Mercuriali F. Compensatory erythropoiesis during autologous blood donation under standard conditions. Transfusion 1998; 38:613.
RBC, red blood cell; IV, intravenous.

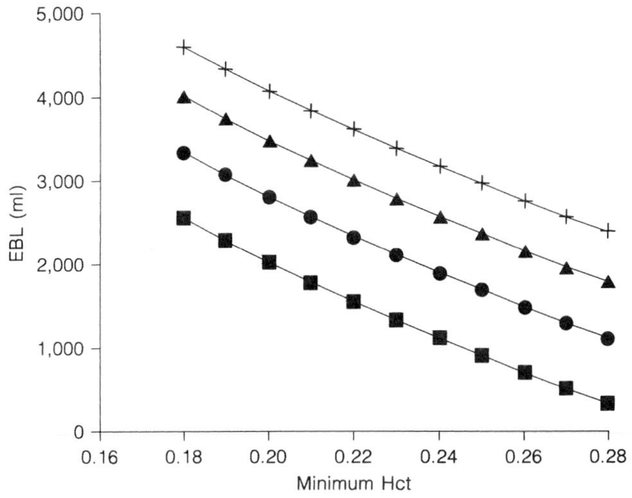

Figure 40–1. Relationship of estimated blood loss (EBL) and minimum (nadir) hematocrit (Hct) during hospitalization at various initial Hct levels in a surgical patient with a whole blood volume of 5000 mL. *Squares* represent Hct of 0.30; *circles* represent Hct of 0.35; *triangles* represent Hct of 0.40; *plus signs* represent Hct of 0.45. (From Cohen JA, Brecher ME. Preoperative autologous blood donation: benefit or detriment? A mathematical analysis. Transfusion 1995; 35:640.)

If the EBL for the procedure exceeds the EBL required for transfusion, then PAD would be beneficial; if not, PAD is not recommended.

ACUTE NORMOVOLEMIC HEMODILUTION

Acute normovolemic hemodilution (ANH) is a technique in which whole blood is removed from a patient while the circulating blood volume is maintained with acellular fluid shortly before an anticipated significant surgical blood loss. Blood is collected in standard blood bags containing anticoagulant on a tilt-rocker with automatic cutoff accomplished by volume sensors. The blood is then stored at room temperature and reinfused in the operating room after major blood loss has ceased, or sooner if indicated. Simultaneous infusions of crystalloid (3 mL of crystalloids to 1 mL of blood withdrawn) and colloid (1 mL of dextrans, starches, gelatin, or albumin to 1 mL of blood withdrawn) have been recommended. The first unit collected, and therefore the last unit transfused, has the greatest red cell mass and the highest concentration of coagulation factors and platelets.

Efficacy

The chief benefit of ANH has been recognized to be the reduction of red cell losses when whole blood is shed perioperatively at lower hematocrit levels after ANH is complete.[31] Mathematical modeling has suggested that severe ANH to preoperative hematocrit levels of less than 20%, accompanied by substantial blood losses, would be required before the red cell volume saved by ANH became clinically important.[32] A case-study analysis of patients who had undergone minimal ANH (representing only 15% of patients' blood volume) estimated that 100 mL of red cells (the equivalent of 0.5 U of blood) is saved under these conditions.[33] With moderate ANH (target hematocrit levels of 28%), the savings becomes more substantial. The removal of 3 U of blood from a 100-kg patient who subsequently undergoes a blood loss of 2600 mL results in an estimated 215 mL in red cell volume savings, or the equivalent of one allogeneic blood unit.[34] The safety and efficacy of more extensive ANH is controversial[35] and may provide little additional blood conservation.

Two prospective, randomized trials[36, 37] and a case-controlled, retrospective comparison[38] of ANH and PAD in patients undergoing radical prostatectomy demonstrated that subsequent allogeneic blood exposure was not different (10% to 20%) for patients undergoing either method of autologous blood procurement. A prospective study of moderate ANH reported that 21% of patients received allogeneic blood[39]; this is comparable to the allogenic blood exposure rates for three units of PAD[27, 40] and to the 17% to 20% allogeneic blood exposure rates in patients undergoing elective surgery, for which PAD is routinely practiced.[27, 39, 41]

The benefits of ANH are illustrated in Figure 40–2. An adult with an initial hematocrit of 40% and surgical blood losses of up to 3000 mL is predicted to have a hematocrit of 25% or higher postoperatively without any autologous blood intervention.[42] This level of hematocrit is generally considered safe for patients without known risk factors.[43] The performance of ANH in patients with initial hematocrit levels of 40% to 45% could allow for 2500 to 3500 mL of surgical blood losses, and yet the nadir level of hematocrit would be maintained $\geq$ 28%. The benefit of ANH is to protect patients who have substantial blood losses that cannot be predicted[44] and to maintain perioperative levels of hematocrit that minimize risks related to ischemia.[45] Blood conservation strategies are needed to address both these issues.[46, 47]

ANH represents "point of care" autologous blood procurement and is less costly than PAD. First, autologous blood units procured by ANH are retransfused before the patient leaves the operating room and require no inventory or testing costs. ANH therefore eliminates the possibility of an administrative error that could lead to an ABO-incompatible blood transfusion and also the risk of bacterial contamination seen with stored blood units. The estimated risk of death from an acute transfusion reaction[48] now approximates the rate of transfusion-related mortality from HIV or hepatitis infection.[15] In addition, ANH and reinfusion is accomplished in the operating room by on-site personnel, and costs are minimized. Blood obtained during ANH does not require the commitment of patient time, transportation, and loss of work associated with PAD. A pro-and-con debate on the merits of ANH has been published.[49, 50] In the future, the availability of blood substitutes for use in the hemodilution process may increase the efficacy of ANH.

INTRAOPERATIVE BLOOD SALVAGE

The term *intraoperative blood salvage* describes the technique of salvaging and reinfusing blood lost by a patient

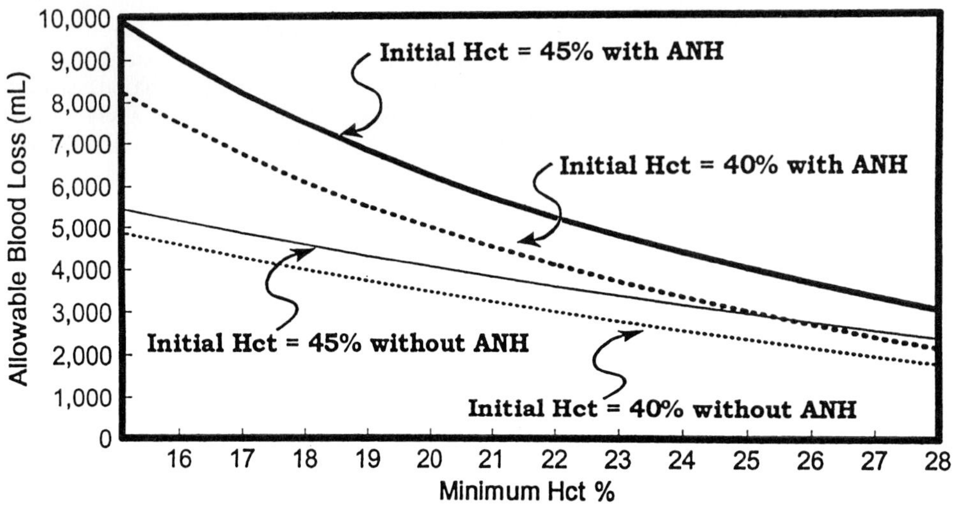

Figure 40–2. The maximum allowable blood loss in a patient with a blood volume of 5000 mL and an initial hematocrit (Hct) level of 45% *(solid lines)* or 40% *(dotted lines)*, with and without acute normovolemic hemodilution (ANH). (From Goodnough LT, Monk TG, Brecher ME. Acute normovolemic hemodilution in surgery. Hematology 1997; 2:413.)

during surgery. The oxygen-transport properties of salvaged red blood cells are equal to or better than those of stored allogeneic red cells, and the survival rate of red blood cells appears to be at least comparable with that of transfused allogeneic red cells.[51] Relative contraindications include malignant neoplasm, infection, and contaminants such as topical collagen in the operative field. Because washing does not remove bacteria from recovered blood, intraoperative salvage should not be used if the operative field has gross bacterial contamination or other body fluids, such as amniotic or ascitic fluid.

Cell-washing devices can provide the equivalent of 12 units of banked blood per hour to a patient with massive bleeding. The incidence of adverse events resulting from reinfusion of salvaged blood is not known, but the procedure is not without risk.[52] Hemolysis of salvaged blood can occur, particularly when blood is aspirated at vacuum settings greater than 100 mm Hg. The clinical importance of free hemoglobin concentration has not been established, although excessive free hemoglobin may indicate inadequate washing.[51] Most programs use machines that collect shed blood and then wash and concentrate the red cells. This process typically results in units of 225 mL of saline-suspended red cells with a hematocrit of 50% to 60%. Dilutional coagulopathy may occur if large volumes of salvaged blood are administered.

Intraoperative autologous blood salvage should, in addition, undergo scrutiny regarding not only safety but also cost effectiveness. A controlled study in cardiothoracic surgery demonstrated a lack of efficacy for intraoperative salvage when transfusion requirements and clinical outcome were analyzed.[52] Although the salvage of a minimum of one blood unit equivalent is possible with less expensive (with unwashed blood) methods, it is generally agreed that at least two blood unit equivalents need to be salvaged by using the cell-saver (with washed blood), in order to achieve cost effectiveness.[53–55]

POSTOPERATIVE BLOOD SALVAGE

Postoperative blood salvage denotes the collection of blood from surgical drains followed by reinfusion, with or without processing. The evolution of cardiac surgery has been accompanied by increased use of postoperative autologous blood salvage and reinfusion, which is widely, but not uniformly, practiced. Prospective and controlled trials have reported discordant results as to the efficacy of postoperative blood salvage in cardiac surgery patients: at least three studies have demonstrated lack of efficacy,[56–58] whereas at least two studies have shown benefit.[59, 60] The disparity of results may be explained, at least in part, by differences in transfusion practices.

In the postoperative orthopedic surgical setting, a number of reports have similarly described the successful salvage and reinfusion of washed[61] and unwashed[62, 63] wound drainage from patients undergoing arthroplasty. The safety of reinfused unwashed orthopedic wound drainage remains controversial. Theoretical concerns regarding infusion of potentially harmful materials in salvaged blood have been expressed. One group concluded that inscrtion of drains for postoperative wound salvage and reinfusion is of no clinical benefit.[64] Prospective identification of patients who can benefit from intraoperative and postoperative autologous blood salvage may be possible if preoperative hematocrit, anticipated surgical blood losses, and the perioperative "transfusion trigger" are taken into account (see Figure 40–1).

PHARMACOLOGICAL ALTERNATIVES TO BLOOD

Erythropoietin and Erythropoiesis Under Normal Conditions

EPO is a glycoprotein growth factor produced by the kidneys in a feedback control system (Fig. 40–3) in which a renal oxygen-sensing mechanism responds to hypoxia or hyperoxia to enhance or reduce the production of the circulating hormone.[65, 66] In turn, EPO interacts with erythroid progenitor cells through a specific receptor site on erythroid colony-forming units (CFU-E) to enhance the manufacture of new red blood cells,[67, 68] completing the feedback loop. The molecular biology of erythropoietin, along with its mechanism of action, has been reviewed previously.[69]

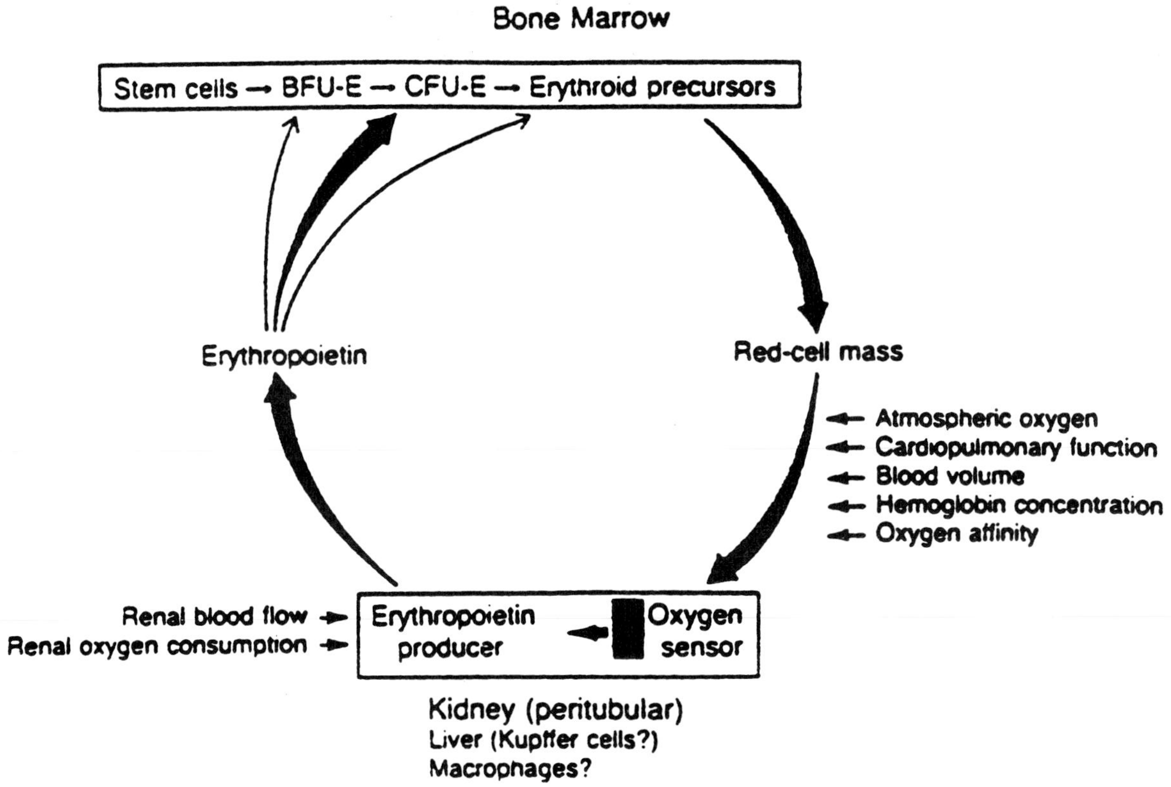

Figure 40–3. The feedback circuit that adjusts the rate of red cell production to the demand for oxygen. BFU-E, erythroid burst-forming units; CFU-E, erythroid colony-forming units, both erythroid progenitor cells. (From Erslev AJ. Erythropoietin. N Engl J Med 1991; 324:1340.)

Under normal steady-state conditions, EPO facilitates the survival of sufficient numbers of erythroid progenitor cells to replace losses of senescent red blood cells, thus ensuring maintenance of a normal red cell mass.[70] The process of programmed red blood cell death, apoptosis,[71] is inhibited by high levels of erythropoietin in erythropoietin-dependent erythroid progenitors, which are responsible for normal red blood cell production.[72, 73] Conversely, when EPO levels are decreased below normal as a result of hypertransfusion or renal disease, EPO-dependent progenitors undergo apoptosis and red blood cell production is reduced.

The relationship between reduction in red cell mass and the endogenous EPO response in patients with chronic iron deficiency anemia[74] and in patients with anemia due to blood loss[75] is semilogarithmic, as illustrated in Figures 40–4*A* and 40–4*B*. In the absence of anemia, plasma levels of EPO range from 10 to 20 μL. With greater degrees of anemia, EPO levels increase exponentially, so that when the hematocrit is less than 20%, the plasma level of EPO increases 100-fold or more.[76]

Pharmacologic Agents to Replace Blood

Erythropoietin Therapy in Surgical Anemia

The current status of approval worldwide for use of recombinant human EPO therapy is shown in Table 40–4. EPO was approved for use in patients undergoing PAD in Japan, the European Union, and Canada in 1993,

Table 40–4. Approval of Status of Recombinant Human Erythropoietin Therapy in Medical and Surgical Anemias

Anemia Related to	United States	Canada	European Union*	Australia	Japan
Chronic renal failure					
Dialysis	1989	1990	1988	1991	1990
Predialysis	1990	1990	1990	1991	1994
HIV infection treated with zidovudine	1990	1990	—	—	—
Cancer or cancer treatment	1993	1995	1994	Under review	—
Autologous blood donation	—	1996	1994	Under review	1993
Surgery	1996†	1996	1998	1996	Under review

*Approval dates for France, Germany, Italy, and the United Kingdom are the same as for other countries of the European Union.
†Noncardiac, nonvascular surgery.
HIV, human immunodeficiency virus.

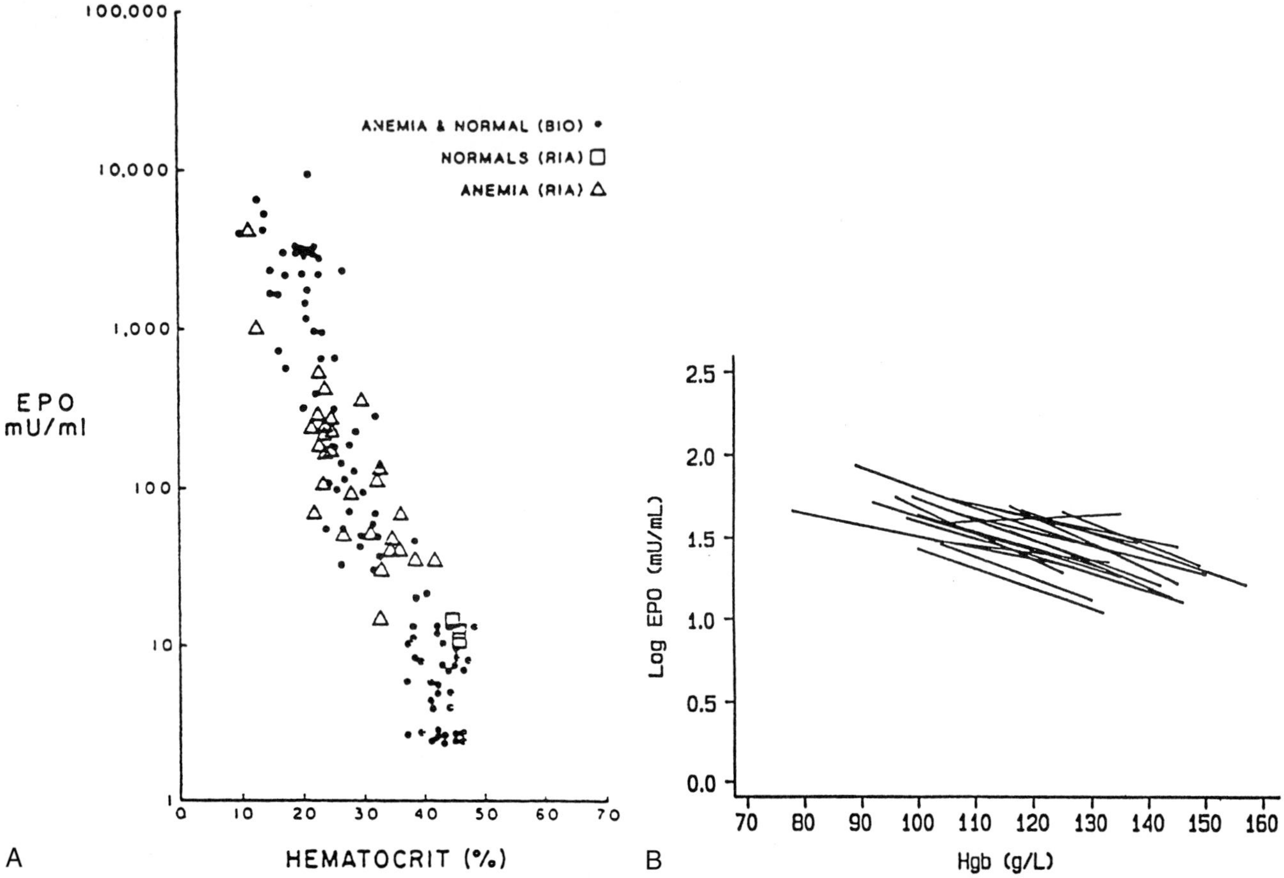

Figure 40–4. *A*, The relationship between packed red blood cell volume and endogenous plasma erythropoietin. (From Erslev AJ, Caro J. Physiologic and molecular biology of erythropoietin. Med Oncol Tumor Pharmacother 1986; 3:159.) *B*, The estimated preoperative linear relationships between log erythropoietin (mU/mL) and hemoglobin (g/L) in the placebo group of autologous donors subjected to aggressive phlebotomy. Eighteen patients had complete data recorded at three preoperative phlebotomy visits (nos. 1, 3, and 6 at days 0, 7.0 ± 0.5, and 17.6 ± 0.6, respectively). The slopes of the individual regression lines among patients were not significantly different. The pooled slope for the group was significantly less than zero. (From Goodnough LT, Price TH, Parvin CA, et al. Erythropoietin response to anemia is not altered by surgery or recombinant human erythropoietin therapy. Br J Haematol 1994; 87:695).

1994, and 1996, respectively. Approval was granted for perisurgical EPO therapy in major surgical procedures without PAD in Canada in 1996 and in the European Union in 1998 and for nonvascular, noncardiac procedures in the United States in 1996.[77] Erythropoietin (along with iron, vitamin B_{12}, and folic acid) therapy "should be used instead of blood transfusion if the clinical condition of the patient permits sufficient time for these agents to promote erythropoiesis."[78]

Patients donating autologous blood under standard conditions (i.e., one blood unit weekly) have an inadequate response of endogenous erythropoietin to anemia,[79] which suggests that EPO therapy might facilitate autologous blood donation by enhancing compensatory erythropoiesis; this was subsequently confirmed in a clinical trial of aggressive autologous blood donation (up to 6 U over a 3-week preoperative interval), with or without EPO therapy, in patients undergoing orthopedic surgery.[80] Subsequent clinical trials[81–83] in orthopedic patients demonstrated no clinical benefit of erythropoietin therapy in autologous blood donors who were not anemic (hematocrit > 39%) at first donation.

For anemic (hematocrit ≤ 39%) autologous blood donors, a European clinical trial demonstrated that EPO therapy reduced exposure to allogeneic blood during orthopedic surgery, but this result was achieved with both intravenous and oral iron supplementation.[23] A subsequent U.S. trial with supplemental oral iron and EPO therapy could not demonstrate reduced allogeneic blood transfusions, in large part because a substantial percentage of the patients were either severely anemic (hematocrit < 33%) or were iron deficient.[84]

Several studies have evaluated perisurgical EPO therapy in nonanemic orthopedic surgical patients without autologous blood procurement. Both a Canadian study[85] and a U.S. study[86] were able to show that EPO-treated patients had approximately half the rate of exposure to allogeneic blood (25%) as the placebo-treated patients (50%). On the basis of these clinical trials, EPO therapy was approved for perisurgical use in anemic (hematocrit < 39%) surgical patients in Canada and the United States in 1996.

The safety of EPO therapy in patients undergoing noncardiac surgery has been demonstrated in more than

1000 patients participating in clinical trials. Thrombotic events attributed to EPO therapy have not been seen in these surgical settings.[81] An unresolved question is the issue of safety for EPO therapy in cardiac surgery patients and its use in this setting. In a European trial,[87] the authors found no differences in mortality rates, thrombotic events, or serious adverse events between the EPO-treated and placebo cohorts. However, adverse events and mortalities in a U.S. study[88] indicated that an uneven distribution of these events between the placebo and the EPO-treated groups could not be excluded.[89] The use of EPO in patients undergoing cardiac or vascular surgery is therefore currently not recommended in the United States.

The costs associated with EPO therapy and the potential impact of reimbursement policies are important issues in the setting of surgical anemias, as has been the case in medical anemias.[89, 90] Costs associated with EPO therapy may be lowered by strategies that improve the dose and response relationship. The pharmacoeconomics of subcutaneous administration are superior to those of intravenous administration.[91] One study[92] demonstrated that four weekly injections of subcutaneous EPO (600 U/kg) was less costly but was just as effective as a daily dose of EPO (300 U/kg for 14 doses). However, perioperative EPO therapy remains expensive and, when unaccompanied by autologous blood procurement, is still associated with an allogeneic transfusion exposure rate of 16% to 25%.[85, 86, 92] Patients undergoing complex operations with substantial blood needs may require a combination of EPO therapy and autologous blood procurement, such as acute normovolemic hemodilution. Low-dose EPO therapy coupled with ANH has been shown to be cost equivalent to the collection of three autologous blood units before elective surgery.[36]

Erythropoietin Therapy in the Medical Setting

Anemia of Chronic Renal Disease

EPO therapy has become standard practice in dialysis patients with the anemia of chronic renal failure; a clinical response is observed in more than 95% of patients who were previously transfusion dependent.[93, 94] The improvement in hematocrit levels in this setting not only reduces transfusion requirements[95] but also is associated with improvement in quality of life.[96, 97] Early experience with EPO therapy in chronic renal failure revealed that up to 30% of patients had exacerbation of hypertension, including hypertensive encephalopathy in 5% of patients.[98] Subsequent studies have indicated that complications associated with EPO therapy in this setting were more likely related to the indirect effects of drug administration on factors such as blood viscosity and changes in vascular resistance than to direct effects of the drug itself.[99]

EPO therapy has also been demonstrated to be effective in patients with chronic renal disease who are not on dialysis[100, 101]; the mean change in hematocrit was from 28% before therapy to 32% after therapy. These patients are not usually transfusion dependent, however, and subjective improvement or increase in exercise capacity has been more difficult to demonstrate.[101] Nevertheless, EPO therapy is approved for patients with chronic renal insufficiency with serum creatinine levels higher than 1.8 mg/dL.

Anemia of Other Chronic Diseases

The use of EPO in patients with medical anemias outside the setting of uremia has been reviewed.[102] One such application for EPO therapy is the treatment of the anemia induced by zidovudine (AZT) in patients who are infected with HIV. Anemia with hemoglobin levels below 7.5 g/dL was reported in 24% of patients with acquired immunodeficiency syndrome (AIDS) who underwent a clinical trial of AZT therapy, in comparison with only 4% of placebo recipients; in this study, 31% of the AZT recipients were given red cell transfusions, in comparison with 11% of the placebo recipients.[103] A subsequent study reported anemia in 18% of asymptomatic HIV-positive patients, 50% of patients with AIDS-related complex, and 75% of patients with AIDS.[104]

A study of the relationship between hemoglobin level and serum-immunoreactive EPO in anemic AIDS patients undergoing AZT therapy demonstrated that the endogenous EPO response was inadequate for the degree of anemia in this setting. This observation led to a trial of EPO therapy in AIDS patients undergoing AZT therapy.[105] A reduction in red cell transfusions, as well as in the number of patients transfused, was observed in patients with initial endogenous EPO levels less than 500 μL. In patients with higher levels of EPO, pharmacological doses of EPO appear to be ineffective.

Similar studies of the relationship between hemoglobin and serum-immunoreactive EPO have been conducted in patients with the anemia of rheumatoid arthritis.[106, 107] In this model of the anemia of chronic inflammatory disease, the endogenous EPO response to anemia was again found to be blunted. A subsequent randomized, placebo-controlled trial of EPO showed that all patients receiving the hormone attained a normal hematocrit.[108] However, no meaningful changes were observed in patients' capacity to perform activities of daily living, nor did subjective amelioration of pain occur in patients receiving EPO. A second study also demonstrated that patients with rheumatoid arthritis have similar erythropoietic responses to EPO therapy in comparison with patients who do not have rheumatoid arthritis.[109] The anemia in chronic disorders caused by other inflammatory conditions, such as cirrhosis, has also been demonstrated to respond to EPO therapy before elective surgery.[110]

Decreased EPO response to anemia has also been reported in patients with cancer, indicating that EPO deficiency contributes to the development of anemia in this setting.[111] A randomized trial of EPO therapy (150 U/kg subcutaneously three times weekly) in cisplatin-treated cancer patients demonstrated that hematocrit levels can be improved and transfusion requirements reduced in this setting.[112, 113] Reports indicate that EPO therapy can also improve the anemia in patients with malignancy involving the bone marrow.[113–115]

Myelodysplastic/Aplastic Anemia Syndromes

Although an overall relationship between the degree of anemia and circulating EPO was observed in myelodysplastic syndromes, the EPO response did not correspond to the degree of anemia.[116] In a randomized, placebo-controlled trial, only 4 (24%) of 17 patients responded to EPO doses of up to 1200 to 1600 U/kg given intravenously twice weekly.[117] Although this study indicated that EPO could be administered safely in very high doses to some patients with myelodysplastic syndromes, the patients most in need of a beneficial response failed to show such a response. A more recent case report was able to demonstrate sustained improvement in anemia in a patient with hypoplastic myelodysplastic syndrome,[118] which suggested that a high initial EPO level does not preclude a clinical response to EPO therapy.[119]

Anemia of Prematurity

Like the anemia seen in adult medical conditions, the anemia of prematurity has been demonstrated to be related to an inadequate endogenous EPO response.[120] Data from clinical trials suggest that EPO therapy can lower transfusion requirements in premature infants weighing more than 1000 g.[121]

Iron Therapy

In the setting of blood loss, normal people have been shown to have difficulty providing sufficient iron to support rates of erythropoiesis that are greater than three times basal rates of erythropoiesis.[122] The variable relationship between EPO blood loss and the erythropoietic response[123] most likely results from iron-restricted erythropoiesis, even with oral iron supplementation.[11] Patients with enhanced plasma iron and transferrin saturation are able to produce an optimal (six- to eightfold) erythropoietic response, such as in hemochromatosis[124] or in patients supplemented with intravenous iron administration.[23] The term *relative iron deficiency* has thus been described as occurring when the iron stores are normal but the increased erythron iron requirements exceed the supply of iron.[125]

A trial of intravenous iron dextran therapy coupled with EPO therapy demonstrated rapid erythropoietic responses in patients undergoing surgical repair of hip fracture.[126] However, intravenous iron dextran therapy can be associated with side effects that may preclude routine use outside the setting of renal dialysis.[127] One study found that side effects related to the toxicity of free iron can be avoided by the slow infusion of 100 mg iron dextran over 4 hours of renal dialysis[128]; this rate of infusion may be impractical, however, in nondialysis patients. The approval, in the United States, of an iron gluconate preparation that appears well-tolerated in dialysis patients may lead to its use as iron therapy in patients outside the dialysis setting.[129]

PHARMACOLOGICAL INTERVENTIONS TO REDUCE BLOOD LOSS

Because a substantial proportion of blood components is used by patients undergoing cardiac surgery, most of the pharmacological blood conservation strategies have arisen in this patient population (Table 40–5).

Pathophysiology of Hemostasis Abnormalities

Patients undergoing cardiac surgery with cardiopulmonary bypass (CPB) are at risk for excessive perioperative blood loss that necessitates transfusion of blood products. This risk is influenced by the duration of CPB.[130, 131] Although excessive perioperative bleeding may occasionally be related to preexisting hemostatic abnormalities,[130, 132, 133] CPB more often causes hemostatic alterations that predispose to excessive bleeding. Crystalloid or colloid solutions used to prime the CPB circuit (and as a component of cardioplegia) cause significant dilution of coagulation factors and platelets.[133, 134] Activation of the hemostatic system during CPB can lead to thrombin- and plasmin-mediated consumption of platelets and labile coagulation factors (Fig. 40–5). This activation is related to the interaction of the contact factors XII and XI, high–molecular weight kininogen, and prekallikrein with extracorporeal surfaces[135, 136] and, of more importance, is related to activation of the extrinsic pathway[137] via release of tissue factor by surgical trauma or retransfusion of pericardial blood.[138] Fibrinolysis can be triggered by CPB-mediated contact system activation of factor XII[139] and the generation of thrombin, hypothermia,[140] the release of tissue plasminogen activator (tPA) from the pericardial cavity[141] or from surgically injured endothelial cells,[142] and through a protamine-mediated mechanism.[143] Even after protamine neutralization, heparin may potentially inhibit coagulation[144] and platelet function[145, 146]; similarly, excess protamine has been shown to inhibit coagulation[147] and affect platelet function.[148–150] Finally, release of elastase from polymorphonuclear leukocytes may affect hemostasis.[151]

Table 40–5. Pharmacologic Agents That Have Been Used to Reduce Blood Loss and Transfusion

Desmopressin acetate (DDAVP)
Topical agents
Fibrin glue
Hemostatic swabs (calcium alginate)
Vasoconstricting agents (oxymetazoline)
Absorbable collagen (INSTAT)
Topical thrombin, oxidized cellulose, and porcine collagen
Platelet gel
Anticoagulation during extracorporeal circulation: therapeutic heparin
Platelet inhibitors
Aspirin
Dipyridamole
Iloprost*
Prostaglandin E_1 (PGE_1)
Antifibrinolytic agents
Epsilon aminocaproic acid (EACA)
Tranexamic acid
Broad-spectrum serine protease inhibitors
Aprotinin
Gabexate (FOY)
Nafamostat (Futhan)

*Withdrawn in 1996.

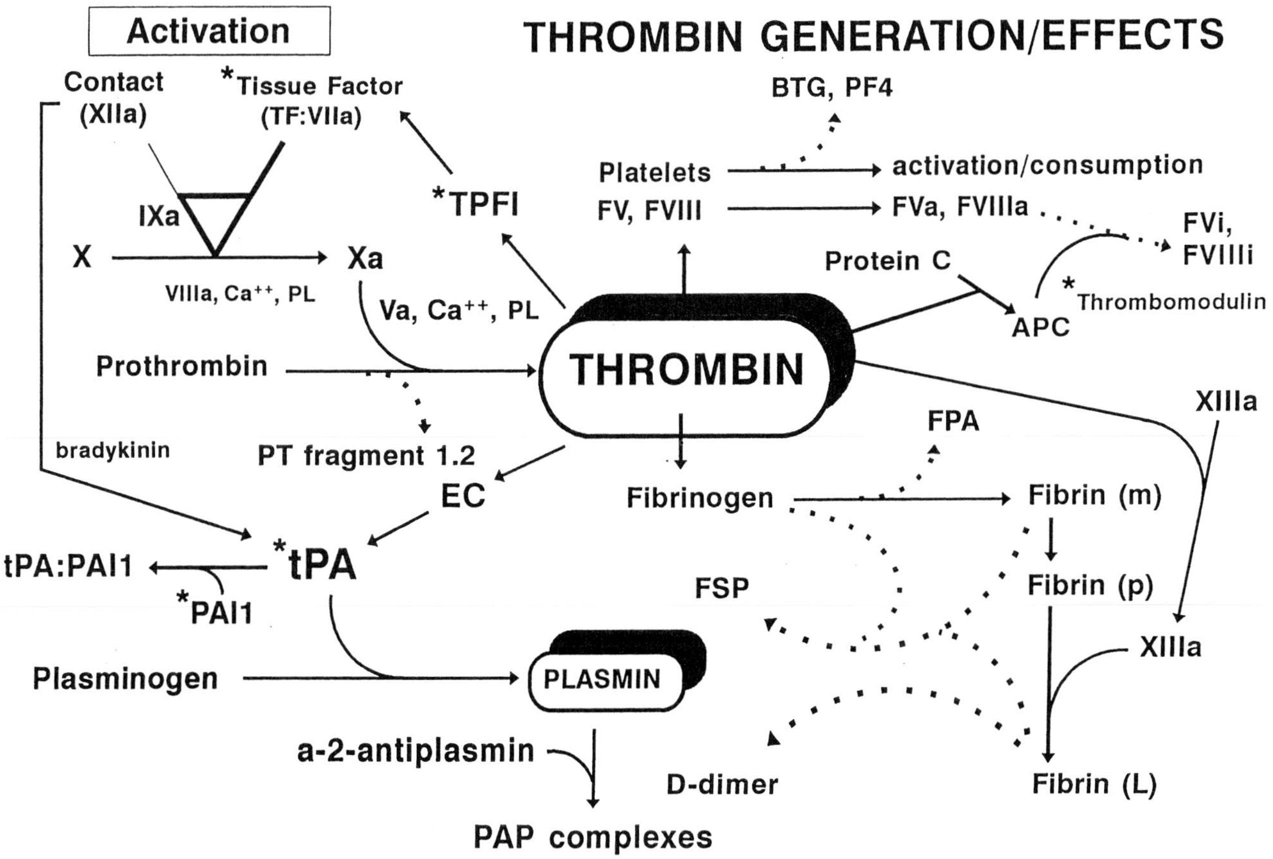

Figure 40–5. Mechanisms and effects of excessive hemostatic activation with cardiac surgery. *Dashed line* designates release of protein cleavage by-products. In abbreviations, activated factors are designated by a lowercase "a," whereas inactivated factors are designated by a lowercase "i." XII, factor XII; VII, factor VII; X, factor X; VIII, factor VIII; IX, factor IX; V, factor V; XIII, factor XIII; PT 1.2, prothrombin fragment 1.2; FPA, fibrinopeptide A; PL, phospholipid; PAP, plasmin-antiplasmin complexes; EC, endothelial cells; tPA:PAI1 = tPA PAI1 complexes; fibrin (m), fibrin monomer; fibrin (p), fibrin polymer; fibrin (L), fibrin crosslinked polymer; PAI1, plasminogen activator inhibitor; tPA, tissue plasminogen activator; FDP, fibrinogen/fibrin degradation products; D-dimers, polymerized fibrin degradation products. (From Despotis GJ, Levy J, Filos K, Gravlee G. Anticoagulation monitoring during cardiac surgery: a survey of current practice and review of current and emerging technologies. Anesthesiology, in press.)

Desmopressin Acetate

Desmopressin acetate (DDAVP [1-deamino-8-D-arginine] vasopressin)[152] is a synthetic analog of antidiuretic hormone (vasopressin) that causes vasodilation.[153] DDAVP increases plasma levels of factor VIII and the high–molecular weight forms of von Willebrand factor.[154] When a dose of 0.3 mg/kg body weight is administered intravenously, factor VIII activity increases three- to fivefold. Receptor-mediated release of von Willebrand factor from endothelial cells may be regulated by monocyte-derived platelet-activating factor.[155] Although increases in von Willebrand factor can enhance platelet-subendothelial[154] and platelet-platelet interactions,[156] other mechanisms may be operative for DDAVP, such as expression of glycoprotein Ib receptors,[157] generation of platelet microparticles/enhanced procoagulant activity,[158] increased release of von Willebrand factor from platelets[159] and expression of P-selectin by endothelial cells.[160] Release of high–molecular weight forms (i.e., largest multimers) of von Willebrand factor may have clinical implications because these forms have been shown to be decreased with aortic stenosis,[161] other congenital or acquired valvular heart disease,[162–164] and CBP.[165–167]

DDAVP can be used to treat patients with mild hemophilia A or von Willebrand's disease and some patients with circulating anticoagulants for factor VIII who are undergoing mild surgical procedures (e.g., dental surgery).[168, 169] DDAVP has been shown to improve or correct the prolonged bleeding times not only in patients with von Willebrand's disease but also in patients with acquired platelet defects such as uremia,[170] cirrhosis,[171, 172] and aspirin ingestion.[173] Although DDAVP is generally considered to be safe, a number of side effects, including facial flushing, headache, hypotension,[153, 174, 175] water retention, and hyponatremia, are well recognized.[176–178] DDAVP should be administered intravenously over 20 to 30 minutes, and excessive free water administration should be avoided. Although early case reports suggested a potential relationship between desmopressin and thrombotic complications,[179, 180] a more recent analysis of 1833 surgical patients did not demonstrate a clear increased risk of thrombotic complications.[181]

DDAVP was initially shown to be effective in reducing perioperative blood loss and transfusion requirements in cardiac surgical patients who undergo complex procedures with prolonged extracorporeal circulation.[182] However, a number of subsequent studies in cardiac surgery showed no significant benefit when DDAVP was administered prophylactically to patients undergoing cardiac surgery.[183–189] Certain patients at high risk for excessive bleeding may benefit from DDAVP,[190–194] such as those with excessive postoperative bleeding (e.g., >1180 mL/24 hours)[192] or those receiving platelet-inhibiting drugs.[191, 193, 195] Patients at increased risk for excessive bleeding may be identified through tests of hemostatic function.[190, 194, 196] Czer and associates demonstrated that DDAVP is beneficial when administered to patients with excessive bleeding and prolonged bleeding times.[194] In a randomized, prospective trial, a thromboelastography-based measurement identified patients who responded to DDAVP therapy.[190] Patients with an abnormal (>50 mm) thromboelastography (TEG) maximum amplitude (MA) treated with placebo had significantly greater mediastinal chest tube drainage than did matched patients who received DDAVP or patients with a normal MA value. DDAVP administration in cardiac surgical patients at risk by TEG evaluation for excessive bleeding was demonstrated to reduce blood product use in the intervention cohort.[197] A point-of-care test has been developed to evaluate platelet activating factor–inducible platelet procoagulant activity. In one clinical trial, 101 patients with abnormal platelet function after discontinuation of CPB were randomly assigned to either receive placebo ($n = 51$) or DDAVP ($n = 50$). DDAVP-treated patients had a 61% reduction in red cell units transfused, a 94% reduction in platelet units transfused, and an 83% reduction in plasma units transfused in comparison with placebo recipients. Cumulative mediastinal chest tube drainage in the first 24 postoperative hours was also significantly less ($p = .001$) in DDAVP-treated patients than in placebo recipients. Finally, DDAVP has reduced operative blood loss in patients with normal platelet function who undergo Harrington rod spinal fusion surgery.[198]

Topical Agents

Fibrin glue and fibrin gel are blood derivatives rather than pharmacological agents and are increasingly being used as an intervention in surgical hemostasis and blood conservation, as a result of approval by the U.S. Food and Drug Administration (FDA) of fibrin glue from commercial pooled plasma. These agents can be applied directly to wounds that display diffuse microvascular bleeding or can be used to seal vascular grafts. Fibrin glue is derived from a source of fibrinogen and factor XIII (fibrin-stabilizing factor), whereby a solution of fibrinogen is mixed with a solution of bovine thrombin and applied to a surgical field.[199] It is important to note that preparations derived from cryoprecipitate, commercial pooled plasma, or single donor plasma[199, 200] represent additional allogeneic blood donor exposure. Alternatively, the source of fibrinogen and factor XIII can be derived from as little as 40 mL of the patient's autologous blood[201] or prepared from an autologous plasma unit.[202] Potential recipients of clinical applications of this intervention include patients undergoing reoperative cardiac surgery,[202, 203] vascular surgery,[204] thoracic surgery,[205] renal surgery,[206] pancreatic injuries/resections,[207] and otologic surgery[208] and patients with a preoperative coagulation disorder undergoing hepatic or splenic procedures.[209] On the basis of data from animal studies, fibrin glue may also be beneficial with regard to tracheal repair,[210] common bile duct anastomosis,[211] and splenic trauma.[212]

The potential use of this product has been reviewed.[213] Patients should be made aware of the potential complications as well as the potential benefits of its use. There has been one case report of an anaphylactic reaction after a total of only 8 mL of fibrin glue administration and one case of HIV transmission.[214, 215] The use of autologous donation as a source of fibrinogen would be the safest, and therefore the preferable, approach. A solvent-detergent treated fibrin glue preparation appears promising.[216] Reports of cardiac surgery patients who presented with acquired bovine thrombin–induced factor V deficiency, each of whom had been previously exposed to bovine thrombin,[217, 218] causes concern over the potential toxic effects associated with the use of both allogeneic and autologous fibrin sealants. Issues of informed consent to administration of these blood products and criteria for utilization review need to be addressed.

Platelet gel consists of platelet-rich plasma that is mixed with a solution of bovine thrombin and applied to a surgical field. Platelet-rich plasma is provided during the intraoperative period from patients through the use of designated pheresis instruments or combined-function cell salvage systems. Preliminary evaluations of its use have been reported.[219, 220] Several other topical hemostatic agents such as hemostatic swabs (calcium alginate),[221] vasoconstricting agents such as oxymetazoline,[222] absorbable collagen,[223] topical thrombin,[224, 225] and topical oxidized cellulose and porcine collagen also enhance hemostasis.[226] Absorbable collagen and vasoconstricting agents have been shown to be effective in otorhinolaryngological procedures, whereas use of calcium alginate swabs has been shown to reduce blood loss with general surgical procedures.[221] A comparison between fibrin glue and collagen powder administered in patients undergoing elective hepatic resection demonstrated a slight advantage of fibrin glue.[227] Fibrin glue was also shown in dogs to reduce perioperative hematoma formation related to sealed vascular grafts in comparison with oxidized regenerated cellulose.[228] In addition, in comparison with oxidized cellulose and microfibrillar or positively charged collagen, fibrin glue was more effective in controlling hemostasis within renal lesions in rats.[229] In summary, no study has been able to show reduction in allogeneic donor exposure with the use of these products; without these data, these agents cannot be considered true pharmacological alternatives.

PHARMACOLOGICAL PRESERVATION OF THE HEMOSTATIC SYSTEM DURING EXTRACORPOREAL CIRCULATION

Heparin Anticoagulation/Reversal Management Strategies

Anticoagulation is used during cardiac surgery to prevent overt thrombosis of the extracorporeal circuit and to minimize excessive CPB-related activation of the hemostatic system. Unfractionated heparin is routinely used because it is immediately reversible with protamine, is generally well-tolerated, and is relatively inexpensive. Clinical benefits of optimal administration of heparin and protamine during CPB have been examined. Patient-specific therapy guided by a point-of-care hemostasis system was prospectively compared to empirical activated clotting time (ACT)–based management in 48 adult patients undergoing primary cardiac surgical procedures.[230] Patient-specific management resulted in more heparin administration and 50% less protamine. These patients exhibited 50% less chest tube drainage and received 80% fewer transfusions in the first 24 postoperative hours than did control patients.

Inadequate anticoagulation during CPB results in activation of the hemostatic system.[231] ACT-based anticoagulation protocols can contribute to a hemostatic consumptive state related to underheparinization, particularly in patients requiring prolonged use of CPB, because ACT values are prolonged by other factors such as hemodilution and hypothermia.[232] Because generation of fibrinopeptide A (FPA)[233, 234] and inhibition of clot-bound thrombin[235] have been shown to be related inversely to heparin concentration, maintenance of heparin concentrations that more effectively inactivate thrombin can preserve hemostasis during prolonged CPB, as confirmed in several studies. In a trial, the impact of heparin and protamine administration, as directed by patient-specific requirements using a point of care, whole blood hemostasis system, on bleeding and blood transfusion was compared to an empirical ACT-based dosing protocol.[236] In this prospective, randomized trial, patients in the intervention cohort received 25% larger total doses of heparin and had lower ratios of protamine to heparin (25%) than did control patients. Patients in the control cohort received more platelets, fresh-frozen plasma, and cryoprecipitate; had 10% longer operative post-CPB closure times; and had 15% greater mediastinal chest tube drainage in the first 4 hours after surgery. Another study involving 31 patients requiring repeat or combined cardiac procedures (i.e., coronary revascularization plus valve repair/replacement) at particularly high risk for excessive bleeding[237] confirmed that maintenance of higher heparin concentrations through patient-specific management preserved consumable antithrombin III and factors I, V, and VIII in comparison to a control cohort. This effect was accompanied by suppression of thrombin (65% reduction in FPA levels) and fibrinolytic (i.e., 50% reduction in D-dimers) activity. Another study also demonstrated that higher heparin doses can suppress thrombin (i.e., lower thrombin-antithrombin III complexes) and fibrinolytic activity (i.e., lower D-dimers) in patients undergoing deep hypothermic arrest.[238] Higher heparin concentrations during CPB have also been shown to preserve platelet function during prolonged CPB, as demonstrated by shorter bleeding times[237] or lower platelet factor 4 (PF4) and β thromboglobulin (BTG) levels.[238]

Agents That Preserve or Enhance Platelet Function

Data from several studies indicate that platelet function can be preserved during CPB with nonspecific platelet inhibitors such as aspirin[239]/dipyridamole,[240–242] Iloprost,[243–246*] or prostaglandin E_1 (PGE_1).[247] Infusion of the antiplatelet agent dipyridamole has been reported to reduce platelet activation and depletion during extracorporeal circulation with cardiac surgery. In a prospective randomized trial of oral and intravenous dipyridamole compared with placebo, significant reductions in postoperative blood loss and transfusion requirements were reported.[239] Prostacyclin (PGI2) was reported to have a platelet-sparing effect during CPB,[244] presumably by inhibition of platelet aggregation[245]; however, another study failed to confirm any platelet-sparing effect of prostacyclin during CPB.[248]

Antifibrinolytic and Serine Protease Inhibitors

Antifibrinolytic Agents

Two antifibrinolytic agents that are currently approved for commercial use include ε-aminocaproic acid (EACA) and tranexamic acid.[249] EACA and tranexamic acid are synthetic inhibitors of fibrinolysis.[250] These agents adhere to the lysine binding sites of plasminogen and plasmin and therefore inhibit the conversion of plasminogen to plasmin and interfere with plasmin's ability to cleave fibrinogen and fibrin. Because antifibrinolytic agents are contraindicated in patients with disseminated intravascular coagulation, their use in the setting of activation of the coagulation system with extracorporeal circulation is of concern. Previous studies have demonstrated comparable rates of perioperative stroke and myocardial infarction between patients treated with antifibrinolytic agents and placebo-treated patients. Although there is currently no evidence that these agents induce a hypercoagulable state, the risk profiles should be further evaluated because perioperative thrombotic events have a multifactorial etiology and low incidence. EACA was initially shown to reduce bleeding and transfusion requirements when hyperfibrinolysis was demonstrated in patients with excessive postperfusion bleeding.[251] More recent studies have also demonstrated that this agent is also effective in reducing bleeding and allogeneic blood transfusions when administered prophylactically during extracorporeal circulation.[252, 253]

Tranexamic acid is the trans-isomer of 4-(aminomethy)-cyclohexanecarboxylic acid and has been shown to have the major inhibitory potency of the two isomers. Although tranexamic acid has a similar mechanism of action as

*Withdrawn in 1996.

EACA, this antifibrinolytic agent is approximately 7 to 10 times as potent. Initial studies have shown that tranexamic acid decreases blood loss and transfusion requirements in comparison placebo in matched patients.[254–258] However, a later retrospective study indicated a weaker effect on blood loss and transfusion when a consistent blood conservation protocol was applied.[259]

Serine Protease Inhibitors

There are several important serine proteases or protease enzymes, such as plasmin, trypsin, thrombin, kallikrein, and elastase, that regulate the hemostatic and inflammatory systems and are inhibited by a variety of endogenous inhibitors (e.g., antithrombin III, α_2-macroglobulin, α_1-antitrypsin, and heparin cofactor II). Aprotinin is an inhibitor of human trypsin, plasmin, and kallikrein that substantially reduces bleeding and blood product utilization in patients undergoing cardiac surgery.[260, 261] In addition, aprotinin has been shown to reduce blood loss in patients receiving aspirin preoperatively,[262, 263] in combination with autotransfusion,[264] or in patients requiring use of cardiac assist devices.[265] At low concentrations (50 kIU/mL), aprotinin is similar to EACA and tranexamic acid in that it inhibits plasmin generation, resulting in reduced fibrinolysis.[249] In contrast to these two antifibrinolytic agents, aprotinin at higher concentrations (200 kIU/mL) also has significant anti-inflammatory properties (e.g., kallikrein and complement inhibition[266]) and may protect von Willebrand factor, platelet glycoprotein Ib,[267] IIb/IIIa receptors,[260] and factors Va/VIIIa[268] from proteolytic degradation. Although aprotinin has some anticoagulant properties,[269, 270] aprotinin can also increase circulating procoagulants by reducing proteolysis[271] and potentially enhance coagulation through plasmin inhibition,[266] reduced heparin-mediated platelet inhibition,[146] decreased heparin anticoagulant effect resulting from heparin-aprotinin binding,[272] and protein C inhibition in patients with[268] or without[268, 273] factor V Leiden. These effects may potentially alter hemostasis toward increased fibrin deposition and thromboembolic complications.

Although there have been a few isolated reports of clot formation on pulmonary artery catheters,[274] of thromboembolic complications,[275–278] and of decreased graft patency[276, 279] another study involving deep hypothermic arrest[280] and several placebo-controlled, blinded prospective trials have not demonstrated an increased incidence of thrombotic complications[281, 282] or reduced graft patency.[281, 283] In addition, a reduced stroke rate has been reported[282, 284] in aprotinin-treated patients.

Because the few isolated reports of thromboembolic complications were initially described in cardiac patients whose heparin administration was based on celite ACT protocols,[275, 276, 279] several investigators have assessed the impact of aprotinin on coagulation assays.[285–293] Of interest is that in three multicenter evaluations, the incidence of thrombotic complications was not increased in aprotinin-treated patients in whom heparin administration was based on either whole blood heparin measurements or a fixed-dose regimen.[281–283]

Cardiovascular collapse after aprotinin administration has been described in four patients.[294–297] An anaphylactic reaction was clearly evident in only one of these patients,[297] whereas the other patients may have had hypotension related to rapid administration of aprotinin, which can cause vasodilation.[266] Nevertheless, true anaphylactic reactions can occur with an estimated incidence of 2.5% in patients who are reexposed to aprotinin.[298]

New synthetic agents such as gabexate (FOY) and nafamostat (Futhan) have been used to attenuate bleeding associated with plasmapheresis,[299, 300] hemodialysis,[301–303] or cardiac assist devices.[304–306] An additional evaluation demonstrated that gabexate mesylate can reduce blood loss after cardiac surgery involving extracorporeal circulation.[307]

Comparative Efficacy of Antifibrinolytic Agents and Aprotinin

The impact of aprotinin on blood conservation after cardiac surgery has been illustrated in large trials performed in both Europe[260, 261] and the United States.[281, 282, 308] Although EACA may be as effective as aprotinin in reducing perioperative blood loss,[309] results from several comparisons suggest that aprotinin has a greater impact on blood conservation.[310–312] These observations were illustrated in a large-scale study that demonstrated that aprotinin is more effective than EACA at reducing blood loss and the need for transfusion.[312] Although red cell requirements were reduced in patients who received tranexamic acid, greater reductions in blood loss were observed in patients who received aprotinin.[310, 311, 313–315] In one analysis, patients treated with tranexamic acid had reduced blood product requirements and bleeding in comparison with control patients and patients treated with EACA.[256]

Use of Serine Protease Inhibitors in Patients Undergoing Noncardiac Surgical Procedures

The impact of aprotinin on blood conservation has also been investigated in patients undergoing noncardiac surgical procedures such as liver/lung transplantation, orthopedic procedures, and peripheral and aortic reconstruction. Reductions in both blood loss (26% to 68%) and transfusion requirements were observed in three studies involving orthopedic procedures,[316–318] whereas another study did not demonstrate a difference.[319] Patients undergoing liver transplantation are at risk for excessive bleeding and have been previously shown to benefit from EACA when hyperfibrinolysis was demonstrated.[320] Of eight studies that have investigated the use of aprotinin with liver transplantation, five have demonstrated a reduction in blood loss[321] and/or a reduction in transfusion requirements (23% to 70%).[321–325] However, two other studies did not demonstrate a difference.[326, 327] Aprotinin has also been shown to reduce blood loss and transfusion in patients undergoing lung transplantation[328, 329] or vascular procedures involving the aorta or peripheral vasculature.[330, 331]

CURRENT INDICATIONS AND GUIDELINES FOR PHARMACOLOGICAL INTERVENTIONS IN PATIENTS UNDERGOING EXTRACORPOREAL CIRCULATION

Until the exact mechanism and incidence of thrombotic complications with antifibrinolytic agents is discerned, a conservative approach would be to restrict use of these agents to patients at increased risk for bleeding complications and to maintain adequate anticoagulation, especially in patients who undergo procedures involving deep hypothermic circulatory arrest. Further studies are needed to define the role of emerging, patient-specific pharmacological thrombin and platelet inhibitors in the prevention and treatment of excessive blood loss with extracorporeal circulation.

REFERENCES

1. Wallace EL, Churchill WH, Surgenor DM, et al. Collection and transfusion of blood and blood components in the United States, 1992. Transfusion 1995; 35:802.
2. Mintz PD, Nordine RB, Henry JB, Weble R. Expected hemotherapy in elective surgery. N Y State J Med 1976; 76:532.
3. Goodnough LT, Monk TG, Brecher ME. A review of autologous blood procurement in the surgical setting: lessons learned in the last 10 years. Vox Sang 1996; 71:133.
4. National Heart, Lung and Blood Institute Expert Panel. Transfusion alert: Use of autologous blood. Transfusion 1995; 35:703.
5. National Heart, Lung and Blood Institute Autologous Transfusion Symposium Working Group. Autologous transfusion: current trends and research issues. Transfusion 1995; 35:525.
6. Consensus Conference on Autologous Transfusion. Final consensus statement. Transfusion 1996; 36:667.
7. British Committee for Standards in Hematology, Blood Transfusion Task Force. Guidelines for autologous transfusion. Transfus Med 1993; 307.
8. Menitove J (ed): Standards for Blood Banks and Transfusion Services, 18th ed. Bethesda, MD: American Association of Blood Banks, 1997.
9. U.S. Food and Drug Administration. Memorandum: Autologous Blood Collection and Processing Procedures. Rockville, MD: Congressional and Consumer Affairs, February 12, 1990.
10. Goodnough LT, Price TH, Rudnick S. Iron restricted erythropoiesis as a limitation to autologous blood donation in the erythropoietin-stimulated bone marrow. J Lab Clin Med 1991; 118:289.
11. Goodnough LT, Marcus RE. Erythropoiesis in patients stimulated with erythropoetin: the relevance of storage iron. Vox Sang 1998; 75:128.
12. Silvergleid AJ. Safety and effectiveness of predeposit autologous transfusions in preteen and adolescent children. JAMA 1987; 257:3403.
13. Mann M, Sacks HJ, Goldfinger D. Safety of autologous blood donation prior to elective surgery for a variety of potentially high risk patients. Transfusion 1983; 23:229.
14. Popovsky MA, Whitaker B, Arnold NL. Severe outcomes of allogeneic and autologous blood donation: frequency and characterization. Transfusion 1995; 35:734.
15. Schreiber GB, Busch MP, Kleinman SH, Korelitz JJ. The risk of transfusion-transmitted viral infections. N Engl J Med 1996; 334:1685.
16. Sayers MH. Controversies in transfusion medicine. Autologous blood donation in pregnancy. Con Transfusion 1990; 30:172.
17. Renner SW, Howanitz PJ, Bachner P. Preoperative autologous blood donation in 612 hospitals. Arch Pathol Lab Med 1992; 116:613.
18. Goodnough LT, Saha P, Hirschler N, Yomtovian R. Autologous blood donation in non-orthopaedic surgery as a blood conservation strategy. Vox Sang 1992; 63:96.
19. Goodnough LT, Mercuriali F. Compensatory erythropoiesis during autologous blood donation under standard conditions. Transfusion 1998; 38:613.
20. Toy PTCY. When should the first of two autologous donations be made? Transfusion 1994; 34:S54.
21. Kasper SM, Gerlich W, Buzello W. Preoperative red cell production in patients undergoing weekly autologous blood donation. Transfusion 1997; 37:1058.
22. Goodnough LT, Price TH, Rudnick S, Soegiarso RW. Preoperative red blood cell production in patients undergoing aggressive autologous blood phlebotomy with and without erythropoietin therapy. Transfusion 1992; 32:441.
23. Mercuriali F, Zanella A, Barosi G, et al. Use of erythropoietin to increase the volume of autologous blood donated by orthopedic patients. Transfusion 1993; 33:55.
24. Cohen JA, Brecher ME. Preoperative autologous blood donation: benefit or detriment? A mathematical analysis. Transfusion 1995; 35:640.
25. Kanter MH, Van Maanen D, Anders KH, et al. Preoperative autologous blood donation before elective hysterectomy. JAMA 1996; 276:798.
26. Goodnough LT, Vizmeg K, Verbrugge D. The impact of autologous blood procurement practices on allogeneic blood exposure in elective orthopaedic surgery patients. Am J Clin Pathol 1994; 101:354.
27. Goodnough LT, Grishaber JE, Birkmeyer JD, et al. Efficacy and cost-effectiveness of autologous blood predeposit in patients undergoing radical prostatectomy procedures. Urology 1994; 44:226.
28. Etchason J, Petz L, Keeler E, et al. The cost-effectiveness of preoperative autologous blood donations. N Engl J Med 1995; 332:719.
29. Birkmeyer JD, Aubuchon JP, Littenberg B, et al. Cost-effectiveness of preoperative autologous blood donation in coronary artery bypass grafting. Ann Thorac Surg 1994; 57:161.
30. Birkmeyer JD, Goodnough LT, Aubuchon JP, et al. The cost-effectiveness of preoperative autologous blood donation for total hip and knee replacement. Transfusion 1993; 33:544.
31. Messmer K, Kreimeier M, Intagliett A. Present state of intentional hemodilution. Eur Surg Res 1986; 18:254.
32. Brecher ME, Rosenfeld M. Mathematical and computer modeling of acute normovolemic hemodilution. Transfusion 1994; 34:176.
33. Goodnough LT, Grishaber JE, Monk TG, Catalona WJ. Acute preoperative hemodilution in patients undergoing radical prostatectomy: a case study analysis of efficacy. Anesth Analg 1994; 78:932.
34. Goodnough LT, Bravo J, Hsueh Y, et al. Red blood cell volume in autologous and homologous units: implications for risk/benefit assessment for autologous blood "crossover" and directed blood transfusion. Transfusion 1989; 29:821.
35. Weiskopf RB. Mathematical analysis of isovolemic hemodilution indicates that it can decrease the need for allogeneic blood transfusion. Transfusion 1995; 35:37.
36. Monk TG, Goodnough LT, Brecher ME, et al. A prospective, randomized trial of three blood conservation strategies for radical prostatectomy. Anesthesiology, in press.
37. Ness PM, Bourke DL, Walsh PC. A randomized trial of perioperative hemodilution versus transfusion of preoperatively deposited autologous blood in elective surgery. Transfusion 1991; 31:226.
38. Monk TG, Goodnough LT, Birkmeyer JD, et al. Acute normovolemic hemodilution is a cost-effective alternative to preoperative autologous blood donation by patients undergoing radical retropubic prostatectomy. Transfusion 1995; 35:559.
39. Monk TG, Goodnough LT, Brecher ME. Acute normovolemic hemodilution can replace preoperative autologous donation as a method of autologous blood procurement in radical prostatectomy. Anesth Analg 1997; 85:953.
40. Toy PTCY, Menozzi D, Strauss RG, et al. Efficacy of preoperative donation of blood for autologous use in radical prostatectomy. Transfusion 1993; 33:721.
41. Goodnough LT, Shaffron D, Marcus RE. The impact of preoperative autologous blood donation on orthopaedic surgical practice. Vox Sang 1990; 598:65.
42. Goodnough LT, Monk TG, Brecher ME. Acute normovolemic hemodilution in surgery. Hematology 1997; 2:413.
43. American Society of Anesthesiology. Practice guidelines for blood component therapy. Anesthesiology 1996; 84:732.
44. Brecher ME, Monk TG, Goodnough LT. A standardized method for the calculation of blood loss. Transfusion 1997; 37:1070.

45. Andreole GL, Smith DS, Rao G, et al. Early complications of contemporary anatomic radical retropubic prostatectomy. J Urol 1994; 152:1858.
46. Faust RJ. Perioperative indications for red cell transfusion. Has the pendulum swung too far? Mayo Clin Proc 1993; 68:512.
47. Goodnough LT, Monk TG. Evolving concepts in autologous blood procurement. Case reports of perisurgical anemia complicated by myocardial infarction. Am J Med 1996; 101:12A.
48. Sazama K. Reports of 355 transfusion-associated deaths: 1975 through 1985. Transfusion 1990; 30:583.
49. Goodnough LT, Monk TG, Brecher ME. Acute normovolemic hemodilution should replace preoperative autologous blood donation before elective surgery. Transfusion 1998; 38:473.
50. Rottman G, Ness PM. Is acute normovolemic hemodilution a legitimate alternative to allogeneic blood transfusions? Transfusion 1998; 38:477.
51. Williamson KR, Taswell HF. Intraoperative blood salvage: a review. Transfusion 1991; 31:662.
52. Linden JV, Kaplan HS, Murphy MT. Fatal air embolism due to perioperative blood recovery. Anesth Analg 1997; 84:822.
53. Solomon MD, Rutledge ML, Kane LE, Yawn DH. Cost comparison of intraoperative autologous versus homologous transfusion. Transfusion 1988; 28:379.
53. Bell K, Stott K, Sinclair CJ, et al. A controlled trial of intraoperative autologous transfusion in cardiothoracic surgery measuring effect on transfusion requirements and clinical outcome. Transfus Med 1992; 2:295.
54. Bovill DF, Moulton CW, Jackson WS, et al. The efficacy of intraoperative autologous transfusion in major orthopaedic surgery: a regression analysis. Orthopedics 1986; 9:1403.
55. Goodnough LT, Monk TG, Sicard G, et al. Intraoperative salvage in patients undergoing elective abdominal aortic aneurysm repair. An analysis of costs and benefits. J Vasc Surg 1996; 24:213.
56. Ward HB, Smith RA, Candis KP, et al. A prospective, randomized trial of autotransfusion after routine cardiac surgery. Ann Thorac Surg 1993; 56:137.
57. Thurer RL, Lytle BW, Cosgrove DM, Loop FD: Autotransfusion following cardiac operations: a randomized, prospective study. Ann Thorac Surg 1979; 27:500.
58. Roberts SP, Early GL, Brown B, et al. Autotransfusion of unwashed mediastinal shed blood fails to decrease banked blood requirements in patients undergoing aorta coronary bypass surgery. Am J Surg 1991; 162:477.
59. Schaff HV, Hauer JM, Bell WR, et al. Autotransfusion of shed mediastinal blood after cardiac surgery. A prospective study. J Cardiovasc Thorac Surg 1978; 75:632.
60. Eng J, Kay PH, Murday AJ, et al. Post-operative autologous transfusion in cardiac surgery. A prospective, randomized study. Eur J Cardiothorac Surg 1990; 4:595.
61. Semkiw LB, Schurman OJ, Goodman SB, Woolson ST. Postoperative blood salvage using the cell saver after total joint arthroplasty. J Bone Joint Surg (Am) 1989; 71:823.
62. Faris PM, Ritter MA, Keating EM, Valeri CR. Unwashed filtered shed blood collected after knee and hip arthroplasties. J Bone Joint Surg (Am) 1991; 73:1169.
63. Martin JW, Whiteside LA, Milliano MT, Reedy ME. Postoperative blood retrieval and transfusion in cementless total knee arthroplasty. J Arthroplasty 1992; 7:205.
64. Ritter MA, Keating EM, Faris PM. Closed wound drainage in total hip or total knee replacement. J Bone Joint Surg (Am) 1994; 76:35.
65. Erslev AJ. Erythropoietin. N Engl J Med 1991; 324:1339.
66. Goldberg MA, Dunning SP, Bunn HF. Regulation of the erythropoietin gene: evidence that the oxygen sensor is a heme protein. Science 1988; 242:1412.
67. Sawada K, Krantz SB, Kans JS, et al. Purification of human erythroid colony-forming units and demonstration of specific binding of erythropoietin. J Clin Invest 1987; 80:357.
68. D'Andrea AD, Zon LT. Erythropoietin receptor: subunit structure and activation. J Clin Invest 1990; 86:681.
69. Krantz SB. Erythropoietin. Blood 1991; 77:419.
70. Lipton JM, Kudisch M, Nathan DG. Response of three classes of human erythroprogenitors to the absence of erythropoietin in vitro as a measure of maturity. Exp Hematol 1981; 9:1035.
71. Wyllie AH. Apoptosis: cell death in tissue regulation. J Pathol 1987; 153:313.
72. Eaves CJ, Humphries RK, Krystal G, Eaves AC. Erythropoietin action: models, data, and speculation. *In* Stamatoyannopoulos G, Neinhuis AW (eds): Hemoglobins in Development Differentiation. New York: AR Liss, 1981, pp 63.
73. Koury MJ, Bondurant MC. Control of red cell production: the roles of programmed cell death (apoptosis) and erythropoietin. Transfusion 1990; 30:673.
74. Erslev AJ, Caro J. Physiologic and molecular biology of erythropoietin. Med Oncol Tumor Pharmacother 1986; 3:159.
75. Goodnough LT, Price TH, Parvin CA, et al. Erythropoietin response to anemia is not altered by surgery or recombinant human erythropoietin therapy. Br J Haematol 1994; 87:695.
76. Erslev AJ, Caro J, Miller O, Silver R. Plasma erythropoietin in health and disease. Ann Clin Lab Sci 1980; 10:250.
77. Goodnough LT, Monk TG, Andriole GL. Erythropoietin therapy. N Engl J Med 1997; 336:933.
78. Joint Council of the American Red Cross, Council of Community Blood Centers, American Association of Blood Banks. Circular of Information for the Use of Human Blood Components. Washington, DC: U.S. Food and Drug Administration, March 1994.
79. Kickler TS, Spivak JL. Effect of repeated whole blood donations on serum immunoreactive erythropoietin levels in autologous donors. JAMA 1988; 260:65.
80. Goodnough LT, Rudick S, Price TH, et al. Increased collection of autologous blood preoperatively with recombinant human erythropoietin therapy. N Engl J Med 1989; 321:1163.
81. Goodnough LT, Price TH, the EPO Study Group. A phase III trial of recombinant human erythropoietin therapy in non-anemic orthopaedic patients subjected to aggressive autologous blood phlebotomy: dose, response, toxicity, and efficacy. Transfusion 1994; 34:66.
82. Beris P, Mermillod B, Levy G, et al. Recombinant human erythropoietin as adjuvant treatment for autologous blood donation. Vox Sang 1993; 65:212.
83. Biesma DH, Marx JJ, Kraaijenhagen RJ, et al. Lower homologous blood requirement in autologous blood donors after treatment with recombinant human erythropoietin. Lancet 1994; 344:367.
84. Price TH, Goodnough LT, Vogler W, et al. The effect of recombinant erythropoietin administration on the efficacy of autologous blood donation in patients with low hematocrits. Transfusion 1996; 36:29.
85. Canadian Orthopedic Perioperative Erythropoietin Study Group. Effectiveness of perioperative recombinant human erythropoietin in elective hip replacement. Lancet 1993; 341:1227.
86. Faris PM, Ritter MA, Abels RI. The effects of recombinant human erythropoietin on perioperative transfusion requirements in patients undergoing major orthopaedic surgery. J Bone Joint Surg (Am) 1996; 78:62.
87. Sowade O, Warnke H, Scigalla P, et al. Avoidance of allogeneic blood transfusions by treatment with epoetin beta (recombinant human erythropoietin) in patients undergoing open heart surgery. Blood 1997; 89:411.
88. D'Ambra MN, Gray RJ, Hillman R, et al. The effect of recombinant human erythropoietin on transfusion risk in coronary bypass patients. Ann Thorac Surg 1997; 64:1686.
89. Sisk JE, Gianfrancesco FD, Costner JM. Recombinant erythropoietin and Medicare payment. JAMA 1991; 266:247.
90. Doolittle RF. Biotechnology—the enormous cost of success. N Engl J Med 1991; 324:1360.
91. McMahon FG, Vargas R, Ryan M, et al. Pharmacokinetics and effects of recombinant human erythropoietin after intravenous and subcutaneous injections in healthy volunteers. Blood 1990; 76:1718.
92. Goldberg MA, McCutchen JW, Jove M, et al. A safety and efficacy comparison study of two dosing regimens of erythropoietin alpha in patients undergoing major orthopedic surgery. Am J Orthop 1996; 25:544.
93. Winnearls CG, Oliver DO, Pippard MJ, et al. Effects of human erythropoietin derived from recombinant DNA on the anemia of patients maintained by chronic haemodialysis. Lancet 1986; 2:1175.
94. Besarab A, Bocton WK, Browne JK, et al. The effects of normal as compared with low hematocrit values in patients with cardiac disease who are receiving hemodialysis and epoietin. N Engl J Med 1998; 339:584.

95. Goodnough LT, Strasburg D, Riddell J, et al. Has recombinant human erythropoietin therapy minimized red cell transfusions in hemodialysis patients? Clin Nephrol 1994; 41:303.
96. Canadian Erythropoietin Study Group. Association between recombinant human erythropoietin and quality of life and exercise capacity of patients receiving haemodialysis. BMJ 1990; 300:573.
97. Evans RW, Rader B, Manninen DL, Cooperative Multicenter EPO Clinical Trial Group. The quality of life of haemodialysis recipients treated with recombinant human erythropoietin. JAMA 1990; 263:825.
98. Eschbach JW, Egrie JC, Downing MR, et al. Correction of the anemia of end-stage renal disease with recombinant human erythropoietin. N Engl J Med 1987; 316:3.
99. Raine AEG. Hypertension, blood viscosity, and cardiovascular morbidity in renal failure: implications for erythropoietin therapy. Lancet 1988; 1:97.
100. Eschbach JB, Kelley MR, Haley NR, et al. Treatment of the anemia of progressive renal failure with recombinant human erythropoietin. N Engl J Med 1989; 32:158.
101. Lim VS, DeGowin RL, Zavala D, et al. Recombinant human erythropoietin treatment in pre-dialysis patients. Ann Intern Med 1989; 110:108.
102. Cazzola M, Mercuriali F, Brugnara C. Use of recombinant human erythropoietin outside the setting of uremia. Blood 1997; 89:4248.
103. Richman DD, Fischz MA, Grieco MH, et al. The toxicity of azidothymidine (AZT) in the treatment of patients with AIDS and AIDS-related complex. N Engl J Med 1987; 317:192.
104. Spivak JL, Barnes DC, Fuchs E, Quinn TC. Serum immunoreactive erythropoietin in HIV-infected patients. JAMA 1989; 261:3104.
105. Fischl M, Galpin JE, Levine JD, et al. Recombinant human erythropoietin for patients with AIDS treated with zidovudine. N Engl J Med 1990; 322:1488.
106. Baer AN, Dessypris EN, Goldwasser E, Krantz SB. Blunted erythropoietin response to anemia in rheumatoid arthritis. Br J Haematol 1987; 66:559.
107. Hochberg MC, Arnold CM, Hogans BB, Spivak JL. Serum immunoreactive erythropoietin in rheumatoid arthritis: impaired response to anemia. Arthritis Rheum 1988; 31:1318.
108. Pincus T, Olsen NJ, Russell J, et al. Multicenter study of recombinant human erythropoietin in correction of anemia in rheumatoid arthritis. Am J Med 1990; 89:161.
109. Goodnough LT, Marcus RE. The erythropoietic response to erythropoietin therapy in patients with rheumatoid arthritis. J Lab Clin Med 1997; 130:381.
110. Thompson FL, Powers JS, Graber SE, Krantz SB. Use of recombinant human erythropoietin to enhance autologous blood donation in a patient with multiple red cell allo-antibodies and the anemia of chronic disease. Am J Med 1991; 90:398.
111. Miller CB, Jones RJ, Piantadosi S, et al. Decreased erythropoietin response in patients with the anemia of cancer. N Engl J Med 1990; 322:1689.
112. Cascinu S, Fedelia A, Del Ferro E, et al. Recombinant human erythropoietin treatment in cis-platin–associated anemia: a randomized, double-blind trial with placebo. J Clin Oncol 1994; 12:1058.
113. Cazzola M, Messinger D, Battistel V, et al. Recombinant human erythropoietin in the anemia associated with multiple myeloma or non-Hodgkin's lymphoma: dose finding and identification of predictors of response. Blood 1996; 86:4446.
114. Ludwig H, Fritz E, Kotzmann H, et al. Erythropoietin treatment of anemia associated with multiple myeloma. N Engl J Med 1990; 322:1693.
115. Oster W, Hermann F, Gamm H, et al. Erythropoietin for the treatment of anemia of malignancy associated with neoplastic bone marrow infiltration. J Clin Oncol 1990; 8:956.
116. Jacobs A, Janowska-Wieczorek A, Caro J, et al. Circulating erythropoietin in patients with myelodysplastic syndromes. Br J Haematol 1989; 73:36.
117. Stein RS, Abels RI, Krantz SB. Pharmacologic doses of recombinant human erythropoietin in the treatment of myelodysplastic syndromes. Blood 1991; 78:1658.
118. Tamai Y, Takami H, Nakahatara R, et al. Sustained improvement in anemia with low-dose recombinant human erythropoietin therapy in a patient with hypoplastic myelodysplastic syndrome and chromosome abnormalities. Intern Med 1998; 37:320.
119. Yoshida Y. Erythropoietin therapy for aplastic anemia. Intern Med 1998; 37:235.
120. Brown MS, Garcia JF, Phibbs RH, Dallman PR. Decreased response of plasma immunoreactive erythropoietin to "available oxygen" in anemia of prematurity. J Pediatr 1984; 105:793.
121. Shannon KM, Keith JF, Mentzer WC, et al. Recombinant human erythropoietin stimulates erythopoiesis and reduces erythrocyte transfusions in very low birth weight preterm infants. Pediatrics 1995; 95:1.
122. Coleman PH, Stevens AR, Dodge HT, Finch CA. Rate of blood regeneration after blood loss. Arch Intern Med 1953; 92:341.
123. Goodnough LT, Price TH, Parvin CA. The endogenous erythropoietin response and the erythropoietic response to blood loss anemia: the effects of age and gender. J Lab Clin Med 1995; 126:57.
124. Crosby WH. Treatment of hemochromatosis by energetic phlebotomy. One patient's response to getting 55 liters of blood in 11 months. Br J Haematol 1958; 4:82.
125. Finch CA. Erythropoiesis, erythropoietin, and iron. Blood 1982; 60:1241.
126. Goodnough LT, Merkel K. The use of parenteral iron and recombinant human erythropoietin therapy to stimulate erythropoiesis in patients undergoing repair of hip fracture. Int J Hematol 1996; 1:163.
127. Fishbane S, Ungureanu VG, Maesaka JK, et al. The safety of intravenous iron dextran in hemodialysis patients. Am J Kidney Dis 1996; 28:529.
128. Zanen AL, Adriaansen HJ, Von Bommel EFH, et al. Oversaturation of transferrin after intravenous ferric gluconate (Ferrlecit®) in haemodialysis patients. Nephrol Dial Transplant 1996; 11:820.
129. Navarro JF, Teruel JL, Ciano F, et al. Effectiveness of intravenous administration of Fe-gluconate–Na complex to maintain adequate body iron stores in haemodialysis patients. Am J Nephrol 1996; 16:268.
130. Khuri SF, Wolfe JA, Josa M, et al. Hematologic changes during and after cardiopulmonary bypass and their relationship to the bleeding time and nonsurgical blood loss. J Thorac Cardiovasc Surg 1992; 104:94.
131. Despotis GJ, Filos KS, Zoys TN, et al. Factors associated with excessive postoperative blood loss and hemostatic transfusion requirements: a multivariate analysis in cardiac surgical patients. Anesth Analg 1996; 82:13.
132. Woodman RC, Harker LA. Bleeding complications associated with cardiopulmonary bypass [Review]. Blood 1990; 76:1680.
133. Despotis GJ, Santoro SA, Spitznagel E, et al. Prospective evaluation and clinical utility of on-site monitoring of coagulation in patients undergoing cardiac operation. J Thorac Cardiovasc Surg 1994; 107:271.
134. Kalter RD, Saul CM, Wetstein L, et al. Cardiopulmonary bypass: associated hemostatic abnormalities. J Thorac Cardiovasc Surg 1979; 77:427.
135. Despotis GJ, Levy J, Filos K, Gravlee G. Anticoagulation monitoring during cardiac surgery: a survey of current practice and review of current and emerging technologies. Anesthesiology, in press.
136. Heimark RL, Kurachi K, Fujikawa K, Davie EW. Surface activation of blood coagulation, fibrinolysis and kinin formation. Nature 1980; 286:456.
137. Boisclair MD, Lane DA, Philippou H, et al. Mechanisms of thrombin generation during surgery and cardiopulmonary bypass. Blood 1993; 82:3350.
138. de Haan J, Boonstra PW, Monnink SH, et al. Retransfusion of suctioned blood during cardiopulmonary bypass impairs hemostasis. Ann Thorac Surg 1995; 59:901.
139. Holloway DS, Summaria L, Sandesara J, et al. Decreased platelet number and function and increased fibrinolysis contribute to postoperative bleeding in cardiopulmonary bypass patients. Thromb Haemost 1988; 59:62.
140. Yoshihara H, Yamamoto T, Mihara H. Changes in coagulation and fibrinolysis occurring in dogs during hypothermia. Thromb Res 1985; 37:503.
141. Tabuchi N, de Haan J, Boonstra PW, van Oeveren W. Activation of fibrinolysis in the pericardial cavity during cardiopulmonary bypass. J Thorac Cardiovasc Surg 1993; 106:828.
142. Stibbe J, Kluft C, Brommer EJ, et al. Enhanced fibrinolytic activity during cardiopulmonary bypass in open-heart surgery in man is caused by extrinsic (tissue-type) plasminogen activator. Eur J Clin Invest 1984; 14:375.

143. Gram J, Janetzko T, Jespersen J, Bruhn HD. Enhanced effective fibrinolysis following the neutralization of heparin in open heart surgery increases the risk of post-surgical bleeding. Thromb Haemost 1990; 63:241.
144. Hirsh J. Heparin [Review]. N Engl J Med 1991; 324:1565.
145. Khuri SF, Valeri CR, Loscalzo J, et al. Heparin causes platelet dysfunction and induces fibrinolysis before cardiopulmonary bypass. Ann Thorac Surg 1995; 60:1008.
146. John LC, Rees GM, Kovacs IB. Inhibition of platelet function by heparin. An etiologic factor in postbypass hemorrhage. J Thorac Cardiovasc Surg 1993; 105:816.
147. Cobel-Geard RJ, Hassouna HI. Interaction of protamine sulfate with thrombin. Am J Hematol 1983; 14:227.
148. Ereth MH, Klindworth JT, Campbell BA, Sill JC. Protamine attenuates agonist induced platelet signaling/adhesion molecule expression [Abstract]. Anesth Analg 1996; 82:5.
149. Mochizuki T, Olson PJ, Ramsay JG, et al. Does protamine reversal of heparin affect platelet function? [Abstract] Anesth Analg 1997; 84:35.
150. Ammar T, Fisher CF. The effects of heparinase 1 and protamine on platelet reactivity. Anesthesiology 1997; 86:1382.
151. Wachtfogel YT, Kucich U, Greenplate J, et al. Human neutrophil degranulation during extracorporeal circulation. Blood 1987; 69:324.
152. Kestin AS, Valeri CR, Khuri SF, et al. The platelet function defect of cardiopulmonary bypass. Blood 1993; 82:107.
153. Bichet DG, Razi M, Lonergan M, et al. Hemodynamic and coagulation responses to 1-deamino[8-D-arginine] vasopressin in patients with congenital nephrogenic diabetes insipidus. N Engl J Med 1988; 318:881.
154. Sakariassen KS, Cattaneo M, van der Berg A, et al. DDAVP enhances platelet adherence and platelet aggregate growth on human artery subendothelium. Blood 1984; 64:229.
155. Hashemi S, Palmer DS, Aye MT, Ganz PR. Platelet-activating factor secreted by DDAVP-treated monocytes mediates von Willebrand factor release from endothelial cells. J Cell Physiol 1993; 154:496.
156. Cattaneo M, Lombardi R, Bettega D, et al. Shear-induced platelet aggregation is potentiated by desmopressin and inhibited by ticlopidine. Arterioscler Thromb 1993; 13:393.
157. Sloand EM, Alyono D, Klein HG, et al. 1-Deamino-8-D-arginine vasopressin (DDAVP) increases platelet membrane expression of glycoprotein Ib in patients with disorders of platelet function and after cardiopulmonary bypass. Am J Hematol 1994; 46:199.
158. Horstman LL, Valle-Riestra BJ, Jy W, et al. Desmopressin (DDAVP) acts on platelets to generate platelet microparticles and enhanced procoagulant activity. Thromb Res 1995; 79:163.
159. Lattuada A, Varanukulsak P, Castaman GC, Mannucci PM. The response of plasma von Willebrand factor to desmopressin (DDAVP) is related to the platelet levels of von Willebrand factor. Thromb Res 1992; 67:467.
160. Kanwar S, Woodman RC, Poon MC, et al. Desmopressin induces endothelial P-selectin expression and leukocyte rolling in postcapillary venules. Blood 1995; 86:2760.
161. Warkentin TE, Moore JC, Morgan DG. Aortic stenosis and bleeding gastrointestinal angiodysplasia: is acquired von Willebrand's disease the link? Lancet 1992; 340:35.
162. Gill JC, Wilson AD, Endres-Brooks J, Montgomery RR. Loss of the largest von Willebrand factor multimers from the plasma of patients with congenital cardiac defects. Blood 1986; 67:758.
163. King RM, Pluth JR, Giuliani ER. The association of unexplained gastrointestinal bleeding with calcific aortic stenosis. Ann Thorac Surg 1987; 44:514.
164. Cappell MS, Lebwohl O. Cessation of recurrent bleeding from gastrointestinal angiodysplasias after aortic valve replacement. Ann Intern Med 1986; 105:54.
165. Perrin EJ, Ray MJ, Hawson GA. The role of von Willebrand factor in haemostasis and blood loss during and after cardiopulmonary bypass surgery. Blood Coagul Fibrinolysis 1995; 6:650.
166. Weinstein M, Ware JA, Troll J, Salzman E. Changes in von Willebrand factor during cardiac surgery: effect of desmopressin acetate. Blood 1988; 71:1648.
167. Bagge L, Lilienberg G, Nystrom SO, Tyden H. Coagulation, fibrinolysis and bleeding after open-heart surgery. Scand J Thorac Cardiovasc Surg 1986; 20:151.
168. Mannucci PM, Canciani MT, Rota L, Donovan BS. Response of factor VIII/von Willebrand factor to DDAVP in healthy subjects and patients with haemophilia A and von Willebrand's disease. Br J Haematol 1981; 47:283.
169. Naorose-Abidi SM, Bond LR, Chitolie A, Bevan DH. Desmopressin therapy in patients with acquired factor VIII inhibitors. Lancet 1988; 1:366.
170. Mannucci PM, Remuzzi G, Pusineri F, et al. Deamino-8-D-arginine vasopressin shortens the bleeding time in uremia. N Engl J Med 1983; 308:8.
171. Burroughs AK, Matthews K, Qadiri M, et al. Desmopressin and bleeding time in patients with cirrhosis. BMJ 1985; 291:1377.
172. Mannucci PM. Desmopressin: a nontransfusional form of treatment for congenital and acquired bleeding disorders. Blood 1988; 72:1449.
173. Kobrinsky NL, Israels ED, Gerrard JM, et al. Shortening of bleeding time by 1-deamino-8-D-arginine vasopressin in various bleeding disorders. Lancet 1984; 1:1145.
174. D'Alauro FS, Johns RA. Hypotension related to desmopressin administration following cardiopulmonary bypass. Anesthesiology 1988; 69:962.
175. Frankville DD, Harper GB, Lake CL, Johns RA. Hemodynamic consequences of desmopressin administration after cardiopulmonary bypass. Anesthesiology 1991; 74:988.
176. Humphries JE, Siragy H. Significant hyponatremia following DDAVP administration in a healthy adult. Am J Hematol 1993; 44:12.
177. Shepherd LL, Hutchinson RJ, Worden EK, et al. Hyponatremia and seizures after intravenous administration of desmopressin acetate for surgical hemostasis. J Pediatr 1989; 114:470.
178. Weinstein RE, Bona RD, Altman AJ, et al. Severe hyponatremia after repeated intravenous administration of desmopressin. Am J Hematol 1989; 32:258.
179. Bond L, Bevan D. Myocardial infarction in a patient with hemophilia treated with DDAVP. N Engl J Med 1988; 318:121.
180. O'Brien JR, Green PJ, Salmon G, et al. Desmopressin and myocardial infarction. Lancet 1989; 1:664.
181. Mannucci PM, Carlsson S, Harris AS. Desmopressin, surgery and thrombosis. Thromb Haemost 1994; 71:154.
182. Salzman EW, Weinstein MJ, Weintraub RM, et al. Treatment with desmopressin acetate to reduce blood loss after cardiac surgery. A double-blind randomized trial. N Engl J Med 1986; 314:1402.
183. Hackmann T, Gascoyne RD, Naiman SC, et al. A trial of desmopressin (1-deamino-8-D-arginine vasopressin) to reduce blood loss in uncomplicated cardiac surgery. N Engl J Med 1989; 321:1437.
184. Lazenby WD, Russo I, Zadeh BJ, et al. Treatment with desmopressin acetate in routine coronary artery bypass surgery to improve postoperative hemostasis. Circulation 1990; 82:IV413.
185. Ansell J, Klassen V, Lew R, et al. Does desmopressin acetate prophylaxis reduce blood loss after valvular heart operations? A randomized, double-blind study. J Thorac Cardiovasc Surg 1992; 104:117.
186. Casas JI, Zuazu-Jausoro I, Mateo J, et al. Aprotinin versus desmopressin for patients undergoing operations with cardiopulmonary bypass. A double-blind placebo-controlled study. J Thorac Cardiovasc Surg 1995; 110:1107.
187. Temeck BK, Bachenheimer LC, Katz NM, et al. Desmopressin acetate in cardiac surgery: a double-blind, randomized study. South Med J 1994; 87:611.
188. de Prost D, Barbier-Boehm G, Hazebroucq J, et al. Desmopressin has no beneficial effect on excessive postoperative bleeding or blood product requirements associated with cardiopulmonary bypass. Thromb Haemost 1992; 68:106.
189. Hackmann T, Gascoyne RD, Naiman SC, et al. A trial of desmopressin (1-deamino-8-D-arginine vasopressin) to reduce blood loss in uncomplicated cardiac surgery. N Engl J Med 1989; 321:1437.
190. Mongan PD, Hosking MP. The role of desmopressin acetate in patients undergoing coronary artery bypass surgery. A controlled clinical trial with thromboelastographic risk stratification. Anesthesiology 1992; 77:38.
191. Sheridan DP, Card RT, Pinilla JC, et al. Use of desmopressin acetate to reduce blood transfusion requirements during cardiac surgery in patients with acetylsalicylic-acid–induced platelet dysfunction. Can J Surg 1994; 37:33.
192. Cattaneo M, Harris AS, Stromber U, Mannucci PM. The effect of

desmopressin on reducing blood loss in cardiac surgery: a meta-analysis of double-blind, placebo-controlled trials. Thromb Hemostas 1995; 74:1064.
193. Gratz I, Koehler J, Olsen D, et al. The effect of desmopressin acetate on postoperative hemorrhage in patients receiving aspirin therapy before coronary artery bypass operations. J Thorac Cardiovasc Surg 1992; 104:1417.
194. Czer LS, Bateman TM, Gray RJ, et al. Treatment of severe platelet dysfunction and hemorrhage after cardiopulmonary bypass: reduction in blood product usage with desmopressin. J Am Coll Cardiol 1987; 9:1139.
195. Dilthey G, Dietrich W, Spannagl M, Richter JA. Influence of desmopressin acetate on homologous blood requirements in cardiac surgical patients pretreated with aspirin. J Cardiothorac Vasc Anesth 1993; 7:425.
196. Despotis GJ, Levine V, Saleem R, et al. DDAVP reduces blood loss and transfusion in cardiac surgical patients with impaired platelet function identified using a point-of-care test: a double blind, placebo controlled trial [Abstract]. Anesthesiology 1998; 89:A209.
197. Mongan PD, Hosking MP. Desmopressin decreases blood loss and transfusion therapy after high risk CPB procedures [Abstract]. Anesth Analg 1994; 78:292.
198. Kobrinsky NL, Letts RM, Patel LR, et al. 1-Deamino-8-D-arginine vasopressin (desmopressin) decreases operative blood loss in patients having Harrington rod spinal fusion surgery. A randomized, double-blinded, controlled trial. Ann Intern Med 1987; 107:446.
199. Baker JW, Spotnitz WD, Matthew TL, et al. Mediastinal fibrin glue: hemostatic effect and tissue response in calves. Ann Thorac Surg 1989; 47:450.
200. Dresdale A, Bowman FO Jr, Malm JR, et al. Hemostatic effectiveness of fibrin glue derived from single-donor fresh frozen plasma. Ann Thorac Surg 1985; 40:385.
201. Silberstein LE, Williams LJ, Hughlett MA, et al. An autologous fibrinogen-based adhesive for use in otologic surgery. Transfusion 1988; 28:319.
202. Hartman AR, Galanakis DK, Honig MP, et al. Autologous whole plasma fibrin gel. Intraoperative procurement. Arch Surg 1992; 127:357.
203. Rousou J, Levitsky S, Gonzalez-Lavin L, et al. Randomized clinical trial of fibrin sealant in patients undergoing resternotomy or reoperation after cardiac operations. A multicenter study. J Thorac Cardiovasc Surg 1989; 97:194.
204. Glimaker H, Bjorck CG, Hallstensson S, et al. Avoiding blow-out of the aortic stump by reinforcement with fibrin glue. A report of two cases. Eur J Vasc Surg 1993; 7:346.
205. Jessen C, Sharma P. Use of fibrin glue in thoracic surgery. Ann Thorac Surg 1985; 39:521.
206. Kram HB, Ocampo HP, Yamaguchi MP, et al. Fibrin glue in renal and ureteral trauma. Urology 1989; 33:215.
207. Kram HB, Clark SR, Ocampo HP, et al. Fibrin glue sealing of pancreatic injuries, resections, and anastomoses. Am J Surg 1991; 161:479.
208. Moretz WH Jr, Shea JJ Jr, Emmett JR, Shea JJ 3d. A simple autologous fibrinogen glue for otologic surgery. Otolaryngol Head Neck Surg 1986; 95:122.
209. Kram HB, Nathan RC, Stafford FJ, et al. Fibrin glue achieves hemostasis in patients with coagulation disorders. Arch Surg 1989; 124:385.
210. Kram HB, Shoemaker WC, Hino ST, et al. Tracheal repair with fibrin glue. J Thorac Cardiovasc Surg 1985; 90:771.
211. Kram HB, Garces MA, Klein SR, Shoemaker WC. Common bile duct anastomosis using fibrin glue. Arch Surg 1985; 120:1250.
212. Kuzu A, Aydintu S, Karayalcin K, et al. Use of autologous fibrin glue in the treatment of splenic trauma: an experimental study. J R Coll Surg Edinb 1992; 37:162.
213. Gibble JW, Ness PM. Fibrin glue: the perfect operative sealant? Transfusion 1990; 30:741.
214. Milde LN. An anaphylactic reaction to fibrin glue. Anesth Analg 1989; 69:684.
215. Wilson SM, Pell P, Donegan EA. HIV-1 transmission following the use of cryoprecipitated fibrinogen as gel/adhesive [Abstract]. Transfusion 1991; 31:51S.
216. Burnouf-Radosevich M, Burnouf T, Huart JJ. Biochemical and physical properties of a solvent-detergent–treated fibrin glue. Vox Sang 1990; 58:77.
217. Cmolik BL, Spero JA, Magovern GJ, Clark RE. Redo cardiac surgery: late bleeding complications from topical thrombin-induced factor V deficiency. J Thorac Cardiovasc Surg 1993; 105:222.
218. Banninger H, Hardegger T, Tobler A, et al. Fibrin glue in surgery: frequent development of inhibitors of bovine thrombin and human factor V. Br J Haematol 1993; 85:528.
219. Hood AG, Potter PS, Keating RF, et al. New techniques for the rapid perioperative sequestration of autologous blood components and preparation of platelet gel. Proc Am Acad Cardiovasc Perf 1993; 13:191.
220. Tawes RL Jr. Reducing homologous blood use in vascular surgery: the promotion of hemostasis. Semin Vasc Surg 1994; 7:82.
221. Blair SD, Jarvis P, Salmon M, McCollum C. Clinical trial of calcium alginate haemostatic swabs. Br J Surg 1990; 77:568.
222. Riegle EV, Gunter JB, Lusk RP, et al. Comparison of vasoconstrictors for functional endoscopic sinus surgery in children. Laryngoscope 1992; 102:820.
223. Green JG, Durham TM. Application of INSTAT hemostat in the control of gingival hemorrhage in the patient with thrombocytopenia. A case report. Oral Surg Oral Med Oral Pathol 1991; 71:27.
224. Ofodile FA, Sadana MK. The role of topical thrombin in skin grafting. J Natl Med Assoc 1991; 83:416.
225. Decker CJ. An efficient method for the application of Avitene hemostatic agent. Surg Gynecol Obstet 1991; 172:489.
226. Blair SD, Backhouse CM, Harper R, et al. Comparison of absorbable materials for surgical haemostasis. Br J Surg 1988; 75:969.
227. Kohno H, Nagasue N, Chang YC, et al. Comparison of topical hemostatic agents in elective hepatic resection: a clinical prospective randomized trial. World J Surg 1992; 16:966.
228. Kram HB, Nugent P, Reuben BI, Shoemaker WC. Fibrin glue sealing of polytetrafluoroethylene vascular graft anastomoses: comparison with oxidized cellulose. J Vasc Surg 1988; 8:563.
229. Raccuia JS, Simonian G, Dardik M, et al. Comparative efficacy of topical hemostatic agents in a rat kidney model. Am J Surg 1992; 163:234.
230. Jobes DR, Schaffer GW, Aitken GL. Increased accuracy and precision of heparin and protamine dosing reduces blood loss and transfusion in patients undergoing primary cardiac operations. J Thorac Cardiovasc Surg 1995; 110:36.
231. Esposito RA, Culliford AT, Colvin SB, et al. Heparin resistance during cardiopulmonary bypass. The role of heparin pretreatment. J Thorac Cardiovasc Surg 1983; 85:346.
232. Despotis GJ, Summerfield AL, Joist JH, et al. Comparison of activated coagulation time and whole blood heparin measurements with laboratory plasma anti-Xa heparin concentration in patients having cardiac operations. J Thorac Cardiovasc Surg 1994; 108:1076.
233. Gravlee GP, Haddon WS, Rothberger HK, et al. Heparin dosing and monitoring for cardiopulmonary bypass. A comparison of techniques with measurement of subclinical plasma coagulation. J Thorac Cardiovasc Surg 1990; 99:518.
234. Hashimoto K, Yamagishi M, Sasaki T, et al. Heparin and antithrombin III levels during cardiopulmonary bypass: correlation with subclinical plasma coagulation. Ann Thorac Surg 1995; 58:799.
235. Weitz JI, Hudoba M, Massel D, et al. Clot-bound thrombin is protected from inhibition by heparin–antithrombin III but is susceptible to inactivation by antithrombin III–independent inhibitors. J Clin Invest 1990; 86:385.
236. Despotis GJ, Joist JH, Hogue CW, et al. The impact of heparin concentration and activated clotting time monitoring on blood conservation: a prospective, randomized evaluation in patients undergoing cardiac operations. J Thorac Cardiovasc Surg 1995; 110:46.
237. Despotis GJ, Joist JH, Hogue CW, et al. More effective suppression of hemostatic system activation in patients undergoing cardiac surgery by heparin dosing based on heparin blood concentrations rather than ACT. Thromb Haemost 1996; 76:902.
238. Okita YO, Takamoto S, Ando M, et al. Coagulation and fibrinolysis system in aortic surgery under deep hypothermic circulatory arrest with aprotinin: the importance of adequate heparinization. Circulation 1997; 96:376.
239. Teoh KH, Christakis GT, Weisel RD, et al. Blood conservation with membrane oxygenators and dipyridamole. Ann Thorac Surg 1987; 44:40.

240. Smith JP, Walls JT, Muscato MS, et al. Extracorporeal circulation in a patient with heparin-induced thrombocytopenia. Anesthesiology 1985; 62:363.
241. Makhoul RG, McCann RL, Austin EH, et al. Management of patients with heparin-associated thrombocytopenia and thrombosis requiring cardiac surgery. Ann Thorac Surg 1987; 43:617.
242. Long RW. Management of patients with heparin-induced thrombocytopenia requiring cardiopulmonary bypass [Letter]. J Thorac Cardiovasc Surg 1985; 89:950.
243. Addonizio VP, Fisher CA, Bowen JC, et al. Prostacyclin in lieu of anticoagulation with heparin for extracorporeal circulation. ASAIO J 1981; 27:304.
244. Fish KJ, Sarnquist FH, van Steennis C, et al. A prospective, randomized study of the effects of prostacyclin on platelets and blood loss during coronary bypass operations. J Thorac Cardiovasc Surg 1986; 91:436.
245. Szczeklik A, Gryglewski RJ, Nizankowski R, et al. Circulatory and anti-platelet effects of intravenous prostacyclin in healthy men. Pharmacol Res Commun 1978; 10:545.
246. Addonizio VP Jr, Fisher CA, Kappa JR, Ellison N. Prevention of heparin-induced thrombocytopenia during open heart surgery with iloprost (ZK36374). Surgery 1987; 102:796.
247. Shorten G, Comunale ME, Johnson RG. Management of cardiopulmonary bypass in a patient with heparin-induced thrombocytopenia using prostaglandin E_1 and aspirin. J Cardiothorac Vasc Anesth 1994; 8:556.
248. DiSesa VJ, Huval W, Lelcuk S, et al. Disadvantages of prostacyclin infusion during cardiopulmonary bypass: a double-blind study of 50 patients having coronary revascularization. Ann Thorac Surg 1984; 38:514.
249. Horrow JC. Desmopressin and antifibrinolytics [Review]. Int Anesthesiol Clin 1990; 28:230.
250. Verstraete M. Clinical application of inhibitors of fibrinolysis [Review]. Drugs 1985; 29:236.
251. Lambert CJ, Marengo-Rowe AJ, Leveson JE, et al. The treatment of postperfusion bleeding using epsilon-aminocaproic acid, cryoprecipitate, fresh-frozen plasma, and protamine sulfate. Ann Thorac Surg 1979; 28:440.
252. DelRossi AJ, Cernaianu AC, Botros S, et al. Prophylactic treatment of postperfusion bleeding using EACA. Chest 1989; 96:27.
253. Vander Salm TJ, Ansell JE, Okike ON, et al. The role of epsilon-aminocaproic acid in reducing bleeding after cardiac operation: a double-blind randomized study. J Thorac Cardiovasc Surg 1988; 95:538.
254. Horrow JC, Van Riper DF, Strong MD, et al. Hemostatic effects of tranexamic acid and desmopressin during cardiac surgery. Circulation 1991; 84:2063.
255. Horrow JC, Hlavacek J, Strong MD, et al. Prophylactic tranexamic acid decreases bleeding after cardiac operations. J Thorac Cardiovasc Surg 1990; 99:70.
256. Karski JM, Teasdale SJ, Norman PH, et al. Prevention of postbypass bleeding with tranexamic acid and epsilon-aminocaproic acid. J Cardiothorac Vasc Anesth 1993; 7:431.
257. Nakashima A, Matsuzaki K, Fukumura F, et al. Tranexamic acid reduces blood loss after cardiopulmonary bypass. ASAIO J 1993; 39:M185.
258. Karski JM, Teasdale SJ, Norman P, et al. Prevention of bleeding after cardiopulmonary bypass with high-dose tranexamic acid. Double-blind, randomized clinical trial. J Thorac Cardiovasc Surg 1995; 110:835.
259. Ovrum E, Am Holen E, Abdelnoor M, et al. Tranexamic acid (Cyklokapron) is not necessary to reduce blood loss after coronary artery bypass operations. J Thorac Cardiovasc Surg 1993; 105:78.
260. Royston D. High-dose aprotinin therapy: a review of the first five years' experience [Review]. J Cardiothorac Vasc Anesth 1992; 6:76.
261. Bidstrup BP, Harrison J, Royston D, et al. Aprotinin therapy in cardiac operations: a report on use in 41 cardiac centers in the United Kingdom. Ann Thorac Surg 1993; 55:971.
262. Murkin JM, Lux J, Shannon NA, et al. Aprotinin significantly decreases bleeding and transfusion requirements in patients receiving aspirin and undergoing cardiac operations. J Thorac Cardiovasc Surg 1994; 107:554.
263. Tabuchi N, Huet RC, Sturk A, Eijsman L, Wildevuur CR. Aprotinin preserves hemostasis in aspirin-treated patients undergoing cardiopulmonary bypass. Ann Thorac Surg 1994; 58:1036.
264. Schonberger JP, Bredee J, Speekenbrink RG, et al. Autotransfusion of shed blood contributes additionally to blood saving in patients receiving aprotinin (2 million kIU). Eur J Cardiothorac Surg 1993; 7:474.
265. Goldstein DJ, Seldomridge JA, Chen JM, et al. Use of aprotinin in LVAD recipients reduces blood loss, blood use, and perioperative mortality. Ann Thorac Surg 1995; 59:1063.
266. Fritz H, Wunderer G. Biochemistry and applications of aprotinin, the kallikrein inhibitor from bovine organs. Arzneimittelforschung 1983; 33:479.
267. van Oeveren W, Harder MP, Roozendaal KJ, et al. Aprotinin protects platelets against the initial effect of cardiopulmonary bypass. J Thorac Cardiovasc Surg 1990; 99:788.
268. Sweeney JD, Blair AJ, Dupuis MP, et al. Aprotinin, cardiac surgery, and factor V Leiden. Transfusion 1997; 37:1173.
269. Dietrich W, Spannagl M, Blumel G, Richter JA. Aprotinin inhibits coagulation during cardiopulmonary bypass in man [Abstract]. Anesthesiology 1992; 77:A154.
270. Royston D. Intraoperative coronary thrombosis: can aprotinin be incriminated? [Editorial]. J Cardiothorac Vasc Anesth 1994; 8:137.
271. Havel MP, Griesmacher A, Weigel G, et al. Aprotinin decreases release of 6-keto-prostaglandin F_1 alpha and increases release of thromboxane B_2 in cultured human umbilical vein endothelial cells. J Thorac Cardiovasc Surg 1992; 104:654.
272. Kiernan JA, Stoddart RW. Fluorescent-labelled aprotinin: a new reagent for the histochemical detection of acid mucosubstances. Histochemie 1973; 34:77.
273. Espana F, Estelles A, Griffin JH, et al. Aprotinin (Trasylol) is a competitive inhibitor of activated protein C. Thromb Res 1989; 56:751.
274. Bohrer H, Fleischer F, Lang J, Vahl C. Early formation of thrombi on pulmonary artery catheters in cardiac surgical patients receiving high-dose aprotinin. J Cardiothorac Anesth 1990; 4:222.
275. Sundt TM, Kouchoukos NT, Saffitz JE, et al. Renal dysfunction and intravascular coagulation with aprotinin and hypothermic circulatory arrest. Ann Thorac Surg 1993; 55:1418.
276. Cosgrove DM, Heric B, Lytle BW, et al. Aprotinin therapy for reoperative myocardial revascularization: a placebo-controlled study. Ann Thorac Surg 1992; 54:1031.
277. Alvarez JM, Goldstein J, Mezzatesta J, et al. Fatal intraoperative pulmonary thrombosis after graft replacement of an aneurysm of the arch and descending aorta in association with deep hypothermic circulatory arrest and aprotinin therapy. J Thorac Cardiovasc Surg 1998; 115:723.
278. Westaby S, Forni A, Dunning J, et al. Aprotinin and bleeding in profoundly hypothermic perfusion. Eur J Cardiothorac Surg 1994; 8:82.
279. Laub GW, Riebman JB, Chen C, et al. The impact of aprotinin on coronary artery bypass graft patency. Chest 1994; 106:1370.
280. Goldstein DJ, DeRosa CM, Mongero LB, et al. Safety and efficacy of aprotinin under conditions of deep hypothermia and circulatory arrest. J Thorac Cardiovasc Surg 1995; 110:1615.
281. Lemmer JH, Jr., Stanford W, Bonney SL, et al. Aprotinin for coronary bypass operations: efficacy, safety, and influence on early saphenous vein graft patency. A multicenter, randomized, double-blind, placebo-controlled study. J Thorac Cardiovasc Surg 1994; 107:543.
282. Levy JH, Pifarre R, Schaff HV, et al. A multicenter, double-blind, placebo-controlled trial of aprotinin for reducing blood loss and the requirement for donor-blood transfusion in patients undergoing repeat coronary artery bypass grafting. Circulation 1995; 92:2236.
283. Bidstrup BP, Underwood SR, Sapsford RN, Streets EM. Effect of aprotinin (Trasylol) on aorta-coronary bypass graft patency. J Thorac Cardiovasc Surg 1993; 105:147.
284. Levy JH, Ramsay JG, Murkin JM. Aprotinin reduces the incidence of stroke following cardiac surgery [Abstract]. Circulation 1996; 94:I-535.
285. Wendel HP, Heller W, Gallimore MJ, et al. The prolonged activated clotting time (ACT) with aprotinin depends on the type of activator used for measurement. Blood Coag Fibrinol 1993; 4:41.
286. Wang JS, Lin CY, Hung WT, et al. In vitro effects of aprotinin on activated clotting time measured with different activators. J Thorac Cardiovasc Surg 1992; 104:1135.
287. Wang JS, Lin CY, Hung WT, Karp RB. Monitoring of heparin-

induced anticoagulation with kaolin-activated clotting time in cardiac surgical patients treated with aprotinin. Anesthesiology 1992; 77:1080.
288. Huyzen RJ, Harder MP, Huet RC, et al. Alternative perioperative anticoagulation monitoring during cardiopulmonary bypass in aprotinin-treated patients. J Cardiothorac Vasc Anesth 1994; 8:153.
289. Hunt BJ, Segal HC, Yacoub M. Guidelines for monitoring heparin by the activated clotting time when aprotinin is used during cardiopulmonary bypass [Letter]. J Thorac Cardiovasc Surg 1992; 104:211.
290. Goodnough LT. Need for aprotinin use notification. J Thorac Cardiovasc Surg 1993; 56:1004.
291. Westaby S. Aprotinin in perspective [Review]. Ann Thorac Surg 1993; 55:1033.
292. Aprotinin Package Insert. West Haven, CT: Bayer, Inc., 1995.
293. Despotis GJ, Joist JH, Joiner-Maier D, et al. Effect of aprotinin on activated clotting time, whole blood and plasma heparin measurements. Ann Thorac Surg 1995; 59:106.
294. Schulze K, Graeter T, Schaps D, Hausen B. Severe anaphylactic shock due to repeated application of aprotinin in patients following intrathoracic aortic replacement. Eur J Cardiothorac Surg 1993; 7:495.
295. Dewachter P, Mouton C, Masson C, et al. Anaphylactic reaction to aprotinin during cardiac surgery [Letter]. Anaesthesia 1993; 48:1110.
296. Diefenbach C, Abel M, Limpers B, et al. Fatal anaphylactic shock after aprotinin reexposure in cardiac surgery. Anesth Analg 1995; 80:830.
297. Ceriana P, Maurelli M, Locatelli A, et al. Anaphylactic reaction to aprotinin [Letter]. J Cardiothorac Vasc Anesth 1995; 9:477.
298. Dietrich W, Spath P, Ebell A, Richter JA. Prevalence of anaphylactic reactions to aprotinin: analysis of two hundred forty-eight reexposures to aprotinin in heart operations. J Thorac Cardiovasc Surg 1997; 113:194.
299. Hosokawa S, Oyamaguchi A, Yoshida O. Clinical evaluation of nafamstat mesilate (FUT 175). A new anticoagulant for plasmapheresis. ASAIO J 1992; 38:59.
300. Kinugasa E, Akizawa T, Nakashima Y, et al. Nafamostat as anticoagulant for membrane plasmapheresis in high bleeding risk patients. Int J Artif Organs 1992; 15:595.
301. Taenaka N, Shimada Y, Hirata T, et al. New approach to regional anticoagulation in hemodialysis using gabexate mesilate (FOY). Crit Care Med 1982; 10:773.
302. Taenaka N, Terada N, Takahashi H, et al. Hemodialysis using gabexate mesilate (FOY) in patients with a high bleeding risk. Crit Care Med 1986; 14:481.
303. Matsuo T, Kario K, Nakao K, et al. Anticoagulation with nafamostat mesilate, a synthetic protease inhibitor, in hemodialysis patients with a bleeding risk. Haemostasis 1993; 23:135.
304. Okamoto T, Chung YK, Choi H, et al. Experimental results using nafamostat mesilate as anticoagulant during extracorporeal lung assist for 24 hours in dogs. Artif Organs 1993; 17:30.
305. Takahama T, Kanai F, Hiraishi M, et al. Application of a prostacyclin analogue (PG) and protease inhibitor (FUT) as anticoagulants with an LVAD system. ASAIO J 1986; 32:253.
306. Takahama T, Kanai F, Hiraishi M, et al. Comparative study of anticoagulation therapy with an LVAD system. ASAIO J 1987; 33:227.
307. Murase M, Usui A, Tomita Y, et al. Nafamostat mesilate reduces blood loss during open heart surgery. Circulation 1993; 88:II432.
308. Lemmer JH, Dilling EW, Morton JR, et al. Aprotinin for primary coronary artery bypass grafting: a multicenter trial of three dose regimens. Ann Thorac Surg 1996; 62:1659.
309. Trinh-Duc P, Wintrebert P, Boulfroy D, et al. Comparison of the effects of epsilon-aminocaproic acid and aprotinin on intra- and postoperative bleeding in heart surgery. Ann Chir 1992; 46:677.
310. de Peppo AP, Pierri MD, Scafuri A, et al. Intraoperative antifibrinolysis and blood-saving techniques in cardiac surgery. Tex Heart Inst J 1995; 22:231.
311. Menichetti A, Tritapepe L, Ruvolo G, et al. Changes in coagulation patterns, blood loss and blood use after cardiopulmonary bypass: aprotinin vs tranexamic acid vs epsilon aminocaproic acid. J Cardiovasc Surg 1996; 37:401.
312. Bennett-Guerrero E, Sorohan JG, Gurevich ML, et al. Cost-benefit and efficacy of aprotinin compared with epsilon-aminocaproic acid in patients having repeated cardiac operations: a randomized, blinded clinical trial. Anesthesiology 1997; 87:1373.
313. Blauhut B, Harringer W, Bettelheim P, et al. Comparison of the effects of aprotinin and tranexamic acid on blood loss and related variables after cardiopulmonary bypass. J Thorac Cardiovasc Surg 1994; 108:1083.
314. Speekenbrink RG, Vonk AB, Wildevuur CR, Eijsman L. Hemostatic efficacy of dipyridamole, tranexamic acid, and aprotinin in coronary bypass grafting. Ann Thorac Surg 1995; 59:438.
315. Pugh SC, Wielogorski AK. A comparison of the effects of tranexamic acid and low-dose aprotinin on blood loss and homologous blood usage in patients undergoing cardiac surgery. J Cardiothorac Vasc Anesth 1995; 9:240.
316. Capdevila X, Calvet Y, Biboulet P, et al. Aprotinin decreases blood loss and homologous transfusions in patients undergoing major orthopedic surgery. Anesthesiology 1998; 88:50.
317. Janssens M, Joris J, David JL, et al. High-dose aprotinin reduces blood loss in patients undergoing total hip replacement surgery. Anesthesiology 1994; 80:23.
318. Murkin JM, Shannon NA, Bourne RB, et al. Aprotinin decreases blood loss in patients undergoing revision or bilateral total hip arthroplasty. Anesth Analg 1995; 80:343.
319. Hayes A, Murphy DB, McCarroll M. The efficacy of single-dose aprotinin 2 million kIU in reducing blood loss and its impact on the incidence of deep venous thrombosis in patients undergoing total hip replacement surgery. J Clin Anesth 1996; 8:357.
320. Kang Y, Lewis JH, Navalgund A, et al. Epsilon-aminocaproic acid for treatment of fibrinolysis during liver transplantation. Anesthesiology 1987; 66:766.
321. Mallett SV, Cox D, Burroughs AK, Rolles K. The intra-operative use of Trasylol (aprotinin) in liver transplantation. Transpl Int 1991; 4:227.
322. Bechstein WO, Riess H, Blumhardt G, et al. Aprotinin in orthotopic liver transplantation. Semin Thromb Hemost 1993; 19:262.
323. Grosse H, Lobbes W, Frambach M, et al. The use of high dose aprotinin in liver transplantation: the influence on fibrinolysis and blood loss. Thromb Res 1991; 63:287.
324. Himmelreich G, Muser M, Neuhaus P, et al. Different aprotinin applications influencing hemostatic changes in orthotopic liver transplantation. Transplantation 1992; 53:132.
325. Patrassi GM, Viero M, Sartori MT, et al. Aprotinin efficacy on intraoperative bleeding and transfusion requirements in orthotopic liver transplantation. Transfusion 1994; 34:507.
326. Groh J, Welte M, Azad SC, et al. Does aprotinin affect blood loss in liver transplantation? [Letter]. Lancet 1992; 340:173.
327. Kratzer MA, Azad SC, Groh J, et al. [The effects of aprotinin. Blood loss and coagulation parameters in orthotopic liver transplantation: a clinical-experimental, prospective and randomized double-blind study.] Anaesthetist 1997; 46:294.
328. Jaquiss RD, Huddleston CB, Spray TL. Use of aprotinin in pediatric lung transplantation. J Heart Lung Transplant 1995; 14:302.
329. Kesten S, de Hoyas A, Chaparro C, et al. Aprotinin reduces blood loss in lung transplant recipients. Ann Thorac Surg 1995; 59:877.
330. Thompson JF, Roath OS, Francis JL, et al. Aprotinin in peripheral vascular surgery [Letter]. Lancet 1990; 335:911.
331. Ranaboldo CJ, Thompson JF, Davies JN, et al. Prospective randomized placebo-controlled trial of aprotinin for elective aortic reconstruction. Br J Surg 1997; 84:1110.

CHAPTER 41

Red Cell Substitutes

Robert M. Winslow

THE NEED FOR O_2 CARRIERS

The idea of a red cell substitute is not new. In Ovid's *Metamorphoses*, the witch Medea restored Jason's aged father, Æeson, by slitting his throat to let out old blood and replacing it with a magic brew she had concocted.[1] Sir Christopher Wren was one of the first to apply William Harvey's theories about the circulation to blood substitutes. In 1656 he infused ale, wine, scammony (a gummy exudate of the plant *Convolvulus scammonia*, a folk-medicine cathartic), and opium into dogs and conceived the idea of transfusing blood from one animal to another, as had been suggested to him by the story of Medea and Jason. However, Wren apparently did no more than suggest the possibility of transfusions to his colleague Richard Lower, who actually carried out the experiments.[2] Wren spent the rest of his long life working in the fields of astronomy and architecture rather than medicine, and he never returned to transfusions or red cell substitutes.

In the 20th century, efforts intensified to find a safe and effective alternative to blood for transfusion. Most of these efforts were spurred by the military, because of the need for blood services in both world wars. Attempts were made during World War II to use cell-free hemoglobin on an experimental basis, without success. In 1966, the dramatic demonstration by Clark and Gollan[3] that animals could breathe liquid perfluorocarbons stimulated a renewed search for artificial oxygen carriers. Experiments continued in an effort to design hemoglobin solutions that would have a prolonged vascular retention, but the growth of blood banks and the availability of donated blood reduced the priority for such products. This changed dramatically in the early 1980s when it was discovered that human immunodeficiency virus (HIV) could be transmitted by blood transfusions.[4]

Unfortunately, the HIV epidemic claimed the lives of many recipients of blood products before rigorous testing was introduced in 1985 by American and western European blood banks. In the wake of that tragedy, new products emerged that could be used as alternatives to blood and other blood-derived plasma expanders such as albumin and starches.[5] Ideally, such transfusion substitutes would carry oxygen, provide rapid expansion of blood volume after hemorrhage, not require typing and crossmatching, and be available for immediate use.

Efforts to develop red cell substitutes were spurred by increased investment by the U.S. military in 1985. The military was concerned about contamination of its blood supply for battlefield use and about the perceived need for a resuscitation solution that could be used immediately after wounding, did not require special storage conditions, and could potentially solve the enormous logistical problems of inventory rotation and supply from U.S. collection centers. Research in military and contract-supported laboratories in the period 1985–1995 led military leaders to conclude that the products currently under development would likely not meet military requirements, and efforts were scaled back significantly.[6]

Nevertheless, a decade of research led to at least nine products that are in various stages of civilian clinical development, and it is likely that some of them may be available for clinicians and patients by the end of the 1990s (Table 41–1). These oxygen carriers represent an exciting new class of therapeutics with the possibility of transporting oxygen to hypoxic tissues in patients with circulatory or metabolic problems and serving in emergencies when blood is not available. Furthermore, they offer the promise that huge populations of the world for whom blood services are not available may have access to surgical procedures that have been dependent on transfused blood. These include transplantation procedures and surgeries that require heart-lung bypass.

Many of the current products can fulfill the essential functions of transfused blood: they can provide expansion of the plasma space and transport oxygen. Their development has been slow, however, and they are not yet available in hospitals and emergency rooms because of the discovery of unexpected properties of cell-free oxygen carriers. These include the side effects of hypertension and gastrointestinal irritability and some unexpected oxygen supply mechanisms. These discoveries have slowed clinical development and required new regulatory procedures, but they have also led to a new understanding of fundamental oxygen physiology that will surely result in new and improved products in the future with applications beyond red cell substitutes.

PRODUCTS

Three general classes of products have been under development, based on hemoglobin, perfluorocarbon emulsions, and liposome-encapsulated hemoglobin. Liposomes are perhaps most like native red blood cells, but the cost and complexity of manufacture have slowed clinical development. Because no liposome-hemoglobin products are currently in human clinical trials, they are not discussed here. Instead, the reader is referred to an excellent

Table 41–1. Transfusion Substitute Products in Clinical Trials (1998)

Product (Manufacturer)	Composition	Indications	Clinical Trial Phase
PHP (Apex Bioscience)	Pyridoxilated human hb conjugated to polyoxyethylene	Septic shock	I/II
PEG-hemoglobin (Enzon)	Bovine hb conjugated to polyethyleneglycol	Radiosensitization of solid tumors	Ib
PolyHeme (Northfield Laboratories)	Glutaraldehyde-polymerized, pyridoxilated human hb	Trauma, surgery	III
Hemopure (Biopure)	Glutaraldehyde-polymerized bovine hb	Hemodilution, sickle cell disease	II
Hemolink (Hemosol)	*o*-Raffinose-polymerized human hb	Trauma, hemodilution	II
HemAssist (Baxter)	Human hb internally cross-linked with bis (3,5-dibromosalicyl) fumarate	Trauma, hemodilution	III
Optro (Somatogen)	Recombinant dialpha human hb	Hemodilution, erythropoiesis	II
Oxygent (Alliance Pharmaceutical)	Emulsified perflubron	Hemodilution, cardiopulmonary bypass	II
Oxyfluor (HemaGen/PFC)	Emulsified perfluorodichlorooctane	Cardiopulmonary bypass	I

hb, hemoglobin.

review on the subject.[7] A detailed description of the specific chemical modifications of various products is beyond the scope of this chapter, and the reader is referred to an overview for details.[5] Representative products that are in clinical trials are listed in Table 41–1.

Hemoglobin-Based Products

Hemoglobin is the natural oxygen carrier of the red blood cell. It is a complex protein made up of four subunit polypeptide chains, two α and two β. One α and one β combine to form a stable αβ dimer, and two dimers are more loosely associated to form the complete hemoglobin tetramer. Each subunit contains a single iron-containing heme group that ultimately binds and releases oxygen. When hemoglobin molecules are contained within red cells, they are protected from metabolic breakdown, and their lifetime is that of the red blood cell, 120 days. When hemoglobin is free in the plasma, it rapidly dissociates to αβ dimers, which are oxidized and subsequently cleared by the kidney. If the plasma concentration is high, kidney toxicity results, as seen, for example, in "crush" injury. Cell-free hemoglobin exerts oncotic pressure in addition to other plasma proteins, and its oxygen affinity is different from that inside the red cell. To circumvent these characteristics, cell-free hemoglobin must be chemically modified to prevent its breakdown in the plasma if it is to be useful as an oxygen carrier (Table 41–2). These modifications accounted for the bulk of the research on red cell substitutes in the 1970s and 1980s, and many useful biochemical strategies have emerged. The general classes into which hemoglobin modifications fall and some representative properties are given in Table 41–2 and Figure 41–1.

Surface-Modified Hemoglobin

Surface-modified hemoglobins are conjugates of hemoglobin and larger molecules, such as dextran or polyethyleneglycol (PEG). The primary reason to modify hemoglobin in this way is to prolong its vascular retention. One such product is human hemoglobin modified first with pyridoxal phosphate to lower its oxygen affinity and then with polyoxyethylene (POE).[8] The derivative has the working name pyridoxilated hemoglobin polyoxyethylene (PHP). Preclinical studies with PHP showed a favorable safety profile, and phase I clinical trials began in 1992. Clinical development has been based on the product's propensity to bind nitric oxide (NO) and has targeted PHP as an agent to raise blood pressure in patients with septic shock. Another product, PEG-hemoglobin, manufactured from bovine hemoglobin, is similar to the human-based PHP, with some differences in the details of the conjugation chemistry.[9] Hemoglobin has also been

Table 41–2. Classes of Hemoglobin-Based Transfusion Substitutes

Class	Examples*	Intravascular Persistence (Hours)	Oncotic Pressure	Viscosity	Vasoactivity
Cross-linked hemoglobin tetramers	HemAssist, Optro	~12	Low	Low	Marked
Polymerized hemoglobin tetramers	Hemopure, Hemolink, PolyHeme	~12–14	Low	Low	Moderate
Surface-modified hemoglobin tetramers	PHP, PEG-Hemoglobin	~24–48	Moderate-high	Moderate-high	Mild

*See Table 41–1.
PEG, polyethyleneglycol; PHP, pyridoxilated hemoglobin polyoxyethylene.

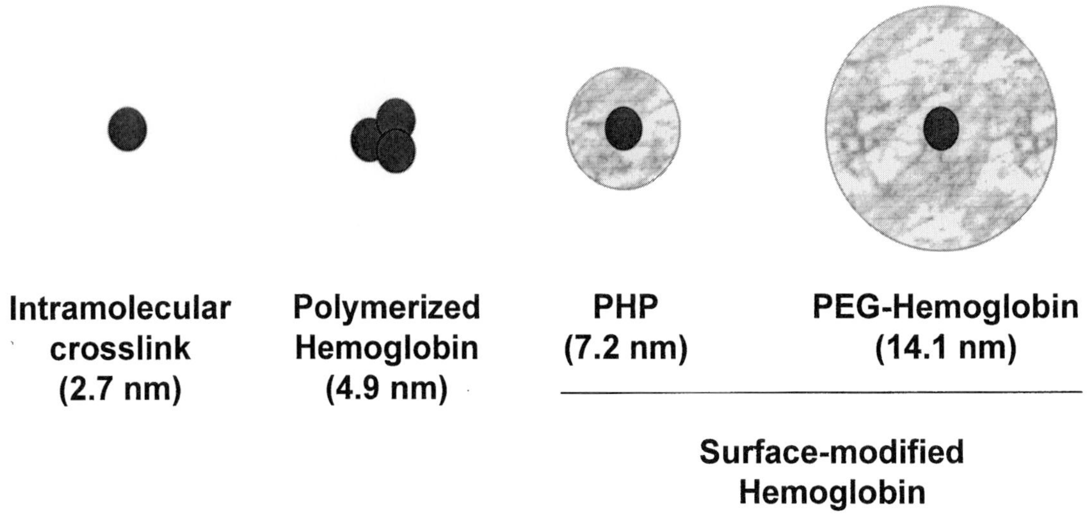

Figure 41–1. Relative sizes of various modified hemoglobins. Intramolecular cross-link products are the same size as native hemoglobin tetramers. Polymerized products have an average of approximately three hemoglobin tetramers per polymer. Surface-modified products are larger because the polyethyleneglycol (PEG) groups attached to their surfaces immobilize a "cloud" of water that increases the effective molecular radius, even though the molecular weight is not increased in proportion to the size of the molecule. The radii of the molecules were calculated from their solution properties.[59] PHP, pyridoxilated hemoglobin polyoxyethylene.

conjugated to dextrans[10, 11] and other polymers in an effort to prolong its intravascular retention.

Conjugation of hemoglobin effectively increases its molecular size and surface characteristics, resulting in a slow rate of removal from the circulation, reduced antigenicity, and reduced "visibility" to the reticuloendothelial system. Unique features of conjugated hemoglobins are their high oncotic pressure and viscosity (see Table 41–2). The former means that they are potent plasma volume expanders. The latter may be important in maintaining microvascular blood flow.[12] Conjugated hemoglobins have longer plasma retention times compared with other modified hemoglobins (Fig. 41–2).

Intramolecular Cross-Linked Hemoglobin

Intramolecular cross-linked hemoglobins are not significantly increased in molecular weight but have specific chemical cross-links between polypeptide chains that prevent dissociation to dimers or monomers. An example is human hemoglobin cross-linked between the chains with bis (3,5-dibromosalicyl) fumarate. The product has been called αα-hemoglobin by the U.S. Army[13] and HemAssist by its manufacturer. The basic chemical reaction is the same for both products.[14] In 1985 the U.S. Army began development of this product as a model compound for research, and the commercial product was subsequently modified by introducing a virus-inactivating heating procedure. This step is possible only because the protein has been stabilized by cross-linking. αα-hemoglobin has been shown to produce significant vasoactivity in animal models of shock and resuscitation.[15] Nevertheless, HemAssist has advanced to phase III clinical trials in the United States and Europe for use in perioperative blood loss and trauma.

A unique product, Optro, is manufactured by means of recombinant technology.[16] Its manufacturer, in collaboration with the Medical Research Council of the United Kingdom, demonstrated that human hemoglobin could be expressed in *Escherichia coli* after the introduction of human genes into that organism.[16] A novel derivative, called "dialpha" hemoglobin, was later expressed in *E. coli*.[17] Dialpha hemoglobin is unique because the two chains are fused, head to tail. The final assembled molecule cannot dissociate into subunits and therefore cannot be cleared rapidly by the kidney. A further mutation has been introduced into dialpha hemoglobin (Presbyterian, β 108(G10) Asn→Lys)[18] to reduce its oxygen affinity,

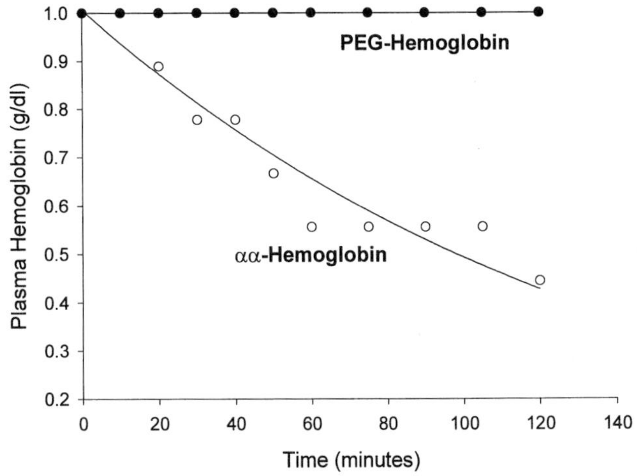

Figure 41–2. Plasma retention of two modified hemoglobins. A 10% (by volume) bolus of product was given to rats, and the plasma hemoglobin concentration was followed for 2 hours. The half-time of disappearance for the αα-hemoglobin is approximately 1 hour in this model, whereas disappearance of the polyethyleneglycol (PEG)–hemoglobin cannot be detected during the observation period (unpublished data).

creating rHb1.1, or Optro. The oxygen-binding curve of Optro is similar to that of normal human blood.

The major obstacles to large-scale production of recombinant hemoglobin were achieving a high yield of product, a high level of gene expression, proper protein folding and assembly, and purification from other *E. coli* products, as well as containing costs to a reasonable level. Impressive advances on these problems have been made, and phase I clinical trials began in 1991. Gastrointestinal side effects were reported in human subjects, complaints that have subsequently been disclosed by many other manufacturers of hemoglobin-based products.[19] This side effect was thought to be due to the well-known propensity of hemoglobin to scavenge NO.[19] Sophisticated nuclear magnetic resonance studies have shown that Optro is capable of delivering oxygen to muscle. Up to 100 g has been administered to patients, with no significant adverse events reported.

Polymerized Hemoglobin

Polymerized hemoglobins are reacted with bifunctional cross-linkers that target surface amino groups and therefore have the propensity to link adjacent molecules, leading to a variety of molecular sizes and configurations. One product based on human hemoglobin obtained from outdated blood, PolyHeme, is the result of polymerization with the cross-linker glutaraldehyde. Much has been published in the open literature about this product,[20] and its development has contributed a substantial amount of information about producing modified hemoglobins and their biochemical and physiological effects. PolyHeme has many properties that are similar to those of human blood, including its oxygen affinity and colloid osmotic pressure.

A similar, product, HemoLink, is a human hemoglobin cross-linked and polymerized with the polyfunctional reagent ring-opened raffinose (*o*-raffinose).[21] This cross-linker also produces hemoglobin polymers of various sizes. Therefore, post-reaction processing is necessary to remove the unreacted hemoglobin molecules and those with relatively low molecular weight (32 and 64 kD). Another polymerized product, Hemopure, is manufactured from purified bovine hemoglobin that is subsequently reacted with glutaraldehyde to form polymers.[22] The reaction mixture is subjected to further fractionation to reduce the amount of unreacted hemoglobin and potentially toxic hemoglobin tetramers (64 kD) and dimers (32 kD). To what extent public concern over transmission of the bovine spongiform encephalitis organism might impact the development of such bovine products is not clear. Preclinical and basic research has shown that this product is able to transport oxygen effectively to tissues and to function as a red cell substitute.[23] However, other studies have shown that even low doses administered to humans raise mean arterial blood pressure and lower cardiac index.[24] One version of this product was approved by the U.S. Food and Drug Administration (FDA) to be marketed for veterinary use.

Perfluorocarbon-Based Products

Perfluorocarbons are chemically synthesized halogenated molecules that are completely inert but dissolve large

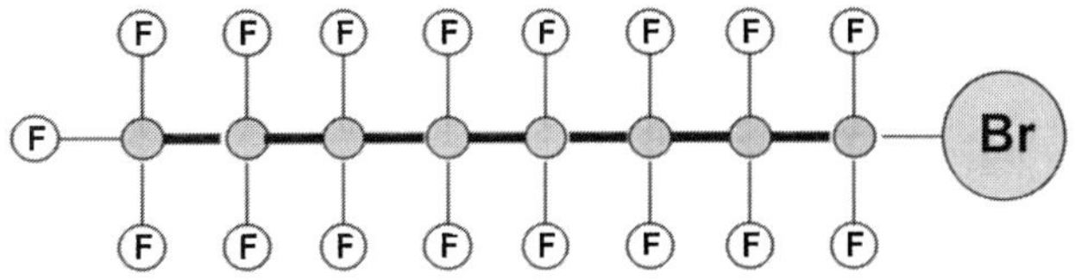

Figure 41–3. Perflubron, an example of a perfluorocarbon. The eight-carbon backbone is fully substituted with fluorine (F) atoms, except for the single bromine (Br). It is the bromine that confers radiopacity.

amounts of gases, including oxygen.[4] An example, perflubron, is shown in Figure 41–3. Under normal arterial conditions, human blood contains only about 0.3 mL/dL of O_2 dissolved in plasma, compared with a total O_2 content of nearly 18 mL/dL. Perfluorocarbons typically can dissolve approximately 50 mL/dL at one atmosphere oxygen partial pressure. This property, plus their nonbiological source and low cost, has made perfluorocarbons attractive as red cell substitutes. They cannot be used directly, however, because they are not miscible with aqueous solutions such as plasma and must be emulsified with lipids before introduction into the blood stream. Recipients of emulsions and particulates such as perfluorocarbons sometimes develop fever and a flulike syndrome that is annoying but not dangerous. Dose-related thrombocytopenia can also be seen after administration, but it is not known whether either of these problems will limit clinical development of perfluorocarbon emulsions.[25]

If a perfluorocarbon emulsion contains 50% (by volume) of the perfluorocarbon, at arterial PO_2 of 100 torr, the maximal capacity for O_2 would be not 50 mL/dL but 6.6 mL/L. If the side effects noted earlier limit the dose that can be administered, the amount of supplemental O_2 carried by the emulsion would be further reduced. As Figure 41–4 shows, red cells are essentially completely saturated at PO_2 of 100 torr, whereas the amount of O_2 that can be carried by a perfluorocarbon emulsion can be

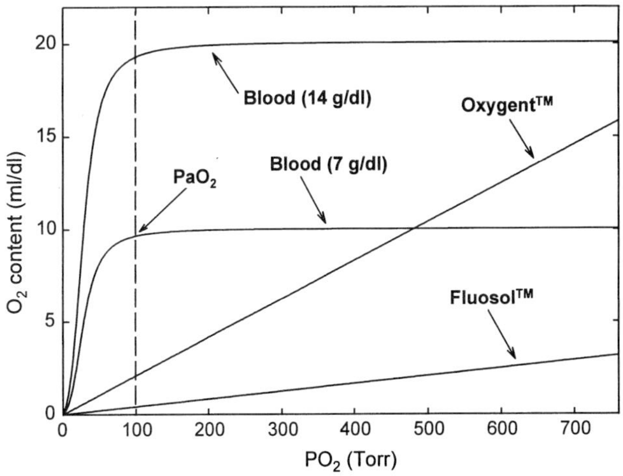

Figure 41–4. Oxygen capacity of Oxygent, Fluosol, and blood. Note that the blood curves are sigmoidal (cooperative), whereas the perfluorocarbon PO_2 is linearly related to the O_2 partial pressure in equilibrium with the emulsion. Oxygent is a 60% (w/v) emulsion.[25]

increased linearly if the arterial Po_2 can be increased. For this reason, perfluorocarbon emulsions may be best exploited in clinical applications in which the inspired Po_2 can be significantly elevated.

A commercial product, Fluosol-DA, was the first (and curently the only) "red cell substitute" product to be approved by the FDA for clinical use. It is composed of perfluorodecalin (14 g/dL) and perfluorotripropylamine (6 g/dL), emulsified with a mixture of the surfactant poloxamer 188 (pluronic F-68), glycerol, egg yolk phospholipids, and oleic acid. The emulsion must be stored frozen and is thawed before use. The maximal dose approved by the FDA is 40 mL/kg of body weight.

A clinical trial of Fluosol-DA was conducted by Gould and colleagues[26] in anemic surgical patients who refused red cell transfusion. Twenty-three patients with hemoglobin levels below 10 g/dL were evaluated, but 15 patients with a mean hemoglobin level of 7.2 g/dL were judged to be hemodynamically compensated and were therefore not treated. The eight patients with a mean hemoglobin of 3 g/dL met the criteria for treatment and were given up to 40 mL/kg of the emulsion. There were no significant hemodynamic or oxygen transport benefits. Fourteen of 15 untreated patients lived, and six of eight treated patients died. The treatment was considered to be ineffective.

The FDA approved Fluosol-DA, however, for adjunctive use during coronary angioplasty. In this application, the fully oxygenated product is pumped through the central lumen of the angioplasty catheter to provide oxygen delivery while the balloon is inflated. Used in this way, small amounts of Fluosol-DA reduce pain,[27] myocardial ischemia, and myocardial dysfunction[28] associated with angioplasty. After a relatively short time on the market, the product was withdrawn by its manufacturer because of poor physician acceptance.

More recent research on perfluorocarbon emulsions has identified materials that permit higher volume fractions of the perfluorocarbon and more stable emulsions. One such product, Oxygent, is a stable emulsion of perflubron (see Fig. 41–3) and egg yolk lecithin.[29] Among perflubron's useful properties are its high solubility for gases such as oxygen and carbon dioxide, high density, radiopacity (a property conferred by the bromine atom), and chemical inertness. This product, in contrast to other red cell substitutes, is relatively inexpensive to manufacture, has a long shelf life, and has an unlimited supply of raw materials. Oxyfluor is a 40% (volume/volume) emulsion of perfluorodichlorooctane stabilized with egg yolk phospholipid and safflower oil.[30] In equilibrium with 100% oxygen, Oxyfluor carries 17.2 volume percent of oxygen, and it has a shelf life of greater than 1 year at room temperature. Preclinical animal studies with Oxyfluor showed efficacy as an oxygen transporter.

CLINICAL APPLICATIONS

Clinical Testing

In the mid-1980s, the need for a blood substitute seemed obvious because of the threat to the blood supply from HIV contamination. In addition, it had been shown many years previously that cell-free hemoglobin and perfluorocarbon emulsions were capable of carrying oxygen. Therefore, demonstration of efficacy was not a concern, and it was assumed that a plasma expander that carries oxygen would be superior to one that does not. These attitudes came into question when it was recognized that cell-free hemoglobin can cause serious renal toxicity and, later, elevated blood pressure. At the same time, the safety of the blood supply was greatly increased by implementation of a number of new measures, including elimination of paid donors and testing for HIV. The FDA, in cooperation with the National Institutes of Health, held two key conferences to address the safety and efficacy of red cell substitutes.[31, 32] These focused attention on the lack of a consensus on the regulatory requirements for new products, and the debate is still not settled.

Table 41–3. Transfusion Substitute Efficacy End Points

Reduced allogeneic blood use
Lowered cost of care
Shortened hospitalization
Reduced symptoms
Fewer complications
Better end-organ function
Better tissue oxygenation

Some of the potential efficacy end points are given in Table 41–3. Most of the end points listed would be difficult to demonstrate for blood transfusions, not to mention red cell substitutes. For example, trials to demonstrate improvement in symptoms, better end-organ function, or better tissue oxygenation for patients who receive red cell substitutes compared with blood would be exceedingly difficult, as well as massive and expensive. Shortened hospitalization and fewer postoperative complications, such as infections or myocardial infarctions, might be quantifiable but would still be difficult to demonstrate. Reduced use of allogeneic blood transfusion is perhaps the most tractable end point and is amenable to quantification in the short term. Lowered cost of medical care is also problematic but important, as managed health care takes a stronger hold on the practice of medicine.

Potential Clinical Applications

Given the problems, the hurdles to development, and the current products, some applications for red cell substitutes seem more viable than others.

Shock and Trauma

The army research program established that αα-hemoglobin produces significant systemic and pulmonary hypertension in some animal species and subsequently abandoned its efforts to develop this product.[6] Among the reasons for this change in direction (besides limited funds) were improved safety of banked blood and the apparent dangers of infusing vasoactive materials into soldiers who might already be volume depleted from dehydration and blood loss.

Clinical trials of PolyHeme in trauma patients began in 1989. According to information from the manufacturer, phase I safety testing of this product was conducted in 21 volunteers and 11 patients. The highest dose administered was 63 g (equal to approximately 1 unit of blood). There was no evidence of kidney toxicity, blood pressure increases or vasoconstriction, fever, liver abnormalities, or other organ system dysfunction in this or subsequent tests. More than 40 trauma patients and emergency surgery patients have been treated with PolyHeme in ongoing trials. To date, 8 patients have received 300 g of hemoglobin (equal to approximately 6 units of blood). Phase III clinical trials began in 1998.

Hemodilution

Perioperative hemodilution[33] is a procedure whereby some volume of the patient's blood is replaced with a diluent before an elective surgical procedure. During surgery, if blood or volume expansion is required, the operating team can choose whether to administer the autologous blood or more of the diluent. The goal of the procedure is to reduce the use of allogeneic blood.

After a successful phase I clinical trial of HemoLink in Canada in 1995 and further refinement of the manufacturing process, the product has returned to clinical trials and is being developed first for hemodilution, then for trauma and emergency indications. Optro was tested in a multicenter trial of intraoperative surgical blood loss, in which doses ranged from 25 to 100 g. No differences were observed between treated patients and controls in acute effects, long-term follow-up, or adverse events, except for transient rises in lipase and amylase levels in the patients who received Optro. In a second trial, 10 patients underwent acute normovolemic hemodilution with Optro before surgery, with doses ranging from 12.5 to 50 g. Again, no adverse events were reported. Oxygent has also been used in trials of acute normovolemic hemodilution. Side effects so far have included mild thrombocytopenia and a transient flulike syndrome caused by release of certain cytokines.[25] Whether the recommended use of relatively small amounts of Oxygent will impact the conservation of blood hoped for by the manufacturer remains to be seen. The product is currently in phase II clinical trials.

Cardiopulmonary Bypass

Oxyfluor is being investigated as an agent to absorb microemboli in patients during cardiopulmonary bypass.[34] It has been known for some time that bypass patients suffer neurological and neuropsychological impairment after bypass and that the severity of the damage is proportional to the time the patient is on bypass.[30] It was shown by retinal angiography that microemboli occur after bypass and that these microemboli could be prevented by pretreatment with Oxyfluor. This effect was seen at very low doses in dogs, which may permit its effective use without significant concern about thrombocytopenia. Although high doses of Oxyfluor do produce thrombocytopenia, the nadir in animal and human studies has been demonstrated to be approximately 4 to 5 days after dosing, whereas the "bypass lesion" in platelets occurs immediately as patients come off the bypass machine.

NO Scavenging

Treatment of septic shock is an intriguing application, because it takes advantage of the ability of cell-free hemoglobin to scavenge NO, which is known to be overproduced in that condition and is presumed to be responsible for vasodilatation and subsequent hypotension. Septic shock has been targeted as the primary application for PHP, after a successful phase I clinical trial in normal volunteers. A U.K. trial of HemAssist in 14 sepsis patients produced a significant vasopressor response in 4 patients who were expected to survive for only 24 hours but subsequently survived for 28 days. Septic shock is an extremely complex clinical entity, but early results with hemoglobin solutions are promising.

Pressure and Perfusion

The manufacturer of HemAssist has focused on the product's ability to raise blood pressure. Sponsored and proprietary research indicated that the mechanism of the vasoactivity was due in part to NO binding but also to upregulation of endothelin and, possibly, adrenergic mechanisms as well.[35] Researchers were able to show improved tissue perfusion in animals in which the shock state had been induced by hemorrhage and that blood pressure could be restored by administration of relatively small amounts of the product. They have also been successful in demonstrating improved reperfusion after cerebral ischemia in animals and therefore have proposed the use of HemAssist immediately after vaso-occlusive strokes.

Erythropoiesis

The FDA has approved clinical trials of Optro in patients with end-stage renal disease and in patients with refractory anemia. The latter is in conjunction with exogenous erythropoietin, which appears to act synergistically with Optro in stimulating erythropoiesis. The mechanism of erythropoietin stimulation in this application is still not understood, and it is possible that the cause is actually reduced renal oxygenation resulting from local vasoconstriction.[36] A clinical trial showed that administration of HBOC-201, closely related to Hemopure, produces increases in serum iron, ferritin, and erythropoietin.[22]

Cancer

Some products have been tested as radiosensitizers in patients with solid tumors. This approach is based on the known increased susceptibility of tumor cells to killing by either irradiation or chemotherapy when tissue oxygen levels are raised.[37] PEG-hemoglobin successfully completed phase I safety trials in normal volunteers, and the product has advanced to phase Ib trials in approximately 20 cancer patients with solid tumors receiving radiation therapy. Perfluorocarbons have also been used in trials with animals with solid tumors, and the results have been promising.[25]

LIMITATIONS OF TRANSFUSION SUBSTITUTES

The side effects of the various products are still not completely understood. Chief among these are gastrointestinal complaints and vasoconstriction with hemoglobin products and thrombocytopenia and dose limitation with perfluorocarbon emulsions. As clinical development continues, additional information will become available, such as whether anesthetized patients exhibit the same side effects or whether new ones arise as a result of interactions with anesthetics.

A universal problem among all red cell substitutes is their short duration of action. The plasma residence times for hemoglobin-based products range from approximately 12 hours for cross-linked hemoglobin to about 2 days for PEG-hemoglobin (see Fig. 41–2). These times are very short compared with a mean residence time of 120 days for human red blood cells. The hope, however, is that the new products will be used in clinical situations in which short-term use of banked blood can be eliminated or reduced, such as in surgical bleeding or hemodilution. None of the current products would be optimal in patients with chronic anemia. A longer plasma persistence is one of the attractive features of liposome-encapsulated hemoglobin.

Development of red cell substitutes has also raised new issues with regard to mechanisms of oxygen transport. When an oxygen carrier is present outside of the red blood cell, the diffusion of oxygen to tissues is predicted to be more efficient because of elimination or reduction of the barrier imposed by the low solubility of O_2 in plasma and the fact that red cells are separated by large plasma gaps.[38] At first consideration, this might seem to be an advantage. However, consider that the mammalian circulation is "engineered" around cellular oxygen delivery and has sophisticated mechanisms in place to regulate the amount of oxygen that reaches tissues (autoregulation). These mechanisms have evolved to ensure maximal oxygen delivery in both anemia and hypoxia. Autoregulation is a complex mechanism that increases blood flow locally to tissue to compensate for too little oxygen, but it also limits flow when excess oxygen is sensed. Development of cell-free O_2 carriers has made understanding of this mechanism essential.[39]

The cost of the new products could be a significant impediment to their widespread use. Companies developing them are not yet in a position to project ultimate cost, because manufacturing scale, source of raw materials, and exact procedures are not yet established. However, it appears that the price of blood substitute products will have to be close to that of banked human blood if such products are to be competitive, unless significant advantages over blood can be demonstrated.

In developing countries, the cost issue is complex. First, it is difficult to ascertain the exact costs of current transfusion practices in many countries, because transfusions are usually provided as part of a socialized medical system. Second, transfusions are often provided in "tiers"—that is, blood obtained from family members, private donors, or hospitals could all have different prices (and safety standards). Finally, the most complex issue is what impact safe transfusion practices would have on the overall economy of the health care system. Any definitive analysis must consider the impact not only of caring for post-transfusion complications, such as hepatitis and HIV infection, but also of caring for patients who are denied surgical procedures. For example, what is the relative cost to support a patient who is disabled and cannot work because of degenerative or other joint disease, compared with the cost of joint replacement by elective surgery and returning the patient to work?

Products that use human blood as their source will be limited by availability of outdated units or collection of blood from paid donors. Some of the manufacturing processes lead to overall yields of only 50%, in which case collection will have to exceed production by a factor of two. This could be problematic, because blood donation is often perceived as a charitable act, and donors might be less willing to give if they know that their blood will be used to manufacture a product for profit. If paid donors are used, the risk of contamination will increase. Animal blood will raise concern about the transmission of animal pathogens. For example, although the risk of transmission of the bovine spongiform encephalitis virus may be remote, it is perceived as a great danger, especially in Europe and Canada.[40] Recombinant or encapsulated hemoglobin may be the ultimate hope, but so far, the processes are limited by low yields, high cost, and challenging technical requirements.

VASOACTIVITY AND THE CONTROL OF TISSUE O_2 DELIVERY

Amberson realized as early as 1947 that cell-free hemoglobin solutions were vasoactive.[41] He noted that when his patients received stroma-free hemoglobin, their blood pressure increased. At the time, this was considered to be a positive quality of the solutions, because they were intended to be used in hypotensive shock states. Studies in the isolated, perfused heart showed that this is a phenomenon of the interaction of hemoglobin with the vasculature itself, rather than a more general neurally mediated mechanism.[42, 43] Direct observations have now shown that hemoglobin solutions actually produce a narrowing of arterioles, which may restrict blood flow to the capillaries.[44]

The problem of vasoconstriction is illustrated by a study done by the U.S. Army in an evaluation of hemoglobin solutions for the battlefield.[15, 45] In these studies, pigs were dehydrated to simulate battlefield conditions, then subjected to a controlled hemorrhage. They were resuscitated with hemoglobin solutions, and hemodynamic and oxygen transport measurements were subsequently made. The studies showed that in spite of increased O_2 carrying capacity conferred by the solutions, the rise in blood pressure (Fig. 41–5) and concomitant fall in cardiac output offset any advantage in the administration of these solutions. These studies established a link between vasoconstriction and O_2 transport that has defined the aims of the present generation of hemoglobin-based products. The capacity of local microcirculatory beds to autoregulate their O_2 supply (Fig. 41–6) is well known,[46] but the mechanism is not. Thus, development of a successful red cell substitute requires knowledge of autoregulatory

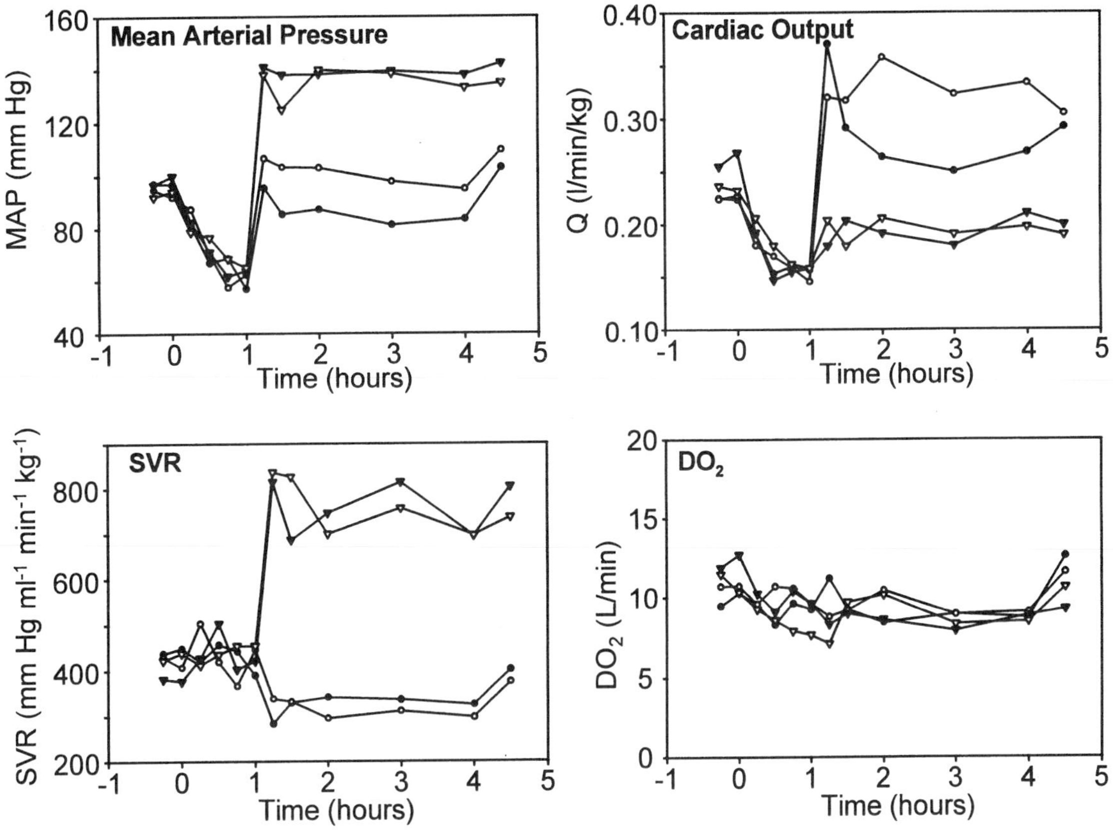

Figure 41–5. Experimental shock resuscitation in swine. The animals were dehydrated before the experiment to simulate battlefield conditions, and hemorrhage was induced over the first hour of the experiment. Resuscitation was carried out with Ringer's lactate *(open circles)*, albumin *(closed circles)*, unmodified hemoglobin *(closed triangles)*, or αα-hemoglobin *(open triangles)*. Note that resuscitation with either hemoglobin solution raised blood pressure to approximately 20 mm Hg higher than baseline, reduced cardiac output, and raised systemic vascular resistance (SVR). The net result was that even though the O_2 capacity was increased in the hemoglobin-treated animals, the O_2 delivery (DO_2) was unchanged.[15, 45]

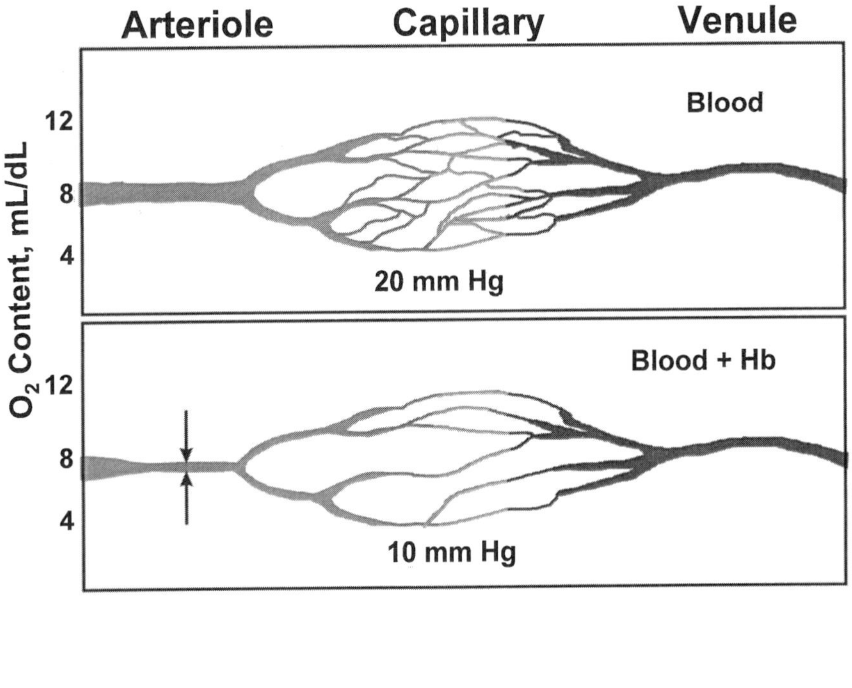

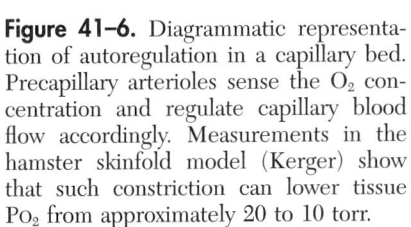

Figure 41–6. Diagrammatic representation of autoregulation in a capillary bed. Precapillary arterioles sense the O_2 concentration and regulate capillary blood flow accordingly. Measurements in the hamster skinfold model (Kerger) show that such constriction can lower tissue Po_2 from approximately 20 to 10 torr.

mechanisms and the design of molecules that do not engage them so that the added O_2 capacity can be effectively used.

At first consideration, facilitated O_2 diffusion might seem to be an advantage.[38, 47] However, the mammalian circulation is "engineered" around cellular oxygen delivery and has sophisticated mechanisms to regulate the amount of oxygen that reaches tissues. These mechanisms imply that the microcirculation can regulate itself locally to maintain O_2 supply to tissues within optimal limits; therefore, regulatory pathways must be in place to sense O_2 supply and match perfusion to the local O_2 requirement. Understanding autoregulation has been advanced by the study of cell-free oxygen carriers.[12] Attempts to show increased O_2 delivery by these products have failed, both for hemoglobin solutions[48, 49] and for perfluorocarbon emulsions,[50] demonstrating the effectiveness of autoregulatory mechanisms.

Two separate views on the role of cell-free hemoglobin in vasoconstriction have emerged. The first builds on early observations in isolated aortic rings that hemoglobin solutions produce constriction by scavenging NO.[51] Assuming this mechanism, research efforts have been undertaken to design hemoglobin molecules with reduced NO binding at the heme sites.[52] A second NO mechanism has been suggested by the discovery that NO can bind reversibly at β93 cysteine of hemoglobin and that this binding is an allosteric effect—that is, NO binding may be linked to O_2 binding in such a way as to be picked up in the lung and unloaded in tissue beds, where it can act as a vasodilator.[53]

The NO affinity of model hemoglobins does not correlate with the effect on mean arterial blood pressure in rats,[54] and it is possible that the autoregulatory mechanism itself is responsible for the vasoconstriction seen with cell-free hemoglobin. That is, oversupply of O_2 due to diffusion of oxyhemoglobin (HbO_2) may be the primary stimulus for the local microcirculation to constrict its flow. Direct experimental evidence for this idea comes from the observation that arterioles, particularly at the A2/A3 level, consume large amounts of O_2,[55] indicating that they are capable of prodigious metabolic activity. Innervation of these arterioles is particularly dense,[56] suggesting that they regulate downstream capillary blood flow. Increasing the O_2 available to these arterioles would be expected to be a potent stimulus to engage autoregulatory mechanisms.

The presence of cell-free hemoglobin predictably engages these mechanisms because of its capacity for facilitated diffusion. HbO_2 free in the plasma space can diffuse freely. Because the solubility of O_2 in plasma is so low, addition of as little as 3 mM HbO_2 (4.8 g/dL plasma hemoglobin) doubles the amount of O_2 present in the plasma at 100 torr O_2 partial pressure. This additional O_2 availability is called facilitated diffusion and is the result of the removal of barriers to diffusion imposed by red cells, their membranes, and the layer of unstirred plasma surrounding them (Fig. 41–7). Similarly, the presence of HbO_2 in plasma makes scavenging NO more efficient and would logically lead to a reduction in local NO concentration, possibly causing vasoconstriction. The exact biochemical mechanisms that underlie these events could

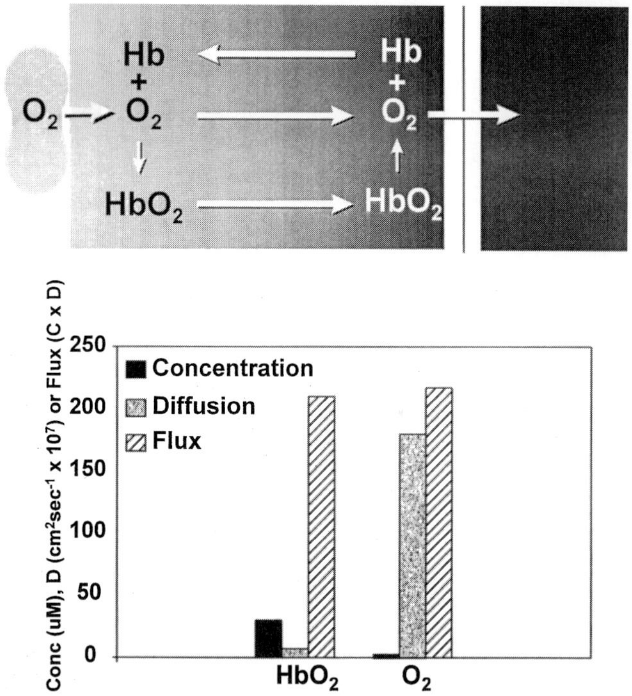

Figure 41–7. Facilitated diffusion. When hemoglobin (Hb) is free in the plasma space, it can diffuse along an oxyhemoglobin (HbO_2) concentration gradient. The solubility of free O_2 in plasma is very low, but its diffusion constant is high. In contrast, the diffusion constant for HbO_2 is relatively low, but addition of as little as 2 g/dL Hb results in a large increase in plasma O_2 concentration, nearly doubling the O_2 available to tissues.

be mediated by pathways that are sensitive to O_2, NO, or both.

Resolution of the mechanism of vasoconstriction produced by cell-free hemoglobin is the central issue in the further development of red cell substitutes. If the primary mechanism is NO binding at heme sites, it is unlikely that cell-free hemoglobin of any type will ever serve as a blood substitute. This is because restriction of NO binding will probably also restrict O_2 binding, given that O_2 and NO are similar in size and in their ability to diffuse into the heme pocket of hemoglobin. If the primary mechanism involves nitrosyl hemoglobin formation, it may be possible to design recombinant hemoglobins that either eliminate this effect or use it to augment local tissue perfusion under appropriate circumstances.[57] If, however, vasoconstriction is a result of normal autoregulatory mechanisms, the correct strategy will be to produce a substitute with reduced facilitated diffusion by increasing the size of the cell-free HbO_2 molecule, increasing the solution viscosity, or altering O_2 affinity so as to reduce O_2 release in precapillary regulatory arterioles (see Fig. 41–6). Whatever the mechanism, unraveling this puzzle will surely lead not only to a better class of O_2 carriers but also to a better understanding of the control of O_2 delivery in the microcirculation.

WORLD HEALTH IMPLICATIONS

Is there a global shortage of blood for transfusion? This question cannot be answered with certainty, but if medical practice were uniform worldwide, and if the U.S. rate of transfusion (0.05 unit per capita per year) were extended to the world's population of 5,863,072,031, a total annual demand for 293 million units of red blood cells could be projected. No firm estimate of the number of units actually transfused is available, but Tomasulo speculated that the number could be as low as 90 million.[58] If this is estimation is accurate, it suggests that the worldwide shortfall is potentially 200 million units per year. Note that this assumes a uniformly sophisticated level of health care, which is certainly not the case presently.

Many of the current products can fulfill the essential functions of transfused blood: they can provide expansion of the plasma space, and they can transport oxygen. Furthermore, development of these products has revealed unexpected properties of cell-free oxygen carriers, such as vasoactivity and autoregulation of oxygen supply.[12] Although these discoveries are exciting, they have slowed clinical development and have necessitated new regulatory procedures. Understanding their physiological effects will surely lead to new and improved products in the future. Whether blood substitutes will be successful in developing countries with serious, and possibly insoluble, problems with blood supply will depend on a number of factors, including local patterns of medical practice and, most importantly, on the willingness and commitment of local governments to improve the state of the public health.

CONCLUSION

Red cell substitutes are a group of oxygen carriers designed to temporarily replace transfused blood. Each product is unique in its limitations and advantages. Research and development has been slow because of the far-reaching consequences of replacing an oxygen carrier outside of the red cell. Nevertheless, a number of products are in advanced clinical trials and nearing the market. When they are available for use, it is likely that development will accelerate and even better products will substantially alleviate the worldwide shortage of blood for transfusion and enable the delivery of medical care to underserved populations. An important consequence of the development of these products has been a better understanding of how oxygen is delivered to tissues.

ACKNOWLEDGMENTS

This work was supported in part by a grant received from the National Institutes of Health, Heart, Lung and Blood Institute (HL48018).

REFERENCES

1. Diamond L. A history of blood transfusion. *In* Wintrobe M (ed): Blood, Pure and Eloquent. New York: McGraw-Hill, 1980, p 659.
2. Hollingsworth M. Blood transfusion by Richard Lower in 1665. Ann Med Hist 1928; 10:213.
3. Clark L, Gollan F. Survival of mammals breathing organic liquids equilibrated with oxygen at atmospheric pressure. Science 1966; 152:1755.
4. Leveton LR, Sox HC Jr, Stoto M. HIV and the Blood Supply: An Analysis of Crisis Decision Making. Washington, DC: National Academy Press, 1995.
5. Winslow R. Hemoglobin-Based Red Cell Substitutes. Baltimore: Johns Hopkins University Press, 1992.
6. Hess J, Riess R. Resuscitation and the limited utility of the present generation of blood substitutes. Transfus Med Rev 1996; 10:276.
7. Rudolph A. Encapsulation of hemoglobin in liposomes. *In* Winslow R, Vandegriff K, Intaglietta M (eds): Blood Substitutes: Physiological Basis of Efficacy. Cambridge: Birkhaüser, 1995.
8. Iwasaki K, Iwashita Y. Preparation and evaluation of hemoglobin-polyethylene glycol conjugate (pyridoxilated polyethylene glycol hemoglobin) as an oxygen-carrying resuscitation fluid. Artif Organs 1986; 10:411.
9. Zalipsky S, Seltzer R, Nho K. Succinimidyl carbonates of polyethylene glycol: useful reactive polymers for preparation of protein conjugates. *In* Dunn RL, Ottenbrite RM (eds): Polymeric Drugs and Drug Delivery Systems. Washington, DC: American Chemical Society, 1991, p 92.
10. Dellacherie E, Bonneaux F, Labrude P, et al. Modification of human hemoglobin by covalent association with soluble dextran. Biochim Biophys Acta 1983; 749:106.
11. Tam S, Blumenstein H, Wong J. Blood replacement in dogs by dextran-hemoglobin. Can J Biochem 1978; 56:981.
12. Intaglietta M, Johnson P, Winslow R. Microvascular and tissue oxygen distribution. Cardiovasc Res 1996; 32:632.
13. Winslow R, Chapman K. Pilot-scale preparation of hemoglobin solutions. *In* Everse J, Vandegriff K, Winslow R (eds): Methods in Enzymology. Hemoglobin, Part B. Biochemical and Analytical Methods, vol 231. San Diego: Academic Press, 1994, p 3.
14. Chatterjee R, Welty E, Walder R, et al. Isolation and characterization of a new hemoglobin derivative crosslinked between chains (lysine 99α_1-lysine 99α_2). J Biol Chem 1986; 261:9929.
15. Hess J, Macdonald V, Brinkley W. Systemic and pulmonary hypertension after resuscitation with cell-free hemoglobin. J Appl Physiol 1993; 74:1769.
16. Hoffman S, Looker D, Roehrich J, et al. Expression of fully functional tetrameric human hemoglobin in *Escherichia coli*. Proc Natl Acad Sci U S A 1990; 87:8521.
17. Looker D, Abbott-Brown D, Cozart P, et al. A human recombinant haemoglobin designed for use as a blood substitute. Nature 1992; 356:258.
18. Kumar R. Recombinant hemoglobins as blood substitutes: a biotechnology perspective. Proc Soc Exp Biol Med 1995; 208:150.
19. Murray J, Ledlow A, Launspach J, et al. The effects of recombinant human hemoglobin on esophageal motor function in humans. Gastroenterology 1995; 109:1241.
20. Gould S, Sehgal L, Sehgal H, et al. The development of hemoglobin solutions as red cell substitutes: hemoglobin solutions. Transfus Sci 1995; 16:5.
21. Hsia J. Pasteurizable, freeze-driable hemoglobin-based blood substitute. United States Patent Number 4,857,636; August 15, 1989.
22. Lee R, Atsumi N, Jacobs E, et al. Ultrapure, stroma-free, polymerized bovine hemoglobin solution: evaluation of renal toxicity. J Surg Res 1989; 47:407.
23. Hughes G, Francom S, Antal E, et al. Hematologic effects of a novel hemoglobin-based oxygen carrier in normal male and female subjects. J Lab Clin Med 1995; 126:441.
24. Kasper S, Walter M, Grune F, et al. Effects of a hemoglobin-based oxygen carrier (HBOC-201) on hemodynamics and oxygen transport in patients undergoing preoperative hemodilution for elective abdominal aortic surgery. Cardiovasc Anesth 1996; 83:921.
25. Flaim S. Perflubron-based emulsion: efficacy as temporary oxygen carrier. *In* Winslow R, Vandegriff K, Intaglietta M (eds): Advances in Blood Substitutes: Industrial Opportunities and Medical Challenges. Cambridge: Birkhaüser, 1997.
26. Gould S, Rosen A, Sehgal L, et al. Polymerized pyridoxilated hemoglobin: efficacy as an oxygen carrier. J Trauma 1986; 26:903.
27. Anderson H, Leimgruber P, Roubin G, et al. Distal coronary artery perfusion during percutaneous transluminal coronary angioplasty. Am Heart J 1985; 110:720.
28. Jaffe C, Wohlgelernter D, Highman H, et al. Oxygenated fluosol

DA-20% distal infusion during coronary angioplasty protects myocardial function. Prog Clin Biol Res 1986; 211:21.
29. Long C, Long D, Riess J, et al. Preparation and application of highly concentrated perfluorooctylbromide fluorocarbon emulsions. Biomat Artif Cells Artif Organs 1988; 16:441.
30. Kaufman R. Clinical development of perfluorocarbon-based red cell substitutes. *In* Winslow R, Vandegriff K, Intaglietta M (eds): Blood Substitutes: Physiological Basis of Efficacy. New York: Birkhaüser, 1995.
31. Center for Biologics Research and Evaluation. Points to consider in the safety and evaluation of hemoglobin-based oxygen carriers. Transfusion 1991; 31:369.
32. Center for Biologics Research and Evaluation. Points to consider on efficacy evaluation of hemoglobin- and perfluorocarbon-based oxygen carriers. Transfusion 1994; 34:712.
33. Stehling L, Zauder H. Acute normovolemic hemodilution. Transfusion 1991; 31:857.
34. Blauth C, Kohner EM, Arnold J, et al. Retinal microembolism during cardiopulmonary bypass demonstrated by fluorescein angiography. Lancet 1986; 11:837.
35. Przybelski R, Daily E, Birnbaum M. The pressor effect of hemoglobin—good or bad? *In* Winslow R, Vandegriff K, Intaglietta M (eds): Advances in Blood Substitutes: Industrial Opportunities and Medical Challenges. Cambridge: Birkhaüser, 1997.
36. Hager S, Gonzales A, Gonzales M, et al. Erythropoietin response to blood substitutes: a model for tissue hypoxia. Blood 1996; 88:184.
37. Suit H. Tumor oxygenation and radiosensitivity. *In* Winslow R, Vandegriff K, Intaglietta M (eds): Blood Substitutes: Physiological Basis of Efficacy. Cambridge: Birkhaüser, 1995.
38. Federspiel W, Popel A. A theoretical analysis of the effect of the particulate nature of blood on oxygen release in capillaries. Microvasc Res 1986; 32:164.
39. Winslow RM, Vandegriff KD. Hemoglobin oxygen affinity and the design of red cell substitutes. *In* Winslow R, Vandegriff K, Intaglietta M (eds): Advances in Blood Substitutes: Industrial Opportunities and Medical Challenges. Boston: Birkhaüser, 1997, p 167.
40. Vaughan P. Creutzfeldt-Jacob disease latest unknown in struggle to restore faith in blood supply. Can Med J 1996; 155:565.
41. Amberson W. Clinical experience with hemoglobin-saline solutions. Science 1947; 106:117.
42. Vogel W, Lieberthal W, Apstein C, et al. Effects of stroma-free hemoglobin solutions on isolated perfused rabbit hearts and isolated perfused rat kidneys. Biomat Artif Cells Artif Organs 1988; 16:227.
43. Macdonald V. Methemoglobin-induced decrease of vascular reactivity to human stroma-free hemoglobin in isolated perfused rabbit hearts. *In* Brewer G (ed): The Red Cell. Seventh Ann Arbor Conference. New York: Alan R. Liss, 1989, p 423.
44. Kerger H, Torres Filho I, Rivas M, et al. Systemic and subcutaneous microvascular oxygen tension in conscious Syrian golden hamsters. Am J Physiol 1995; 268:H802.
45. Hess J, Macdonald V, Murray A, et al. Pulmonary and systemic hypertension after hemoglobin administration. Blood 1991; 78:356A.
46. Johnson P. Brief review: autoregulation of blood flow. Circ Res 1986; 59:483.
47. Homer L, Weathersby P, Kiesow L. Oxygen gradients between red blood cells in the microcirculation. Microvasc Res 1981; 22:308.
48. Hogan M, Kurdak S, Richardson R, et al. Partial substitution of red blood cells with free hemoglobin does not improve maximal O_2 uptake of working in situ dog muscle. Adv Exp Med Biol 1994; 361:375.
49. Biro G, Anderson P, Curtis S, et al. Stroma-free hemoglobin: its presence in plasma does not improve oxygen supply to the resting hindlimb vascular bed of hemodiluted dogs. Can J Physiol Pharmacol 1991; 69:1656.
50. Hogan M, Wilford D, Keipert P, et al. Increased plasma O_2 solubility improves O_2 uptake of in situ dog muscle working maximally. J Appl Physiol 1992; 361:2470.
51. Furchgott R, Martin W, Cherry P. Blockade of endothelium-dependent vasodilation by hemoglobin: a possible factor in vasospasm associated with hemorrhage. Adv Prostaglandin Thromboxane Leukot Res 1985; 15:499.
52. Doherty DH, Doyle MP, Curry SR, et al. Rate of reaction with nitric oxide determines the hypertensive effect of cell-free hemoglobin. Nat Biotech 1998; 16:672.
53. Jia L, Bonaventura J, Stamler J. S-nitrosohaemoglobin: a dynamic activity of blood involved in vascular control. Nature 1996; 380:221.
54. Rohlfs R, Bruner E, Chiu A, et al. Arterial blood pressure responses to cell-free hemoglobin solutions and the reaction with nitric oxide. J Biol Chem 1998; 273:12128.
55. Torres F, Intaglietta M. Microvessel PO_2 measurement by phosphorescence decay method. Am J Physiol 1993; 265:H1434.
56. Saltzman D, DeLano F, Schmid-Schonbein G. The microvasculature in skeletal muscle. VI. Adrenergic innervation of arterioles in normotensive and spontaneously hypertensive rats. Microvasc Res 1992; 44:263.
57. Stamler J, Jia L, Eu J, et al. Blood flow regulation by S-nitrosohemoglobin in the physiological oygen gradient. Science 1997; 276:2034.
58. Tomasulo P. Transfusion alternatives: impact on blood banking worldwide. *In* Winslow R, Vandegriff K, Intaglietta M (eds): Blood Substitutes: Physiological Basis of Efficacy. Cambridge: Birkhaüser, 1995.
59. Vandegriff K, McCarthy M, Rohlfs R, et al. Colloid osmotic properties of modified hemoglobins: chemically cross-linked versus polyethylene glycol surface-conjugated. Biophys Chem 1997; 69:23.

CHAPTER 42

Viral Clearance Methods Applied to Blood Products

Thomas J. Lynch
Joseph C. Fratantoni

In the 1994 edition of this book, this chapter opened with the statement that "blood transfusion is now safer than it has ever been." The same statement can be made today, but the safety of blood components and products has notably and significantly improved since 1994. Significant improvements are expected to be made in the future, and so the level of success achieved by current safety measures has not dampened the effort to develop new technologies and strategies for further reducing the risk associated with the transfusion of blood components (red blood cells, platelets, plasma) or the use of plasma derivatives (albumin, immunoglobulin, coagulation factors).[1, 2]

This chapter presents an overview of the methods of viral clearance that are now either in use or under investigation. The term *viral clearance* is used here in a broad sense to encompass procedures that employ physical and chemical agents designed to disrupt viruses or otherwise render them noninfectious (viral inactivation), as well as processes that separate viruses from blood products (viral removal). A number of excellent reviews of this subject are available.[3–9]

It must be emphasized that viruses do not constitute the only risks associated with the use of blood products or plasma derivatives. Transfusion-associated infections from bacteria or more complex parasites continue to be a significant problem, associated primarily with the transfusion of blood components.[10, 11] In addition, there is considerable concern over the potential risk of transmitting the causative agents of transmissible spongiform encephalopathies, such as Creutzfeldt-Jakob disease, by transfusion or through the use of plasma derivatives.[12–14] However, a comprehensive treatment of these other infectious agents is beyond the scope of this chapter, which is restricted to procedures effective against viruses.

NATURE OF THE RISKS

Bloodborne Viruses

The risks of transmitting disease by transfusion are currently estimated to be approximately 1:500,000 for human immunodeficiency virus (HIV), 1:60,000 for hepatitis B virus (HBV), and 1:100,000 for hepatitis C virus (HCV).[15] The low risks of transmitting these agents by transfusion are the result of donor screening for high-risk behaviors and by medical history, testing of individual donations for evidence of current or prior infections, and deferring individuals thought to be at high risk from future donations. The risks just noted remain after these precautionary measures are taken, primarily because of "window donations," which are made by persons soon after an infection and before the tests performed on the donated unit yield positive results. Much effort is being directed to improving test methods to reduce the window periods associated with these viruses.

Although HBV, HCV, and HIV have been responsible for most clinically significant transmissions of disease for both blood components and plasma derivatives, they are not the only viruses of consequence.[16, 17] For example, human T cell lymphotropic virus (HTLV) types I and II are found only intracellularly and therefore do not pose a serious risk with regard to plasma derivatives. However, HTLV may be transmitted by cellular components, and so whole blood donations (but not source plasma) are tested for antibodies against HTLV. Similarly, cytomegalovirus (CMV) may pose risks to recipients of blood components but is not significant for plasma derivatives.[18] In contrast, hepatitis A virus (HAV) and human parvovirus (HPV) B19 are rarely transmitted by transfusion of components, presumably because the antibodies that are elicited soon after infection are neutralizing in each case.[19, 20] One report of a possible transmission of HPV B19 by an immunoglobulin product suggests that antibodies may not be completely protective in all cases.[21] However, HAV[22–24] and HPV B19[25–30] have been transmitted by plasma derivatives, especially coagulation factors, but no test exists for screening blood or plasma donations for either virus. Finally, there is ongoing concern about viruses and other agents that may emerge in the blood supply in the future. The recognition of agents such as human herpesvirus type 6 (HHV-6)[31] and hepatitis G (HGV)[32, 33] illustrate this potential risk.

HBV, HCV, HIV, and HTLV are all *enveloped viruses;* that is, they include an outer lipid coating analogous to the plasma membrane of a cell. Consequently, these viruses are of rather substantial size (40 to 120 nm in diameter). The presence of the lipid envelope also renders these viruses susceptible to physical or chemical methods that disrupt the envelope and render the virus noninfectious. On the other hand, HAV and HPV B19 lack a lipid coating and are termed *nonenveloped viruses.* Both are small (~20 nm) and are highly resistant to physical and chemical inactivation; hence HAV and HPV

B19 pose particular challenges to the viral clearance methods considered later in this chapter.[34]

In the case of contamination with most viral agents, the infectious particle is suspended in plasma, although virus may be physically adherent to cells. In the special case of retroviruses, such as HIV and HTLV, infectious particles may persist in an intracellular location, and sequences of viral nucleic acid may be incorporated into the host cell genome. Viral inactivation of cellular blood products therefore presents a special challenge, and documenting the efficacy of inactivation requires recognition of this complex biology.[35]

Transfusable Components Versus Plasma Derivatives

The risks of HBV, HCV, and HIV transmission are calculated from studies of volunteer donors of whole blood. Whole blood donations are the source for transfusable components, including plasma, and the plasma derived from these donations ("recovered plasma") is also used to manufacture 20% to 25% of the plasma-derived products used in the United States. The majority of plasma-derived products, however, are manufactured from "source plasma" collected from remunerated donors by plasmapheresis. Comparable risk data are not currently available for source plasma donations.

More important than the risk associated with any given donation is the difference in how donations are used for transfusion and for the manufacture of plasma derivatives. Transfusable blood components are administered as single units (or units pooled from several donations) given one or a few at a time. The recipient of the transfusion is thus exposed to the risk that one or more of the donors of the component was harboring an infectious agent at the time of the donation. The same multiplication of risk applies to manufactured products, but most plasma derivatives are manufactured from pools of plasma that comprise many thousands of donations. Hence, the possibility that a product was manufactured from plasma that included a potentially infectious unit is greatly amplified.[36]

Because of their potentially enhanced risk, the safety of plasma-derived products depends largely on viral clearance methods (inactivation and removal) incorporated into the manufacturing process. Moreover, because the residual risk associated with any single donation (e.g., a window donation) can never be entirely eliminated, there is great interest in extending viral clearance methods to transfusable components.[37]

CLASSIFICATION OF METHODS

Table 42–1 summarizes the various approaches to viral inactivation and elimination now in use or under investigation. The application of these methods to a particular product is not always straightforward because there is a need to balance desirable injury to contaminating viruses against unwanted damage to the blood product. There are also significant differences in how viral clearance methods may be applied to transfusable components and manufactured plasma derivatives. For example, it is unlikely that inactivation methods based on heat or the use of solvent/detergent can be applied to cellular components. Finally, the fact that the cells most often transfused (red cells and platelets) are nonreplicating is of prime importance in the choice of agents directed against nucleic acids.

Table 42–1. Viral Inactivation and Elimination Procedures

Viral Inactivation Methods	
Physical Methods	
Heat	Heating in solution
	Dry heating in final containers
	Vapor heating
	Heating under organic solvent
Radiation	Ionizing
	Ultraviolet
Chemical Agents	
Nucleic acid target	Alkylating agents
Membrane lipid target	Solvent/detergent
Combined	Photosensitizers plus irradiation
	Acidic pH (with or without protease)
	Sodium thiocyanate
Virus Removal Methods	
Specific Methods	
Nanofiltration	Various porosities, materials, and configurations
Purification Steps	
Partitioning	Cold ethanol fractionation
	Other precipitation methods (PEG, cryoprecipitation)
Chromatography	Anion and cation exchange
	Affinity (especially immunoaffinity)

HISTORICAL BACKGROUND

Albumin

Treatment of blood products before transfusion in order to reduce infectivity preceded the development of satisfactory tests for hepatitis. The stabilization of liquid albumin against heat denaturation was initially intended to permit the long-term storage of the product under adverse conditions during World War II. But it was soon recognized that "stabilized" albumin could be heated, thereby reducing the risk of transmitting "serum hepatitis."[38] Heat treatment of albumin has been standard practice since 1948. All albumin products licensed for use in the United States today are heated at 60°C for 10 hours in the presence of chemical stabilizers to prevent denaturation of the protein. Heat treatment of albumin is also performed in the final container; since this practice was mandated, there have been no transmissions of HBV, HCV, or HIV by U.S.-licensed albumin.[39]

Plasma

Heating proved difficult to adapt to whole plasma; early attempts resulted in either protein denaturation when sufficient heat was applied or failure to prevent transmission of hepatitis when less rigorous heating regimens were employed.[40, 41] Similarly, attempts were made to decrease the plasma-associated transmission of hepatitis by ultraviolet (UV) irradiation of the plasma.[42] It was found that the doses required for significant viral inactivation resulted in unacceptable levels of protein denaturation.

Coagulation Factor Concentrates

Coagulation factor concentrates were developed in the 1970s for the treatment of hemophilia A (antihemophilic factor, or factor VIII) and hemophilia B (factor IX). These products offered great improvements in the care of these patients, but because they were manufactured from pools of many units of plasma, the risk of transmitting hepatitis was greatly increased. Because the clinical significance of infection with HBV and HCV (responsible for the majority of what was then known as non-A, non-B hepatitis) was not fully realized at the time, the improved quality of life that the coagulation factor concentrates offered was thought to outweigh the risk of contracting hepatitis.[43] Moreover, there was concern that heat treatment of the coagulation factor concentrates (then the only well-established method of viral clearance) would increase the immunogenicity of the products, rendering the recipients untreatable by conventional means.

This point of view changed abruptly in 1983 when the transmission of acquired immune deficiency syndrome (AIDS) by transfusion and by the use of coagulation factor concentrates was recognized.[44] By early 1984, the major producers of U.S.-licensed factor VIII had approved viral inactivation steps incorporated into their manufacturing processes; all involved heating of the products under various conditions, and the use of heat-treated products was recommended.[45, 46] However, not all the earliest heat-inactivation methods proved sufficiently effective.[47] In 1984, donor screening was also instituted, and in 1985 a serological test for anti-HIV antibodies was introduced. By 1987, all coagulation products licensed in the United States were subjected to "effective" viral inactivation procedures during their manufacture and the transmission of HBV, HCV, and HIV by these products was all but eliminated.[48–50] In contrast, the prevalence of HBV and HCV infection among hemophiliacs before 1984 had reached as high as 90%, and about half had been infected with HIV.[47, 51]

Immunoglobulins

Until the early 1990s, the clinical safety record of immunoglobulin did not indicate a need to incorporate viral inactivation methods into their manufacturing processes.[52, 53] Intramuscular preparations of immunoglobulin (IMIG) manufactured by the conventional cold ethanol procedure have never transmitted HCV or HIV, even before the introduction of screening methods for these viruses. There has been only one instance in which HBV was transmitted by IMIG before the introduction of screening for hepatitis B surface antigen (HBsAg),[54] and there has been none since. (However, there have been reports of HCV transmission by specific immunoglobulins produced by chromatographic methods.[55–57]) Consequently, IMIG was considered a low-risk product with regard to viral infections. Intravenous preparations of immunoglobulin (IVIG) have never transmitted HBV or HIV, but before 1993, there were several isolated reports of HCV transmission by IVIG.[58–62] Nevertheless, IVIG was also considered to be a reasonably safe product even though manufactured without specific viral inactivation procedures.

However, in 1993, there was an outbreak of hepatitis C among recipients of one particular IVIG product after the introduction of the second generation (multiantigen) assays for anti-HCV antibodies in blood and plasma donations.[63] It was established that the outbreak could be ascribed to the introduction of the multiantigen test for anti-HCV, which removed from the plasma pools antibodies that hitherto had formed complexes with HCV and facilitated the removal of the virus during manufacturing.[64–66] In response to this situation, testing of IVIG for HCV RNA by the polymerase chain reaction method was instituted as an interim measure (later extended to IMIG). Since then, all manufacturing processes for IVIG (and all but two for IMIG) either have been modified to incorporate effective viral clearance steps or have been validated as effective in clearing HCV.

VIRUS REMOVAL FROM PLASMA DERIVATIVES

During the manufacturing of plasma derivatives, viruses may become physically separated from the products without necessarily being inactivated. The particular steps responsible for removing viruses may have been intentionally included in the manufacturing scheme to remove viruses (e.g., nanofiltration), or the removal of virus may be the result of a manufacturing step originally intended to purify the product from contaminating proteins (e.g., ethanol fractionation and chromatography). Strategies for removing viruses from cellular components have also been developed, but these are discussed separately.

Partitioning by Ethanol Fractionation

All albumin products currently licensed in the United States, most immunoglobulin products (IMIG and IVIG), and several other plasma proteins are purified by the Cohn-Oncley cold ethanol fractionation process.[67, 68] European manufacturers use a similar procedure, the Kistler-Nitschmann method,[69] which operates on the same principles as the Cohn-Oncley process. During the isolation of these proteins by fractionation, significant reductions in the amounts of viruses initially present in plasma may also be accomplished.[65, 70–74] The effect of ethanol is probably mediated by two processes: partitioning of virus particles during phase separation of the proteins in ethanol and destruction of the virus particle as a result of denaturation of virus lipid, protein, and nucleic acid.[75, 76] However, the virucidal effect of the ethanol is probably attenuated by the low temperatures at which the procedure is carried out and the fact that the concentration of ethanol never exceeds 40%. It should be noted that factor

VIII and fibrinogen (a component of fibrin sealant) are produced from cryoprecipitate that is drawn off from freshly thawed plasma before the addition of ethanol. Also, the factor IX products are typically produced by chromatographic capture from plasma or "cryodepleted" plasma before ethanol fractionation begins.

The safety of albumin preparations (albumin and plasma protein fraction [PPF]) with regard to transmission of virus is due in large part, but not exclusively, to processing by ethanol fractionation. For instance, HIV titers have been reported to be reduced by more than 15 $\log_{10}$ ($>10^{15}$) during the production of fraction V, from which albumin is made by the Cohn-Oncley method.[77] This clearance factor, referred to as a log reduction factor (LRF), is probably sufficient alone to render albumin safe from HIV transmission. However, more modest levels of removal have been reported for HCV,[65, 78] and it is well established that unheated albumin or PPF, or albumin heated at 60°C for less than 10 hours, is capable of transmitting HBV if prepared from unscreened plasma.[79–82] Therefore, the viral safety of albumin and PPF depends on the combined effect of the fractionation process and heat treatment of the final containers.

Even before the introduction of specific viral inactivation steps in the manufacture of immunoglobulins (IMIG and IVIG), these products were never implicated in the transmission of HIV. Piszkiewicz and associates,[83] using 20% ethanol at −5°C to simulate early steps of a common fractionation procedure, demonstrated a reduction in infectivity of HIV-spiked cryodepleted plasma. In 1986, Wells and colleagues[84] evaluated the cumulative effect of the fractionation steps in the reduction of the viral load of plasma treated with the Cohn-Oncley process. They reported that HIV infectivity was reduced by a factor of 10^{15} between the starting plasma and the final fraction (precipitate II) used in the production of the immunoglobulins. Immunoglobulins produced by the Kistler-Nitschmann method have had an equally good safety record with regard to HIV transmission. The safety of immunoglobulin with regard to HBV transmission results from reduced titers of infectious HBV by as much as 7.5 logs.[85] The overall clearance factor may result from the combined effect of cold ethanol fractionation and the complexing of antibodies (anti-HBs) with HBsAg in the final product.[86] Indeed, the one outbreak of hepatitis B associated with the use of immunoglobulin was attributed to batches of IMIG that had atypically low titers of anti-HBs and measurable levels of HBsAg.[54]

The role of antiviral antibodies was brought into sharp focus by the outbreak of hepatitis C in association with the use of IVIG after the introduction of the multi-antigen test for anti-HCV antibodies in blood and plasma donations. The fractionation process was shown to reduce HCV titers by about 4.7 $\log_{10}$ when plasma positive for anti-HCV antibodies was used as the starting material.[65] However, when plasma screened by the multiantigen test, and thereby depleted of anti-HCV antibodies, was fractionated by the same method, only 3.5 $\log_{10}$ of virus were removed.[87] These results, the isolated reports of transmission of HCV by IVIG preparations, and other viral clearance experiments using bovine viral diarrhea virus as a model virus for HCV[78] indicate that the fractionation process alone is not sufficient to render IVIG safe from viral transmission. Consequently, additional viral clearance steps have since been incorporated into and/or validated for all IVIG products licensed in the United States.

It is notable that the same risk of transmitting HCV has not been associated with IMIG preparations prepared by ethanol fractionation. This fact seems somewhat counterintuitive because the production of IVIG entails additional manufacturing steps applied to the same ethanol fraction (fraction II) that gives rise to IMIG. In any event, additional precautions have also been included in the production processes for most U.S.-licensed IMIG products.

Chromatography

Various chromatography steps used in the production of several plasma derivatives may also serve to remove viruses from the products.[88] Those shown to be most effective in removing viruses include methods based on ion exchange (diethylaminoethanol [DEAE] for factors VIII and IX and for IVIG) and affinity (immobilized heparin for factor VIII and immobilized monoclonal antibodies for factors VIII and IX). Hydrophobic interaction chromatography was also thought at one time to be effective in removing HBV, HCV, and HIV from factor IX concentrates, but this proved not to be the case.[89] Gel filtration (size exclusion) chromatography probably lacks the resolution necessary to achieve significant reductions in viral contamination in most cases.

Under various conditions, DEAE chromatography has been validated to remove 3.5 to 5 $\log_{10}$ of HBV[90, 91] and 2 to 5 $\log_{10}$ of other viruses, including HIV.[88] However, transmission of HCV by IGIV products manufactured by DEAE chromatography (without prior ethanol fractionation) has been documented.[55–57] Affinity chromatography on resins to which monoclonal antibodies against the product of interest (factor VIII or IX) have been immobilized has also been validated to remove 2 to 6 $\log_{10}$ of various model viruses.[92] Thus, in general, chromatographic procedures provide moderate viral safety margins. There has been a novel application of monoclonal affinity chromatography, with sodium thiocyanate as the eluent, that combines the partitioning of the chromatographic step with the virucidal activity of the elution buffer.[93]

The effectiveness of chromatographic procedures depends on the specific context in which they are applied, identification of the operating parameters within which viral clearance is effected, and strict adherence to those parameters during routine manufacturing. Although safety margins achieved are typically modest, these techniques play an important role in reducing the risk posed by viruses such as HAV and HPV B19 that resist physical or chemical methods of inactivation.[34, 94, 95]

Nanofiltration

Small-pore-size filters (most commonly 15 to 75 nm) have come into use for the removal of viruses from plasma derivatives and other biological products. These filters may be made of multilayered cellulose[96] or polyvinylidene fluoride (PVDF)[97] and are typically operated by passing the fluid to be filtered over the surface of the membranes (tangential flow). Of course, the effectiveness of these filters depends at least partly on their pore size.[98, 99] For example, membranes with a mean pore size of 50 nm have been reported to be capable of clearing 6 $\log_{10}$ or more of viruses that have diameters greater than 40 to 50 nm (e.g., HBV, HCV, HIV) while permitting more than 85% to 90% recovery of albumin or immunoglobulin G (IgG).[97, 100] Significant removal of smaller viruses (e.g., poliovirus, 28 to 30 nm in diameter) may require filters of smaller pore sizes (on the order of 15 nm).[101] Although there have been reports of efficient removal of small viruses such as parvovirus (~20 nm in diameter),[102] the effectiveness of nanofiltration in removing HCV (35 to 65 nm in diameter) has been questioned.[103]

It is likely that the effectiveness of nanofiltration methods in removing a given virus depends on the milieu in which the virus is suspended and the conditions under which the filtration is performed. This necessitates careful validation of the effectiveness of the method and its routine application in each case in which it is employed. In addition, nanofiltration, although adaptable to the manufacture of moderate-sized proteins (factor IX and immunoglobulin), may not be applicable to larger or more asymmetric proteins such as factor VIII, fibrinogen, or von Willebrand factor. Nevertheless, nanofiltration has the advantages of being easily integrated into existing manufacturing processes and of being relatively nonselective, whereby viral size is apparently the primary determinant of the effectiveness of depletion.

VIRAL INACTIVATION OF PLASMA DERIVATIVES

Heat Treatment

Thermal inactivation of microorganisms is chiefly the result of protein denaturation. Many viruses are heat labile because the protein capsid is denatured after a few minutes of heating to temperatures of 55°C to 60°C.[104] Plasma proteins such as albumin, immunoglobulins, and clotting factors are also heat labile. Therefore, conditions of heating that reduce virus titers in these products while maintaining an acceptable level of protein concentration and activity had to be developed. Heat treatment methods have generally proved effective against enveloped viruses, but the nonenveloped viruses HAV and HPV B19 are more resistant to heat inactivation.

Three prevalent schemes for applying heat to plasma derivatives have emerged: (1) heating the product in solution (which nearly always equates to 60°C for 10 hours); (2) heating the final containers of a lyophilized product, termed "dry heat" or "terminal dry heat"; (3) heating of a lyophilized bulk intermediate in the manufacturing process at elevated pressure and under controlled humidity, termed "vapor heating."

Heating in Solution

Final containers of albumin and PPF are heated at 60°C for 10 to 11 hours in the presence of chemical stabilizers (caprylate and tryptophanate) to reduce the denaturing effects of heating. The effectiveness of this method in preventing hepatitis and HIV infections has already been considered; two points remain to be made here. First, heat treatment of albumin and PPF is performed in the final containers because of an incident in which two lots of PPF that had been heated in bulk (i.e., before filling into final containers) transmitted HBV.[105, 106] The cause of this incident was traced to a cold spot on the tank, in which during the heating the temperature failed to reach 60°C for the full incubation period. Today, this would be considered a breakdown of acceptable standards for manufacturing a biological drug (Current Good Manufacturing Practices) because the tank was inadequate for its intended use. In any event, since 1977 all albumin and PPF products licensed in the United States are heated only in their final containers. The second important point to be made is that the heat treatment of albumin and PPF is probably not sufficient to completely inactivate all virus present in the plasma from which the products are made.[40, 107] It is only in combination with the viral clearance attained by the fractionation process that heat inactivation achieves the level of safety that has been observed with these products.

Heating in solution at 60°C for 10 hours has been applied to coagulation factors VIII and IX, to IGIV, and to several other plasma derivatives.[108] Because of the heat lability of these proteins, stabilizers (amino acids, citrate, sugars) must be used to preserve the activity of the product, but they may also reduce the sensitivity of virus to the inactivation process.[109] Several prospective clinical trials of factor VIII heat-treated by this method revealed no transmissions of HBV, HCV, or HIV,[110–113] but there have been several individual reports of HBV and HCV transmissions associated with the use of factor VIII that had been heated in solution.[114–116] It is possible that these reports reflect errors in manufacturing, rather than an inherent limitation in the effectiveness of the heating procedure. In this regard, it is useful to bear in mind that these products, unlike albumin and PPF, are heated as bulk intermediates because the final containers are lyophilized. Transmission of HPV B19 has also been associated with the use of factor VIII heated as a liquid at 60°C for 10 hours.[117]

Dry Heat

In the wake of early reports of the heat lability of HIV,[118–120] several methods of heat-treating clotting factor concentrates, such as factor VIII and factor IX, were developed. Some involved heating of the final vials containing the lyophilized product at various temperatures for different times. However, the less severely heated products (e.g., below 68°C for 30 to 72 hours) were still capable of transmitting hepatitis[121–123] and HIV.[124–127]

Dry heating procedures that proved ineffective were abandoned for more robust methods. A greater appreciation also developed for the importance of residual moisture, composition of the dried product, and how the product was handled before and during drying with regard to the overall effectiveness of any given dry heat inactivation procedure.[4, 109, 128]

One procedure used for factor VIII in the United States (and various products in Europe) is the heating of the final containers at 80°C for 72 hours.[129] Clinical studies have revealed no instances of hepatitis transmission through products heated by this procedure,[130–132] and there have been no other confirmed reports of transmission of HBV, HCV, or HIV. Preclinical data also suggest that this method is effective against HAV,[133] and clinical data suggest that the risk of HPV B19 infection is reduced as well.[134] Nevertheless, HPV B19 transmission has been reported in association with the use of coagulation factor concentrates dry-heated at 80°C for 72 hours.[135, 136]

A second dry heating procedure entails heating the final containers at 60°C for 144 hours. This method is used for a factor IX complex concentrate and an anti-inhibitor coagulation complex (a mixture of partially activated coagulation factors used to treat patients who develop inhibitory antibodies to factor VIII) licensed in the United States. No published clinical data are available as to the safety of these products; the authors are unaware of any confirmed reports of viral transmissions by either.

In Europe, extreme temperature (100°C) for short durations (up to 1 hour) has been applied to some products already treated with solvent/detergent.[137, 138] The goal has been to improve the safety of these products with regard to the nonenveloped viruses (HAV and HPV B19). Nevertheless, transmission of HPV B19 by at least one of these products has been reported.[139]

Vapor Heating

This procedure is applied to an anti-inhibitor coagulation complex and the components of fibrin sealant (thrombin and fibrinogen), both licensed in the United States, as well as to other plasma derivatives available in Europe. The procedure entails the lyophilization of a bulk intermediate in the manufacturing process and then heating the bulk under controlled humidity and at elevated pressure. The current procedure includes two stages: the first at 60°C and 1190 milliBar (mBar) for 10 hours, followed by 1 hour at 80°C and 1375 mBar. Clinical studies have been performed on patients receiving products made with a predecessor process (single stage, 60°C and 1190 mBar for 10 hours). In the first, evidence of HBV transmission was detected in 4 of 28 enrolled patients.[140] A subsequent trial, however, revealed no transmission of HBV to any of 50 patients.[141] No transmission of HIV or HCV was detected in either trial. Clinical data also substantiate the effectiveness of the two-stage procedure with regard to HCV and HIV transmission,[142] and in vitro data suggest its effectiveness against HAV and parvoviruses.[143]

Miscellaneous Heating Procedures

Because of the evidence that organic solvents could inactivate enveloped viruses, particularly HCV, methods were developed that combined heat and exposure of the product to organic solvents (chloroform or n-heptane). In one process applied to factor VIII and IX products licensed in the United States, bulk intermediates in the manufacturing process were lyophilized, suspended in n-heptane, and heated for 20 hours at 60°C. Preclinical evidence (chimpanzee studies) had suggested that this method was effective against HCV; however, clinical trials showed that transmission of HCV was still possible.[144, 145] These methods are no longer used for products marketed in the United States.

Chemical Inactivation of Viruses

General Chemical Agents

Inactivation of viruses by chemical means is often performed for purposes of disinfection and sterilization in a clinical setting, disinfection of the water supply, and manufacture of inactivated vaccines. The concentration of the chemical agent, exposure time, and temperature all influence the inactivation capacity of chemical disinfectants. General chemical agents with demonstrated virucidal activity are listed in Table 42–2. Chemicals such as alcohols, sodium hypochlorite, glutaraldehyde, and formaldehyde are useful in the disinfection of surfaces and equipment. Chlorine-based compounds are also used for disinfection of public water supplies, swimming pools, and industrial process water. Typical means of inactivating viruses in the production of vaccines include treatment with formaldehyde or β-propiolactone plus UV radiation.[146]

Ethyl alcohol and isopropyl alcohol are generally effective against enveloped viruses. Inactivation of nonenveloped viruses depends on protein denaturation and requires higher concentrations of alcohol.[104] The susceptibility of HIV to inactivation by alcohol has been demonstrated[147, 148] and probably plays a role in reducing virus activity from albumin and other plasma proteins purified by the Cohn-Oncley cold ethanol fractionation process.

Common chlorine-based disinfectants, including sodium hypochlorite, calcium hypochlorite, and chlorinated trisodium phosphate, act as oxidizing agents. The biocidal activity is mediated by hypochlorous acid (HOCl), formed in solution at a pH of 5 to 8, and the endproducts of the reaction with biological material are inactive chlorides.[104] Enveloped viruses are more susceptible to inactivation than nonenveloped viruses. It has been reported that HIV activity is undetectable after treatment with 0.1% household bleach (52.5 ppm of sodium hypochlorite), and

Table 42–2. Chemical Agents With Virucidal Activity

Alcohols	Ethyl alcohol
	Isopropyl alcohol
Alkylating agents	Formaldehyde
	Glutaraldehyde
	β-Propiolactone
Lipid solvents	Chloroform
	Ether
	Tri(n-butyl)phosphate
Oxidizing agents	Sodium hypochlorite
	Calcium hypochlorite
	Hydrogen peroxide
Other agents	Peracetic acid
	Sodium hydroxide
	Phenolics
	Iodophors

a concentration of at least 5000 ppm (10% bleach) is recommended for laboratory use.

Glutaraldehyde and formaldehyde are effective alkylating agents against enveloped viruses. The aldehydes interact with viral nucleic acid, as well as induce crosslinking and denaturation of proteins.[104] Formaldehyde is used in the production of influenza vaccine and Salk polio vaccine.[146] HIV is highly sensitive to low concentrations of glutaraldehyde (0.01%),[148] 0.5% paraformaldehyde, and 1% neutral buffered formalin[149]; these concentrations are typically used for fixation of cells. The inactivation of non-A, non-B hepatitis virus (HCV) by formalin has also been reported.[150]

Other chemical disinfectants for which virucidal activity has been demonstrated include nonspecific agents such as peracetic acid, sodium hydroxide, hydrogen, phenolics, and iodophors.[104, 147] Chemicals with specificity for the lipid envelope of bloodborne viruses include lipid solvents such as chloroform,[151] ether,[152] and tri(n-butyl)-phosphate (TNBP).[153, 154] The combined treatment of blood products with lipid solvents and nonionic detergent is discussed in detail in the following section. In addition, the treatment of blood products with β-propiolactone and with UV radiation for the inactivation of hepatitis viruses and HIV has been reviewed.[155] Several methods of chemical inactivation of viruses currently applied to the purification of plasma proteins are listed in Table 42–3.

Solvent/Detergent Methods

Mixtures of solvents and detergents have been used to identify enveloped viruses and to inactivate viruses for the production of rabies and influenza vaccines.[156] Solvent/detergent extraction of essential enveloped lipids renders the virus noninfective. Because many of the transfusion-transmitted viruses (e.g., HBV, HCV, HIV) possess a lipid envelope, solvent/detergent treatment is an effective means of reducing viral infectivity of plasma protein products.[157, 158] Solvent/detergent, although effective against enveloped viruses, has virtually no effect on nonenveloped viruses, and several reported transmission of HAV and HPV B19 have been associated with the use of solvent/detergent–treated products. On the other hand, the solvent/detergent method as practiced has proved quite benign to proteins and adaptable to a variety of plasma derivatives. Factor VIII concentrate prepared by the solvent/detergent viral inactivation method has been licensed in the United States since 1985, and the solvent/detergent method has since been extended to other products.

Table 42–3. Methods of Viral Clearance Applied to U.S.-Licensed Plasma Derivatives

Method	Manner	Plasma Derivative
Heat	Heating in solution	Albumin, PPF, factor VIII, IVIG, IMIG
	Dry heating in final containers	Factor IX complex, anti-inhibitor coagulation complex, factor VIII
	Vapor heating	Anti-inhibitor coagulation complex, fibrin sealant (fibrinogen and thrombin)
Chemical agents	Solvent/detergent	Various products, whole plasma
	Sodium thiocyanate	Factor IX
Nanofiltration	Various	Factor IX
Partitioning	Cold ethanol fractionation	Albumin, PPF, IVIG, IMIG
	Other precipitation methods	Factor VIII
Chromatography	Ion exchange	Factors VIII and IX, IVIG
	Affinity	Factors VIII and IX

PPF, plasma protein fraction; IVIG, intravenous immunoglobulin; IMIG, intramuscular immunoglobulin.

It was known for some time that enveloped viruses are inactivated by membrane solubilization procedures with ethyl ether and other organic solvents, detergents, or solvent/detergent combinations. In 1984, Prince and colleagues[152] reported that stocks of HBV and a strain of HCV were inactivated by a combined treatment with 20% ether plus 1% Tween 80 at 4°C for 18 hours. The treated virus suspensions did not cause viral disease in inoculated chimpanzees. Factor VIII procoagulant activity was reduced by 30% by ether plus Tween 80 treatment.

Because of the hazardous nature of ethyl ether, an alternative nonexplosive solvent, TNBP, was tested for virucidal activity in combination with detergent. Horowitz and associates[153] examined the inactivation by TNBP in combination with detergent of several marker viruses added to antihemophilic factor (AHF) concentrates. Three enveloped viruses—vesicular stomatitis virus (VSV), Sindbis virus, and Sendai virus—were inactivated by 0.1% TNPB plus 1% Tween 80 at 4°C. This method proved to be more efficient than treatment with 20% ethyl ether plus 1% Tween 80. The nonenveloped encephalomyocarditis virus was unaffected by either method. In addition, the three enveloped viruses were treated at 30°C with 0.3% TNBP plus 0.2% sodium cholate instead of Tween 80, and all three were inactivated to undetectable levels (5 to 7 $\log_{10}$ reduction in titer). Triton X-100 has also been used as a detergent in combination with TNBP, often resulting in more rapid kinetics of inactivation than those produced by sodium cholate or Tween 80.[158]

TNBP/detergent combination treatments have been shown to be effective against marker viruses added to many products derived from blood, including whole plasma, cryoprecipitate, AHF, prothrombin complex concentrate, immunoglobulin, antithrombin III, and hemoglobin. Good recovery of functional activity has been recorded for factors VII, VIII, IX, and XIII and for fibrinogen, fibronectin, immunoglobulin, haptoglobin, and hemoglobin.[159]

HIV is very sensitive to solvent/detergent treatment.[154, 159] The combination of 0.3% TNBP plus 0.2% sodium cholate is effective in inactivating $10^{4.2}$ or more tissue culture infectious doses ($TCID_{50}$) of HIV added to factor VIII preparations, within 20 minutes at 24°C.[154] VSV at a similar initial titer is inactivated under the same conditions in 1 to 2 hours. Effective inactivation of at least 10^4 chimp infectious doses (CID_{50}) of HBV and HCV (Hutchinson strain) in plasma was also achieved in this study.

The safety of AHF treated with 0.3% TNBP plus 0.2% sodium cholate was assessed in a multicenter clinical study.[160] Patients with hemophilia A were enrolled in the study if they had no prior exposure to blood products prepared from pooled plasma. No transmission of HCV or HIV has been documented thus far with this product.[157, 158]

This viral inactivation process has been extended to the treatment of whole plasma.[161–163] Complete inactivation of marker viruses resulted from the treatment of plasma with 2% TNBP at 37°C, with 1% TNBP plus 1% Tween 80 at 30°C, and with 1% TNBP plus 1% Triton X45 at 30°C for 4 hours. Good recoveries of factors VIII, IX, and V were reported after treatment with TNBP plus detergent. In addition, subsequent fractionation of desired proteins from plasma was unaffected by prior solvent/detergent treatment of the plasma.[161, 164] Significant reduction of the infectivity of marker viruses HIV, HBV, and HCV was also reported for solvent/detergent treatment, with 1% TNBP and 1% Triton X-100 at 30°C for 4 hours, of fresh-frozen plasma.[162, 163] Coagulation factor activity appeared to be minimally affected, and there were no transmissions of HBV, HCV, and HIV during clinical trials of solvent/detergent–treated plasma.

Solvent/detergent–treated plasma is licensed in the United States and available in several countries in Europe. In order to perform the inactivation step, many units of fresh-frozen plasma are pooled together, treated, extracted to remove the solvent and detergent, and refilled into individual bags. Thus the treated plasma is no longer a single donor product but is derived from a pool of plasma traced to as many as 2500 donors. There is some concern that this practice may increase the risk of transmitting infectious agents that are not susceptible to inactivation by the solvent/detergent procedure. One alternative inactivation method that can be performed on individual plasma units, abrogating the need for pooling, is the addition of phenothiazine dyes, such as methylene blue, followed by illumination with visible light.[165]

β-Propiolactone

Another chemical means of viral inactivation utilizes the alkylating agent β-propiolactone (β-PL). β-PL destroys the infectivity of a wide variety of viruses by interacting with nucleic acid; it has been used in the preparation of inactivated vaccines.[91, 146] In addition to affecting nucleic acid, β-PL can cause protein denaturation. In the manufacture of human rabies vaccine, however, immunogenicity of the viral protein is maintained. Typically, chemical inactivation by β-PL is coupled with photochemical inactivation by UV radiation in vaccine production and treatment of human plasma for purified plasma derivatives.[91, 155] β-PL is unstable in solution and is rapidly degraded in plasma to a relatively nontoxic compound, β-hydroxypropionic acid, by the action of plasma hydrolases. Concerns remain, however, as to the carcinogenicity of the parent compound.

The combined treatment of plasma with β-PL and UV (254 nm) irradiation was first proposed by LoGrippo and Hartmann[166] in the 1950s. A 6.9 $\log_{10}$ reduction in HBV titers, a 4.5 $\log_{10}$ reduction in HCV titers, and a 4.2 $\log_{10}$ reduction in HIV titers were demonstrated for human plasma treated with β-PL plus UV.[91, 155, 167] However, there were reports of transmission of HIV to recipients of a factor IX product inactivated by treatment with β-PL and UV,[168] and the procedure is not used for any product currently marketed in the United States.

Other Chemical Methods

Iodine has a long history of use as a sterilizing agent and possesses significant virucidal properties.[169] However, the potential reactivity of iodine with proteins and the need to remove the chemical from the final product has limited its use in parenterals, including plasma derivatives. However, it has been reported that immobilizing iodine onto a substrate reduces damage to proteins and the amounts of iodine introduced into solution while preserving activity against both enveloped and nonenveloped viruses.[170]

The processing of some IVIG products includes incubating the protein at low pH (~4), with or without the addition of pepsin.[74, 171, 172] This manufacturing step, intended primarily to reduce anticomplementary activity, confers additional protection against viral transmission.

RADIATION-MEDIATED INACTIVATION OF VIRUSES

Inactivation of Viruses by Ionizing Radiation

Ionizing radiation, such as gamma rays from a cobalt 60 source or x-rays, is often used for sterilization of products that might be damaged by heating.[104] Ionizing radiation kills all types of microorganisms and is usually of high enough energy to penetrate solids and liquids. Gamma radiation was viewed for some time as a low-energy, safe method of killing viruses with the advantage of minimal molecular change in viral proteins, which is especially important in the manufacture of vaccines or viral antigen reagents.[173] Gamma radiation is also in use as a means of inactivating viruses and microorganisms in sewage, waste water, and foods.

DNA is the main cellular target of ionizing radiation, simply because of the volume it occupies in the cell. Proteins are less sensitive than nucleic acid to ionizing radiation, but significant protein damage can occur at very high doses. The action of radiation on living cells involves direct and indirect effects of ionization. Absorbed radiation excites electrons, yielding active radicals that may react with cell components such as DNA. Double-strand breaks can occur if the free radicals are produced directly in the DNA molecule.[174] The indirect effects of ionizing radiation are manifested by free radicals produced in the aqueous medium. Products of irradiated water include hydroxyl radical and peroxide. Their effects on both nucleic acids and proteins are evident when the biological material is irradiated in dilute solution, at temperatures above freezing, or when organic materials have been eliminated from the medium. Damage to nucleic acid includes cleavage of phosphodiester bonds and nucleic acid conversions. Cells with an enhanced capacity for DNA repair require a large increase in the dose of radiation to inactivate repair enzymes. Protein damage involves deamination, decarboxylation, and other covalent bond cleavage.[174] In addition, crosslinking of protein to

DNA may occur as a result of indirect free radical effects.[174]

Microorganisms are much more resistant to ionizing radiation than are higher forms of life. Viruses are highly resistant, and very high doses of radiation (5 to 10 Mrad) are required, because the nucleic acid represents the smallest target. Bacterial viruses and "slow viruses" (e.g., the causative agents of Creutzfeldt-Jakob disease) are the most resistant.[104] The inactivation of viruses by ionizing radiation occurs as a first-order reaction when the suspending medium contains free radical scavengers or is in a frozen state.[174] Inactivation of viruses with single-stranded nucleic acid by ionizing radiation is highly efficient, because almost every ionization causes a lethal strand break. In viruses with double-stranded nucleic acid, however, only some single-strand breaks are lethal, inasmuch as some repair mechanisms may operate in double-stranded DNA viruses.[173]

Inactivation of many human viruses, including HIV, has been achieved with gamma radiation.[173, 175–177] Spire and associates irradiated HIV in a medium containing 10% fetal calf serum and then inoculated normal T cells with the viral suspension.[118] Viral infectivity was measured as reverse transcriptase activity in cell supernatants over 25 days. Doses of gamma radiation (0.1 Mrad) caused a lag in expression of virus activity. HIV was completely inactivated by 0.25-Mrad irradiation.

The dose of gamma radiation required to inactivate most viruses, including HIV, would be expected to damage the cellular components of blood. However, several investigators have examined radiation treatment of plasma and coagulation factor concentrates as an alternative to heat or solvent/detergent treatment of these products. Horowitz and colleagues treated lyophilized AHF with gamma radiation at room temperature.[109] Acceptable AHF activity was recovered after radiation with a maximum 1-Mrad dose, whereas for the marker viruses, VSV and Sindbis virus, there were 6.0 $\log_{10}$ and 3.3 $\log_{10}$ titer reductions, respectively. It was noted that minor protein changes, including albumin aggregation, were detectable by crossed immunoelectrophoresis.

Kitchen and associates studied the effect of gamma radiation on HIV and factors VIII and IX. HIV in plasma was irradiated at $-40°C$ with doses as high as 4 Mrad.[176] The frozen state reduced the indirect effects of radiation on labile plasma proteins and favored direct effects on the larger target, the viral nucleic acid. These investigators demonstrated inactivation of $10^{6.5}$ infectious doses per milliliter of HIV with 4 Mrad of gamma radiation. Loss of coagulation factor activity was 14.6% for factor VIII:C (procoagulant), 38.8% for factor VIII:vWF (von Willebrand factor), and 23.3% for factor IX. No gross changes in the plasma proteins were detected by electrophoretic analyses. Therefore, freezing the plasma sample afforded protection to the protein components but did not interfere with virus inactivation. In comparison, Horowitz and colleagues reported a significant loss of AHF activity and major protein alterations after treatment of AHF in the lyophilized state with 2-Mrad gamma radiation.[109]

Inactivation of Viruses by Ultraviolet Radiation

Viral inactivation of blood products has also been attempted with UV radiation. UV radiation is often used in the laboratory for sterilization of exposed surfaces and air within closed spaces, such as biological hoods. Disinfection of waste water with UV radiation is a practical alternative to chlorine in that it does not have potentially toxic and mutagenic by-products.[104, 146]

The UV region of the electromagnetic spectrum covers the wavelength range of 200 to 400 nm and is divided into three regions: UVA (320 to 400 nm, near-UV), which is not strongly absorbed by protein and nucleic acids; UVB (290 to 320 nm, midrange); and UVC (200 to 290 nm, far-UV), which kills bacteria and other microorganisms.[178]

For UV radiation to cause a chemical change, a photon or quantum of light energy must first be absorbed by a light-absorbing molecule or chromophore. Nucleic acid and protein are the chief chromophores absorbing light in the UV region. As with ionizing radiation, energy absorption results in elevation of the molecule to the short-lived excited, or singlet, state. The single-state molecule may convert to a longer lived triplet state. Photoproducts form if a chemical change occurs in excited-state molecules. Complex biochemical processes are initiated, such as induction of repair enzymes, and the accumulation of photoinduced effects may result in damage at the cellular level.[179]

Because molecular structure dictates the efficiency of absorption of radiation, a range of sensitivity to UV would be expected to exist for different biological moieties. The most important UV chromophores are those with conjugated bonds.[179] Molecules with six-membered carbon rings, molecules with conjugated rings containing nitrogen, and structures with double, triple, and quadruple rings absorb strongly in the far UV portion of the spectrum. Triple-ringed molecules, such as riboflavin, and quadruple-ringed porphyrins absorb light in the near-UV region. The UV-absorbing components of proteins are the aromatic amino acids and the peptide bond. In nucleic acids, all the bases are aromatic and absorb strongly in the far-UV region. Pyrimidines are approximately 10-fold more sensitive to UV than are purines. In the region of 240 to 290 nm, nucleic acids absorb up to 20 times the UV radiation absorbed by equal weights of protein.[179]

Major photoproducts in DNA after far UV irradiation are dimers formed between adjacent pyrimidine bases, especially cyclobutylthymidine dimers, cytosine-thymine dimers, and DNA hydrates. Dimerization occurs within a single strand, and only pyrimidines adjacent in a chain dimerize to form cyclobutane linkages. The frequency of formation of pyrimidine dimers in DNA is a function of the DNA sequence and of the dose of applied UV radiation.[180] Unrepaired dimers can block nucleic acid replication and result in a lethal event for the cell or virus if the blocked DNA is essential.

Pyrimidine dimers are induced by near-UV (365 nm) radiation.[181] Near-UV radiation also produces single-strand breaks in bacterial DNA by an oxygen-dependent mechanism. The rate of single-strand break formation in relation to that of pyrimidine dimer formation increases from 254 to 405 nm.[181] Another class of photoproducts that may play a significant role in the lethal and mutagenic consequences to cells exposed to UV radiation involves covalent crosslinking of proteins to DNA.[182]

Other photoinduced changes in proteins are free radical formation and amino acid oxidation. Aromatic amino acids, histidine, and cystine serve as the major UV targets in proteins.[178]

The inactivation of many bacterial, animal, and human viruses by far-UV radiation has been previously demonstrated.[179, 183, 184] Kallenbach and associates reported that the "target theory" holds for most viruses: that is, the larger the viral genome, the easier the inactivation of the virus.[185] Viruses with single-stranded nucleic acid are, on the average, 10 times more sensitive to UV than are double-stranded viruses.[186] In viruses with double-stranded genomes, one strand may serve as a template for repairing damage to the other. Viral protein susceptibility to UV and host cell repair mechanisms also influence the extent of viral inactivation by UV radiation.

The AIDS crisis brought a renewed examination of UV radiation as a potential means of sterilizing labile blood derivatives and cellular blood products. Spire and associates demonstrated that HIV is moderately sensitive to UV radiation and that infectivity was eliminated only at UV doses higher than those routinely used for disinfection in the laboratory.[118] The susceptibility of HIV in blood products to UV radiation (254 nm) was also investigated by Stephan as part of a study of β-PL–UV sterilization of plasma derivatives.[155] UV irradiation alone inactivated 2.5 $\log_{10}$ of HIV titers in plasma and more than 4.5 $\log_{10}$ reduced in titer in cryoprecipitate.

Kallenbach and associates examined the effect of virucidal doses of UV radiation on factor VIII activity.[185] These authors showed that the UV dose required to inactivate 5 $\log_{10}$ of SV40 titers also reduced factor VIII activity by approximately 50%. Using a genome target size model for estimating UV efficacy, they suggested that the similarity in size of SV40 and HBV and the moderate resistance of SV40 to UV inactivation correlate with the size and resistance in previous reports of HBV resistance to UV radiation. Although UV irradiation does not introduce additives or by-products to the treated blood products, Kallenbach and associates concluded that significant protein damage may preclude its use as a procedure for sterilization of blood.

In another study, UV radiation was suggested as an agent that could inactivate viruses that contaminate cellular blood components.[187] A reduction of poliovirus titers by 4 to 6 $\log_{10}$ was demonstrated with a range of UVB doses that only moderately affected platelet and plasma protein function. Higher UVB doses resulted in significant damage to platelet and plasma proteins, without enhancing viral killing. In addition, it has been reported that UVB doses similar to the low-intensity laser-UVB doses used in this study may induce damage to platelets that is measurable only after several days of storage of platelet concentrates under blood-banking conditions.[188] Finally, UVB radiation has been used with platelet concentrates as a means of inactivating cells bearing alloantigens that cause alloimmunization in recipients of this product.[189]

Photo-oxidative damage to proteins by short-wavelength UV light has been addressed by the inclusion of a quencher of reactive oxygen species, the flavonoid rutin, in the solution being irradiated. The presence of 0.5 mmol of rutin was shown not to affect the efficiency of UVC inactivation of various viruses, while protecting plasma and factor VIII,[190] fibrinogen,[191] albumin, and IVIG[192] from aggregation or denaturation. In the presence of rutin, 0.1 J/cm^2 of UVC irradiation inactivated about 6 $\log_{10}$ of titers of the enveloped HIV type 1 and VSV, as well as several nonenveloped viruses, including HAV and porcine parvovirus.

PHOTOSENSITIZED INACTIVATION OF VIRUSES

Background

Another approach to the inactivation of viruses involves the use of photosensitizing compounds that, when activated by light, mediate the transfer of absorbed energy to an acceptor molecule such as nucleic acid, protein, lipid, water, or oxygen.[193] As was outlined for direct absorption of UV radiation, absorption of energy indirectly through the light-activated compound elevates target molecules to the excited state and may result in chemical changes within the molecules, the formation of photoproducts, and cellular damage.[178, 194] Photosensitizers currently under consideration for use with blood products and the viruses shown to be susceptible to treatment with these compounds are listed in Table 42–4.

The mechanism of photodamage induced by a photosensitizer and light may be classified as either a type I or a type II reaction.[195] In a type I reaction (also called a free radical or direct reaction), the photosensitizer reacts directly with the biomolecule through an electron or hydrogen atom transfer. The reaction results in a semireduced free radical form of the photosensitizer and a semioxidized free radical form of the molecule. These free radicals can react further to form oxidized substrate and reaction products, including superoxide anion and hydrogen peroxide, as a result of free radical photosensitizer reactions with oxygen. In other cases, photosensitizer and substrate radicals can interact to form covalent photoadducts. This type of reaction (cycloaddition after energy transfer) occurs with the photosensitizer psoralen.[194] A type II or indirect reaction involves singlet oxygen.[195]

Table 42–4. Photosensitizers With Virucidal Activity Proposed for Use With Cellular Blood Products

Photosensitizer	Radiation	Target(s)
Psoralens		
8-Methoxypsoralen (8-MOP)	UVA	Nucleic acid
4′ Aminomethyl-4,5′, 8-trimethylpsoralen (AMT)	UVA	Nucleic acid
Hematoporphyrin derivative		
Dihematoporphyrin ether	630 nm	Lipid
Benzoporphyrin derivative (BPD)		
BPD-monoacid, ring A	692 nm	Lipid
Cyanine dyes		
Merocyanine 540	520–550 nm	Lipid, protein
Aluminum phthalocyanine	670 nm	Lipid
Phenothiazine dyes		
Methylene blue	620–670 nm	Lipid, protein
Toluidine blue	620–670 nm	Lipid, protein

UV, ultraviolet.

Absorbed energy is transferred from the singlet excited-state photosensitizer to the more stable triplet state. Transfer of energy to ground-state molecular oxygen, $^3O_2$, results in ground-state sensitizer and the singlet excited-state of oxygen, $^1O_2$. Singlet oxygen is highly reactive and cytotoxic, reacting rapidly with electron-rich regions of DNA, RNA, proteins, and lipids, resulting in oxidized forms of the molecules. A type II reaction occurs with the membrane-active photosensitizers, hematoporphyrin, and benzoporphyrin derivatives.[196]

Photosensitizers Specific for Nucleic Acid

Psoralens

Psoralens are naturally occurring tricyclic furocoumarins that display photosensitizing activity when activated by UV radiation at wavelengths of 320 to 380 nm (UVA). Psoralens, in general, readily penetrate cells, bacteria, and enveloped and nonenveloped viruses.[197] These compounds interact with DNA and, to a lesser extent, with RNA by intercalating in the double-stranded or single-stranded structure.[198] The intercalated psoralen molecule forms covalent cyclobutane-type adducts with nearby pyrimidine bases when activated by UVA radiation. Psoralen adds across the 5,6 carbon-carbon double bond of the pyrimidine (usually thymine) and can form crosslinks in the DNA by cycloaddition of the 3,4 and 44,54 double bonds of the psoralen. This reaction is 4′,5′-dependent and is essentially a type I or direct reaction, proceeding through energy transfer from photosensitizer to DNA.[198]

Psoralen-photosensitized reactions have many effects on cells, most of which are the results of effects on DNA and DNA synthesis. In the presence of oxygen, however, psoralens can also damage cellular constituents other than nucleic acids by production of singlet oxygen generated by furocoumarin excitation.[199]

Treatment of psoriasis with psoralen (8-methoxypsoralen [8-MOP]) and UVA was introduced in 1974 by Parrish and coworkers.[200] Psoralen probably blocks DNA synthesis in the rapidly proliferating keratinocytes within the epidermal lesions seen in patients with psoriasis. Administration of 8-MOP may be topical or oral. Typically, 2 hours after ingestion, patients receive whole-body exposure to UVA radiation.

Psoralen photochemotherapy is also effective in the treatment of cutaneous T cell lymphoma. Edelson and colleagues described the extracorporeal photosensitization of peripheral blood lymphocytes in the presence of psoralen and UVA as a method of lethally damaging the malignant T cells.[201] Psoralen (8-MOP) is administered orally. Leukocyte-enriched blood obtained by leukapheresis is irradiated by UVA in a flow cell and then returned to the patient.

Psoralen inactivation of viruses has been effective in the production of vaccines and viral antigens for immunodiagnostics.[146, 197] In many cases, the antigenicity of viral proteins is unaffected by even extremely high doses of psoralen and UVA. The water-soluble synthetic psoralen derivative 4′-aminomethyl-4,5′,8-trimethylpsoralen hydrochloride (AMT) is a potent photoinactivator of RNA viruses.[197] The positively charged amino group on the molecule enhances the ability of AMT to bind nucleic acid.[202] Trioxsalen (4,5′,8-trimethylpsoralen [TMP]) is more photoreactive toward DNA viruses such as herpesvirus.[197]

Psoralen-UVA treatment is also effective for the inactivation of retroviruses.[203] In one study, suspensions of HIV containing 10^6 in vitro infectious units per milliliter were inactivated to undetectable levels after a 30-minute exposure to AMT and UV radiation at 365 nm.[120]

The application of photochemical treatment with psoralen to the decontamination of cellular blood products was first described by Lin and coworkers.[204] These investigators, using 8-MOP and UVA, developed a system of inactivation of viruses in platelet concentrates. Standard platelet concentrates inoculated with marker viruses were treated with 300 μg/mL of 8-MOP and irradiated for 6 hours with UVA in an atmosphere of 2 psi of 5% CO_2 and 95% N_2. Marker viruses, chosen on the basis of similarity of genomic size to that of common human viruses, were inactivated by combined 8-MOP–UVA treatment but not by either agent alone. Platelets were not adversely affected by the psoralen-UVA procedure, as judged by a number of in vitro assays of function and morphology, but platelets stored for 18 hours after 8-MOP–UVA treatment were slightly activated, as demonstrated by surface expression of the activation-dependent glycoprotein GMP-140. Further storage of treated platelet concentrates for 96 hours did not result in damage other than that displayed by untreated stored platelets.

Lin and coworkers subsequently reported that 8-MOP and UVA were active against cell-associated HIV in platelet concentrates.[205] They correlated inhibition of HIV type 1 infectivity with 8-MOP–DNA adduct formation in contaminating nucleated cells and measured the inhibition of polymerase chain reaction (PCR)–mediated amplification of cellular DNA sequences as a surrogate for inactivation of integrated proviral nucleic acid sequences. The authors concluded that high titers of cell-associated HIV type 1 in platelet concentrates were inactivated by the system and that the numbers of 8-MOP-DNA adducts in nucleated cells were sufficient to inhibit amplification of DNA segments that encode for as few as 80 amino acids. More recently, this group used a synthesized analog of 8-MOP, designated S-59, which they contended is less mutagenic than 8-MOP.[206] Activity against various viruses were (all as $\log_{10}$) more than 6.6 plaque-forming units (pfu)/mL of HIV (cell-free and cell-associated), more than 6.8 ID50/mL of duck hepatitis B virus, and more than 6.5 pfu/mL of bovine viral diarrhea virus. Activity against bacteria and contaminating leukocytes was also shown. In vitro and in vivo platelet function were adequately maintained after antiviral and antibacterial treatment.

Photosensitizers Specific for Viral Lipid Envelope

Hematoporphyrin Derivative

Hematoporphyrin derivative (HPD), a complex mixture of ringed tetrapyrroles derived from hematoporphyrin, is a fluorescent photosensitizer used for both the localization and eradication of neoplasms.[196] In 1988, Matthews and colleagues reported that HPD and 630-nm light readily inactivated herpes simplex virus (HSV) type 1, cytomegalovirus (CMV), and measles virus in culture medium but did not inactivate two nonenveloped viruses: Echovirus type 21 and adenovirus type 6.[207] These researchers concluded that the major site of the photodamage by HPD is the viral envelope and proposed that HPD and light might be effective in inactivating viruses that contaminate blood. The proposal was based on the demonstrated affinity of HPD for lipid-containing membranes and the fact that the most common viruses found in blood are lipid enveloped: HBV, CMV, HIV, and probably HCV.

The photoinactivation of viruses in blood by a preparation of HPD enriched with dihydroergotamine (DHE) was examined by diluting HSV type 1 in whole blood to an initial titer of 10^5 to 10^6 pfu/mL.[207] Treatment with 2.5 to 20 mg/mL DHE and light reduced HSV titers to approximately 10 pfu/mL. The effect of 2.5 mg/mL of DHE and 630-nm light on whole blood was determined by assaying fibrinogen levels, clotting times, plasma protein electrophoresis, sodium and potassium levels, glucose level, and cell number. The only reported adverse effect of phototreatment with DHE was a significant drop in platelet count.

In a later report, Matthews and colleagues described the photoinactivation of cell-free HIV type 1 by 20 mg/mL of DHE when the virus was prepared in culture medium or in whole blood.[208] A 10- to 20-fold higher concentration of DHE had no effect on red cell fragility, 2,3-diphosphoglycerate (2,3-DPG), or adenosine triphosphate (ATP) or on whole blood potassium concentrations.

Benzoporphyrin Derivative

Another membrane-active photosensitizer, benzoporphyrin derivative (BPD), is activated by light at a peak wavelength of 692 nm. BPD has been shown to be much more phototoxic than HPD, and its cytotoxic effects are also mediated by singlet oxygen.[209] Synthesis of BPD yields four structural analogs, one of which (BPD-monoacid, ring A [BPD-MA]) has been described as a candidate for photodynamic eradication of tumors.[210] Like HPD, BPD has been shown to inactivate enveloped viruses.[211] In this study, BPD-MA at concentrations of 2 to 4 mg/mL inactivated up to 7 $\log_{10}$ of VSV titers in whole blood. Hemolysis of red blood cells did not occur during the 48 hours after treatment. It has been reported that the presence of increasing concentrations of serum competed for binding of leukemic cells to the porphyrin.[209] The efficient binding of many hydrophobic photosensitizers by lipoproteins or albumin is an issue that must be addressed for the inactivation of viruses in blood products that have a high plasma protein concentration. Experience with merocyanine 540 provides another example of this problem.[212]

Other Photosensitizers

Phthalocyanine Dyes

Other photosensitizers have been identified as possible candidates for photodynamic therapy and photoinactivation of viruses on the basis of their absorption characteristics in the red region of the spectrum. Treatment at wavelengths of 630 nm or more—the wavelength used with HPD—would allow better light penetration of the target tissue. Photosensitizers that absorb in this region include the phthalocyanines.[213, 214] These molecules typically contain a ring system of four isoindole structures linked by azo nitrogen atoms. Metal atoms are readily inserted into the central ring, and the addition of amino, carboxylic, nitrogen or sulfonic acid groups to the isoindole units may confer water solubility.[214]

Horowitz and coworkers[215] studied the inactivation of viruses in blood with aluminum phthalocyanine (AlPc) and its sulfonated derivatives and demonstrated the specificity of this photosensitizer for enveloped viruses. A cell-free form of VSV was inactivated to undetectable levels in whole blood and in red cell concentrates with 10 mmol of aluminum phthalocyanine and visible light (>570 nm). Virucidal activity was also demonstrated against cell-free HIV and cell-associated forms of VSV and HIV but not against encephalomyocarditis virus, a nonenveloped virus. The disulfonated and tetrasulfonated derivatives of AlPc were more active against VSV than the nonsulfonated forms. Lysis of red blood cells was reported to be minimal both immediately after treatment with AlPc and after storage of treated whole blood for 17 days at 4°C.

Phenothiazine Dyes

Cationic phenothiazine dyes, such as methylene blue, toluidine blue, and neutral red, have been shown to inactivate viruses.[165, 181, 216, 217] The dyes bind to viral nucleic acid and to the virus surface as well. Activation of the dye by visible light results in destruction of viral components by a process involving oxygen radicals.[216]

The treatment of red blood cells with methylene blue was described by Wagner and colleagues.[218] Conditions of methylene blue and light treatment shown to inactivate 5 to 6 $\log_{10}$ of VSV or Sindbis virus titers did not affect red cell ATP and 2,3-DPG levels or cause membrane lipid peroxidation. Hemolysis was minimal. Damage to the red cell surface was manifested, however, as an increase in Na^+ and K^+ permeability and binding of immunoglobulin G. There is also one report of the treatment of human thrombocyte concentrates with methylene blue.[219]

The photodynamic inactivation of viruses has also been accomplished in fresh plasma by treatment with low doses of methylene blue (typically 1 μmol) and visible light.[220–223] The methylene blue procedure has been shown to inactivate 5 to 7 $\log_{10}$ of model enveloped virus titers[224] and at least 6 $\log_{10}$ of HIV type 1 titers.[225] Methylene blue is potentially effective against some, but not all, nonenveloped viruses.[224] Methylene blue treatment has also been reported to cause photo-oxidative damage to fibrinogen, resulting in alterations of fibrin polymerization[221] and decreases in the activities of several coagulation factors.[226] No other major changes in protein composition or antigenicity are apparent.[227, 228] Methylene blue–treated plasma has been available in Europe since 1992.

Other phenothiazine dyes, such as 1,9-dimethylmethylene blue, have also been found to be effective virucidal agents upon illumination. It appears that the relative effectiveness of these compounds is directly correlated with their yield of singlet oxygen.[229] Practical utility may be limited by other properties such as solubility or toxicity.

OTHER TREATMENTS

Ozone

Ozone, the triatomic form of oxygen (O_3), is a more rapid oxidizing agent than molecular oxygen (O_2) and has been used as a germicidal and virucidal agent in medicine, water purification, and sewage treatment.[230] Ozone treatment is effective in inactivating human viruses that contaminate the water supply, including HAV[231] and poliovirus.[232]

A preliminary report described the effect of ozone on human blood contaminated with HIV-infected lymphocytes.[233] Ozone eliminated HIV from blood at a dosage range of 45 to 55 mg/mL. The effect of ozone on the blood cells was not described. Wells and associates[234] demonstrated the inactivation of more than 11 $\log_{10}$ of titers of cell-free HIV treated with ozone in cell culture medium. HIV-infected factor VIII preparations that were similarly treated maintained 90% or more factor activity. Significant adverse effects on red blood cells have been described in another study,[235] which suggests that ozone damage would not be specific for viruses in a cellular blood product.

WASHING AND FILTRATION

The possibility of physically removing free virus particles and virus associated with lymphocytes has been explored with washing and filtration techniques, respectively.[236] In one study, leukocyte-depleted red cell units were spiked with 10^7 pfu/mL of VSV, Sindbis virus, or $+\phi 6$ and extensively washed by established automated procedures.[237] The reduction of viral activity was less than 2 $\log_{10}$, indicating that the association of virus particles with the red cells is not disrupted by washing.

Rawal and associates[238] evaluated filters designed for the removal of leukocytes to reduce cell-associated HIV infectivity in red blood cells and whole blood. Filtration of the blood products resulted in a mean leukocyte removal of 2.75 $\log_{10}$ titers and a mean reduction of virus infectivity of 5.9 $\log_{10}$ titers. In another study, these filters were shown to remove both intact HIV-infected cells and the infectious particulate debris that forms during storage of blood.[239] In several instances, however, the effluent still contained infected cells and cell-free virus; it was therefore recommended that leukocyte depletion by filtration be accompanied by a method of virus inactivation to reduce virus transmission by these products.

Sadoff and colleagues[240] described the removal of 6 $\log_{10}$ of white blood cells from red blood cell products through the use of experimental filters. Red blood cell recovery was 85% or greater, and in vitro storage parameters were not significantly affected. Filtration of red blood cells was performed within 8 hours of blood collection in an effort to lessen the potential for release of viral particles from contaminating cells.

More recently, there has been a randomized trial in CMV-seronegative marrow recipients to determine whether filtration of leukocytes from blood products was as effective as CMV-seronegative blood products for the prevention of transfusion-transmitted CMV infection after marrow transplantation.[241] In this multicenter study, 502 patients were randomly assigned to receive either filtered or seronegative blood products. Endpoints included the development of CMV infection and tissue-documented CMV disease between days 21 and 100 after transplantation. In the primary analysis of evaluable infections, there were no significant differences in the probabilities of CMV infection (1.3% versus 2.4%, $p = 1.00$) and disease (0% versus 2.4%, $p = 1.00$) between the seronegative and filtered product recipients, respectively, or in probability of survival ($p = .6$). Further analysis showed that although the infection rates were similar, the probability of CMV disease in the filtered product recipients was greater (2.4% versus 0% in the seronegative product recipients, $p = .03$). The authors concluded that filtration is an effective alternative to the use of seronegative blood products for prevention of transfusion-associated CMV infection in marrow transplant recipients.

KEY ISSUES REGARDING VIRAL INACTIVATION

In selecting and implementing viral inactivation strategies, three critical factors must be taken into account: (1) the method to be used must be shown to be effective against the target viruses; (2) the method to be used must not introduce undesirable changes in the product; and (3) the method must be implemented under appropriate controls so that it is applied reliably and effectively on a day-to-day basis.

The effectiveness of an inactivation procedure is demonstrated by spiking experiments, wherein the product or an intermediate in its manufacture is spiked with high titers of relevant or model viruses and the removal or inactivation of those viruses is measured. Relevant viruses—those that can be expected to be encountered in the product or source material (e.g., HIV or the hepatitis viruses)—are preferred; however, for HBV and HCV there are no reliable in vitro assays for measuring infectivity. Model viruses are useful in this regard because they are adapted for use in the laboratory. However, in selecting model viruses to be used in these studies, care must be taken to ensure that the characteristics of the models reflect those of the viruses of interest.

For plasma derivatives, which are produced on very large scales, the demonstration that a viral clearance step is effective is done on scaled-down laboratory models of the manufacturing process. These scaled-down models introduce a degree of uncertainty, and so care must be taken to verify that the laboratory model chosen reflects the full-scale process in all material respects.

Finally, standards to ensure the adequacy and reliability of the experimental design have been set for performing experiments to demonstrate the effectiveness of the clearance method. It is generally accepted that a given viral clearance method will not necessarily perform identically in all settings, and so its effectiveness must be shown each time it is applied to a new blood product.

With regard to the effect of a clearance method on the product itself, several considerations are important. The introduction of chemical agents into products for transfusion creates risks associated with the toxicity and mutagenicity of the original and residual chemical and its by-products. For example, solvent/detergent treatment of clotting factor concentrates involves the use of chemicals that are potentially toxic and must be removed after the inactivation step. Immunoaffinity chromatography for the production of factor VIII provides a very pure product but may contaminate the product with monoclonal antibody leached from the affinity column. The alkylating agent β-propiolactone has demonstrated carcinogenic activity, although it has been shown to degrade rapidly in plasma. Finally, all of the photosensitizers proposed for use with cellular blood components present a risk associated with intravenous administration of the native compound as well as potentially toxic by-products.

Minimal modification of the activity and function of the transfused blood product by physical or chemical treatment is always an important consideration. For example, pasteurization methods that include protein stabilizers have been developed for the protection of albumin and factor VIII during processing. It is also important to assess the influence of any denaturing technique on soluble and cellular protein structure, in order to guard against the creation of neoantigens. Even a procedure that has been used successfully for one product may render a similar product immunogenic under slightly different circumstances.[242]

The preservation of cellular protein activity presents a significant challenge to designers of viral inactivation methods, such as UV irradiation and photosensitization, for use with cellular products. The susceptibility of cellular proteins and lipids to oxidative damage may effectively eliminate from consideration the photosensitizers that inactivate viruses through singlet oxygen or oxygen radical mechanisms. In many cases, it would be pointless to use plasma proteins to protect the cells, because protein protects the viruses as well. Treatment of products with psoralens under reduced oxygen tension may ameliorate protein damage caused by secondary singlet oxygen effects, leaving only the specific action of the photosensitizer on viral nucleic acid. Any agent with demonstrated activity against nucleic acid, however, must be closely examined for carcinogenic and mutagenic potential.

Another important consideration in the treatment of cellular products is level of contamination by virus-infected lymphocytes. These cells serve as a potential reservoir of intact virus particles, a supply of repair machinery for restoration of virus production, and a source of genomic and inducible virus. Expression of HIV and other viruses with a latent state may be induced by agents that damage DNA.[243] The damage, which may occur via a mechanism that involves cellular DNA repair, transcription of the viral genome, and virus production, is seen with some agents (e.g., UV radiation and 8-MOP) but not others (e.g., phthalocyanine Pc 4).[244]

Finally, once an effective method that has no adverse effects on a product has been identified, the method must be applied on a routine basis so that the procedure reliably accomplishes its purpose. This is done by establishing carefully defined procedures and appropriate controls that govern the operation as applied in a real-world setting. The standards under which this is done are known as Current Good Manufacturing Practices. Because the viral clearance procedures implemented for plasma derivatives are so effective, the major risk today derives from the possibility of manufacturing errors that compromise those procedures. Adherence to the Current Good Manufacturing Practices minimizes the chance of such errors.

CONCLUSION

The combination of donor screening for markers of virus exposure and use of methods of viral inactivation has been instrumental in reducing the transmission of viruses by purified plasma-derived products. At present, research in the area of inactivation techniques to be applied to cellular blood components continues. The important step in this endeavor is a rigorous assessment of the risk imparted to the recipient by additional physical or chemical treatment of the product, weighed against the low risk of exposure to viruses that have thus far been identified as transmitted by transfusion.

REFERENCES

1. Fricke WA, Lamb MA. Viral safety of clotting factor concentrates. Semin Thromb Hemost 1993; 19:54.
2. Sloand EM. Viral risks associated with blood transfusion. Photochem Photobiol 1997; 65:428.
3. Horowitz B. Specific inactivation of viruses which can potentially contaminate blood products. Dev Biol Stand 1991; 75:43.
4. Cuthbertson B, Reid KG, Foster PR. Viral contamination of human plasma and procedures for preventing virus transmission by plasma products. *In* Harris JR (ed): Blood Separation and Plasma Fractionation. New York: Wiley-Liss, 1991, pp 385–435.
5. Suomela H. Inactivation of viruses in blood and plasma products. Transfus Med Rev 1993; 7:42.
6. Horowitz B, Ben-Hur E. Strategies for viral inactivation. Curr Opin Hematol 1995; 2:484.
7. Friedman LI, Stromberg RR. Viral inactivation and reduction in cellular blood products. Rev Fr Transfus Hemobiol 1993; 36:83.
8. Dodd RY. Viral inactivation in platelet concentrates. Transfus Clin Biol 1994; 1:181.
9. Horowitz B, Ben-Hur E. Viral inactivation of blood components: recent advances. Transfus Clin Biol 1996; 3:75.
10. Krishnan LA, Brecher ME. Transfusion-transmitted bacterial infection. Hematol Oncol Clin North Am 1995; 9:167.
11. Wagner S. Transfusion-related bacterial sepsis. Curr Opin Hematol 1997; 4:464.
12. Brown P. Can Creutzfeldt-Jakob disease be transmitted by transfusion? Curr Opin Hematol 1995; 2(6):472.
13. Brown P. Donor pool size and the risk of blood-borne Creutzfeldt-Jakob disease. Transfusion 1998; 38:312.
14. Busch MP, Glynn SA, Schreiber GB. Potential increased risk of virus transmission due to exclusion of older donors because of concern over Creutzfeldt-Jakob disease. The National Heart, Lung, and Blood Institute Retrovirus Epidemiology Donor Study. Transfusion 1997; 37:996.
15. Schreiber GB, Busch MP, Kleinman SH, Korelitz JJ. The risk of transfusion-transmitted viral infections. N Engl J Med 1996; 334:1685.

16. Sayers MH. Transfusion-transmitted viral infections other than hepatitis and human immunodeficiency virus infection. Cytomegalovirus, Epstein-Barr virus, human herpesvirus 6, and human parvovirus B19. Arch Pathol Lab Med 1994; 118(4):346.
17. Chamberland M, Khabbaz R. Emerging issues in blood safety. Infect Dis Clin North Am 1998; 12:217.
18. Bowden RA. Transfusion-transmitted cytomegalovirus infection. Hematol Oncol Clin North Am 1995; 9:155.
19. Lemon SM. The natural history of hepatitis A: the potential for transmission by transfusion of blood or blood products. Vox Sang 1994; 67(suppl 4):19.
20. Brown KE, Young NS. Parvovirus B19 in human disease. Annu Rev Med 1997; 48:59.
21. Erdman DD, Anderson BC, Török TJ, et al. Possible transmission of parvovirus B19 from intravenous immune globulin. J Med Virol 1997; 53(3):233.
22. Mannucci PM, Gdovin S, Gringeri A, et al. Transmission of hepatitis A to patients with hemophilia by factor VIII concentrates treated with organic solvent and detergent to inactivate viruses. Ann Intern Med 1994; 120(1):1.
23. Lawlor E, Johnson Z, Thornton L, Temperley I. Investigation of an outbreak of hepatitis A in Irish haemophilia A patients. Vox Sang 1994; 67(suppl 1):18.
24. Centers for Disease Control and Prevention. Hepatitis A among persons with hemophilia who received clotting factor concentrate—United States, September–December 1995. MMWR 1996; 45:29.
25. Mortimer PP, Luban NLC, Kelleher JF, Cohen BJ. Transmission of serum parvovirus-like virus by clotting factor concentrates. Lancet 1983; 2:482.
26. Lyon DJ, Chapman CS, Martin C, et al. Symptomatic parvovirus B19 infection and heat-treated factor IX concentrate. Lancet 1989; 1:1085.
27. Morfini M, Longo G, Rossi Ferrini P, et al. Hypoplastic anemia in a hemophiliac first infused with a solvent/detergent treated factor VIII concentrate: the role of human B19 parvovirus. Am J Hematol 1992; 39:149.
28. Groβe-Bley A, Eis-Hübinger AM, Kaiser R, et al. Serological and virological markers of human parvovirus B19 infection in sera of hemophiliacs. Thromb Haemost 1994; 72:503.
29. Luban NLC. Human parvoviruses: implications for transfusion medicine. Transfusion 1994; 34:821.
30. Erdman DD, Anderson BC, Török TJ, et al. Possible transmission of parvovirus B19 from intravenous immune globulin. J Med Virol 1997; 53:233.
31. Penchansky L, Jordan JA. Transient erythroblastopenia of childhood associated with human herpesvirus type 6, variant B. Am J Clin Pathol 1997; 108:127.
32. Thomas HC, Pickering J, Karayiannis P. Identification, prevalence and aspects of molecular biology of hepatitis G virus. J Viral Hepat 1997; 4(suppl 1):51.
33. Alter HJ, Nakatsuji Y, Melpolder J, et al. The incidence of transfusion-associated hepatitis G virus infection and its relation to liver disease. N Engl J Med 1997 Mar 13;336(11):747–754.
34. Lemon SM. Hepatitis A virus and blood products: virus validation studies. Blood Coagul Fibrinolysis 1995; 6(suppl 2):S20.
35. Dodd RY. Viral contamination of blood components and approaches for reduction of infectivity. Immunol Invest 1995; 24:25.
36. Lynch TJ, Weinstein MJ, Tankersley DL, et al. Considerations of pool size in the manufacture of plasma derivatives. Transfusion 1996; 36:770.
37. Sherwood WC. The significance of the blood-borne viruses: blood banking and transfusion medicine. Dev Biol Stand 1993; 81:25.
38. Gellis SS, Neefe JR, Stokes J Jr, et al. Inactivation of the virus of homologous serum hepatitis in solutions of normal human serum albumin by means of heat. J Clin Invest 1948;27:239.
39. Tabor E. The epidemiology of virus transmission by plasma derivatives: clinical studies that support lack of transmission. Transfusion, in press.
40. Shikata T, Karasawa T, Abe K, et al. Incomplete inactivation of hepatitis B virus after treatment at 60°C for 10 hours. J Infect Dis 1978; 138:242.
41. Burnouf-Radosevich M, Burnouf T, Huartt JJ. A pasteurized therapeutic plasma. Infusionstherapie 1992; 19:91.
42. Murray R, Oliphant JW, Trip JT, et al. Effect of ultraviolet irradiation on the infectivity of icterogenic plasma. JAMA 1955; 157:814.
43. Hughes-Jones NC. Risk assessment and factor VIII concentrates. Lancet 1995; 345:502.
44. Desforges JF. AIDS and preventive treatment in hemophilia. N Engl J Med 1983; 308:94.
45. National Hemophilia Foundation Medical and Scientific Advisory Council. Recommendations Concerning AIDS and Therapy of Hemophilia (revised October 13, 1984). New York: National Hemophilia Foundation, 1984.
46. Centers for Disease Control. Update: acquired immunodeficiency syndrome (AIDS) virus in persons with hemophilia. MMWR 1985; 33:589.
47. Epstein JS, Fricke WA. Current safety of clotting factor concentrates. Arch Pathol Lab Med 1990; 114(3):335.
48. Fricke W, Augustyniak L, Lawrence D, et al. Human immunodeficiency virus infection due to clotting factor concentrates: results of the Seroconversion Surveillance Project. Transfusion 1992; 32:707.
49. Mannucci PM. Clinical evaluation of viral safety of coagulation factor VIII and IX concentrates. Vox Sang 1993; 64:197.
50. Mannucci PM. Viral safety of plasma-derived and recombinant products used in the management of hemophilia A and B. J Am Blood Res Assoc 1995; 4:8.
51. Gomperts ED. Procedures for the inactivation of viruses in clotting factor concentrates. Am J Hematol 1986; 23:295.
52. Morgenthaler J-J. Workshop of the safety of IVIG preparations with respect to transmission of hepatitis and AIDS viruses. Vox Sang 1986; 51:25.
53. Finlayson JS. Safety and efficacy of immune globulins. *In* Krijnen HW, Strengers PWF, van Aken WG (eds): Immunoglobulins: Proceedings of an International Symposium. Central Laboratory of the Netherlands Red Cross Blood Transfusion Service, 1988, pp 231–246.
54. Tabor E, Gerety RJ. Transmission of hepatitis B by immune serum globulin. Lancet 1979; 2:1293.
55. Foster PR, McIntosh RV, Welch AG. Hepatitis C infection from anti-D immunoglobulin. Lancet 1995; 346:372.
56. Meisel H, Reip A, Faltus B, et al. Transmission of hepatitis C virus to children and husbands by women infected with contaminated anti-D immunoglobulin. Lancet 1995; 345:1209.
57. Power JP, Lawlor E, Davidson F, et al. Molecular epidemiology of an outbreak of infection with hepatitis C virus in recipients of anti-D immunoglobulin. Lancet 1995; 345:1211.
58. Webster ADB, Lever AML. Non-A, non-B hepatitis after intravenous gammaglobulin. Lancet 1986; 1:322.
59. Ochs HD, Fischer SH, Virant FS, et al. Non-A, non-B hepatitis after intravenous gammaglobulin. Lancet 1986; 1:322.
60. Lee M, Courter S, Tai D, et al. A long term evaluation of an intravenous immunoglobulin preparation (Gammagard) with regard to non-A, non-B hepatitis safety. J Med Virol 1987; 21:44.
61. Björklander J, Cunningham-Rundles C, Lundin P, et al. Intravenous immunoglobulin prophylaxis causing liver damage in 16 of 77 patients with hypogammaglobulinemia or IgG subclass deficiency. Am J Med 1988; 84:107.
62. Williams PE, Yap PL, Gillon J, et al. Transmission of non-A, non-B hepatitis by pH 4–treated intravenous immunoglobulin. Vox Sang 1989; 57:15.
63. Bresee JS, Mast EE, Coleman PJ, et al. Hepatitis C virus infection associated with administration of intravenous immune globulin: a cohort study. JAMA 1996; 276:1563.
64. Finlayson JS, Tankersley DL. Anti-HCV screening and plasma fractionation: the case against. Lancet 1990; 335:1274.
65. Yei S, Yu MW, Tankersley DL. Partitioning of hepatitis C virus during Cohn-Oncley fractionation of plasma. Transfusion 1992; 32:824.
66. Yu MW, Mason BL, Guo ZP, et al. Hepatitis C transmission associated with intravenous immunoglobulins. Lancet 1995; 345:1173.
67. Cohn EJ, Strong LE, Hughes WL Jr, et al. Preparation and properties of serum and plasma proteins IV: a system for the separation into fractions of the protein and lipoprotein components of biological tissues and fluids. J Am Chem Soc 1946; 68:459.
68. Oncley JL, Melin M, Richert DA, et al. The separation of the antibodies, isoaggulinins, prothrombin, plasminogen and b-lipoprotein into subfractions of human plasma. J Am Chem Soc 1949; 71:541.

69. Kistler P, Nitschmann H. Large scale production of human plasma fractions. Vox Sang 1962; 7:414.
70. Pennell RB. The distribution of certain viruses in the fractionation of plasma. *In* Hartman FW, LoGrippo GA, Mateer JG, Barron J (eds): Hepatitis Frontiers. Boston; Little, Brown, 1957, pp 297–310.
71. Holland PV, Alter HJ, Purcell RH, et al. Hepatitis B antigen (HB Ag) and antibody (anti–HB Ag) in cold ethanol fractions of human plasma. Transfusion 1972; 12:363.
72. Trepa C, Hantz O, Jacquier MF, et al. Different fates of hepatitis B virus markers during plasma fractionation. Vox Sang 1978; 35:143.
73. Mitra G, Wong MF, Mozen M, et al. Elimination of infectious retroviruses during preparation of human plasma fractions. Transfusion 1986; 26:39.
74. Morgenthaler J-J, Omar A. Partitioning and inactivation of viruses during isolation of albumin and immunoglobulins by cold ethanol fractionation. Dev Biol Stand 1993; 81:185.
75. Morgenthaler J-J. Effect of ethanol on viruses. *In* Morgenthaler J-J (ed): Virus Inactivation in Plasma Products. Basel: Karger, 1989, pp 109–121.
76. Henin Y, Marechal V, Barre-Sinoussi F, et al. Inactivation and partition of human immunodeficiency virus during Kistler and Nitschmann fractionation of human blood plasma. Vox Sang 1988; 54:78.
77. Zuck TF, Preston MS, Tankersley DL, et al. More on partitioning and inactivation of AIDS virus in immune globulin preparations. N Engl J Med 1986; 314:1454.
78. Scheiblauer H, Nubling M, Willkommen H, Lower J. Prevalence of hepatitis C virus in plasma pools and the effectiveness of cold ethanol fractionation. Clin Ther 1996; 18(suppl B):59.
79. Murray R, Diefenbach WCL. Effect of heat on the agent of homologous serum hepatitis. Proc Soc Exp Biol Med 1953; 84:230.
80. Murray R, Diefenbach WCL, Geller H, et al. The problem of reducing the danger of serum hepatitis from blood and blood products. N Y State J Med 1955; 55:1145.
81. Pennell RB. The distribution of certain viruses in the fractionation of plasma. *In* Hartman FW, LoGrippo GA, Matteer JG, Barron J (eds): Hepatitis Frontiers. Little, Brown, 1957, pp 297–310.
82. Barker LF, Murray R. Relationship of virus dose to incubation time of clinical hepatitis and time of appearance of hepatitis-associated antigen. Am J Med Sci 1971; 263:27.
83. Piszkiewicz D, Kingdom H, Apfelzweig R, et al. Inactivation of HTLV-III/LAV during plasma fractionation. Lancet 1985; 2:118.
84. Wells MA, Wittek AE, Epstein JS, et al. Inactivation and partition of human T-cell lymphotrophic virus, type III, during ethanol fractionation of plasma. Transfusion 1986; 26:2103.
85. Murray R, Ratner F. Safety of immune serum globulin with respect to homologous serum hepatitis. Proc Soc Exp Biol Med 1953; 84:230.
86. Hoofnagle JH, Wagonner JG. Hepatitis A and B markers in immune serum globulin. Gastroenterology 1980; 78:259.
87. Tankersley DL, Mason BL, Guo Z-P, Yu MW. Viral safety of intravenous immunoglobulin. *In* Kazatchkine MD, Morell A (eds): Intravenous Immunoglobulin: Research and Therapy. New York: Parthenon, 1996, pp 3–9.
88. Burnouf T. Chromatographic removal of viruses from plasma derivatives. Dev Biol Stand 1993; 81:199.
89. Manucci PM, Colombo M. Virucidal treatment of clotting factor concentrates. Lancet 1988; 2:782.
90. Suomela H, Myllylä G, Raaska E. Preparation and properties of a therapeutic factor IX concentrate. Vox Sang 1977; 33:37.
91. Prince AM, Stephan W, Brotman B. β-propiolactone/ultraviolet irradiation: a review of its effectiveness for inactivation of viruses in blood derivatives. Rev Infect Dis 1983; 5:92107.
92. Schreiber AB, Hriuda ME, Newman J, et al. Removal of viral contaminants by monoclonal antibody purification of plasma proteins. Curr Stud Hematol Blood Transfus 1989; 56:146.
93. Kim HC, McMillan CW, White GC, et al. Purified factor IX using monoclonal immunoaffinity technique: clinical trials in hemophilia B and comparison to prothrombin complex concentrates. Blood 1992; 79:568.
94. Hamman J, Zou J, Horowitz B. Removal and inactivation of hepatitis A virus (HAV) during processing of factor VIII concentrates. Vox Sang 1994; 67(suppl 1):72.
95. Lemon SM, Murphy PC, Smith A, et al. Removal/neutralization of hepatitis A virus during manufacture of high purity, solvent/detergent factor VIII concentrate. J Med Virol 1994; 43:44.
96. Hamamoto Y, Harada S, Kobayashi S, et al. A novel method for removal of human immunodeficiency virus: filtration with porous polymeric membranes. Vox Sang 1989; 56:230.
97. Oshima KH, Evans-Strickfaden TT, Highsmith AK, Ades EW. The use of a microporous polyvinylidene fluoride (PVDF) membrane filter to separate contaminating viral particles from biologically important proteins. Biologicals 1996; 24:137.
98. DiLeo AJ, Allegrezza AE Jr, Builder SE. High resolution removal of virus from protein solutions using a membrane of unique structure. Biotechnology (N Y) 1992; 10:182.
99. Meltzer TH. The significance of sieve-retention to the filter validation process. PDA J Pharm Sci Technol 1995; 49:188.
100. Roberts P. Efficient removal of viruses by a novel polyvinylidene fluoride membrane filter. J Virol Methods 1997; 65:27.
101. O'Grady J, Losikoff A, Poiley J, et al. Virus removal studies using nanofiltration membranes. Dev Biol Stand 1996; 88:319.
102. Burnouf-Radosevich M, Appourchaux P, Huart JJ, Burnouf T. Nanofiltration, a new specific virus elimination method applied to high-purity factor IX and factor XI concentrates. Vox Sang 1994; 67:132.
103. Eibl J, Barrett N, Hammerle T, Dorner F. Nanofiltration of immunoglobulin with 35-nm filters fails to remove substantial amounts of HCV. Biologicals 1996; 24:285.
104. Gardner JF, Peel MM. Introduction to Sterilization and Disinfection. New York: Churchill Livingstone, 1986.
105. Pattison CP, Klein CA, Leger RT, et al. An outbreak of type B hepatitis associated with transfusion of plasma protein fraction. Am J Epidemiol 1976; 103:398.
106. Pattison CP, Klein CA, Leger RT, et al. Field studies of type B hepatitis associated with transfusion of plasma protein fraction. *In* Sgouris JT, Renee A (eds): Proceedings of the Workshop on Albumin. Bethesda, MD: National Institutes of Health, 1976, pp 315–319.
107. Soulier J-P, Blatix C, Courouce AM, et al. Prevention of virus B hepatitis (SH hepatitis). Am J Dis Child 1972; 123:429.
108. Heimburger N, Karges HE. Strategies to produce virus-free blood derivatives. Curr Stud Hematol Blood Transfus 1989; 56:23.
109. Horowitz B, Wiebe ME, Lippin A, et al. Inactivation of viruses in labile blood derivatives: II. Physical methods. Transfusion 1985; 25:5237.
110. Kreuz W, Brackmann HH, Auerswald G, et al. Absence of hepatitis after treatment with a pasteurized factor VIII. N Engl J Med 1987; 316:918.
111. Schimpf K, Brackmann HH, Kreuz W, et al. Absence of anti-human immunodeficiency virus types 1 and 2 seroconversion after the treatment of hemophilia A and B or von Willebrand's disease with pasteurized factor VIII concentrate. N Engl J Med 1989; 321:1148.
112. Mannucci PM, Schimpf K, Brettler DB, et al. Low risk for hepatitis in hemophiliacs given a high-purity, pasteurized factor VIII concentrate. The International Study Group. Ann Intern Med 1990; 113:27.
113. Kreuz W, Auerswald G, Bruckmann C, et al. Prevention of hepatitis C virus infection in children with hemophilia A and B and von Willebrand's disease. Thromb Haemost 1992; 67:184.
114. Brackmann HH, Egli H. Acute hepatitis B infection after treatment with heat-inactivated factor VIII concentrate. Lancet 1988; 2:967.
115. Schulman S, Lindgren ACH, Petrini P, Allander T. Transmission of hepatitis C with pasteurized factor VIII. Lancet 1992; 2:305.
116. Gerritzen A, Schneweis KE, Scholt B, et al. Acute hepatitis C in hemophiliacs due to virus inactivated clotting factor concentrates. Thromb Haemost 1992; 68:781.
117. Azzi A, Ciappi S, Zakvrezeska K, et al. Human parvovirus B19 infection in hemophiliacs first infused with two high-purity virally attenuated factor VIII concentrates. Am J Hemat 1992; 39:228.
118. Spire B, Dormont D, Barre-Sinoussi F, et al. Inactivation of lymphadenopathy-associated virus by heat, gamma rays and ultraviolet light. Lancet 1985; 1:1889.
119. McDougal JS, Martin LS, Cort SP, et al. Thermal inactivation of the acquired immunodeficiency syndrome virus, human T lymphotrophic virus–III/lymphadenopathy–associated virus, with special reference to antihemophilic factor. J Clin Invest 1985; 76:8757.

120. Quinnan GV Jr, Wells MA, Wittek AE, et al. Inactivation of human T-cell lymphotrophic virus, type III by heat, chemicals and irradiation. Transfusion 1986; 26:4813.
121. Lush CJ, Chapman CS, Mitchell VE, Martin C. Transmission of hepatitis B by dry-heat treated factor VIII and IX concentrates. Br J Haematol 1988; 69:421.
122. Blanchette VS, Vorstman E, Shore A, et al. Hepatitis C infection in children with hemophilia A and B. Blood 1991; 78:285.
123. Pistello M, Leccherini-Nelli L, Cecconi N, et al. Hepatitis C virus prevalence in Italian hemophiliacs infected with virus-inactivated concentrates: 5-year follow-up and correlation with antibodies to other viruses. J Med Virol 1991; 33:43.
124. Mariani G, Ghirardini A, Mandelli F, et al. Heated clotting factor and seroconversion for human immunodeficiency virus in three hemophiliac patients. Ann Intern Med 1987; 107:113.
125. Centers for Disease Control. Safety of therapeutic products used for hemophilia patients. MMWR 1988; 37:441.
126. Dietrich SL, Mosley JW, Lusher JM, et al. The Transfusion Safety Study Group. Transmission of human immunodeficiency virus type 1 by dry-heated clotting factor concentrates. Vox Sang 1990; 59:129.
127. Remis RJ, O'Shaughnessy MV, Tsoukas C, et al. HIV transmission to patients with hemophilia by heat-treated, donor-screened factor concentrates. Can Med Assoc J 1990; 142:1247.
128. Piszkiewicz D, Thomas W, Lieu MY, et al. Virus inactivation by heat treatment of lyophilized coagulation factor concentrates. Curr Stud Hematol Blood Transfus 1989; 56:44.
129. Winkelman L, Owen NE, Evans DR, et al. Severely heated therapeutic factor VIII concentrate of high specific activity. Vox Sang 1989; 57:97.
130. Colvin BT, Rizza CR, Hill FGH, et al. Effect of dry-heating of coagulation factor concentrates at 80°C for 72 hours on transmission of non-A, non-B hepatitis. Lancet 1988; 2:814.
131. Skidmore SJ, Pasi KJ, Mawson SJ, et al. Serological evidence that dry-heating of clotting factor concentrates prevents transmission of non-A, non-B hepatitis. J Med Virol 1990; 30:50.
132. Bennett B, Dawson AA, Gibson BS, et al. Study of viral safety of the Scottish National Blood Transfusion Service factor VIII/IX concentrates. Transfus Med 1993; 3:295.
133. Hart HF, Hart WG, Crossley J, et al. Effect of terminal (dry) heat treatment on non-enveloped viruses in coagulation factor concentrates. Vox Sang 1994; 67:345.
134. Williams MD, Cohen BJ, Beddall AC, et al. Transmission of human parvovirus B19 by coagulation factor concentrates. Vox Sang 1990; 58:177.
135. Lyon DJ, Chapman CS, Martin C, et al. Symptomatic parvovirus B19 infection and heat treated factor IX concentrate. Lancet 1989; 1:1085.
136. Yee TT, Lee CA, Pasi KJ. Life-threatening human parvovirus B19 infection in immunocompetent haemophilia. Lancet 1995; 345:795.
137. Rubenstein, AI, Rubenstein DB, Coughlin J. Combined solvent-detergent and 100°C (boiling) sterilizing dry-heat treatment of factor VIII concentrates to assure sterility. Vox Sang 1991;60:60
138. Arrighi S, Rossi R, Borri MG, et al. "In vitro" and in animal model studies on a double virus-inactivated factor VIII concentrate. Thromb Haemost 1995; 74:868.
139. Santagostino E, Mannucci PM, Gringeri A, et al. Eliminating parvovirus B19 from blood products. Lancet 1994; 343:798.
140. Mannucci PM, Zanetti AR, Colombo M. Prospective study of hepatitis after factor VIII concentrate exposed to hot vapour. Br J Haematol 1988; 68:427.
141. Mannucci PM, Schimpf K, Abe T, et al. Low risk of viral infection after administration of vapour heated factor VIII concentrates. Transfusion 1992; 32:134.
142. Shapiro A, Abe T, Aledort LM, et al. Low risk of viral infection after administration of vapor-heated factor VII concentrate or factor IX complex in first-time recipients of blood components. International Factor Safety Study Group. Transfusion 1995; 35:204.
143. Barrett PN, Meyer H, Wachtel I, et al. Inactivation of hepatitis A virus in plasma products by vapor heating. Transfusion 1997; 37:215.
144. Kernouf PBA, Miller EJ, Savidge GF, et al. Reduced risk of non-A, non-B hepatitis after first exposure to 'wet heated' factor VIII concentrate. Br J Hemat 1987; 67:207.
145. Carnelli V, Gomperts ED, Friedman A. Assessment for evidence of non-A, non-B hepatitis in patients given n-heptane suspended heat-treated clotting factor concentrates. Thromb Res 1987; 46:827.
146. White DO, Fenner F. Medical Virology. New York: Academic Press, 1986.
147. Martin LS, McDougal JS, Loskoski SL. Disinfection and inactivation of the human T lymphotrophic virus type III/lymphadenopathy–associated virus. J Infect Dis 1985; 152:400.
148. Spire B, Barre-Sinoussi F, Montagnier L, Chermann JC. Inactivation of lymphadenopathy-associated virus by chemical disinfectants. Lancet 1984; 2:899.
149. Martin LS, Loskoski SL, McDougal JS. Inactivation of human T-lymphotrophic virus type III/lymphadenopathy–associated virus by formaldehyde-based reagents. Appl Environ Microbiol 1987; 53:70.
150. Tabor E, Gerety RJ. Inactivation of an agent of human non-A, non-B hepatitis by formalin. J Infect Dis 1980; 142:767.
151. Feinstone S, Mihalik KB, Kamimura T, et al. Inactivation of hepatitis B virus and non-A, non-B hepatitis by chloroform. Infect Immunol 1983; 41:816.
152. Prince AM, Horowitz B, Brotman B, et al. Inactivation of hepatitis B and Hutchinson strain non-A, non-B hepatitis viruses by exposure to Tween 80 and ether. Vox Sang 1984; 46:36.
153. Horowitz B, Wiebe ME, Lippin A, Stryker MH. Inactivation of viruses in labile blood derivatives I: disruption of lipid-enveloped viruses by tri(n-butyl)phosphate–detergent combinations. Transfusion 1985; 25:516.
154. Prince AM, Horowitz B, Brotman B. Sterilization of hepatitis and HTLV-III viruses by exposure to tri(n-butyl)phosphate and sodium cholate. Lancet 1986; 1:706.
155. Stephan W. Inactivation of hepatitis viruses and HIV in plasma and plasma derivatives by treatment with β-propiolactone/UV irradiation. *In* Morgenthaler J-J (ed): Virus Inactivation in Plasma Products. Basel: Karger, 1989, pp 12–27.
156. Horowitz B. Investigations into the application of tri(n-butyl)phosphate–detergent mixtures to blood derivatives. *In* Morgenthaler J-J (ed): Virus Inactivation in Plasma Products. Basel: Karger, 1989, pp 83–96.
157. Horowitz B, Prince AM, Horowitz MS, Watklevicz C. Viral safety of solvent-detergent treated blood products. Dev Biol Stand 1993; 81:147.
158. Horowitz B, Prince AM, Hamman J, Watklevicz C. Viral safety of solvent/detergent–treated blood products. Blood Coagul Fibrinolysis 1994; 5(suppl 3):S21.
159. Edwards CA, Piet MPJ, Chin S, et al. Tri(n-butyl)phosphate–detergent treatment of licensed therapeutic and experimental blood derivatives. Vox Sang 1987; 52:539.
160. Horowitz MS, Rooks C, Horowitz B, Hilgartner MW. Virus safety of solvent/detergent–treated antihaemophilic factor concentrate. Lancet 1988; 2:1869.
161. Piet MPJ, Chin S, Prince AM, et al. The use of tri(n-butyl)phosphate–detergent mixtures to inactivate hepatitis viruses and human immunodeficiency virus in plasma and plasma's subsequent fractionation. Transfusion 1990; 30:5918.
162. Horowitz B, Bonomo R, Prince AM, et al. Solvent/detergent–treated plasma: a virus-inactivated substitute for fresh frozen plasma. Blood 1992; 79:826.
163. Hellstern P, Sachse H, Schwinn H, Oberfrank K. Manufacture and in vitro characterization of a solvent/detergent–treated human plasma. Vox Sang 1992; 63:178.
164. Keeling DM, Luddington R, Allain JP, et al. Cryoprecipitate prepared from plasma virally inactivated by the solvent detergent method. Br J Haematol 1997; 96:194.
165. Lambrecht B, Mohr H, Knuver-Hopf J, Schmitt H. Photoinactivation of viruses in human fresh plasma by phenothiazine dyes in combination with visible light. Vox Sang 1991; 60:207.
166. LoGrippo GA, Hartmann FW. Chemical and combined methods for plasma sterilization. Bibl Haematol 1958; 7:225.
167. Prince AM, Stephan W, Dichtelmueller H, et al. Inactivation of the Hutchinson strain of non-A, non-B hepatitis virus by combined use of β-propiolactone and ultraviolet irradiation. J Med Virol 1985; 16:119.
168. Klein JP, Bailly E, Schneweis KE, et al. Acute HIV-1 infection in patients with hemophilia B treated with beta-propiolactone UV-inactivated clotting factor. Thromb Haemost 1990; 64:336.

169. Highsmith F, Xue H, Chen X, et al. Iodine-mediated inactivation of lipid- and nonlipid-enveloped viruses in human antithrombin III concentrate. Blood 1995; 86:791.
170. Highsmith FA, Xue H, Caple M, et al. Inactivation of lipid-enveloped and non–lipid-enveloped model viruses in normal human plasma by crosslinked starch-iodine. Transfusion 1994; 34(4):322.
171. Kempf C, Jentsch P, Poirier B, et al. Virus inactivation during production of intravenous immunoglobulin. Transfusion 1991; 31:423.
172. Louie RE, Galloway CJ, Dumas ML, et al. Inactivation of hepatitis C virus in low pH intravenous immunoglobulin. Biologicals 1994; 22:13.
173. Thomas FC, Davies AG, Dulac GC, et al. Gamma ray–inactivation of some animal viruses. Can J Comp Med 1981; 45:39.
174. Ginoza W. Inactivation of viruses by ionizing radiation and by heat. *In* Maramorosch K, Koprowski H (eds): Methods in Virology, vol IV. New York: Academic Press, 1968, pp 139–179.
175. Horowitz B, Piet MPJ, Prince AM, et al. Inactivation of lipid-enveloped viruses in labile blood derivatives by unsaturated fatty acids. Vox Sang 1988; 54:14.
176. Kitchen AD, Mann GF, Harrison JF, Zuckerman AJ. Effect of gamma irradiation on the human immunodeficiency virus and human coagulation proteins. Vox Sang 1989; 56:22.
177. Hiemstra H, Tersmette M, Vox AHV, et al. Inactivation of human immunodeficiency virus by gamma radiation and its effect on plasma and coagulation factors. Transfusion 1991; 31:3.
178. Kochevar IE. Photobiology. Dermatol Clin 1986; 4:17.
179. Jagger J. Introduction to Research in Ultraviolet Photobiology. Englewood Cliffs, NJ: Prentice-Hall, 1967.
180. Cadet J, Voituriez L, Grand A, et al. Recent aspects of the photochemistry of nucleic acid and related model compounds. Biochimie 1985; 67:277.
181. Webb RB. Lethal and mutagenic effects of near-ultraviolet radiation. *In* Smith KC (ed): Photochemical and Photobiological Reviews. New York: Plenum Press, 1991, pp 169–261.
182. Kittler L, Lober G. Photochemistry of the nucleic acids. *In* Smith KC (ed): Photochemical and Photobiological Reviews, vol 1. New York: Plenum Press, 1991, pp 39–132.
183. McLaren AD, Shugar D. Photochemistry of Proteins and Nucleic Acids. New York: Macmillan, 1964.
184. Chang JCH, Ossoff SF, Lobe DC, et al. UV inactivation of pathogenic and indicator microorganisms. Appl Environ Microbiol 1985; 49:1361.
185. Kallenbach NR, Cornelius PA, Negus D, et al. Inactivation of viruses by ultraviolet light. *In* Morgenthaler J-J (ed): Virus Inactivation in Plasma Products. Basel: Karger, 1989, pp 70–82.
186. Rauth AM. The physical state of viral nucleic acid and the sensitivity of viruses to ultraviolet light. Biophys J 1965; 5:257.
187. Prodouz KN, Fratantoni JC, Boone EJ, Bonner RF. Use of laser-UV for inactivation of virus in blood products. Blood 1987; 70:589.
188. Snyder E, Beardsley D, Smith B, et al. Storage of platelet concentrate after ultraviolet B irradiation. Transfusion 1991; 31:491.
189. The Trial to Reduce Alloimmunization to Platelets Study Group. Leukocyte reduction and ultraviolet B irradiation of platelets to prevent alloimmunization and refractoriness to platelet transfusions. N Engl J Med 1997; 337:1861.
190. Chin S, Williams B, Gottlieb P, et al. Virucidal short wavelength ultraviolet light treatment of plasma and factor VIII concentrate: protection of proteins by antioxidants. Blood 1995; 86:4331.
191. Marx G, Mou X, Freed R, et al. Protecting fibrinogen with rutin during UVC irradiation for viral inactivation. Photochem Photobiol 1996; 63:541.
192. Chin S, Jin R, Wang XL, et al. Virucidal treatment of blood protein products with UVC radiation. Photochem Photobiol 1997; 65:432.
193. Ben-Hur E, Moor ACE, Margolis-Nunno H, et al. The photodecontamination of cellular blood components: mechanisms and use of photosensitization in transfusion medicine. Trans Med Rev 1996; 10:15.
194. Kochevar IE. Basic concepts in photobiology. *In* Parrish JA (ed): Photoimmunology. New York: Plenum Press, 1983, pp 257–265.
195. Spikes JD. Photosensitization in mammalian cells. *In* Parrish JA (ed): Photoimmunology. New York: Plenum Press, 1983, pp 23–49.
196. Kessel D. Hematoporphyrin and HPD: photophysics, photochemistry and phototherapy. Photochem Photobiol 1948; 39:851.
197. Hanson CV, Riggs JL, Lennette EH. Photochemical inactivation of DNA and RNA viruses by psoralen derivatives. J Gen Virol 1978; 40:345.
198. Song PS, Tapley KJ Jr. Photochemistry and photobiology of psoralens. Photochem Photobiol 1979; 29:117.
199. Moreno G. Cell photosensitization by psoralens and porphyrins. *In* Bensasson RV, Jori G, Land EJ, Truscott TG (eds): Primary photoprocesses in biology and medicine. New York: Plenum Press, 1985, pp 37–80.
200. Parrish JA, Fitzpatrick TB, Tannenbaum L, Pathak MA. Photochemotherapy of psoriasis with oral methoxypsoralen and long-wave ultraviolet light. N Engl J Med 1974; 291:120.
201. Edelson R, Berger C, Gasparro F, et al. Treatment of cutaneous T-cell lymphoma by extracorporeal photochemotherapy. N Engl J Med 1987; 316:297.
202. Isaacs ST, Shen CKJ, Hearst JE, Rapoport H. Synthesis and characterization of new psoralen derivatives with superior photoreactivity with DNA and RNA. Biochemistry 1977; 16:105.
203. Watson AJ, Klaniecki J, Hanson CV. Psoralen/UV inactivation of HIV-1–infected cells for use in cytologic and immunologic procedures. AIDS Res Hum Retroviruses 1990; 6:50.
204. Lin L, Wiesehahn GP, Morel PA, Corash L. Use of 8-methoxypsoralen and long-wavelength ultraviolet for decontamination of platelet concentrates. Blood 1989; 74:517.
205. Lin L, Londe H, Hanson CV, et al. Photochemical inactivation of cell-associated human immunodeficiency virus in platelet concentrates. Blood 1993; 82:292.
206. Lin L, Cook DN, Wiesehahn GP, et al. Photochemical inactivation of viruses and bacteria in platelet concentrates by use of a novel psoralen and long-wavelength ultraviolet light. Transfusion 1997; 37:423.
207. Matthews JL, Newman JT, Sogandares-Bernal F, et al. Photodynamic therapy of viral contaminants with potential for blood banking applications. Transfusion 1988; 28:813.
208. Matthews JL, Sogandares-Bernal F, Judy MM, et al. Preliminary studies of photoinactivation of human immunodeficiency virus in blood. Transfusion 1991; 31:636.
209. Richter AM, Kell B, Chow J, et al. Preliminary studies on a more effective phototoxic agent than hematoporphyrin. J Natl Cancer Inst 1987; 19:1327.
210. Richter AM, Waterfield E, Jain A, et al. In vitro evaluation of phototoxic properties of four structurally related benzoporphyrin derivatives. Photochem Photobiol 1990; 52:495.
211. Neyndorff HC, Bartel DL, Tufaro F, Levy JG. Development of a model to demonstrate photosensitizer-mediated viral inactivation in blood. Transfusion 1990; 30:485.
212. Prodouz KN, Lytle CD, Keville EA, et al. Inhibition by albumin of merocyanine 540–mediated photosensitization of platelets and viruses. Transfusion 1991; 31:415.
213. van Lier JE. New sensitizers for photodynamic therapy of cancer. *In* Douglas RH (ed): Light in Biology and Medicine, vol 1. New York: Plenum Press, 1988, pp 133–141.
214. Spikes JD. Phthalocyanines as photosensitizers in biological systems and for the photodynamic therapy of tumors. Photochem Photobiol 1986; 43:691.
215. Horowitz B, Williams B, Rywkin S, et al. Inactivation of viruses in blood with aluminum phthalocyanine derivatives. Transfusion 1991; 31:10.
216. Schnipper LE, Lewin AA, Swartz M, Crumpacker CS. Mechanisms of photodynamic inactivation of herpes simplex viruses. J Clin Invest 1980; 65:432.
217. Walis C, Melnick JL. Photodynamic inactivation of animal viruses: a review. Photochem Photobiol 1965; 4:159.
218. Wagner SJ, Storry J, Mallory D, et al. Red cell surface alterations resulting from virucidal photochemical treatment. Photochem Photobiol 1991; 53(suppl):54s.
219. Klein-Struckmeier A, Mohr H. Photodynamic virus inactivation of thrombocyte concentrates by phenothiazine dyes. Beitr Infusionsther Transfusionsmed 1997; 34:43.
220. Mohr H, Lambrecht B, Knuver-Hopf J. Virus inactivated single-donor fresh plasma preparations. Infusionsther Transfusionsmed 1992; 19:79.
221. Wieding JU, Hellstern P, Kohler M. Inactivation of viruses in fresh-frozen plasma. Ann Hematol 1993; 67:259.
222. Williamson LM, Allain JP. Virally inactivated fresh frozen plasma. Vox Sang 1995; 69:159.

223. Mohr H, Bachmann B, Klein-Struckmeier A, Lambrecht B. Virus inactivation of blood products by phenothiazine dyes and light. Photochem Photobiol 1997; 65:441.
224. Mohr H, Lambrecht B, Schmitt H. Photo-inactivation of viruses in therapeutical plasma. Dev Biol Stand 1993; 81:177.
225. Lambrecht B, Norley SG, Kurth R, Mohr H. Rapid inactivation of HIV-1 in single donor preparations of human fresh frozen plasma by methylene blue/light treatment. Biologicals 1994; 22:227.
226. Zeiler T, Riess H, Wittmann G, et al. The effect of methylene blue phototreatment on plasma proteins and in vitro coagulation capability of single-donor fresh-frozen plasma. Transfusion 1994; 34:685.
227. Mohr H, Knuver-Hopf J, Lambrecht B, et al. No evidence for neoantigens in human plasma after photochemical virus inactivation. Ann Hematol 1992; 65:224.
228. Tissot JD, Hochstrasser DF, Schneider B, et al. No evidence for protein modifications in fresh frozen plasma after photochemical treatment: an analysis by high-resolution two-dimensional electrophoresis. Br J Haematol 1994; 86:143.
229. Wagner SJ, Skripchenko A, Robinette D, et al. Factors affecting virus photoinactivation by a series of phenothiazine dyes. Photochem Photobiol 1998; 67:343.
230. Wickramanayake GB. Disinfection and sterilization by ozone. *In* Block SS (ed): Disinfection, Sterilization and Preservation. Philadelphia: Lea & Febiger, 1991, pp 182–190.
231. Vaughn JM, Chen YS, Novotny JF, Strout D. Effects of ozone treatment on the infectivity of hepatitis A virus. Can J Microbiol 1990; 36:557.
232. Herbold K, Flehmig B, Botzenhart K. Comparison of ozone inactivation, in flowing water, of hepatitis A virus, poliovirus, and indicator organisms. Appl Environ Microbiol 1989; 55:2949.
233. Wagner K, Mayers D, Toro L, Baker JR Jr. The effect of ozone on lymphocyte populations in normal and HIV-1–infected blood [Abstract]. Int Conf AIDS 1990, p 656.
234. Wells KH, Latino J, Gavalchin J, Poiesz BJ. Inactivation of human immunodeficiency virus type I by ozone in vitro. Blood 1991; 78:1882.
235. Wagner SJ, Wagner K, Friedman L, Benade LE. Virucidal levels of ozone induce hemolysis and hemoglobin degradation. Transfusion 1991; 31:748.
236. Wagner SJ, Friedman L, Dodd RY. Approaches to the reduction of viral infectivity in cellular blood components and single donor plasma. Transfus Med Rev 1991; 5:18.
237. Stromberg R, Cole M, Sadoff BJ, et al. Viral depletion in red cells by cell washing [Abstract]. *In* Proceedings of the ISBT/American Association of Blood Banks. International Society of Blood Transfusion, 1990, p 196.
238. Rawal BD, Busch MP, Endow R. Reduction of human immunodeficiency virus–infected cells from donor blood by leukocyte filtration. Transfusion 1989; 29:460.
239. Rawal BD, Yen TSB, Vyas GN, Busch MP. Leukocyte filtration removes infectious particulate debris but not free virus derived from experimentally lysed HIV-infected cells. Vox Sang 1991; 60:21.
240. Sadoff BJ, Stromberg R, Miller K, et al. Experimental 6 $\log_{10}$ white cell-reduction filters for red cells. Transfusion 1992; 32:129.
241. Bowden RA, Slichter SJ, Sayers M, et al. A comparison of filtered leukocyte-reduced and cytomegalovirus (CMV) seronegative blood products for the prevention of transfusion-associated CMV infection after marrow transplant. Blood 1995; 86:3598.
242. Peerlinck K, Arnout J, Di Giambattista M, et al. Factor VIII inhibitors in previously treated haemophilia A patients with a double virus-inactivated plasma derived factor VIII concentrate. Thromb Haemost 1997; 77:80.
243. Zmusdzka BZ, Beer JZ. Activation of human immunodeficiency virus by ultraviolet irradiation. Photochem Photobiol 1991; 52:1153.
244. Zmudzka BZ, Strickland AG, Beer JZ, Ben-Hur E. Photosensitized decontamination of blood with the silicon phthalocyanine Pc 4: no activation of the human immunodeficiency virus promoter. Photochem Photobiol 1997; 65:461.

CHAPTER 43

Somatic Gene Therapy

Kenneth Cornetta
Thomas Moritz
David A. Williams

After the introduction of recombinant DNA technology into medicine, the 1980s and 1990s were a period of enormous growth in the understanding of the fundamental biology that defines a wide variety of diseases at the molecular level. An expanding number of inherited diseases have been shown to arise from single gene mutations, and the ability to diagnose these diseases early at the molecular level is rapidly increasing (Table 43–1). For many diseases, a complementary DNA (cDNA) sequence of the causative gene has been cloned. In addition, for diseases not clearly inherited, such as malignancies and acquired immune deficiency syndrome (AIDS), the molecular mechanisms underlying these fatal disorders have become clearer. Many of the genes involved in the pathogenesis of clinically significant diseases are now cloned, and theoretically, there exists a method for introducing the functional counterparts of these genes into mammalian cells. This progress in the understanding of disease at the molecular level has generated increasing interest and greater efforts to establish gene therapy as a treatment modality.

Since the late 1980s, advances in technology have allowed the first use of gene transfer technology in human studies. These studies include the first clinical safety studies with marker genes in humans; the first introduction of a therapeutic gene, adenosine deaminase (ADA), into lymphocytes of children suffering from severe combined immunodeficiency disease (SCID); and the use of "suicide" genes in T lymphocyte transductions to abrogate graft-versus-host disease. It is now clear that significant progress in transduction of repopulating hematopoietic stem cells in large animals has occurred. These advances have led to new enthusiasm for the ultimate goal of using gene transfer technology to treat human diseases. Overall progress in the field in the 1990s was incremental but consistent. The main forces behind this progress are (1) a refined recombinant DNA technology and increasing knowledge about the human genome, both promoted by the large-scale efforts of the human genome project; (2) greater accuracy of disease diagnosis at the molecular level, including prenatal diagnosis; and (3) significant progress in the field of cell biology, allowing infection of cells in vitro and transplantation of these cells into organisms in a functional state (ex vivo infection). This chapter gives an overview of principles, definitions, and methods relevant to gene therapy; describes retrovirus-mediated gene transfer, which is so far the standard technology for clinical gene transfer; summarizes the current achievements and problems encountered in the attempt to transfer genes to the human hematopoietic system (especially hematopoietic stem cells); discusses the current and potential future role of gene transfer in selected diseases, including current clinical gene therapy protocols; and discusses safety aspects of gene therapy.

PRINCIPLES, DEFINITIONS, AND METHODS

General Considerations for Gene Therapy

For the purpose of this chapter, *gene therapy* is defined as the introduction of new genetic material into the cells of an organism for therapeutic purposes. Genes may be introduced either into the whole organism, including the germ line, usually during the embryonic or fetal state, or

Table 43–1. Inherited Diseases Caused by Single Gene Defects*

Disease	Gene Defect
Chronic granulomatous disease	GP 91 phox, GP 22 phox, p47, p67
Cystic fibrosis	Cystic fibrosis transmembrane conductor
Fanconi's anemia	Fanconi's anemia group A and C complementing genes
Gaucher's disease	Glucocerebrosidase
Hemophilia	Factor IX, factor VIII
Hypercholesterolemia	Low-density lipoprotein (LDL) receptor
Immunodeficiency disease	Adenosine deaminase, purine nucleoside phosphorylase
Lesch-Nyhan syndrome	Hypoxanthineguanine phosphoribosyltransferase
Leukocyte adhesion deficiency	CD18
Mucopolysaccharidosis	β-glucuronidase
Muscular dystrophy	Dystrophin
Phenylketonuria	Phenylalanine hydroxylase
Sickle cell anemia	β globin
Thalassemia	β globin, α globin

*This table lists some inherited diseases for which cure through gene therapy may be possible and that are focuses of research. The table is not complete. In several diseases (e.g., Fanconi's anemia, chronic granulomatous disease), the listed gene is only one of several gene defects that may cause the disease.

only into a group of specialized somatic cells, usually in later life. In the former, called *germ line gene therapy*, the introduced genes would be passed on to subsequent generations and would be integrated into the common human gene pool, whereas in the latter, called *somatic gene therapy*, the presence of the introduced gene sequence is limited to the lifetime of an individual. Both forms are theoretically able to cure serious inherited diseases. Because of the experimental nature of the technique and the potential nonreversibility of germ line therapy, a moratorium on germ line therapy is in effect in the United States, and only somatic gene therapy is justified.

The ultimate goal of gene therapy for inherited diseases is replacement of a defective gene and advances in the ability to achieve targeting of gene sequences to specific sites of the mammalian genome by homologous recombination suggest that this aim may ultimately be achievable.[1, 2] In situ correction of a mutant gene might better ensure that the repaired gene would be adequately regulated by the *cis*-regulatory genetic elements required for its expression (promoter, enhancer, and intervening sequences). However, gene replacement is at present an impractical approach for clinical gene therapy. Currently available technology, particularly retrovirus-mediated gene transfer, leads to random integration of the gene of interest into the genome with reasonable efficiency. Thus an attractive alternative, at least for recessive disorders (which usually result from deficient protein activity), is the introduction of an appropriately regulated intact gene into a cell, without replacement of the defective gene. Because of the still rudimentary knowledge of the precise regulation of individual human genes and because of the size limitations of the currently available retroviral vectors (which transfer DNA sequence only up to the size of ~7 kb), only cDNAs lacking most *cis*-regulatory elements other than promoters have been used for gene transfer to date. In these vectors, enhancer elements that may be situated upstream, downstream, or within introns of the genes are missing. Obviously, this approach is imperfect by design, in as much as the introduced gene is not subject to normal regulation of expression. In addition, cell dysfunction caused by the remaining mutant gene may be problematic in some cases. Therefore, inherited disorders in which the defective gene requires a high degree of regulation for normal function, such as sickle cell anemia and the thalassemias, are at this time difficult to consider for curative gene therapy.

In view of the random integration of the introduced gene, disruption of an important gene or *cis*-regulatory elements of a gene may occur through the integration process of retrovirus vectors. The risk that the introduced gene sequences may integrate near an oncogene or a tumor suppressor gene and cause nonphysiological activation or inactivation of such genes and subsequent tumor formation (insertional mutagenesis) is a possibility that must be considered when safety aspects of retroviral gene transfer are discussed.

Initially, the pluripotent hematopoietic stem cell, with its capacity for long-term reconstitution and differentiation into a large variety of mature progeny, seemed to be the perfect target for gene therapy, and it obviously still holds much therapeutic promise. However, the low efficiency of gene transfer into this rare cell has generated interest in other target tissues. More differentiated hematopoietic progenitor cells, lymphocytes, liver cells, muscle cells, fibroblasts, lung epithelium, and even tumor cells as targets of manipulation have been the subjects of intensive research and have led to the first clinical studies performed in humans.[3–5]

Possible Applications of Gene Therapy

Although inherited diseases are the obvious targets for which somatic gene therapy holds the promise of cure, the wide variety of new options available for treatment with gene transfer has begun to affect many other fields of medicine. Only a few of the clinical trials that are being conducted or have been approved by the Recombinant Advisory Committee (RAC) of the National Institutes of Health (NIH) and the U.S. Food and Drug Administration (FDA) have dealt with inherited diseases. Many of the clinical trials to date are not aimed at therapy but rather use transfer of marker genes, usually neomycin phosphotransferase (NEO) or β-galactosidase (β-gal), in an effort to obtain new information about biological or pathological mechanisms. This approach is especially common with regard to normal or abnormal (leukemic) hematopoiesis. The purpose of these trials is to improve the understanding about hematopoietic stem cell biology, about clonal hematopoietic recovery after bone marrow transplantation, or about identification of the source of relapse after autologous bone marrow transplantation used as a therapy in hematological malignancies.

The use of gene therapy has reached clinical trials most often in oncology. The approach taken by several trials has been augmentation of host antitumor responses through overexpression of immunoregulatory cytokines or through genetic alteration of the tumor cell. Other approaches are to use gene transfer technology to make tumor cells more susceptible to specific drugs or make tumor cells susceptible to drugs that have no effect on other mammalian cells. Some strategies are more indirect and aim to reduce hematological side effects of chemotherapy by introducing drug resistance genes into hematopoietic progenitor and/or stem cells. This approach may allow further dose intensification in treatment protocols for drug-sensitive tumors. In the case of hematological malignancy (such as chronic myelogenous leukemia), the latter approach may be combined with selection for normal hematopoiesis, if it is possible to restrict the gene transfer to nonmalignant cells. Another disease for which the use of gene transfer technology is being considered is AIDS. Although at present no single gene transfer option is completely defined, several of the new approaches to this disease offer some long-term potential for therapy.

METHODS OF INTRODUCING DNA INTO CELLS

There are two principal approaches to introducing DNA into mammalian cells. One approach is to use different physical and chemical methods; the other is to use biological methods (i.e., different viral vectors).

Physical and Chemical Methods

A wide variety of physical and chemical methods have been established, leading to more or less efficient introduction of DNA into cells in vitro. Although some methods, such as calcium phosphate precipitation, liposome-mediated gene transfer, and electroporation, have important applications in generating vectors for gene transfer in the laboratory, only a few techniques appear directly applicable to somatic gene therapy, and none to date offers the efficiency of biological vectors. Nevertheless, both liposome-mediated gene transfer and electroporation have been envisioned by some researchers as means to transfer genes encoding antigens into human tumors. A more elaborate approach involves complexing DNA with polylysine, transferrin, and inactivated adenovirus, achieving transferrin receptor–mediated endocytosis of this complex, with subsequent endosome lysis by the adenovirus-inherited endosome disruption activity. Although the method allows incorporation of large pieces of DNA (up to 40 kb) into target cells, expression thus far has been only transient.[6, 7]

Biological (Virus-Based) Gene Transfer Systems

Table 43–2 summarizes viral vector systems and the advantages and limitations of each vector system.

Retrovirus-Based Vectors. The viruses most commonly used for vectors to date have been retroviruses. Retroviruses are the only vector system for which relatively extensive in vivo experience exists, and most human gene therapy protocols already in progess or approved by the RAC involve this vector system. To date, retrovirus vectors are usually based on the Moloney murine leukemia virus (MoMLV), although exciting new approaches with lentivirus and foamy virus vectors have been described and are in development (see Table 43–2).

Adeno-Associated Virus-Based Vectors. Adeno-associated virus (AAV) is a defective parvovirus that requires coinfection with a helper virus (adenovirus or herpesvirus) to undergo a complete reproductive cycle. AAV does not require helper virus to infect host cells, where it integrates in a site-specific manner and remains latent until the cells are superinfected with helper virus. AAV has a broad host range (e.g., human, monkey, mouse), is ubiquitous among humans, can be concentrated to very high infectious titers (10^6 to 10^9 units/mL), and seems to be a completely nonpathogenic integrating virus, all of which make it an attractive candidate vector system for gene therapy. Two further advantages of AAV over the retrovirus vector system, especially for infection of hematopoietic cells, are that the viral life cycle does not seem to require (although it prefers) actively cycling cells for integration and that packaging systems using lineage-specific adenovirus as helper virus have been developed, allowing lineage-specific infection and expression of the transferred gene. In the past, these systems have been hampered by poor expression, but vectors allowing high-level expression of the gene of interest in target cells in vitro have been developed.[8, 9] Other problems that are still associated with AAV-based vectors are (1) the restriction in size of the introduced sequence to less than 5 kb; (2) the rather low frequency of integration into the genome of primary cells; and (3) the difficulties in obtaining adenovirus-free helper virus stocks.[10]

Despite these problems, transduction of human CD34 positive cells from marrow, peripheral blood, and umbilical cord blood has been demonstrated by several groups by using marker or therapeutic genetic sequences.[11–13] As with other vector systems, however, unequivocally positive data on efficient transduction of long-lived stem cells are missing. Even for the well-characterized mouse system, only sporadic reports of relatively inefficient gene transfer into transplantable stem cells have been thus far published.[14]

Table 43–2. Properties of Various Viral Vectors

Property	Murine Retrovirus (MLV)	Adeno-Associated Virus (AAV)	Adenovirus	Herpesvirus	Lentivirus	Foamy Virus
Titer	10^6–10^7/mL	10^6–10^{12}/mL	10^{11}–10^{12}/mL	10^4–10^{10}/mL	10^6–10^8/mL; no stable producer lines	10^4–10^5/mL (wild type, 10^9/mL); no stable producer lines
Genome	RNA	ssDNA	dsDNA	dsDNA	RNA	RNA
Integration	Yes	Sometimes	No	No	Yes	Yes
Insert size	6–7 kb	2–4.5 kb	7–36 kb	10–100 kb	8–9 kb	9–10 kb
Cell proliferation	Requires mitosis	Prefers S phase	Not required	Not required	Not required but helpful	Not required but helpful
Helper virus pathogenicity	Potentially dangerous	Not pathogenic	Mild pathogen	Varies	Probably dangerous	Not pathogenic
Host response	Complement inactivates	?	Immunogenic and inflammatory	? (latency)	?	?

ss, single-stranded; ds, double-stranded.

Modified from Williams DA, Levitsky HI, Dinauer MD, Russell DW. Genetic Therapies in Hematology: Human Diseases, Educational Program, American Society of Hematology, 1997, p 71.

Herpesvirus-Based Vectors. Gene delivery systems involving defective herpes simplex type I (HSV-I) viruses have been described.[15] One obvious advantage of these vectors is the size of the HSV gene, which may allow packaging of much larger gene sequences (up to 100 kb) than are currently achievable with retroviral vectors. In addition, HSV infects nonreplicating cells and has a natural tropism for neuronal cells (e.g., neurons and glial cells), which makes this viral vector system an interesting option for attempts to deliver genes to the human central nervous system. To be useful for gene transfer, these vectors must address issues related to generation of helper-free virus stock, virus-induced cell toxicity, and stable transgene expression. These characteristics can potentially be achieved by deleting mutants of HSV, in which single or combined deletion of viral "immediate-early" genes, necessary for viral replication, lead to replication-defective vectors and, in addition, to a major reduction in cellular toxicity.[16, 17] The feasibility of such an approach in transduction of hematopoietic cells has been demonstrated.[18] The vector system may be well suited for situations in which high-level but transient expression of the transgene is needed.

Adenovirus-Based Vectors. Progress has been made in the use of an adenovirus-based vector system, which may be especially suited for infection of lung tissue. In addition to the capacity to infect nonreplicating cells in vivo, advantages of adenovirus-based vectors include their potential to carry very large DNA fragments (7 to 36 kb) as well as to generate very high titers (up to 10^{11} U/mL). From early studies, it is clear that the major blood lineages are relatively resistant to adenovirus infection; only CD34$^+$ progenitor cells or glycophorin A positive erythroid cells are permissive. Relatively high viral concentrations have been necessary to transduce clonogenic cells with up to 45% efficiency.[19, 20] Major problems with these vectors are uncertainty about long-term gene expression (especially as these vectors do not integrate into chromosomal DNA) and the fact that the adenovirus vectors still carry many adenovirus genes that have the potential for serious side effects in patients and elicit a rapid, strong immune response in humans. In addition, subsequent infection with wild-type adenovirus can reactivate a productive infection with recombinant vector.[21] Adenovirus vectors have been used in clinical trials targeting tumor cells in which inflammatory reaction may be beneficial.

Vectors Based on Other Viruses. Vectors based on simian virus 40 (SV40), bovine papillomavirus, *Vaccinia* virus, and other poxviruses have been investigated for gene therapy. All these systems still have major problems that have not been solved, and they currently have little use in the preclinical and clinical evaluation of gene therapy.

Non-Oncovirinae Retroviruses. In contrast to retroviruses of the Oncovirinae subfamily, lentiviruses such as human immunodeficiency virus type 1 (HIV-1) are capable of infecting noncycling cells (see Table 43–2). This capacity is conferred to lentiviruses at least in part by nuclear localization sequences present within the *gag* protein encoded by this virus, which allow the viral preintegration complex to pass through the intact nuclear membrane.[22] On the basis of these data, investigators have speculated that lentivirus vectors may allow the infection of noncycling cells, such as long-lived stem cells. Current lentivirus vectors are based on the genome of HIV-1, and initial constructs using the HIV-1 envelope protein were restricted in their tropism to CD4$^+$ cells. Like MoMLV-based retrovirus vectors, however, pseudotyped lentivirus vectors can be generated with amphotropic, ecotropic, vesicular stomatitis virus (VSV), or human T cell lymphoma/leukemia virus type 1 (HTLV-1) envelope proteins, thereby extending the host range of these vectors considerably.[23–26] These pseudotyped vectors have been used to infect human CD34$^+$ hematopoietic cells, and transduction rates of up to 90% have been reported.[23, 25] Although there are no available data at present on transduction efficiency for long-lived stem cells, studies are currently under way and will most likely determine the future usefulness of lentivirus vectors for hematopoietic gene therapy.

A significant obstacle to the development of lentiviral vectors has been (and still is) the generation of safe and efficient packaging cell lines, as several of the HIV-1 proteins, such as *gag, rev,* and *vpr,* display considerable cellular toxicity. In addition, current lentivirus vectors still need to contain large parts of the HIV-1 genome, including several functioning genes. Therefore, a number of issues, especially safety concerns, need to be addressed before these vectors can be considered for clinical studies on any larger scale.

Foamy viruses, or spumaviruses, are a class of retroviruses different from lentiviruses or Oncovirinae.[27] Although these viruses have not been associated with human diseases, they have been isolated from hematopoietic tissue in primates, and studies with wild-type virus have demonstrated the capacity of foamy virus to infect hematopoietic cells in vitro.[28] Like lentiviruses, foamy viruses can transduce noncycling cells, and nuclear localization signals have been identified in their *gag* protein.[29] Vectors based on the genome of human foamy virus have been constructed, and efficient transduction of primary hematopoietic cells from different animal species, including humans, has been achieved with these vectors.[30, 31] The major drawback at present is the lack of high-titer helper-free packaging systems for foamy virus vectors. Once these are established, it should be possible to investigate the potential of foamy virus–based vectors in clinically relevant models in more detail.

RETROVIRUS VECTORS

Retroviral Structure and Life Cycle

Retroviruses are small RNA viruses composed of an outer glycoprotein envelope and an inner RNA- and protein-containing core (Fig. 43–1). The retroviral genome consists of three coding regions, termed *gag, pol,* and *env,* which encode viral capsid proteins, reverse transcriptase and integrase, and the envelope proteins, respectively. The noncoding sequences include the psi-region, located 5′ of the *gag* gene, which directs packaging of the viral RNA and is required in *cis* to allow production of infec-

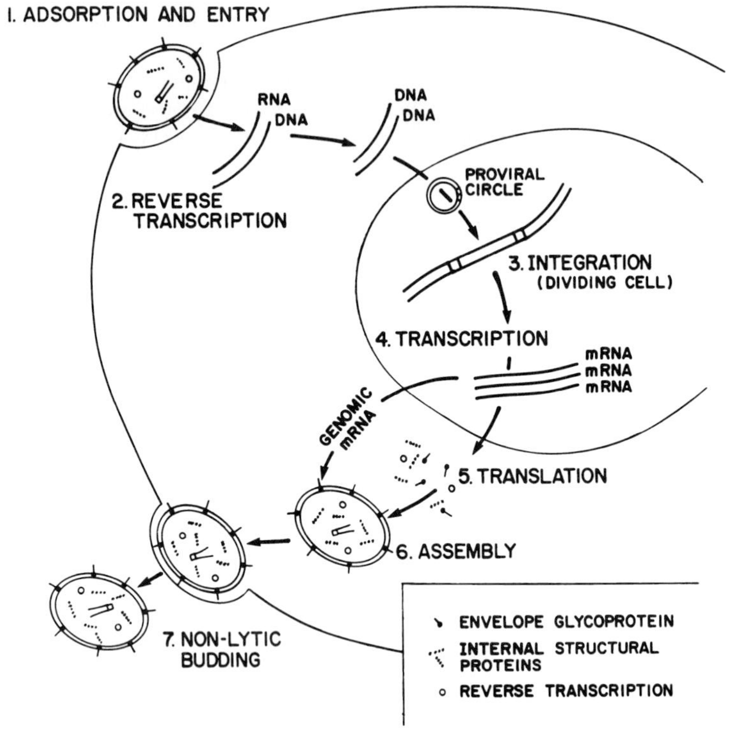

Figure 43–1. Life cycle of prototype retrovirus. See text for details. (From Williams DA, Orkin SH. Molecular techniques in hematopoiesis: retroviral-mediated gene transfer into hematopoietic stem cells. Hematol Rev 1987; 2:1.)

tious viral particles. The whole genome is contained within two repeated sequences: the long terminal repeats (LTRs), which contain promoter/enhancer elements and which direct the integration and replication of the viral genome and transcription of viral-encoded proteins. Ecotropic, xenotropic, and amphotropic retroviruses (among others), which differ in host range, can be differentiated according to envelope gene sequence. *Ecotropic* viruses infect and replicate only in cells of a specific species (e.g., the mouse). *Xenotropic* viruses are endogenous in one species (e.g., the mouse) but do not replicate well in this species; they do, however, replicate well in a different species (e.g., primates). *Amphotropic* viruses infect and replicate in a wide variety of species. Since the cloning of the receptor for amphotropic retrovirus,[32, 33] it has become increasingly clear that primitive hematopoietic cells constitutively express this receptor only at low levels.[34] Similar results have been reported for the receptor of Gibbon ape leukemia virus (GALV), an envelope gene used alternatively in some retroviral constructs. The low receptor density found on these cells appears to be one of the limiting factors preventing efficient retroviral transduction of hematopoietic stem cells (HSCs). This observation is supported by murine studies, in which use of ecotropic retrovirus leads to transduction of long-lived stem cells with relatively high efficiency. The receptor density of the ecotropic receptor on murine stem cells appears to be considerably higher than the density of amphotropic or GALV receptors on human stem cells.

To circumvent these problems, heterotypical, or "pseudotyped," vectors that combine characteristics of different viruses or viral subgroups have been generated. One such pseudotype combines the MoMLV *gag* and *pol* genes with the envelope protein of GALV, a closely related retrovirus. These vectors have been shown to compare favorably with standard amphotropic vectors with regard to infection efficiency of monkey respiratory epithelial cells.[35] However, like those of the amphotropic receptor, GALV receptor levels on HSCs are low. Nevertheless, there have been reports of increased transduction efficiency of hematopoietic cells with the use of GALV pseudotypes in comparison with amphotropic vectors.[36] Another heterotypical retroviral vector system uses the VSV envelope protein in combination with the MoMLV *gag/pol* genes.[37] This vector has the wide host range of VSV and, in addition, can be concentrated by density centrifugation to titers of up to 10^9 virions/mL. However, to date this system has not led to any improvements in stem cell transduction rates, most likely because of the toxicity of membrane fusion that is associated with uptake of VSV or VSV-pseudotyped vectors. Therefore, ecotropic viruses are currently used to infect mouse cells, whereas amphotropic or GALV virus is necessary to infect cells from other species, including humans.

Figure 43–2 shows the life cycle of a retrovirus. After binding to receptors at the cell surface of host cells, viruses are internalized into the cells and uncoat (lose their envelope proteins). Virus-encoded reverse transcriptase is released at this point and, with host cell DNA polymerases, produces a double-stranded DNA copy of the viral genome. The proviral DNA copy integrates, probably at random, into the host genome, becoming a *cellular gene* (which depends completely on the host cell metabolism for subsequent expression). The integrated proviral DNA is transmitted within the genome to all subsequent progeny of this cell. Viral RNA and proteins are produced by the host cell. During this process, the 5′ LTR serves as a transcriptional promoter/enhancer, whereas the 3′ LTR leads to polyadenylation of transcribed messenger RNA (mRNA). Viral RNA and pro-

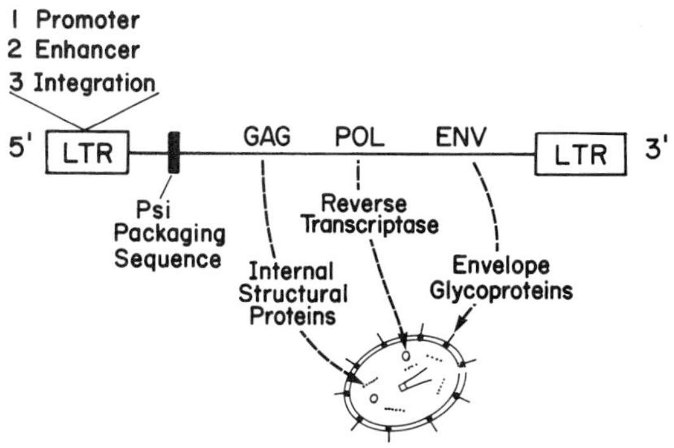

Figure 43–2. Genome of prototype retrovirus. LTR, long terminal repeat; GAG, core proteins; POL, reverse transcriptase; ENV, envelope protein. (From Williams DA, Orkin SH. Molecular techniques in hematopoiesis: retroviral-mediated gene transfer into hematopoietic stem cells. Hematol Rev 1987; 2:1.)

teins assemble into infectious virus particles inside the host cell, which are subsequently budded nonlytically from the cell membrane.

Recombinant Retroviruses and Packaging Lines

The *gag, pol,* and *env* genes, coding for the viral proteins and making up approximately 80% of a retroviral genome, can be deleted and replaced by DNA sequences coding for a gene of interest. If this recombinant virus is then inserted into the genome of a host cell, the foreign gene is transcribed in place of the missing viral genes. However, because essential viral genes are absent, no new viral particles can be produced, although recombinant retroviral RNA is present. Thus the recombinant retrovirus is incapable of producing infectious particles (i.e., is replication defective) unless the necessary viral proteins are supplied in *trans*.

Gene transfer requires infection with an intact but replication-defective virus. This can be achieved in one of two ways. Replication-defective virus can be introduced into a cell line containing a wild-type (replication-competent) retrovirus. These cells then produce both replication-defective and replication-competent virus, because the wild-type proteins *gag, pol,* and *env* can be used by both wild-type and recombinant RNA for packaging virions. A major disadvantage of this system is the persistence of replication-competent virus. To obviate the disadvantage, special cell lines that allow packaging of the recombinant viral RNA (*packaging cell lines*) have been constructed. These cell lines contain *gag, pol,* and *env* genes in a retrovirus genome from which the packaging signal (psi) has been deleted. The *gag, pol,* and *env* proteins encoded by this genome can be used to package the defective recombinant viral genome. In theory, only the recombinant retroviral RNA, not the psi-deleted wild-type RNA, is packaged. The resulting replication-defective recombinant virus is capable of only one infection cycle.[38]

Several packaging cell lines capable of producing high-titer recombinant retrovirus have been constructed through this approach. Some amount of replication-competent helper virus has been generated, in addition to the recombinant virus, through the use of some of these cell lines. The reason for this is twofold: (1) the lack of packaging as a result of deletion of the psi sequence is not absolute, and some replication-competent helper virus is still packaged (although at a rate less than one-thousandth that of the intact wild-type virus)[39]; and (2) recombination events can occur in the packaging lines as a result of considerable sequence homology between the replication-defective genome and the psi-deleted retrovirus, thus supplying the wild-type genome with an intact psi sequence.[40–42] The risk of generating replication-competent helper virus from packaging cell lines has been further reduced by making deletions and mutations in the helper virus genome, which then require two or more independent recombination events before intact helper virus can be generated.[43–45]

Further improvement in generating helper virus–free producer lines has come from the idea of generating lines that contain two psi-deleted retroviruses, one of which encodes the *gag* and *pol* genes only, and the other the *env* gene only (split-coding-region vectors). Early packaging cell lines constructed along this approach still released some intact helper virus after prolonged culture periods, probably because a nearly complete genome was used to synthesize the *gag* and *pol* proteins or because extensive stretches of homology between the two vectors were present, facilitating more than one recombination event. The multiple and extensive mutations and deletions in these split-coding-region vectors, however, has made the generation of intact helper virus highly unlikely and has led to the generation of safer producer cell lines (such as GP + *env* AM 12, GP + E86, DSN, and DAN[46–49]) that have been maintained in tissue culture for several years without helper virus detection.[50]

Depending on the infection protocol, target cells can be exposed to large numbers of retrovirus either by cocultivation with adherent producer cells or by exposure to filtered supernatant harvested from these cells. In both cases, it has been shown that efficiency of infection increases with increasing infectious viral titer.[51] One way to achieve higher infectious titers has been to use a retroviral vector construct that contains a relatively large amount of *gag* sequence downstream of the 5′-LTR (gag^+ vector). Inclusion of this sequence results in a 10- to 40-fold increase in the titer of the produced virus after introduction into a packaging cell line.[52] The initial impression that gag^+ vectors also improve long-term expression of transferred retroviral sequence in target cells, however, is still controversial.

Another frequently used method to increase retroviral titers is "ping-pong" amplification. In this method, amphotropic and ecotropic packaging lines, one of them already expressing the vector of interest at lower titer, are cocultured for a limited time. The ensuing superinfection of amphotropic cells by ecotropic cells and vice versa often leads to a 100- to 1000-fold increase over the original titer. With this "ping-pong" method, virus producer cell lines generating 1×10^7 infectious particles per milliliter have been generated.[53, 54]

In wild-type retroviruses, the *gag* and *pol* genes are expressed from genomic mRNA, whereas the *env* gene is translated from a subgenomic (spliced) message. Transcription of both messages is regulated by sequences within the 5′-LTR; the *env*-mRNA represents approximately 50% of the level of the genomic RNA. Genes introduced into the retroviral vectors may be transcribed with the viral LTR as promoter, or they may be introduced in combination with a heterologous (internal) promoter. Recombinant retroviruses carrying two genes commonly express the first gene from the unspliced message and the second gene from the spliced message.[55] However, for reasons not completely understood at present, expression of the second gene product is highly variable.[56] It is also possible to express one or both genes from internal promoters. One disadvantage of this approach is potential transcriptional interference between the LTR and the internal promoters. The introduced genes and their promoters are therefore commonly inserted in reverse orientation in relation to that of LTR transcription. It has been postulated, however, that any advantage obtained from this approach may be neutralized by antisense messages produced by the 5′-LTR. To overcome this limitation, the enhancer of the retrovirus can be deleted from the 3′-LTR (U3 region),[57, 58] because this deletion is replicated, and thereby inactivates, the 5′-LTR during the process of retroviral replication within the infected host cell. Although there is some evidence that vectors containing only one gene sequence may lead to better expression in primary hematopoietic cells, no one vector design is universally accepted as superior. It seems likely that vector design may be very specific as to use and sequence in the future. In the past, most investigators used vectors based on MoMLV, and the problems encountered in expressing transferred genes from these vectors led to a widespread use of very simple vectors, expressing only one gene from the 5′-LTR or an internal promoter ("simplified vectors"). Although some of these vectors, such as those using the human phosphoglycerate kinase (PGK) promoter,[54, 57] have achieved high-level and long-lived gene expression in cells of hematopoietic origin, promoters from other viruses such as the myeloproliferative sarcoma virus (MPSV) and the Friend murine leukemia virus (FLV) may more reliably express genes in hematopoietic tissues.[59–62] MPSV vectors have been shown to facilitate the expression of exogenous genes in undifferentiated, totipotent embryonic stem cells[63] and have successfully been used for gene transfer into hematopoietic cells from a variety of species, including human progenitor cells.[64, 65] Also, vectors that combine elements of MPSV and FLV (called FMEV and MPEV), which may further improve gene expression in HSCs, have been developed.[66] Extensive work characterizing *cis*-regulatory elements of retrovirus vectors that affect expression of *trans*-genes has led to progressively more sophisticated versions of MPSV- and MoMLV-based vectors[67a] (Fig. 43–3). For instance, alterations in the primer binding site, an SP-1 binding site, the upstream control region, and the LTR direct sequence all affect expression from the 5′-LTR.[67b, 67c]

Safety Aspects

In the application of any proposed treatment, the risks and benefits of the therapy and the severity of the underlying illness must be weighed. First, in the case of retroviral gene therapy, attempts to express an exogenous gene may prove pathogenic if the gene in question is overexpressed or inadvertently expressed in certain cell types. Second, contaminants may be introduced during vector manufacture. The former problems may be addressed by careful toxicology studies in animals; the latter risk may be minimized by careful manufacturing methods and stringent product certification. Beyond these issues, retroviral vectors themselves pose a variety of theoretical safety concerns. To better understand the risks associated with these vectors, the way in which the retroviruses from

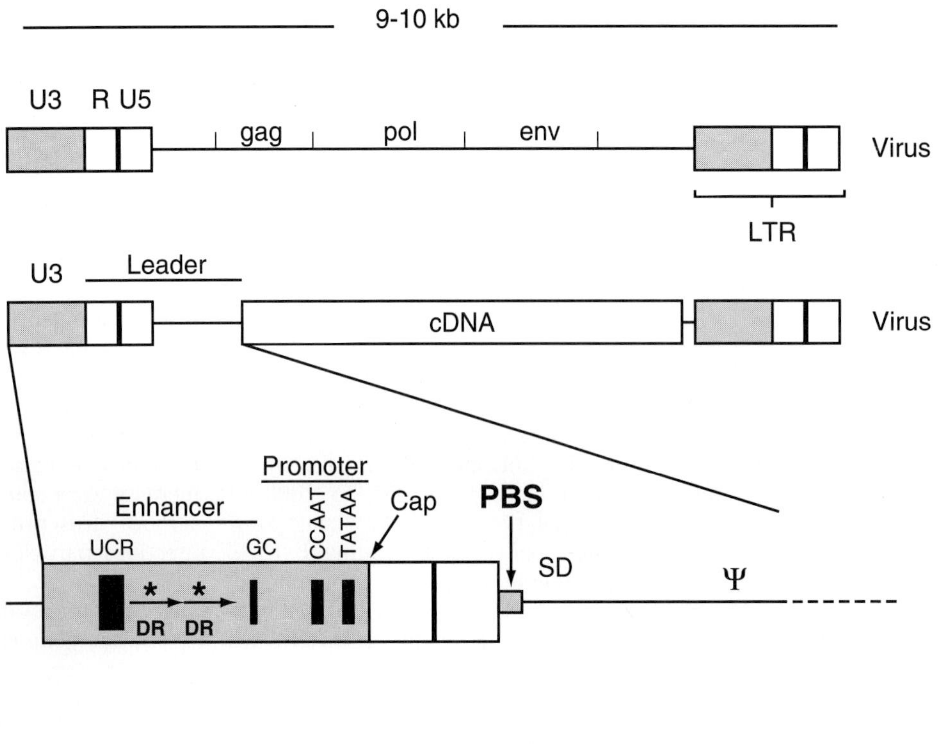

Figure 43–3. *Cis*-regulatory elements affecting expression from vector constructs. UCR, upstream control region; DR, direct repeat; GC, GC-box (Sp1); PBS, primer binding site; SD, splice donor. (Modified from Baum C, Ostertag W, Stocking C, Von Laer D. Retroviral vector design for cancer gene therapy. *In* Lattime EC, Gerson SL [eds]: Gene Therapy of Cancer: Translational Approaches from Preclinical Studies to Clinical Implementation. San Diego: Academic Press, 1998.)

which they are derived cause disease in mice must be considered.

Retroviruses and retroviral vectors insert essentially randomly throughout the genome.[67, 68] Disruption of a gene required for cell viability is a relatively rare occurence in diploid cells, and cell death should not lead to clinically significant sequelae. Of greater concern is the potential for abnormal gene regulation, alteration in cell growth, and the subsequent development of malignancy as the result of retroviral vector insertion, a phenomenon known as insertional mutagenesis. Many retroviral vectors intended for human clinical use are derived from the MoMLV, a retrovirus which is known to produce murine T cell lymphomas. The maturing thymus permits recombination between MoMLV and endogenous retroviral sequences, leading to the generation of recombinant viruses, known as mink cell focus-forming (MCF) viruses.[69] It is these highly leukemogenic MCF viruses, not MoMLV, that are believed to be the proximal cause of MoMLV-associated T cell lymphoma.[70–72] The *pim*-1 domain, encoding a lymphocyte-specific protein with homology to serine-protein kinases, is most often disrupted by insertion of the viral LTR into the 3′ exon of *pim*-1.[73, 74] The major determinants for MoMLV tropism (the propensity of a particular virus to cause a specific malignancy) are located in the U3 region of the LTR (see Fig. 43–3). Exchanging the U3 regions of MoMLV with that of the Friend MLV (which causes erythroleukemia) also exchanges tropism (i.e., the altered MoMLV produces erythroleukemia).[75–78] These findings suggest that specific interaction between viral sequences and unique factors in the target cell are required for tumor formation.

Although MoMLV does not generally cause disease in adult mice, Shen-Ong and Wolff and associates have shown that pristane-induced inflammation permits tumor development in adult mice exposed to MoMLV.[79–81] These mice developed promonocytic leukemia with MoMLV (not MCF), which disrupted the *c-myb* proto-oncogene. Tumor development was strain dependent and could be prevented by suppressing the inflammatory response with indomethacin. This observation suggests that genetic background and concurrent disease states may enhance the risk of MoMLV-associated disease.

In mice, malignant transformation by MoMLV is a rare event. Tumor development occurs in the setting of active viral infection, permitting multiple integrations into a single target cell. In contrast to retrovirus exposure, retroviral vectors integrate, on average, a single copy of their genome into each target cell. This difference is important in view of the multistep process of malignant transformation, because as many as 10 genetic alterations may be involved in the generation of certain de novo human tumors.[82–84] MoMLV-induced tumor also appears to require multiple gene alterations in as much as transgenic mice expressing the *pim*-1 gene have a low incidence of T cell lymphoma.[85] When these mice are injected with MoMLV, they have accelerated development of lymphoma, and each tumor has demonstrated a proviral integration into the *c-myc* or *n-myc* gene. The probability of affecting all the genes required for cell transformation, when human gene therapy protocols are designed to insert one vector per cell, appears to be exceedingly low. Therefore, the major risk of insertional mutagenesis is related to the risk of exposure to replication-competent retrovirus.

Intravenous injection of amphotropic murine retrovirus into immunocompetent or moderately immunosuppressed rhesus monkeys results in rapid clearance of infectious virus from serum (within 15 minutes). Primate serum is known to inactivate murine retroviruses, which likely explains the rapid viral clearance.[86, 87] Despite this rapid clearance, peripheral blood mononuclear cells are infected at very low frequencies. This infection is not associated with viremia or clinical illness.[87] Two studies have evaluated monkeys exposed to replication-competent virus during periods of severe immunosuppression (autologous bone marrow transplantation). Donahue and colleagues attempted gene transfer into rhesus monkeys by coculturing bone marrow on a packaging cell line that had generated replication-competent retrovirus in addition to vector. Three of 10 animals developed lethal lymphoma of T cell origin, which resembled the disease produced by MoMLV in mice. Two viruses were detected within lymphoma cells that arose from recombination between vector sequences, packaging sequences, and endogenous murine retroviral genome sequences.[88, 89, 89a] In a retrospective study of four animals exposed to replication-competent retrovirus in a similar transplantation model, animals were clinically well more than 6 years after exposure.[90] In both studies, animals that did not develop lymphoma had detectable antiviral antibodies, whereas those with disease failed to mount an antibody response and had persistent viremia. These findings indicate that retroviruses are pathogenic in primates in the setting of severe immunosuppression.

Two steps have been taken to decrease the chance of accidental exposure to replication-competent retrovirus. First, packaging cell lines and retroviral vectors have been redesigned to decrease the likelihood of recombination.[91, 92] Second, careful screening methods have been developed to test vector preparations for replication-competent retrovirus.[93, 94] Guidelines for testing vectors before use have been published[95] and continue to be refined. To date, exposure to replication-competent retrovirus, or malignancies arising as a result of insertional mutagenesis, have not been reported during clinical gene therapy trials.

The potential for recombination of gene therapy vectors with human endogenous retroviral sequences (HERV) is also a theoretical concern with retroviral gene transfer. The human genome contains many HERV. However, known HERV contain numerous mutations, making them replication defective.[96–98] The risk of recombination between HERV and retroviral vectors appears low because murine-based vectors and HERV share little homology, differing in the enhancer, promoter, and transfer RNA binding sites. Also, the same regions deleted in the construction of retroviral vectors are frequently deleted in HERV sequences. The factors limiting recombination between retroviral vectors and HERV also apply to human retroviruses, such as HIV and HTLV.

On rare occasions, virions inadvertently package cellular mRNA. A more common event, but still at least 0.001% as likely as the transfer of retroviral vector sequences, is the transfer of virus-like 30s elements (VL30, ~ 200 copies/haploid genome)[99, 100] and the intracisternal A-type particles (IAP, ~ 1000 copies/haploid genome)[101, 102] contained within retroviral packaging cell lines. VL30 sequences have been shown to be transmitted into a monkey developing lymphoma after exposure to replication-competent virus, although RNA was not transcribed.[89] Although transfer of these sequences during retroviral-mediated gene transfer has been documented, it is not believed to be of significance, because both VL30 and IAP genomes are defective and noninfectious.[103–105]

GENE TRANSFER INTO HEMATOPOIETIC CELLS

Vectors and Genes Used for Gene Transfer Into Hematopoietic Cells

The longevity and extensive self-renewal capacity of progenitor cells and especially of stem cells make human hematopoietic cells one of the most attractive target cell populations for gene therapy. The first successful retrovirus-mediated gene transfer into murine hematopoietic cells was described in 1983, when the marker gene NEO was introduced into granulocyte-macrophage colony-forming unit (CFU-GM) progenitor cells.[106] This was followed, in 1984, by the first report of transfer of the NEO gene into a transplantable multilineage stem cell, the spleen colony-forming unit (CFU-S).[107] In 1985, the feasibility of successful gene transfer into a pluripotent stem cell capable of long-term and multilineage reconstitution was further verified by retroviral integration pattern analysis, which showed clonally derived NEO gene–containing cells in bone marrow, thymus, and spleen after gene transfer experiments in bone marrow transplantation.[108, 109]

Since these early reports, a wide variety of different genes have been introduced into bone marrow cells from mice, humans, primates, and other animals. The genes include marker genes such as NEO and β-gal,[110] drug resistance genes such as mutants of the dihydrofolate reductase (mDHFR) gene[111] and the multidrug resistance gene (MDR-1),[112] growth factor genes such as interleukin-3 (IL-3),[113] and a wide variety of potentially therapeutic genes such as hypoxanthine phosphoribosyltransferase (HPRT),[114] purine nucleoside phosphorylase (PNP),[115] ADA,[116, 117] glucocerebrosidase,[118, 119] and β-globin.[120, 121] Despite these successes, the difficulties that must be overcome before HSC gene transfer therapy can be regarded as a therapeutic option for lifelong cure of a larger variety of diseases have become more clear.

It is now well established that predicting the efficiency of infection and expression of any specific vector in primary hematopoietic cells from in vitro testing is impossible. For instance, retroviral producer clones selected on the basis of expression in a murine fibroblast cell line, such as NIH/3T3, or in hematopoietic cell lines are not necessarily well expressed in primary hematopoietic cells.[58, 117] This fact was shown particularly for vectors generated to express the ADA gene off the SV40, thymidine kinase, metallothionein, *c-fos*, cytomegalovirus, and adenovirus E1A promoters.[40, 57, 115] To further complicate matters, promoters that are seemingly inefficient in murine hematopoietic cells, such as the cytomegalovirus promoter, function well in human cells.[122]

Poor expression of these promoters in primary hematopoietic cells parallels reports that retroviral constructs are also expressed poorly in primitive embryonic carcinoma cells.[123, 124] These reports suggested that the MoMLV promoter/enhancer contained in the LTR was not active in totipotent stem cells[125] and raised doubts about the use of this promoter in HSCs. It was later shown that highly conserved sequences near the 5′ end of the MoMLV LTR exhibit a regulatory role in viral transcription.[126, 127] Other *cis*-regulatory elements have also been implicated in poor expression of retroviral constructs in hematopoietic cells (see Fig. 43–3). In spite of these concerns, long-term expression of both NEO and ADA of the MoMLV LTR has since been demonstrated in murine models.[40, 109] To this point, most investigators have used vectors based on MoMLV, although LTRs from other viruses, such as the MPSV and the Friend MLV, might more reliably express genes in hematopoietic tissues.[59–61] The problems with the expression of transferred genes has led to a growing trend to use very simple vectors and to incorporate internal promoters. Some of these vectors, especially those using the human PGK promoter,[54, 57] have been noted to direct high-level and long-lived expression of genes in cells of hematopoietic origin in vitro and in vivo.

LONG-TERM GENE EXPRESSION IN HEMATOPOIETIC CELLS IN VIVO

In early reports showing reconstitution of lethally irradiated mice with bone marrow cells infected with retroviral vectors, expression of the transferred genes tended to be low, was present in only a minority of cells, and was often of relatively short duration.[57, 120, 121] However, through a better understanding of the regulation of gene expression, identification of promoter/enhancer elements with specificity for hematopoietic cells, and new insights into basic HSC biology, expression of foreign genes in mouse bone marrow is now a well-established technique in a number of laboratories. The success rate for gene expression of some introduced gene sequences at 6 months (i.e., after complete reconstitution) approaches 100%.[54, 112, 118, 119, 128, 129]

Retroviral integration within the target cell genome requires active division of the infected cell.[130] Among the hematopoietic population derived from normal bone marrow, the most primitive cells divide less frequently than more differentiated progenitor cells.[3] Several investigators have developed methods of increasing the number of stem cells in cycle at the time of infection. Chemotherapeutic agents such as 5-fluorouracil (5-FU) increase cycling of otherwise dormant stem cells during recovery from chemotherapy.[131] Pretreatment of donor animals with 5-FU is now a routine part of murine gene transfer protocols targeting hematopoietic cells.[132] In addition, a variety of hematopoietic growth factors have been shown to enhance gene transfer into mouse stem cells in addition to the chemotherapy pretreatment. IL-1, IL-3, and IL-6, Steel factor (SLF) (also called stem cell factor [SCF]), leukemia inhibitory factor (LIF), and various combinations of these factors[54, 128, 132, 134] have all been shown to be effective when incubated with bone marrow cells before and during infection by retrovirus in vitro. The optimal factor combination remains controversial at present.

Cycling rates do not seem to be the only determinant for retroviral infectivity, because studies using cells known to have a large cycling fraction (fetal liver cells, chronic myeloid leukemia cells, or hematopoietic cells from dogs with cyclic neutropenia) have not shown major increases in infection efficiency over normal bone marrow.[51, 134] Although protocols designed to optimize stem cell cycling rates improved gene transfer efficiency substantially, other strategies to improve long-term gene expression have met with only limited success. Selectable marker genes such as NEO and mDHFR have been introduced into retroviral vectors, allowing selection of infected hematopoietic cells before injection into recipient mice. Although increasing the relative number of transduced cells infused into recipients, these protocols did not improve long-term expression in recipients.[121, 135]

In addition, investigators using vectors containing two genes have shown that expression of one gene results in poor expression of the second gene to various degrees.[136, 137] Also, when retroviruses expressing two genes (one from the LTR and one from an internal SV40 promoter) are used, the genes are poorly transcribed in vivo despite intact proviral integration.[60] Impaired expression of a second gene sequence in hematopoietic cells in vivo has also been shown when no selection pressure is applied before infusion of transduced cells.[138] An alternative approach that has been used with some success in the murine system has been in vivo selection for cells expressing transduced and selectable genes such as mDHFR and MDR-1.[111, 112] However, this approach is limited to the few genes for which in vivo selection therapies are possible.

Despite successful long-term gene expression in the murine hematopoietic system, extension of gene transfer technology to larger outbred animals has had only very limited success. Early experiments in monkeys documented very low level expression of NEO and ADA after transplantation of bone marrow cells infected with retroviral vector carrying these genes.[139] With a higher titer vector, these results were improved, with expression of the transduced genes in approximately 1% of peripheral blood cells for up to 3 months and, in later experiments, for even longer periods.[53] However, interpretation of these experiments was complicated by the presence of helper virus in the vector preparations used, which led to active viremia and subsequent lymphoma formation in some of the animals.[140] The presence of replication-competent virus in these monkeys makes interpretation of the pluripotency of the infected cells and of the stability of expression from this retrovirus impossible. Expression of the clinically relevant ADA gene for at least 1 year in approximately 1% of PBMCs, through the use of a producer cell line clone demonstrated to be free of any detectable helper virus, has been reported.[141, 142]

Similar data have been generated in a canine bone marrow transplantation gene transfer model. Using a helper-free viral vector containing both NEO and ADA genes to transduce bone marrow, investigators have detected expression of NEO but not ADA sequences intermittently in 1% to 10% of myeloid progenitors (CFU-GM) grown from transplanted bone marrow of dogs for 2 years.[143]

Present and Future Directions in Hematopoietic Gene Therapy

In the past, nearly all successful in vivo gene transfer protocols in the mouse, as well as in larger animals, have used cocultivation of virus producer lines rather than supernatant infection. The data have generated increasing interest in the role of stroma during retroviral infection protocols. Experiments in vitro have shown that the presence of stromal layers (usually bone marrow fibroblasts) during supernatant infection can increase gene transfer into hematopoietic cells significantly[144, 145]; most recently, this approach has been successfully applied to hematopoietic cells transplanted into primates and dogs.[142, 146] Long-term expression of transferred ADA cDNA in hematopoietic cells in these experiments is similar to that in previous experience with coculture infection protocols (approximately 1%). This approach may ultimately allow identification of the minimum factors necessary for optimal infection of stem cells with retroviral vectors. Several groups are already experimenting with stromal cells genetically engineered to express high levels of specific growth factors.[147, 148] Supernatant infection on stromal layers is potentially safer because it would reduce the risk of exposure of patients to virus producer cells contaminating hematopoietic cells after retroviral coculture infection.

Many problems in transducing pluripotent and long-lived reconstituting stem cells are related to the fact that phenotypic identification of these cells is in its infancy. Considerable improvements have been achieved in the enrichment of primitive cells through the use of cell density and various combinations of cell surface antigens, especially the CD34 antigen.[149, 150] Although infection efficiency of hematopoietic cells is not necessarily better after enrichment in comparison with nonpurified cells, the enormous reduction in numbers of cells required during the retroviral infection protocol (depending on the selection procedure, 0.05% to 10% of total bone marrow mononuclear cell number) is of practical importance.

Two other sources of HSCs capable of long-term reconstitution after bone marrow transplantation have been defined and may be useful targets for gene transfer: peripheral blood stem cells, often collected after chemotherapy and growth factor administration,[151] and human umbilical vein cord blood–derived stem cells,[152] which are available at birth for every infant. Both are currently under study for potential use in transplantation, including gene therapy. Stem cells from both sources have biological characteristics that suggest a higher proliferative potential than do bone marrow–derived stem cells.[153–155] Interestingly, in vitro data concerning gene transfer into committed progenitor cells, precursors of colony-forming units, and long-term culture-initiating cells (an in vitro model of stem cell function) from both peripheral blood and cord blood have demonstrated greater gene transfer efficiency through retroviral vectors in comparison with adult human bone marrow.[156, 157]

Because of the problems encountered with efficient infection of long-term reconstituting HSCs, some groups have looked for alternative target populations to deliver genes to the hematopoietic system. Lymphocytes, which have a long lifespan (up to several months) and are more easily infected by retroviral vectors, have been an obvious target. The first "therapeutic" gene therapy trial used repeated infusion of transduced lymphocytes to deliver the ADA cDNA into patients with SCID. Another possible target population is that of committed hematopoietic progenitor cells.[158] The use of hematopoietic growth factors allows large numbers of these cells to be generated in vitro. One reasonable approach would be to target these cells with vectors encoding drug resistance genes before chemotherapy; chemotherapy intensity might be increased because side effects on bone marrow would be reduced.

ROLE OF GENE THERAPY IN SELECTED DISEASES

SCID Caused by ADA Deficiency

Deficiency of ADA is the molecular basis for approximately 30% of cases of SCID in children. The pathophysiological processes result mainly from the deficiency of enzyme in lymphocytes. Because the disease has been corrected by allogeneic bone marrow transplantation, gene transfer into autologous HSCs could provide a lifelong cure. Allogeneic bone marrow transplantation is the treatment of choice, if a human leukocyte antigen (HLA)–matched donor is available. An alternative treatment is regular infusion therapy with polyethylene glycol–modified ADA (PEG-ADA). Although this treatment is very effective, it usually does not normalize the disease symptoms completely, and its effectiveness lessens with time in some cases because of the development of anti-ADA antibodies. ADA deficiency is a rare disease, but several features have made it an attractive model for gene therapy. First, the ADA cDNA was cloned and fits easily within the size constraints of retroviral vectors. Second, expression of the ADA protein over a wide range of activity (5% to 100% ADA expression in normal people) is associated with normal immune phenotype. Third, lymphocytes expressing ADA have a selection advantage in vivo over ADA-deficient cells.

Stable long-term expression of human ADA in mice has been demonstrated in all hematopoietic lineages after full hematopoietic reconstitution with transduced bone marrow by several laboratories.[128, 159, 160] The levels of human ADA expression achieved in these studies were comparable with endogenous (murine) levels of ADA protein. Although application of this technology to larger animals (primates in particular) has suffered the same problems noted previously, successful gene transfer into primate stem cells and long-term expression of introduced human or murine ADA cDNA have been reported by two groups. Expression in approximately 1% of peripheral blood cells has been shown at the mRNA and protein levels.[141, 142] It is currently unclear whether this level of gene transfer and expression is sufficient to affect the phenotypic abnormalities of SCID patients.

In addition to work on curative gene therapy (i.e., the use of reconstituting HSCs as targets), a strategy has been developed at the NIH that targets lymphocytes, the cells apparently most affected in SCID.[161] The approach closely follows a protocol that had proved successful in the first human gene-marking trials with tumor-infiltrating lymphocytes (TILs).[162] Two ADA-deficient children received infusions of autologous lymphocytes infected with an ADA-containing retrovirus. The children were maintained on PEG-ADA therapy throughout the gene transfer protocol. To decrease the risk of oligoclonal reconstitution by the infected T cell population, repeated blood samples were used for infection. The first patient received eight infusions over 10 months, after which ADA levels in circulating peripheral blood cells increased significantly (from below 2% to approximately 20% of normal), and circulating T cell number increased from below normal into the normal range. Immune function, as measured by isohemagglutinin titers, skin test for antigen sensitivity, and cytotoxic T cell assays, improved significantly. Large numbers of the transduced T lymphocytes persisted without further treatment for over 6 months. The half-life of transduced T lymphocytes increased from between 30 and 35 days before treatment to between 3 and 5 months after transduction with the ADA gene. The second patient showed similar results. Both children are receiving maintenance treatment with ADA-transduced autologous lymphocytes every 3 to 5 months in addition to the continued PEG-ADA infusions. Both are currently asymptomatic, with no adverse side effects detected to this point.

Bordignon and associates[163] transduced peripheral blood lymphocytes (PBLs) or bone marrow cells (after T cell depletion) from ADA-SCID patients either with multiple exposure to cell-free supernatant or by cocultivation with irradiated packaging cells. Gene transfer efficiency increased 1% to 2.5% with cell-free retroviral supernatant and up to 40% by cocultivation. Gene transfer efficiency into CFU-GM and erythroid burst-forming units (BFU-E) hematopoietic progenitors averaged 30% to 40%. In this study, the contribution of PBLs and bone marrow stem and progenitor cells was evaluated by transducing them with two similar but molecularly distinguishable retroviral vectors. It was shown in vivo that the transduced PBLs made up 0.8% to 8.5% of the circulating PBLs and provided an immediate reserve of immunocompetent lymphocytes before maturation of bone marrow–derived lymphocytes. However, the contribution of these PBL-derived transduced cells was not long-lived. Kohn and colleagues[164] transduced CD34-enriched cord blood cells from three neonates with ADA SCID in three infection cycles, which resulted in gene transfer efficiency of 12% to 21%. In the absence of cytoablative therapy, 0.03% to 0.001% of peripheral blood leukocytes contained vector-derived sequences at 18 months after transplantation.

β-Globin Gene Transfer

Although most of the inherited diseases described in this chapter are relatively rare, genetic diseases involving β-globin mutations, such as β-thalassemia and sickle cell disease, are common throughout the world. However, cure of these diseases by gene therapy is more difficult than that of diseases such as ADA deficiency. Tissue-specific and precisely regulated expression of the introduced β-globin sequence is required. Thus the introduced gene should be expressed only in erythroid cells and at a level balanced with regard to expression of the paired globin chain. In view of the required high degree of regulation of expression and the relatively small size of the gene, transfer of the β-globin gene has usually been accomplished through the use of genomic DNA rather than cDNA, which is used for most other genes.

Genomic DNA contains several *cis*-regulatory sequences, including introns, that are required for normal transcriptional regulation and RNA processing. The importance of these intronic gene sequences has been demonstrated by comparing expression of genomic β-globin vectors with vectors containing the β-globin minigene (lacking introns). Only the genomic β-globin vectors led to expression of β-globin mRNA in mouse erythroleukemia cells.[165, 166] Several studies have demonstrated successful retrovirus-mediated gene transfer of β-globin into murine HSCs using vectors in which the β-globin gene is expressed in the antisense direction (related to the 5′ LTR).[120, 121, 167, 168] However, levels of β-globin mRNA were very low (0.4% to 4% of mouse endogenous β-globin expression) and limited to a minority of cells in the peripheral blood. Expression of the α-globin gene was tissue specific in these studies. Slightly better results have been reported in W/W^V mice, in which transduced normal cells have a competitive advantage during reconstitution over endogenous (W/W^V) stem cells.[167]

Gene Therapy for Gaucher's Disease

Gaucher's disease is an inherited recessive disorder caused by deficiency of a single enzyme, glucocerebrosidase. As with ADA deficiency and diseases involving the β-globin gene, the pathological manifestations of this disease involve defects in the hematopoietic system. Deficiency of the gene product leads to increasing accumulation of the substrate glucocerebroside, with subsequent damage to the bone marrow, liver, spleen, brain, lungs, and heart. Early allogeneic bone marrow transplantation is at present the treatment of choice if an HLA-compatible donor is available.

Genetic engineering for Gaucher's disease has advanced considerably since the early 1990s. In the murine system, retrovirus-mediated gene transfer of glucocerebrosidase into HSCs and stable expression of the enzyme for longer than 6 months at four to five times the level of the endogenous (murine) enzyme has been reported.[118, 119] In addition, it has been possible to achieve correction of the gene defect in short-term macrophage cultures by using cells derived from patients with Gaucher's disease.

GENE THERAPY FOR CYSTIC FIBROSIS

Since identification and cloning of the causative gene, cystic fibrosis transmembrane conductant regulator (CFTR),[169] gene therapy of cystic fibrosis has been an anticipated goal of the future. Cystic fibrosis is a common recessive disorder (1 per 2000 births in the white population). Transfer of a normal CFTR gene in vitro into respiratory epithelial cells from patients with cystic fibrosis restores the ability of these cells to secrete chloride, a lack of which is the basic defect in cystic fibrosis.

A major problem facing this field is the delivery of genetic sequences to the respiratory epithelium, the cells thought to be most affected in patients with cystic fibrosis. Adenovirus, which has a natural tropism for respiratory epithelial cells and does not require host cell proliferation for infection, may be a useful vector system in cystic fibrosis. Adenovirus-based vectors have been used extensively to introduce the CFTR gene into respiratory epithelial cells in animal models. The most successful experiment so far has involved intratracheal instillation of vector in rats.[170] The transferred human CFTR gene was detected for 6 weeks by RNA Northern blot analysis and for 11 to 14 days by anti–human CFTR antibodies. Up to 30% of the epithelial cells of alveolar surfaces were apparently infected. These results have generated interest in beginning human treatment with adenoviral vectors, and clinical trials with treatment of patients with cystic fibrosis every 2 to 3 months with CFTR vectors have been approved.

GENE THERAPY IN ONCOLOGY

Original safety studies were performed for retrovirus-mediated gene transfer by using marker genes introduced into TILs. Thereafter, potentially therapeutic genes were used in retroviral vectors. Tumor necrosis factor (TNF), a cytokine with extensive antiproliferative and immunomodulatory potential, has been limited in applications in vivo because of severe systemic toxicity. Therefore, the objective of the first therapeutic trial using genetically modified TILs was to deliver high doses of TNF locally to the tumor and thereby enhance the antitumor effects of TIL cell therapy. This trial in patients with malignant melanoma is currently under way at the NIH.[171]

Another approach to augmenting the antitumor effect of TIL cells by using gene transfer is also currently being evaluated. Either TNF or IL-2 gene sequences are introduced into tumor cells in vitro, and the transduced cells are then injected into patients either subcutaneously or intradermally. The goal is to generate a large number of TIL cells locally. After 3 weeks, the injection site (including the adjacent lymph nodes) is removed surgically. T cells present in the specimen are isolated and expanded in vitro, and the cells are subsequently infused back into the patient in combination with systemic IL-2.[172, 173]

One novel approach to using gene therapy in the treatment of cancer has been approved by the RAC for clinical trials. These trials are based on experiments in animals. In these studies, retroviral producer cells for the gene herpes simplex thymidine kinase (TK) were injected in vivo into rat brain gliosarcoma and murine fibrosarcoma or adenosarcoma. Expression of TK renders cells sensitive to the antiherpes drug ganciclovir. Subsequent treatment of the animals with ganciclovir was associated with complete regression of the tumors and long-term survival.[174] Not all tumor cells had been infected with the retrovirus, and this "bystander effect" on uninfected cells was confirmed in in vitro studies with several carcinomas in humans. In one case, such effects were demonstrated when only 1% of melanoma tumor cells were infected.

The HSV-TK/ganciclovir suicide system has also successfully been used to control the severity of graft-versus-host disease in allogeneic transplantation. When the HSV-TK gene was introduced ex vivo into the T lymphocytes contained in the graft, exposure to ganciclovir effectively abrogated severe graft-versus-host disease in two of three patients tested.[175]

Another application for gene therapy that could be envisioned in the field of oncology is the generation of chemotherapy-resistant hematopoietic cells to protect the hematopoietic system against therapy-induced myelosuppression. Despite the use of hematopoietic growth factors and autologous progenitor cell rescue, hematopoietic toxicity is still an important obstacle to dose intensification, especially in heavily pretreated patients. The strategy suggested in this context might be the infusion of autologous hematopoietic cells that have been modified ex vivo to express specific drug resistance genes. A number of these genes have been identified and cloned, the most well-known of which are mDHFR, MDR-1, O^6-methylguanine DNA methyltransferase (MGMT), aldehyde dehydrogenase (ALDH), and glutathione-S-transferase (GST); these actions confer resistance to a wide variety of commonly used chemotherapeutic agents. While most genes are currently under preclinical investigation, MDR-1 and MGMT are already being tested in clinical trials.[176, 177]

GENE THERAPY FOR AIDS

Gene therapy has been investigated as an alternative therapy for treatment of AIDS. The aim of most approaches is to disrupt the function of key HIV-encoded gene products in infected cells. One target has been the *tat* gene, which activates expression of other HIV-1–encoded genes primarily at the level of transcription. Multimerized (TAR-RNA) elements that bind and inactivate the *tat* protein have been developed. Overexpression of these elements in HIV-infected cell lines in vitro substantially reduces HIV replication in these cells.[178] However, there is some evidence that this effect may decrease over time.

Another approach is the delivery of genes encoding ribozymes, which can specifically cleave HIV-1 RNA. Ribozymes are pieces of RNA that play an important role in post-transcriptional gene regulation and have the dual property of sequence-specific recognition and site-specific cleavage of RNA. This approach is undergoing in vitro testing.

An important problem that must be addressed before gene therapy for AIDS can be performed clinically is to target the therapeutic gene sequences to the HIV-1–infected cells in vivo. One approach is the construction of retroviral vectors, which infect cells universally but are activated only in HIV-infected cells. The HIV-1–encoded *rev* gene, which is required for expression of structural viral proteins and viral replication, may be useful in this context. The function of *rev* depends on interaction of the protein with specific HIV-1 sequences, *rev* response elements (RREs) located in the HIV-1 *env* gene introns. Incorporation of these RREs into other genes may allow expression of these genes specifically in HIV-infected cells at the time of HIV replication, when *rev* expression normally takes place. Use of an HIV-derived, recombinant vector that has conserved the cell-type specificity of HIV-1 infection has been suggested as another way to target therapeutic genes into HIV-infected cells.

All these approaches require extensive work with in vivo animal models before they reach the stage of gene therapy protocols in humans. However, another strategy for tackling AIDS is already in clinical testing: fibroblasts are recovered from the skin of HIV-infected patients, transduced ex vivo with the HIV *env* gene, irradiated to prevent further proliferation, and then injected back into the patient. Experiments in animals have shown that these fibroblasts survive for several weeks and are able to trigger a cytotoxic T lymphocyte response against HIV-infected and *env* gene–expressing cells. Analogous ongoing studies in humans may offer a new therapeutic approach for patients with HIV infection.

INFECTION PROTOCOLS: RECENT IMPROVEMENTS AND STRATEGIES FOR FUTURE IMPROVEMENTS

In spite of considerable progress in the understanding of retroviral vector design, stem cell enrichment methods, and alternative gene transfer systems, the frequency of stem cell transduction still appears to be the major limitation in the application of gene transfer technology to disease therapy in humans. Strategies currently being employed to address this overriding issue are shown in Table 43–3. As previously mentioned, the expression and density of receptors for different viral envelope proteins are being examined. This basic information will be used in two ways to improve gene transfer: (1) to direct the use of new pseudotypes in vector constructs, such as GALV[32] and VSV,[37] and (2) in attempts to manipulate the expression of the receptor in hematopoietic cells.[34] Exploitation of viruses that do not require cell mitosis for integration appears to be a promising although as yet largely untested approach. Preliminary results suggest that both lentivirus[23–25] and foamy virus[28, 30, 31] vectors may prove useful for transduction of nondividing cell populations. In addition to continued studies on optimal cytokines to be used in ex vivo manipulation (before and

Table 43–3. Strategies for Improved Gene Transfer

Use of different viral pseudotypes in an effort to utilize viruses with increased receptor density on the target cells
Use of viruses that do not require cell division for integration
Use of in vivo selection methods to select and amplify a small population of transduced cells
Methods to increase the level of viral receptor expression on target cells
Methods to improve ex vivo manipulation of cells and/or modify virus/cell interactions

during infection), it has been appreciated that cytokine treatment in vivo before stem cell harvest may also affect gene transfer efficiency.[179, 180] Finally, inclusion of the peptides derived from the extracellular matrix protein fibronectin,[181] which has been shown to colocalize virus particles and target cells,[182] increases transduction of both hematopoietic progenitor[183] and stem cells,[184] and primary human T lymphocytes.[185] Using all of these advances, both Kiem and associates[186] and Wu and colleagues[187] reported transduction of primate repopulating cells at markedly improved frequencies of 10% to 20%. If such methods improve gene transfer into human repopulating cells to the same degree, the prospects for therapeutic success in future human gene therapy trials will be greatly enhanced.

REFERENCES

1. Smithies O, Gregg RO, Boggs SS, et al. Insertion of DNA sequences into the human chromosomal β-globin locus by homologous recombination. Nature 1985; 317:230.
2. Thomas KR, Capecchi MR. Site-directed mutagenesis by gene targeting in mouse embryo–derived stem cells. Cell 1987; 51:503.
3. Miller DA. Human gene therapy comes of age. Nature 1992; 357:455.
4. Anderson WF. Human gene therapy. Science 1992; 256:808.
5. Weissman SM. Gene therapy. Proc Natl Acad Sci U S A 1992; 89:11111.
6. Wagner E, Zatloukal K, Cotten M, et al. Coupling of adenovirus to transferrin-polylysine/DNA complexes greatly enhances receptor-mediated gene delivery and expression of transfected genes. Proc Natl Acad Sci U S A 1992; 89:6099.
7. Cotten M, Wagner E, Zatloukal K, et al. High-efficiency receptor-mediated delivery of small and large (48 kilobase) gene constructs using the endosome-disruptive activity of defective or chemically inactivated adenovirus particles. Proc Natl Acad Sci U S A 1992; 89:6094.
8. Chatterjee S, Wong KK, Podsakoff G, et al. Adeno-associated virus vectors for high efficiency gene transfer into primary human hematopoietic cells [Abstract]. Blood 1992; 80:167a.
9. Goodman S, Walsh C, Hirshman J, et al. Recombinant adeno-associated virus-mediated gene transfer into hematopoietic progenitor cells [Abstract]. Blood 1992; 80:167a.
10. Chatterjee S, Wong KK Jr. Adeno-associated virus vectors for gene therapy of the hematopoietic system. Curr Top Microbiol Immunol 1996; 218:61.
11. Chatterjee S, Wong KK, Lu D, et al. Novel approaches for efficient gene transfer into hematopoietic progenitor cells: the use of adeno-associated virus vectors. Bone Marrow Transplant 1995; 15:5309.
12. Walsh CE, Nienhuis AW, Samulski RJ, et al. Phenotypic correction of Fanconi anemia in human hematopoietic cells with a recombinant adeno-associated virus vector. J Clin Invest 1994; 94:1440.
13. Zhou SZ, Broxmeyer HE, Cooper S, et al. Adeno-associated virus 2–mediated high efficiency gene transfer into immature and mature subsets of hematopoietic progenitor cells in human umbilical cord blood. J Exp Med 1994; 179:1867.
14. Ponnazhagan S, Yoder M, Srivastava A. Adeno-associated virus type 2–mediated transduction of murine hematopoietic cells with long-term repopulating ability and sustained expression of a human globin gene in vivo. J Virol 1997; 71:3098.
15. Geller AI, Keyomarsi K, Byran J, Pardee AB. An efficient deletion mutant packaging system for defective herpes simplex virus vectors: potential applications to human gene therapy and neuronal physiology. Proc Natl Acad Sci U S A 1990; 87:8950.
16. Deluca NA, McCarthy AM, Schaffer PA. Isolation and characterization of deletion mutants of herpes simplex virus type 1 in the gene encoding immediate-early regulatory protein ICP. J Virol 1985; 56:558.
17. Johnson PA, Wang MJ, Friedmann T. Improved cell survival by the reduction of immediate-early gene expression in replication-defective mutants of herpes simplex virus type 1 but not by mutation of the virion host shutoff function. J Virol 1994; 68:6347.
18. Dilloo D, Rill D, Enwistle C, et al. A novel herpes vector for the high efficiency transduction of normal and malignant human hematopoietic cells. Blood 1997; 89:199.
19. Watanabe T, Kuszynski C, Ino K, et al. Gene transfer into human bone marrow hematopoietic cells mediated by adenovirus vectors. Blood 1996; 87:5032.
20. Neering SJ, Hardy SF, Minamoto D, et al. Transduction of primitive human hematopoietic cells with recombinant adenovirus vectors. Blood 1996; 88:1147.
21. Nienhuis AW, Walsh CE, Liu J. Viruses as therapeutic gene transfer vectors. *In* Young NS (ed): Viruses and Bone Marrow. New York: Marcel Dekker, 1993, pp 353–414.
22. Bukrinsky MI, Haggerty S, Dempsey MP, et al. A nuclear localization signal with HIV-1 matrix protein that governs infection of non-dividing cells. Nature 1993; 365:666.
23. Akkina RK, Walton RM, Chen ML, et al. High-efficiency gene transfer into $CD34^+$ cells with a human immunodeficiency virus type 1–based retroviral vector pseudotyped with vesicular stomatitis virus envelope glycoprotein G. J Virol 1996; 70:2581.
24. Naldini L, Blomer U, Gallay P, et al. In vivo gene delivery and stable transduction of nondividing cells by a lentiviral vector. Science 1996; 272:263.
25. Reiser J, Harmison G, Kluepfel-Stahl S, et al. Transduction of nondividing cells using pseudotyped defective high-titer HIV type 1 particles. Proc Natl Acad Sci U S A 1996; 93:15266.
26. Landau NR, Page KA, Littman DR. Pseudotyping with human T-cell leukemia virus type 1 broadens the human immunodeficiency virus host range. J Virol 1991; 65:162.
27. Flugel RM. Spumaviruses: a group of complex retroviruses. J Acquir Immune Defic Syndr 1991; 4:739.
28. Yu SF, Stone J, Linial ML. Productive persistent infection of hematopoietic cells by human foamy virus. J Virol 1996; 70:1250.
29. Schliephake AW, Rethwilm A. Nuclear localization of foamy virus *gag* precursor protein. J Virol 1994; 68:4946.
30. Russell DW, Miller AD. Foamy virus vectors. J Virol 1996; 70:217.
31. Hirata RK, Miller AD, Andrews RG, Russell DW. Transduction of hematopoietic cells by foamy virus vectors. Blood 1996; 88:3654.
32. Miller DG, Edwards RH, Miller AD. Cloning of the cellular receptor for amphotropic murine retroviruses reveals homology to that for gibbon ape leukemia virus. Proc Natl Acad Sci U S A 1994; 91:78.
33. van Zeijl M, Johann SV, Closs E, et al. A human amphotropic retrovirus receptor is a second member of the gibbon ape leukemia virus receptor family. Proc Natl Acad Sci U S A 1994; 91:1168.
34. Orlic D, Girard LJ, Jordan CT, et al. The level of mRNA encoding the amphotropic retrovirus receptor in mouse and human hematopoietic stem cells is low and correlates with the efficiency of retrovirus transduction. Proc Natl Acad Sci U S A 1996; 93:11097.
35. Bayle J-Y, Johnson LG, St. George JA, et al. High-efficiency gene transfer to primary monkey airway epithelial cells with retrovirus vectors using the gibbon ape leukemia virus receptor. Hum Gene Ther 1993; 4:161.
36. Kiem HP, Heyward S, Winkler A, et al. Gene transfer into marrow repopulating cells: comparison between amphotropic and gibbon ape leukemia virus pseudotyped retroviral vectors in a competitive repopulation assay in baboons. Blood 1997; 90:4638.
37. Burns JC, Friedmann T, Driever W, et al. Vesicular stomatitis virus G glycoprotein pseudotyped retroviral vectors: concentration to very high titer and efficient gene transfer into mammalian and nonmammalian cells. Proc Natl Acad Sci U S A 1993; 90:8033.
38. Lehn DM. Gene therapy using bone marrow transplantation. Bone Marrow Transplant 1987; 1:243.
39. Mann R, Baltimore D. Varying the position of a retrovirus packaging sequence results in the encapsidation of both unspliced and spliced RNAs. J Virol 1985; 54:401.
40. Belmont JW, MacGregor GR, Wager-Smith K, et al. Expression of human adenosine deaminase in murine hematopoietic cells. Mol Cell Biol 1988; 8:5116.
41. Karlsson S, Papayannopoulou T, Schweiger SG, et al. Retroviral-mediated transfer of genomic globin genes leads to regulated production of RNA and protein. Proc Natl Acad Sci U S A 1987; 84:2411.

42. Stoker AW, Bissell MJ. Development of avian sarcoma and leukosis virus–based vector-packaging cell lines. J Virol 1988; 62:1008.
43. Miller AD, Buttimore C. Redesign of retrovirus packaging cell lines to avoid recombination leading to helper virus production. Mol Cell Biol 1986; 6:2895.
44. Sorge J, Wright D, Erdman VD, Cutting AE. Amphotropic retrovirus vector system for human cell gene transfer. Mol Cell Biol 1984; 4:1730.
45. Savatier P, Bagnis C, Thoraval P, et al. Generation of a helper cell line for packaging avian leukosis virus–based vectors. J Virol 1989; 63:513.
46. Markowitz D, Goff S, Bank A. A safe packaging line for gene transfer: separating viral genes on two different plasmids. J Virol 1988; 62:1120.
47. Danos O, Mulligan RC. Safe and efficient generation of recombinant retroviruses with amphotropic and ecotropic host ranges. Proc Natl Acad Sci U S A 1988; 85:6460.
48. Markowitz D, Goff S, Bank A. Construction and use of a safe and efficient amphotropic packaging cell line. J Virol 1988; 167:400.
49. Dougherty JP, Wisniewski R, Yang S, et al. New retrovirus helper cells with almost no nucleotide sequence homology to retrovirus vectors. J Virol 1989; 63:3209.
50. Miller AD. Retrovirus packaging cells. Hum Gene Ther 1990; 1:5.
51. Hogge DE, Humphries RK. Gene transfer to primary normal human hematopoietic progenitors using recombinant retroviruses. Blood 1987; 69:611.
52. Armentano D, Yu SF, Kantoff PW, et al. Effect of internal viral sequences on the utility of retroviral vectors. J Virol 1987; 61:1647.
53. Bodine DM, McDonagh KT, Brandt SJ, et al. Development of a high-titer retrovirus producer cell line capable of gene transfer into rhesus monkey hematopoietic stem cells. Proc Natl Acad Sci U S A 1990; 87:3738.
54. Luskey BD, Rosenblatt M, Zsebo K, Williams DA. Stem cell factor promotes retroviral-mediated gene transfer into murine hematopoietic stem cells. Blood 1992; 80:396.
55. Cepko CL, Roberts RE, Mulligan RC. Construction and applications of a highly transmissible murine retrovirus shuttle vector. Cell 1984; 37:1053.
56. Bowtell DD, Johnson GR, Kelso A, Cory S. Expression of genes transferred to hematopoietic stem cells by recombinant retroviruses. Mol Biol Med 1987; 4:229.
57. Lim B, Williams DA, Orkin SH. Retrovirus-mediated gene transfer of human adenosine deaminase: expression of functional enzyme in murine hematopoietic stem cells in vivo. Mol Cell Biol 1987; 7:3459.
58. Magli MC, Dick JE, Huszar D, et al. Modulation of gene expression in multiple hematopoietic cell lineages following retroviral vector gene transfer. Proc Natl Acad Sci U S A 1987; 84:789.
59. Stocking C, Kollek R, Bergholz U, Ostertag W. Long terminal repeat sequences impart hematopoietic transformation properties to the myeloproliferative sarcoma virus. Proc Natl Acad Sci U S A 1985; 82:5746.
60. Bowtell DD, Cory S, Johnson GR, Gonda TJ. Comparison of expression in hematopoietic cells by retroviral vectors carrying two genes. J Virol 1988; 62:2464.
61. Holland CA, Anklesaria P, Sakakeeny MA, Greenberger JS. Enhancer sequences of a retroviral vector determine expression of a gene in multipotent hematopoietic progenitors and committed erythroid cells. Proc Natl Acad Sci U S A 1987; 84:8662.
62. Baum C, Ostertag W, Stocking C, vonLaer D. Retroviral Vector Design for Cancer Gene Therapy. San Diego: Academic Press, 1998.
63. Grez M, Akgun E, Hilberg F, Ostertag W. Embryonic stem cell virus, a recombinant murine retrovirus with expression in embryonic stem cells. Proc Natl Acad Sci U S A 1990; 87:9202.
64. Hawley RG, Fong AZC, Ngan BY, et al. Progenitor cell hyperplasia with rare development of myeloid leukemia in interleukin 11 bone marrow chimeras. J Exp Med 1993; 178:1175.
65. Baum C, Hegewisch-Becker S, Eckert H-G, et al. Novel retroviral vectors for efficient expression of the multidrug resistance *(MDR-1)* gene in early hematopoietic cells. J Virol 1995; 69:7541.
66. Eckert H-G, Stockschlader M, Just U, et al. High-dose multidrug resistance in primary human hematopoietic progenitor cells transduced with optimized retroviral vectors. Blood 1996; 88:3407.
67. Shin C, Stoye JP, Coffin JM. Highly preferred targets for retrovirus integration. Cell 1988; 53:531.
67a. Hawley RG, Lieu FHL, Fong AZC, Hawley TS. Versatile retroviral vectors for potential use in gene therapy. Gene Ther 1994; 1:136.
67b. Baum C, Hegewisch-Becker S, Eckert H-G, et al. Novel retroviral vectors for efficient expression of the multidrug resistance (MDAR-1) gene in early hematopoietic cells. J Virol 1995; 69:7541.
67c. Baum C, Itoh K, Meyer J, et al. The potent enhancer activity of $SFFV_p$ in hematopoietic cells is governed by a binding site for Sp1 in the upstream control region and by a unique enhancer core creating an exclusive target for PEBP/CBF. J Virol 1997; 71:6323.
68. Rohdewohld H, Weihen H, Reik W, et al. Retrovirus integration and chromatin structure: Moloney murine leukemia proviral integration sites map near DNase I–hypersensitivity sites. J Virol 1987; 61:336.
69. Cloyd MW, Hartley JW, Rowe WP. Lymphomagenicity of recombinant mink cell focus-forming murine leukemia viruses. J Exp Med 1980; 151:542.
70. Chattopadhyay SK, Cloyd MW, Linemeyer DL, et al. Cellular origin and role of mink cell focus-forming viruses in murine thymic lymphomas. Nature 1982; 295:25.
71. Evans LH, Cloyd MW. Friend and Moloney murine leukemia viruses specifically recombine with different endogenous retroviral sequences to generate mink cell focus-forming viruses. Proc Natl Acad Sci U S A 1985; 82:459.
72. Laigret F, Repaske R, Boulukos AB, et al. Potential progenitor sequences of mink cell focus-forming (MCF) murine leukemia viruses: ecotropic, xenotropic and MCF-related viral RNA's are detected concurrently in thymus tissue of AKR mice. J Virol 1988; 62:376.
73. Cuypers HT, Selten G, Quint W, et al. Murine leukemia virus–induced T-cell lymphomagenesis: integration of proviruses in a distinct chromosomal region. Cell 1984; 37:141.
74. Selten G, Cuypers HT, Boelens W, et al. The primary structure of the putative oncogene *pim*-1 shows extensive homology with protein kinases. Cell 1986; 46:603.
75. Chatis PA, Holland CA, Hartley JW, et al. Role for the 3′ end of the genome in determining disease specificity of Friend and Moloney murine leukemia viruses. Proc Natl Acad Sci U S A 1983; 80:4408.
76. Chatis PA, Holland CA, Silver JE, et al. A 3′ end fragment encompassing the transcriptional enhancers of nondefective Friend virus confers erythroleukemogenicity on Moloney leukemia virus. J Virol 1984; 52:248.
77. Li Y, Golemis E, Hartley JW, Hopkins N. Disease specificity of nondefective Friend and Moloney murine leukemia viruses is controlled by a small number of nucleotides. J Virol 1987; 61:693.
78. Golemis E, Li Y, Fredrickson TN, et al. Distinct segments within the enhancer region collaborate to specify the type of leukemia induced by nondefective Friend and Moloney viruses. J Virol 1989; 63:328.
79. Shen-Ong GLC, Wolff L. Moloney murine leukemia virus–induced myeloid tumors in adult BALB/c mice: requirements of *c-myb* activation but lack of v-abl involvement. J Virol 1987; 61:3721.
80. Wolff L, Mushinski JF, Shen-Ong GLC, Morse HCI. A chronic inflammatory response: its role in supporting the development of *c-myb* and *c-myc* related promonocytic and monocytic tumors in BALB/c mice. J Immunol 1988; 14:681.
81. Wolff L, Nason-Burchenal K. Retrovirus-induced tumors whose development is facilitated by a chronic immune response: a comparison of two tumors committed to the monocytic lineage. Curr Top Microbiol Immunol 1989; 149:79.
82. Liu E, Dollbaum C, Scott G, Rochlitz C. Molecular lesions involved in the progression of a human breast cancer. Oncogene 1988; 3:323.
83. Vogelstein B, Fearson ER, Kern SE, et al. Allelotype of colorectal carcinoma. Science 1989; 244:207.
84. Weston A, Willey JC, Modali R, et al. Differential DNA sequence deletions from chromosomes 3, 11, 13 and 17 in squamous-cell carcinoma, and adenocarcinoma of the human lung. Proc Natl Acad Sci U S A 1989; 86:5099.
85. Van Lohuizen M, Merbeek S, Krimpenfurt P, et al. Predisposition to lymphomagenesis in *pim*-1 transgenic mice: cooperation with *C-myc* and *N-myc* in murine leukemia virus-induced tumors. Cell 1989; 56:673.
86. Banapour B, Sernatinger J, Levy JA. The AIDS associated retrovi-

rus is not sensitive to lysis or inactivation by human serum. J Virol 1986; 152:268.
87. Cornetta K, Moen RC, Culver K, et al. Amphotropic murine leukemia retrovirus is not an acute pathogen for primates. Hum Gene Ther 1990; 1:13.
88. Donahue RE, Kessler SW, Bodine D, et al. Helper virus induced T cell lymphoma in nonhuman primates after retroviral mediated gene transfer. J Exp Med 1992; 176:1125.
89. Vanin EF, Kaloss M, Broscius C, Nienhuis AW. Characterization of replication-competent retroviruses from non-human primates with virus-induced T cell lymphomas and observations regarding the mechanism of oncogenesis. J Virol 1994; 68:4241.
89a. Purcell DFJ, Broscius CM, Vanin EF, et al. An array of murine leukemia virus–related elements is transmitted and expressed in a primate recipient of retroviral gene transfer. J Virol 1996; 70:887.
90. Cornetta K, Morgan RA, Gillio A, et al. No retroviremia in long-term follow-up of monkeys exposed to a murine amphotropic retrovirus. Hum Gene Ther 1991; 2:215.
91. Mann R, Mulligan RC, Baltimore D. Construction of a retrovirus packaging mutant and its use to produce helper-free defective retrovirus. Cell 1983; 33:153.
92. Watanabe S, Temin HM. Construction of a helper cell line for avian reticuloendotheliosis virus cloning vectors. Mol Cell Biol 1983; 3:2241.
93. Cornetta K, Nguyen N, Morgan RA, et al. Infection of human cells with murine amphotropic replication-competent retroviruses. Hum Gene Ther 1993; 4:579.
94. Forestell SP, Dando JS, Bohnlein E, Rigg RJ. Improved detection of replication-competent retrovirus. J Virol Methods 1996; 60:171.
95. Wilson CA, Ng T, Miller AE. Evaluation of recommendations for replication-competent retrovirus testing associated with use of retroviral vectors. Hum Gene Ther 1997; 8:869.
96. Bonner TI, O'Connell C, Cohen M. Cloned endogenous retroviral sequences from human DNA. Proc Natl Acad Sci U S A 1982; 79:4709.
97. Rabson AB, Hamagishi Y, Steele PE, et al. Characteristics of human endogenous retroviral envelope RNA transcripts. J Virol 1985; 56:176.
98. Repaske R, Steele PE, O'Neill RR, et al. Nucleotide sequence of a full-length human endogenous retroviral segment. J Virol 1985; 54:764.
99. Courtney MG, Elder PK, Steffen DL, Getz MJ. Organization and expression of endogenous virus-like (VL30) DNA sequences in nontransformed and chemically transformed mouse embryo cells in culture. Cancer Res 1982; 42:569.
100. Hatzoglou M, Hodgson CP, Mularo F, Hanson RW. Efficient packaging of a specific VL30 retroelement by 2 cells which produce MoMLV recombinant retroviruses. Hum Gene Ther 1990; 1:385.
101. Lueders KK, Kuff EL. Intracisternal A-particle genes: identification in the genome of *Mus musculus* and comparison of multiple isolates from a mouse gene library. Proc Natl Acad Sci U S A 1980; 77:3571.
102. Ono M, Cole MD, White AT, Huang RC. Sequence organization of cloned intracisternal A-particle genes. Cell 1980; 21:465.
103. Mietz JA, Grossman Z, Lueders KK, Kuff EL. Nucleotide sequence of a complete mouse intracisternal A-particle genome: relationship to known aspects of a particle assembly and function. J Virol 1987; 6:3020.
104. Adams SE, Rathjen PS, Stanway CA, Fulton SM. Complete nucleotide sequence of a mouse VL30 retro-element. Mol Cell Biol 1988; 8:2989.
105. Morgan RA, Cornetta K, Anderson WF. Application of polymerase chain reaction in retroviral-mediated gene transfer and the analysis of gene-marked human TIL cells. Hum Gene Ther 1990; 1:136.
106. Joyner A, Keller G, Phillips RA, Bernstein A. Retrovirus transfer of a bacterial gene into mouse haematopoietic progenitor cells. Nature 1983; 305:556.
107. Williams DA, Lemischka IR, Nathan DG, Mulligan RC. Introduction of new genetic material into pluripotent haematopoietic stem cells of the mouse. Nature 1984; 310:476.
108. Dick JE, Magli MC, Huszar D, et al. Introduction of a selectable gene in primitive stem cells capable of long-term reconstitution of the hemopoietic system of W/Wv mice. Cell 1985; 42:71.
109. Keller G, Paige C, Gilboa E, Wagner EF. Expression of a foreign gene in myeloid and lymphoid cells derived from multipotent haematopoietic precursors. Nature 1985; 318:149.
110. Clapp DW, Dumenco LL, Hatzoglou M, Gerson SL. Fetal liver hematopoietic stem cells as a target for in utero retroviral gene transfer. Blood 1991; 78:1132.
111. Corey CA, DeSilva A, Holland C, Williams DA. Serial transplantation of methotrexate-resistant bone marrow: protection of murine recipients from drug toxicity by progeny of transduced stem cells. Blood 1990; 75:337.
112. Sorrentino BP, Brandt SJ, Bodine D, et al. Selection of drug-resistant bone marrow cells in vivo after retroviral transfer of human *MDR1*. Science 1992; 257:99.
113. Wong PM, Chung S-W, Nienhuis AW. Retroviral transfer and expression of the interleukin-3 gene in hemopoietic cells. Genes Dev 1987; 1:358.
114. Miller AE, Eckner RJ, Jolly DJ, et al. Expression of a retrovirus encoding human HPRT in mice. Science 1984; 225:630.
115. McIvor RS, Johnson MJ, Miller AD, et al. Human purine nucleoside phosphorylase and adenosine deaminase: gene transfer into cultured cells and murine hematopoietic stem cells by using recombinant amphotropic retroviruses. Mol Cell Biol 1987; 7:838.
116. Valerio D, Duyvesteyn MG, van der Eb AJ. Introduction of sequences encoding functional human adenosine deaminase into mouse cells using a retroviral shuttle system. Gene 1984; 34:163.
117. Williams DA, Orkin SH, Mulligan RC. Retrovirus-mediated transfer of human adenosine deaminase gene sequences into cells in culture and into murine hematopoietic cells in vivo. Proc Nat Acad Sci U S A 1986; 83:2566.
118. Ohashi T, Boggs S, Robbins P, et al. Efficient transfer and sustained high expression of the human glucocerebrosidase gene in mice and their functional macrophages following transplantation of bone marrow transduced by a retroviral vector. Proc Natl Acad Sci U S A 1992; 89:11332.
119. Correll PH, Colilla S, Dave HPG, Karlsson S. High levels of human glucocerebrosidase activity in macrophages of long-term reconstituted mice after retroviral infection of hematopoietic stem cells. Blood 1992; 80:331.
120. Dzierzak EA, Papayannopoulou T, Mulligan RC. Lineage-specific expression of a human β-globin gene in murine bone marrow transplant recipients reconstituted with retrovirus-transduced stem cells. Nature 1988; 331:35.
121. Karlsson S, Bodine DM, Perry L, et al. Expression of the human alpha-globin gene following retroviral-mediated transfer into multipotential hematopoietic progenitors of mice. Proc Natl Acad Sci U S A 1988; 85:6062.
122. Hock RA, Miller AD, Osborne WR. Expression of human adenosine deaminase from various strong promoters after gene transfer into human hematopoietic cell lines. Blood 1989; 74:876.
123. Stewart CL, Stuhlmann H, Jahner D, Jaenisch R. De novo methylation, expression and infectivity of retroviral genomes introduced into embryonal carcinoma cells. Proc Natl Acad Sci U S A 1982; 79:4098.
124. Barklis E, Mulligan RC, Jaenisch R. Chromosomal position or virus mutation permits retrovirus expression in embryonal carcinoma cells. Cell 1986; 47:391.
125. Gorman CM, Rigby PWJ, Lane DP. Negative regulation of viral enhancers in undifferentiated embryonic stem cells. Cell 1985; 42:512.
126. Sassone-Corsi P, Duboule D, Chambon P. Viral enhancer activity in teratocarcinoma cells. *In* Cold Spring Harbor Symposium on Quantitative Biology. Cold Spring Harbor, NY: Cold Spring Harbor Press, 1986, p. 747.
127. Flanagan JH, Krieg AM, Max EE, Khan AS. Negative control region at the 5′ end of murine leukaemia virus long terminal repeats. Mol Cell Biol 1989; 9:739.
128. Einerhand MPW, Bakx TA, Kukler A, Valerio D. Factors affecting the transduction of pluripotent hematopoietic stem cells: long-term expression of a human adenosine deaminase gene in mice. Blood 1993; 81:254.
129. Moore KA, Fletcher FA, Villalon DK, et al. Human adenosine deaminase expression in mice. Blood 1990; 75:2085.
130. Weiss R, Teich N, Varmus H, Coffin J. RNA tumour viruses. Cold Spring Harbor 1982.
131. Hodgson GS, Bradley TR. Properties of haematopoietic stem cells surviving 5-fluorouracil treatment: evidence for a pre–CFU-S cell? Nature 1979; 281:381.

132. Bodine DM, McDonagh KT, Seidel NE, Nienhuis AW. Survival and retrovirus infection of murine hematopoietic stem cells in vitro: effects of 5-FU and method of infection. J Exp Hematol 1991; 19:206.
133. Fletcher FA, Moore KA, Ashkenazi M, et al. Leukemia inhibitory factor improves survival of retroviral vector–infected hematopoietic stem cells in vitro, allowing efficient long-term expression of vector-encoded human adenosine deaminase in vivo. J Exp Med 1991; 174:837.
134. Eglitis MA, Kantoff PW, Jolly JD, et al. Gene transfer into hematopoietic progenitor cells from normal and cyclic hematopoietic dogs using retroviral vectors. Blood 1988; 71:717.
135. Lemischka IR, Raulet DH, Mulligan RC. Developmental potential and dynamic behavior of hematopoietic stem cells. Cell 1986; 45:917.
136. Emerman M, Temin HM. Genes with promoters in retrovirus vectors can be independently suppressed by an epigenetic mechanism. Cell 1984; 39:459.
137. Emerman M, Temin HM. Quantitative analysis of gene suppression in integrated retrovirus vectors. Mol Cell Biol 1986; 6:792.
138. Apperley JF, Luskey BD, Williams DA. Retroviral gene transfer of human adenosine deaminase in murine hematopoietic cells: effect of selectable marker sequences on long-term expression. Blood 1991; 78:310.
139. Kantoff PW, Gillio AP, McLachlin JR, et al. Expression of human adenosine deaminase in nonhuman primates after retrovirus-mediated gene transfer. J Exp Med 1987; 166:219.
140. Donahue RE, Kessler SW, Bodine D, et al. Helper virus induced T cell lymphoma in nonhuman primates after retroviral mediated gene transfer. J Exp Med 1992; 176:1125.
141. van Beusechem VW, Kukler A, Heidt PJ, Valerio D. Long-term expression of human adenosine deaminase in rhesus monkeys transplanted with retrovirus-infected bone-marrow cells. Proc Natl Acad Sci U S A 1992; 89:7640.
142. Bodine D, Moritz T, Luskey B, et al. Expression of the adenosine deaminase (ADA) gene after transduction into rhesus monkey repopulating stem cells [Abstract]. Blood 1992; 80:72a.
143. Schuening FG, Kawahara K, Miller AD, et al. Retrovirus-mediated gene transduction into long-term repopulating marrow cells of dogs. Blood 1991; 78:2568.
144. Moore KA, Deisseroth AB, Reading CL, et al. Stromal support enhances cell-free retroviral vector transduction of human bone marrow long-term culture-initiating cells. Blood 1992; 79:1393.
145. Schuening FG, Storb R, Stead RB, et al. Improved retroviral transfer of genes into canine hematopoietic progenitor cells kept in long-term marrow culture. Blood 1989; 74:152.
146. Carter RF, Abrams-Ogg ACG, Dick JE, et al. Autologous transplantation of canine long-term marrow culture cells genetically marked by retroviral vectors. Blood 1991; 79:356.
147. Toksoz D, Zsebo KM, Smith KA, et al. Support of human hematopoiesis in long-term bone marrow cultures by murine stromal cells selectively expressing the membrane-bound and secreted forms of the human homolog of the *Steel* gene products, stem cell factor. Proc Natl Acad Sci U S A 1992; 89:7350.
148. Otsuka T, Thacker JD, Hogge DE. The effects of interleukin 6 and interleukin 3 on early hematopoietic events in long-term cultures of human marrow. J Exp Hematol 1991; 19:1042.
149. Williams DA. In search of the self-renewing hematopoietic stem cell. Blood Cells 1991; 17:296.
150. Brandt J, Srouf EF, van Besian K, et al. Cytokine-dependent long-term culture of highly enriched precursors of hematopoietic progenitor cells from human bone marrow. J Clin Invest 1990; 86:932.
151. Gianni AM, Siena S, Bregni M, et al. Granulocyte-macrophage colony-stimulating factor to harvest circulating haemopoietic stem cells for autotransplantation. Lancet 1989; 2:580.
152. Gluckman E, Broxmeyer HE, Auerbach AD, et al. Hematopoietic reconstitution in a patient with Fanconi's anemia by means of umbilical-cord blood from an HLA-identical sibling. N Engl J Med 1989; 321:1174.
153. Broxmeyer HE, Hangoc G, Cooper S, et al. Growth characteristics and expansion of human umbilical cord blood and estimation of its potential for transplantation in adults. Proc Natl Acad Sci U S A 1992; 89:4109.
154. Hows JM, Bradley BA, Marsh JC, et al. Growth of human umbilical-cord blood in longterm haemopoietic cultures. Lancet 1992; 340:73.
155. Tarella C, Ferrero D, Bregni M, et al. Circulating hemopoietic precursors after high-dose cyclophosphamide and rhGM-CSF: evidence for a preferential expansion of early progenitor cells. Eur J Cancer 1991; 27:22.
156. Bregni M, Magni M, Siena S, et al. Human peripheral blood hematopoietic progenitors are optimal targets of retroviral-mediated gene transfer. Blood 1992; 80:1418.
157. Moritz T, Williams D. Retroviral mediated gene transfer into human cord blood hematopoietic cells [Abstract]. Blood 1992; 80:178a.
158. Moritz T, Williams DA. Transfer of drug-resistance genes to hematopoietic precursors. *In* Bertino J (ed): Encyclopedia of Cancer, vol. 3. San Diego: Academic Press, 1997, pp 1765–1776.
159. Lim B, Apperley JF, Orkin SH, Williams DA. Long-term expression of human adenosine deaminase in mice transplanted with retrovirus-infected hematopoietic stem cells. Proc Natl Acad Sci U S A 1989; 86:8892.
160. Wilson JM, Danos O, Grossman M, et al. Expression of human adenosine deaminase in mice reconstituted with retrovirus-transduced hematopoietic stem cells. Proc Natl Acad Sci U S A 1990; 87:439.
161. Treatment of severe combined immunodeficiency disease (SCID) due to adenosine deaminase (ADA) deficiency with autologous lymphocytes transduced with a human ADA gene. Hum Gene Ther 1990; 1:327.
162. Rosenberg SA, Aebersold P, Cornetta K, et al. Gene transfer into humans—immunotherapy of patients with advanced melanoma, using tumor-infiltrating lymphocytes modified by retroviral gene transduction. N Engl J Med 1990; 323:570.
163. Bordignon C, Notarangelo LD, Nobili N, et al. Gene therapy in peripheral blood lymphocytes and bone marrow for ADA-immunodeficient patients. Science 1995; 270:470.
164. Kohn DB, Weinberg KI, Nolta JA, et al. Engraftment of gene-modified umbilical cord blood cells in neonates with adenosine deaminase deficiency. Nat Med 1995; 1:1017.
165. Bender MA, Miller AD, Gelinas RE. Expression of the human β-globin gene after retroviral transfer into murine erythroleukemia cells and human BFU-E cells. Mol Cell Biol 1988; 8:1725.
166. Rixon MW, Harris EAS, Gelinas RE. Expression of the human globin gene after retroviral transfer to transformed erythroid cells. Biochemistry 1990; 29:4393.
167. Bender MA, Gelinas RE, Miller AD. A majority of mice show long-term expression of a human β-globin gene after retrovirus transfer into hematopoietic stem cells. Mol Cell Biol 1989; 9:1426.
168. Li CL, Dwarki VJ, Verma IM. Expression of human α-globin and mouse/human hybrid β-globin genes in murine hemopoietic stem cells transduced by recombinant retroviruses. Proc Natl Acad Sci U S A 1990; 87:4349.
169. Riordan J, Rommens JM, Kerem BS, et al. Identification of the cystic fibrosis gene: cloning and characterization of the complete DNA. Science 1989; 245:1066.
170. Rosenfeld MA, Yoshimura K, Trapnell BC, et al. In vivo transfer of the human cystic fibrosis transmembrane conductance regulator gene to the airway epithelium. Cell 1992; 68:143.
171. Gene therapy of patients with advanced cancer using tumor infiltrating lymphocytes transduced with the gene coding for tumor necrosis factor. Hum Gene Ther 1990; 1:441.
172. Immunization of cancer patients using autologous cancer cells modified by insertion of the gene for tumor necrosis factor. Hum Gene Ther 1992; 3:57.
173. Immunization of cancer patients using autologous cancer cells modified by insertion of the gene for interleukin-2. Hum Gene Ther 1992; 3:75.
174. Culver KW, Ram Z, Wallbridge S, et al. In vivo gene transfer with retroviral vector-producer cells for treatment of experimental brain tumors. Science 1992; 256:1550.
175. Bonin C, Ferrari G, Verzeletti S, et al. HSV-TK gene transfer into donor lymphocytes for control of allogeneic graft-versus-leukemia. Science 1997; 276:1719.
176. Hesdorffer C, Ayello J, Ward M, et al. Phase I trial of retroviral-mediated transfer of the human MDR1 gene as marrow chemoprotection in patients undergoing high-dose chemotherapy and autologous stem-cell transplantation. J Clin Oncol 1998; 16:165.

177. Hanania EG, Giles RE, Kavanagh J, et al. Results of MDR-1 vector modification trial indicate that granulocyte/macrophage colony-forming unit cells do not contribute to posttransplant hematopoietic recovery following intensive systemic therapy. Proc Natl Acad Sci U S A 1996; 93:15346.
178. Sullenger BA, Gallardo HF, Ungers GE, Gilboa E. Overexpression of TAR sequences renders cells resistant to human immunodeficiency virus replication. Cell 1990; 63:601.
179. Bodine DM, Seidel NE, Gale MS, et al. Efficient retrovirus transduction of mouse pluripotent hematopoietic stem cells mobilized into the peripheral blood by treatment with granulocyte colony-stimulating factor and stem cell factor. Blood 1994; 84:1482.
180. Dunbar CE, Seidel NE, Doren S, et al. Improved retroviral gene transfer into murine and rhesus peripheral blood or bone marrow repopulating cells primed in vivo with stem cell factor and granulocyte colony-stimulating factor. Proc Natl Acad Sci U S A 1996; 93:11871.
181. Moritz T, Patel VP, Williams DA. Bone marrow extracellular matrix molecules improve gene transfer into human hematopoietic cells via retroviral vectors. J Clin Invest 1994; 93:1451.
182. Hanenberg H, Xiao XL, Dilloo D, et al. Colocalization of retrovirus and target cells on specific fibronectin fragments increases genetic transduction of mammalian cells. Nat Med 1996; 2:876.
183. Hanenberg H, Hashino K, Konishi H, et al. Optimization of fibronectin-assisted retroviral gene transfer into human $CD34^+$ hematopoietic cells. Hum Gene Ther 1997; 8:2193.
184. Moritz T, Dutt P, Xiao XL, et al. Fibronectin improves transduction of reconstituting hematopoietic stem cells by retroviral vectors: evidence of direct viral binding to chymotryptic carboxy-terminal fragments. Blood 1996; 88:855.
185. Pollok KE, Hanenberg H, Noblitt TW, et al. High-efficiency gene transfer into normal and adenosine deaminase–deficient T-lymphocytes is mediated by transduction on recombinant fibronectin fragments. J Virol 1998; 72:4882.
186. Kiem HP, Morris J, Heyward S, et al. Gene transfer into baboon hematopoietic repopulating cells using recombinant human fibronectin fragment Ch-296 [Abstract]. Blood 1997; 90:236a.
187. Wu T, Sellers SE, Kim HJ, et al. The use of cytokines active on primitive hematopoietic cells and stromal or fibronectin support during transduction improves stable retroviral gene transfer into primate $CD34^+$ hematopoietic cells to clinically relevant levels [Abstract]. Blood 1998; 92:689a.

INDEX

Note: Page numbers in *italics* refer to illustrations; page numbers followed by t refer to tables.

A

B

D

H

I

J

K

L

M

N

O

P

ISBN 0-7216-7684-7
90038
9 780721 676845